Advanced Concepts of
Personal Training
SECOND EDITION

Brian Biagioli, Ed.D

University of Miami

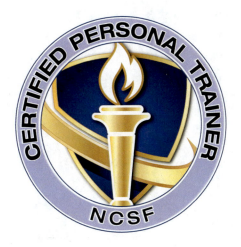

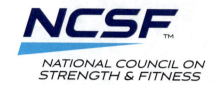

Contributing Authors

Arturo Leyva, PhD
Davy Levy, MS
Jennifer Maher, PhD
Lafayette Watson, PhD
Robert Silver, MS
Craig Flanagan, PhD
Steven Hicks, MS
Sean Grieve, MS
Steven Wermus, MS
Ozgur Alan, PhD
Taylor Snook, MS

Library of Congress Catalog Card Number: 2019931496
ISBN: 978-0-9791696-5-6

Copyright © 2019 National Council on Strength & Fitness (NCSF)
All rights reserved. Except for use in a review, the reproduction or utilization of this work in any form or by any electronic, mechanical, or other means, now known or hereafter invented, including xerography, photocopying, and recording, and in any information retrieval system, is forbidden without the written permission of the National Council on Strength & Fitness.

Printed in the United States of America
Our printing requirements use a mix of recycled and environmentally sustainable (FSC and COC) papers.

Distributed by:
National Council on Strength & Fitness
5915 Ponce de Leon Blvd., Suite 60
Coral Gables, FL 33146
800-772-NCSF(6273)
www.NCSF.org

Table of Contents

◆ Chapter 1
Introduction to Personal Training 1
    Personal Training: Past, Present and Scope of Practice 2
    Understanding Health and Wellness 5
    Health-Related Components of Fitness 13
    Performance-Related Components of Fitness 18

◆ Chapter 2
Functional Anatomy and Training Instruction 25
    Bones and Joints 26
    Muscle Tissue and Contraction Types 32
    Spatial and Directional Terminology 44
    Anatomical Movements 48
    Training Instruction 66

◆ Chapter 3
Kinetic Chain Function, Dysfunction and Corrective Exercise 113
    Local and Global Systems 114
    The Integrated Model of Function 117
    Muscular Units 121
    Common Postural Distortions and Muscular Imbalances 125
    Corrective Exercise 132

◆ Chapter 4
Human Physiology 141
    Anaerobic Energy Systems 142
    Aerobic Metabolism 151
    Muscular Fatigue 157
    Cardiac Physiology 163
    The Endocrine System 182

◆ Chapter 5
Evaluating Health and Physical Fitness 201
    Factors that Affect Fitness 202
    Considerations for Pre-Exercise Screening 206
    Pre-Exercise Screening 208
    Compiling the Data 221

Chapter 6

Physical Activity & Risk for Disease 225
    Cardiovascular Disease, Stroke, Hypertension and Physical Activity 228
    Obesity & Physical Activity 242
    Diabetes & Physical Activity 245
    Osteoarthritis, Osteoporosis and Physical Activity 250
    Cancer & Physical Activity 254
    Mental Health & Physical Activity 256

Chapter 7

Resting and Active Fitness Assessments 265
    Resting Cardiovascular Tests 266
    Body Composition and Anthropometrics 270
    Exercise Participation Clearance 292
    Exercise Testing 295
    Testing Considerations 298
    Exercise Testing 306
    Testing for Muscular Fitness 319
    Flexibility and Mobility Assessments 336

Chapter 8

Understanding Nutrition 347
    Energy Value of Food 348
    Carbohydrates 351
    Fats 366
    Protein 372
    Vitamins and Minerals 380
    Water 388

Chapter 9

Exploring Dietary Supplements 401
    Reading a Food Label 403
    Exploring Dietary Supplements 406
    Mass and Strength Gains 410
    Weight Loss Supplements 420

Chapter 10

Body Composition 433
    Obesity: A Worldwide Health Issue 434
    Stature-Weight Indices 438
    Body Composition Assessment 442

Chapter 11
Weight Management 455
    Factors that Impact Weight Management 456
    Energy Balance and Weight Management Strategies 461
    Stress, Social Behaviors, and Weight Management 473
    Eating Disorders 476

Chapter 12
Exercise Program Components 481
    Warm-ups 484
    Metabolic System and Programming Considerations 489
    Exercise Program Components 491
    Exercise Program Safety Factors 503

Chapter 13
Anaerobic Resistance Training 507
    Training for a Desired Outcome 513
    Training Systems 531
    Exercise Considerations 538
    Common Injuries Associated with Training 545

Chapter 14
Cardiorespiratory Fitness 557
    Assessing Cardiorespiratory Fitness 558
    Types of Aerobic Training 565
    Modes of Aerobic Training 573
    Aerobic Training Considerations 576
    Preventing Common Overuse Injuries 581

Chapter 15
Flexibility 587
    Introduction to Flexibility 588
    Properties of Soft Tissues 591
    Factors Affecting Joint Range of Motion 592
    Testing and Types of Flexibility Training 601
    Common Flexibility Techniques 609

Chapter 16

Introduction to Exercise Programming 617
    Program Design 618
    Prioritizing Needs 619
    Preparation Phase 622
    Anaerobic Endurance Phase 627
    Hypertrophy-Strength 630
    Strength-Power 634
    Duration of Program Phases and Cycles 638

Chapter 17

Working with Special Populations 641
    Exercise & Asthma 642
    Diabetes & Exercise 645
    Exercise & Cardiovascular Disease 649
    Exercise during Pregnancy 657
    Children & Exercise 662
    Exercise & the Elderly 666

Chapter 18

Ethics and Professional Practice 675
    What Makes a Professional 676
    Professional Principles 678
    Duty of the Profession 682

Glossary of Terms 690

Index 704

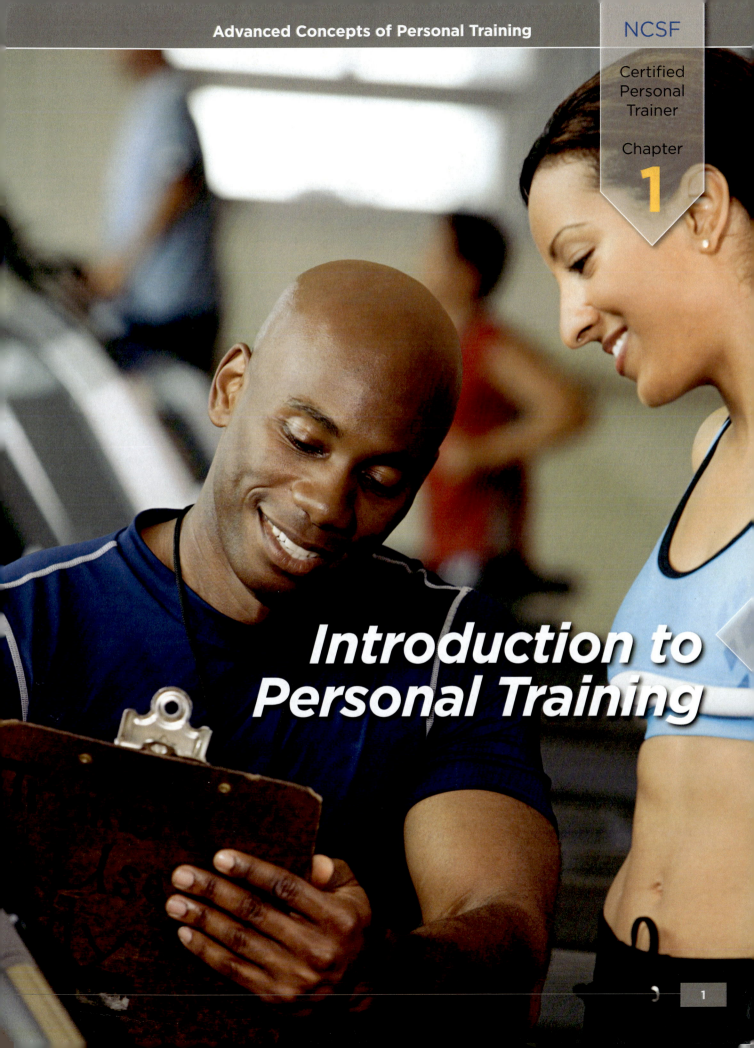

Personal Training: Past, Present and Scope of Practice

◆ Personal Training: The Beginning

Personal training began to mature into a profession in the 1980s as the fitness industry gradually found an identity. Rooted in the weight rooms popularized by bodybuilders and arenas where athletes trained for performance, the idea of regular exercise using an instructor became *en vogue*. Jogging and cycling were established fitness activities, but the increasing popularity of weight training was paralleled by growing interest in group "exercise to music" classes. Unlike jogging and cycling, these exercise choices required an increased level of technical knowledge for safe participation. Research interests brought validity to the health benefits of these activities, and the medical profession found interest in the systematic improvements exhibited by those adopting exercise routines [11, 23, 26]. The idea of hiring an experienced "weight trainer" or "exercise leader" gained merit, both from a social and health perspective. At this point, organizations started to form to help enthusiasts learn the fledgling fitness trade, which also brought like-minded educators together to establish standards and guidelines. Early on, traditional bodybuilding programs comprised the majority of personal training routines, while spending time on the increasingly-popular stationary aerobic equipment became a casual complement. This meant everyone needed to exercise in a gym, and facilities like Bally Total Fitness benefited from the social movement, reaching more than 400 club sites during the company's peak.

Today, personal training has mostly shed its foundational skin, as both the concept and profession have grown in scope and diversity. The original notion has remained somewhat consistent, but the landscape, services, and professionals that provide those services have transformed to better reflect a broader and more beneficial influence on society. Whereas early training emphasized vanity outcomes over health, today's imperatives are the maintenance of function, disease-prevention, and life quality. Service interests' expansion has also created new environments where these benefits are offered.

The original idea that personal trainers work in gyms and health clubs still holds true today, but now, personal trainers also practice in small boutiques, wellness centers, medical clinics, schools, and corporate environments. They are also entrepreneurs traveling to clients' homes and providing training services in parks and on recreational fields. As one would expect, if trainers leave the gym, they must have new methods or skills to help their clients attain fitness goals without traditional equipment; thus, this diversity in environments has fueled corresponding variation in the tools used by personal trainers on the job. Both novel and traditional examples of exercise equipment have become mainstream aids to facilitate fitness. Ropes, tires, medicine balls, kettlebells, and similar devices now join the more traditional appliances used in personal training. And while the equipment may be novel and the environments less traditional, the human element remains the same. The adage "old science in new spaces" holds true and continues to chart the course for exercise programming.

Unfortunately, however, the linear growth of the personal training profession has been mirrored by a decline in population health. Obesity rates from the 1970-80s have now tripled in some states [15, 16]. Expectedly, more competent trainers are needed to address this growing demand. Because of the rise in preventable "first-world" diseases, such as diabetes and heart disease, the role of the personal trainer continues to evolve as the industry enters the debate about ways to address this health care crisis. Essentially, the inevitable change from the sick-care model, which emphasizes medicine, to the preventative health-care model will require a workforce that can serve this role.

◆ Personal Training: Modern Concept

The 21st-century exercise professional will be expected to place greater emphasis on health and behavior changes as neither exercise nor diet alone represent viable solutions. Additionally, the total number of individuals who need the professional help of a personal trainer far exceeds the total number of actual professionals in the United States. In 2016, the Department of Labor suggested there were 279,100 personal trainers, while, in 2017, the Center for Disease Control (CDC) announced the incidence of diabetes and pre-diabetes in the population had reached 114 million [1, 3]. This group represents those in real need of behavioral support for their medical conditions. Based on this information, the demand for exercise professionals offering healthcare-oriented services would be over 1000 hours per trainer each week. This unworkable scenario suggests something must change to resolve this growing problem. A novel concept involves moving from the traditional one-on-one scenario to a trainer-client management scheme. This model provides a refreshing approach to the trainer-client relationship, allowing the knowledge of a personal trainer, through innovative technology and social media, to effectively reach more people to help manage their lifestyle habits. Tech-savvy professionals who adopt this model can provide more interactive education, guidance, and motivation with less face-to-face, individualized contact time in the gym. Trainer-client management demonstrates the progression of the field and the need for well-qualified practitioners to fill these emerging new roles.

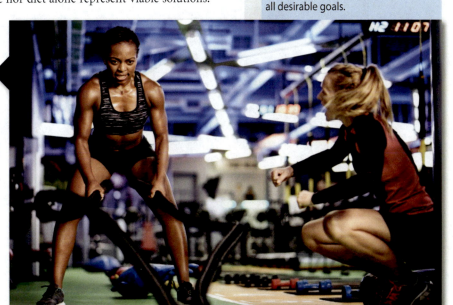

Today's exercise professionals are expected to place greater emphasis on health, fitness, and complementary behavior changes as neither exercise nor diet alone can help a client reach all desirable goals.

◆ Scope of Practice and Legal Ramifications

Each career field has a defined scope which embodies the primary services provided by an eligible professional and extends to the boundaries of the individual's qualification. At the time of this text's publication, the fitness industry enjoyed, for better or worse, no regulatory oversight by any municipality in the United States. Instead of federal or state regulations, credible organizations, including the NCSF, provide accredited, third-party certifications by role as defined by the Department of Labor, for stakeholder protection. Professionals take legally-defensible board exams and, upon passing, become certified and then registered with the United States Registry of Exercise Professionals (USREPS.org). Employers can be confident the professional has been properly vetted against a validated standard. Consumers can hire with confidence, knowing they've retained a trainer properly qualified to provide the appropriate services.

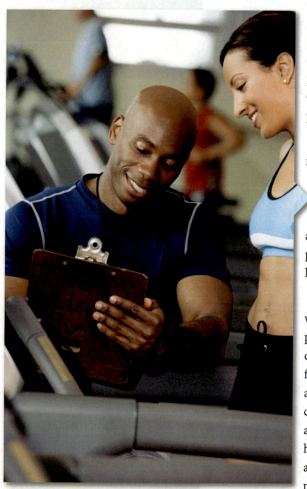

To appropriately define the scope of a profession, a role delineation study is employed. This tool surveys stakeholders of the profession to determine what the job requires for effective and appropriate implementation. Academics who teach the curriculums, employers who hire the professionals, and the professionals themselves all identify the important aspects of the profession. This process also includes surveying aligned professions, so boundaries are established in a manner that is suitable and legally defensible.

In some cases, aligned professions overlap in what they do but differ in where, when, and how they deliver the services. For instance, several professions employ exercise modalities for a purpose appropriate to the discipline. Physical therapists will use exercise for rehabilitation in medical facilities, athletic trainers will use exercise in return-to-play scenarios in athletic facilities, and strength coaches will use exercise to enhance athletic capabilities and help prevent injury on the field or court. None of the aforementioned professions is qualified to function as a personal trainer however, and would need to add a personal trainer certification to serve appropriately as one. Similarly, a personal trainer is not qualified to be a physical therapist, athletic trainer, or a strength coach without the proper education and credentialing. In fact, if someone were to assume such a role in a state that regulates one of these professions, the act would be criminal.

In many cases, professional status goes beyond the technical skill needed to accomplish tasks. Qualified and credentialed individuals should also meet certain industry standards and hold to elevated personal expectations. In fields where an imbalance of power exists, ethics and practice standards become crucial cornerstones. All legitimate credentials in the fitness field have a code of ethics and principles (or standards) of appropriate practice, which should be used to guide decisions and evaluate behavior. If professionals fail to comply with such standards, they run the risk of sanctioning, which may include removal of earned credential. Essentially, practice standards represent the essentials of established expectations, based on agreement within a consortium of professional organizations or governing bodies; whereas ethics reflect the principles of conduct governing an individual to protect interests of all stakeholders.

Understanding Health and Wellness

People commonly engage in certain behaviors, begin physical activity, and hire personal trainers because they want to be healthy: however, the definition of health or being healthy is somewhat vague because the term **"health"** has been conceived in so many ways. Even today, not everyone agrees on a universally accepted meaning. Traditionally, the concept of health applied to a person's susceptibility for disease. If a person did not have any diagnostic criteria for disease or present any known "health" problems, that person was considered "healthy."

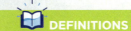

Health –

The condition of being sound in body, mind, or spirit and free from physical pain, illness, or disease.

The Merriam–Webster dictionary [2] suggests that health is:

1) the condition of being sound in body, mind, or spirit; especially freedom from physical disease or pain

2) the general condition of the body

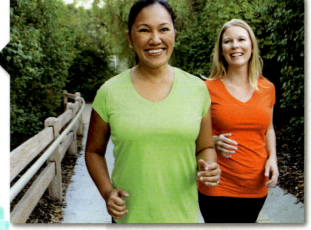

Both aspects of this definition merit attention: namely, the spirit, mind, and (physical) body arise from the general condition of the body. Historically, health professionals have determined health status based on specific, quantifiable health measurements, such as blood pressure, and any self-reported issues, such as pain or discomfort. Viewing health from this narrow diagnostic perspective poses a problem in that it fails to consider disease or symptomatic criteria that is unknown to the individual. In addition, it does not view the person's overall well-being as a defining characteristic. During the late seventies and early eighties, a broadened philosophy of health emerged, suggesting that people be viewed holistically rather than by independent physiological measures.

An Evolved Concept of Wellness Includes

| Physical health | Mental health | Emotional health | Intellectual health | Social health | Environmental health |

The rationale for wellness' evolution was that each health-related component had potential implications for overall well-being. When individuals control these physiological and psychological areas, they minimize the negative impact each may have on health. For instance, good social health entails meaningful relationships and confident social interaction. Both contribute to reduced stress and depression risk. While fitness professionals are familiar with the concept of wellness, it is not clearly understood among the general population. Rarely will the term wellness be applied in conversation. Instead, people more often use "healthy" to describe an overall condition. Therefore, the term health is better understood as both the physical and mental state of a person and the assortment of lifestyle behaviors that affect either state, rather than simply freedom from disease.

It is well-known and documented that health is affected by what enters and leaves the body, what the body is exposed to, and what the body is required to do each day. Therefore, lifestyle largely determines the outcome of these collectively applied factors. Healthy lifestyle is defined as a group of actions and behaviors that positively affect a person's overall well-being, suggesting that wellness is the culmination of healthy behaviors.

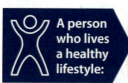

A person who lives a healthy lifestyle: Avoids stress and negative health behaviors → Eats nutritionally appropriate foods → Enjoys positive relationships → Engages in routine physical activity

The Office of Disease Prevention and Health Promotion, through the U.S. Department of Health and Human Services (HHS), lists objectives to encourage healthy lifestyles by Americans in the *Healthy People 2020* initiative. Through this initiative, Americans are asked to take personal responsibility for their health through lifestyle management. Under the title 'Objectives A-Z', the initiative lists the numerous aspects every person should consider when attempting to maintain good health. The government website Healthypeople.gov provides a catalogue of all the topic areas, which includes the objectives and supportive data and evidence-based resources for consumers. The topics range from vision and hearing to mental health to nutrition, anthropometrics, and physical activity. New topics include health-related quality of life and well-being, as well as social determinants of health, further reflecting the trend towards wellness and the broadening definition of health.

Health Risk Behaviors – *Connecting the Dots*

Common contributors to premature health decline:	Common health disorders and disease:
• Physical inactivity	• Hypertension
• Inadequate sleep	• Hyperlipidemia
• Chronic stress	• Arteriosclerosis/Atherosclerosis
• Poor diet	• Diabetes
• Dehydration	• Chronic obstructive pulmonary disease (COPD)
• Obesity	• Cancer
• Tobacco use	• Depression
• Alcohol consumption	• Stroke
• Poor emotional health	• Systemic inflammation

Expectedly, routine engagement in physical activity features importantly in the plan. According to the HHS, the physical activity objectives for Healthy People 2020 mirror the significant scientific evidence supporting the health benefits of regular physical activity among youth and adults. The data is operationalized in the 2008 Physical Activity Guidelines for Americans (PAG) with new updates expected in the 2018 Physical Activity Recommendations [4]. Even though strong scientific support and documented medical outcomes demonstrate the benefits of physical activity, the HHS suggests nearly 80% of adults do not meet the guidelines for both aerobic and muscle-strengthening activities [5]. Similarly, more than 80% of adolescents do not perform enough aerobic physical activity to meet the guidelines for youth [33].

Among adults and older adults, physical activity can lower the risk of:	Among children and adolescents, physical activity can improve:
• Early death • Coronary heart disease and stroke • High blood pressure • Type 2 diabetes • Breast and colon cancer • Falls • Depression	• Bone health • Cardiorespiratory fitness • Muscular fitness • Body composition if overweight • Social development and confidence

According to HHS, regular physical activity can improve the health and quality of life of Americans of all ages, regardless of the presence of a chronic disease or disability [1,2]. The recommendations appropriately cite that regular "physical activity" includes participation in moderate and vigorous actions and muscle-strengthening activities, but this necessitates clarification for consumers. The term "physical activity" means different things to different people and often aligns with interests and experiences. For some, physical activity means exercise, but for others, the idea calls to mind sports participation or recreational activities. Regardless, **exercise** and **physical activity** have two distinctly different meanings. Physical activity refers to a period of time in which physical acts are performed. The definition is independent of the quantity of work, oxygen demand, and resultant energy expenditure. Examples of physical activity include hiking, gardening, walking the dog, and cleaning the house. Exercise, on the other hand, is defined as planned, structured, and repetitive bodily movements performed to improve or maintain one or more components of physical fitness. Thus, exercise qualifies as physical activity, but physical activity may not be exercise. All types of physical activity can improve overall health, but exercise entails physical activity with specific parameters that, properly applied, allow an individual to achieve defined outcomes.

> **DEFINITIONS**
>
> **Physical activity –**
> *Any purposeful and repeated bodily movement produced by voluntary skeletal muscle actions that increase metabolism.*
>
> **Exercise –**
> *Planned, structured, and repetitive bodily movements performed to improve or maintain one or more components of physical fitness.*

QUICK FACT: *Physical inactivity has been identified as the fourth leading risk factor for global mortality, causing an estimated 3.2 million deaths globally.*

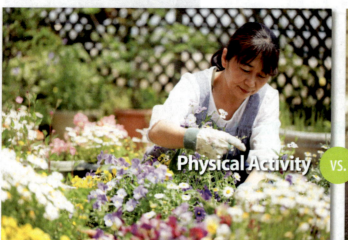
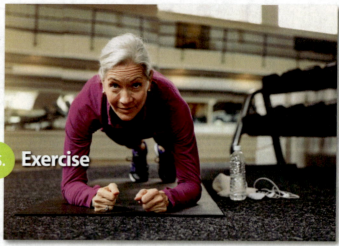

Physical Activity vs. Exercise

In 2015* the Surgeon General issued a call to action for public engagement in routine walking [6]. This is valuable from a "Get America Moving" perspective but can be confusing for those trying to understand how to achieve health and fitness because an interesting dichotomy exists between physical activity and exercise. For one person, walking may function as both physical activity and beneficial exercise, but for another, it may only be a physical activity with no exercise benefit. To realize the difference, one must first understand what constitutes exercise. Exercise, as defined above, produces a stress that stimulates a cellular response, generating the potential for a new or sustained adaptation. The adaptation may occur in specific tissues or affect multiple systems. For instance, those who routinely engage in cardiovascular exercise will not produce enough stress while walking to stimulate a new adaptation because the body already tolerates the level of stress involved. If, however, a sedentary person walks continuously, this movement would be perceived by the body as a new, unaccustomed level of stress and, therefore, could function as exercise if performed routinely. When stress is applied beyond what the body is accustomed to, it is termed "overload".

When the body experiences an unaccustomed level of stress, it exhibits an acute response to the overload, but that does not mean the stress will stimulate new adaptations. Whereas physical activity can occur in a single episode, exercise specifically requires a defined frequency for a sustained change to occur. The exposure to the stress must be adequate to stimulate the body to adapt. If a sedentary person walks once, the act will not have a significant impact on the individual's health or fitness. Certainly, the person's heart rate will increase, body temperature will rise, and muscles will metabolize energy for the duration of the event, but no discernable adaptive response will follow. This acute phenomenon is termed an "elastic" response. During elastic responses, the body changes temporarily due to the specific circumstances it is exposed to; however, it then reverts to its starting condition when the environment returns to its baseline, similar to a rubber band that is stretched and then allowed to return to its initial state. Conversely, when a person walks every day, the repeated stress causes improvements in system function due to recurring exposure. These chronic changes or adaptations become a semi-permanent characteristic of the body. This is known as a "plastic" response, and adaptations are sustained as long as the stress remains present at an appropriate level.

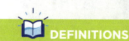 **DEFINITIONS**

Overload –

A principle of exercise programming, overload is stress applied beyond that which the body is accustomed for the promotion of fitness improvements.

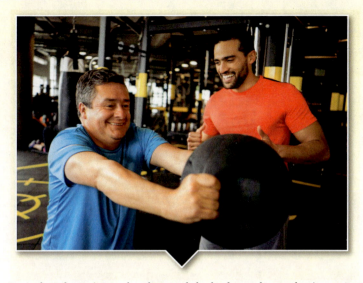

Once the adaptations take place and the body reaches a plastic state, a new stress must occur to promote further adaptation. This concept is referred to as progressive stress or simply **"progression"**. It functions with overload (progressive overload) to stimulate the plastic response. Importantly, different stress promotes different body responses and subsequent adaptation. The third element to consider when employing exercise for body improvements is the **specificity** of the stress. Creating an exercise program that causes a specific adaptation requires knowledge of the body systems and their responses to different stresses. Specificity refers to the idea that different stress is controllable and can be used in quantified measures to elicit desirable responses from the body. Routine performance of a weighted bicep curl, for instance, can make an exerciser stronger when the person flexes their arm against resistance; however, weighted bicep curls will do nothing to improve leg strength. Likewise, running long distances may increase leg endurance but does not improve flexibility in the same manner. In sum, specific stress causes specific adaptations when presented in a consistent and appropriate manner. When stress is inadequate, it can lead to physical decline, but too much stress will cause overtraining and injury. Therefore, personal trainers, in a sense, use thoughtful applications to manage stress in proper dosages to create desirable outcomes.

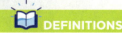

DEFINITIONS

Progression –

A principle of exercise programming, once the body has adapted to a level of stress, additional or novel stress is needed to promote further adaptations. This principle is normally combined with overload (progressive overload) for ongoing adaptation planning.

Specificity –

A principle of exercise programming. A desired adaption must match the specific stresses placed upon the body; controlled stress applied in quantified measures to elicit desirable responses from the body.

This begs the question of how stress is properly quantified. The physical fitness guidelines describe activity as a measure of time and self-quantified effort. For sustaining health, these parameters recommend a total of 150 minutes of moderate intensity exercise (described as brisk walking) per week or 75 minutes of vigorous exercise (described as jogging or running) per week. Alternately, they advocate an equivalent mix of the two at doses of at least 10 minutes at a time combined with muscle strengthening activities twice a week. For greater health benefits, the duration of physical activity at moderate, vigorous, or combined intensity of exercise is simply doubled (300 min moderate exercise or 150 min vigorous exercise); the strengthening requirements though remain the same. From an energy perspective, this essentially suggests that exercisers exert 1,000 purposeful calories a week when looking for basic health improvements from physical activity and 2,000 calories a week for fitness-related benefits[38].

Americans Need More Physical Activity

Less than half of all adults get the recommended amount of physical activity:

- Adults need at least 2 and 1/2 hours (150 minutes) a week of aerobic physical activity. This should be at a moderate level, such as a fast-paced walk, for no less than 10 minutes at a time.
- Women and older adults are not as likely to get the recommended level of weekly physical activity.
- Inactive adults have a higher risk for early death, heart disease, stroke, type 2 diabetes, depression, and some cancers.
- Regular physical activity helps people achieve and maintain a healthy weight.
- Walkable communities result in more physical activity.

Fundamental Physical Activity Guidelines

Moderate-intensity physical activity: On an absolute scale, physical activity that is done at 3.0-5.9 times the intensity of rest. On a scale relative to an individual's personal capacity, moderate-intensity physical activity usually rates at a 5 or 6 on a scale of 0-10.

Vigorous-intensity physical activity: On an absolute scale, physical activity done at 6.0 or more times the intensity of rest. On a scale relative to an individual's personal capacity, vigorous-intensity physical activity usually ranks at a 7 or 8 on a scale of 0-10.

Muscle-strengthening activity (strength training, resistance training, or muscular strength and endurance exercises): Physical activity, including exercise that increases skeletal muscle strength, power, endurance, and mass.

Examples of Different Physical Activities Based on Intensity

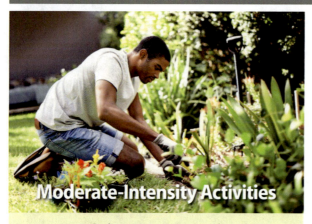
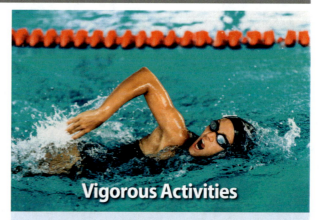

Moderate-Intensity Activities	Vigorous Activities
Cycling at a pace <10 mph	Jogging, running, or repeat sprinting
Water Aerobics	Swimming laps
Gardening	Aerobic dance class
Walking at ≤3 mph	Cycling at a pace > 10 mph
Tennis (doubles)	Downhill skiing
Snorkeling or recreational swimming	Jumping Rope
Yoga	Heavy, continuous yardwork
Golf while wheeling clubs	Karate/martial arts class participation
Playing frisbee	Circuit weight training
Shoveling light snow	Team sport play (soccer, basketball)

Note: The table above is not exhaustive but provides several examples of common activities classified as moderate-intensity or vigorous-intensity

The physical activity recommendations for Americans originate from scientific evidence and can be effective if adopters understand and implement these endorsements properly; however, their message may be a bit oversimplified to yield actual success. Indeed, walking will help one to be healthy, and jogging will help one to be fit, but exercise devoted towards specific adaptations requires much more detailed planning and implementation. Here the difference between physical activity for health and that appropriate for fitness becomes clearly evident. Health is measured by consistent systemic normalcy, whereas fitness is measured by quantified applications of physical function that serve a purpose for either health or performance. Again, a healthy person may not be fit, and a fit person may not be healthy. To make matters more confusing, health tends to encompass the big picture while fitness necessitates a categorical, system-specific view. A person may be fit in one category but extremely unfit when measured in another category. Likewise, an individual may be athletic and do well in performance-related fitness tasks but fail to score well on health-related assessments. These statements suggest the need to apply both holistic efforts towards being *healthy* and specific efforts towards being *fit* [38].

Figure 1.1 Percentage of U.S. Adults Who Met the 2008 Federal Physical Activity Guidelines for Aerobic and Strengthening Activity, by Sex
– National Health Interview Survey, 2000–2014 [5].

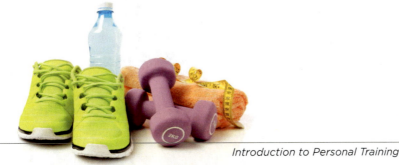

◆ Physical Fitness

Physical fitness embraces two categories: health-related physical fitness and performance-related physical fitness. The first category comprises factors that quantifiably affect health, while the second category affects performance outcomes. The health-related components of fitness include cardiorespiratory fitness, muscular strength, muscular endurance, flexibility, and body composition. In some cases, metabolic fitness also qualifies as a supplementary health-related component because it affects risk for metabolic diseases, including obesity and diabetes. The performance-related components of physical fitness include power, speed, coordination, balance, and agility. Each plays an important role in human performance and should be considered a secondary health component for youth and adults but a primary consideration for older adults. Those in this demographic require appropriate measures of performance emphasis compared to their younger counterparts for two reasons: first, power declines with age and can lead to loss of independence; second, movement speed is associated with function, fall risk increases with age, and both relate to balance. Thus, exercise professionals are often surprised by the fact that programs aimed at older adults warrant promoting strength, power, and dynamic balance over cardiovascular exercise; however, due to the high incidence of cardiovascular and metabolic disorders, the latter remains important as well. These facts indicate the need for strategic program offerings that prevent disease and promote active-aging.

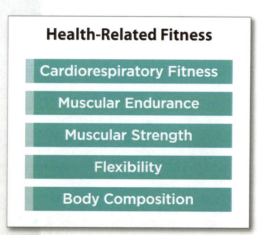

Health-Related Fitness
- Cardiorespiratory Fitness
- Muscular Endurance
- Muscular Strength
- Flexibility
- Body Composition

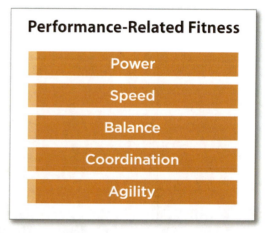

Performance-Related Fitness
- Power
- Speed
- Balance
- Coordination
- Agility

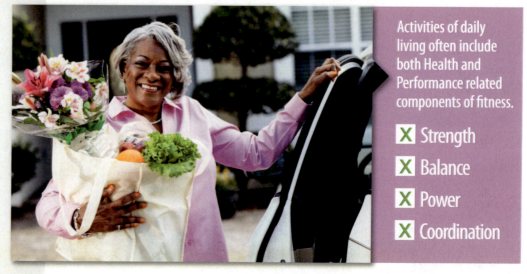

Activities of daily living often include both Health and Performance related components of fitness.

- X Strength
- X Balance
- X Power
- X Coordination

Health-Related Components of Fitness

Health-related components of fitness are fundamental to a person's overall well-being. They reflect quantifiable measures of efficiency and proper function of both the movement and metabolic systems of the body. Appropriate values or improvements in each of the components promote positive health. High scores in these same categories will benefit the individual beyond that of basic health and also apply directly to improved capabilities in all physical activities. Whereas high ranks in certain categories may be more desirable for specific goal-related outcomes, such as a low body fat or significant strength, all individuals should strive to maintain an acceptable level of fitness within each of the five areas. Individuals who score very well in only one or two components of fitness may experience health consequences or higher risk for problems when compared to those who maintain a moderate level of fitness in all the health categories.

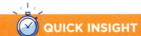
QUICK INSIGHT

Health vs. Fitness

Many people believe that health and fitness are synonymous, but this may not always be the case. Health is a disease-free state of well-being that allows an individual to experience improved quality of life and independence. Fitness is a criterion-based measure of physical performance. A person does not have to be fit to be healthy nor is a person guaranteed health because they are fit. Certainly, the two are interrelated, but distinct differences exist, and emotional, psychological, and physical assessments reveal these differences. A person who scores satisfactorily in the health-related components of fitness may meet a definition of fitness according to certain criteria; however, if this same person experiences high stress on the job, eats a diet high in saturated fats, and suffers from hypertension and hyperlipidemia, the person may be fit but not necessarily healthy. Conversely, a person may not score well on assessments of physical fitness; however, if he or she eats a very healthy diet, gets enough physical activity to maintain functional performance levels, has low blood pressure, and a reasonable lipid profile, the person is classified as healthy, though not physically fit.

In measures of skill or performance-related fitness, this difference can be even more significant. A person may show respectable scores in measures of speed or power but be unhealthy in several other categories. Genetics, exercise, and physical activity affect performance-related fitness, but the activities that improve performance may not necessarily improve health. For instance, a weightlifter may exhibit high levels of strength but low levels of cardiorespiratory fitness. Likewise, a person may have excellent balance and coordination but be categorically obese. The key point: skill measures indicate health poorly, even though people who score well on them often do so because they participate in sports and related physical activities.

When the level of physical activity is assessed in relation to health and fitness, two different criteria are used to define acceptable values. Health simply requires routine physical activity of appropriate frequency and duration. Fitness requires a regimented program designed to emphasize the specific components of health-related physical fitness. In general, moderate fitness may be attained from exercise performed 3 days a week at an intensity level of 60-70% of maximum. High-level fitness, however, often requires 4-6 days a week at 75-90% intensities.

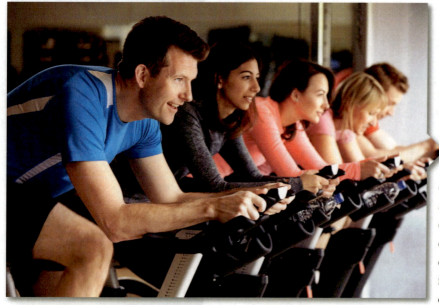

Cardiorespiratory Fitness

Cardiorespiratory fitness (**CRF**) includes several synonymous terms: aerobic fitness, aerobic endurance, cardiovascular efficiency, cardiovascular fitness or cardiovascular endurance, and cardiorespiratory efficiency. These all represent the same thing – the body's ability to consume and utilize oxygen and are determined by a person's **VO_2max**. CRF reflects the synergistic efficiency of the body's systems and includes the cardiopulmonary system (heart and lungs), cardiovascular system, and muscular system. CRF is the single most important health-related component of fitness because of its link to risk for disease and death. Low measures of VO_2max are a risk factor for heart disease, diabetes, and obesity [20, 27, 34]. On the contrary, high levels of CRF associate with positive health, including improved self-reported quality of life and longer lifespan [8, 14, 27]. Unfortunately, cellular limitations create a natural decline of ~ 1% per year in cardiorespiratory fitness with age, and this decline is accelerated after 45 years-old; therefore, it is important to emphasize oxygen utilization enhancements during the years of youth through young adulthood [19]. This makes sense for two reasons: first, routine behaviors established in youth tend to persist, and second, attaining a high level of oxygen consumption and efficiency is much easier to attain before age 30 and, thus, comparably easier to sustain in adulthood, making lifetime fitness an easier undertaking.

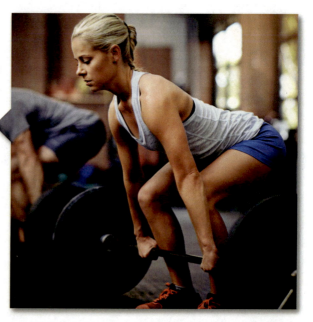

Muscular Fitness

Muscular fitness is the body's ability to produce and sustain force output via neuromuscular characteristics. It encompasses two of the health-related components of fitness: **muscular strength** and **muscular endurance**. Muscular strength is defined as the body's ability to exert a single, maximal contractile force, whereas muscular endurance reflects the ability of muscle tissue to sustain force output or apply force for an extended period of time. Muscular fitness is essential for health because it determines movement capabilities, affects joint health, and is responsible

DEFINITIONS

Cardiorespiratory fitness –

A health-related component of physical fitness, defined as the ability of the circulatory, respiratory, and muscular systems to supply oxygen during sustained physical activity.

VO_2max –

Measure of an individual's cardiorespiratory fitness as indicated by maximal oxygen use - measured by milliliters of oxygen per kilogram of body weight per minute of work.

Muscular strength –

A health-related component of fitness, defined as the measure of an individual's maximal contractile force production against a resistance.

Muscular endurance –

A health-related component of fitness, defined as the measure of muscle force decline over time.

for posture and **stability**. Poor muscular fitness associates with increased risk of injury in youth sports [21] and links to functional decline and loss of independence in the elderly [9]. Beyond functional demands, the specific activities an individual routinely participates in will determine the actual amount of muscular strength and endurance that individual needs to support the task. Therefore, no single metric exists that defines muscular fitness. Unlike cardiorespiratory fitness, the muscular system cannot be optimally assessed using a single action or test. The literature cites grip strength as a correlate to overall strength, but all movements entail different muscle actions and the respective joints require specific **strength balance** relationships for proper function. For these reasons, muscular strength and endurance should be tested using movements that measure different muscle groups and account for joint stabilization.

Flexibility

Despite the participation of many in dance, yoga, Pilates or martial arts, **flexibility** is probably the most undervalued and least-emphasized component of health-related fitness among physically active adults.

Anecdotally, this is likely due to three factors:

1) Improvements in flexibility do not satisfy those motivated by vanity, as they are not obvious.

2) Most normal activities do not require high levels of flexibility.

3) Flexibility training is often viewed as time consuming, boring, and uncomfortable.

> **DEFINITIONS**
>
> **Stability –**
>
> *The synergistic ability of muscles, nerves, proprioceptors, and connective tissues to maintain firm positioning and offset disruptive forces.*
>
> **Flexibility –**
>
> *A health-related component of fitness, indicated by the ability of a muscle to move through a range of motion at a single joint in a single plane.*
>
> **Mobility –**
>
> *The ability to move cooperative body segments through a full, unrestricted range of motion.*

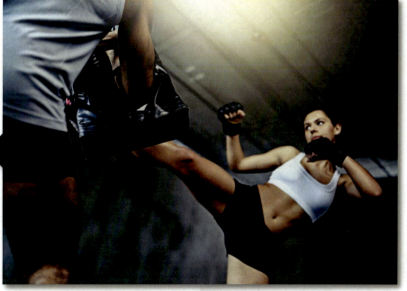

Informed analysis demonstrates the irony of all three of these statements: flexibility affects posture and therefore, appearance; those with better flexibility experience less movement restriction and demonstrate improvements in performance; and to the third point, individuals can employ a variety of techniques beyond traditional static stretching which are well-tolerated, engaging, and less time consuming. Of note, flexibility is defined as the range of motion at a single joint and is specific to direction. This means it is independently measured by specific movements at specific joints, similar to strength. Flexibility ties directly into joint function, movement capabilities, risk for injury, and chronic pain. This is why flexibility has earned its place next to CRF, muscular fitness, and body composition as an important component of health-related physical fitness. A decrease in flexibility is also associated with a decline in bodily function and is both a direct and indirect variable for health problems that can lead to disability in older adults [30]. However, flexibility does not equate to **mobility**, an important distinction when considering range of motion. Though these terms are often used interchangeably, an important distinction exists between them: mobility entails being able to move the body through full range of motion without undesirable restriction or change in proper joint biomechanics. Mobility is different than flexibility because multiple joints are employed during the movements. Joint angles change during quantifying activities which cause variation in muscle fascia tension across fascial lines. For example, raising one's arm overhead would represent shoulder-joint range of motion, or flexibility at the shoulder, whereas performing an overhead squat would test one's mobility, or proper joint position and biomechanics, across multiple joints (e.g., shoulder, spine, and hip). The difference between flexibility and mobility helps explain why a person can raise an arm up overhead when standing or seated, exhibiting appropriate flexibility of the shoulder, but cannot maintain the same overhead position when squatting, leading to a failed mobility test.

> **DEFINITIONS**
>
> **Body composition –**
>
> *A health-related component of fitness, indicated by the ratio of fat mass to fat-free mass within the body, often expressed as a percentage of body fat.*
>
> **Fat-free mass –**
>
> *All tissues within the human body that contain no fat.*

Flexibility –vs– Mobility

Shoulder Flexion – **PASS** ✓   Overhead Squat – **FAIL** ✗

Body Composition

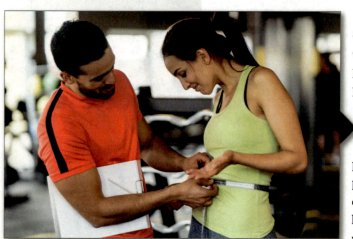

Most people erroneously view **body composition** as the amount of fat in a person's body; but body composition is the ratio of fat mass to **fat-free mass** (FFM). While it is often expressed as a percentage of body fat, this ratio is the important factor for health purposes because tissue mass can change: a person may add or lose muscle and fat throughout a lifespan. Clinically, the body is viewed as being composed of five components: water, minerals, protein, and glycogen make up FFM, with fat as the 5th component. If a person adds muscle mass, he or she increases the body's protein and glycogen, and therefore, water content, which positively changes the body composition ratio even if the individual did not lose any fat. The quantified value is expressed as a mathematical percentage, so if one body constituent goes up (muscle), the other (fat) goes down, even though the absolute amount did not change: it always must equal

100% of body weight. In terms of health risk, the percentage of body fat is evaluated, not the actual pounds of fat on the body. For example, a 200 lb. man with 40 lbs. of fat in his body would be 20% body fat, whereas a 140 lb. woman with 40 lbs. of fat in her body would be 28.5% body fat, respectively. Here, a difference in body fat percentage exists even though both people have the same amount of fat weight. Obesity describes a person possessing an unhealthy quantity of fat mass relative to a person's lean mass or weight. Obesity may be defined as an excess percentage of body fat based on the sex of an individual or by body mass index (BMI) which employs indices of stature and weight but does not measure body fat.

Importantly, the quantity of lean mass, along with body fat distribution, is as significant as total fat mass when considering health. This occurs because both lean and fat mass can affect metabolic function [13, 17, 24]. **Normal-weight obesity** represents a relatively new classification describing individuals who maintain population normal weight but carry too much fat compared to relative muscle content. Lean mass is crucial because greater quantities of muscle mass relative to size links with better metabolic fitness and lower overall body fat [31]. Since body composition directly correlates to risk for disease, individuals who maintain high levels of body fat dramatically elevate their risk for disease and premature mortality; conversely, low body fat percentages correlate with longer lifespans and higher quality of life [34]. The CDC suggests more than one-third (34.9% or 78.6 million) of U.S. adults qualify as obese based on BMI values. When obesity rates are added to the percentage of Americans who are overweight, the number jumps to 70%. According to the CDC, non-Hispanic Blacks have the highest age-adjusted rates of obesity (47.8%), followed by Hispanics (42.5%), non-Hispanic whites (32.6%), and non-Hispanic Asians (10.8%) [28].

QUICK FACT

Lean Mass vs. Fat-free Mass

Lean body mass differs from fat-free mass. It consists of bones, ligaments, tendons, internal organs, and muscles: almost everything that is not fat. Due to essential fat within the bone marrow and internal organs, lean mass does include a small amount of fat.

DEFINITIONS

Normal-weight obesity –

Classification indicated by normal weight by population norms, but high body fat percentage.

Diet factors associated with obesity and specific health risks:

- Over-sufficiency – excess caloric intake
- High in sugar and processed carbohydrates
- High in saturated fat
- Low in potassium and high in sodium
- Low in fruits and/or vegetables
- Excessive red and/or processed meat consumption
- Low in water
- High in alcohol

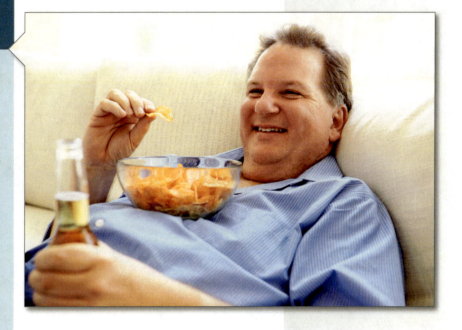

Performance-Related Components of Fitness

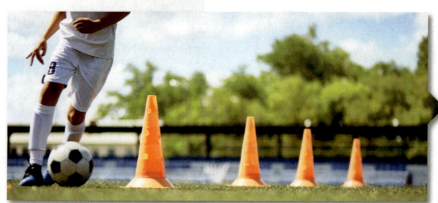

For obvious reasons, performance-related components of fitness have traditionally been the emphasis of sports-related conditioning programs. Individuals looking to excel in competitive sports often train to improve system-specificity for a particular performance component such as speed or power, based on the sport's requirements. Recently however, greater emphasis has been placed on training for improvements in the performance-related areas for all populations as they affect overall physical function. Power, speed, balance, coordination, and agility all have implications for health, as they indirectly affect the health-related components. Without power, a person cannot rise from a chair; poor balance and coordination increase the risk of falls; and gait speed decline correlates to functional deterioration of both mind and body [36]. The most effective exercise professionals will recognize the importance of integrating the performance components of fitness into exercise prescriptions for improved health. Even those clients who are not training for sport performance, especially older individuals, will benefit greatly from this type of training. This is not to suggest all people should perform ballistic movements, like Olympic weightlifting, and engage in high-speed sprints; rather, training should emphasize the benefit of utilizing activities that encourage improvements in human performance.

Power

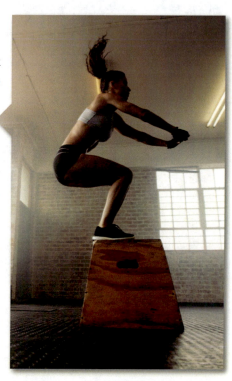

Power means the speed at which work is performed (force x distance/time). To enhance power, training focuses on acceleration, rather than on the amount of resistance moved (as is the case when one is training for strength). Performing a very heavy back squat is a relatively slow movement, so while it requires high force, thereby improving strength, it yields low power because of the slow performance velocity. On the other hand, a squat jump would be considered a high-power activity: it uses rapid acceleration to perform the jump. Olympic lifts, plyometrics, sled drives, and ballistics – such as weighted jumps and throws, all emphasize acceleration by calling on recruitment patterns that elicit the fastest

DEFINITIONS

Power –

The rate at which work is performed: (force x velocity) = (force x distance/time) = (work/time).

development of force to promote power. When power is viewed from a functional standpoint, it suggests muscles maintain an adequate force-velocity relationship for specific power-based tasks. For instance, getting up from a seated position requires powerful movements by the hip flexors to bring the center of mass over the base of support so that the hip extensors and the knee extensors can propel the body to an upright position. Individuals who lose this ability, as a result of their loss of power, increase the risk of losing independence [12, 30]. Many older adults find it difficult to get out of chairs or cars because of age-related decline in muscular power output. Losses in fast-twitch protein structures lead to an inability to produce adequate acceleration forces. Individuals experiencing **sarcopenia** and other age-related declines in fitness may attempt to thrust forward to get up from a seated position; however, when the force generation rate falls below a certain threshold, they become unable to move the mass an appropriate distance. Thus, exercise professionals should encourage power development in their exercise programs with age appropriate recommendations [10, 29, 35].

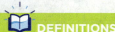

DEFINITIONS

Sarcopenia –

A muscular disease indicated by the loss of total skeletal muscle mass, with particular significance in reduction of fast-twitch muscle fibers.

Speed –

The time to perform a movement in one direction: the rate of positional change.

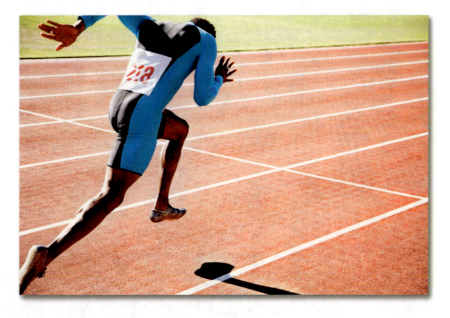

Speed

Speed entails the ability to move the body or body parts (rate of positional change) over a distance in a measured period of time. Like power, speed of movement also depends upon neural recruitment patterns and adequate muscular capability. Speed is crucial to successful athletic performance and is often considered to be the most valued performance measure in many sports. It is also relevant for normal function. Loss of speed capabilities correlate to both function and age-related decline [7, 36]. The rate of decline with age depends upon several health-related factors. Individuals who maintain higher levels of activity experience a slower rate of decline in speed compared to their non-active counterparts. Stability, dynamic balance, and flexibility all affect movement speed. These aspects of training should be appropriately addressed in activities designed for improved movement proficiency, regardless of age. Interestingly, when older adults perform routine power and strength training activities, both total movement and movement speed improve [37].

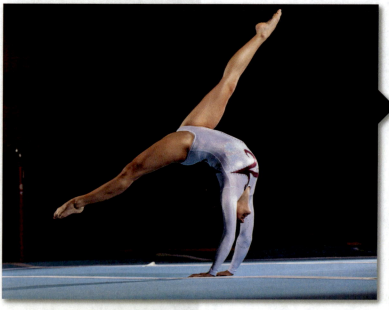

Balance

Balance can be described as the ability to manage forces which act to disrupt stability. Consistent with the other performance components, the nervous system plays the largest role in manipulating muscle tension to accommodate the demand. Balance is needed on many occasions for sport and daily activities as individuals attempt to manage disruptive forces. The stabilizing function of the muscles translates to efficient posture, movement, and body control during dynamic applications. To improve balance, a person must attain adequate strength, a synergy of force, and education of proprioceptors through neural familiarity. When the body is challenged by disruptive environments, the applied stress promotes improved neuromuscular coordination. This in turn, enhances equilibrium through increases in **proprioception** in both static and dynamic conditions. Employing balance training across population segments encourages improved function and performance on several levels [18, 22, 25, 32]. For the athlete, this means better management of force at higher speeds; for the general public, it suggests reduced risk of injury from falls or related accidents. Of note, proper muscle **strength balance** across a joint is required to improve static and dynamic balance in addition to more efficient activation patterns during movement.

DEFINITIONS

Balance –

The ability to manage forces which act to disrupt stability.

Proprioception –

The cumulative input to the CNS from receptors that relay body and positional movement: physical awareness of the body's position in space.

Strength Balance –

The functional strength ratio of opposing muscle groups across a joint: also referred to as agonist/antagonist muscle ratio or muscle balance ratio.

Coordination –

The ability to control and use multiple body parts and/or senses at the same time efficiently.

Coordination

Coordination is synonymous with neural efficiency. The better an individual manages force, the easier the body performs tasks. Webster's dictionary defines coordination as *"the regulation of diverse elements into an integrated and harmonious operation."* For instance, hand-eye coordination combines processing visual data with the neuromuscular control of the hands. High levels of coordination are associated with the proficient execution of complicated or rapidly performed tasks integral to sports performance. Undeniably, athletes need coordination to succeed in sports; however, adequate levels of coordination are also needed to perform daily tasks safely and in a controlled manner. Although all activities require coordination, high levels are not necessary for health improvements. Exercise professionals should recognize that selecting activities appropriate for a client's coordination level will make for a safer exercise experience.

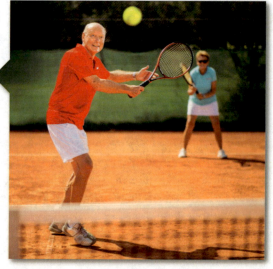

Agility

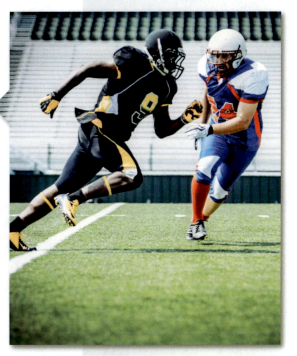

Agility is often erroneously identified as the ability to change direction, but that is not independently true. A better definition of agility is the performance of a movement involving a rapid change, of direction or velocity, in reaction to an analysis of the environment. True agility is challenged using **open skill** development. An open skill is one where the environment changes in some way; whereas a **closed skill** is performed in a static environment where all aspects never change and are completely predictable. In object-based sports, agility allows the athlete to physically pursue a ball, puck, or another implement that is constantly changing direction under varying conditions. Agility is often a defining quality in athletic pursuits as it is necessary for success in many sports. While the average person does not experience the same need for agility as a football running back or a point guard on a basketball team, all people need to be able to evaluate a situation and manage directional change without losing balance. For example, a person may have to navigate a busy city sidewalk and get out of the way of an oncoming cyclist. Agility often necessitates the ability to move quickly; therefore, it applies most in situations involving fast movement speeds in which the environment constantly changes. Individuals with low levels of agility have difficulty moving rapidly to manage offsetting forces when high movement velocities are present. This is of particular concern for older adults, who must be able to manage forces to avoid falls and injury from unplanned situations.

◆ Integrating Physical Fitness

Humans are predictable when it comes to physical fitness. In fact, significant commonalities exist among first-world nations that collect physical activity data on their populations. Regardless of the country evaluated, a fairly constant percentage of people engage in physical activity, along with a smaller but equally consistent number of those who exercise regularly; however, the largest percentage of data-supported populations around the world are sedentary. Though humans demonstrate diverse interests regarding things they enjoy, most fall into homogeneous groups when it comes to physical activity. In America, six areas of interest stand out, representing the top ten reported activities. These include bipedal locomotion (i.e., walk/jog/run/hike), cycling, swimming, weight training, flexibility training/stretching, and bowling. This data demonstrates that people gravitate towards specific activities. Anecdotally, most people who exercise regularly tend to participate heavily in one type of modality and may or may not engage in any other form. Weightlifters prefer to lift weights, those who like stretching gravitate to yoga or related activities, and endurance enthusiasts tend to run, bike, or swim for the majority of the time they engage in physical activity. While most forms of physical activity are beneficial, few promote all of the health-related components of fitness, and even fewer employ the performance-related components. Exercise professionals must understand that for someone to be optimally healthy and fit, the person must adopt a program which incorporates activities that promote complementary adaptations in multiple systems. The interaction of system engagement and specific adaptations will be covered later in the text, but for now, the idea of integrating aerobic and anaerobic activities as part of a more comprehensive plan is emphasized to achieve lifelong health goals.

DEFINITIONS

Agility –

A rapid whole-body movement with change of velocity or direction in response to a stimulus.

Open skills –

Motor skills requiring the participant to react to changes in an unpredictable environment (e.g., playing basketball).

Closed skills –

Motor skills performed in a stable or predictable environment (e.g., bowling).

Most Popular Physical Activities in the United States

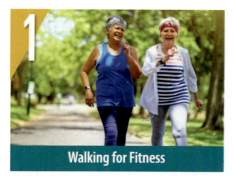
1. Walking for Fitness

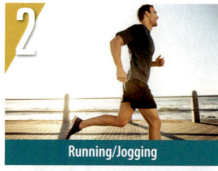
2. Running/Jogging

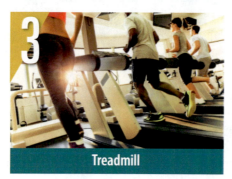
3. Treadmill

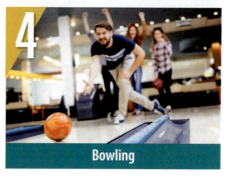
4. Bowling

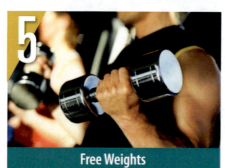
5. Free Weights

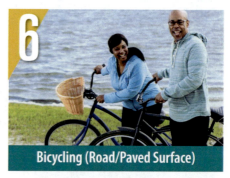
6. Bicycling (Road/Paved Surface)

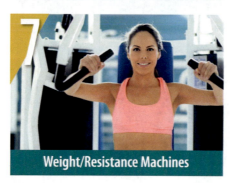
7. Weight/Resistance Machines

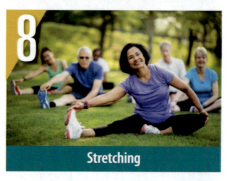
8. Stretching

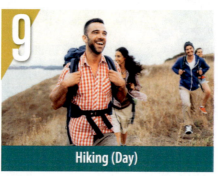
9. Hiking (Day)

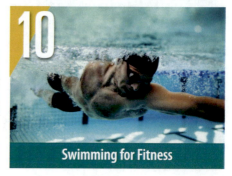
10. Swimming for Fitness

REFERENCES:

1. Centers for Disease Control and Prevention. National Diabetes Statistics Report, 2017. Atlanta, GA: Centers for Disease Control and Prevention, U.S. Dept of Health and Human Services.

2. Health. In: *Merriam-Webster Dictionary*, 2017.

3. Occupational Outlook Handbook, 2016-17 Edition, Fitness Trainers and Instructors, 2017., edited by Statistics UDoLBoL.

4. Physical Activity Guidelines Advisory Committee report, 2008. To the Secretary of Health and Human Services. Part A: executive summary. *Nutr Rev* 67: 114-120, 2009.

5. QuickStats: Percentage of U.S. Adults Who Met the 2008 Federal Physical Activity Guidelines for Aerobic and Strengthening Activity,* by Sex - National Health Interview Survey,(dagger) 2000-2014. *MMWR Morb Mortal Wkly Rep* 65: 485, 2016.

6. U.S. Dept. of Health and Human Services. Step It Up! The Surgeon General's Call to Action to Promote Walking and Walkable Communities. U.S. Dept. of Health and Human Services, Office of the Surgeon General; 2015., 2015.

7. Beavers KM, Beavers DP, Houston DK, Harris TB, Hue TF, Koster A, Newman AB, Simonsick EM, Studenski SA, Nicklas BJ, and Kritchevsky SB. Associations between body composition and gait-speed decline: results from the Health, Aging, and Body Composition study. *Am J Clin Nutr* 97: 552-560, 2013.

8. Bosnes I, Almkvist O, Bosnes O, Stordal E, Romild U, and Nordahl HM. Prevalence and correlates of successful aging in a population-based sample of older adults: the HUNT study. *Int Psychogeriatr* 29: 431-440, 2017.

9. Brill PA, Macera CA, Davis DR, Blair SN, and Gordon N. Muscular strength and physical function. *Med Sci Sports Exerc* 32: 412-416, 2000.

10. Byrne C, Faure C, Keene DJ, and Lamb SE. Ageing, Muscle Power and Physical Function: A Systematic Review and Implications for Pragmatic Training Interventions. *Sports Med* 46: 1311-1332, 2016.

11. Colberg SR, Sigal RJ, Yardley JE, Riddell MC, Dunstan DW, Dempsey PC, Horton ES, Castorino K, and Tate DF. Physical Activity/Exercise and Diabetes: A Position Statement of the American Diabetes Association. *Diabetes Care* 39: 2065-2079, 2016.

12. De Luca CR, Wood SJ, Anderson V, Buchanan JA, Proffitt TM, Mahony K, and Pantelis C. Normative data from the CANTAB. I: development of executive function over the lifespan. *J Clin Exp Neuropsychol* 25: 242-254, 2003.

13. Dulloo AG, Jacquet J, Solinas G, Montani JP, and Schutz Y. Body composition phenotypes in pathways to obesity and the metabolic syndrome. *Int J Obes (Lond)* 34 Suppl 2: S4-17, 2010.

14. Duscha BD, Slentz CA, Johnson JL, Houmard JA, Bensimhon DR, Knetzger KJ, and Kraus WE. Effects of exercise training amount and intensity on peak oxygen consumption in middle-age men and women at risk for cardiovascular disease. *Chest* 128: 2788-2793, 2005.

15. Flegal KM, Carroll MD, Kit BK, and Ogden CL. Prevalence of obesity and trends in the distribution of body mass index among US adults, 1999-2010. *JAMA* 307: 491-497, 2012.

16. Flegal KM, Carroll MD, Kuczmarski RJ, and Johnson CL. Overweight and obesity in the United States: prevalence and trends, 1960-1994. *Int J Obes Relat Metab Disord* 22: 39-47, 1998.

17. Grundy SM. Adipose tissue and metabolic syndrome: too much, too little or neither. *Eur J Clin Invest* 45: 1209-1217, 2015.

18. Hrysomallis C. Balance ability and athletic performance. *Sports Med* 41: 221-232, 2011.

19. Jackson AS, Sui X, Hebert JR, Church TS, and Blair SN. Role of lifestyle and aging on the longitudinal change in cardiorespiratory fitness. *Arch Intern Med* 169: 1781-1787, 2009.

20. Kodama S, Saito K, Tanaka S, Maki M, Yachi Y, Asumi M, Sugawara A, Totsuka K, Shimano H, Ohashi Y, Yamada N, and Sone H. Cardiorespiratory fitness as a quantitative predictor of all-cause mortality and cardiovascular events in healthy men and women: a meta-analysis. *JAMA* 301: 2024-2035, 2009.

21. Lloyd RS, Faigenbaum AD, Stone MH, Oliver JL, Jeffreys I, Moody JA, Brewer C, Pierce KC, McCambridge TM, Howard R, Herrington L, Hainline B, Micheli LJ, Jaques R, Kraemer WJ, McBride MG, Best TM, Chu DA, Alvar BA, and Myer GD. Position statement on youth resistance training: the 2014 International Consensus. *Br J Sports Med* 48: 498-505, 2014.

22. Low DC, Walsh GS, and Arkesteijn M. Effectiveness of Exercise Interventions to Improve Postural Control in Older Adults: A Systematic Review and Meta-Analyses of Centre of Pressure Measurements. *Sports Med* 47: 101-112, 2017.

23. MacDonald HV, Johnson BT, Huedo-Medina TB, Livingston J, Forsyth KC, Kraemer WJ, Farinatti PT, and Pescatello LS. Dynamic Resistance Training as Stand-Alone Antihypertensive Lifestyle Therapy: A Meta-Analysis. *J Am Heart Assoc* 5, 2016.

24. Magkos F, Fraterrigo G, Yoshino J, Luecking C, Kirbach K, Kelly SC, de Las Fuentes L, He S, Okunade AL, Patterson BW, and Klein S. Effects of Moderate and Subsequent Progressive Weight Loss on Metabolic Function and Adipose Tissue Biology in Humans with Obesity. *Cell Metab* 23: 591-601, 2016.

25. McKeon PO, Ingersoll CD, Kerrigan DC, Saliba E, Bennett BC, and Hertel J. Balance training improves function and postural control in those with chronic ankle instability. *Med Sci Sports Exerc* 40: 1810-1819, 2008.

26. Mu L, Cohen AJ, and Mukamal KJ. Resistance and aerobic exercise among adults with diabetes in the U.S. *Diabetes Care* 37: e175-176, 2014.

27. Nauman J, Nes BM, Lavie CJ, Jackson AS, Sui X, Coombes JS, Blair SN, and Wisloff U. Prediction of Cardiovascular Mortality by Estimated Cardiorespiratory Fitness Independent of Traditional Risk Factors: The HUNT Study. *Mayo Clin Proc* 92: 218-227, 2017.

28. Ogden CL, Carroll MD, Kit BK, and Flegal KM. Prevalence of childhood and adult obesity in the United States, 2011-2012. *JAMA* 311: 806-814, 2014.

29. Peterson MD, Sen A, and Gordon PM. Influence of resistance exercise on lean body mass in aging adults: a meta-analysis. *Med Sci Sports Exerc* 43: 249-258, 2011.

30. Puggaard L. Effects of training on functional performance in 65, 75 and 85 year-old women: experiences deriving from community based studies in Odense, Denmark. *Scand J Med Sci Sports* 13: 70-76, 2003.

31. Saltin B and Pilegaard H. [Metabolic fitness: physical activity and health]. *Ugeskr Laeger* 164: 2156-2162, 2002.

32. Sherrington C, Whitney JC, Lord SR, Herbert RD, Cumming RG, and Close JC. Effective exercise for the prevention of falls: a systematic review and meta-analysis. *J Am Geriatr Soc* 56: 2234-2243, 2008.

33. Song M, Carroll DD, and Fulton JE. Meeting the 2008 physical activity guidelines for Americans among U.S. youth. *Am J Prev Med* 44: 216-222, 2013.

34. Stewart KJ, Bacher AC, Turner K, Lim JG, Hees PS, Shapiro EP, Tayback M, and Ouyang P. Exercise and risk factors associated with metabolic syndrome in older adults. *Am J Prev Med* 28: 9-18, 2005.

35. Straight CR, Lindheimer JB, Brady AO, Dishman RK, and Evans EM. Effects of Resistance Training on Lower-Extremity Muscle Power in Middle-Aged and Older Adults: A Systematic Review and Meta-Analysis of Randomized Controlled Trials. *Sports Med* 46: 353-364, 2016.

36. Teixeira-Salmela LF, Santiago L, Lima RC, Lana DM, Camargos FF, and Cassiano JG. Functional performance and quality of life related to training and detraining of community-dwelling elderly. *Disabil Rehabil* 27: 1007-1012, 2005.

37. Tschopp M, Sattelmayer MK, and Hilfiker R. Is power training or conventional resistance training better for function in elderly persons? A meta-analysis. *Age Ageing* 40: 549-556, 2011.

38. United States. Department of Health and Human Services. *2008 physical activity guidelines for Americans: be active, healthy, and happy!* Washington, DC: U.S. Dept. of Health and Human Services, 2008.

Advanced Concepts of Personal Training

NCSF

Certified Personal Trainer

Chapter 2

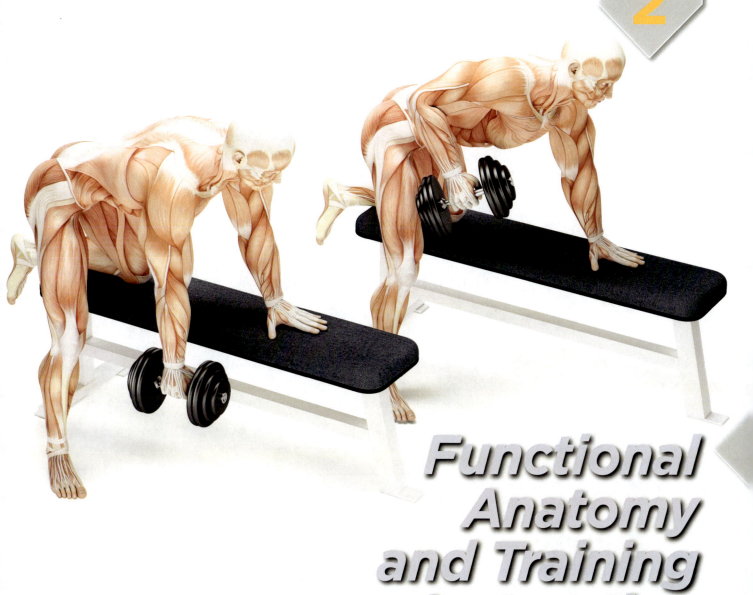

Functional Anatomy and Training Instruction

Human Movement

Many biomechanists refer to the body as a living machine. Machines and the human body are comprised of a frame with levers acting on movable and structural joints. The integrity of the parts, efficiency of the structural system, and the economy of the applicable movements often determine how well and for how long a machine can perform proficiently. In humans, a strong skeletal system, efficient joints, and capable movements predict a healthy body. Therefore, a personal trainer's main responsibility is to keep the "human machine" running optimally. Knowledge of functional anatomy features critically in this effort, as it allows identification of issues and is vital for creating a prescription for improvement. Because voluntary movement stems from the application of force produced by a muscle on the attached bone, having a clear comprehension of musculoskeletal structures and their function underlies an understanding of human movement. Again, a working knowledge of the body's structures and how they coordinate allows personal trainers to use appropriate decision-making criteria for individual exercise prescription.

◆ Composition of Bones

The skeletal system serves as the body's framework, providing shape, protection, and support. The structures of the skeleton are comprised of a mineral component, which provides rigidity, and a protein component, which attenuates bone tension. The organic compounds of bone are formed mainly by collagen, which makes up 33% of bone mass, while the mineral component represents the other 67% [1]. Together, these tissues function to systematically produce and control motor function by managing internal and external forces.

Bone tissue is hardened by calcium salts, which represent approximately 98% of the calcium storage in the body. Although it is the most significant location of calcium in the body,

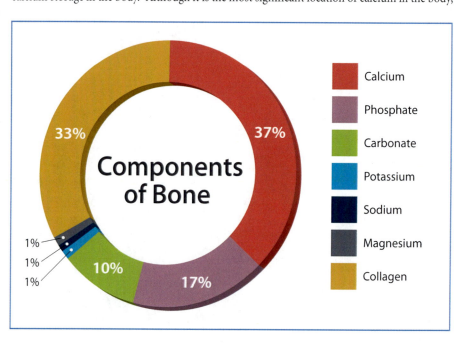

bone is not simply a mineral composite. Bone is living tissue and actually very dynamic. It has a fairly complex vascular system, which serves as a vehicle for calcium mobility and allows calcium and other minerals to enter and leave the bone, based on internal signaling. For instance, when extracellular calcium levels fall too low, calcium is recruited from bone storage and mobilized to the physiological destination of need. This is part of the self-regulating process the body uses to maintain a constant desirable range of conditions called **homeostasis**. When daily calcium intake is insufficient for prolonged periods of time, bone stores of calcium become compromised as the mineral density declines. A significant reduction in **bone mineral density** (**BMD**) causes a pre-disease condition called osteopenia. If **osteopenia** is untreated, it may progress to the pathological disease state known as **osteoporosis**, which is the most common bone disease in humans[7].

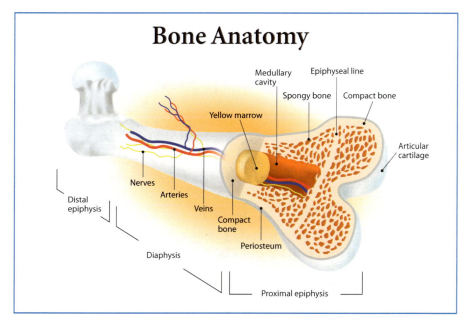

As stated earlier, the skeleton is a system of levers, support structures, and struts, which allow the body to maintain postural control, perform movement through varied ranges, and protectively house vital organs. It consists of two segments, the axial skeleton and the appendicular skeleton. The axial skeleton frames the body and consists of the skull, hyoid bone, vertebral column, and rib cage, while the peripheral attachments are referred to as the appendicular skeleton. For the most part, the axial skeleton protects the central nervous system, heart, and lungs and is the structural segment for body posture; on the other hand, the appendicular skeleton supports locomotion and everyday movements through its limbs and girdles. Each segment contains various bones to support its respective role and function.

Bones come in several shapes and sizes that are specific to their purpose and define how they are classified. The proximal bones of the arms and legs are long bones; in the hands and feet, they are called short bones. The unique shape of the vertebrae yields the term, irregular bones, while bones with a broad connective surface, like that of the scapulae, are called flat bones. The kneecap, or patella, is classified as a sesamoid bone. As stated above, each bone's shape has distinctions that support the role it serves within the body. Long bones, for instance, function as levers that allow for bipedal movement and include an elongated diaphysis (shaft), which contains a significant marrow cavity where 2.5 million red blood cells are formed every second. The short bones make up intricate formations in the hands (providing for dexterity)

DEFINITIONS

Homeostasis –

The body's tendency to seek a constant, desirable range of conditions that maintain equilibrium within all physiological systems.

Bone mineral density (BMD) –

The mineral content in a given volume of bone, used as a measure of bone health as well as to diagnose diseases, such as osteoporosis.

Osteopenia –

A pre-disease condition, which indicates bone mineral density is lower than normal for a given individual's age and sex, but is not yet low enough to be classified as osteoporosis. In other words, it is a precursor for osteoporosis.

Osteoporosis –

A bone disease in which a decrease in mineral density causes skeletal structures to become brittle and fragile, often leading to fractures and disability; this condition is typically caused by negative hormonal changes, sedentary behaviors over the lifespan, and/or a deficiency of energy, calcium and/or Vitamin D.

Human Skeletal System

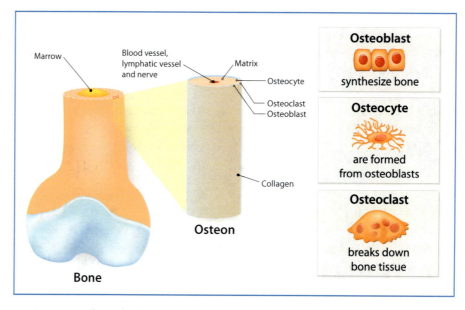

and feet (serving as a platform for postural balance). The flat bones allow for broad muscular attachments, which are often used to support significant force requirements, as seen with the insertion sites of the rhomboids on the scapula and pectoralis major on the sternum. Irregular bones manage uniquely designed muscle arrangements, as seen with the spiny process of the vertebrae. These bones support the numerous muscular attachments to the spine and function to accommodate the specific actions of the trunk.

◆ Bone Growth

The skeleton begins as a cartilaginous structure and is replaced by bone through a maturation process called ossification. Increases in bone mass (width or diameter) occur from the formation of new bone on the surface of existing bone tissue, called appositional growth. During normal maturation, a bone increases in size and is remodeled by the removal and replacement of bone. Bone length is attributed to endochondral growth, where cartilage is ossified at the **epiphyseal plates** at the epiphysis of long bones. As humans age, new hyaline cartilage is formed to promote growth but eventually turns to bone. Vertical growth ceases when no further cartilage is formed, and the present cartilage becomes fully ossified. In most humans, peak bone mass is reached by age 18 in females and 20 in males and peak bone density is achieved between the ages of 20 and 30 for both men and women [17, 48]. The integrity of bone is often measured by mass and density. A low **bone mass** is associated with osteopenia and increases the risk of fractures and osteoporosis while BMD provides a t-score which reflects the difference in mineral concentration between one's relative bone density and the average bone density of young healthy adults of the same sex. Diagnoses of osteopenia or osteoporosis are made based on this t-score.

DEFINITIONS

Epiphyseal plates –

The transverse cartilage plates, located near the end of long bones and responsible for increases in vertical growth during childhood and adolescence.

Bone mass –

This represents the surface area of bone and total tissue volume.

Weight-bearing physical activity –

Activities where the skeleton must bear the weight of the body while performing the movement; these activity types are favored for improvements in bone mass, strength, and resilience.

To promote bone development, children and adolescents must consume adequate calories, vitamin D, magnesium, calcium and also participate in regular **weight-bearing physical activity**. An important fact regarding bone development is that bone mass reaches maturity before BMD.

Changes in bone mass are normally complete by age 20, but BMD can be positively affected for another full decade. BMD is subject to variations over a person's lifespan based on genetics, diet, and behaviors, which combine to dictate the rate of decline [3]. For instance, the application of resisted movement activities represents one key factor in maintaining healthy bones. The correlation between BMD and the strength of the attached musculature suggests that resistance training can be an important activity used to maintain bone health at all ages and is recommended for both young and old alike via routine, age-appropriate strengthening activities [7, 45]. It is important to note that children and adolescents have the greatest risks to bone health from malnutrition, disease, and trauma.

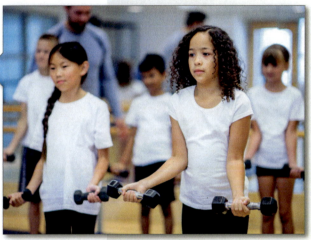

Resistance training activities performed by children and adolescents have raised concerns due to the potential risk of damage or premature ossification of the epiphyseal plates of long bones [24]. The evidence of epiphyseal fractures in children performing resistance exercise is equivocal, as no clinical trials have demonstrated any adverse effects [22]. However, due to the developmental stage of the bone and the stress associated with resisted movement, there may be some increased vulnerability. Premature cessation of bone growth may represent another potential adverse event associated with intense resistance training in children. The epiphyseal plates close naturally in response to high levels of sex hormones that exist during post-pubescence. Some theorize that the increased androgenic hormones produced in response to intense resistance training may promote a premature ossification of the epiphyseal plates, attenuating natural bone growth. Others suggest the stress of high-intensity training (HIT) is inappropriate for developing bones. Nevertheless, no clear evidence exists to support either notion except that anabolic steroid abuse has been associated with premature ossification in youth [10, 22, 25]. In fact, most physicians will encourage age-appropriate resistance activity when performed under supervision of a prudent professional. The International Weightlifting Federation (IWF) and USA Weightlifting's youth age category is recognized as 13-17, which are clearly developmental years. No clinical trial to date has indicated that appropriately applied resisted movements damage the epiphyseal plates of long bones [22, 25]. Analysis of bone stress shows that the impact of activities such as playing, jumping, and landing, exceeds that of controlled resisted activities, such as squatting and pressing, when performed with 10 RM resistance [10, 28].

◆ Joint Classifications

The intersection of two bones is called an articulation or a **joint**. Depending on the role and structure of the joint, its movement may have a broad range, such as the shoulder's glenohumeral joint, or it may be limited for structural purposes, such as the acromioclavicular joint at the clavicle. The more movement afforded to a joint, the greater the requirements for soft tissue support to manage stability.

The three major classifications of joints are fibrous, cartilaginous, and **synovial**. The connective tissue characteristics determine classification. Fibrous joints are not intended to move, or exhibit very little movement, so they are tightly connected by fibrous tissue and do not possess a joint cavity. Cartilaginous joints unite articular surfaces with **hyaline cartilage**, which allows for very slight movement, or **fibrocartilage**, which has slightly greater movement capabilities due to the tissue's flexible nature. The aforementioned joints primarily support the skeletal

DEFINITIONS

Joint –

A point of articulation between two or more bones that allows for a functional connection and various amounts of motion, depending on local anatomical features.

Synovial joint –

A type of joint that uses synovial fluid to reduce frictional stresses and allow for considerable movement between the associated articulating bones.

Hyaline cartilage –

Tough yet elastic connective tissue found in various parts/joints of the body which allows for minimal movement, depending on the surrounding anatomy.

Fibrocartilage –

Tough connective tissue composed of a dense matrix of fibers serving as a shock absorber for structures exposed to high forces.

system's structural integrity or serve as connectors for growth. In contrast, synovial joints manage movement. Thus, to allow for the considerable movement range between articulations, synovial joints are more anatomically complex than fibrous and cartilaginous joints and are also subject to more injuries.

◆ Synovial Joints

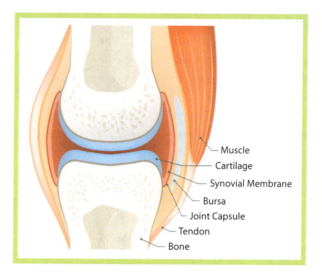

The joints of the appendicular skeleton are predominantly synovial to accommodate locomotion and daily activity needs. Synovial joints rely on several mechanisms to reduce friction and maintain the joint's integrity under the duress of applied forces. Hyaline cartilage covers the articular surfaces, providing a smooth coating layer at the site where the bones meet. In areas subject to compressive or shock forces, the surfaces feature the additional support of fibrocartilage and fat pads. The fibrocartilage forms articular discs, which provide added strength and support to the joint, as is the case for the menisci in the knee. The fat pads are often found around the edges of joints to provide protection for the cartilage. Each joint is enclosed by a dual-layer **joint capsule**. The joint capsule is made up of fibrous tissue extending from the **periosteum**, the fibrous external membrane covering the bone. The fibrous capsule may have thickened regions which provide ligamentous support to the joint. A **synovial membrane** lining the joint capsule secretes synovial fluid to form a thin lubricating film which covers the articular surfaces to further reduce the frictional co-efficient created by movement. In some synovial joints, the lining extends to form a pocket or sac called a **bursa**, which serves as a fluid-filled cushion between surfaces to prevent contact or the rubbing of connective tissues during movement. **Ligaments** and **tendons** external to the joint capsule may further add structural support to the joint.

Types of Synovial Joints

There are several types of synovial joint classifications, defined according to the adjoining articular surfaces' shapes. The six types of synovial joints include the following: ball-and-socket joints, consisting of a rounded articular surface of one bone that fits into the socket (cup-shaped depression) of the corresponding bone and allows for complementary movements (shoulder and hip); plane or gliding joints, consisting of two opposed flat surfaces that are relatively equal in size and may glide across or twist slightly over each other (spinal vertebrae); hinge joints,

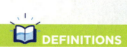

DEFINITIONS

Joint capsule –

A connective tissue enclosure that surrounds specific joints and consists of an outer fibrous membrane and an inner synovial membrane, assisting in joint protection and stability.

Periosteum –

A dense fibrous membrane covering the surface of bones that serves as an attachment site for tendons to connect muscle to bone.

Synovial membrane –

A special membrane that lines synovial joints and secretes synovial fluid to lubricate the articulating surfaces.

Bursa –

A small fluid-filled sac that reduces friction between connective and bony tissues during movement.

Ligaments –

Tough fibrous bands of connective tissue that support internal organs and attach adjacent bones at articulation sites; due to limited blood supply, self-repair is difficult following an injury.

Tendons –

Tough fibrous bands of connective tissue that connect muscles to bones; tendons positively adapt to flexibility and resistance-based exercise.

Synovial Joints

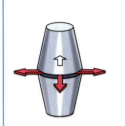 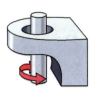 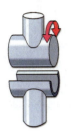 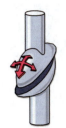 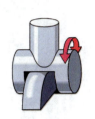 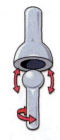

PLANE JOINT	PIVOT JOINT	HINGE JOINT	CONDYLOID JOINT	SADDLE JOINT	BALL-AND-SOCKET JOINT
A plane joint allows bones to slide past each other. Midcarpal and midtarsal joints are plane joints.	A pivot joint allows rotation around an axis. Pivot joints are found in the neck and forearm.	A hinge joint allows extension and retraction of an appendage. Hinge joints are found in the knees, elbows, fingers, and toes.	A condyloid joint is similar to ball and socket but with less movement. The wrist is a condyloid joint.	A saddle joint allows movement back and forth and up and down. The only saddle joint in the human body is the thumb.	A ball and socket joint allows for radical movement in almost any direction. Ball-and-socket joints are found in the shoulders and hips.

which work by fitting a convex cylinder inside a concave articular surface, allowing for movement in a single plane (elbow and knee); pivot joints, which restrict movement to rotation around a single axis (radius/ulna); saddle joints, which have similarly shaped (saddle) articular surfaces and fit into one another, allowing for two planes of movement (thumb); and condyloid joints, which form a uniquely structured, shallow ball-and-socket with limited movement range (wrist).

The joint's ability to move depends upon several factors, including the locations of the muscular attachment insertion sites, the type of joint, and the shape of the articular surface. The joints that have the greatest mobility have the least stability and are often considered to be "weak" when compared to range-limited synovial or non-moving fibrous and cartilaginous joints. Comparing the shoulder and hip joints provides a good example. Although a freely moving ball-and-socket joint, the shoulder loses stability when fully abducted, flexed, or externally rotated due to the scapula's limited surface area. In the shoulder, the joint's socket portion is formed from the glenoid fossa of the scapula, which is a shallow cup. The hip, on the other hand, better exemplifies a true ball-and-socket joint due to the amount of articulating (contact) surface. The hip provides for less range of motion (ROM) but much greater stability, explaining its reduced risk for injury compared to the shoulder. The body has created defense mechanisms to help manage the risk for injury in highly moveable joints by attempting to limit movement range. This is accomplished by the following: location of fibrous connective fibers in and around the joint capsule; the particular shape of the articulating surface in relation to the muscle attachment sites; the presence of other structures, including disks and fat pads; and the activity of **proprioceptors** that manage muscle and tendon tension. When these mechanisms cannot manage an external force, a joint may dislocate, causing the articular surfaces to come apart. This may damage the joint capsule, articular cartilage, and/or ligaments. Individuals with extremely mobile joints may be diagnosed with joint laxity or **hypermobility** [20]. If too much flexibility compromises the joint's stability, it should be strengthened and no longer stretched. It is important that the surrounding tissues are bolstered in a manner that promotes stability, and individuals with hypermobility should be cautious to avoid injury during high-force activities [20, 33, 51].

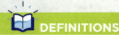

DEFINITIONS

Proprioceptors –

Special sensory receptors found in joints and connective tissues that send signals concerning body position and movement to motor neurons in the spinal cord, thereby effectively managing muscle and tendon tension.

Hypermobility –

Also known as "joint laxity", this term indicates joint movement capabilities which surpass a normal, healthy range; addressing hypermobility usually requires an emphasis on strength and stability, while avoiding flexibility activities to reduce the risk for injury.

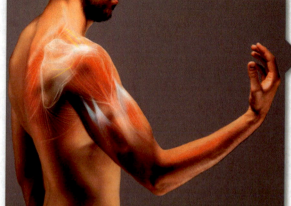

◆ How Joints Work

Joints move when internal or external forces are applied to the skeleton. Voluntary movements require coordinated muscle contraction to produce internal forces, which act on the bone via its tendons. A muscle's tendons extend from the musculotendinous junction to the periosteum of the bone. The periosteum isolates the bone from surrounding tissues and encases a network of nerves and vessels, which provide blood flow and nutrients to the interior. Near joints, the periosteum becomes continuous with connective tissue to hold bones together and form the joint capsule. The fibers of the periosteum are also interwoven with the tendons that attach to the bone, forming strong attachment sites. Collagen fibers further secure these tissues to the bone, profoundly increasing the attachment strength. These attachments are so strong that when a force beyond the tissue's strength is applied, it will most often break a bone before snapping the collagen fibers at the bone's surface. To attenuate this risk, the body monitors tension via special proprioceptive cells called **golgi tendon organs** (**GTOs**), which send signals back to the spinal cord to decrease tension. When muscle tension on the bone reaches a critical threshold, the GTOs' protective mechanism is activated and inhibitory signals are responsively sent to the spinal cord to "turn off" motor output to the muscle, effectively eliminating the muscle's tension.

On the other end of the tendon, muscle connective tissue is structured in a way that produces and manages efficient force development. Muscle anatomy is organized to serve several purposes. Obviously, skeletal muscle's first role is to pull on the tendons to move or stabilize the skeleton during physical actions. The skeletal muscles must also produce tension to maintain posture and sustain body positions when not moving. In addition, skeletal muscles serve to support soft tissues, such as the visceral organs, guard entrances and exits, including the digestive and urinary tracts for swallowing, defecation, and urination, and finally, assist the maintenance of body temperature by releasing heat.

◆ Types of Muscle Tissue

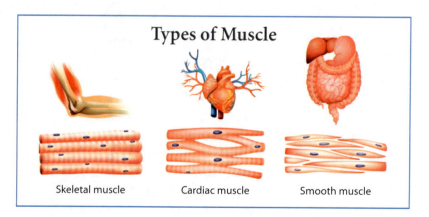

Three types of muscle tissue comprise the muscular system: **skeletal**, **cardiac**, and **smooth**. Each performs specialized functions within the body. Skeletal muscle acts on the skeleton to maintain posture, create voluntary movement, manage force transfer, and prevent undesirable body actions. The cardiac muscle tissue, located only in the heart, pushes blood through the circulatory system. Smooth muscle is integrated in the walls of blood vessels as well as the

---

DEFINITIONS

Golgi tendon organs (GTOs) –

Special kinesthetic receptors located near muscle-tendon junctions which send reflexive signals to the spinal cord to regulate muscle tension; they function to protect tissue from overstraining and injury using autogenic inhibition.

Skeletal muscle –

A type of striated muscle which attaches to the skeleton to facilitate movements by applying force to bones and joints via contractions.

Cardiac muscle –

A type of involuntary, mononucleated, striated muscle found exclusively within the heart.

Smooth muscle –

A type of involuntary, non-striated muscle found within the walls of organs and vascular structures.

gastrointestinal tract, which includes the esophagus, stomach, small intestine, large intestine, and rectum. Smooth muscle affects blood flow through the dilation and constriction of small blood vessels, moves fluids and solids, and performs a variety of other functions to help keep the body in a state of homeostasis. For the purposes of personal training, this chapter will focus on the functions and adaptations of skeletal muscle.

◆ Skeletal Muscle Architecture

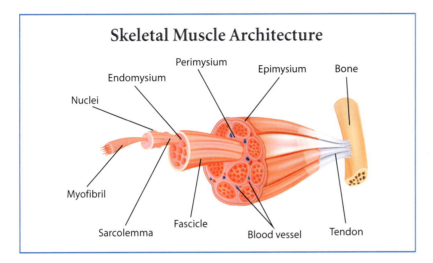

> **DEFINITIONS**
>
> **Fascia –**
>
> *The most superficial layer of muscle composed of a fibrous connective tissue that encapsulates the underlying layers to form individual muscles; fascia provides shape consistent with the arrangement of the muscle tissue to enhance intramuscular tension and regulate transfer of force across joints.*
>
> **Epimysium –**
>
> *A dense collection of collagen fibers that covers the entire surface of muscle.*
>
> **Perimysium –**
>
> *A layer of tissue below the epimysium that encompasses bundles of fibers.*
>
> **Fascicle –**
>
> *A bundle of wrapped muscle fibers.*
>
> **Endomysium –**
>
> *A thin sheath of connective tissue that covers each separate muscle fiber within a fascicle.*
>
> **Sarcolemma –**
>
> *The external lamina of each single muscle fiber.*

Skeletal muscle is organized into several layers. The most superficial layer, the **fascia**, is composed of a fibrous connective tissue that encapsulates the underlying layers to form individual muscles. It provides shape consistent with the arrangement of the muscle tissue to enhance intramuscular tension. Just beneath the fascia is the **epimysium**: a dense collection of collagen fibers that cover the entire muscle surface. Inside the epimysium lies the **perimysium**, a layer of tissue that encompasses bundles of fibers called **fascicles**. A fascicle is made up of individual muscle fibers, each separated by a thin sheath called the **endomysium**.

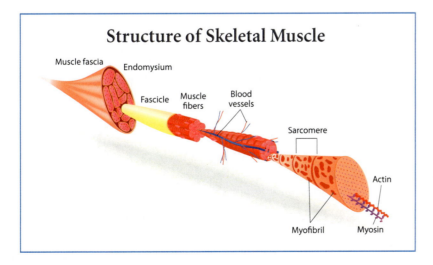

The muscle fiber, or muscle cell, is generally thought of as the functional element of the muscle; while this is true, muscle tissue can be analyzed even more deeply. The **sarcolemma**, a delicate external lamina of reticular fibers, serves as an extension of the muscle fiber. It contains the **sarcoplasm**, **mitochondria**, and **myofibrils**. Myofibrils are made up of long cylinder-like protein elements called **myofilaments**, which, operationally, set the actions of the muscle into motion. Under the microscope, myofilaments have discernibly different thicknesses. The thick myofilaments, called **myosin**, and the thin filaments, **actin**, are arranged in a functional sequence along the myofibril and are used to create tension inside the muscle tissue when activated by a nerve.

◆ How Muscles Contract

To produce internal tensile and compressive forces, skeletal muscles must contract. For this to happen, the body requires multiple systems to work concurrently and synergistically. Signals initiated by the **central nervous system** (**CNS**) stimulate muscle through an electrical and chemical signal, causing it to shorten and produce tension. If the force requirements continue, the muscle will need a continuous supply of energy and blood. The interwoven muscle layers of the epimysium and perimysium contain the nerves and blood vessels that support muscular contractions to produce force. These networks of nerves and blood vessels are extremely important, as they carry the motor information via **action potentials** from the CNS and allow the vascular system not only to deliver energy and oxygen, but also to remove the waste that builds up as a by-product of metabolic energy production (analogous to the exhaust of a car). The **peripheral nervous system** (**PNS**) and vascular system run together through the muscle tissue, branching into smaller units all the way down to the muscle fiber, where **capillaries** and nerve fibers interact with the contractile proteins.

A muscle fiber is arranged like a small factory, with each structure serving a particular function to create contractile tension. The **sliding filament theory** explains the molecular

DEFINITIONS

Sarcoplasm –

The cytoplasm within each single muscle fiber.

Mitochondria –

An organelle responsible for significant energy production and metabolic processes within each cell.

Myofibrils –

The sectional units found within each muscle fiber which contain bundles of myofilaments.

Myofilaments –

The long, cylinder-like protein elements in muscle tissue which operationally set the action of contraction into motion; these are the smallest fiber components in muscle, composed of actin and myosin.

Sarcoplasm –

The cytoplasm within each single muscle fiber.

Actin –

The thin myofilament within sarcomeres used to create tension inside muscle cells.

Myosin –

The thick myofilament within sarcomeres used to create tension inside muscle cells.

Central nervous system (CNS) –

The central processing unit for the nervous system, consisting of the brain and spinal cord; the CNS is responsible for integrating all sensory information and sending nerve impulses that regulate appropriate responses.

Action potential –

A wave-like change in the electrical properties of a cell membrane that functions as a signal to promote a cascade of events including muscular contraction.

Peripheral nervous system (PNS) –

The portion of the nervous system outside of the brain and spinal cord; the PNS connects the central nervous system to the limbs and organs to regulate sensory and motor control as well as other functions via somatic (voluntary) and autonomic subsystems.

Capillaries –

The tiny vascular structures that connect arteries and veins; they form an intricate network within bodily tissues to ensure adequate distribution of oxygen and nutrients as well as waste removal.

Sliding filament theory –

This explains the molecular mechanisms surrounding the multi-step interaction between actin (thin myofilament) and myosin (thick myofilaments) during a muscular contraction.

mechanisms of multistep interaction between actin (thin filament) and myosin (thick filaments) during a contraction. If the body needs to create tension in a group of muscle fibers, the CNS initiates a signal, called an action potential. The action potential travels via electrical current from the CNS to the PNS. From the spinal cord, the electrical current runs within the **motor neuron**, through outer levels of the muscle tissue toward a specific group of muscle fibers. The motor neuron and all the muscle fibers it innervates collectively form a **motor unit**. The motor neuron extends branches of individual nerve fibers to all of the individual muscle fibers within that motor unit. The action potential travels down to the motor endplate, where it reaches the **neuromuscular junction**. Here, the signal is converted from an electrical current to a chemical signal in the form of the neurotransmitter acetylcholine. Acetylcholine is released from the motor end-plate across the neuromuscular junction to bind to its receptor on the post-synaptic cleft. Here, the chemical signal creates a new electrical signal, this time along the sarcolemma, that travels along the sarcolemma and deep into invaginations in the muscle fiber known as the T-tubules. This process is referred to as **excitation-contraction coupling**.

Inside the muscle fiber, near the T-tubules are large holding tanks of calcium known as the sarcoplasmic reticulum (SR). When the action potential reaches the individual muscle fiber, the SR is triggered to rapidly release calcium. In a relaxed state, the myosin heads of the thick myofilaments inside the **sarcomere** are blocked from binding to actin by a protein complex consisting of troponin and tropomyosin. When calcium is released from the SR, it binds to troponin, causing a conformational change in the tropomyosin molecule which exposes the attachment sites of actin to myosin. When the calcium unlocks the bond, the **troponin-tropomyosin complex** rotates out of the way of the binding site, just like opening a door.

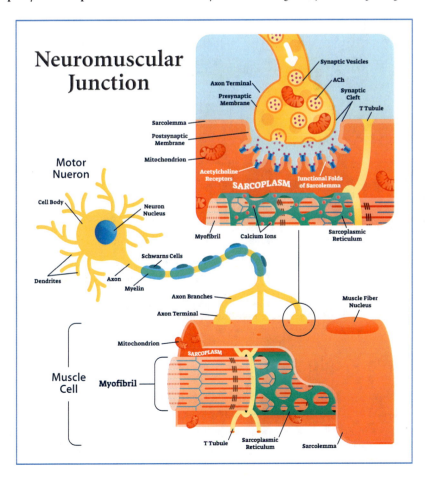

DEFINITIONS

Motor neuron –

A nerve cell within the peripheral nervous system that propagates electrical impulses to working musculature to regulate contractions and bodily movement.

Motor unit –

A motor neuron and all of the muscle fibers it innervates.

Neuromuscular junction –

This is also known as the motor end plate: a junction where a motor neuron and muscle cells interact via chemo-electrical impulses to facilitate the stimulation of muscle cell contraction.

Excitation-contraction coupling –

This describes the process in which an action potential propagates across the sarcolemma triggering release of calcium by the sarcoplasmic reticulum to initiate a muscular contraction.

Sarcoplasmic reticulum (SR) –

The tubular network that surrounds each individual muscle fiber and acts as a storage site for calcium to play its part in facilitating contractions.

Sarcomere –

The repeating functional units of a muscle fiber, consisting of contractile myofilaments; sarcomeres are the muscle components which shorten and re-lengthen during contractions.

Troponin-tropomyosin complex –

A connection site within separate muscle fibers which allows for the myosin heads to attach to actin and form a cross-bridge for muscular contraction; the attachment site is opened via the unlocking action of calcium ions released from the sarcoplasmic reticulum.

Calcium essentially acts as a key and unlocks the bond between the actin filament and tropomyosin, revealing a binding site to allow myosin heads to attach and form cross-bridges. At the site of attachment, **adenosine triphosphate (ATP)** is split, releasing energy, thereby allowing the muscle fiber to contract and produce force. When a new molecule of ATP binds to the myosin head, the attachment between myosin and actin is released. This complex chain of interactions permits the actin and myosin filament proteins to slide over each other, which is why this process is described as the sliding filament theory.

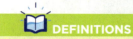

DEFINITIONS

Adenosine triphosphate (ATP) –

The primary energy source created within the mitochondria of muscle cells via various metabolic processes. ATP facilitates performance of mechanical work.

Cross bridges –

These consist of a myosin head that projects from the surface of the thick myofilament and binds to the surface of the thin myofilament (actin) in the presence of calcium ions.

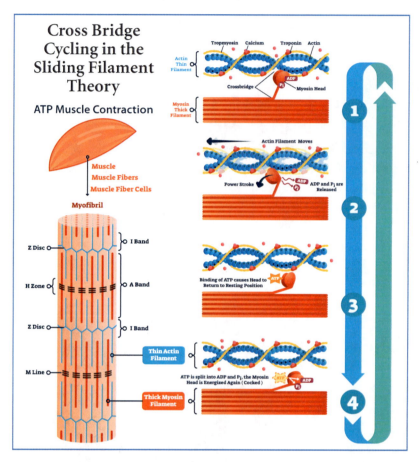

The sliding force is directed by a power-stroke action of the myosin head, which resembles the movement of an oar when rowing a boat. An oar enters the water, is pulled across the surface of the water, and is removed from the water, before being repositioned for the next rowing cycle; similarly, the myosin head attaches, pulls, detaches, re-cocks, and starts the process again. If the excitation is maintained by the nervous system and adequate ATP exists to supply energy, this process can be repeated up to five times per second. The amount of tension produced depends on the resting length of the fiber and the frequency of stimulation; it is proportionate to the number of active **cross bridges** along the myofibril.

◆ Force Production

A muscle fiber exists in a state either of producing maximum tension or not producing any tension at all. This is often referred to as the "all-or-none" principle. It suggests that the tension produced by a muscle depends on the number of fibers stimulated and the frequency of the stimulation, rather than by how much tension each individual fiber produces. When a muscle fiber is stimulated through a single contraction-relaxation cycle, this is called a **twitch**. Individual twitches in a skeletal muscle are too minute to accomplish anything useful. To produce movement, a muscle can either activate more individual fibers to increase force production or not allow the muscle to relax between twitches, an event called **summation**. The duration and force of a twitch are contingent upon the type of fiber producing the action. Fibers are generally defined as one of two types: fast-twitch or slow-twitch. Fast-twitch fibers twitch quickly (10 milliseconds), whereas slow-twitch fibers take more time to complete the contraction-relaxation cycle (100 milliseconds) [8, 39]. It takes multiple sustained muscle contractions to affect movement. This summation of muscle contractions occurs when the rate of stimulation of the twitches increases to the point that there is no longer a relaxation phase. This is called **complete tetanus**. Normal muscle contractions occur due to complete tetanus or the recruitment of more individual muscle fibers.

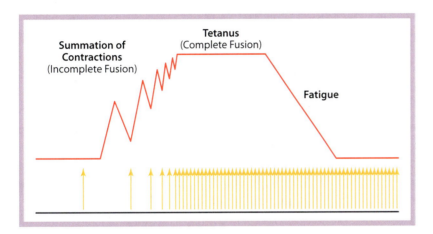

Muscle Tone

Muscle tone occurs because some of the motor units are always active even when the muscle is not voluntarily contracted. The motor unit activation does not produce enough tension to cause any external movement but provides a degree of firmness to the tissue. This tone relates to the number of motor units firing to stabilize the position of the bones and joints. The motor units are stimulated in varying patterns to prevent fatigue. When external forces act on the body, the tissue tension provides data to the nervous system via proprioceptors, which better enable the skeletal muscles and tendons to function in response to sudden changes in tension or body position [37]. The major type of these proprioceptors are the specialized intrafusal fibers called **muscle spindles**, which detect the length and velocity of the muscle and help the tissue manage forces [37].

Muscle spindles function as clusters of intrafusal fibers that lie in the muscle belly and run parallel to the normal muscle fibers (extrafusal fibers) [5]. The muscle spindles relay information regarding changes in the tissue length and the rate of length change to sensory neurons. When stretched, these tissues respond using reflex action, called the stretch reflex, to initiate a stronger contraction to reduce the imposed stretch in a shock-absorbing fashion. The excitatory impulses activate **agonist** muscles to contract and **antagonist** muscles to relax in a process of rapid self-regulation. Agonist/antagonist muscles cause opposite movement trajectories across a joint, exemplified by the biceps

DEFINITIONS

Twitch –

A single contraction-relaxation cycle within skeletal muscle fibers.

Summation –

A neuromuscular response that does not allow the muscle to relax between twitches; sequential summation responses lead to complete tetanus.

Complete tetanus –

This indicates the achievement of a sustained muscular contraction due to a rate of repeated stimulation (twitches), which prevents relaxation.

Muscle tone –

Always present to some degree in skeletal muscle, as motor units are active even when the muscle is not voluntarily contracted; the motor unit activation does not produce enough tension to cause any external movement but provides firmness to the tissue to maintain the integrity of connective structure and force closure in joints.

Muscle spindles –

A specialized type of proprioceptor in muscle fibers which aids in managing tension via the detection of tissue length and movement velocity, sending information to the nervous system in response to muscle stretching.

Agonist –

The muscle that contracts and shortens during a given movement/exercise to resist/accelerate the load (e.g., biceps during a biceps curl).

Antagonist –

The muscle that relaxes and lengthens during a given movement/exercise to allow full contraction of the working muscle(s) (e.g., triceps during a biceps curl).

and triceps muscles at the elbow joint. As the biceps muscle receives excitatory signals to contract, the triceps muscle receives inhibitory signaling to relax, thus allowing the full contraction of the agonist.

Regionalization of stretch reflex is possible through preferential (localized) activation of motor units via intrafusal fibers [12]. The reflex action aids in automatic tone adjustment, which supports control of body position and posture. Because it is a reflex, the process does not require input from the brain, but rather occurs at the level of the spinal cord, allowing for immediate compensatory adjustments during activities requiring balance and coordination. The constant supply of information from the muscle spindles through the stretch reflex is fundamental to neuromuscular regulation.

As alluded to earlier, GTOs complement muscle spindles in regulating muscle and connective tissue tension [16]. The GTOs are tiny sensory receptors which exist at the ends of the muscle fibers at the tendons. They rapidly communicate information to the motor neurons in the muscles they serve to prevent excessive tension that could be potentially dangerous to tissue integrity. If tension becomes too great, the GTOs send inhibitory signals to reduce motor neuron activity, which immediately lowers the muscular contraction's force. By inhibiting tension in the muscle, the GTOs serve to prevent tissue injury that would likely occur from excessive stress [19]. An example of this process occurs in the masseter muscle in the jaw. Contraction of the masseter muscle causes closure of the jaw bone when one chews, but the masseter muscle can produce enough force in the jaw to cause fracturing of the teeth. However, the GTOs embedded in the masseter's musculotendinous tissue sense the amount of tension in the muscle and prevent the muscle from attaining this level of force, preventing damage.

To produce the tension necessary for movement, groups of motor units are stimulated as directed by the CNS. The greater the number of motor units stimulated via total recruitment, the more tension is produced. The total force exerted by a skeletal muscle is a factor of how many muscle fibers are recruited for the contraction. Peak tension occurs when all the motor units in the muscle are contracting without a relaxation phase due to summation, producing complete tetanus.

Motor units generally work in a tag-team fashion by firing alternately. Because most actions are not performed under peak tension, the muscle can reduce the incidence of fatigue by using the alternating technique for lower force requirements. When maximal outputs are required, all the motor units are recruited at a high rate to produce tension. Due to its high energy demand, this level of tension can only occur for a short period of time, as the muscle will start to fatigue after a few seconds. When activities require force for prolonged periods, the motor units take turns firing; this allows some fibers to recover while others contribute to the work. This phenomenon suggests that firing patterns are specific to the activity's demand [4]. This makes sense when you consider an endurance activity such as jogging, which takes advantage of **asynchronous motor unit firing** to attenuate fatigue, and compare it to a 100m sprint, which requires maximal motor unit recruitment, higher firing rates, and greater **synchronicity** to produce the most force output the muscle can attain relative to the action [4]. High-output demands use synchronized firing of fast-twitch fibers and a high number of motor units, whereas endurance activity uses asynchronous firing patterns of slow-twitch fibers to conserve

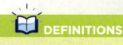

DEFINITIONS

Asynchronous motor unit firing –

A neuromuscular adaptation presenting itself within type I muscle fibers in response to repeated bouts of prolonged activity which helps preserve energy and prevent premature fatigue.

Synchronicity –

The performance of multiple actions in unison, which often results in improved force production.

motor-unit potential, thereby allowing for longer periods of sustained work [26].

Muscle force potential, as it relates to the motor unit, is analogous to a crew team rowing a boat. Muscle's peak tension requires sustained tetanus: the sustained firing of all muscle fibers recruited. This is comparable to everyone on the crew team rowing at a non-stop rate. The more teammates who contribute (recruitment) and the faster they row (frequency), the more force they will produce to move the boat across the water. The same idea applies to force production in muscle tissue. The more muscle tissue recruited, the greater the force potential of the contraction. Referring again to the example, if one can get the rowers to stroke faster (increased firing-rate frequency), the boat will accelerate due to greater total force production. If the firing rate in the motor neurons increases so does the resultant muscle contraction's force. If all of the rowers are recruited to put forth an effort (increased recruitment), and they are coordinated to row at precisely the same time (improved synchronicity) they will attain the best performance and fastest boat speed. The motor unit works the same way. With training, the nervous system learns to recruit the fibers more efficiently, the motor unit's firing rates are enhanced due to the frequency of the action potentials, and firing will occur in unison, creating synchronized tension and greater force outputs. It is important to understand that these actions are functions of the nervous system, which adapts specifically to the training experience. The ability to increase force production within a muscle through training depends on adaptations that occur to both the muscle fibers and the nervous system together [23].

The example of the crew team rowing a boat explains improvements in maximal tension development. But what if the rowers want to travel long distances rather than moving at an extremely fast rate? In this case, it would make more sense for the rowers to use an alternating rowing pattern and slower stroke. If two rowers perform a synchronized stroke and then recover while two other rowers perform their stroke in an alternating fashion, the boat's momentum will be maintained without any particular rower becoming overly fatigued. This illustrates the asynchronous motor-unit firing pattern for endurance activities described above. An interesting fact illustrating the neural influence on force production is that improvements in the development of force occur without the need for new muscle tissue; essentially, due to the CNS, a muscle may become stronger without becoming any larger. The efficiency changes related to motor-unit recruitment make this possible. As the body experiences situations which require force production, it learns the most efficient methods to meet the new demands through "motor learning." In essence, the body learns how to maximize the use of the tissue it already has via improved nervous system regulation [23, 34]. This underscores the fact that most improvements in strength are related to changes in the nervous system, not the muscular system. With this said, a muscle that increase its cross-sectional area will always be stronger than when it was smaller.

◆ Types of Muscle Contractions

The muscle contractions produced by the stimulation of motor units contribute to different internal forces within the body. Three contraction types occur in the body: **isotonic**, **isometric**, and **isokinetic**. These are categorized by the actions they produce. A tonic action, during which a lengthening (**eccentric**) or shortening (**concentric**) occurs within the muscle, is called an isotonic contraction. The term isotonic is derived from

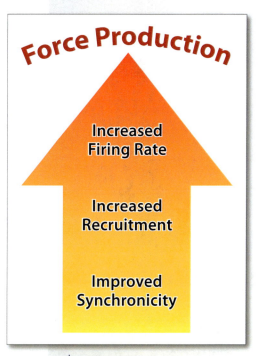

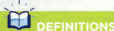 **DEFINITIONS**

Isotonic contraction –

Tension remains while joint angles change; this contraction is seen during most exercises/activities that include a concentric (acceleration) and eccentric (deceleration) component.

Isometric contraction –

Tension is created but no changes in joint angles occur; it often occurs in stabilizers during movement to regulate body segment/joint positioning.

Isokinetic contraction –

This signifies a constant speed of movement regardless of the muscular force applied; training requires specialized laboratory equipment, which is primarily used for rehab and research purposes.

Eccentric –

A muscle contraction where the resistive force is greater than the force applied by the muscle so that it lengthens as it contracts; this contraction often occurs among the muscles decelerating resistance during a lift.

Concentric –

A muscle contraction where the working tissues apply enough force to overcome applied resistance so that the tissues shorten as they contract; this process often occurs among the muscles involved during the acceleration phase of a lift.

the Greek *isotonos* (*iso*, meaning equal, and *tonos*, meaning tension). Many use this term erroneously to describe dynamic muscle actions in which the muscle's force production actually changes across the different joint angles and portions of the movement. These contraction types are visible in all movements. The shortening (concentric) phase, when muscles are shortening under tension, occurs when muscle tension force exceeds the resistance force applied to it, so positive work is attained. This can be demonstrated with a bicep curl. As the bicep muscle contracts concentrically, the elbow flexes, causing the bones of the lower portion of the limb to be pulled closer to the humerus, the upper portion of the arm. When the arm returns to the start position of the curl movement, the bicep lengthens eccentrically because the muscle produces less tension than is necessary to accelerate the resistance in the direction of the force or to hold the resistance in place. When the muscle lengthens under tension, it produces an eccentric contraction called negative work. An important concept to grasp here is that concentric contractions accelerate joint movements, while eccentric contractions decelerate movements.

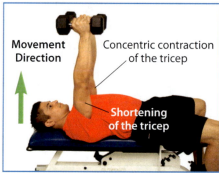 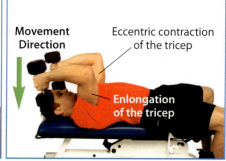

If the force created to accelerate a resistance equals the resistance force, the energy sums cancel out, and no movement will occur. Although the motor units fire and contractile units contract, the total muscle tension remains insufficient to accelerate the object in the direction of the force, so the position is held. This contraction type is called an isometric contraction. The joint angle does not change, even though the attached musculature contracts and exerts force. Isometric contractions, though used in laboratory and rehabilitation settings, are not commonly employed in training programs to strengthen prime movers or develop athletic movements. However, any time the body performs a movement, isometric contractions are necessary to prevent undesirable actions of the body. Most often, isometric contractions are exerted by the neutralizing and stabilizing muscles that act upon a joint segment. These control skeletal positioning and ensure that the force the prime mover produces transfers to perform the desired action. When the body is in a stationary position for example, the muscles acting on the skeleton must contract isometrically to prevent it from collapsing under the pull of gravity. The same contraction types maintain posture and joint position during dynamic activities, such as the isometric contractions of the trunk necessary to properly perform a push-up. In effect, we use and train with isometric contractions all of the time, as they contribute to system stability. The last type of contraction, mainly seen in a laboratory setting, is an isokinetic contraction. Isokinetic signifies that there is a constant speed throughout the ROM. Though helpful in identifying risk for injury, the equipment necessary to control the speed of the movement throughout the ROM is very expensive. The cost of equipment, and the fact that movements in everyday life and in sports are rarely, if ever, performed at one constant speed, make such training's applicability very limited in most exercise environments.

◆ Muscle Fiber Types

The type of muscle fiber recruited to produce a contraction depends upon the amount of force needed for the desired outcome. Muscle fibers and their respective motor units are classified by their physiological and mechanical properties. These properties include the fiber contractile speed (twitch characteristics), force output (tension-generating capacity), total cross-sectional area, potential for growth, and ability to resist fatigue. The particular characteristics gear the motor units for either power or endurance. Motor units are either classified as fast-twitch fatigable (FF), fast-twitch fatigue-resistant (FR), or slow-twitch fatigue-resistant (S). Consistent with the motor-unit classifications, humans exhibit three major skeletal-muscle fiber types: two fast-twitch fiber types and a slow-twitch fiber type. The fiber-type classifications are sometimes expressed using type-distinction abbreviations or labeled according to the energy system they prefer to utilize. The high-force producing fibers are called **Type IIX fibers** or fast glycolytic fibers (FG). The intermediate force producing fibers are called **Type IIA fibers** or fast oxidative-glycolytic fibers (FOG). The low-power output fibers are called **Type I** or slow oxidative fibers (S). The glycolytic or oxidative annotation refers to the predominant type of metabolism utilized to generate ATP for use by the muscle fiber upon recruitment.

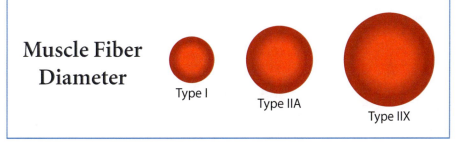

Fast-twitch fibers (Type IIA and IIX) are recognized by their characteristically large diameter, densely packed myofibrils, well developed sarcoplasmic reticulum, and substantial glycogen reserves. They are preferentially recruited for activities requiring high power outputs, providing between 20-50 grams of force per motor unit. Additionally, they are subject to dramatic improvements in size and strength when trained under conditions of short duration and high intensity. They preferentially function using the **anaerobic** metabolic systems, which depend upon high-energy phosphates or carbohydrates. Slow-twitch muscle fibers (Type I), on the other hand, are 50% smaller than their fast twitch counterparts and produce peak force at one third the rate upon stimulation. Slow-twitch motor units provide about 5 grams of sustainable force during activation. They preferentially employ the **aerobic** metabolism and are far better suited for endurance, as they contain an extensive capillary network to deliver oxygenated blood to the working muscle, as well as high mitochondrial density, necessary for the aerobic production of ATP. Notably, they also possess a relatively higher amount of myoglobin, which increases oxygen reserves in the cell and characterizes these units as red muscle. These characteristics make it ideal for activities of prolonged duration.

Conceptually, it is easy to view muscle as either strong or enduring, but humans experience diverse force requirements and often rely on both characteristics simultaneously. When an activity requires the combination of elevated force and prolonged duration, the intermediate fibers, Type IIA, provide significant support. Due to the fact that these fibers maintain properties of both fast and slow fibers, they are well suited to support both anaerobic and aerobic activities. In fact, with the commencement of a training program, all fast-twitch fibers initially shift

---

DEFINITIONS

Type IIX fibers –

The fast-twitch glycolytic fibers that possess the highest power output capabilities, largest fiber diameter, and lowest resistance to fatigue; they provide significant support during intense strength and power activities.

Type IIA fibers –

The fast-twitch, oxidative-glycolytic fibers that possess intermediate power output capabilities, intermediate fiber diameter, and a moderate resistance to fatigue; these fibers provide support during intense strength/power activities as well as prolonged work, making them the most versatile from a metabolic standpoint.

Type I fibers –

The slow-twitch oxidative fibers that possess the lowest power output, smallest fiber diameter, and the highest resistance to fatigue; these fibers are well suited for prolonged aerobic work and possess the highest capillary and mitochondrial densities.

Anaerobic –

Metabolic processes of energy production that do not require the presence of oxygen.

Aerobic –

Metabolic processes of energy production that require the presence of oxygen, also known as oxidative metabolism.

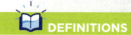

DEFINITIONS

Myoglobin –

The oxygen-transporting protein found in muscle that contains heme iron; myoglobin is structurally similar to the hemoglobin found in red blood cells in circulation.

Size principle –

The idea that muscle fiber types are recruited sequentially based on their size and force output capacities; recruitment occurs in the following order based on need – type I → type IIa → type IIx.

towards the Type IIA intermediate fiber. Intermediate fibers are classified as fast-twitch fibers because they can produce significant force and contain small quantities of **myoglobin**. But, like the slow-twitch fibers, they have an extensive blood supply and are more resistant to fatigue, making them useful for varied types of work. During high-intensity actions, they supply up to 30 grams of force per motor unit, which provides for several minutes of time under high tension. They also can drop the force output to 4-5 grams to support ongoing aerobic activities at a low fatigue rate.

FIBER TYPE	FATIGUE POWER/NERVE CHARACTERISTICS	METABOLIC CHARACTERISTICS
TYPE I	Fatigue Resistant/Slow Twitch Low Power Output Small Fiber Diameter	High Oxidative Capacity Low Glycolytic Capacity High Mitochondrial Density
TYPE IIA	Fatigue Resistant/Fast Twitch Intermediate Power Output Intermediate Fiber Diameter	Medium/High Oxidative Capacity High Glycolytic Capacity Moderate Mitochondrial Density
TYPE IIX	Fast Fatigue/Fast Twitch High Power Output Large Fiber Diameter	High Glycolytic Capacity Low Oxidative Capacity Low Mitochondrial Density

QUICK INSIGHT

When an individual begins training with resistance or velocity, the tissue actually experiences changes that cause a percentage of fast-twitch Type X fibers to become fast-twitch Type A. Thus, the fast-twitch fibers (IIX) tend to shift characteristics towards the more enduring (IIA) fiber. The conversion seems to be counterintuitive to anaerobic demands, but anaerobic activities lasting more than 5 seconds warrant an improvement in endurance characteristics and energy system efficiency. Type IIA fibers can produce high force outputs and resist fatigue, features which enable support of actual daily demands. Even with the characteristic adjustments in some motor units, adequate IIX fibers remain to support high amounts of force for five seconds or less.

In the previous section, we identified that the motor-recruitment patterns respond to muscle tension demands. This fact illustrates that the fiber types selected for activation depend upon the speed and magnitude of the tension an activity requires. Slow-twitch fibers often function for stability or enduring work, and even though they are recruited first, the **size principle** dictates that they do not generate tension at a rate needed to meet the demand of high power output. Instead, they function in anticipatory contractions promoting stability and activities of low force. During fast and powerful activities, selective recruitment adds fast-twitch fibers for a greater magnitude of force production. During activities of varying intensity, such as those found with soccer, basketball, and interval training, slow-twitch fibers serve the lower force outputs aerobically, while fast-twitch fibers dominate the high-intensity

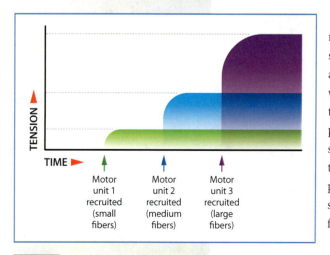

anaerobic segments of the activity. The recruitment patterns match the fiber characteristics and harmonize to accommodate any situation.

Fiber Type Distribution

Fiber type distribution is genetically predetermined, so no method exists to manipulate how the fibers are proportionately concentrated in the body. The distribution of fiber types within a particular skeletal muscle can vary considerably. Although certain muscles, such as those used primarily for posture, maintain higher concentrations of slow-twitch fibers. These muscles, including the soleus, tibialis anterior, deep muscles of the back, and the rectus abdominis, must contract continuously to maintain upright posture. They are not designed for rapid, high-force output, and therefore, experience limited improvements in activities aimed at speed, strength, power, or **hypertrophy**. This explains the relative difficulty in training a slow-twitch dense muscle like the soleus for improvements in size, as it may, proportionately, be 80% slow-twitch fibers. Conversely, muscles that are predominantly composed of fast-twitch fibers, like the biceps brachii, which has a density of fast-twitch fibers closer to 60%, see significant improvements in lean mass with training. Observationally, it is much easier to induce hypertrophy for the biceps compared to the calf.

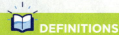

Hypertrophy –

An increase in muscle fiber size.

This would also explain the adage "you don't pick your sport, your sport picks you," suggesting that certain people are designed to succeed in a particular sport, whereas others are not. While the nervous system remains a key contributing factor to athleticism, fiber-type distribution also plays a role in this determination. Muscle biopsies of the leg demonstrate that individuals who perform well in sprint or burst-power activities have higher concentrations of fast-twitch fibers in the respective prime movers necessary for sprinting. Endurance athletes show higher concentrations of slow-twitch fibers in these same muscle groups. If a highly trained sprinter and marathoner switched roles for a day, neither would be very successful in the other's event. However, when the body experiences prolonged exposure to any type of training, it will begin to adapt accordingly; a person that begins to do long endurance activities will see muscle-fiber transitions that favor more oxidative fiber types [15, 31, 35, 40, 43, 46, 49, 50]. This is why training must be specific to the types of activities that one wants to prepare the body to perform. Although training in a particular event will certainly cause anyone to improve, practice alone is not enough for a person to reach an elite status. Genetic predisposition is a powerful factor [32], as are the types of activities one partakes in while a young child [44]. Ultimately, the percentage of any particular fiber type within a muscle is based on the tissue's role in movement and the genetically determined distribution pattern assigned to the muscle. Among individuals in similar sports, distinctions in performance advantage by muscle-fiber-type distribution seem to be specific to the most elite levels. However, fiber distribution patterns determine only one component of performance capacity. They do provide an advantage in activities that match the fiber-specific characteristics, but do not define performance outcomes because measurable performance is based on a blend of many physiological systems.

Training for an activity will cause improvements in many of the physiological systems that affect individual performance. In response to training stress, several components of the motor unit adapt to become better suited to the conditions. The motor units begin to more closely reflect the desired skeletal tissue type, making the demands of the training less "stressful" through modifications in properties and characteristics. The actual fiber type, however, does not change. To this date, research studies have been equivocal on the possibility of a complete slow to fast, or fast to slow, fiber-type transition [1, 6, 13, 35, 40, 50]. Some studies suggest that the transitions occur on a spectrum due to specific contraction velocities; however, regardless of whether a complete fiber-type transition is possible, other mechanical and physiological adaptations have been proven. Changes in patterns of neural stimulation, capillary density, mitochondrial density, and enzyme concentration cause muscle fiber to become better suited to the training stimulus [46, 50]. Changes in performance with training exemplify this principle. Although a person may not be born with a muscle-fiber-type distribution that is best suited for a given activity, through specific training, he or she can experience adaptations that allow improved performance despite his or her genetic predisposition [1, 13, 27, 32].

◆ Spatial and Directional Terminology

Movement of the musculoskeletal system requires contractile forces that extend from the myofilaments through the muscle fibers to the muscle's outer layers and tendons. This process, in turn, applies pulling force at the attachment site of the bone. When these forces attain enough magnitude to move the bone, action is transferred across the associated joint, causing motion. When voluntary movement occurs at a given joint, it will be specific to the contractile force's location, the joint's shape, and the structures that act on it. In most cases, anatomical movement occurs either to move a body segment away from or back to the body. This pattern sounds simple enough, but describing the actions or motions of synovial joints requires specific anatomical terminology. Anatomical and spatial terms allow for proper illustration of direction, which indicates the muscles responsible for the movement as well as those involved in the outcome. For instance, "lifting the arm" could apply to abduction, flexion, extension, and even rotation, depending on the starting position, the direction, and the plane of movement in which the end action occurs. These terms are applied to anatomical structures and serve as the standard to indicate the tissue requirements for a desirable performance. Due to the assembly of forces involved, all voluntary movements (i.e. acceleration, deceleration, and stabilization) require a coordination of structural components.

Describing movement anatomically requires knowledge of the starting position, axis of joint rotation, anatomical structures involved, and the plane in which the movement occurs. Anatomical position is the standard reference position for the body when describing locations, positions, and movements of limbs or other anatomical structures. Anatomical position assumes the body is standing in an erect posture, facing forward with both feet aligned parallel under the hips with the toes forward, the arms and hands hanging below the shoulders at the side with the elbows and fingers extended, and the palms facing forward. From this reference position, spatial and directional terms can be easily described. Certainly, movement occurs from numerous postures and positions, but for the purposes of building foundational knowledge, anatomical position will be referenced in this chapter.

ANATOMICAL POSITION

◆ Positional Lines and Movement Planes

Comprehending spatial terms and accurately applying them can be enhanced by defining lines of origin along the anatomical position. These lines correspond with movement planes. The line that dissects the body down the center, splitting it into left and right halves, is called the **midline**, which lies along the **sagittal plane**. The line that dissects the body into front and back halves is called the **midaxillary line**, which runs along the **frontal plane**. When that line is shifted forward to align with the anterior crease of the armpit, it is referred to as the anterior axillary line; when moved backwards to align with the posterior crease of the armpit, it is referred to as the posterior axillary line. While no dissection line is acknowledged for top and bottom halves, there does exist a plane for movement reference. The **transverse plane** runs parallel to the floor, dissecting the body into superior (top) and inferior (bottom) parts. Sometimes the terms cardinal or cross planes are used to identify the body's center of gravity. Planes will be reviewed further under movement terminology.

DEFINITIONS

Sagittal plane –

A plane of movement split by the midline which breaks the body into left and right halves; applicable actions often involve flexion and extension and require a forward-backward movement of the body or joints (e.g., lunge).

Frontal plane –

The plane of movement split by the midaxillary line which breaks the body into front and back halves; applicable actions often involve abduction and adduction and require side-to-side movement of the body or joints (e.g., lateral lunge).

Transverse Plane –

The plane of movement which breaks the body into top and bottom halves (no dissection line is acknowledged); applicable actions often involve rotational movement of the body or joints (e.g., oblique twists).

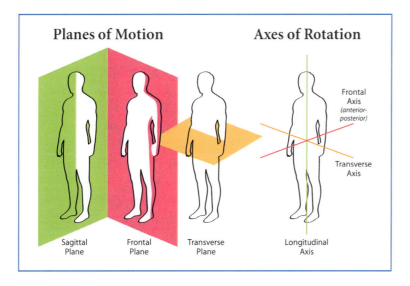

◆ Spatial Terms

When spatial terms are used, they may be referencing location or direction. They function to describe the area of space relative to the body's anatomical position. If something is in front of the body or the body segment moves forward, the space descriptor for the movement or location would be **anterior**. If the location of space is behind the body or a segment of the body moves backward, the space location would be **posterior**. In some cases, other words can be used to designate the same area of space For instance, anterior is synonymous with **ventral** and posterior is synonymous with **dorsal**. This situation may also occur when spatial terms are used as directional movement terms, as is the case with medial, internal, and inward rotation, or lateral, external, and outward rotation. **Medial** and its rotational synonyms refer to the direction or location toward, or closer to, the midline of the body, while **lateral** and its alternatives refer to a position or movement away from, or further from the midline.

When locating a point or direction along a limb, the terms **proximal** and **distal** are used. Proximal refers to the direction or location close to where the limb attaches to the body. Distal refers either to the point toward the end of the limb, a location farthest away from the body, or the limb's skeletal attachment site. When

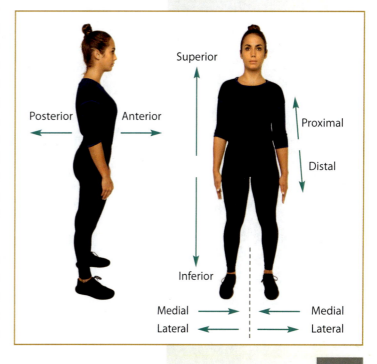

Positional Terms

- **Anatomical position** – A reference posture used in anatomical description in which the subject stands erect with feet parallel and arms adducted and supinated, with palms facing forward.

- **Midline** – The median plane of the body.

- **Anterior axillary line** – Crease of the axilla (underarm).

- **Midaxillary line** – A perpendicular line drawn downward from the apex of the axilla.

- **Anterior** – Placed before or in front.

- **Posterior** – Located behind a part or toward the rear of a structure.

- **Ventral** – Synonymous with anterior.

- **Dorsal** – Synonymous with posterior.

- **Proximal** – Situated nearest to point of attachment or origin.

- **Distal** – Situated farthest from point of attachment or origin, as of a limb or bone.

- **Medial** – At, in, near, or being the center; dividing a person into right and left halves.

- **Lateral** – Situated or extending away from the medial plane of the body.

- **Ipsilateral** – On, or relating to, the same side of the body.

- **Contralateral** – On, or relating to, the opposite side of the body.

- **Superficial** – Shallow proximity in relation to a surface.

- **Deep** – Extending inward in relation to a surface layer.

---

the limbs are viewed from a particular side, instead of left or right, they are often referenced by the terms **ipsilateral** (same side) or **contralateral** (opposite side). The terms **superficial** and **deep** also refer to locations on (or within) the body. These location descriptors refer to positions relative to the body's exterior surfaces. Deep tissues are internally located as opposed to the superficial layers, which refer to tissues closer to the skin. So, one might refer to the deep muscles of the spine or identify the trapezius as superficial to the rhomboids. Another way these location descriptors are used is to describe wounds, whether they refer to superficial/surface or deep damage.

When terms are used to describe movement, the planes and axes of motion are applied to the anatomical positions, and often reference spatial descriptors to make the movement description concise. The three movement planes that dissect the body each have a corresponding axis that passes perpendicularly through the plane. The sagittal plane is probably the most referenced due to the number of activities and movements the body performs in this plane. The two-dimensional surface connects anterior to posterior and superior to inferior: in layman's terms it runs front to back and top to bottom. The axis that corresponds with the sagittal plane is the transverse axis. The frontal, or coronal, plane dissects the body into front and back. It runs side to side and superior to inferior (top to bottom). The respective axis of movement is the anteroposterior axis. The transverse plane runs perpendicular to the sagittal plane, splitting the body into top and bottom segments. The axis of rotation for the transverse plane is called the longitudinal axis. Sometimes the technical concepts of planes and axes seem to become far removed from practical considerations, but that is not at all the case. For instance, an alignment issue in one plane will disturb its corresponding axis, compromising proper movement and often joint function. This is commonly seen in injury or movement compensation associated with musculoskeletal imbalances.

When planes and rotational axes are defined, the application of movements can be referenced and described accurately. The movements can be categorized by the plane in which they occur or the direction of force they produce. Movements that occur in the sagittal plane (around the transverse axis) include **flexion**, **extension**, **hyperextension**, **plantarflexion**, and **dorsiflexion**. The joint movements that occur around the anteroposterior axis in the frontal plane include **abduction**, **adduction**, **lateral flexion**, **inversion**, **eversion**, **elevation**, **depression**, **radial deviation**, and **ulnar deviation**. The joint movements around the longitudinal axis that take place in the transverse plane perpetuate different types of rotational movements. These include **internal** and **external rotation**, **supination**, **pronation**, **horizontal abduction**, and **horizontal adduction**.

Movement Terms

- **Flexion** – To bend; in hinge joints, the articulating bones move closer together; in ball-and-socket joints, the limb moves anterior to the midaxillary line.
- **Extension** – To straighten or extend; in hinge joints the articulating bones move away from each other; in ball-and-socket joints, the limb moves posterior to the midaxillary line.
- **Lateral flexion** – Spinal movement to the left or right, occurs at the neck and trunk.
- **Protraction** – Movement of a structure toward the anterior surface in a straight horizontal line.
- **Retraction** – Movement back to the anatomical position or additionally, posterior to functional range of motion.
- **Dorsiflexion** – Movement of the ball of the foot towards the shin.
- **Plantarflexion** – Foot movement towards the plantar surface.
- **Pronation** – Unique rotation of the forearm which crosses the radius and ulna; the palm faces posterior (prone means lying face down).
- **Supination** – Unique rotation of the forearm where the radius and ulna uncross; the palms face anteriorly (supine means lying face up).
- **Inversion** – Confined to the ankle; consists of turning the ankle so the plantar surface of the foot faces medially.
- **Eversion** – Confined to the ankle; consists of turning the ankle so the plantar surface of the foot faces laterally.
- **Abduction** – Movement away from the midline.
- **Adduction** – Movement toward the midline.
- **Hyperextension** – Extension of a joint beyond a range that surpasses full extension; can be safe as seen at the shoulder during a row, or unsafe as seen at the spine during activities involving the lower back (depending on the force vectors and loading involved).
- **Ulnar deviation** – Joint action at the wrist that causes the hand to move medially towards the little finger in the frontal plane.
- **Radial deviation** – Joint action at the wrist that causes the hand to move laterally towards the thumb in the frontal plane.
- **External rotation** – Action at the shoulder and hip joint where the articulating bone is rotated away from the body from anatomical position.
- **Internal rotation** – Action at the shoulder and hip joint where the articulating bone is rotated towards the body from anatomical position.
- **Circumduction** – Circular movement of an extremity at which the distal end allows 360° of movement while the proximal end remains fixed.
- **Elevation** – Superior movement of a bone or tissues.
- **Depression** – Inferior movement of a bone or tissues.
- **Horizontal abduction** – Movement away from the midline in the transverse plane.
- **Horizontal adduction** – Movement towards the midline in the transverse plane.
- **Rotation** – The turning of a structure around its long axis.

Anatomical Movements

Trunk and Neck

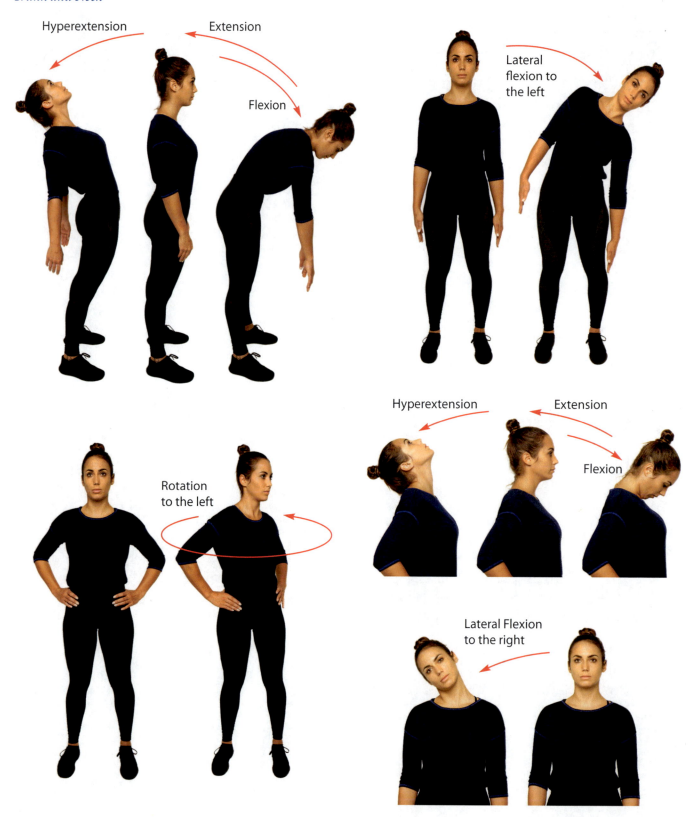

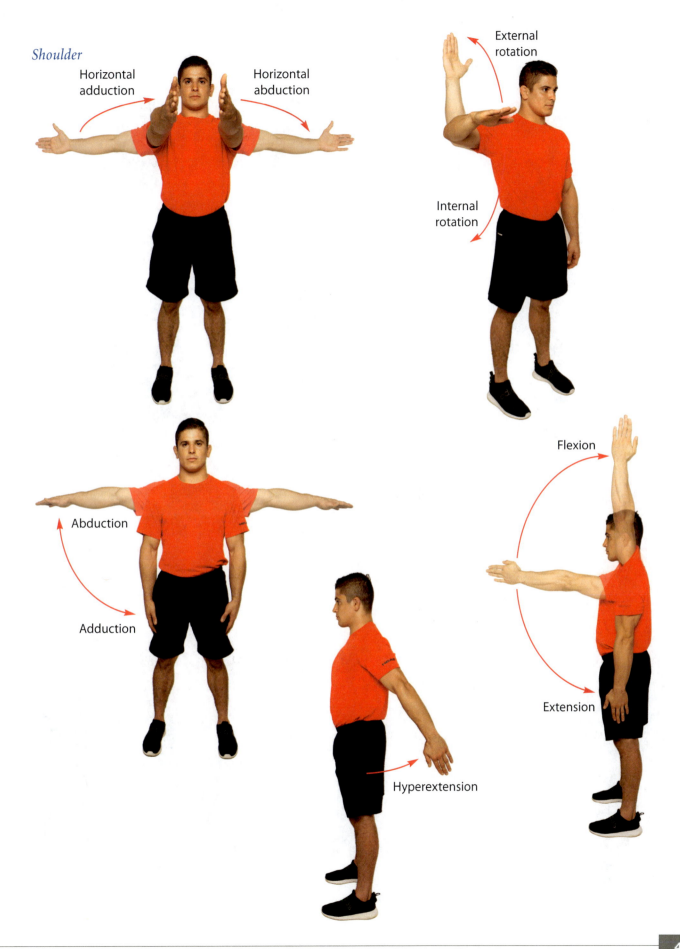

Functional Anatomy and Training Instruction

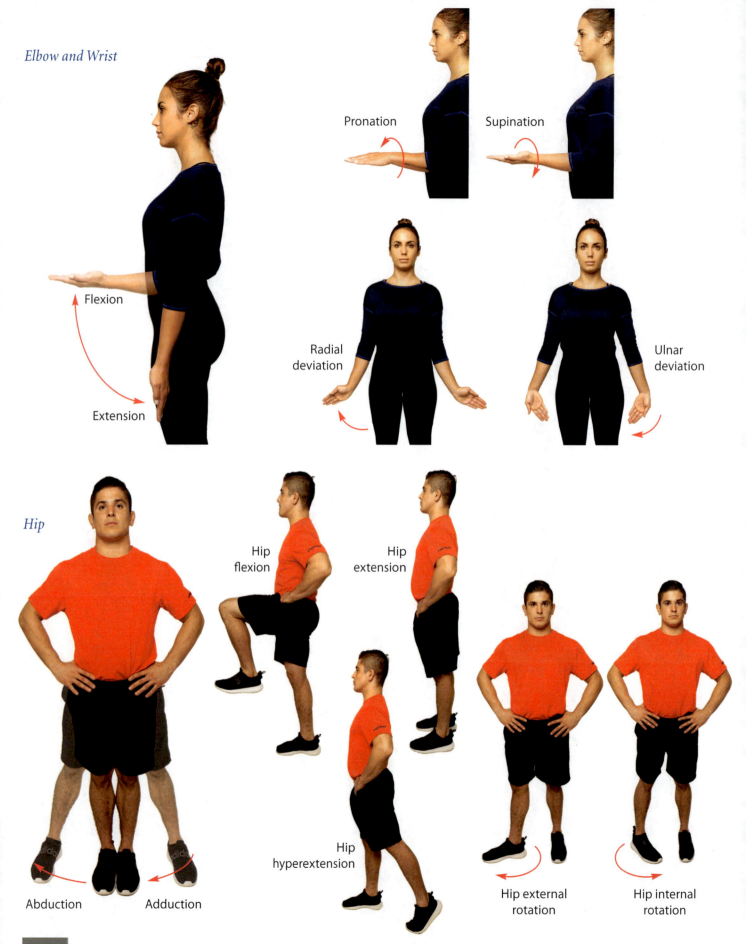

Knee and Ankle

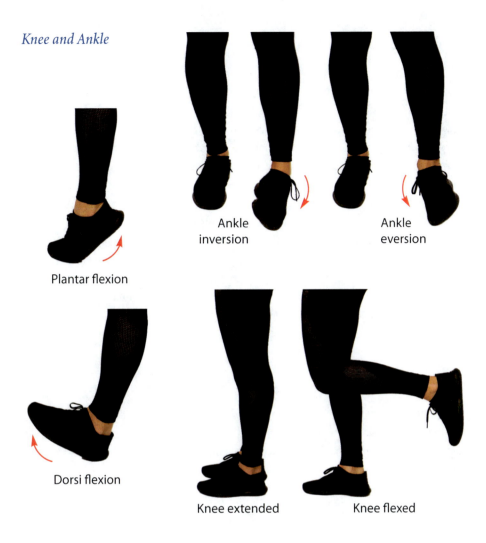

Due to the diverse movement capabilities of the body, a single plane of movement may or may not always be precise when describing a joint action of the body. For example, suggesting that a bicep curl occurs in the sagittal plane would be accurate, as the elbow joint is a hinge capable of flexion and extension; with a fixed humeral position, the arm flexes to a terminal position and then extends back to the starting position. The weight simply moves forward and backward. It would seem that the bench press functions in the same way as the resistance moves forward and backward in reference to the body. However, the body employs more than one joint, even while performing these seemingly simple movements. When performing a bench press, the shoulder complex and elbow must function together, requiring movement of the scapula, humerus, and the radius/ulna. The humerus moves in the transverse plane, but the forearm moves in the sagittal plane. However, unless each joint is individually examined for movement during **compound exercises**, the external resistance or the center of mass is referenced. In the case of the bench press, the movement would be classified as a sagittal-plane one because the weight moves forward and backward.

> **DEFINITIONS**
>
> **Compound exercises –**
>
> *Exercises that involve more than one joint and multiple muscle groups.*

> **DEFINITIONS**
>
> **Prime movers –**
>
> *The muscle required to perform the majority of mechanical work necessary to overcome the load during a given exercise; these may not necessarily contribute more than 50% of the necessary force but will contribute to the greatest extent relative to all tissues involved.*
>
> **Kyphotic –**
>
> *A convex curvature of the spine, as seen in the thoracic segment.*
>
> **Lordotic –**
>
> *A concave curvature of the spine, as seen in the lumbar segment.*

SPINAL CURVES

(Kyphotic / Lordotic)

◆ Muscle Identification

More than 600 muscles work together to operate the human body. Some of these muscles are voluntary, while others are not. During movement, muscles may accelerate, decelerate, neutralize, or stabilize. Therefore, to properly develop a comprehensive exercise program, it is important to identify the voluntary muscles' role relative to position and movement. For this purpose, the following text provides an overview of the joint segments and the respective muscles that act upon them to support proper anatomical position and proper biomechanical movements. The following lists of muscles that act upon the joint are by no means exhaustive but do represent the universally recognized **prime movers** for each action. Importantly, with any joint action, several muscles contribute to the movement; so to better understand and discuss the muscles and their functions, the prime mover, or the muscle contributing the highest acceleration force for the movement, is usually identified with the specific joint action. Thus, the distinction of prime mover is a factor of contribution. The muscle that does the most work over the designated range is so termed, even if the maximal contribution is only 30%. People erroneously assume the prime mover does all the work, which is not the case. This concept supports active training movements over the isolation of muscles for improvements in human function.

Spine and Neck

The human body's vertebral column, or spine, has five regions which serve independent and cooperative functions. Its curvilinear, boney chain provides support and allows for movement of the head and trunk. It also protects the spinal cord while providing routes for nerve outlets and extends out spiny processes for efficient muscle attachments. The five segments of the human spine, from top to bottom, include seven cervical vertebrae, twelve thoracic vertebrae, and five lumbar vertebrae and terminate at a single sacral bone (sacrum: five fused vertebrae) with its tail, the coccygeal bone. The respective spinal regions allow for varied amounts of movement based on the interactions and shape of the vertebral joints: these segments are called the articular processes. The 12 thoracic vertebrae articulate with the 12 ribs, making it the sturdiest, most stable region; however, because of the stable attachments to the ribs through costotransverse and costovertebral joints, it is far less mobile compared to the cervical or lumbar spine [18, 38]. The thoracic spine not only differs in its stability and mobility when compared to its counterparts, but also in its **kyphotic** (convex from the posterior) curvature. This is distinct from the cervical and lumbar spine's **lordotic** (concave from the posterior)

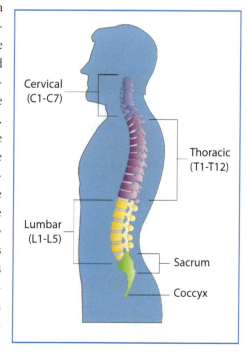

curvatures, which provide more efficient flexion and extension. Conversely, the thoracic spine's kyphotic shape enables for energy transfer management and posture while also serving to encase the major cardiopulmonary organs [38].

The four major curvatures that make up the entire spine assist in shock absorption, movement, and posture maintenance. The general reference term describing the state of proper postural position is **neutral spine**. In this position, the cervical and lumbar regions present with a lordotic curvature and the thoracic and sacral regions maintain a kyphotic curvature. When the lordotic curvature is exaggerated or overextended in an undesirable manner, such as in hyperextension, it is termed **lordosis**. When the thoracic spine experiences an exaggerated curvature, or is overly flexed when at rest, it is referred to as being in a state of **kyphosis**. Kyphosis is common in elderly populations and those whose thoracic extensors have become weak over time due to chronically poor posture. The vertebral column's exaggerated curves impede the function of the articulations within the area, as well as those joints that depend on spinal position for proper function. The upper spine position affects the neck, shoulder, and scapular rhythm, and extends that influence to the lower spine and pelvic joints. A person experiencing a chronic "rounding of the upper back" will lose the ability to flex or externally rotate the shoulder and will often present with low back pain due to the changes at the lumbo-pelvic region. When the body experiences chronic lordosis, the condition is often referred to as **lower-cross syndrome**. Observationally, it looks like an arched back with hip flexion. This undesirable curvature is associated with low back pain but even more significantly impacts hip action.

DEFINITIONS

Neutral spine –

A state of proper postural positioning for the spine that includes four major curvatures for shock absorption and efficient movement.

Lordosis –

An exaggerated lordotic (anterior) curvature of the spine which can lead to postural issues and injury.

Kyphosis –

Exaggerated kyphotic (posterior) curvature of the spine which can lead to postural issues and injury.

Lower cross syndrome –

Refers to chronic lordosis in the lumbar region, demonstrated by an arched back with hip flexion; it is associated with lower back pain, various injuries, and lumbo-pelvic muscular imbalances.

Intervertebral disc –

A fibrocartilaginous disc that serves as a cushion between the vertebra of the spinal column.

Nucleus-pulposus –

A gelatinous, fluid-filled component found in the center of each intervertebral disc.

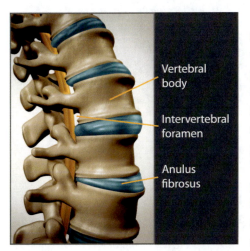

The spine's joints are separated by a fibrocartilaginous **intervertebral disc**, which provides support and stability and prevents contact between the bony surfaces of the vertebrae. From a top-down view, the disc looks much like a fried egg and is comprised of an outer annulus encasing a gelatinous, fluid-filled **nucleus-pulposus**. With age, the discs become more compressed and gradually lose water decreasing their cushioning capabilities and reducing stability during high-speed actions. This decline, in part, explains the shortening phenomenon that occurs as a person gets older [36]. In addition, if the disc is compressed from repetitive microtrauma or blunt trauma, it may bulge or herniate [11]. This often causes a partial or complete release of the nucleus pulposus and annulus fibrosus. The bulging or herniated portion may also impinge upon the spinal nerves, compromising their function and causing pain, which may radiate unilaterally or bilaterally down the legs, sometimes manifesting as a burning pain in the foot. In terms of motion, spinal segment design facilitates several dynamic processes. The spine can flex and extend (hyperextend), laterally flex the neck and trunk, and rotate the trunk and head. In many cases, the spinal movements are segmentally joined with appendicular skeletal movements to allow completion of numerous actions. Limitations in the movement of the spinal articulations often lead to premature functional decline [36]. With age, the ability to extend and rotate the spine often declines due to lack of use. Historically, this seemed to be a problem after age 50; however, today young people experience musculoskeletal limitations before the age of 20 due to the lack of natural physical activity and technology-induced forward posture [29].

SPINAL & TRUNK MUSCULATURE

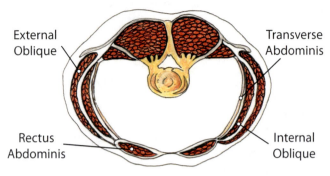

Cross Sectional View

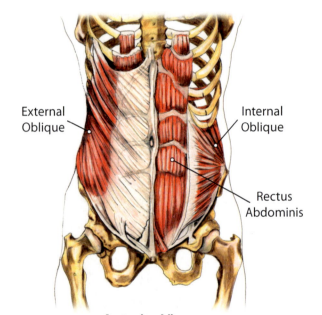

Anterior View

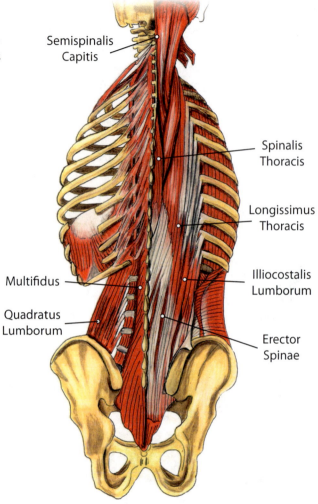

Posterior View

Trunk Muscles	Movement Function	Example Exercise
Rectus Abdominis	Trunk flexion	Ab curl-up
External Oblique	Flexes and rotates vertebral column	Diagonal chop
Internal Oblique	Flexes and rotates vertebral column	Cable torso twist
Transverse Abdominis	Compresses abdomen	Draw in
Erector Spinae Group	Extends vertebral column	Good morning
Quadratus Lumborum	Abducts vertebral column	Lateral flexion

Pelvic Positioning

The pelvis has an intimate relationship with the spine, based mainly on the movements that occur at the lumbosacral joint, formed by the sacrum (pelvis) and lowest lumbar vertebrae. When the iliac spine rotates forward, the movement is termed an **anterior pelvic tilt**. When the iliac crest rotates backwards, the pelvis assumes a **posterior pelvic tilt**. When either of these pelvic tilts exists, the spine's curvature changes. An anterior pelvic tilt increases the extension (lordosis) of the lumbar spine, which consequently, may place excessive stress on the posterior aspect of the vertebrae and discs in the region. A posterior pelvic tilt reduces the lordotic curvature, causing the spine to flex, flattening its natural lordotic curvature, sometimes even rounding the lumbar spine. This pelvic and spinal interaction points to the need to properly control the pelvis and the natural curvature of the spine when lifting resistance or maintaining posture for prolonged time periods. Weakness or tightness in the muscles that attach to the pelvis and spine can lead to pelvic instability, often manifesting in low back pain.

> **DEFINITIONS**
>
> **Anterior pelvic tilt –**
>
> *A forward rotational movement of the iliac crests of the pelvis, originating from the lumbosacral joint, which impacts the curvature of the spine.*
>
> **Posterior pelvic tilt –**
>
> *A backward rotational movement of the iliac crests of the pelvis, originating from the lumbosacral joint, which impacts the curvature of the spine.*

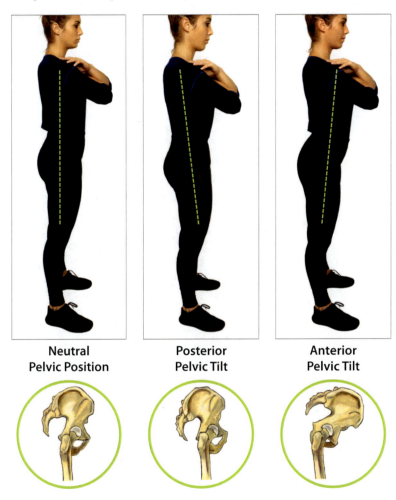

Neutral Pelvic Position | Posterior Pelvic Tilt | Anterior Pelvic Tilt

Shoulder

The glenohumeral joint is a ball-and-socket joint, which allows for the most movement of any articulation. As previously mentioned, the shallow glenoid fossa allows for substantial dynamic capabilities in the humerus at the expense of stability. The hip allows for the same movements as the shoulder, but they are more closely limited by the articulating surfaces of the

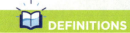

DEFINITIONS

Rotator cuff –

A set of various ligaments and four muscles including the supraspinatus, infraspinatus, teres minor, and subscapularis which function to counteract the relative lack of stability in the shoulder joint and regulate proper movement.

joint, reducing ROM but providing more stability. For instance, abduction at the shoulder joint far surpasses the 45 degrees attainable at the hip. During unrestricted shoulder flexion, the arm can be raised far above the shoulder when the hand maintains a neutral position. Additionally, the joint allows for movement in all planes, including flexion, extension, hyperextension, abduction, adduction, horizontal adduction, horizontal abduction, internal and external rotation, and circumduction. As mentioned, these vast movement capabilities come at the cost of stability due to a reduced contact area between the scapula and the humerus. To counteract the lack of stability, the body uses three sets of ligaments and four muscles, which collectively make up the **rotator cuff**. The rotator cuff is comprised of the supraspinatus, infraspinatus, teres minor, and subscapularis muscles. These muscles serve to assist and manage movement at the shoulder. The teres minor and infraspinatus extend and externally rotate the humerus; the supraspinatus stabilizes and abducts the humerus to 30°, while the subscapularis extends and medially rotates the humerus.

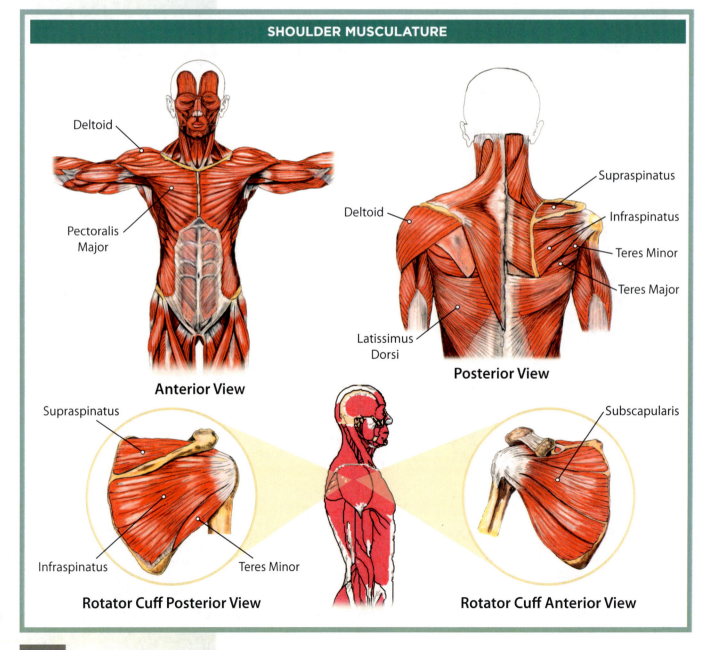

SHOULDER MUSCULATURE

Shoulder Muscles	Movement Function	Example Exercise
Deltoids	Horizontally abduct, flex, extend, and rotate humerus	Side raise
Latissimus dorsi	Adduct, medially rotate, and extend humerus	Pull-up
Pectoralis major	Horizontally adduct, flex, extend, and medially rotate humerus	Bench press
Teres major	Adduct, extend, and medially rotate humerus	Single-arm row
Coracobrachialis	Adduct and flex humerus	Front raise
Infraspinatus	Extend and externally rotate humerus	External band rotation
Subscapularis	Extend and internally rotate humerus	Internal band rotation
Supraspinatus	Abduct humerus	Empty can raise
Teres minor	Adduct and externally rotate humerus	External band rotation

Shoulder Girdle

Rather than a single joint, the **shoulder girdle** is a joint complex that includes the articulations between the sternum and clavicle (sternoclavicular joint) and the clavicle and the scapula (acromioclavicular joint). The prior joint mentioned functions to connect the axial and appendicular skeleton and the latter allows for the ability to raise the arm above the head. The shoulder girdle movements complement the actions of the glenohumeral joint. These movements, which are defined by scapular action, can be performed without shoulder-joint motion, but most often are employed to enhance arm movements. Although slight gliding movements do occur at the respective articulations of the sternoclavicular and acromioclavicular joints, the actual joint movement terms applied describe the actions of the scapula. The scapula can be elevated and depressed, abducted (protracted) and adducted (retracted), and rotated upward and downward. As mentioned, these movements are often combined with movements at the shoulder. For instance, the scapula may be downwardly rotated and adducted while the humerus is hyperextended to allow for the action of a seated row; in addition, the scapula may be depressed and rotated downward while the arm is adducted to accommodate a pull-up. Interestingly, these movements need to be instructed for correct exercise performance. Scapular movement proficiency is not innate to most humans, who often rely heavily on shoulder and elbow actions to accomplish tasks. For instance, in rowing exercises, the action of the shoulder and scapula should be synchronized to encourage proper activation of the back musculature and joint ROM. Most exercisers erroneously dominate the exercise performance with arm

DEFINITIONS

Shoulder girdle –

A joint complex that includes the articulations between the sternum and clavicle (sternoclavicular joint) and the clavicle and the scapula (acromioclavicular joint).

flexion, effectively training the biceps and elbow flexors, contrary to the rationale for this "back" exercise in the first place.

SHOULDER GIRDLE

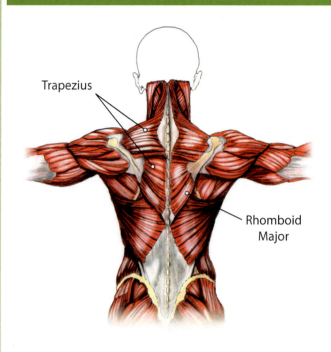

Shoulder Girdle Muscles	Movement Function	Exercise
Trapezius	Elevates, depresses, rotates, and fixes scapula; extends cervical spine	Shoulder shrug
Rhomboid major	Retracts, rotates, and fixes scapula	Seated row
Pectoralis minor	Depresses scapula	Chest flyes
Levator scapulae	Elevates and retracts scapula; laterally flex cervical spine	High row

Posterior View

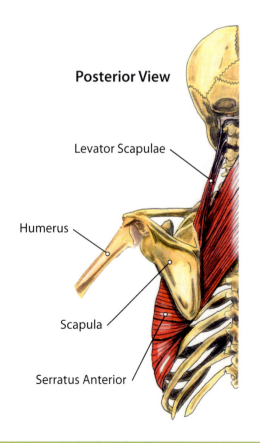

Anterior View

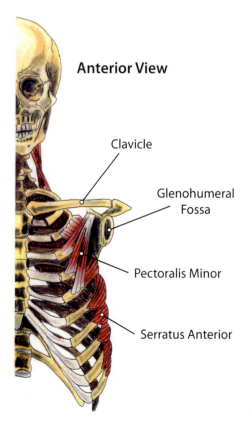

Functional Anatomy and Training Instruction

Elbow

The elbow joint, like the knee, is a hinge joint which allows for arm flexion and extension. The biceps muscle attaches to the humerus and the radius, crossing the elbow to function as the prime mover for arm flexion. The triceps muscle similarly crosses the elbow, but attaches the humerus to the ulna, functioning to extend the arm. The elbow exhibits stability because the surface of the humerus and ulna interlock when the elbow fully extends; if a person can hyperextend the arm, this is due to the irregular shape of their articulating surfaces and/or joint laxity. The elbow incurs the most risk for injury when a person falls and uses an extended arm position to brace the impact. Although the elbow can become dislocated in traumatic injuries, in most cases, injuries are often related to overuse or poor movement mechanics during ballistic activities such as throwing.

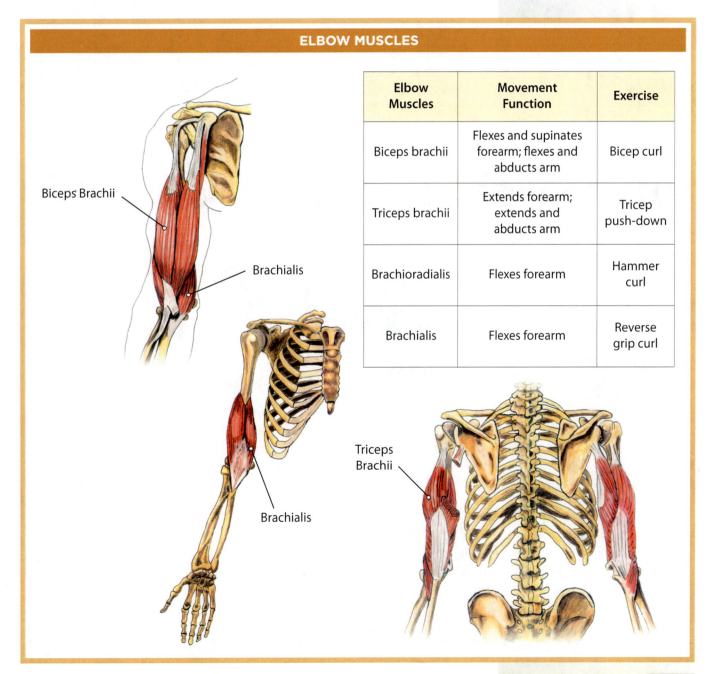

ELBOW MUSCLES

Elbow Muscles	Movement Function	Exercise
Biceps brachii	Flexes and supinates forearm; flexes and abducts arm	Bicep curl
Triceps brachii	Extends forearm; extends and abducts arm	Tricep push-down
Brachioradialis	Flexes forearm	Hammer curl
Brachialis	Flexes forearm	Reverse grip curl

Radioulnar Joint

The radius and ulna of the forearm come together to form a pivot joint, which allows the bone to cross and uncross so the hand is supinated (facing forward) or pronated (facing backward) from anatomical position. When supinated, the radius and ulna are parallel; when pronated, the radius lies across the top of the ulna. Hand position variations when lifting will change the application of the resistive load to different structures. For instance, if the arm is flexed and hand pronated, the brachioradialis, which is always active in arm flexion, performs more work. If the hand is supinated during arm flexion, as seen in the traditional bicep curl, the bicep brachii experiences greater resistive force. The brachialis also flexes the arm at the elbow joint, but unlike the biceps, the brachialis does not insert on the radius and does not participate in pronation and supination of the forearm.

Wrist

Wrist movements generally occur in three planes: from the anatomical position, these allow for radial and ulnar deviation, also called abduction and adduction, in the frontal plane, circumduction in the transverse plane, and flexion and extension in the sagittal plane. The wrist can hyperextend, which occurs as the back of the hand moves closer to the top of the forearm from a neutral wrist position. Forceful extension of the wrist over time can result in wrist-extensor inflammation called tennis elbow [47].

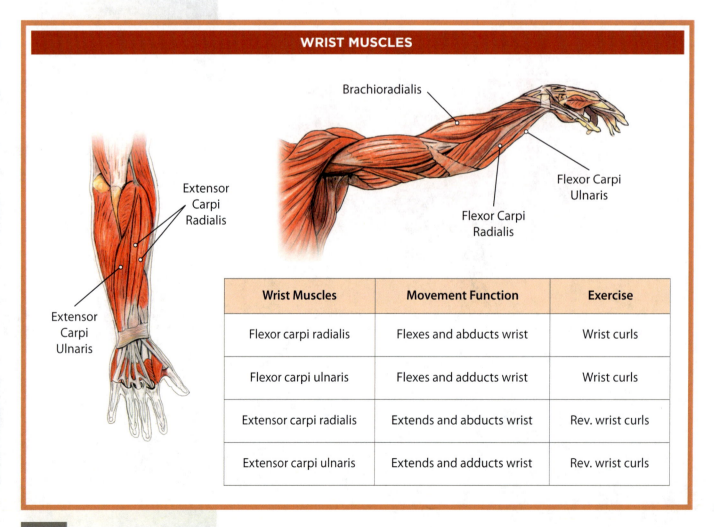

WRIST MUSCLES

Wrist Muscles	Movement Function	Exercise
Flexor carpi radialis	Flexes and abducts wrist	Wrist curls
Flexor carpi ulnaris	Flexes and adducts wrist	Wrist curls
Extensor carpi radialis	Extends and abducts wrist	Rev. wrist curls
Extensor carpi ulnaris	Extends and adducts wrist	Rev. wrist curls

Hip

Hip movements occur at the articular surface of the acetabulum and femoral head. Due to its connective make-up, the hip's joint capsule is very dense, providing for strength and stability. The joint's shape, organization of the articular capsule, and four broad ligament attachments supporting the ball-and-socket joint ensure the femoral head stays securely inside the acetabulum. As mentioned, the hip joint allows for similar movements as the shoulder joint but often to a lesser ROM. The hip can flex, extend, hyperextend, abduct, adduct, and internally and externally rotate. The greater limitation to its specific ROM results from its deeper socket and supportive connective structures. For instance, bone impingement limits true hip abduction to about 45° and hip hyperextension is limited in range compared to that of the shoulder. In young adults and adolescents, the hip is injured less frequently than the shoulder because the comparable decrease in mobility encourages greater stability [14, 42].

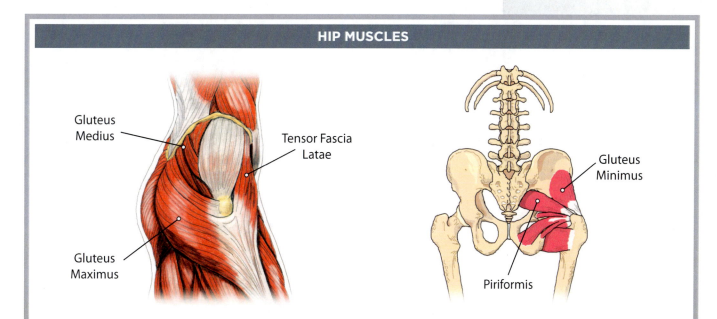

HIP MUSCLES

Hip Muscles	Movement Function	Example Exercise
Psoas major	Flexes thigh (hip)	Knee raise
Iliacus	Flexes and medially rotates thigh (hip)	Diagonal knee raise
Gluteus maximus	Extends, adducts, and laterally rotates thigh	Squat
Gluteus medius	Abducts and medially rotates thigh	Lateral squat
Gluteus minimus	Abducts and medially rotates thigh	Lateral squat
Tensor fascia latae	Abducts and medially rotates thigh	Supine leg abduction
Piriformis	Laterally rotates and abducts thigh	Rotational step-outs
Quadratus femoris	Laterally rotates and abducts thigh	Rotational step-outs

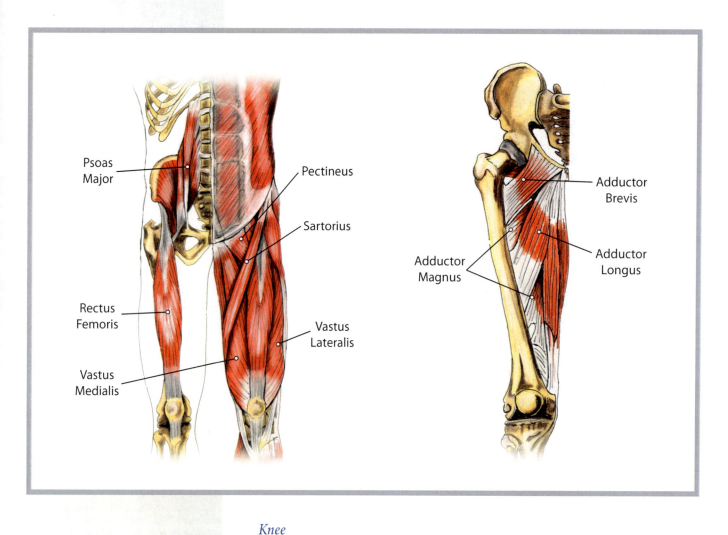

Knee

The movement relationship between the shoulder and hip resembles that of the knee and the elbow. The elbow and knee are both hinge joints and perform flexion and extension, but the knee is far more complex. The femoral condyles allow for variations in contact with the tibia. These change during movement, and the patella-femoral relationship further differentiates this special joint. Additionally, the knee does not have a unified capsule or common synovial cavity. Rather, it uses fibrocartilage discs called menisci for cushioning, shape, and lateral stability, as well as fat pads to reduce friction. In addition, a fairly complex organization of ligaments assists stability. Due to the dynamic nature of physical activity, these ligaments and menisci are subject to high force and increased risk for injury [2]. In activities that use resistance, the risk of ligament injury is decreased compared to sport participation because the movements are slower and more directionally controlled. Risk still exists however, when the knee does not follow proper biomechanical patterns. When the knee passes the plane of the toe during flexion for instance, the action forces undesirable tibial motion, called **tibial translation**, which disrupts normal patellar tracking. When this occurs frequently, the patellar tendon and ligament are subject to pain from inflammation, termed patellar tendinopathy, "jumper's knee," or chondromalacia patella, an overuse state called "runner's knee." The knee joint can also lock in place to allow for prolonged periods of standing without contracting the knee extensors. This action is undesirable during lifting activities because the mechanism requires the meniscus to be compressed between the tibia and femur to maintain the position.

DEFINITIONS

Tibial translation –

This describes potentially harmful translational forces created by the tibia that are placed upon the patellar tendon and knee joint due to migration of the knees in front of the toes during lower-body movements, such as stepping and lunging.

MUSCLES OF THE HIP AND KNEE

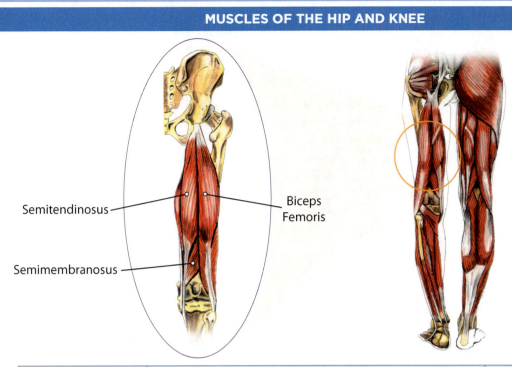

Muscles	Movement Function	Example Exercise
Rectus Femoris	Extends leg, flexes thigh (hip)	Front squat
Vastus Lateralis	Extends leg	Lunge
Vastus Intermedius	Extends leg	Leg press
Vastus Medialis	Extends leg	Leg extension
Sartorius	Flexes hip and leg, rotates leg medially and thigh laterally	Lateral step-ups
Biceps Femoris	Extends thigh (hip); flexes and laterally rotates leg	Romanian deadlift
Semitendinosus	Extends thigh (hip); flexes and medially rotates leg	Supine leg curl
Semimembranosus	Extends thigh (hip); flexes and medially rotates leg	Standing leg curl
Adductor Brevis	Adducts, flexes, and laterally rotates thigh	Lateral lunge
Adductor Longus	Adducts, flexes, and laterally rotates thigh	Side step-ups
Adductor Magnus	Adducts, extends, and laterally rotates thigh	Seated adduction
Pectineus	Adducts and flexes thigh	Cable adduction

Under load, the risk for damage dramatically increases compared to unloaded standing with the knee in the same position [21, 41]. Related concerns have also been raised about the deep-flexed (squat) position and the potential for cartilage and meniscus injury. Early research suggested deep squatting to be hazardous to knee structures, but some newer research suggests this may not be true when the tibia-spine angles are parallel [9, 30, 41]. A major issue with biomechanical and electromyography-related exercise studies is the variability in the technique used to perform the exercises, which often compromises the data.

Ankle

The ankle joint is also a hinge joint and provides for two primary movements: plantarflexion (extended ankle) and dorsiflexion (flexed ankle). The gastrocnemius attaches to the femur and the calcaneus (heel bone), crossing both the knee and ankle, thereby serving two functions: as prime mover for standing plantarflexion and assistive mover in knee flexion. The soleus also supports plantarflexion, but in a seated position, as it does not cross the knee; it mainly functions as a postural muscle and a neutralizer during locomotion. The anterior tibialis functions to dorsiflex and invert the ankle as well as help control the tibial angle during walking and running. In addition to flexing and extending at the ankle, the foot can also be inverted and everted through a limited range at the intertarsal joints (gliding joints). Injuries can occur when the foot is inverted or everted under load. This commonly occurs during jumping or running activities when body weight is applied to an uneven surface, such as landing on a person's foot during a rebound in a basketball game or stepping in a divot when running. Damage to feedback structures in the ankle are a concern with most ankle injuries and can lead to repeated or chronic injury. Ankle mechanoreceptors require re-education following injury and need proprioceptive training as part of return to play exercise plan.

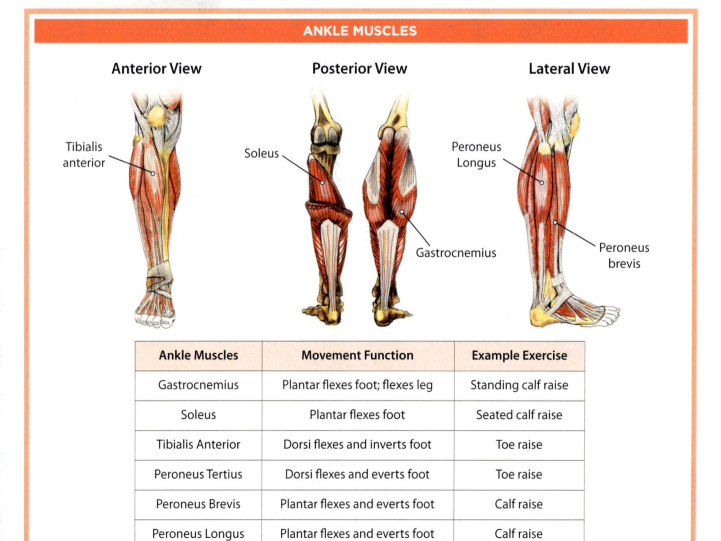

ANKLE MUSCLES

Ankle Muscles	Movement Function	Example Exercise
Gastrocnemius	Plantar flexes foot; flexes leg	Standing calf raise
Soleus	Plantar flexes foot	Seated calf raise
Tibialis Anterior	Dorsi flexes and inverts foot	Toe raise
Peroneus Tertius	Dorsi flexes and everts foot	Toe raise
Peroneus Brevis	Plantar flexes and everts foot	Calf raise
Peroneus Longus	Plantar flexes and everts foot	Calf raise

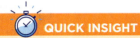
QUICK INSIGHT

The ankle is often involved in two tri-planar motions, supination and pronation. As a result of this characteristic, feet can present a very high arch (supination), or no arch at all, flat feet (pronation). Supination combines dorsiflexion, abduction, and eversion, whereas a pronated foot is inverted, adducted, and plantarflexed.

Deformation of the foot

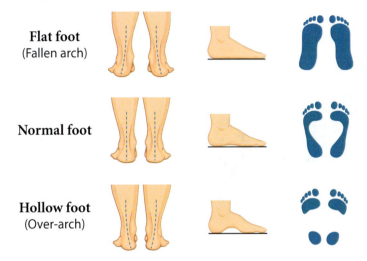

Flat foot (Fallen arch)

Normal foot

Hollow foot (Over-arch)

◆ Training Instruction

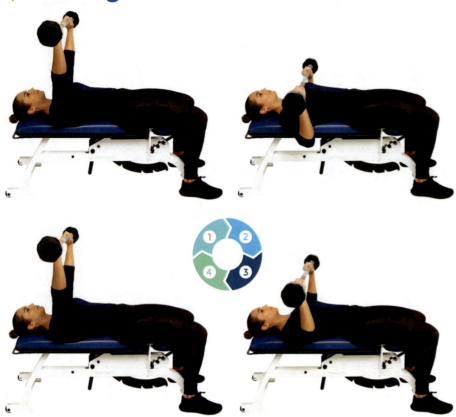
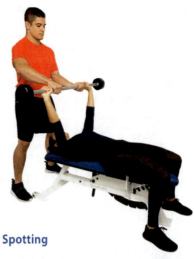

Exercise: **Barbell Bench Press**

Joint Action: Shoulder horizontal adduction, shoulder flexion, elbow extension

Muscles Involved: Pectoralis major, anterior deltoid, triceps brachii

Modifications: Barbells, dumbbells, cables, bands, medicine ball (MB) throws on a bench/physioball

Starting Position

- Begin supine with both feet flat on the ground, and grasp the bar just outside shoulder width, using a closed grip (thumbs wrapped around bar); the wrist should align with the elbow at the bottom of the eccentric phase.
- The shoulders and gluteals remain in contact with the bench, and the spine is neutral.
- Lift the bar off the rack and position it over the chest with the arms fully extended.

Movement Phase

- Lower the bar in a controlled manner toward the chest while limiting any other bodily movements.
- The bar descends at a constant speed until it contacts the chest (or reaches the functional range for the lifter).
- From the lowest point, press the bar in the same plane of motion used during the descent phase until the arms are extended.

Spotting

- Lift the bar off the rack, assisting the client to the start position. This reduces shoulder stresses during the lift-off.
- Focus on the client and movement of the bar during the descent but do not contact the bar.
- Monitor the upward movement with the hands in an alternate grip, inside the lifter's grip position; provide assistance to the bar as needed.
- When re-racking the bar, use an alternate grip to guide it securely onto the rack.
- If the rack has low-positioned arms, use caution when replacing the barbell; this is of particular concern with long-limbed clients.

Training Considerations

- Do not bounce the bar off the chest, as this can cause injury to the sternum; use a "touch-and-go" method.
- Do not raise the hips off the bench during the ascent to increase mechanical advantage.
- If the lifter must compensate to perform the exercise, the weight is too heavy and should be lowered.
- Ensure the bar is not uneven during the eccentric or concentric phase; this commonly indicates asymmetrical stabilizer fatigue or a muscle strength imbalance issue: e.g., rotator cuff imbalance/weakness, triceps brachii imbalance, or previous injury.
- Using lighter loads with higher repetitions can remedy many problems.

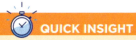

QUICK INSIGHT

GRIP VARIATIONS

Even the smallest refinements to a resistance training program can provide for significant differences in adaptation over time. A good example of this is the employment of varying gripping methods during applicable lifts. Utilizing the proper grip for a given exercise will keep joint angles aligned in a manner that will not cause undue stress to major junctions, such as the wrist, elbow, and shoulder. The primary hand positions, or grips, used in weightlifting include:

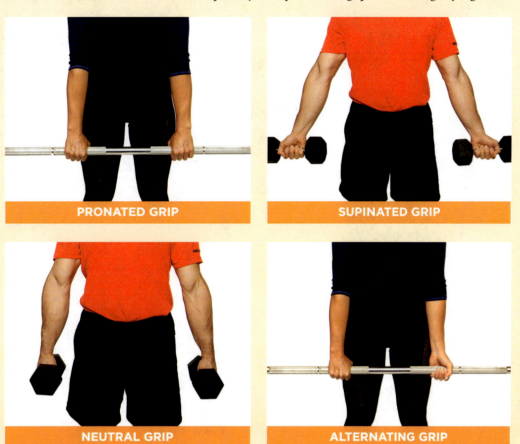

PRONATED GRIP

SUPINATED GRIP

NEUTRAL GRIP

ALTERNATING GRIP

Variations in grip can alter activation of musculature during a number of pulling and pressing actions that challenge the hips, shoulders, and upper back. For example, if a wide, pronated grip is used during lat pull-downs or pull-ups; the load is resisted primarily through shoulder adduction. This grip variation is used to promote latissimus dorsi activity due to the angle of stress. Conversely, if a supinated grip is used with relatively narrow hand placement during pull-downs or pull-ups the biceps brachii will assist the movement to a greater degree and the latissimus dorsi will be challenged through shoulder extension.

Lower and upper-body pulls and presses using the pronated or supinated grips will change muscle activation patterns, depending on the action performed and the joints involved. Supinated grip positions tend to increase biceps brachii activation and promote greater sagittal plane musculature, while pronated grip position will cause various changes in muscle activation depending on whether the action is performed in the frontal, sagittal, or transverse plane. The neutral grip can be used during curls to increase brachioradialis activation, as will be seen with the hammer curl, as well as during various other movements, such as overhead presses, swings, and rows. The neutral grip is sometimes used as a variation when flexibility does not allow for proper form using a standard grip for the given exercise (e.g., during dumbbell overhead presses vs. pronated grip). The alternated grip is primarily used to increase grip/pulling strength for spotting or heavy pulls from the floor.

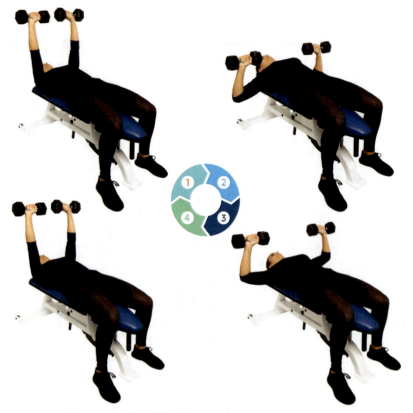
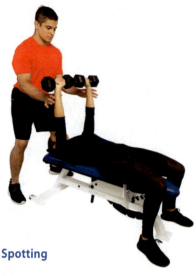

Exercise: ## Dumbbell Chest Press

Joint Action: Shoulder horizontal adduction, elbow extension
Muscles Involved: Pectoralis major, anterior deltoid, triceps brachii
Modifications: Cable, performed on a physioball, bench, Bosu

Starting Position

- Start supine with the shoulders and gluteals in contact with the bench, spine should be neutral with feet flat on the floor.
- Make sure the wrists, elbows, and shoulders are aligned, with the arms fully extended and the hands/dumbbells positioned over the shoulders.
- A pronated grip should be used (palms facing the feet).

Movement Phase

- Lower the resistance under control toward the lateral aspects of chest by simultaneously flexing the arms and horizontally abducting the humerus so that the wrists maintain alignment with the elbows.
- The body remains in a fixed, stable position with no extraneous movements.
- The weight descends until the dumbbells are in a position lateral to the sides of the chest.
  - Avoid any internal and/or external rotation, abduction of the shoulder, or excessive elbow flexion.
- Once a full, functional ROM is met, the client presses the weight upward in the same plane of motion.
- The resistance is pressed until the elbows are extended with the wrist, elbow, and shoulder joints in line.

Spotting

- A wrist assist may be needed to help get the client to a proper start position if the load is very heavy.
- If necessary, lightly grasp the lifter's wrists to help stabilize the dumbbells in the appropriate descent position.
- During the ascent, if necessary, apply upward force as needed to the wrist until the lift is complete.
- If fatigue or loss of arm/shoulder control occurs, grasp the forearms/wrist to help lower the weight down to the bottom position, and have the client lower the dumbbells to the floor.

Training Considerations

- Proper wrist and elbow positioning is important to proper execution.
- Using an open-circuit system, such as dumbbells, as opposed to a closed-circuit system, like a bar, requires the lifter to possess a higher amount of motor control and stability, explaining why the weight is lighter.
- Performing the exercise on a physioball protects the shoulder, allowing the scapula to more easily retract, but this adds to the balance requirements.
- The most common error is excessive elbow flexion, reducing the lateral position of the load.

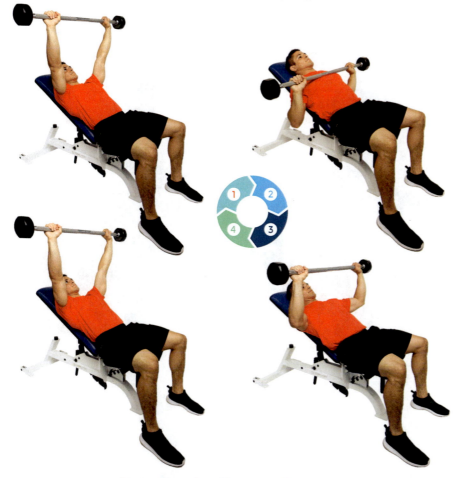

Exercise: **Incline Barbell Bench Press**

Joint Action: Shoulder horizontal adduction and elbow extension

Muscles Involved: Pectoralis major (clavicular head), anterior deltoid, triceps brachii

Modifications: Barbell, dumbbell, cable, bands, MB throws from a bench or physioball

Starting Position

- Start supine on an incline bench (30-75°) with both feet flat on the ground.
- Each joint segment should closely align, the spine is neutral, and the hips are securely positioned in the seat.
- Position the hands just outside shoulder-width using a closed grip and lift the bar off the rack to position it over the chest with the arms fully extended (spotter assistance from the rack is recommended).

Movement Phase

- Lower the bar with control toward the superior portion of the chest.
- The body remains fixed during the eccentric portion of the exercise with no extraneous movements, and the bar descends at a constant speed until it contacts the chest (or the defined functional range of the client).
- From the lowest point, exert concentric force in the same plane of motion used during the eccentric phase.

Spotting

- The spotter assists with the lift-off to the start position to reduce shoulder stress.
- During the eccentric phase, monitor the bar without using contact; cue controlled deceleration to the chest.
- Monitor the upward movement with the hands in a supinated grip inside the lifter's hand position. Provide assistance at the bar if needed.
- If the bar stops under assistance, switch to an alternate grip to rack it.
- Ensure a secure re-rack. If the rack has low-positioned arms, use caution when replacing the barbell; this is of particular concern with long-limbed clients.

Training Considerations

- Do not bounce the bar off the chest due to risk for injury to the ribcage/sternum.
- Do not raise the hips off the bench during the ascent to increase mechanical advantage; if this occurs, lower the weight.
- Monitor uneven bar extension, which can be due to diminished motor control, asymmetrical stabilizer fatigue, or a muscle strength imbalance issue (similar to the situation mentioned regarding the bench press).
- Using lighter loads with further practice should correct most problems.

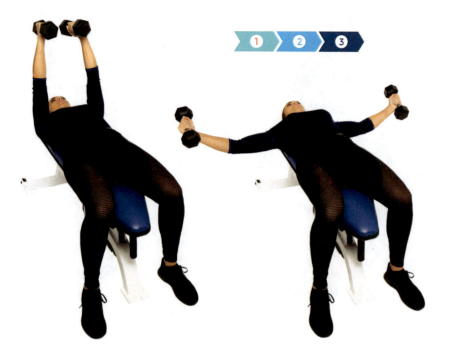
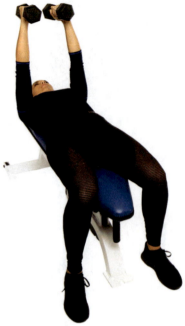

Exercise: **DB Chest Fly**

Joint Action: Shoulder horizontal adduction

Muscles Involved: Pectoralis major, anterior deltoid

Modifications: Cable, bands performed standing/seated on a physioball, bench, or Bosu

Starting Position

- Start supine on a bench with a neutral spine and feet flat on the floor.
- Hold dumbbells with a closed, neutral-grip with the arms extended above the shoulders.

Movement Phase

- Start by slightly flexing the elbows and horizontally abducting the shoulders.
- In a slow, arching motion, eccentrically lower the weight until a full, functional ROM is reached.
- Horizontally adduct the arms, maintaining a slightly flexed elbow position throughout the movement, until the dumbbells are back to the starting position.
- Both phases of the lift follow the same plane of motion.

Spotting

- Provide spotting assistance at the wrist or forearm, depending on arm length.
- Do not spot from the elbow as it reduces flexion control, may cause arm hyperextension or loaded external rotation, and can contribute to stability loss.

Training Considerations

- Potential injuries stem from performing the chest fly incorrectly or with too much weight; this exercise is only used if the client has healthy shoulder joint structures.
- Do not externally rotate the shoulder during the decent, which places excessive stress on the joint.
- Other common errors are over-flexing or extending the elbow, performing excessive scapular protraction, or lowering the weights too aggressively.

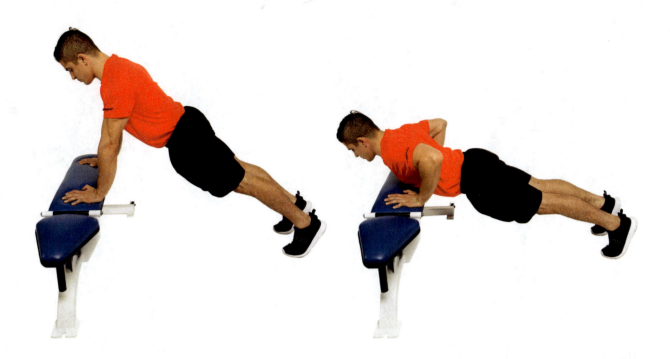

Exercise: Bench Push-up

Joint Action: Shoulder horizontal adduction, elbow extension

Muscles Involved: Pectoralis major, anterior deltoid, triceps brachii

Modifications: Performed on a Smith machine, physioball, the floor, or Bosu

Starting Position

- Place both hands on the bench with the arms extended and walk the feet back to an extended, straight-body position.
- The hands are placed just outside the chest just wider than shoulder-width apart.
- A straight bodyline should exist through the shoulders, hips, knees and ankles; the feet are spaced in-line with the hips.

Movement Phase

- Lower the body in a controlled manner toward the bench by retracting the scapulae, flexing the arms, and horizontally abducting the humerus so that the wrists are horizontally aligned with the elbows.
  - During the eccentric phase, the body remains in a fixed, stable position, similar to a plank, with no extraneous body movement.
- Descend evenly until the xyphoid process reaches a position at or near the bench; once full functional ROM is attained, concentrically press the whole body upward in the same plane of motion.
- Press upward until the arms are fully extended but not locked.

Spotting

- The push-up is not commonly spotted. For weaker clients, use a higher bench level, as an incline provides a mechanical advantage.
- Use cuing during the movement to maintain a stable torso and hip positioning.

Training Considerations

- Proper wrist and elbow positioning ensures safe execution and minimizes wrist and shoulder stress.
- Novice exercisers commonly use improper hand placement that is either superior to the shoulder or too narrow, causing increased shoulder abduction.
- Force should be maintained in the bottom portion of the palm to avoid subjecting the wrist to loaded extension.

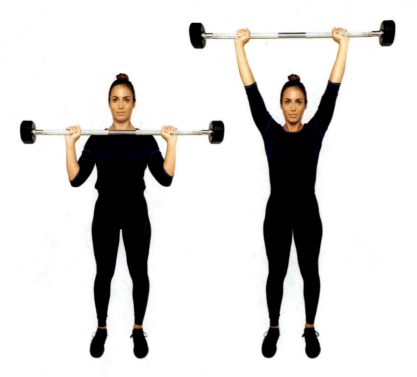
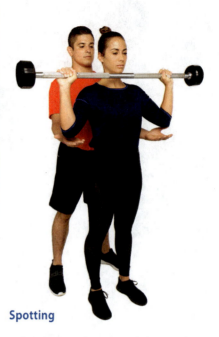

Exercise: **Military Press**

Joint Action: Shoulder flexion transition into shoulder abduction, shoulder flexion, elbow extension

Muscles Involved: Anterior deltoid, medial deltoid, supraspinatus, triceps brachii

Modifications: Seated on a machine or bench

Starting Position

- The movement is preferably performed standing to optimize improvements in total-body strength and central stability through closed-chain activation and stabilization, but it can be performed from a seated position.
- Start in an upright posture with feet underneath the hips and the spine neutral with wrists and elbows aligned.
- Hold the bar using a pronated grip that is lateral to the shoulders, at approximately the sub-clavicular level, and keep the neck slightly retracted to avoid bar-chin contact.
- Make sure the wrists are aligned, perpendicular to the floor, and not in an excessively extended position.

Movement Phase

- Start by contracting the deltoids while extending the elbows to press the resistance off the upper chest.
- As the resistance travels near the chin and the bar passes the forehead, re-establish a neutral neck position.
- Press the resistance upwards until the arms are fully extended.
- Once the arms are fully extended, lower the bar back to the starting position in the same plane of motion.
- Once a full, functional ROM is met, the client presses the weight upward in the same plane of motion.

Spotting

- Seated position: if using a straight bar or machine, spot the bar as opposed to the appendage performing the lift.
- Standing position: spot at the distal end of each humerus, not the elbow, during both the concentric and eccentric phases.

Training Considerations

- Do not perform this exercise with inadequate latissimus dorsi ROM; this can cause a backward lean, which places stress on the lumbar spine.
- Do not perform the lift behind the head: this causes excessive stress on the anterior capsule of the shoulder and is considered contraindicated.
- Do not allow the weight to bounce at the bottom of the movement, or flex the hip, as this natural tendency employs momentum and hip extension rather than the targeted muscle groups.

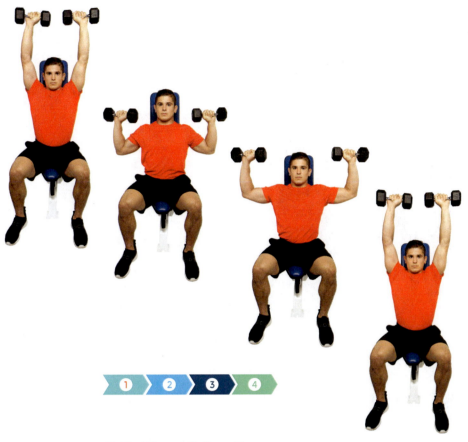
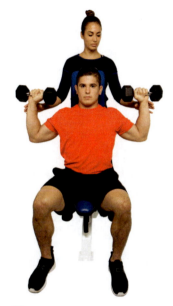

Exercise: **DB Shoulder Press**

Joint Action: Shoulder abduction, scapular rotation, elbow extension

Muscles Involved: Medial deltoid, anterior deltoid, triceps brachii, trapezius

Modifications: Cable, kettlebell, or bands performed standing or seated on a physioball or bench

Starting Position

- Can be performed in either a seated or standing position.
- Stand upright with the feet in neutral positions, separated to approximately hip width.
- Flex the arms against the midaxillary line with the wrists aligned above the elbows.
- Hold dumbbells using a pronated grip (palms facing away) above the height of the shoulders.

Movement Phase

- Contract the deltoids while extending the elbows to press the resistance upwards in a vertical line directly above the shoulders; maintain a neutral spine position at all times.
- Press the dumbbells upward until the arms are fully extended with the wrists, elbows, and shoulders aligned.
- Once the arms are fully extended, lower the resistance back to the starting position in the same plane of motion.

Spotting

- Seated position: spotting is consistent with the dumbbell bench press: assistance is given via support at the wrists.
- Standing position: provide assistance at the distal end of each humerus during both the concentric and eccentric phases.

Training Considerations

- Do not press the weight upward and outward: a common error among novices.

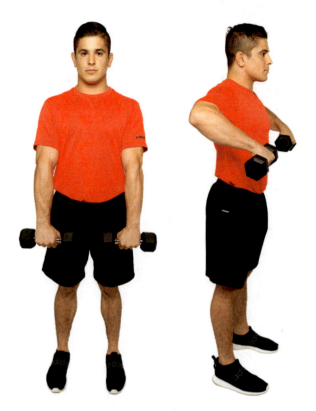

Exercise: **Dumbbell Upright Row**

Joint Action: Shoulder abduction, scapular elevation/rotation, elbow flexion

Muscles Involved: Medial deltoid, anterior deltoid, supraspinatus, levator scapulae, rhomboids, trapezius, brachialis, brachioradialis

Modifications: Kettlebell, cable, bands

Starting Position

- Stand in an upright posture with the feet in neutral positions, separated to approximately hip width.
- Extend the arms downward with the wrists and elbows aligned.
- Turn palms to face the body while using a pronated dumbbell grip.

Movement Phase

- Contract the deltoids and flex the arms to begin an upward and outward ascent and maintain thoracic extension by keeping the chest elevated.
- The elbows remain superior to the wrists and the spine remains neutral during all phases of the lift.
- The resistance travels along the front of the body until the upper arms are approximately parallel to the floor.
- Once functional ROM is attained, the resistance is lowered back to the starting position.

Spotting

- This exercise is not spotted. Select an appropriate weight and use verbal cuing so the lifter can complete all repetitions with proper form.

Training Considerations

- Do not allow the client to use momentum to bounce or jerk the weight to the end point.
- Do not shrug the shoulders during the concentric phase.
- If the exerciser cannot maintain proper shoulder abduction or excessive shoulder elevation occurs, decrease the resistance.
- Some individuals are susceptible to shoulder impingement or rotator-cuff issues if the arms are abducted beyond 90°.
- If pain is present during the lift, discontinue the movement.

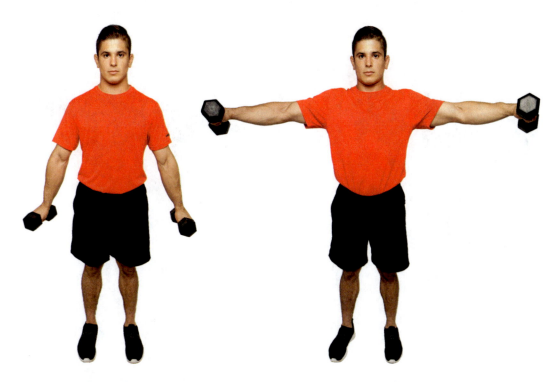

Exercise: **Lateral Deltoid Raise**

Joint Action: Shoulder abduction

Muscles Involved: Medial deltoid, supraspinatus, levator scapulae, trapezius, rhomboids, brachialis, brachioradialis

Modifications: Kettlebells, cable, bands in a seated or standing position, manual resistance

Starting Position

- Stand upright with the feet in neutral positions, separated to approximately hip width.
- Extend the arms downward along the midaxillary lines with the palms facing the body while using a neutral grip.
- The arms are extended and held approximately 4-6 inches from the sides of the body to start; the abducted position (30 degrees) removes supraspinatus activation and concentrates the resistance on the deltoid.

Movement Phase

- For the concentric phase, abduct the arms while maintaining stiff, straight wrist positions in the frontal plane.
- The arms remain extended with little to no elbow flexion while maintaining a neutral spine at all times.
- Abduct the shoulders until the upper arms are parallel with the floor; once attaining full ROM, lower the arms back to the starting position in the same plane of motion.
- To maximize deltoid recruitment, the lowest point should be approximately 30° from the hip.

Spotting

- Stand behind the lifter and apply assistance to the proximal forearm area when needed.

Training Considerations

- Poor technique and cheating with hip extension is common for this lift.
- Common errors include bending the elbows (reduces the resistance arm), using hip flexion and extension for momentum, or using the upper trapezius to shrug the weight up.
- This exercise can also be performed using manual resistance applied by the trainer.

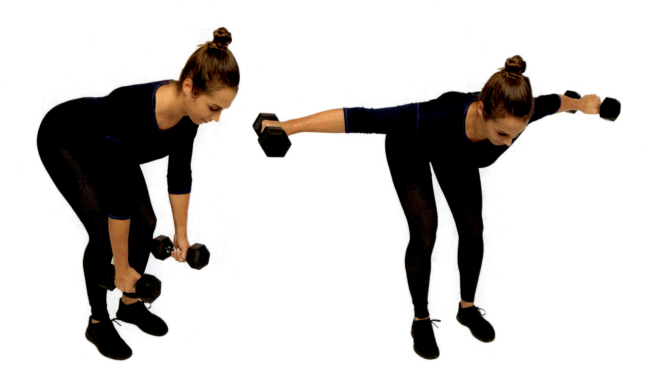

Exercise: **Rear Deltoid Raise**

Joint Action: Horizontal shoulder abduction (90 degrees of abduction)

Muscles Involved: Posterior deltoid

Modifications: Dumbbells, cable, bands in a seated or standing position

Starting Position

- Assume a standing, flexed-hip position with a neutral spine and pelvis so that the torso is parallel with the floor and the feet are in neutral positions, hip-width apart.
- Tight hamstrings may warrant a slightly wider stance or more knee flexion.
- Extend the arms downward under the shoulder just outside the feet; hold the dumbbells using a neutral grip.

Movement Phase

- While maintaining a flat back, horizontally abduct the arms until parallel with the floor with the wrists in line with the clavicles.
- The path of motion is slightly anterior to the superior aspect of the shoulders.
- Once end ROM is attained, lower the arms back to the starting position, following the same plane of motion.

Spotting

- Spot from the front of the client, providing assistance to the forearms.
- Use cuing to ensure the lift is performed with the torso in a position parallel to the floor to maintain true shoulder horizontal abduction (extension). Also ensure that the resistance is being moved against full vertical (gravitational) force.

Training Considerations

- Poor technique and cheating with hip extension is common for this lift.
- Common errors include bending the elbows (reduces the resistance arm), using hip flexion and extension for momentum, or using the upper trapezius to shrug the weight up.
- This exercise can also be performed using manual resistance applied by the trainer.

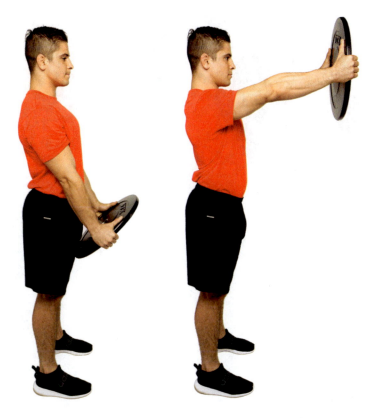

Exercise: **Front Raise**

Joint Action: Shoulder flexion

Muscles Involved: Anterior deltoid

Modifications: Dumbbells, plate, MB, sand bag

Starting Position

- Stand upright with the feet shoulder-width apart, holding a weight plate at waist height using a neutral grip.
- Extend the elbows with little to no elbow flexion (flexion should never exceed 15°).

Movement Phase

- Flex the shoulders while simultaneously depressing the scapula: all while maintaining neutral spine and pelvic positions with the feet flat on the floor.
- Flex the shoulders to at least 90°, or until the upper arms are parallel with the floor; to perform the exercise through a greater ROM, adopt a neutral grip.
- Upon reaching a full, functional ROM, lower the resistance under control until it reaches the starting position.

Spotting

- There is normally no spotting used for this exercise.
- Use cuing to help the client maintain a stable body position throughout the movement.

Training Considerations

- Avoid any forward or backward movement to generate momentum or swing the weight.
- Using a pronated grip can be detrimental when performed at ROM that exceeds 90° of shoulder flexion due to shoulder stress and impingement risk.
- The neutral grip is always favored, as it lowers the risk for injury and allows for a greater functional ROM.

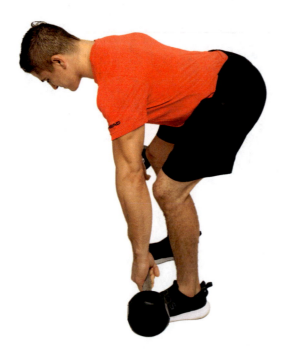
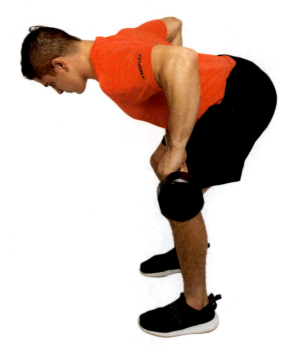

Exercise:	**Bent-Over Row**

Joint Action: Shoulder horizontal abduction/extension, scapular retraction, elbow flexion

Muscles Involved: Latissimus dorsi, rhomboids, trapezius, infraspinatus, posterior deltoid, brachialis, biceps brachii, brachioradialis

Modifications: Barbell, dumbbell, Smith machine

Starting Position

- Assume a flat back position with flexed-hips so that the torso is parallel with the floor.
- The feet are approximately hip-width apart with the knees flexed; a slightly wider stance may be needed for those with tight hamstrings.
- Position the bar so that the arms are extended downward, perpendicular to the floor and directly over the shoelaces.
- Keep the arms under the shoulders with the hands in a pronated position (neutral grip for dumbbells) slightly wider than the chest.

Movement Phase

- Retract the scapula and simultaneously extend the humerus to pull the weight upward in a vertical line.
- Maintain a flat back position, ensuring that the torso remains parallel to the floor at all times.
- Continue the upward movement phase until the bar reaches the trunk between the umbilicus and the xyphoid process, the scapulae are fully retracted, and the shoulders can no longer hyperextend.
- Maintaining a flat back, lower the weight as the arms extend and the scapula protracts back to a neutral position.

Spotting

- There is no spot for this movement; assign appropriate weight and use verbal cuing.

Training Considerations

- Do not extend the hips, legs, or spine to gain mechanical advantage.
- If performed correctly, the bent-over row is excellent for developing the back and central stability.
- It is imperative that no "rounding" of any spinal segments occurs.
- The most common error is a spinal angle that is too high due to use of excess resistance and poor posterior mobility.

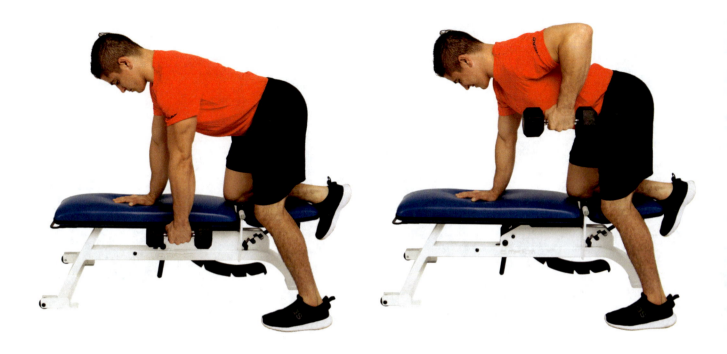

Exercise: ## Single-Arm Row

Joint Action: Shoulder horizontal abduction, shoulder extension, scapular retraction, arm flexion

Muscles Involved: Latissimus dorsi, trapezius, posterior deltoid, rhomboids, brachialis, biceps brachii, brachioradialis

Modifications: Place hand and knee on bench or execute with no support, two dumbbells, kettlebell(s)

Starting Position

- Assume a flexed hip/knee position on a bench with the torso parallel with the floor.
- Place one arm on the bench in an extended position to support the upper body; extend the other arm downward, holding the dumbbell in a neutral grip.
- Keep the spine and pelvis neutral.

Movement Phase

- Simultaneously retract the scapula, extend the shoulder, and flex the arm
- Continue until the scapula is fully retracted, shoulder hyperextended, elbow flexed, and the dumbbell is at a point lateral to the rib cage with arm flexed at 90 degrees.
- Lower the resistance back to the start by extending the arm and protracting the scapula while maintaining a flat back position.

Spotting

- Spotting is achieved using verbal cues; watch the position of the spine to avoid rotation and rounding of the back.

Training Considerations

- Do not extend the hip or rotate the spine to create momentum; this is common when using too much resistance.
- Do not bring the torso downward to meet the rising dumbbell during the concentric phase.
- Do not pull the dumbbell toward the shoulder solely through elbow flexion, the emphasis is shoulder hyperextension.

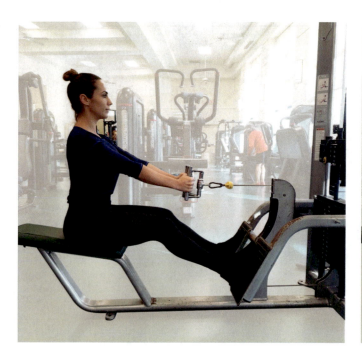
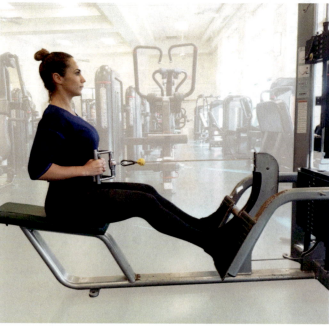

Exercise:	**Seated Cable Row**
Joint Action:	Shoulder horizontal abduction, shoulder extension, scapular retraction, elbow flexion
Muscles Involved:	Rhomboids, latissimus dorsi, trapezius, teres major, brachialis, biceps brachii, brachioradialis
Modifications:	Unilateral or bilateral

Starting Position

- Assume a seated position with the knees slightly flexed.
- Grasp the handles using a neutral grip with the arms extended, scapula slightly protracted, spine in a neutral position and the shoulders aligned directly above the hips.

Movement Phase

- While maintaining a neutral spine, simultaneously retract the scapula while extending and horizontally abducting the shoulders and flexing the elbows.
- Pull the handle to the mid-point of the abdomen while keeping the back flat and chest elevated; the scapulae are fully retracted at the end ROM.
- Once a full range is attained, extend the arms, flex the shoulders, and protract the scapula back to the starting position following the same plane of motion as the pulling phase.
- Maintain a flat back; do not allow the weight to accelerate forward during the eccentric phase.

Spotting

- Verbal and tactile cues are used to maintain proper body alignment.
- Ensure the lifter's scapula retract during the pulling phase and prevent trunk extension, and/or shoulder elevation.

Training Considerations

- Do not lean forward (flexing the hip and then extending the hip and spine) to generate momentum forces similar to that of rowing ergometry.
- The hip angle should be relatively unchanged while the spine remains in a neutral position throughout the lift.
- Another common mistake is primarily performing arm flexion with minimal scapular retraction.

NCSF Advanced Concepts of Personal Training

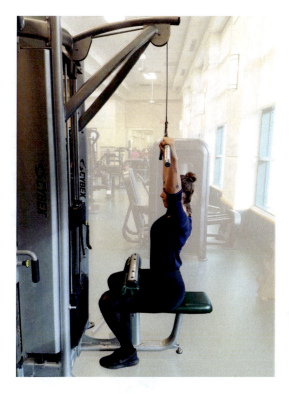
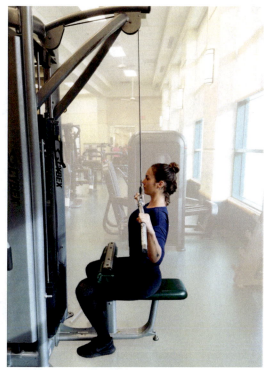

Exercise: ## Lat Pull-Down

Joint Action: Shoulder adduction, scapular medial rotation, elbow flexion

Muscles Involved: Latissimus dorsi, teres major, brachialis, biceps brachii, brachioradialis

Modifications: Cables, bands, using one arm or two, kneeling, or half-kneeling

Starting Position

- Grasp the bar with a closed, pronated grip; for normal execution grasp a few inches wider than shoulder-width, but grip widths can vary.
- Securely position the legs under the kneepad for stability and keep the hips in contact with the seat.

Movement Phase

- Pull the bar downward by simultaneously depressing/adducting the scapulae and flexing the arms while adducting the humerus.
- Maintain the initial torso position and pull the bar to the upper chest.
- Once the bar has traveled through a full ROM, allow the upper arms to abduct while also outwardly rotating the scapula and extending the arms to decelerate the bar back to the start position.
- The upward and downward phases should follow the same plane of motion with limited to no movement in the hips or spine.

Spotting

- Assistance can be applied to the bar while standing behind the lifter.
- Watch for undesirable movements such back extension for increased mechanical advantage and provide verbal cues as needed.

Training Considerations

- Do not lean backwards to generate momentum forces.
- Do not pull the bar to a position behind the head; this motion places excessive stress on the shoulder joint, reduces activation of the latissimus dorsi, and increases the risk of cervical spine injury.
- Allow the scapula to rotate downward and adduct; many exercisers only flex the elbows during the lift, effectively training the biceps in lieu of the back musculature.

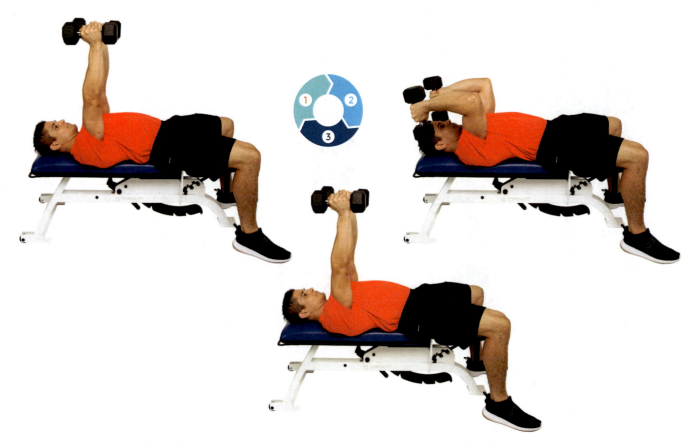

Exercise: **Supine Triceps Extension**

Joint Action: Elbow extension

Muscles Involved: Triceps brachii

Modifications: Dumbbell, barbell, cable, bands

Starting Position

- Start supine on a bench with the feet flat on the floor.
- Fully extend the arms so the elbows and wrists align with the shoulder joints.
- The hands are maintained in a neutral position when using dumbbells and pronated if using a bar.

Movement Phase

- Flex only the elbows to lower the resistance until the forearms reach a position that is approximately parallel, or just below parallel, to the floor.
- The upper arms and shoulder remain still and perpendicular to the floor at all times.
- Once the descent has reached a full ROM, extend the arms by contracting the triceps without extending the shoulders.
- Maintain a neutral spine and upper arm position as the resistance is extended back to the start position.

Spotting

- Spot from a position above the client by providing assistance as needed to the load itself.
- Establish an end ROM and guard against movements past this position; guard vigilantly against the resistance making contact with the client's head.

Training Considerations

- Some people may experience discomfort in the wrist or elbow region, particularly if the shoulder is abducted during execution.
- Look for technical errors, and decrease or change the resistance to accommodate the client if technique has been compromised.
- Do not allow the gluteals to lift off the bench as the weight approaches the eccentric end-point ROM.
- Attention to safety is paramount due to the positioning of the load as it decelerates towards the face: hence the layman's terms commonly used: nosebreakers/skullcrushers.
- The exercise can be modified to a triceps-pullover if the shoulders flex before the arms, and can reach 150° of flexion.

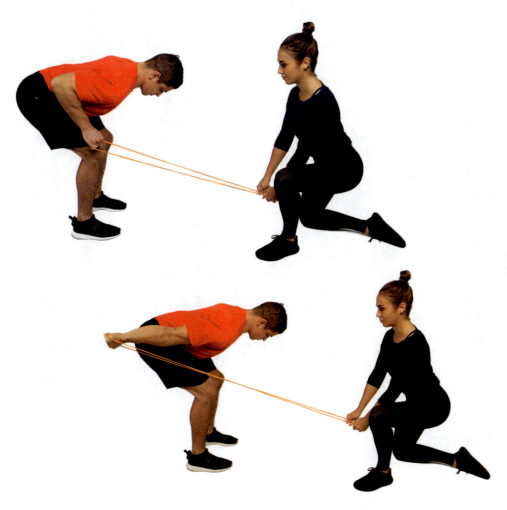

Exercise:	**Triceps Kickback**
Joint Action:	Elbow extension
Muscles Involved:	Triceps brachii
Modifications:	Cables, bands, using one or two arms

Starting Position

- Assume a flexed-hip position with the feet about hip-width apart; the spine is neutral and approximately parallel to the floor.
- Using a pronated grip, grasp a cable or band in one or both hands and extend the shoulders.

Movement Phase

- While maintaining a stable body position, extend the elbow to move the resistance backward and upward; shoulder movement does not occur at any point.
- The humerus remains close to the body, and the elbow positioning remains unchanged.
- The elbow is fully extended at the end-point ROM; at this point, return to the start position by eccentrically flexing the arm through the same plane of motion.

Spotting

- Spot from the side of the client by applying necessary assistance to the forearm while providing mild support to the upper arm.

Training Considerations

- Cables and bands are ideal for this exercise, considering the movement travels across the downward vector of gravitational pull, causing constant resistance.
- Using dumbbells causes the load to cross-gravitational pull and encourages swinging.
- Maintain a neutral spine, and do not swing the weight to take advantage of momentum forces.

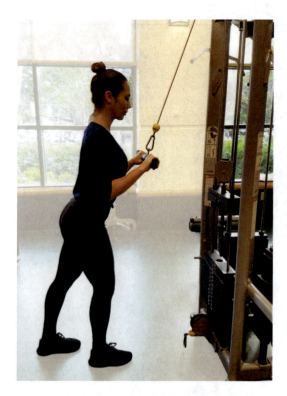
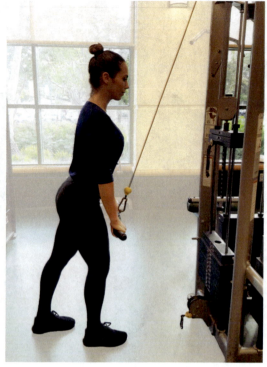

Exercise: **Standing Triceps Push-down**

Joint Action: Elbow extension

Muscles Involved: Triceps brachii

Modifications: Single or double arm, rope/various other attachments

Starting Position

- Stand upright with a neutral spine with feet shoulder-width apart.
- Grasp the bar with a closed, pronated grip.
- The hands are shoulder-width apart, the scapulae are neutral, and the upper arms are kept against the lateral aspects of the body along the anterior-axillary line.

Movement Phase

- Extend the elbows to push the resistance downward towards the floor. Keep the elbows fixed against the sides of the body at all times; the arms are fully extended but not locked.
- Keep the shoulders back and maintain a flat back position while eccentrically flexing the arms in a controlled manner to return to the start position.
- Raise the bar while keeping the elbows in the same position.

Spotting

- Use verbal cues to help the lifter maintain proper body position, especially at the shoulders.

Training Considerations

- Do not generate momentum by flexing the hips and/or flexing and extending the shoulder.
- Perform the lift in a controlled (very isolated) manner with appropriate resistance to limit improper movements. Elbows should remain fixed.
- This exercise can be performed using a wide variety of accessories; it is recommended to periodically change the accessory to stimulate different tricep (head) muscle recruitment with varied training angles.

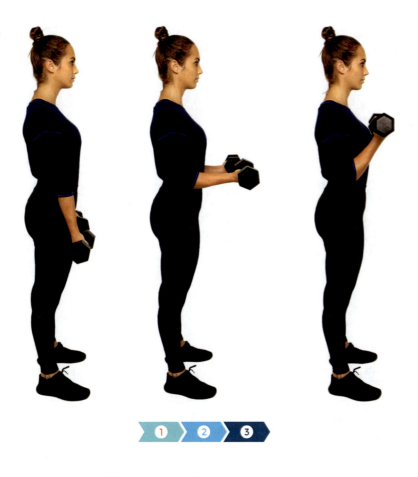
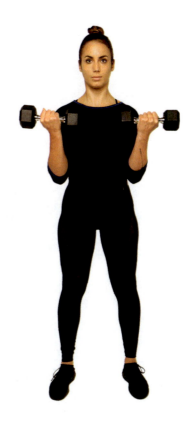

Exercise: **Bicep Curls**

Joint Action: Elbow flexion

Muscles Involved: Biceps brachii, brachialis, brachioradialis

Modifications: Dumbbells, barbell, cable, bands

Starting Position

- Stand upright with the feet shoulder-width apart and grasp a dumbbell in each hand.
- Extend the elbows with the upper arms aligned along the anterior-axillary line.

Movement Phase

- Contract the biceps to flex the elbows while keeping the humerus adducted and fixed to the side of the body.
- Supinate the wrist as the weight ascends to a full ROM without any shoulder flexion or extension.
- Once full ROM is attained, lower the resistance to the starting position under control and through the same plane of motion.
- Maintain a flat back position as the weight is lowered eccentrically.

Spotting

- Spot from the front of the lifter by providing assistance to the dumbbells/hands or bar.
- Use verbal cues to ensure the lifter maintains an erect posture with a neutral spine.

Training Considerations

- Avoid using excess loads and "cheating" by swinging the weight while failing to go through a full eccentric phase.
- Do not flex and extend the hips or shoulders, or lean backwards to generate momentum forces instead of using the biceps to accomplish the lift.

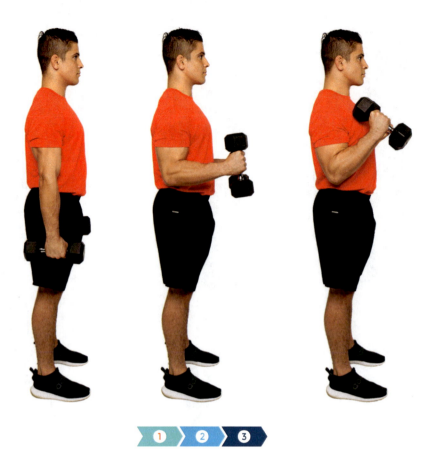

Exercise:	**Hammer Curls**
Joint Action:	Elbow flexion
Muscles Involved:	Brachialis, biceps brachii, brachioradialis
Modifications:	Kettlebells, cable, bands

Starting Position

- Stand upright with the feet shoulder-width apart, and grasp a dumbbell in each hand with a neutral grip.
- Extend the elbows with the upper arm aligned along the midaxillary line.

Movement Phase

- With the palms facing inward, contract the elbow flexors while maintaining the upper arm in a stable position along the midaxillary line.
- Maintain neutral hip and spinal positioning to avoiding generating momentum forces.
- The arms are flexed through a full ROM, and the resistance is lowered under control until the elbows are fully extended.
- Maintain a flat back position as the weight is decelerated to the start position.

Spotting

- Spot from the front of the lifter by providing assistance to the bottom of the dumbbells as needed.

Training Considerations

- Avoiding using excess weight during bicep curl exercises and "cheating" by swinging the weight.
- Do not flex and extend the hips to generate momentum forces: always emphasize no shoulder or hip movement, and avoid internal rotation.

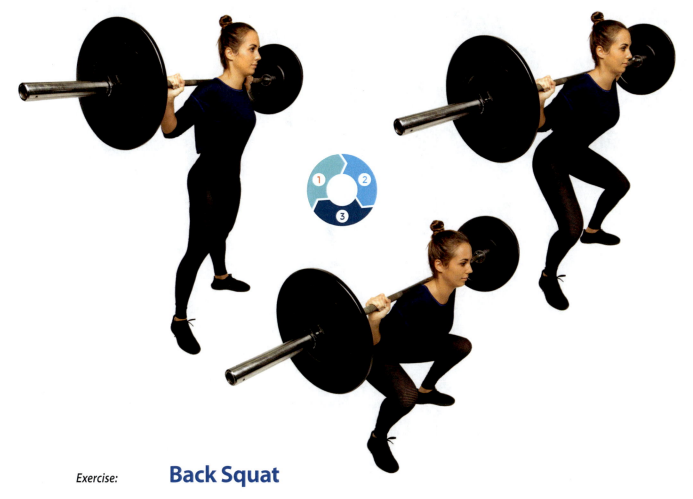

Exercise: **Back Squat**

Joint Action: Hip extension, knee extension, back extension

Muscles Involved: Gluteus maximus, rectus femoris, vastus lateralis, vastus intermedius, vastus medialis, biceps femoris, semimembranosus, semitendinosus

Modifications: Barbell, Smith machine, or cable, performed on a stable or unstable surface

Starting Position

- Prior to the exercise, the correct bar height must be established so the client can safely position the bar across the upper trapezius/posterior deltoids and step clear of the rack.
  - To do this, the bar height should be set at approximately the height of the client's upper chest.
- Face the bar, and grasp it with a closed, pronated grip with the hands placed slightly wider than shoulder-width apart.
- Step under the bar, depress the scapulae, and adduct the shoulders/upper arms; this creates a "shelf-like" position between the upper trapezius and the posterior deltoid where the bar can sit securely.
  - The bar is never placed across the cervical spine.
- Extend the hips and knees to lift the bar off the rack. If plantar flexion is required for this action, the rack should be lowered.
- A position is established a full step away from the rack, with control of the resistance.
- A shoulder-width (to just outside shoulder-width) stance is used with the feet facing forward and turned slightly outward.
  - The degree of outward rotation will be determined by the angle of hip abduction, but should be consistent with the stance width and natural standing gait of the individual.

Back Squat

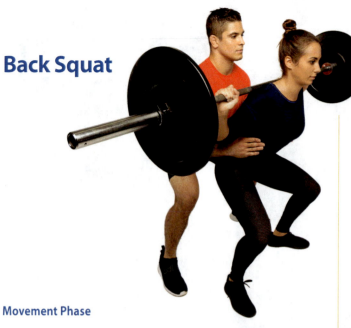

Movement Phase

- Initiate the downward movement by flexing the hips and knees simultaneously under control.

- The muscles of torso and inner unit remain isometrically contracted, the head remains forward, and the chest remains elevated while flexing the hips and knees during the descent phase.

- The ideal end-point ROM to ensure gluteus maximus recruitment is the top of the thighs parallel with the floor, but this will be client specific and vary to a degree.

- The depth of the squat does not go beyond functional ROM, nor should the weight used compromise the movement range.

- The knees never cross the plane of the toes and should be directed toward the pinkie toes for proper knee alignment. This technique helps mitigate anterior and lateral shear forces across the joint.

- Once the end-point ROM is attained, push on the bar to extend the knees and hips while maintaining a stable spinal position at a constant angle to the floor.

- The femurs should not adduct (knee valgus) or rotate, and the knees, hips, and back should extend at an equal rate.

- Upon returning to the starting position, do not lock the knees. Maintain a flat back position while engaging the glutes for full hip extension.

- Once the designated number of repetitions has been completed, re-rack the bar and ensure it rests safely on the rack.

Spotting

- Spotting utilizes an upper-trunk hand placement technique.

- The spotter's hands should be readied outside of the rib cage, just under the chest, with the trainer standing behind the lifter in a stance slightly wider than the lifter's feet.

- Assume the position right at the lift-off from the rack and walk back with the lifter to the starting position. Mirror the client's form and speed at all times.

- When assistance is needed, ensure the client's torso maintains a constant position in relation to the floor by spotting and lifting upward on the rib cage to raise the torso. This allows the lifter's hips to extend and move into an upright position, without compromising the lower back.

Training Considerations

- The term "squat" does not always reflect an externally loaded activity; the movement is one of the most functional actions to perform, regardless of the load.

- A multitude of muscle groups must work synergistically with one another to produce the desired outcome.
  - Whether helping an elderly person more efficiently rise from a seated position or attempting to increase strength for an athlete, the squat exercise promotes useful functions.

- Do not place objects under the heels, as this causes biomechanical shifts that place increased shear stress on the knees.

- If a client cannot attain a proper squat position, a movement screen can establish movement limitations, which are addressed before programming the bilateral squat.

- Many potential technique errors exist; listed below are some common examples fitness professionals should look for and correct:
  - The knees travel forward beyond the toes during the descent phase.
  - Movement is back-dominant rather than glute-dominant.
  - The weight is centered over the front portion of feet (heels come up).
  - The bar is positioned too high on the cervical spine or too low below the shoulders.
  - An anterior pelvic tilt is used to stabilize the spine.
  - The lumbar spine does not remain isometrically contracted (flexion of the spine is observed).
  - Excess forward leaning causes limited knee extension (vertical tibial angles).
  - The knees abduct/adduct during the descent or onset of the concentric movement.
  - The pelvis posteriorly rotates at the bottom of the movement ("butt-wink").

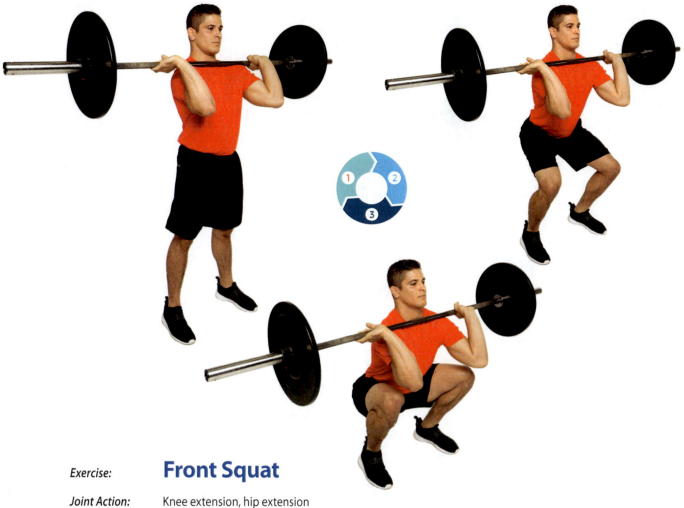

Exercise: **Front Squat**

Joint Action: Knee extension, hip extension

Muscles Involved: Rectus femoris, vastus lateralis, vastus intermedius, vastus medialis, biceps femoris, gluteus maximus, semimembranosus, semitendinosus

Modifications: Dumbbell, barbell, kettlebell, MB performed on a stable or unstable surface

Starting Position

- The correct bar height must be established, so the client can safely position the bar across the shoulders. The bar is set at approximately the height of the client's upper chest.

- Face the bar, and grasp it with a closed, pronated grip just slightly wider than the shoulders. With the elbows fully flexed, step under the bar, and position it across the shoulders and upper chest.

- Extend the hips and knees to lift the bar off the rack, establish control under the load, and gain a position away from the rack to avoid unintentional contact (one full step away).

- The stance is under the shoulders with the feet facing forward; due to the anterior position of the load, the stance used is narrower than during the back squat.

Movement Phase

- Initiate the downward phase by flexing the knees and hips simultaneously under control.

- The torso muscles remain isometrically contracted, the scapulae are retracted, the head remains forward, the upper arms and elbows remain parallel to the floor, and the trunk remains vertical as the lifter flexes the hips and knees through the descent.

Front Squat

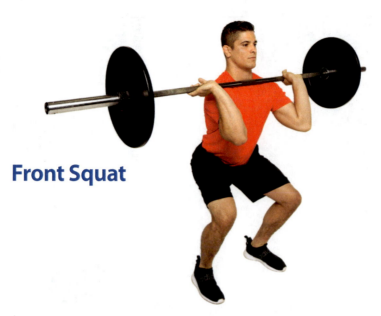

- The ideal end-point ROM is the top of the thighs parallel with the floor, but this will be client specific.
- The knees will migrate forward to the ends of the feet or toes; front squats involve relatively less knee stress due to the position of the load, which is better centered over the base of support.
- Once the end-point ROM is attained, extend the knees and hips simultaneously, pushing specifically on the bar so that neither movement dominates in contributing to vertical bar ascension.
- The spinal position is maintained, the scapulae remain retracted, the femurs should not adduct, and the hips and knees should extend at an equal rate.
- Upon returning to the starting position, do not fully lock the knees, and maintain a flat back.
- Once the designated number of repetitions is complete, re-rack the bar, and ensure it rests safely on the rack.

Spotting

- Spotting utilizes an upper-trunk hand placement technique.
- The spotter's hands should be readied outside of the rib cage, just under the chest, with the trainer standing behind the lifter in a slightly wider stance.
- Assume the position right at the lift-off from the rack and walk back with the lifter to the starting position. Mirror the client's form and speed at all times
- When assistance is needed, lift upward to raise the torso; this allows the hips to extend and move the client safely into an upright position.

Training Considerations

- This exercise is often avoided, as many do not possess the requisite latissimus dorsi and triceps mobility to hold the bar properly at the shoulders, relying instead on excessive wrist extension with upright elbows.
- Some lifters forgo proper racking technique and use a cross-arm method or straps.
- Do not migrate the hips backward, as this impacts the proper torso position and over-stresses the back.
- A lack of ankle dorsiflexion is another major limitation in performing squats correctly.

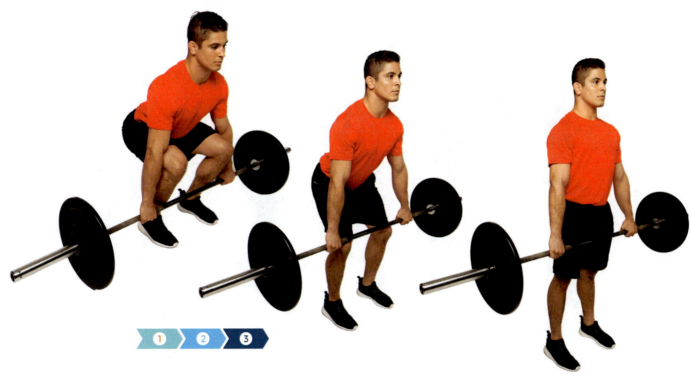

Exercise:	**Traditional Deadlift**
Joint Action:	Hip extension, knee extension, back extension
Muscles Involved:	Gluteus maximus, rectus femoris, vastus lateralis, vastus intermedius, vastus medialis, biceps femoris, semimembranosus, semitendinosus, erector spinae
Modifications:	Barbell, dumbbell, Smith machine, MB

Starting Position

- Assume a hip-width stance in front of the bar, which contacts the shins only at the start.
- Descend into the bottom position by flexing both the knees and hips (resembles the bottom position of a vertical jump).
- Grip the bar with a closed, pronated, or alternating, closed grip, just under the shoulders.
- The shoulders are positioned over the bar and a flat-back, retracted position is maintained with a neutral pelvis.

Movement Phase

- Once the muscles of the torso are isometrically contracted, and the "slack" is pulled out of the arms, begin the lift by simultaneously extending all body segments equally.
  - Press with the knee extensors and pull with the hip extensors at the same time the back is extending to move the bar vertically.
- The back must remain in a flat position throughout the movement
- Continue to extend all body segments until an erect standing posture is attained with all joint segments aligned: shoulders, hips, and knees.
- Different strategies can be employed for the descent phase:
  - In Olympic and sports environments, the lift is concentric only and the bar is dropped using bumper plates; this spares the back extensors.
  - If a controlled descent is used, all segments must be synchronized to ensure they move at the same pace, and the spine does not experience undue stress.

Spotting

- Do not spot the deadlift; it is cued both physically and verbally.
- Using proper loads is the most effective means of attaining proper technique.

Training Considerations

- The deadlift is a very functional movement but is commonly performed incorrectly.
- Common mistakes:
  - Rounding of the back due to a weak trunk
  - Extending the hips, causing a Romanian deadlift position
  - Unsynchronized knee, hip, and/or back extension
  - Dragging the bar up the shins: no contact should be made
  - Leaning too far back or pulling the bar backwards using posteriorly directed force

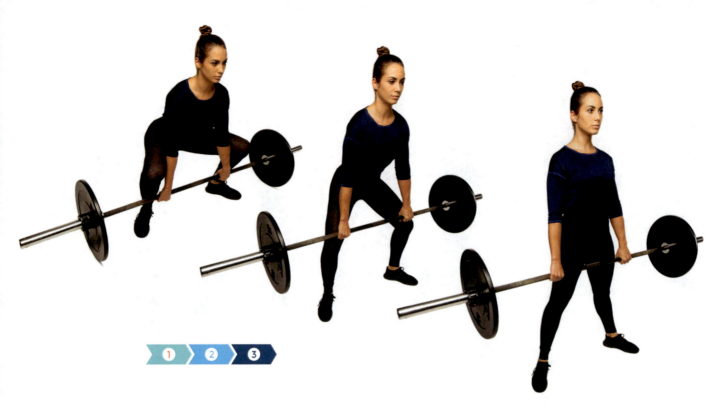

Exercise: **Modified Deadlift**

Joint Action: Hip extension, knee extension, back extension, hip adduction

Muscles Involved: Gluteus maximus, rectus femoris, vastus lateralis, vastus intermedius, vastus medialis, biceps femoris, semimembranosus, semitendinosus, erector spinae, short adductors (adductor magnus, adductor longus, adductor brevis, pectineus), gluteus medius

Modifications: Barbell, dumbbell, MB using one or two arms

Starting Position

- If a client has a weak trunk or poor flexibility, the deadlift can be modified.
- Assume a squat jump position, using a slightly wider than shoulder-width stance (not unlike the back squat) with the bar in front of the shins
- Grip the bar with a closed, pronated, or alternating, closed grip on the knurling, just inside the knees.
- The shoulders are positioned over the bar, and the back is flat.

Movement Phase

- Simultaneously extend the knees and hips while keeping the back in a flat, vertical position as the bar is lifted from the floor.
- Extend the knees and hips until an erect standing posture is attained; the descent is made in the same plane of motion as the ascent.
- If only a concentric lift is performed, "pop & drop" the bar, which requires slightly bouncing the bar forward off the thighs to clear the knees and riding it safely to the ground.
- If an eccentric component is used, the client flexes the hips and knees to lower the bar in a slow, controlled manner, while keeping the back flat.
- No rounding of any spinal segment should occur, as injury may result.

Spotting

- Like the traditional deadlift, spotting is not common; it is cued both physically and verbally.
- Using appropriate loads represents the most effective means of attaining proper technique.

Training Considerations

- The modified deadlift is easier for new exercisers, as the vertical torso position is easier to maintain, and the wider base requires less trunk stability providing greater access to the glutes and adductors.
- Common mistakes are somewhat similar to the traditional deadlift but are less significant.
- Never allow rounding of the back and ensure synchronized knee, hip, and back extension.

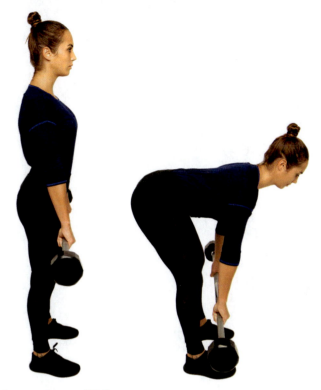

Exercise: Romanian Deadlift

Joint Action: Hip extension, back extension

Muscles Involved: Gluteus maximus, biceps femoris, semimembranosus, semitendinosus, erector spinae

Modifications: Dumbbells, kettlebell, cable, MB using one or two arms, or one or two legs

Starting Position

- Stand upright with the feet placed under the hips, toes pointed forward.
- Grasp the resistance using a closed, pronated, or alternating grip at shoulder width with the arms and knees extended.

Movement Phase

- Initiate the movement by flexing the hips, allowing the knees to flex slightly as the hips and thighs migrate posteriorly.
- The back remains flat throughout the lift, with a neutral pelvis:
  - An anterior pelvic tilt places extra stress on the lumbar spine and presents as an arched back.
  - A posterior pelvic tilt will appear if the spine flexes or "rounds."
- The bar descends in a straight downward path directly toward the end of the shoelaces. This occurs in a slow, controlled manner predominantly through flexion of the hips via the hamstrings. The knees should remain in their initial, slightly flexed position.
- The back remains flat as the resistance is lowered until the greatest functional ROM (or shoulder-hip alignment) is reached. Hamstring flexibility will ultimately define functional range.
- At the terminal position, reverse the lift by elevating the torso and concentrically contracting the hip extensors (hamstrings and glutes).
- The knees remain slightly flexed while returning to the start.

Spotting

- Spotting via verbal cuing rather than manual assistance.
- Key points include maintaining a flat back, keeping the knees slightly flexed (never locked), and executing the lift via action of the glutes and hamstrings, not the back extensors.

Training Considerations

- Many mistake this lift for a lower back exercise because the torso leans forward as the legs move backwards.
- An excellent teaching cue is to advise the lifter to push the bar straight down and not lean forward; this requires "driving" the hips backward as far as possible.
- Common errors include a rounded back, locked knees, protracted scapula, and excessive knee flexion.
- To achieve a greater ROM, the back must not round or arch and the knees are not bent.
- Once initially flexed, the hips do not drop at any point during the descent.

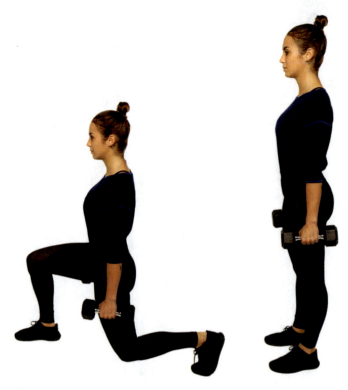

Exercise: **Dumbbell Lunge**

Joint Action: Hip extension, knee extension

Muscles Involved: Gluteus maximus, rectus femoris, vastus lateralis, vastus intermedius, vastus medialis, sartorius, biceps femoris, semimembranosus, semitendinosus

Modifications: Barbell, MB held at different locations while static or walking

Starting Position

- Stand upright with arms extended along the midaxillary line.
- Hold the dumbbells using a neutral grip.

Movement Phase

- Take a large step forward and flex (drop) the back knee to attain a 90°/90° split stance.
  - Direct the force of the forward step through the forward heel.
  - The tibia of the front leg dorsiflexes over the foot but should not cross the knee as the rear knee simultaneously descends toward to the floor.
  - At no time should the front knee cross the plane of the toes (anterior tibial translation), nor should the back knee touch the floor.
  - The top of the forward thigh should now be parallel to the floor.
- Maintaining balance and an upright torso position, extend the knee of the front leg into extension of the hip.
- The majority of the resistance is overcome by the front leg's extension as the back hip helps stabilize the action; maintain balance and an upright posture as the ascent is made to the start position.

Spotting

- Spotting is managed using physical and verbal cues.
- To avoid excessive anterior knee movement, use verbal cues to ensure that knee flexion of the back leg occurs simultaneously as the lifter descends toward the floor.

Training Considerations

- Can be performed a number of ways: stationary, walking, reverse, diagonal.
- Lunge complexity is dictated by movement ability, particularly balance and coordination.
- The forward lunge is knee-extensor dominant, the reverse lunge is glute dominant, and the walking lunge is a combination of decelerated, eccentric knee-extensor work with concentric hip extension.
- Early flexion of the back knee controls the movement lowering the hips to limit the risk for tibial translation.
- The most common error in this exercise is excessively moving the front knee in the sagittal plane (excess dorsiflexion).

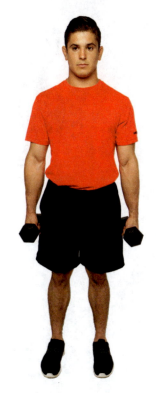
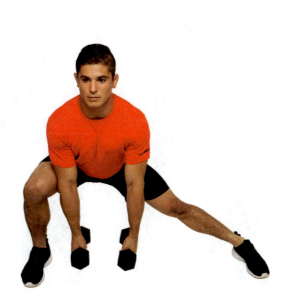

Exercise: **Lateral Lunge**

Joint Action: Hip extension, hip abduction, hip adduction, knee extension

Muscles Involved: Gluteus maximus, glute medius, tensor fascia latae, hip adductors

Modifications: Dumbbell, barbell, MB

Starting Position

- Stand upright with the feet positioned under the hips.
- The arm position depends on the resistance used, but generally will fall within the base of support.

Movement Phase

- Simultaneously and unilaterally abduct and then flex the hip and knee while maintaining an upright torso position. The hip will move laterally and posteriorly.
- The flexed knee moves in the frontal and sagittal planes to a position above the heel of the step foot, and the flexed knee is directed towards the pinky toe.
- The knee of the stance leg remains extended as the body descends to a point of attainable ROM: ideally the point at which the femur of the flexed leg parallels to the floor.
- Once full functional ROM is attained, ascend through the same line of motion by extending and adducting the hip.
- The back should remain flat at all times.

Spotting

- Cuing is most commonly employed.
- Perform the movement in a static, wide stance, to practice before adjusting to make the lift more dynamic.
- Cuing adequate and posteriorly directed hip flexion will prevent excessive frontal plane translation.

Training Considerations

- The The lateral lunge encourages closed-chain movement in the frontal plane.
- It encourages muscle activation of the hip abductors while stretching the long adductors.
- Lateral hip translation must be controlled to reduce the risk of knee injury.
- The most common mechanical error is excess movement of the flexed knee in the frontal plane, caused by not having a wide enough stance and/or inadequate hip flexion.
- To increase the intensity, use an external load and/or add an upper body activity.

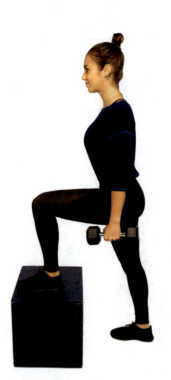
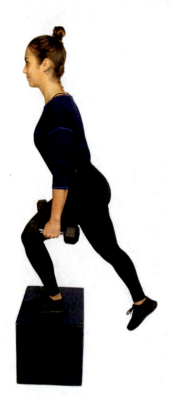
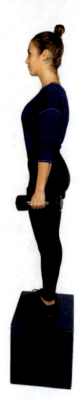

Exercise: **Dumbbell Step-ups**

Joint Action: Knee extension, hip extension

Muscles Involved: Gluteus maximus, rectus femoris, vastus lateralis, vastus intermedius, vastus medialis, sartorius, biceps femoris, semimembranosus, semitendinosus

Modifications: Barbell, sand bags, MB

Starting Position

- Stand in front of the step, box, or bench, placing one foot on top of the platform with the heel fully supported by the step.
- The front knee is flexed at about 90° and directly over the heel while the back leg starts at the length of the femur.
- The arms are extended under the shoulders, holding the dumbbells in a neutral grip.

Movement Phase

- Initiate the upward movement by shifting the center of gravity forward, bringing the chest over top of the flexed leg's thigh.
- Extend the hip and leg on the step by applying force through the heel.
- The back remains flat and the torso upright as the hip is extended and the body is elevated to a standing position on the box with all joint segments aligned: shoulders, hips, and knees.
- Once the end-point ROM and balance are established, flex the knee and the hip, and slowly return one foot to the floor. The feet can be alternated if desired.
- The descent is eccentrically controlled and should follow the same path of motion as the ascent.

Spotting

- Spotting is accomplished via verbal and tactile cuing to ensure the client drives upward through the heel and positions the body so that the full foot remains on the box.

Training Considerations

- Force is directed through the heel of the foot on the platform, which helps to avoid excessive dorsiflexion and anterior tibial translation (seen when the heel of the foot on the box is elevated).
- The knees must not break the plane of the toes during the upward movement; broaden the step backwards and ensure the front heel is fully on the step to correct translation.
- Do not generate force with the back leg, which diminishes the role of the quadriceps and glutes of the leg on the platform.
- Lower steps employ more hamstrings.
- Can be performed with a variety of loads – barbells, dumbbells, MB, or sand bags – and combined with any number of upper body movements.

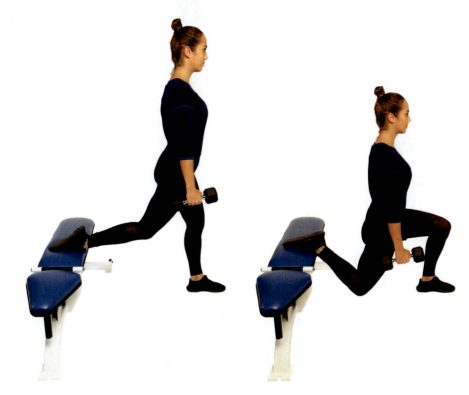

Exercise:	**Single-leg (Bulgarian) Squat**
Joint Action:	Hip extension, knee extension
Muscles Involved:	Gluteus maximus, rectus femoris, vastus lateralis, vastus intermedius, vastus medialis, sartorius, biceps femoris, semimembranosus, semitendinosus
Modifications:	Dumbbell, barbell, MB, sandbag, kettlebell

Starting Position

- Begin by placing one foot on a bench located behind the body. The knee of the front leg is extended, with the foot positioned just anterior to the hip.
- The arms are extended at the sides of the body in line with the hips when dumbbells are used. Arm position may vary depending on the type of resistance used and balance requirements.
- Pelvic and spinal positions are neutral, with the head facing forward.

Movement Phase

- Flex the knee of the back leg while simultaneously flexing the hip and knee of the front leg to descend toward the floor without any extraneous hip or trunk movements.
- Approximately 70% of the lifter's bodyweight is directed through the heel of the forward foot.
- The front knee is flexed and located directly above the heel; the back knee continues to flex towards the ground, until the thigh of the front leg is at least parallel to the floor.
- At no time should the trunk flex, the front knee cross the plane of the toes, or the heel of the front foot be allowed to elevate causing tibial translation.
- Maintain balance and an upright torso, concentrically extend the hip and knee of the front leg to return to the start position.

Spotting

- Spotting is managed using physical and verbal cues.
- In most cases, balance and lateral stability represent the greatest challenges.

Training Considerations

- The single-leg squat is a difficult exercise, which challenges the body through increased stability requirements via mechanical disadvantages.
- It encourages increased neuromuscular coordination, balance, strength, and ROM.
- It requires adequate preparation and practice and should only be used with suitable clients.

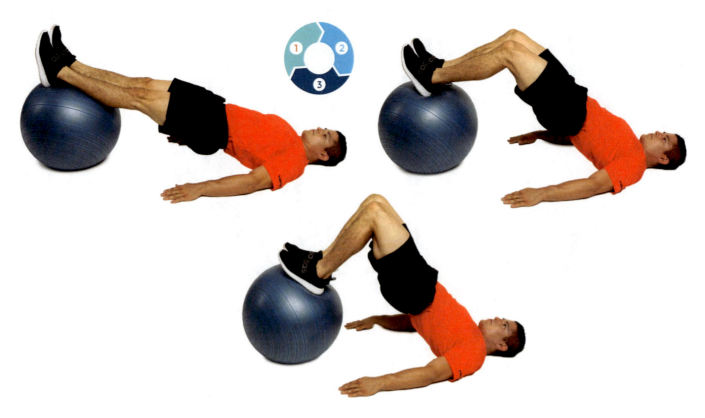

Exercise:	**Physioball Leg Curl**
Joint Action:	Knee flexion with isometric hip extension
Muscles Involved:	Biceps femoris, semimembranosus, semitendinosus, gastrocnemius
Modifications:	Single leg or double leg

Starting Position

- Assume a supine position on the ground with the calves on the ball and the arms extended at the sides of the body.
- A stable, supine bridge position is established by fully extending the hips, with the distal aspect of the lower legs on the ball.
- The ankles and femurs are held neutrally, and the legs are positioned straight and parallel to each other while maintaining a neutral pelvis.

Movement Phase

- Flex the knees and pull the heels towards the body while fully extending the hips in a controlled manner.
- The knees are flexed to the full attainable ROM while the hips remain extended, and a neutral pelvic position is maintained.
- Once full ROM is accomplished the body is eccentrically lowered back to the bridge position, where the hips remain extended off the ground and the knees are extended.

Spotting

- Spot by standing in front of the ball to provide stabilizing assistance at the ball's lateral aspect.

Training Considerations

- Can be performed with one or two legs to increase stability and force requirements.
- The most common error is not fully extending the hips while the knees are flexed; the hips remain extended at all times.
- The ankles and femurs remain neutral during the concentric phase; do not allow external rotation or abduction.

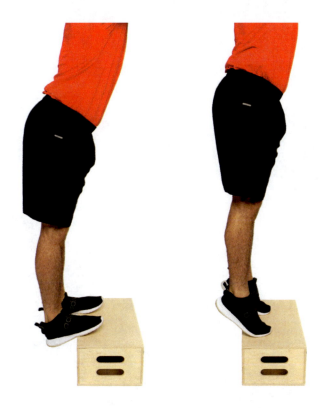

Exercise:	**Heel Raise**
Joint Action:	Plantarflexion
Muscles Involved:	Gastrocnemius, soleus, plantaris
Modifications:	Single or double leg, performed seated or standing

Starting Position

- Place the forefoot (ball of the foot) of one or both feet on an elevated surface near a stabilizing object.
- The height of the elevated surface and the foot position should allow the ankle(s) to be fully dorsiflexed.
- The toes point straight ahead with the knees straight, which are not locked or hyperextended (slight flexion is allowed).

Movement Phase

- Concentrically plantarflex the ankles, transferring the resistance through the balls of the feet to the point of full plantarflexion.
- Maintain a neutral spine and straight leg position throughout the ROM.
- Descend back to the starting position by dorsiflexing the ankles using a controlled speed; no bouncing should be permitted at any point of the movement.

Spotting

- Spotting is usually performed using verbal cues to ensure the client achieves a full ROM through both plantar and dorsiflexion.

Training Considerations

- In a knee-extended (standing) position, the gastrocnemius is emphasized over the soleus, as the soleus muscle does not cross the knee joint.
- When the knee is in a flexed position, as seen during the seated calf raise exercise, soleus activation is the goal, as it does not cross the knee.
- Do not use ballistic movements, and make sure excessive resistance does not limit ROM.

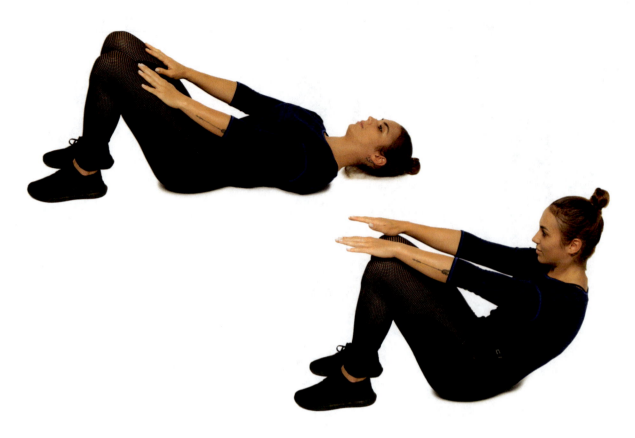

Exercise: **Abdominal Curl-up**

Joint Action: Trunk flexion

Muscles Involved: Rectus abdominis

Modifications: Place legs in air, change resistance arm length, add resistance to movement

Starting Position

- Lie in a supine position with the knees flexed and feet flat on the floor.
- The arms should be extended forward with both hands placed on the thighs.

Movement Phase

- Draw in the umbilicus and posteriorly tilt the pelvis, then flex the abdominals while sliding the hands up the thighs to the top of the knees.
- Once the palms have reached the knees, or 30° of spinal flexion is attained, descend in a controlled manner toward the starting position.
- The descent ends when the upper back and scapulae contact the ground as the abdominals contract continuously.

Spotting

- Spotting is performed using verbal cues to ensure the client reaches a full ROM in a controlled manner.

Training Considerations

- A common error is not initiating the movement using a posterior pelvic tilt, but rather emphasizing hip-flexor activation while trying to perform the exercise with an anterior pelvic tilt.
- Do not use momentum by increasing the rate of the movement and lifting the hips off the ground for mechanical advantage.
- Holding the feet, or hooking the feet under an object, increases hip flexor contribution, effectively decreasing abdominal activation during this movement.

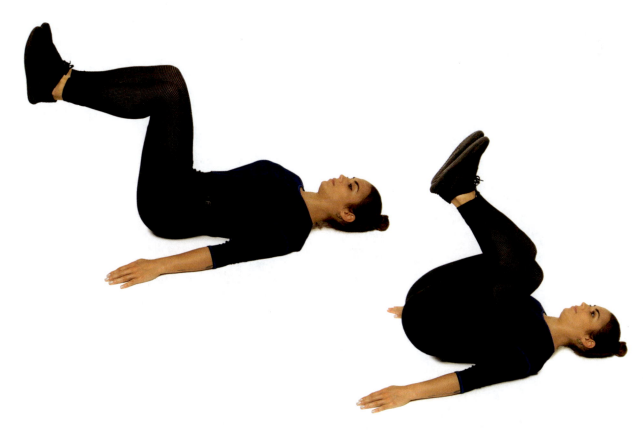

Exercise: ## Reverse Abdominal Curl-up

Joint Action: Trunk flexion

Muscles Involved: Rectus abdominis

Modifications: Perform on an incline or from hanging position

Starting Position

- Lie in a supine position with the knees and hips flexed.
- The arms are extended at the sides of the body with the palms facing down.

Movement Phase

- Draw in the umbilicus and posteriorly tilt the pelvis. Flex the abdominals while pulling the glutes off the ground until full spinal flexion is attained.
- The flexed-knee position remains unchanged throughout the movement. Once full ROM is attained, the client descends in a controlled manner.
- The descent phase ends once the upper gluteals contact the ground.

Spotting

- Spotting is performed using verbal cues to ensure the client reaches a full ROM in a controlled manner.

Training Considerations

- The most common error is using momentum from hip flexion and leg extension.
- To ensure proper activation, the hip flexion angle should not change.
- The exercise can be made more difficult by performing the movement with the knees extended or on an incline.
- The exercise can be done from a decline bench or hang position to increase resistive stress.

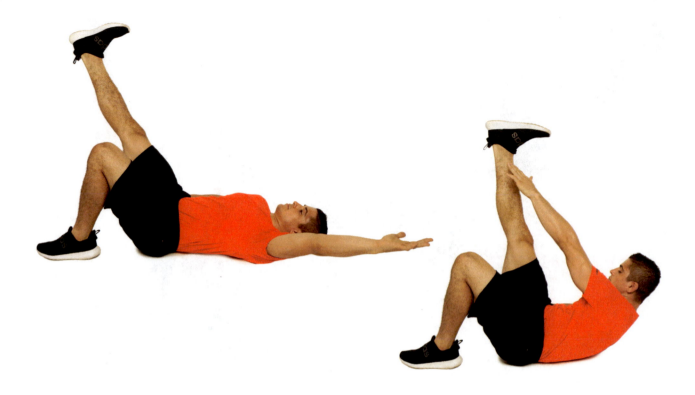

Exercise:	**Alternating Ankle Touches**

Joint Action: Trunk flexion and rotation

Muscles Involved: Rectus abdominis, lateral obliques

Modifications: Add cable or band resistance, on Bosu

Starting Position

- Lie supine with the hips flexed. One knee is flexed with the foot flat on the floor while the other leg extends upward.
- The contralateral arm is extended/abducted in a position lateral and superior to the top of the shoulder.

Movement Phase

- Draw in the umbilicus and posteriorly tilt the pelvis, then flex the abdominals and rotate the thoracic spine by reaching the extended arm upward and across the body toward the toes of the extended leg.
- Once full attainable ROM is reached, descend in a controlled manner toward the starting position.
- The descent lasts until the upper back contacts the ground; the abdominals remain contracted throughout the movement.
- To add rotation, reach to a lateral point further outside the foot of the extended leg.

Spotting

- Spot using verbal cues to ensure the client reaches a full ROM in a controlled manner.

Training Considerations

- Do not initiate the movement using an arm swing to generate momentum. Abdominal exercises are controlled to prevent undesirable actions and optimize activation.
- Providing a hand target can improve technique.

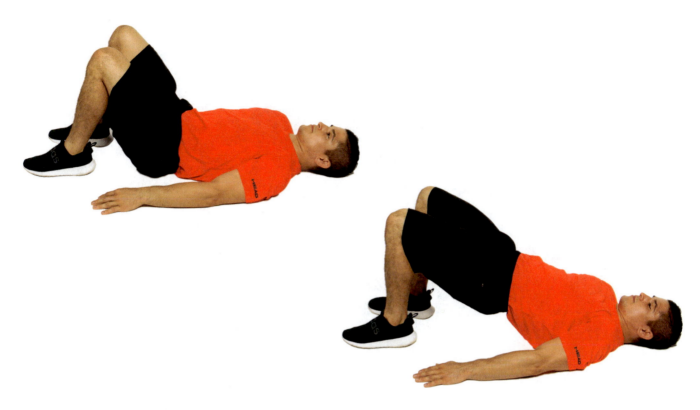

Exercise:	**Floor Bridging**
Joint Action:	Back extension, hip extension
Muscles Involved:	Back extensors (spinalis group), hip extensors (proximal hamstring and glutes maximus)
Modifications:	Ground, physioball, Bosu, or bench performed unilaterally or bilaterally

Starting Position

- Lie supine with the knees flexed and feet flat on the floor.
- The arms are extended forward with both hands (pronated) on the ground.

Movement Phase

- Initiate the movement by contracting the pelvic floor and ensuring a neutral pelvis.
- Press through the heels to extend the hip while contracting the glutes, hamstrings, and low back.
- Once a fully extended (straight) hip and neutral trunk position is attained, descend in a controlled manner back to the start position, right before making ground contact with the glutes.
- The descent lasts until the glutes are in close proximity to the ground. The inner unit of the trunk should remain contracted throughout the movement.

Spotting

- Spot using verbal cues to ensure the client reaches a full ROM in a controlled manner.

Training Considerations

- Placement of the feet changes the emphasis of the movement; more knee flexion increases glute activity, while less knee flexion promotes greater hamstring activation.
- The exercise can be made more difficult by using one leg or performing the movement on a physioball or other stability device.
- Common errors include anterior pelvic tilting, hyperextension of the low back, and directing the force through the forefoot rather than the heel.

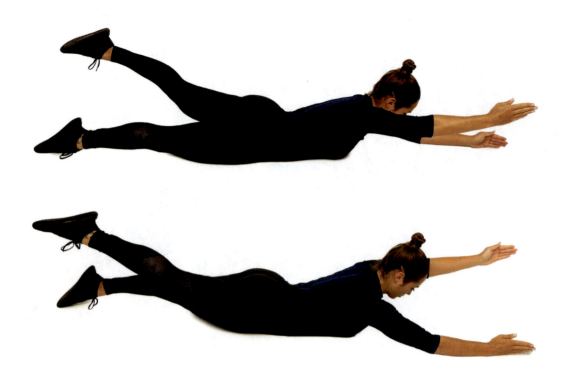

Exercise:	**Opposite Raise**
Joint Action:	Hip extension, spinal extension, shoulder flexion
Muscles Involved:	Gluteus maximus, back extensors, deltoids, mid-trapezius
Modifications:	Floor, kneeling, plank, physioball

Starting Position

- Lie prone with the arms extended forward in shoulder flexion.
- The legs lie parallel to each other in an extended position, with the feet hip-width apart.
- The head should be held neutrally.

Movement Phase

- Lift the leg of one side off the ground via extension of the hip, while simultaneously flexing the shoulder of the contralateral arm and extending the thoracic spine.
- Move the limbs through a full, pain-free ROM.
- Once full ROM is attained, return to the starting position, and perform the same action using the contralateral limbs.

Spotting

- Spot using verbal cues to ensure the client reaches a full ROM in a controlled manner.

Training Considerations

- The opposite raise should be performed in a slow, controlled fashion with smooth transitions between contralateral movements.
- Can be made more challenging by performing it from a kneeling (quadruped) or plank position.

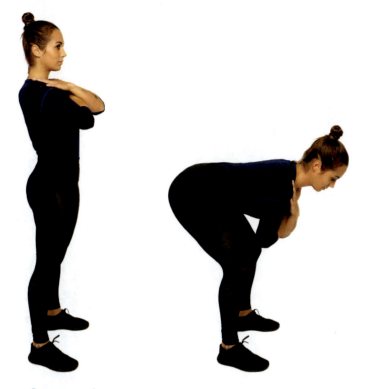

Exercise:	**Goodmorning**
Joint Action:	Back extension, hip extension
Muscles Involved:	Gluteus maximus, biceps femoris, semimembranosus, semitendinosus, erector spinae
Modifications:	Barbell, dumbbell, MB, physioball, plate

Starting Position

- Stand upright with the feet shoulder-width apart.
- The arms are crossed over the chest if no additional resistance is being used.
- The spine and pelvis are in neutral positions.

Movement Phase

- Eccentrically extend the hip, and slightly flex the knees while pushing the hips backward and upwards as far as possible and maintaining a flat back.
- Once the back is parallel to the floor, or full functional ROM is reached, concentrically extend the hips to return to the start position.
- A flat back must be maintained at all times as the movement is performed at a controlled pace.
- The knees remain fixed in the initial slightly flexed position, until they are extended at the end of the movement.

Spotting

- Spot using verbal cues to ensure a full ROM in a controlled manner and that the back remains flat.

Training Considerations

- A common error stemming from hamstring tightness is rounding the back and/or excessively flexing the knees and "squatting" towards the floor.
- Like all low-back exercises, it is performed in a controlled manner through a full ROM to maximize recruitment and safety.
- To make the exercise more difficult, the arms can be extended and the shoulders flexed to lengthen the resistance arm.

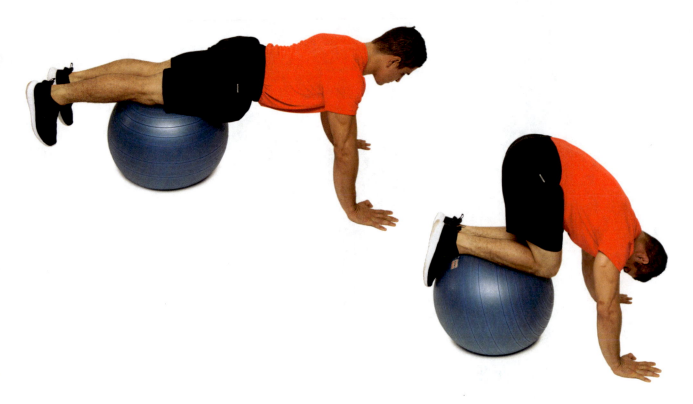

Exercise:	**Physioball Roll-up**
Joint Action:	Trunk flexion
Muscles Involved:	Rectus abdominis
Modifications:	Performed using towels or slide disks, transitioning to a pike

Starting Position

- Assume a prone position with the knees on the ball.
- Walk the arms out into a push-up position until the thighs are held parallel to the floor on the ball.
- The torso and hips remain neutral with the shoulders flexed and elbows extended.

Movement Phase

- Flex the trunk, hips, and knees simultaneously; the back will round and be directed upwards as the pelvis rolls into a posterior tilt and the knees flex under the body.
- The physioball will roll forward toward the arms as the knees fully flex.
- The shoulders and arms remain in the same position throughout the movement.
- Once full ROM is attained, the client extends the trunk, hips, and knees to roll the ball back to the starting position; the back is still flat and the pelvis neutral.

Spotting

- Spot using verbal cues to ensure the client reaches a full ROM in a controlled manner and that the back remains flat.
- Ball management may be needed if it drifts laterally.

Training Considerations

- Adequate upper body strength is needed for this exercise, as the client will have to hold and stabilize the body position at all times; shoulder weakness or instability can lead to injury.
- Common errors are improper start position (knees too far forward to the ball) and reliance on hip flexion more than trunk flexion, which decreases abdominal contribution.

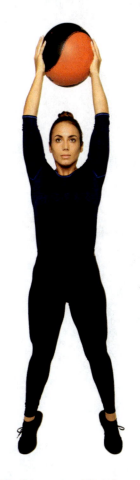
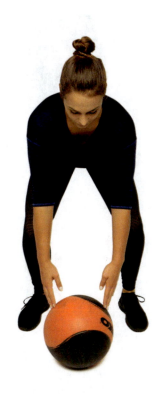

Exercise: ## Medicine Ball Chops (slams)

Joint Action: Trunk and hip flexion

Muscles Involved: Rectus abdominis, hip flexors

Modifications: Change direction, partner passes

Starting Position

- Stand upright with the feet shoulder-width apart.
- Grasp the MB using a neutral grip, and place it overhead by flexing the shoulders. Keep the elbows slightly flexed.

Movement Phase

- Flex the trunk and hips while extending the shoulders.
- The arms remain in the slightly flexed position as the ball accelerates toward the floor.
- Once the ball is either released to the ground or decelerated to a terminal ROM, return to the start position in the same plane as the descent by extending the body.

Spotting

- Spot using verbal cues to ensure the client reaches full ROM with trunk and hip flexion/extension.

Training Considerations

- The MB chop can be performed at different angles and used for bounce-pass activities for increased horizontal work.
- When bouncing is used, be sure the ball is not overly reactive: it may bounce back too quickly and hit the client's face.

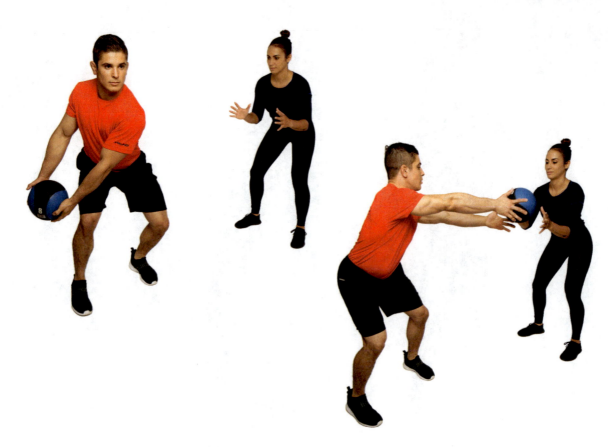

Exercise: Medicine Ball Rotation Pass

Joint Action: Trunk rotation

Muscles Involved: Obliques and hip extensors

Modifications: Change angles, stand on one or two legs

Starting Position

- Stand upright with the feet shoulder-width apart, holding the MB with a neutral grip, arms extended.
- Rotate the trunk posteriorly through to terminal position according to mobility with moderate hip flexion.

Movement Phase

- Rotate the trunk and extend the hips while keeping the arms extended as the ball moves through the transverse plane across the body.
- Once the trunk is fully rotated, the ball is released to a partner who catches and rapidly returns it (a wall can also be used).
- Upon receiving the ball, rotate the opposite side and repeat the action in the same plane as the initial throw.

Spotting

- Verbally cue to ensure the client reaches full ROM with trunk rotation and properly decelerates the ball in a controlled manner.

Training Considerations

- Clients often compensate during the lateral movement by using excess horizontal shoulder action, foot movement, and/or hip rotation.
- The ball is thrown and received in a controlled manner; if the ball is too heavy, it may force a ROM beyond the client's control and lead to injury.
- Be aware of undesirable knee rotation, which can be observed in those who do not direct the energy through the hips and trunk.
- This exercise differs from the cable rotation as the accelerating force is forward, not backward.

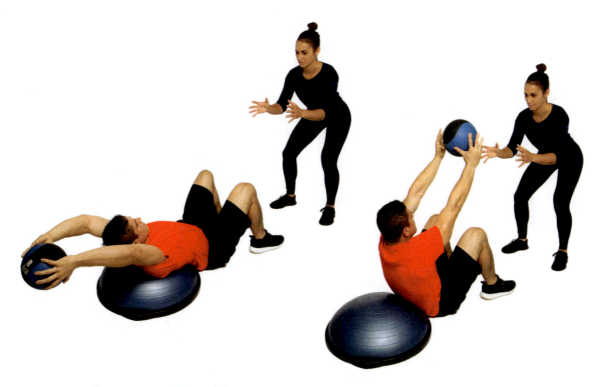

Exercise: **Medicine Ball Pullover**

Joint Action: Trunk flexion, shoulder extension

Muscles Involved: Rectus abdominis, latissimus dorsi

Modifications: Perform to standing position

Starting Position

- Lie in a supine position on a Bosu or similar object with the arms overhead in full shoulder flexion.
- The MB is held with a neutral grip; the hips and knees are flexed with the feet flat on the floor.

Movement Phase

- Flex the trunk and simultaneously extend the shoulders; the arms remain extended as the ball moves through the sagittal plane over the body.
- The movement is dominated by shoulder extension and trunk flexion, although hip flexion will contribute.
- Once the trunk is fully flexed, reach the ball to the ground or throw to a partner, who quickly returns it.
- Return to the start position in the same plane as the forward movement, but decelerate the ball in a controlled manner, maintaining abdominal contraction to avoid hyperextension.

Spotting

- Use verbal cues to ensure the client reaches full ROM with trunk flexion and properly decelerates the ball in a controlled manner to the start position.

Training Considerations

- Ballistic activities increase eccentric stress; be cautious and practice the throwing motion if this mode is used.
- If the ball is too heavy or thrown too hard, it may force excessive ROM and lead to injury.
- Focus on abdominal contraction, so the hips do not assume a primary role.

REFERENCES:

1. Aagaard P, Andersen JL, Bennekou M, Larsson B, Olesen JL, Crameri R, Magnusson SP, and Kjaer M. Effects of resistance training on endurance capacity and muscle fiber composition in young top-level cyclists. *Scand J Med Sci Sports* 21: e298-307, 2011.

2. Adirim TA and Cheng TL. Overview of injuries in the young athlete. *Sports Medicine* 33: 75-81, 2003.

3. Beck BR and Snow CM. Bone health across the lifespan – exercising our options. *Exerc Sport Sci Rev* 31: 117-122, 2003.

4. Bergquist AJ, Babbar V, Ali S, Popovic MR, and Masani K. Fatigue reduction during aggregated and distributed sequential stimulation. *Muscle Nerve*, 2016.

5. Bewick GS and Banks RW. Mechanotransduction in the muscle spindle. *Pflugers Arch* 467: 175-190, 2015.

6. Booth FW, Laye MJ, and Spangenburg EE. Gold standards for scientists who are conducting animal-based exercise studies. *J Appl Physiol (1985)* 108: 219-221, 2010.

7. Cosman F, de Beur SJ, LeBoff MS, Lewiecki EM, Tanner B, Randall S, Lindsay R, and National Osteoporosis F. Clinician's Guide to Prevention and Treatment of Osteoporosis. *Osteoporos Int* 25: 2359-2381, 2014.

8. Dahmane R, Djordjevic S, Simunic B, and Valencic V. Spatial fiber type distribution in normal human muscle Histochemical and tensiomyographical evaluation. *J Biomech* 38: 2451-2459, 2005.

9. Escamilla RF, Fleisig GS, Zheng N, Lander JE, Barrentine SW, Andrews JR, Bergemann BW, and Moorman CT, 3rd. Effects of technique variations on knee biomechanics during the squat and leg press. *Med Sci Sports Exerc* 33: 1552-1566, 2001.

10. Faigenbaum AD and Myer GD. Pediatric resistance training: benefits, concerns, and program design considerations. *Curr Sports Med Rep* 9: 161-168, 2010.

11. Fardon DF, Williams AL, Dohring EJ, Murtagh FR, Gabriel Rothman SL, and Sze GK. Lumbar disc nomenclature: version 2.0: Recommendations of the combined task forces of the North American Spine Society, the American Society of Spine Radiology and the American Society of Neuroradiology. *Spine J* 14: 2525-2545, 2014.

12. Gallina A, Blouin JS, Ivanova TD, and Garland SJ. Regionalization of the stretch reflex in the human vastus medialis. *J Physiol*, 2017.

13. Gehlert S, Weber S, Weidmann B, Gutsche K, Platen P, Graf C, Kappes-Horn K, and Bloch W. Cycling exercise-induced myofiber transitions in skeletal muscle depend on basal fiber type distribution. *Eur J Appl Physiol* 112: 2393-2402, 2012.

14. Gelber AC, Hochberg MC, Mead LA, Wang NY, Wigley FM, and Klag MJ. Joint injury in young adults and risk for subsequent knee and hip osteoarthritis. *Ann Intern Med* 133: 321-328, 2000.

15. Gonzalez-Freire M, de Cabo R, Studenski SA, and Ferrucci L. The neuromuscular junction: aging at the crossroad between nerves and muscle. *Frontiers in aging neuroscience* 6, 2014.

16. Hwang IS and Cho CY. Muscle control associated with isometric contraction in different joint positions. *Electromyogr Clin Neurophysiol* 44: 463-471, 2004.

17. Khosla S and Riggs BL. Pathophysiology of age-related bone loss and osteoporosis. *Endocrinol Metab Clin North Am* 34: 1015-1030, xi, 2005.

18. Kindig M, Li Z, Kent R, and Subit D. Effect of intercostal muscle and costovertebral joint material properties on human ribcage stiffness and kinematics. *Comput Methods Biomech Biomed Engin* 18: 556-570, 2015.

19. Kistemaker DA, Van Soest AJ, Wong JD, Kurtzer I, and Gribble PL. Control of position and movement is simplified by combined muscle spindle and Golgi tendon organ feedback. *J Neurophysiol* 109: 1126-1139, 2013.

20. Kumar B and Lenert P. Joint Hypermobility Syndrome: Recognizing a Commonly Overlooked Cause of Chronic Pain. *Am J Med* 130: 640-647, 2017.

21. Lian OB, Engebretsen L, and Bahr R. Prevalence of jumper's knee among elite athletes from different sports: a cross-sectional study. *Am J Sports Med* 33: 561-567, 2005.

22. Lloyd RS, Faigenbaum AD, Stone MH, Oliver JL, Jeffreys I, Moody JA, Brewer C, Pierce KC, McCambridge TM, Howard R, Herrington L, Hainline B, Micheli LJ, Jaques R, Kraemer WJ, McBride MG, Best TM, Chu DA, Alvar BA, and Myer GD. Position statement on youth resistance training: the 2014 International Consensus. *Br J Sports Med* 48: 498-505, 2014.

23. Maffiuletti NA, Aagaard P, Blazevich AJ, Folland J, Tillin N, and Duchateau J. Rate of force development: physiological and methodological considerations. *Eur J Appl Physiol* 116: 1091-1116, 2016.

24. Maffulli N and Bruns W. Injuries in young athletes. *Eur J Pediatr* 159: 59-63, 2000.

25. Malina RM. Weight training in youth-growth, maturation, and safety: an evidence-based review. *Clin J Sport Med* 16: 478-487, 2006.

26. Maneski LZ, Malesevic NM, Savic AM, Keller T, and Popovic DB. Surface-distributed low-frequency asynchronous stimulation delays fatigue of stimulated muscles. *Muscle Nerve* 48: 930-937, 2013.

27. McGlory C, Devries MC, and Phillips SM. Skeletal muscle and resistance exercise training; the role of protein synthesis in recovery and remodeling. *J Appl Physiol (1985)* 122: 541-548, 2017.

28. Micheli LJ. Sports injuries in children and adolescents. Questions and controversies. *Clin Sports Med* 14: 727-745, 1995.

29. Mullerova D, Langmajerova J, Sedlacek P, Dvorakova J, Hirschner T, Weber Z, Muller L, and Brazdova ZD. Dramatic decrease in muscular fitness in the Czech schoolchildren over the Last 20 years. *Cent Eur J Public Health* 23 Suppl: S9-S13, 2015.

30. Myer GD, Kushner AM, Brent JL, Schoenfeld BJ, Hugentobler J, Lloyd RS, Vermeil A, Chu DA, Harbin J, and McGill SM. The back squat: A proposed assessment of functional deficits and technical factors that limit performance. *Strength Cond J* 36: 4-27, 2014.

31. Nilwik R, Snijders T, Leenders M, Groen BB, van Kranenburg J, Verdijk LB, and van Loon LJ. The decline in skeletal muscle mass with aging is mainly attributed to a reduction in type II muscle fiber size. *Experimental gerontology* 48: 492-498, 2013.

32. Norman B, Esbjornsson M, Rundqvist H, Osterlund T, Glenmark B, and Jansson E. ACTN3 genotype and modulation of skeletal muscle response to exercise in human subjects. *J Appl Physiol (1985)* 116: 1197-1203, 2014.

33. Pacey V, Nicholson LL, Adams RD, Munn J, and Munns CF. Generalized joint hypermobility and risk of lower limb joint injury during sport: a systematic review with meta-analysis. *Am J Sports Med* 38: 1487-1497, 2010.

34. Park JH and Stelmach GE. Effect of combined variation of force amplitude and rate of force development on the modulation characteristics of muscle activation during rapid isometric aiming force production. *Exp Brain Res* 168: 337-347, 2006.

35. Pette D. The adaptive potential of skeletal muscle fibers. *Can J Appl Physiol* 27: 423-448, 2002.

36. Pfirrmann CW, Metzdorf A, Elfering A, Hodler J, and Boos N. Effect of aging and degeneration on disc volume and shape: A quantitative study in asymptomatic volunteers. *J Orthop Res* 24: 1086-1094, 2006.

37. Proske U. The role of muscle proprioceptors in human limb position sense: a hypothesis. *J Anat* 227: 178-183, 2015.

38. Saker E, Graham RA, Nicholas R, D'Antoni AV, Loukas M, Oskouian RJ, and Tubbs RS. Ligaments of the Costovertebral Joints including Biomechanics, Innervations, and Clinical Applications: A Comprehensive Review with Application to Approaches to the Thoracic Spine. *Cureus* 8: e874, 2016.

39. Sanchez GN, Sinha S, Liske H, Chen X, Nguyen V, Delp SL, and Schnitzer MJ. In Vivo Imaging of Human Sarcomere Twitch Dynamics in Individual Motor Units. *Neuron* 88: 1109-1120, 2015.

40. Schiaffino S and Reggiani C. Fiber types in mammalian skeletal muscles. *Physiol Rev* 91: 1447-1531, 2011.

41. Schoenfeld BJ. Squatting kinematics and kinetics and their application to exercise performance. *J Strength Cond Res* 24: 3497-3506, 2010.

42. Schroeder AN, Comstock RD, Collins CL, Everhart J, Flanigan D, and Best TM. Epidemiology of overuse injuries among high-school athletes in the United States. *J Pediatr* 166: 600-606, 2015.

43. Shoepe TC, Stelzer JE, Garner DP, and Widrick JJ. Functional adaptability of muscle fibers to long-term resistance exercise. *Med Sci Sports Exerc* 35: 944-951, 2003.

44. Simoneau JA and Bouchard C. Genetic determinism of fiber type proportion in human skeletal muscle. *FASEB J* 9: 1091-1095, 1995.

45. Suominen H. Muscle training for bone strength. *Aging Clin Exp Res* 18: 85-93, 2006.

46. Tegtbur U, Busse MW, and Kubis HP. [Exercise and cellular adaptation of muscle]. *Unfallchirurg* 112: 365-372, 2009.

47. Tosti R, Jennings J, and Sewards JM. Lateral epicondylitis of the elbow. *Am J Med* 126: 357 e351-356, 2013.

48. Weaver CM, Gordon CM, Janz KF, Kalkwarf HJ, Lappe JM, Lewis R, O'Karma M, Wallace TC, and Zemel BS. The National Osteoporosis Foundation's position statement on peak bone mass development and lifestyle factors: a systematic review and implementation recommendations. *Osteoporos Int* 27: 1281-1386, 2016.

49. Williamson DL, Gallagher PM, Carroll CC, Raue U, and Trappe SW. Reduction in hybrid single muscle fiber proportions with resistance training in humans. *J Appl Physiol* (1985) 91: 1955-1961, 2001.

50. Wilson JM, Loenneke JP, Jo E, Wilson GJ, Zourdos MC, and Kim JS. The effects of endurance, strength, and power training on muscle fiber type shifting. *J Strength Cond Res* 26: 1724-1729, 2012.

51. Wolf JM, Cameron KL, and Owens BD. Impact of joint laxity and hypermobility on the musculoskeletal system. *J Am Acad Orthop Surg* 19: 463-471, 2011.

Advanced Concepts of Personal Training

NCSF Certified Personal Trainer

Chapter 3

Kinetic Chain Function, Dysfunction and Corrective Exercise

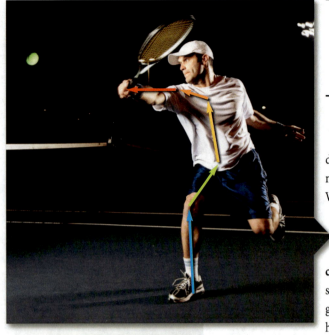

Local and Global Systems

Muscles and joints interact constantly to move and stabilize the body during physical activity. While some segments are recruited for rapid movement, others are employed simultaneously to inhibit undesirable body actions. When these recruitments patterns harmonize via the central nervous systems (CNS), energy transfers fluidly across stable joint segments, and the body effectively manages high levels of force. This occurs through the coordinated actions of three systems, independently referred to as passive (**form closure**), active (**force closure**), and control (neural) systems. Consider this scenario: when a person swings a tennis racquet, the energy derives from ground reaction forces that must transfer from the feet through the legs to the hips; this energy then accelerates through the trunk and transfers across the shoulder to the arm, ultimately manifesting in the hands at the racquet. Any loss in energy along the **kinetic chain** reduces the quantity of kinetic force the player can apply to the ball.

◆ Major Factors Influencing the Transfer of Force

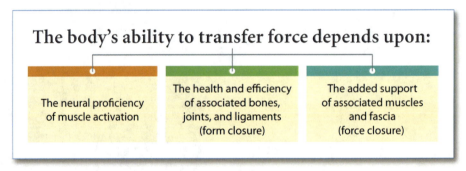

DEFINITIONS

Form closure –

The efficiency of the structural aspects of articulating segments; primarily consists of skeletal and connective tissues.

Force closure –

The support of soft tissues which help maintain positional integrity of a joint.

Kinetic chain –

The chain of force transfer across motion segments of the body.

Local muscle systems –

Musculature essential for localized joint stability and neutral joint positioning.

Global muscle systems –

Larger muscles responsible for motion and regional stability that tend to function in a phasic manner.

The interaction between structures of the musculoskeletal system dictates the proficiency of movement. Muscle contractions make up for deficiencies in structural form, adding to stabilization and energy transfer in a joint, such as the shoulder, or joint system, such as the spine. While the interplay of connective tissue is relevant, the muscular system possesses the greatest potential to promote or resist movement. A muscle's function at any given time may be to stabilize, neutralize, accelerate, or decelerate a body segment, depending on the action required. To ensure that all roles are appropriately accounted for within and between systems, the body maintains specific muscular arrangements at each joint and between joint segments. These arrangements provide each muscle or muscle group with specific responsibilities, which change from time to time depending on the action being performed. In terms of their role, muscles fall under two categories: **local systems** or **global systems** [5]. Local systems pertain to those essential to segmental stability; these smaller, internally-located muscles aid the ligaments in holding bony segments in place. Examples include the multifidus, supraspinatus, vastus medialis, soleus, and pelvic floor. Global system musculature fosters regional stability and motion and tends to function in a phasic manner, suggesting the activation is not constant but, rather, cooperative with other muscles. Some muscles, depending on the task, serve both groups. Global system muscles may aid in stability through phasic actions or function as global movers (mobilizers), depending on variables such as the type of action or direction of forces. Inexperienced personal trainers often oversimplify the function of a muscle to its prime mover role; however, these tissues account for a number of actions beyond simply accelerating linear movement in a single plane, as seen in a leg extension. Consider the role of the same muscles when receiving a pass during a flag football game or pulling on a rope in a tug-o-war. During primal actions, muscles work as part of a system, rather than independently.

Local stabilizing systems tend to be more role-specific [9]. They are continuously active throughout a movement, often across a single joint, functioning to reduce segment translation (or articular sliding). They do not control range of motion, but rather prepare a body segment for oncoming force through a mostly **isometric contraction**. Therefore, they function in an anticipatory manner, preceding movement, impact or a loading condition. This requirement is particularly important for the spine, underscoring the importance of the local stabilizing system of the trunk. Due to the anticipatory response and early activation, a significant neurophysiological difference exists in the timing of contractions between the local muscle system that stabilizes the spine (inner unit) and the global muscle system that acts upon it. The slow-twitch muscles that provide stability to the joint segments do so by firing earlier than the fast-twitch fibers of the global system. This allows the local system to anchor a motion segment before the global system pulls upon it [9]. In healthy individuals, the activity of the trunk musculature precedes that of the muscle(s) responsible for limb movement, thus contributing to what is referred to as the feed-forward postural response. Simply put, the trunk must first brace, creating stability at the joints of the spine to supersede any material force that will be placed upon them. This provides for adequate rigidity during the encounter with the global forces. On the other hand, when these muscles experience a delayed firing response, forces go unmanaged, ultimately leading to injury [21]. In normal function, local stabilizers perform rapid contractions to anticipate multi-directional limb and trunk movements, such as a running back changing direction. This also occurs under conditions of predictable loading in a system where the local stabilizers function normally, such as a back squat. In the spine, anticipatory actions prepare the vertebrae for unexpected perturbations, regardless of the direction of the movement [22-27]. The global system responds more slowly and is therefore directionally-dependent [3, 37]. Individuals with dysfunction demonstrate inefficiency at the local level, ultimately affecting the global level. These individuals present with an increased risk for injury and reduced performance relative to movement potential.

> **DEFINITIONS**
>
> **Isometric contraction –**
>
> *A type of muscle contraction providing for no change in a joint angle; a static muscle contraction.*

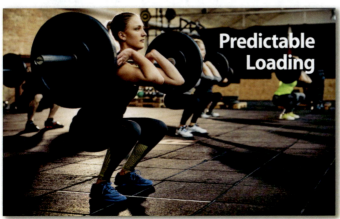

Predictable Loading

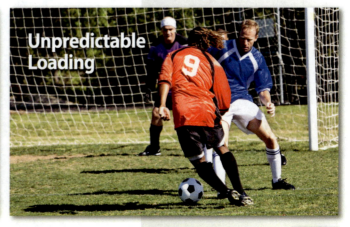

Unpredictable Loading

Kinetic Chain Function, Dysfunction and Corrective Exercise

Local and Global Stability Summary

Local Stabilizers

- **Role** - increase muscle stiffness to control segmental movement
- **Functions** - control neutral joint position; contraction does not produce change in muscle length or movement
- **Characteristics** - fulfill proprioceptive functions; activity is independent of the direction of movement; activation is continuous in nature but reactive to offset forces
- **Examples**
  Transverse Abdominis
  Pelvic Floor
  Diaphragm
  Deep Lumbar
  Multifidus
  Posterior Fibers of Internal Obliques
  Vastus Medialis
  Supraspinatus
  Soleus

Global Stabilizers

- **Role** - generate force to control range of movement
- **Functions** - control the inner and outer ranges of movement; tend to contract eccentrically for low-load deceleration of momentum and for rotational control
- **Characteristics** - activity is direction dependent; activation is non-continuous
- **Examples**
  Quadratus Lumborum
  Psoas Major
  External and Internal Obliques
  Rectus Abdominis
  Hip Adductors
  Trapezius
  Levator Scapula
  Serratus Anterior
  Rhomboids

Global Mobilizers

- **Role** - generate torque to produce movement
- **Functions** - produce joint movement, especially movements in the sagittal plane; tend to contract concentrically and absorb shock forces from impacts
- **Characteristics** - activity is direction dependent; activation is non-continuous
- **Examples**
  External Oblique
  Rectus Abdominis
  Erector Spinae
  Psoas Major
  Latissimus Dorsi
  Gluteus Maximus
  Hip Adductors
  Hamstrings
  Gastrocnemius

Examples of Phasic and Postural Muscles of the Spine

Local Stabilizers	Global Stabilizers	Global Mobilizers
Transverse Abdominis	Internal Obliques	Hamstrings
Deep Lumbar Multifidus	Spinalis	Rectus Abdominis
Supraspinatus	Gluteus Medius	Latissimus Dorsi

The Integrated Model of Function

Isolating muscles and muscle groups is useful to practice joint movements, to remedy strength imbalances, or to recover from an injury, but the body does not function in isolation. Rather, the body integrates mechanisms to manage forces for static positioning and movement. The integrated model of function describes the internal condition of cooperation and coordination between systems and structures of the body [32]. From a biological perspective, the concept of function suggests the body's ability to manage environments and conditions efficiently, without undue stress or restriction. Conversely, poor posture, faulty movement patterns, and incorrect biomechanics due to musculoskeletal deficiencies or imbalances all contribute to known dysfunction, ultimately reducing performance and increasing the risk of injury [55]. A primary role of the exercise professional is to reduce the risk for injury; therefore, promoting musculoskeletal function should be a foundational emphasis in all programs. The idea of proper movement mechanics begins at the skeleton but also includes aspects of both the musculoskeletal and neuromuscular systems. For the skeleton to function correctly, the joints must first properly align. This means all the attached structures must maintain relationships that promote an optimal position. Connective tissues that are too tight may move the joint out of position; likewise, if the muscles that serve to maintain the joint alignment are not in (strength) balance, the joint may migrate in the direction of the dominant pull. When the body moves, this becomes even more relevant due to increases in applied force and the need for proper activation patterns. If the muscles do not fire in synch or compensatory actions occur due to neuromuscular inefficiency, joints will suffer from undue stress and the action loses proficiency. In terms of training, this fact underscores that fundamental work toward movement efficiency must be a priority. This is accomplished by focusing on adequate ROM, muscle balance, passive and active elements of stabilization, and effective muscle activation and neuromuscular contraction patterns.

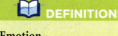

DEFINITIONS

Emotion –

A component of the integrated model of function which relates to the impact of psychological condition on movement efficiency.

The integrated model of function differentiates the role of each bodily system in terms of how they work together to accomplish a given physical outcome. This concept highlights the fact that the human body is really not composed of separate groups of parts but rather works as an integrated ensemble. The efficiency with which these parts work together ultimately determines the level of performance.

There exist three physical components to human function:

1) how well a joint aligns, called *form closure*
2) the ability of connective tissue to maintain joint integrity, called *force closure*
3) the proficiency of the neuromuscular system to anticipate and react through *motor control*

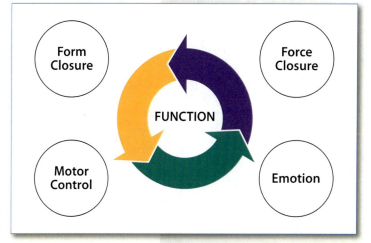

A fourth component stems from the psychological orientation involving **emotion**. One could compare the overall concept to a symphony orchestra: the separate sections overlap together to

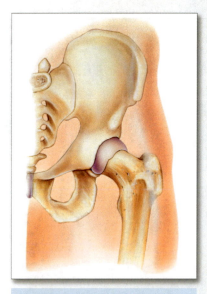

The hip joint's greater form closure provides for superior loading and stress application but limits ROM. On the contrary, the limited form closure of the shoulder joint reduces the joint's stability but provides for greater mobility.

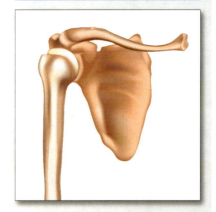

create a particular sound. In the case of physiological integration, functioning systems harmonize, providing specific characteristics to create an intended outcome, whether that is standing still, running, or lifting a weight.

Form Closure

The keystone for joint function is form closure, which describes the structural aspects of the body and the specific architecture of articulating segments. In a sense, form closure frames the human machine, including the bones, joints, and connective tissues that support and move the body. Whereas bones and connective tissue form all joints, the defining characteristics of individual joints stem from their structure, orientation, and shape [52, 53]. These factors ultimately determine the mobility and stability of each movement segment. All joints maintain a level of form closure via contact support between articulating surfaces. In some cases, the joint segments fit together like a puzzle providing a high degree of support, as in the hip. In other cases, the connecting surface area limits the joint's form closure by placing greater reliance on additional tissues to provide stability, as in the case of the glenohumeral joint of the shoulder.

Force Closure

Where form closure originates from the integrity of hard contact between articulating surfaces, force closure comes from soft tissue support (muscles and fascia) that helps maintain the contact position. Consider putting together a cardboard box. The cardboard provides the requisite form for the sides, top, and bottom, but it still requires tape to seal it together. Using one piece of tape may be enough to connect the parts and hold its form, but it will likely not be enough to hold the box together when contents are added. The image seen here of the inner unit, which will be covered in greater detail shortly, demonstrates this "box example" for force closure.

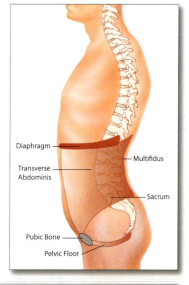

Joints work in a similar fashion. When a joint has weak support attachments, the integrity becomes compromised. Force closure originates from myofascial pull that provides further stabilization and support. Variable stress and loading conditions warrant different levels of stability at different times and at different angles. Force closure supports the deficiency of form closure by increasing compressive force across the joint surface to counter any offsetting forces. The quantity of force closure needed to

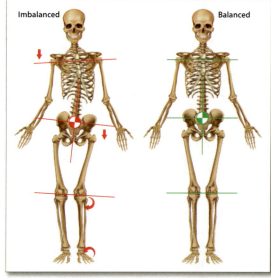

Kinetic Chain Function, Dysfunction and Corrective Exercise

adequately ensure support is a product of the individual's form closure and the overall magnitude of the load (e.g., a cardboard box with heavy contents requires more tape to support the disruptive force). The efficiency of associated ligaments, muscle, and fascia determines the resultant stability. Due to changes in the joint angle, the degree of force closure will vary. The joint most efficiently resists shear stress when the joint angle reaches a close-packed position, as it has maximized both congruence of the articulating surface and tension of associated ligaments [52, 53]. This explains why stability requirements across a movement or joint angle vary when the relative mass and base remain consistent. Weightlifters refer to this position during an exercise as the **sticking point**: the resistance is harder to move at certain joint angles due to inefficiency in the acting joints' stability and mechanical disadvantage.

Form and force closure also depend upon the integrity of associated tissues. When connective tissues are healthy, elastic, strong, and force-balanced there is limited disruption to an area, suggesting no undue resistive stress. When agonist and antagonist muscles lose their functional relationship, or tissues shorten, the internal environment experiences added stress, and these musculoskeletal changes will, over time, offset the skeletal position. When joints are misaligned, the support of form closure is reduced, placing increasing demands on soft tissues for force closure to maintain the same level of stability. In exaggerated conditions, these changes are referred to as **postural syndromes** or distortion patterns (e.g., forward chin, upper or lower cross syndromes). These dysfunctions, while surprisingly common among people, add significant resistance to movement and stability. Due to the compromise in movements and proper biomechanical technique, a new battery of exercises designed to correct these issues has become a staple of many competent performance-based programs. These concepts will be addressed in greater detail later in the text.

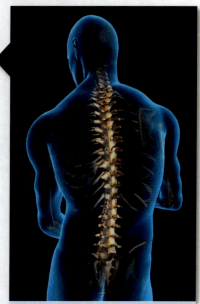

Muscular imbalances can lead to skeletal distortions and postural imbalances which add significant resistance to stability and movement.

DEFINITIONS

Sticking point –

The specific joint angle where the resistance becomes harder to overcome due to inefficiency in stability during a given lift; usually occurs at a transitional point between working joints.

Postural syndromes –

Static or dynamic malalignment of one or more skeletal segments.

Motor Control

The integrated model of function's third component is motor control. Specifically, it refers to neural activation of the motor units within muscle tissue. Most people think of muscles only as movers, but the role of muscle contractions extends well beyond the need to produce force for acceleration alone. Motor control implies the regulation of internal forces created to either cause or resist movement. This is supported by the different types of contractions and their timing.

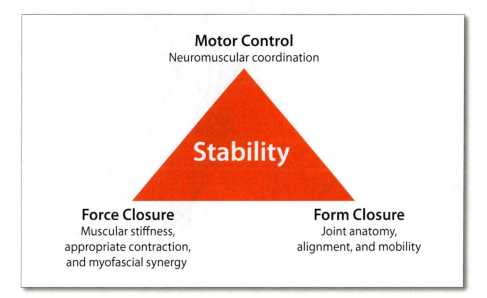

Concentric contractions accelerate movement, eccentric contractions decelerate movement, and isometric contractions stabilize or neutralize a joint position to manage energy efficiently. In most cases, they cooperate to accomplish a task. Importantly, the timing of activation and deactivation of motor units provides motor control not the magnitude of a force applied. When the timing of contractions counters offsetting forces, the body becomes more efficient at producing desired outcomes. Thus, familiarity and rehearsal is key in the process of improving function and motor patterning. Motor control develops through continued exposure to an environment or a condition. A body well-acquainted with a particular environment can more effectively control its actions when encountering this familiar scenario. This is often referred to as motor learning, as the nervous system learns intelligently by rehearsing movement or actions within a specific environment. This explains why practice improves performance. Laymen refer to this concept as "muscle memory," but, in fact, it is nervous system recall, as muscle tissue is useless without direction from the CNS.

Emotion

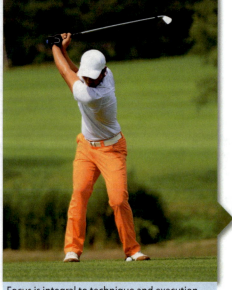

Focus is integral to technique and execution, and is psychomotor-dependent.

The fourth domain of the integrated system does not pertain directly to the body but factors in physical performance nonetheless. Focus is integral to technique and execution and is psychomotor-dependent, which clearly identifies the intimate role of the brain and muscle tissue in physical actions. New research indicates that repetitive practice that incorporates higher elements of visual focus and rehearsal improves brain interaction for finite adjustments in movement efficiency. The use of targeting, location stimuli, and other focal interactions with trained movements improve performance. These improvements have been demonstrated at the elite level, suggesting that although rehearsal leads to quality patterns, greater stimulus of the brain can further improve movement efficiency [16, 30, 31, 44, 49].

To suggest a person is functional means the following:

1 The musculoskeletal system maintains proper symmetry for appropriate form and force closure.

2 Activation is orderly and efficient with proper anticipatory signaling.

3 Local stability balance is attained through appropriate agonist and antagonist muscle relationships acting upon each joint.

4 Overall force development occurs without restriction through effective force couples, resulting in energy conservation during static and dynamic activities.

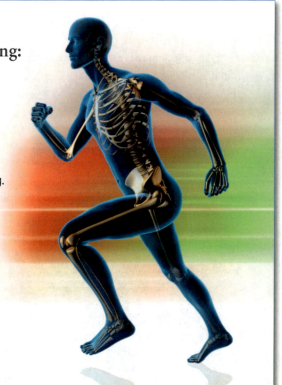

Muscular Units

The aforementioned characteristics suggest that the body's ability to operate proficiently relies upon several factors: the integrity, mechanics, function, and architecture of the joint (form closure); the coordinated tensile and compressive force produced by muscle tissues to manage the other forces acting on the joint (force closure); the appropriate neural activity needed to orchestrate the pattern of motor control. Thus, for the body to become more efficient, the objective should be to improve the control of desired movement as a whole rather than addressing the independent parts, since the coordination of the parts ultimately enhances movement proficiency and function.

Exercise professionals should attempt to recognize where the inefficiencies exist in the body's joint segments to improve force transfer across kinetic chains [6, 19, 28, 51]. Smooth energy transition to, from, and between the upper and lower limb segments of the body depends on the proficiency of the multiple segments of the spine and pelvis. This emphasizes the trunk's importance as a key point of central stability and its role in transferring force throughout the body [6, 7, 17, 33, 47, 56]. Related to this concept is bidirectional force transfer from central to peripheral and peripheral to central areas. For example, standing while performing dumbbells presses overhead requires central to peripheral transfer for stable force application, whereas hanging from a bar to perform leg raises requires peripheral to central stability to perform the exercise through full ROM while preventing undesirable swing.

The significance of the trunk's required stability is further demonstrated when increased limb velocities require the transfer of angular momentum [20]. Physics dictates that a motion segment must become stable to pass its angular momentum to another segment. If the trunk cannot attain an adequate level of stability, the force cannot be effectively transferred from the bottom to the top or from the top down. Throwing, running, kicking, and jumping, as with most dynamic movements, require force transfer from the limbs through the trunk or the trunk through the limbs [57]. Anytime energy transfers to a new segment, energy is lost; however, if the region through which energy passes possesses greater stability, more energy is maintained, allowing for more efficient movement (e.g., throwing harder, running faster, kicking farther, jumping higher).

Joint segment efficiency in the trunk cannot be overstated, especially as it relates to energy transfer and stability at the most centrally located lumbo-pelvic region or lumbo-pelvic-hip complex. When it comes to this area, the body has two primary stability systems that

Force can be lost at various segments of the kinetic chain:

- Cervical spine
- Thoraco-lumbar spine
- Sacroiliac joints
- Hip joints
- Knee joints
- Foot and ankle joints

Ground reaction force

> **DEFINITIONS**
>
> **Inner unit –**
>
> *Collective group of local spinal and pelvic stabilizers: includes the transverse abdominis, diaphragm, posterior internal oblique, pelvic floor, and multifidus.*

allow for energy transfer. The term "muscles of the **inner unit**" describes the tissues that stabilize the joints from deep within the body and act as local stabilizers of this segment; the muscles of the outer unit are global stabilizers and work reactively, along with the global movers, to stabilize and control body segments using the superficial prime mover musculature. The inner unit is comprised of the transverse abdominis (TVA), pelvic floor, multifidus, posterior internal oblique, and the diaphragm. These muscles work synergistically to create internal forces that support the spine and pelvis [17]. The outer unit is composed of groups of tissues that make up the four major independent movement systems of the body, sometimes referred to as myofascial slings or sling systems. These work via the continuity of fascial attachment to provide force closure. They include the posterior oblique, deep longitudinal, anterior oblique, and lateral sling systems.

◆ The Inner Unit

The inner unit manifests force through a feature referred to as hoop tension that is created by the TVA and the deep multifidus muscles; these muscles represent two of the primary local stabilizers of the lumbo-pelvic region [2, 10, 17]. The TVA has a large attachment to the middle layer and the deep lamina of the posterior layer of the thoracolumbar fascia and is recruited in an anticipatory manner prior to any upper or lower extremity movements [2, 57]. When the TVA contracts, tension increases in thoracolumbar fascia, and intra-abdominal pressure increases as the relatively non-compressible viscera pushes against the supportive structures of the diaphragm and pelvic floor. The increased tension of the thoracolumbar fascia initiates a hydraulic amplifier effect that is observed when the spinal musculature contracts, creating an anti-flexion effect; this effect combined with increased intra-abdominal pressure enhance stability of the lumbo-pelvic and upper spinal regions [7, 18]. This represents the "natural weight belt" concept. Similar to a belt, a rigid posterior position counterbalances the drawback forces of the muscles to support the spine from the front, while a sturdy pelvic floor helps hold the pelvis in a neutral position.

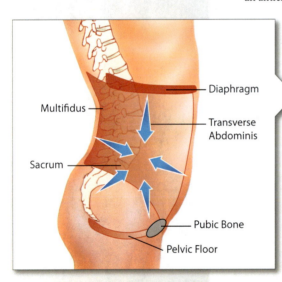

During upper body movements, TVA anticipatory contractions should occur at least 30 milliseconds prior to the movement; for a lower body movement, these should begin 110 milliseconds before initiation for sufficient stability [18]. TVA activation requirements seem to be consistent across varying environmental conditions, regardless of the movement pattern or the plane in which the movement is performed [39, 40]. According to studies, individuals with inner unit activation deficits have an increased risk for low back pain [40, 42]. This explains the popular attention to one's "core muscles." It is suggested that a significant motor control deficit exists in people experiencing chronic low back pain. This deficit is primarily associated with the control of the contraction of the transverse abdominis, which worsens when there is atrophy of the multifidus [50]. However, motor control training has been shown to improve system recruitment [14, 46].

◆ The Outer Unit

The ability of the outer unit, or global muscles systems, to work efficiently depends on stability created by the inner unit. Each sling system consists of connective tissues that stabilize or move body segments common to primal actions (i.e., walking, running, throwing, stepping, climbing).

Posterior Oblique Sling System

The posterior oblique system is comprised of the latissimus dorsi, gluteus maximus, and intervening thoracolumbar fascia, which may further extend to the hamstrings over broad ranges. These muscles integrate with the superficial layer of the trapezius, transverse abdominis, deep layer of the internal oblique, multifidus, and erector spinae muscles to form a structural "force bridge." This lumbar spine and pelvic girdle bridge, created by these active tissues, is fundamental to safe exercise performance because these muscles contribute significantly to the transference of load through the pelvic girdle [19].

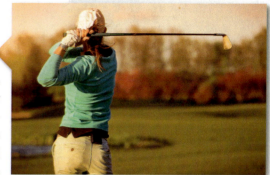

Issues with the Posterior Oblique Sling System can have an adverse effect on power, strength, speed, and ultimately performance.

Anterior Oblique Sling System

On the opposing side of the body, the anterior oblique system combines the abdominal obliques, the adductor muscles of the thigh, and the intervening abdominal fascia, which may extend into the pectoral muscles to create a cross-joint effect. This system contributes importantly to phasic actions, such as the initiation of movement and control of high load activities. In addition, it is integral to bipedal and throwing motions [1, 7]. The oblique muscles operate whenever actions of the trunk, upper, and lower extremities occur [1, 39].

The Anterior Oblique Sling System creates cross-stabilization, much like a cross beam of a bridge, to stabilize the pelvis for sagittal plane locomotion.

Deep Longitudinal Sling System

The deep longitudinal system includes the erector spinae group, deep lamina of the thoracolumbar fascia, multifidus, and sacrotuberous ligament (continuous to the biceps femoris muscle) and extends to the lower extremities. This system serves as an inner unit extension by contributing to tension in the thoracolumbar fascia and facilitating compression through form closure of the sacroiliac joint [41]. This support mechanism adds to dorsal and inferior lumbo-pelvic stabilization. The deep longitudinal system contributes to power and speed in acts such as sprinting, as it facilitates both horizontal and vertical ballistic capabilities.

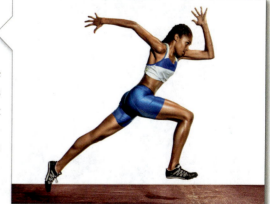

The Deep Longitudinal Sling System connects multiple joints segments allowing for efficient sprinting mechanics.

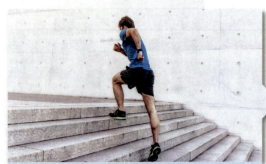

The Lateral Sling System functions to stabilize a loaded hip on an anchored base for actions such as climbing and stepping.

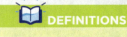

Functional-based activities –

Activities aimed at improving the body's ability to efficiently manage various aspects of daily living, including physical activity, without undue resistance.

Lateral Sling System

The final system of the outer unit is called the lateral system and includes the hip abductors (gluteus medius, gluteus minimus, and the tensor fascia latae) the quadratus lumborum, and the adductors of the thigh. These muscles provide frontal plane stability and aid vertical and horizontal bipedal and climbing motions. As with all systems of the outer unit, the phasic actions of this system depend upon internal stabilizing force. If the inner unit cannot manage the forces produced by the outer unit, not only will force be lost due to inefficiency of the congruent systems, injury is likely to occur due to compensatory movements which try to make up for the inner unit's inability to manage forces properly.

The relationship between the inner and outer unit provides excellent supporting evidence for the inclusion of **functional-based activities** for performance enhancement. The concept of harmonized movement suggests that stability is efficiently attained and the appropriate forces are transferred effectively through body segments for desired outcomes. Any exercise program targeting optimal stability and body function should emphasize training to improve inner unit stability, while utilizing resisted movements consistent with the natural functional systems of the outer unit. [2, 46, 57].

Sample Exercises For Each Sling System

Posterior Oblique Sling
Reverse lunge w/row

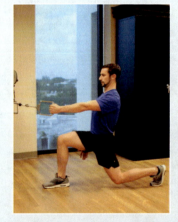
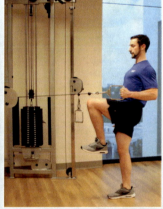

Anterior Oblique Sling

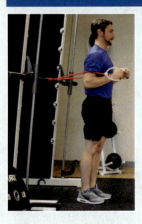
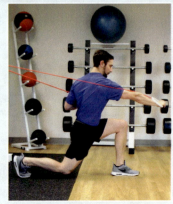
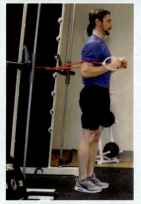
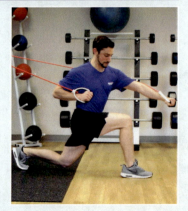

Forward lunge w/ contralateral forward cable press

Sample Exercises For Each Sling System

Lateral Sling
Ballistic Side Step-Overs

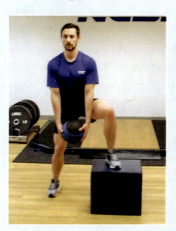
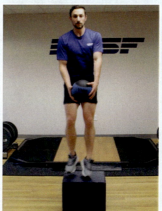
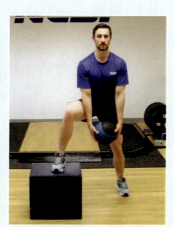

Deep Longitudinal Sling
Ballistic Extension

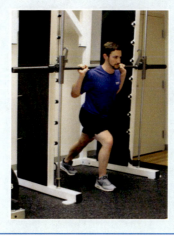
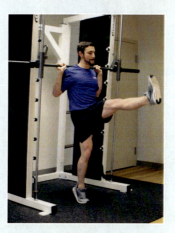

Common Postural Distortions and Muscular Imbalances

Clearly, the body maintains an established process for stability and force management, but the efficiency of the interactions actually determines performance potential. Individuals predisposed to or who develop postural or muscular imbalances often experience impaired joint function, which compromises the coordination between systems and increases the risk for injury.

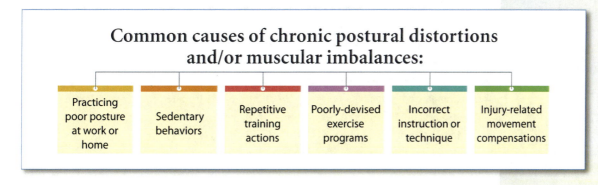

Common causes of chronic postural distortions and/or muscular imbalances:
- Practicing poor posture at work or home
- Sedentary behaviors
- Repetitive training actions
- Poorly-devised exercise programs
- Incorrect instruction or technique
- Injury-related movement compensations

DEFINITIONS

Winged scapulae –

A lifted and outwardly-rotated scapular position; the scapula appears to protrude posteriorly away from the ribcage.

Upper cross syndrome –

Upper body postural distortion that presents as a forward head, raised, internally-rotated, or rounded shoulders, and an exaggerated thoracic curvature.

Kyphosis –

Excessive convex curvature of the thoracic spine presenting as a bowed or rounded back.

Lordosis –

Excessive concavity or inward curvature of the lumbar spine.

Lower cross syndrome –

Lower body distortion characterized by an undesirable anterior tilt of the pelvis.

Plumb line –

Linear assessment tool used to evaluate posture and observe variations in anatomical positions.

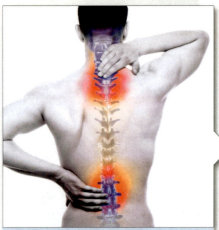

Many clients will possess postural distortions or imbalances which greatly impede their ability to safely and effectively engage in a comprehensive exercise program.

Many of the conditions that lead to postural deviations can cause muscular imbalances and vice versa, as these systems are interrelated and directly affect a joint's efficiency. While localized dysfunction explains some of these factors, others result from interaction between segments within a specified kinetic chain. For instance, a muscular imbalance between the anterior and posterior muscles of the shoulder that pull the shoulder forward will likely cause shoulder impingement syndrome, a localized dysfunction. On the other hand, plantar fasciitis that develops from gait malalignment, associated with running on an uneven surface, exemplifies a kinetic chain disturbance. Common postural distortions include forward head posture, rounded shoulders, symmetrical and asymmetrical **winged scapulae**, **upper cross syndrome**, **kyphosis** of the thoracic spine, **lordosis** of the lumbar spine, as well as **lower cross syndrome**, and fixed anterior, posterior, and lateral pelvic tilts. Additionally, knee and ankle joints may also deviate due to local and global muscle imbalances. These and other examples will be covered in greater detail shortly.

QUICK INSIGHT

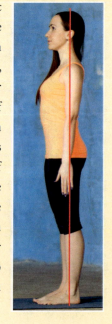

A postural assessment is an easy way to identify basic skeletal issues. This can be accomplished by using a simple **plumb line** to observe variations in anatomical positions from different viewpoints. When assessing posture from the side, initiation of the observation requires the line be placed anterior to the lateral malleolus through the calcaneocuboid joint. If there are no postural deviations, the plumb line will align vertically running from top to bottom through the individual's external auditory meatus (ear hole), acromioclavicular joint of the shoulder, central vertebral bodies, greater trochanter of the hips, slightly anterior to the midline of the knee, and end at the anterior portion of the lateral malleolus of the ankle through the calcaneocuboid joint. The alignment must start at the floor to accurately identify the postural variations. Variations to proper postural alignment suggest a possible consequence in musculoskeletal function.

Genetic predisposition may increase one's propensity toward postural distortions, but in general conditions developed over time explain most occurrences. For example, repetitive forward shoulders and round back posture when seated at work may lead to an anterior migration of the shoulder. Tightness in the hip flexors from excessive sitting or endurance activities, such as running or cycling, can rotate the pelvis anteriorly, while weakness or underactive gluteals and/or imbalances in the knee extensors vs. knee flexors may result in an inclination for the knees to lean inward. Often, multiple joints are affected due to the interdependent relationship of the kinetic chain. When joints become misaligned, the resultant asymmetries can lead to several additional problems down the chain. This is commonly seen when the hip flexors take on a greater role in pelvic stability, resulting in inhibition of the abdominals and hip extensors through reciprocal inhibition. This can also be observed in the glenohumeral joint when tightness in the latissimus dorsi and pectoralis musculature exists, resulting in limitations to shoulder movement. When these issues reach a level that causes joint deficiency, the body experiences greater resistance to movement of the joint, as well as reduced stability and energy transfer.

◆ Training Implications and Considerations

Exercise program models based solely on load or resistance may fail based on two common oversights. The first occurs when loads are applied to a body that has skeletal limitations. Without proper force and form closure, compensatory stabilization occurs, as global movers are recruited to manage the effort. This leads to the rehearsal of faulty recruitment patterns, resulting in undesirable adaptations: the body improperly learns to recruit global movers to compensate for the under-performing stabilizers to move the external load. The second occurs in response to a poor progressive training model. Too often, prime movers are trained initially in stable environments where the demands on the local and global stabilizers are low, and then immediately progressed to loaded, closed chain, compound movements. These movements incur much higher stability requirements, but in this case, an efficient kinetic chain has not been established. This is analogous to learning addition and subtraction in math class, then skipping immediately to algebra. A more informed developmental approach would employ training techniques that first emphasize a properly functioning system before focusing on load or advanced movement requirements.

> **DEFINITIONS**
>
> **Reciprocal inhibition –**
> *Describes neuromuscular regulation of agonist-antagonist contraction patterns; reciprocal innervation provides a reduced resistance to opposing muscle contractions.*

QUICK INSIGHT

Each individual client should be evaluated for musculoskeletal efficiency to detect flaws in static and dynamic postures. After an assessment, a program can be constructed to correct the observed postural distortions. The first step in the process of fixing static and dynamic postural faults involves understanding the underlying characteristics that perpetuate the limitations. Commonly, the postural and phasic muscles are either too tight and/or overactive or too weak and/or underactive, depending on the chronic conditions that apply. While the groupings, such as tight and overactive, are not synonymous, opposing sets generally reflect one strong and inflexible side, while the other is weak and underactive. Interestingly, postural muscles tend to exhibit tightness and increased resistance from over-activity, whereas phasic muscles progressively weaken [29].

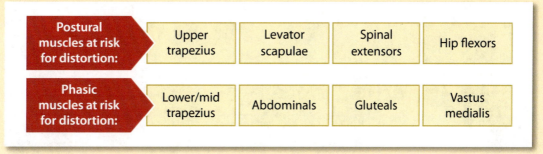

| Postural muscles at risk for distortion: | Upper trapezius | Levator scapulae | Spinal extensors | Hip flexors |
| Phasic muscles at risk for distortion: | Lower/mid trapezius | Abdominals | Gluteals | Vastus medialis |

Without efficiency in joint function, postural muscles will incur increasing demands. In response, phasic muscles experience reduced stress and become weakened over time, inhibited by compensatory actions [29]. In order to influence phasic muscle activity while inhibiting postural muscle activation, traditional programs must be redesigned to emphasize specific activation patterns.

A functional system's deterioration into a postural distortion becomes most obvious when it is required to move at increased velocities or under loads. Issues worsen when system efficiency relies on simultaneous joint alignment from cooperative body segments. For instance, in upper body actions, shoulder function depends on the position of the scapula and thoracic spine, while lower body actions depend on the relationship of the pelvis and lumbar spine (lumbo-pelvic hip complex). Independent joint systems, such as the knee or ankle, are also affected by the position and function of central joints. As such, a deficiency in the central musculature can affect efficiency within the limbs. This further demonstrates the relevance of addressing the kinetic chain in its entirety.

◆ Categories of Postural Distortions

Postural distortions negatively impact health, so they have been categorized into clinically diagnosed musculoskeletal problems. These include upper-extremity postural distortion, lumbo-pelvic hip postural distortion, and lower-extremity postural distortion. Upper-extremity distortions are often classified at one of three progressive levels among individuals. These include forward chin, rounded shoulders, and upper-cross syndrome. In the elderly, exaggerated kyphosis may also occur, which along with structural changes, coincides with osteoporotic microfractures, presenting as a Dowager's Hump. While Dowager's Hump often involves a systematic structural deformation, the other three upper-body distortions can be corrected with exercise therapy. Interestingly, upper-body problems tend to occur in the sagittal plane, whereas lower body distortions manifest in the sagittal and frontal plane. Lower-extremity distortions affect both the hip and limb joints. They include lower-cross syndrome, lumbar lordosis, lateral pelvic tilt at the lumbo-pelvic hip complex, outward rotation seen at the ankle, and/or foot pronation (flat feet).

Upper Body Postural Distortions

Upper body distortions

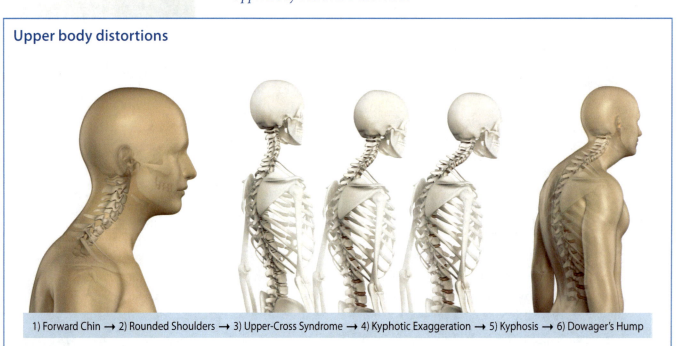

1) Forward Chin → 2) Rounded Shoulders → 3) Upper-Cross Syndrome → 4) Kyphotic Exaggeration → 5) Kyphosis → 6) Dowager's Hump

In upper body distortions, the anatomical segments commonly migrate forward. In the case of a forward chin, the postural muscles acting upon the superior axial skeleton become overactive; these postural muscles include the cervical protractors (splenius muscles, scalenes, sternocleidomastoids), upper trapezius, and levator scapulae, with a coinciding underactive group of deep cervical flexors. Sometimes referred to as a level one upper-body distortion, initial changes in posture begin at the cervical spine. If ignored, this issue can progress into a kyphotic exaggeration: the mid/lower trapezius becomes less active, while the serratus anterior becomes overactive, responding to the chronically forward posture. The progressive forward migration begins to affect the retractors and horizontal abductors as the rhomboids and the external rotators lengthen, adding to the existing mid/lower trapezius dysfunction. This progressive cascade of events ultimately leads to rounded or forward shoulders, an occurrence common to both inactive individuals and athletes alike.

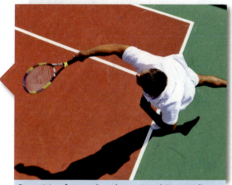

Repetitive forward and rotational (internal) acceleration at the shoulder common to baseball, tennis, swimming, and volleyball may lead to anterior migration of the shoulder.

Among sedentary individuals, rounded shoulders generally stem from poor daily posture, weak central and anterior trunk muscles, and general physical decline; athletes, on the other hand, have a tendency to participate in activities that overemphasize the musculature that mobilizes the arms in the anterior-sagittal and transverse planes. When this occurs, the glenohumeral head is pulled anteriorly, as the latissimus dorsi, teres major, subscapularis, and pectoralis muscles become shortened, strong and overactive. In addition, the infraspinatus, teres minor, rhomboids, and mid/low trapezius become lengthened and weak. Finally, the shoulder's posterior joint capsule tends to tighten, limiting the ability of the glenohumeral head to migrate posteriorly, further fueling an anterior glenohumeral position.

Upper-cross syndrome, a level three upper-body distortion, presents in the anterior view with raised, internally rotated, and/or horizontally adducted shoulders. In the lateral view of both erect and seated posture, presentation involves an exaggerated, kyphotic thoracic spine and rounded shoulders. These upper body distortions not only create significant dysfunction during movement but perpetuate injury during training and physical activity. Common issues include shoulder complex dysfunction, winged scapulae, impingement syndrome, and kinetic chain disturbances. Prior to pain, an exercise professional should recognize the tell-tale signs of limited spinal function, shoulder positioning, reduced shoulder complex efficiency, and poor ROM.

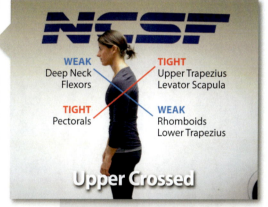

Lower-Body Postural Distortions

A natural hip hike is expected during locomotion, but in some cases, frontal plane disturbances occur as muscles lateral to the spine and hip become imbalanced, resulting in a fixed lateral tilt. Lateral pelvic displacement is one of the five major kinetic determinants of gait, but when stuck in a fixed position, it creates postural dysfunction, problems with locomotion, perceptual leg length disparity, and movements involving combined knee and hip flexion. When functional, the pelvis tilts laterally to synchronize the rhythmic movements of walking, stepping and climbing. This response is produced by either the horizontal shift of the pelvis or relative hip abduction. Dysfunction often presents as a hip elevating, or "hiking up," on one side of the pelvic spine, while the opposing side is depressed. These changes in the pelvic position lead to increased hip adduction on the raised side and subsequent increased hip abduction on the lowered side. The elevated hip causes adaptive shortening of the quadratus lumborum, erector spinae,

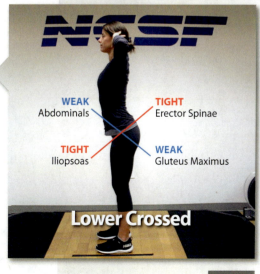

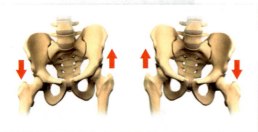

Dysfunction often presents as a hip elevating, or "hiking up," on one side of the pelvic spine, while the opposing side is depressed.

multifidi, obliques, rectus abdominis, iliopsoas, and hip abductors on the high side. The often overlooked and under-treated muscles include the entire adductor group on the depressed side of the lateral lumbo-pelvic tilt. A lateral tilt is commonly attributed to repeated actions in the same plane, such as running, or single-side dominant postures, such as shifting the body's weight to one side while standing, which is sometimes attributed to a unilateral lower limb injury.

Muscles become progressively imbalanced in the associated stabilizers and are often cited as the primary problems; in particular, the quadratus lumborum, psoas group, and illiacus on the elevated side, and hip abductors, including the gluteus medius, on the dropped side. Lateral pelvic tilts can often be visibly diagnosed from the posterior view during squatting movements and, in more exaggerated conditions, present during walking as dysfunctional gait. Athletes commonly present with sacroiliac joint (SI joint), hip, and mid-back pains. Complaints may also arise from translation problems which radiate from the hip as a result of compensatory kinetic chain actions (i.e., lateral thigh pain, sacroiliac (SI) pain, or femoral acetabular impingement (FAI) syndrome). Exercise professionals should also be mindful of iliotibial (IT) band tightness, which can occur due to consequent myofascial deformation and repeated sagittal plane activities. This often occurs from excessive training volumes applied in a single plane without adequate preparation or an overaggressive return to play.

Lower Body Distal-Extremity Distortions

Below the hip, additional **lower body distal-extremity distortions** may exist. Tibial-femoral dysfunction is a collective term used to refer to the various distortions seen at the knee and ankle joints. These issues can include flat pronated feet that may or may not include **knee valgus** and/or internal rotation of the knees (knees in), or externally rotated feet (toes pointed outward - heels in). Certainly, tightness specific to the joint may be the problem, but in many cases the disturbances originate along the kinetic chain. This occurs in response to changes in force that act on a misaligned femur. Essentially, biomechanical adjustments in the hip create a sub-optimal pelvic-femoral position which distorts the ground chain. Consequently, changes in the length-tension relationship due to muscular imbalances affect the static and dynamic positions of the knee. To further emphasize the relevance of the kinetic chain in the lower limbs, when the hip flexors become too tight, the ability of the gluteals and hamstring to rotate the pelvis posteriorly to a neutral position becomes limited, presenting an anterior pelvic tilt. Since these muscles are integral to pelvic position and subsequent knee stability, weakness leads to femoral-tibial adjustments and postural dysfunction.

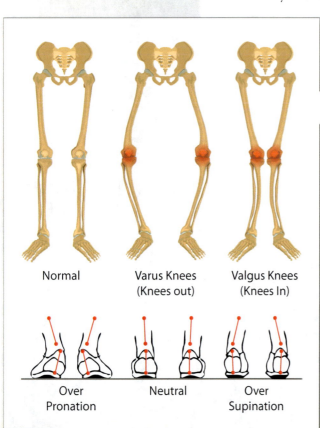

In the anterior view, when the feet are pronated and the knees move in, the probable overactive muscles are the vastus lateralis, short head of the biceps femoris, and adductor complex. The distortion occurs in response to weak gluteal muscles and inefficiency within the vastus medialis. Similarly, when the feet "turn out" and heels rotate inward, the issues likely lie in the calves and hamstrings: the soleus, lateral gastrocnemius, and short head of the biceps femoris may have become overactive, while the medial gastrocnemius, medial hamstring, and long adductors have become underactive. Other muscles worth evaluating when faulty movements occur in the lower limb segments are the peroneals, adductors, ITB, iliopsoas, rectus femoris, sartorius, tibialis posterior, and popliteus. Common injuries associated with adjustments in the knee position during flexion and extension includes plantar fasciitis, shin splints, **IT band syndrome**, and **patellar tendonitis (jumper's knee)**.

DEFINITIONS

Iliotibial (IT) band syndrome –

Common overuse injury that causes inflammation of the IT band due to chronic friction against the femur and lateral aspect of the knee joint.

Patellar tendonitis –

Commonly referred to as "jumper's knee": an overuse injury to the patellar tendon with the accumulation of microtrauma due to repetitive jumping or rapid changes of direction.

Segmental Problem	Issues	Limitations
Forward chin	**Overactive:** Upper trapezius, scalenes, sternocleidomastoids, levator scapulae **Underactive:** Serratus anterior, mid-low trapezius, deep cervical muscles	Contributes to upper cross/upper thoracic hump, limits spinal function, reduces shoulder complex efficiency and ROM *Training issues* – vertical transfer from pulls, overhead pressing limitations, difficulty in receive positions of cleans and snatches and compromised core stability during front squats
Kyphotic exaggeration (Upper cross)	**Overactive:** Upper trapezius, pectoralis muscles, subscapularis, latissimus dorsi, teres major **Underactive:** Rhomboids, mid-lower trapezius, serratus anterior, teres minor, infraspinatus, posterior deltoid	Shoulder complex dysfunction, impingement and kinetic chain disturbances leading to injury *Training issues* – inability to perform overhead lifts, receives, and proper bilateral row position; compromise to spinal position during pulls and squats
Lumbo-pelvic-hip postural distortion (Lower cross)	**Overactive:** Calves, hip adductors, hamstrings, erector spinae, rectus femoris, latissimus dorsi, iliopsoas **Underactive:** Glutes, abdominals, spinal stabilizers	Hamstring strains, groin strains, and low back pain *Training issues* – compromise to bilateral hip and knee flexion activities such as squats, inability to access core musculature, inhibition to glute-driven hip extension, and knee position during heavy loading
Lumbo-pelvic-hip postural distortion (Fixed lateral pelvic tilt)	**Overactive:** *High side:* Quadratus lumborum, iliopsoas, adductors *Low side:* Gluteus medius, tensor fascia latae (TFL) **Underactive:** *High side:* Gluteus medius, TFL *Low side:* Quadratus lumborum, erector spinae, adductors	Unilateral low and/or mid-back pain, hamstrings strains, adductor strains, IT band friction syndrome, lateral hip pain *Training issues* – compromise to all squatting actions, compensatory dominance in leg exercises and ballistic hip extension, difficulty with spinal stabilization
Distal extremity postural distortion	**Overactive:** Calves, peroneals, posterior tibialis, adductors, iliotibial band, iliopsoas, and rectus femoris	Plantar fasciitis, shin splints, and patellar tendonitis (jumper's knee) *Training issues* – improper activation during squats and compromised pull position, difficulty with single-leg balance exercises

Kinetic Chain Function, Dysfunction and Corrective Exercise

Corrective Exercise

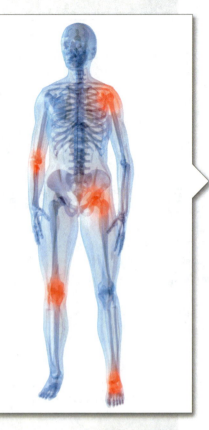

Most middle-age and older adults present with some level of physical dysfunction regardless of their activity status. Comprehensive evaluation by an exercise professional will often reveal patterns of dysfunction commonly due to strength imbalances and deficiencies in utility that are associated with poor mobility and/or faulty activation patterns that develop over time. In most cases, the soft tissues of the musculoskeletal system are at fault, due to chronic seated postures and inadequately balanced physical activity. These and the other common agitators require addressing in a manner that facilitates improvements to joint efficiency, or they will progressively worsen over time. An initial evaluative goal should be to identify as many potential problems as possible. This process allows not only for identification of issues which are independent but also for those associated with interrelated problems. Once the primary dysfunctions have been identified, the initial program design should focus on correcting these issues as an initial goal.

Consider the following rationale:

1) Biomechanical issues negatively affect proper posture and movement.
2) Mechanical deficiencies promote faulty patterns and activation problems.
3) Ongoing postural changes affect form and force closure of a joint and lead to pathology.
4) Dysfunction inhibits health and performance-oriented behavior.
5) Physical discomfort and pain originate from common biomechanical limitations.
6) Biomechanical dysfunctions can predispose one to injury, which can present one with major setbacks to any goals associated with the body.

From the onset of training with a new client, the exercise professional should emphasize addressing all obstacles that may limit the rate of physical health improvement, especially those that present risk for injury.

The preventative and restorative concept is developmental by nature: Remove limitations → Establish function → Enhance health-related fitness → Improve performance

Changing the physical order of this adaptation sequence is counterproductive and will often be detrimental to health. Purposeful exercise selection, proper technique instruction, and when necessary, modifications that are employed for correcting limitations will help maintain (and many times improve) physical capabilities while also progressing towards achieving a client's desired goals.

◆ Quantifying the Level of Dysfunction

When no pathology exists, any identified dysfunction should be managed just as any other adaptation, with the aim of improving health or performance. The level or grade of dysfunction and its consequent effects on movement efficiency should guide the exercise selection process. If the client has back pain associated with pelvic instability and poor muscle strength balance, these issues become prioritized. It is advantageous for exercise professionals to commit time and effort towards concurrent goals; however, the body must first function properly to reach these goals. Thus, training for strength-balance, flexibility, and central stability to reduce related symptoms and restore function should become priorities.

The **prioritization model** should be implemented based on the client's specific needs and level of dysfunction. Significant dysfunction impedes task performance, so addressing it should be a primary focus. These problems warrant immediate corrective strategies as the main emphasis of the exercise program. Lumbo-pelvic instability and varied levels of lower cross and upper cross syndromes are common among adults. When identified within the **needs analysis**, these primary issues should be strategically addressed during all phases of the training program. Secondary limitations may tend to reduce a client's ability to perform certain tasks but generally, do not cause any major discomfort. They pertain to a single plane of motion and tend not to impact all movement applications. These limitations can usually be fixed using combinations of exercise. If the level of dysfunction is isolated to a joint or does not prevent the individual from performing safe movement using acceptable technique or form, it still will require specific attention but usually will not alter the programming plan. These types of issues tend to be isolated to specific ROM limitations and specific strength imbalances, so they are fairly easy to rectify.

Effective programs for attaining or re-attaining basic stability and mobility prioritize function-based work in the early phases of training. Stability and mobility are paramount because muscle activation depends upon the joints' positions when loaded. If a client cannot execute movements properly, compensation in motor firing patterns occurs, and if left unaddressed, these become thoroughly ingrained through practice and rehearsal. Essentially, lack of stability and mobility compromises movement technique, causing the body to learn to move using improper firing patterns and technique to compensate, corrupting biomechanical foundations. Rehearsal of an action creates motor learning and familiarity with environmental stressors, and this repetition of compensatory movements proves detrimental. Fortunately, most tendencies are correctable. When instruction cannot correct the problem, this issue is called a **fixed compensation**: in other words, it will always occur in response to the environment regardless of cueing. To prevent tendencies from becoming a fixed compensation, exercise professionals must require exacting form from the onset of training.

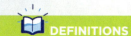

DEFINITIONS

Prioritization model –

Strategy which dictates that areas/issues of greatest need are addressed as a priority in the training program.

Needs analysis –

Inventory of adaptation requirements for an individual as determined by screening and evaluation protocols; includes the identification, organization, and prioritization of physiological needs.

Fixed compensation –

Chronic biomechanical compensation which cannot be alleviated with proper instruction or cueing.

Prioritization Model and Corrective Programming:

Primary Limitations	Secondary Limitations
■ Issue is significant, may be painful, and impedes overall function and performance; it warrants immediate corrective strategies and emphasis in the program	■ Issue tends to reduce the ability to perform certain tasks but generally does not cause major discomfort; warrants adjunct corrective work and attention to proper movement form
■ **Example** *Upper cross syndrome*	■ **Example** *Slight hamstring tightness*

◆ Programming Corrective Exercise

Rehearsal

The early phases of **corrective exercise** training are characteristically high in volume but feature lower resistance, making for ideal teaching environments. **Motor rehearsal**, or repeat exposure to a movement, enhances proficiency and the body's ability to transfer what has been learned into other movements. Emphasizing gross movements when training provides many more benefits when compared to isolated muscle exercises and can also increase movement competency when actions are compounded. Research indicates improved efficiency with practice that continues beyond what is necessary to simply accomplish a task; conversely, limited exposure to an action or environment creates easily disrupted pathways [15]. For instance, if an individual repeatedly performs the lunge using flawed technique without being corrected, the action will be patterned incorrectly. As soon as it is progressed, the increased stress will lead to more error in movement performance. Individuals who have patterned movement and exercise incorrectly are the most difficult to correct because the patterns are ingrained in the nervous system. If proper movement execution is constantly rehearsed and reinforced, the movement pattern will occur correctly every time, which underscores the need to emphasize proper technique.

Kinetic Chains and Circuits

Most training programs lean toward traditional methods aimed at body-part training that emphasizes isolated muscle actions. Training using isolated actions compromises muscle integration in areas such as mobility, force coupling, dynamic stabilization, and improvement in energy transfer across kinetic chains. Programming exercises that unite functional couples can quickly take advantage of established strength and direct it toward more coordinated actions to execute functional movement.

Traditional	Functional
Barbell Reverse Lunge	Reverse Lunge with Contralateral Row

Building upon the force couple concept, activities should be selected based on the adaptation they promote. Primal movements employ closed kinetic chains, which normally require the integration of ground reaction force and internal energy management [8, 36]. Unless the goal is bodybuilding or isolated strength for localized muscle balance or rehabilitation, the foundations of movement-based training should emphasize client-appropriate, **closed kinetic chain exercises**. In a closed kinetic chain, force is applied to a distally-fixed position (usually the ground), forcing the body to stabilize segments so that it may accelerate and transfer the energy from limbs to trunk and vice versa to accomplish tasks. However, not all closed chain exercises use the ground as the fixed force anchor. The pull-up is also closed chain as the body moves around a distally-fixed bar position, increasing the requirements for stability and activation. On the contrary, a cable lat pull-down is an **open kinetic chain exercise**. While the movement looks similar and targets the same muscle groups, the hands pull the bar toward a fixed body, stabilized by the machine, thereby decreasing the trunk's central stability requirents. The open chain consequently reduces the stability and activation requirements of the body but often allows for increased isolated loading.

DEFINITIONS

Corrective exercise –

Activities aimed at restoring or improving joint function via neuromuscular and musculoskeletal system improvements.

Motor rehearsal –

Repeated exposure to a movement pattern which enhances efficiency over time due to increased neuromuscular proficiency.

Closed kinetic chain exercise –

Exercise in which force is applied to a distally-fixed position or object.

Open kinetic chain exercise –

Exercise in which force is applied to a movable object.

When analyzed by electromyographical response, the pull-up exercise encourages much higher muscle activation compared to the lat pull-down exercise [12, 34]. Importantly, the increased activation benefits of closed chain exercises depend upon properly managing the stability requirements needed to produce the force. Stability is the weakest link in the kinetic chain and thus, the greatest limiter to executable force production. This concept explains why most people cannot perform the same number of pull-ups as they can lat pull-down using bodyweight equated loads. In general, machines and external support equipment decrease the stability requirements placed on the body, making them easier. Military press, pull-ups, push-ups, dips, hanging leg raises, lunges, squats, and deadlifts are all closed chain exercises that systematically improve central-peripheral stabilization and provide documented improvements in adaptation-based transfer to other activities [4, 11, 38, 45].

Changing the physical connection to the load, or kinetic circuit, represents another strategy that can be employed to add or change the stress of an exercise. Kinetic circuits determine the stability demands which are dominated either by central or peripheral stabilizers. Open circuits employ independent limb loading or single-sided loads that require increased localized stability relative to the weight. A common example would be the seated dumbbell overhead press. Each shoulder must function independently; whereas, in a closed kinetic circuit, as demonstrated by the seated military press, the joints function cooperatively, because both limbs control the same external load. Chains and circuits can be manipulated and integrated to create the desired level of stability, ROM, and load, based on the adaptations one wishes to elicit. To summarize, closed chain exercises generally require more stability (central) and employ more force couples than do their open chain counterparts. Open circuits promote localized joint stability (peripheral) and increased movement range, whereas closed circuits lessen this burden and tend to place more stress on central stabilizers, and provide for higher loading capacity. This is very obvious when comparing the dumbbell bench press to the barbell bench press. The dumbbell bench press weight (combined total) is always less than the weight attainable using the barbell bench press. Therefore, if range and stability are the goal, employ closed chain, open circuit exercises; maximal strength requires closed chain, closed circuit exercises; whereas body building employs open chains with open and closed circuits to maximize the load with the muscles in isolation with specified **time-under-tension** (TUT).

> **DEFINITIONS**
>
> **Time-under-tension** –
>
> *The total amount of time a given muscle experiences tension during structured exercise; maybe calculated in segments (sets) or in totality (bout).*

Chain and Circuit Summary

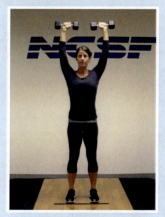

closed chain –
open circuit

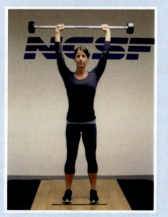

closed chain –
closed circuit

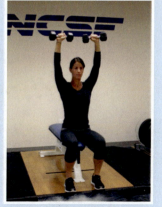

open chain –
open circuit

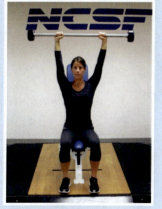

open chain –
closed circuit

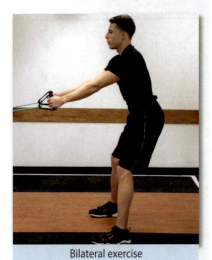

Bilateral exercise

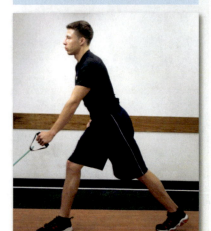

Unilateral exercise

> 📖 **DEFINITIONS**
>
> **Asymmetrical loading –**
> Loading is not symmetrical in the sagittal and frontal plane.

◆ Integrated Corrective Exercise Strategies

Earlier it was identified that when muscle imbalances promote postural distortions, traditional mechanics become compromised. Pelvic instability and forward migration of the shoulder joints often lead to an inability to safely perform compound movements, such as squats and presses, and various ballistic activities, including the Olympic lifts. Most of the problems exist during bilateral closed chain exercises with closed circuits where deficits to mobility are most exposed. An exercise professional must employ strategies to correct these problems in a manner that progresses towards improved movement efficiency. As mentioned previously, the initial phases of training are ideal for emphasizing these areas.

In most cases, open circuit techniques can fix many issues and tend to be predominantly unilateral, particularly in the lower body. Unilateral exercises function well for correcting issues because they can isolate a motion segment to advance movement system stabilization while promoting maximal ROM. Unilateral activities increase local muscle activation, stability, and ROM optimally because they provide less offsetting stress from muscle imbalances. Though the cumulative loading employed is notably lower than the weight used in comparable bilateral lifts, these exercises are more effective when the specific goals are considered. Comparing the overhead squat versus the overhead lunge exemplifies this applied concept. In the overhead squat exercise, the shoulder joints and pelvis are subjected to forward pulling stress based on the insertion sites of the hip flexors and latissimus dorsi. An individual with upper or lower cross syndrome will have a much harder time performing the overhead squat properly. However, these same forward forces do not occur during split stance positions, due to changes in the spinal angle and cross stabilization of the sling systems. An individual with ROM limitations in the latissimus dorsi and/or hip flexors will have a much easier time with the overhead lunge compared to the overhead squat, as the unilateral exercise allows for much easier attainment of the full movement ranges.

In addition to using unilateral actions for improving ROM and stability, changing the load location can also be employed to address specific needs. Changes to load position can provide for varied purposes with the goals of higher loading capacity, specific activation, increased stability, or increased force coupling across the kinetic chain. The axial-loaded position increases resistance potential but often reduces core requirements due to increased back activation. Overhead or contralateral, **asymmetrical loading** increases central trunk and core activation and augments medial-lateral stability requirements; on the other hand, ipsilateral loading increases prime mover activation and often lateral muscle activity.

The following exercises show effective application of loading variations for specific issues:

Underactive glutes and core

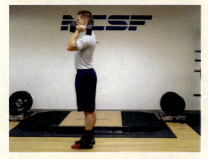 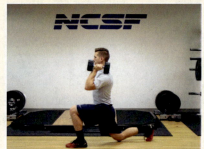

Ipsilateral/asymmetrical reverse lunge

Tight lats and hip flexors

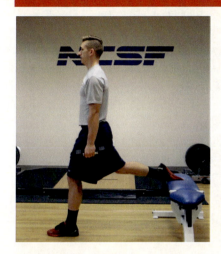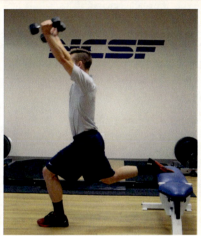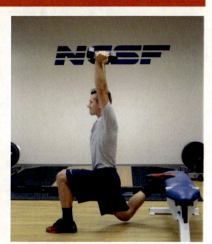

DB Bulgarian swings

Overactive lower back and hip flexors, underactive core

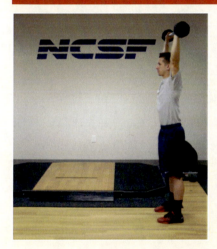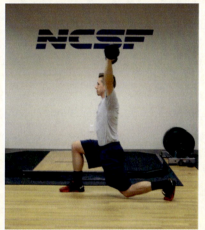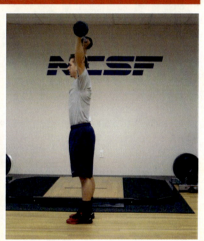

OH walking lunges

Tight internal rotators and shoulder flexors

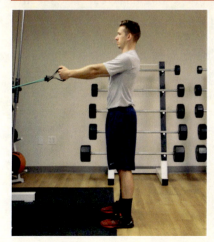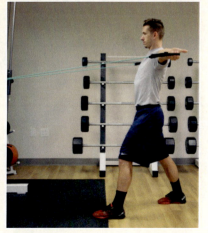

Step-back with T-pull

Kinetic Chain Function, Dysfunction and Corrective Exercise

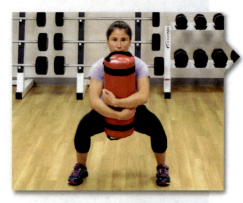

Programming unfamiliar loading may be a useful modification for enhancing adaptations. "Unfamiliar" suggests the resistance is placed in a location to which the body is not accustomed, or that the load is awkward and cumbersome. Unfamiliar loading conditions can create variations in the activation of stabilizing musculature [48]. A front-loaded diagonal lunge exemplifies symmetrical unfamiliar loading; bear-hugging a heavy bag during lateral squats represents another. Both increase force coupling and stability based on the specificity of the conditions. If, however, difficulty in load management causes faulty movement patterns, the load should be adjusted or reduced. A common theme in quality instruction is to pay close attention to the details. The most effective exercise professionals will provide for correct technique and will be discriminatively strict to ensure quality movements are performed all of the time.

Problem Solving with Corrective Exercise

Issue	Problems	Corrective Exercises	Traditional Activities
Forward chin	UA upper back muscles	Good morning, T/Y reaches	Single-arm row
Kyphotic exaggeration	OA cervical flexors	Scapular push-up	U-bar high row Suspension T-pulls
Kyphosis	Tight joint capsule	IYT reaches	2-bench push-ups
Upper cross syndrome	OA internal rotators OA pectoralis, lats	Band T-pulls Reverse lunge w/ cont. reach	Reverse back flys Suspension wide row
Lordosis	OA hip flexors OA low back	Reverse lunge Wide leg back reach	Knee rolls on ball MB pullover to stand
Lower cross syndrome	OA hip flexors/low back UA abdominals/glutes	Field lunge w/ cont. cross reach Slide disc speed lunges	SA OH Bulgarian squat Ipsilateral reverse lunge
Inward knees	UA glutes OA quads	Floor bridge w/ ceiling reach OH Bulgarian reach	Bench leg march Ipsilateral step-ups
Outward knees	OA calves OA glute medius	Single-leg floor reach Split-stance toe reach	Dorsiflexed bridge Single-leg pistol squat

UA = underactive   OA = overactive   MB = medicine ball   DB = dumbbell   OH = overhead   cont. = contralateral   SA = single arm

REFERENCES:

1. Ainscough-Potts AM, Morrissey MC, and Critchley D. The response of the transverse abdominis and internal oblique muscles to different postures. *Man Ther* 11: 54-60, 2006.

2. Akuthota V and Nadler SF. Core strengthening. *Arch Phys Med Rehabil* 85: S86-92, 2004.

3. Allison GT, Morris SL, and Lay B. Feedforward responses of transversus abdominis are directionally specific and act asymmetrically: implications for core stability theories. *J Orthop Sports Phys Ther* 38: 228-237, 2008.

4. Augustsson J, Esko A, Thomeé R, and Svantesson U. Weight training of the thigh muscles using closed versus open kinetic chain exercises: a comparison of performance enhancement. *Journal of Orthopaedic & Sports Physical Therapy* 27: 3-8, 1998.

5. Bergmark A. Stability of the lumbar spine. A study in mechanical engineering. *Acta Orthop Scand Suppl* 230: 1-54, 1989.

6. Blazkiewicz M, Lyson B, Chmielewski A, and Wit A. Transfer of mechanical energy during the shot put. *J Hum Kinet* 52: 139-146, 2016.

7. Chang M, Slater LV, Corbett RO, Hart JM, and Hertel J. Muscle activation patterns of the lumbo-pelvic-hip complex during walking gait before and after exercise. *Gait Posture* 52: 15-21, 2017.

8. Cochrane DJ and Barnes MJ. Muscle activation and onset times of hip extensors during various loads of a closed kinetic chain exercise. *Research in Sports Medicine* 23: 179-189, 2015.

9. Comerford MJ and Mottram SL. Functional stability re-training: principles and strategies for managing mechanical dysfunction. *Man Ther* 6: 3-14, 2001.

10. Danneels LA, Vanderstraeten GG, Cambier DC, Witvrouw EE, Stevens VK, and De Cuyper HJ. A functional subdivision of hip, abdominal, and back muscles during asymmetric lifting. *Spine (Phila Pa 1976)* 26: E114-121, 2001.

11. Davies GJ. Individualizing the Return to Sports After Anterior Cruciate Ligament Reconstruction. *Operative Techniques in Orthopaedics*, 2017.

12. Doma K, Deakin GB, and Ness KF. Kinematic and electromyographic comparisons between chin-ups and lat-pull down exercises. *Sports Biomech* 12: 302-313, 2013.

13. Draovitch P, Edelstein J, and Kelly BT. The layer concept: utilization in determining the pain generators, pathology and how structure determines treatment. *Current reviews in musculoskeletal medicine* 5: 1-8, 2012.

14. Ferreira PH, Ferreira ML, Maher CG, Refshauge K, Herbert RD, and Hodges PW. Changes in recruitment of transversus abdominis correlate with disability in people with chronic low back pain. *Br J Sports Med* 44: 1166-1172, 2010.

15. Gabriel DA, Kamen G, and Frost G. Neural adaptations to resistive exercise: mechanisms and recommendations for training practices. *Sports Med* 36: 133-149, 2006.

16. Gould D, Dieffenbach K, and Moffett A. Psychological characteristics and their development in Olympic champions. *Journal of applied sport psychology* 14: 172-204, 2002.

17. Granata KP and England SA. Stability of dynamic trunk movement. *Spine (Phila Pa 1976)* 31: E271-276, 2006.

18. Granata KP, Orishimo KF, and Sanford AH. Trunk muscle coactivation in preparation for sudden load. *J Electromyogr Kinesiol* 11: 247-254, 2001.

19. Heiss DG and Pagnacco G. Effect of center of pressure and trunk center of mass optimization methods on the analysis of whole body lifting mechanics. *Clin Biomech (Bristol, Avon)* 17: 106-115, 2002.

20. Herr H and Popovic M. Angular momentum in human walking. *J Exp Biol* 211: 467-481, 2008.

21. Hodges PW. Is there a role for transversus abdominis in lumbo-pelvic stability? *Man Ther* 4: 74-86, 1999.

22. Hodges PW and Richardson CA. Contraction of the abdominal muscles associated with movement of the lower limb. *Phys Ther* 77: 132-142; discussion 142-134, 1997.

23. Hodges PW and Richardson CA. Delayed postural contraction of transversus abdominis in low back pain associated with movement of the lower limb. *J Spinal Disord* 11: 46-56, 1998.

24. Hodges PW and Richardson CA. Feedforward contraction of transversus abdominis is not influenced by the direction of arm movement. *Exp Brain Res* 114: 362-370, 1997.

25. Hodges PW and Richardson CA. Inefficient muscular stabilization of the lumbar spine associated with low back pain. A motor control evaluation of transversus abdominis. *Spine (Phila Pa 1976)* 21: 2640-2650, 1996.

26. Hodges PW and Richardson CA. Relationship between limb movement speed and associated contraction of the trunk muscles. *Ergonomics* 40: 1220-1230, 1997.

27. Hodges PW and Richardson CA. Transversus abdominis and the superficial abdominal muscles are controlled independently in a postural task. *Neurosci Lett* 265: 91-94, 1999.

28. Hof AL, Nauta J, van der Knaap ER, Schallig MA, and Struwe DP. Calf muscle work and segment energy changes in human treadmill walking. *J Electromyogr Kinesiol* 2: 203-216, 1992.

29. Janda V. Muscles in the pathogenesis of musculoskeletal disorders. *Oxford Textbook of Musculoskeletal Medicine*: 121, 2015.

30. Jones G. What is this thing called mental toughness? An investigation of elite sport performers. *Journal of applied sport psychology* 14: 205-218, 2002.

31. Kimiecik JC and Jackson SA. Optimal experience in sport: A flow perspective. 2002.

32. Lee D, Lee L-J, and Lee D. An integrated approach to the assessment and treatment of the lumbopelvic-hip region. Canada: s.n. ,, 2004.

33. Lee PJ, Rogers EL, and Granata KP. Active trunk stiffness increases with co-contraction. *J Electromyogr Kinesiol* 16: 51-57, 2006.

34. Leslie KL and Comfort P. The effect of grip width and hand orientation on muscle activity during pull-ups and the lat pull-down. *Strength & Conditioning Journal* 35: 75-78, 2013.

35. Louw M and Deary C. The biomechanical variables involved in the aetiology of iliotibial band syndrome in distance runners–A systematic review of the literature. *Physical Therapy in sport* 15: 64-75, 2014.

36. Lutz GE, Palmitier RA, An KN, and Chao EY. Comparison of tibiofemoral joint forces during open-kinetic-chain and closed-kinetic-chain exercises. *J Bone Joint Surg Am* 75: 732-739, 1993.

37. Masse-Alarie H, Beaulieu LD, Preuss R, and Schneider C. Task-specificity of bilateral anticipatory activation of the deep abdominal muscles in healthy and chronic low back pain populations. *Gait Posture* 41: 440-447, 2015.

38. McMullen J and Uhl TL. A kinetic chain approach for shoulder rehabilitation. *Journal of athletic training* 35: 329, 2000.

39. Ng JK, Parnianpour M, Richardson CA, and Kippers V. Effect of fatigue on torque output and electromyographic measures of trunk muscles during isometric axial rotation. *Arch Phys Med Rehabil* 84: 374-381, 2003.

40. Ng JK, Richardson CA, Parnianpour M, and Kippers V. Fatigue-related changes in torque output and electromyographic parameters of trunk muscles during isometric axial rotation exertion: an investigation in patients with back pain and in healthy subjects. *Spine (Phila Pa 1976)* 27: 637-646, 2002.

41. Pool-Goudzwaard AL, Vleeming A, Stoeckart R, Snijders CJ, and Mens JM. Insufficient lumbopelvic stability: a clinical, anatomical and biomechanical approach to 'a-specific' low back pain. *Man Ther* 3: 12-20, 1998.

42. Radebold A, Cholewicki J, Panjabi MM, and Patel TC. Muscle response pattern to sudden trunk loading in healthy individuals and in patients with chronic low back pain. *Spine (Phila Pa 1976)* 25: 947-954, 2000.

43. Redmond JM, Chen AW, and Domb BG. Greater Trochanteric Pain Syndrome. *JAAOS - Journal of the American Academy of Orthopaedic Surgeons* 24: 231-240, 2016.

44. Schinke RJ, Stambulova NB, Si G, and Moore Z. International society of sport psychology position stand: Athletes' mental health, performance, and development. *International Journal of Sport and Exercise Psychology*: 1-18, 2017.

45. Schoenfeld BJ. Squatting kinematics and kinetics and their application to exercise performance. *The Journal of Strength & Conditioning Research* 24: 3497-3506, 2010.

46. Searle A, Spink M, Ho A, and Chuter V. Exercise interventions for the treatment of chronic low back pain: a systematic review and meta-analysis of randomised controlled trials. *Clin Rehabil* 29: 1155-1167, 2015.

47. Shojaei I, Nussbaum MA, and Bazrgari B. Age-related differences in trunk muscle reflexive behaviors. *J Biomech* 49: 3147-3152, 2016.

48. Smith JD, Royer TD, and Martin PE. Asymmetrical loading affects intersegmental dynamics during the swing phase of walking. *Hum Mov Sci* 32: 652-667, 2013.

49. Swann C, Crust L, Jackman P, Vella SA, Allen MS, and Keegan R. Psychological states underlying excellent performance in sport: Toward an integrated model of flow and clutch states. *Journal of Applied Sport Psychology*: 1-27, 2017.

50. Teyhen DS, Rieger JL, Westrick RB, Miller AC, Molloy JM, and Childs JD. Changes in deep abdominal muscle thickness during common trunk-strengthening exercises using ultrasound imaging. *J Orthop Sports Phys Ther* 38: 596-605, 2008.

51. Umberger BR, Augsburger S, Resig J, Oeffinger D, Shapiro R, and Tylkowski C. Generation, absorption, and transfer of mechanical energy during walking in children. *Med Eng Phys* 35: 644-651, 2013.

52. Vleeming A, Stoeckart R, Volkers AC, and Snijders CJ. Relation between form and function in the sacroiliac joint. Part I: Clinical anatomical aspects. *Spine (Phila Pa 1976)* 15: 130-132, 1990.

53. Vleeming A, Volkers AC, Snijders CJ, and Stoeckart R. Relation between form and function in the sacroiliac joint. Part II: Biomechanical aspects. *Spine (Phila Pa 1976)* 15: 133-136, 1990.

54. Ward MM, Deodhar A, Akl EA, Lui A, Ermann J, Gensler LS, Smith JA, Borenstein D, Hiratzka J, and Weiss PF. American College of Rheumatology/Spondylitis Association of America/Spondyloarthritis Research and Treatment Network 2015 recommendations for the treatment of ankylosing spondylitis and nonradiographic axial spondyloarthritis. *Arthritis & rheumatology* 68: 282-298, 2016.

55. Watson AW. Sports injuries related to flexibility, posture, acceleration, clinical defects, and previous injury, in high-level players of body contact sports. *Int J Sports Med* 22: 222-225, 2001.

56. Williams SJ, Barron TR, Ciepley AJ, and Ebben WP. Kinetic Analysis of the Role of Upper Extremity Segmental Inertia on Vertical Jump Performance. *Journal of Exercise Physiology Online* 20: 28-35, 2017.

57. Zazulak B, Cholewicki J, and Reeves NP. Neuromuscular control of trunk stability: clinical implications for sports injury prevention. *J Am Acad Orthop Surg* 16: 497-505, 2008.

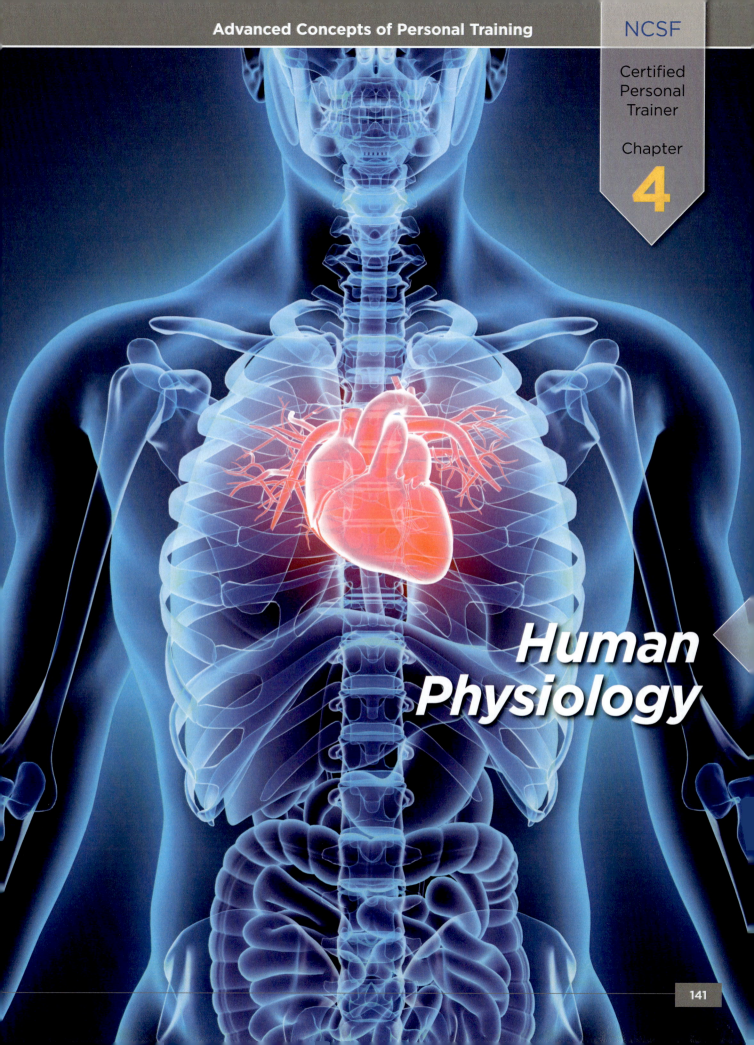

Anaerobic Energy Systems

> **DEFINITIONS**
>
> **Bioenergetics –**
>
> *Describes the various processes of energy/macronutrient use within the body and relates to the function of various energy systems for fuel provision during exercise.*

Bioenergetics represents the flow of energy within organisms. From a simplistic perspective, cars and humans offer a comparison that illustrates the principles of bioenergetics. Consider the following:

1) Both a car's motor and muscle cells derive their respective energy from organic, carbon-based products. Carbon is the key element in fossil fuels for the car and in organic food for humans.

2) In both cases, the fuel product begins as a complicated molecular structure that must be refined and broken down to a usable energy form. In the car's case, oil goes through a refinement process to form gasoline to fuel the car's combustion motor; in the human body, carbohydrates (CHO), fats, and proteins are broken down into smaller usable molecules to fuel the cellular activity.

3) Both processes create varied byproducts after the breakdown of the original structure. These byproducts must be managed and removed, or they will clutter and impede the ongoing refinement process.

4) Both the car motor and human cells produce work based on a single driving fuel. A gasoline motor can only run on gasoline. Muscle cells can only run on adenosine triphosphate (ATP).

5) Both a car's motor and a human's cells have low mechanical efficiencies: the majority of the chemical energy dissipates as heat while being converted for mechanical work.

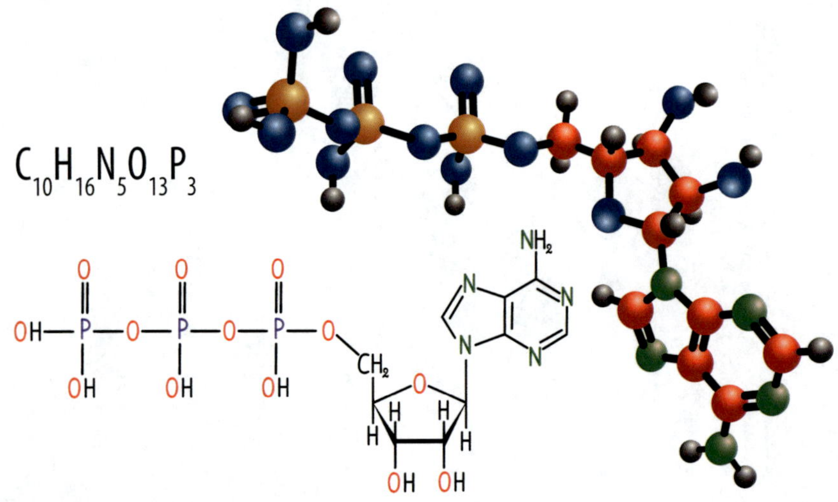

ATP

ATP represents the only form of energy that can be directly used for muscular contractions and, therefore, must be present for any internally controlled action. The fuel for mechanical, chemical, and transport work relies on the energy released from the phosphate bonds stored within the ATP molecule. Similar to the gasoline combustion of the car's motor, when the covalent bonds of phosphagen are broken, energy is released into the system and directed towards a particular action. ATP can be thought of as being "spring-loaded" with energy, which is

Adenosine triphosphate

$C_{10}H_{16}N_5O_{13}P_3$

released when **enzymes** break phosphagen bonds. Enzymatic hydrolysis separates the bonds that connect the phosphate molecules together, releasing energy. Enzymes serve as biological catalysts, which function by speeding up cellular reactions. In many cases, the enzymes are identified by the functions they perform. ATPase is the enzyme responsible for the breakdown of the ATP molecule inside the cell. The common suffix (–ase) specifically identifies the substance as an enzyme. When ATP is split for mechanical work, the action takes place deep within the muscle fiber at the myofilament level. The thick myofilament, myosin, and, more specifically, the myosin head, contains the ATPase enzyme.

> **DEFINITIONS**
>
> **Enzymes –**
> *Protein-based components produced by cells that function to catalyze (speed up) a biochemical reaction.*

Recall the process of cross-bridge cycling: in the presence of calcium, the head of the myosin molecule binds with actin, forming cross-bridges. Once the cross-bridges form, the ATPase of the myosin head acts as a catalyst in which the enzyme cleaves off an inorganic phosphate ion from the ATP molecule, which releases energy, leaving a by-product of adenosine diphosphate (ADP) and an inorganic phosphate. The energy released causes the myosin to detach from the actin filament. This permits the movement of the myosin head, the power stroke, so it can expel the energy by-products and reattach to actin further along the filament. This process allows myofilaments within the sarcomeres of muscle fibers to contract by lengthening and shortening to produce force. The quantity and duration of force depends on the number of fibers recruited, the amount of energy available at a given time, and the concentration of by-products within the environment.

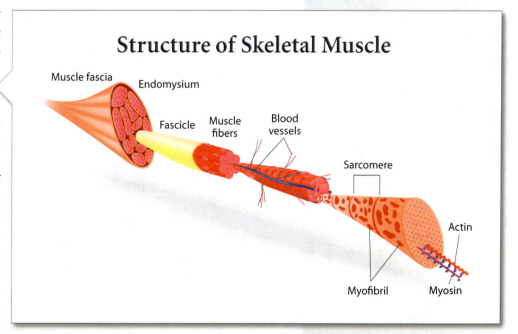

Structure of Skeletal Muscle

ATP derives from the metabolism of carbohydrate (CHO), fat, and protein fuel substrates. However, the cell independently stores small quantities of ATP for immediate work. The location of this ATP inside the cell makes it readily-usable and mechanically more efficient. It is the primary source of energy for immediate, fast, and powerful work [59]. The energy potency of the molecule allows for high-speed reactions and considerable force production. Maximal muscular work, lasting 1-3 seconds, will exploit stored ATP for energy. Examples of activities relying on stored ATP include a maximal vertical jump, pitching a fast ball, a tennis serve, or swinging a driver on the golf course.

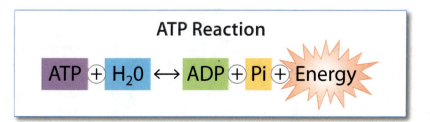

ATP Reaction

$$ATP + H_2O \longleftrightarrow ADP + Pi + Energy$$

> **DEFINITIONS**
>
> **Creatine phosphate (CP) –**
>
> *An inorganic compound found in skeletal muscle tissue capable of storing and providing high-energy phosphate elements to fuel muscular contractions; along with ATP, it comprises an immediate substrate of the phosphagen system.*
>
> **Creatine kinase –**
>
> *An enzyme which can catalyze creatine phosphate into creatine and a free phosphate ion to liberate immediate energy within the phosphagen energy system.*

Phosphagen Energy System

Because stored ATP depletes rapidly, the muscle maintains an additional pool of high-energy phosphate storage in the form of intracellular phosphocreatine. Creatine is phosphorylated with an inorganic phosphate ion to form a molecule with high-energy-yield bonds called **creatine phosphate (CP)** or phosphocreatine (PCr). Phosphorylation occurs when a phosphate group is added to a molecule. When ATP stores begin to plunge, the first reaction that replenishes the energy needed to continue muscular work occurs by splitting CP via the enzyme **creatine kinase (CK)**. CK breaks the high-energy creatine phosphate bond, which releases energy to re-phosphorylate intracellular ADP molecules. During the re-phosphorylation process, ADP binds with an inorganic phosphate molecule to resynthesize ATP for energy. After this occurs, the newly formed ATP molecule is split, and the energy yielded continues to drive the muscle cell. Creatine phosphate concentrations in the cell measure 4-6x that of ATP and provide for 10-15 seconds of high-power energy for burst activities, such as a 3RM (3 maximal repetitions) in weight lifting, a 60-yard shuttle, or a 100-meter sprint. Because the ATP and CP systems represent immediate energy and flow unabatedly, the two processes are generally referred to singly as the phosphagen system or immediate energy system.

CP Energy Sequence Summary

1) Creatine phosphate is split into creatine and an inorganic phosphate (P) by creatine kinase, producing energy.

2) The liberated phosphate uses the released energy to bind (phosphorylate) ADP and P to form ATP.

3) The new ATP molecule is then split into ADP and P, and energy is released.

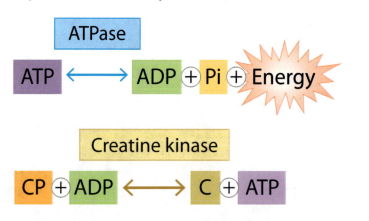

Phosphates are connected by very high energy bonds. As such when they are phosphorylated into ATP or CP, they become heavy molecules. A human body uses the equivalent of 50-70 kg of ATP a day. That means if all the ATP needed for daily biological work were stored, a human would weigh twice as much; however, the body will always aim to be as efficient as possible, which explains why it does not maintain high phosphagen storage levels. Excessive storage would weigh down the body tissue significantly. Instead, once the body begins to use the stored ATP and those levels decrease, the body resynthesizes ATP after ATPase separates the bonds through the CK reaction. This process creates a situation where, for a period of time, perpetual energy can be formed from lighter molecules (CP) rather than relying on higher storage levels of the heavy molecules (ATP) in the cell. When exercise discontinues after a single maximal effort, it takes the body at least 90 seconds to fully refuel ATP storage [120]. It does so by re-phosphorylating the ADP with the liberated phosphagen ions.

When longer durations of high force are exerted, CP continues fueling the mechanical work. However, after a prolonged time, it too becomes depleted. Consequently, the high-power phosphagen energy system fails and can no longer support the same high work output. At the end of a 3RM back squat, for instance, the duration of time for CP stores to replenish can take between 2-5 minutes, constituting maximal recovery time [120]. The phosphorylation periods required to re-establish ATP and CP stores in the muscle ultimately determine the rest periods needed between heavy resistance training and sprinting activities. During maximal lifts or running speeds, the period of rest time needed between repeat sets of equal work output depends on the interval necessary to replenish the energy. Power exercises, such as Olympic lifts and plyometrics, and heavy strength training utilize low repetition numbers and longer rest periods to maximize the performance of the phosphagen energy system [120]. Increases in performance, in part, relate to adaptation of the specified energy system. The intensity, load, and speed of the movement all play roles in determining which system will be the primary driver of energy production. If near-maximal loads or velocities are used, then longer rest will be required for the re-synthesis and re-phosphorylation of ATP and CP, respectively. However, if lighter weights are used for a short duration, the recovery period need not be as long because the action does not fully exhaust the immediate phosphagen stores [40]. For instance, a medicine ball slam drill using a 12 lb. ball performed at maximal speed for 10 seconds would seem to be in line with the phosphagen energy system parameters: high output for less than 15 seconds; however, when it comes to recovery, does the exercise require two or more minutes before a repeat act at the same intensity is performed? The answer is no: due to the load-speed relationship, recruitment patterns, and exercise-induced depletion, the drain on the phosphagen system is not maximal; therefore, a shorter recovery period can be used for repeat performance [30]. An exception to this strategy would be made, however, if the goal is to optimize performance in the phosphagen system: in this case, longer rest is more beneficial. The longer rest increases the amount of phosphocreatine re-synthesis and enhances the system-specific adaptations, again underscoring the importance of goal-specific programming [5, 66].

◆ Intermediate Energy – Glycolysis

The phosphagen system efficiently maintains ATP because phosphagen is simply being mobilized from one molecule to another. As ATP and CP stores yield energy, their form changes to dysfunctional byproducts (ADP, Pi, +H), which build up in the cell. ADP can be split to adenosine mono-phosphate (AMP) to fuel enzymes, but its form can no longer drive contractions. If more energy is required to produce work, the source of the energy will shift from the cell's phosphagen stores to CHO. Phosphagen enzyme activities adjust as CP availability declines. This change signals to the cell that it must initiate support from sugar or CHO metabolism. However, this energy must be derived from **glucose**, a 6-carbon sugar molecule. The CHOs stored in the muscle are made from glucose and water, referred to as **glycogen**; when phosphagen can no longer support work, glycogen must be broken down to glucose to create ATP. Because of the added complexity of the molecule, the process takes several steps and numerous catalysts to produce ATP. In this anaerobic process, known as **glycolysis** (sugar-splitting), ten controlled chemical reactions occur so that ATP synthesizes, and energy metabolites become available for ongoing work.

DEFINITIONS

Glucose –

A simple sugar molecule that provides the primary source of metabolized fuel for the glycolytic energy system.

Glycogen –

Storage form of carbohydrates in the body which is broken down to fuel mechanical work: primary storage sites include skeletal muscles and the liver.

Glycolysis –

Metabolic process involving the breakdown of sugars (glucose) through a series of reactions to provide energy (ATP) during anaerobic work.

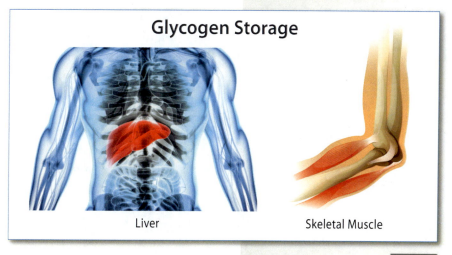

Glycogen Storage — Liver — Skeletal Muscle

Reaction Number	Reaction	Enzyme
1	Glucose + ATP → glucose 6-phosphate + ADP + H$^+$	Hexokinase
2	Glucose 6-phosphate ⇌ fructose 6-phosphate	Phosphoglucose isomerase
3	Fructose 6-phosphate + ATP → fructose 1,6-bisphosphate + ADP + H$^+$	Phosphofructokinase
4	Fructose 1,6-bisphosphate ⇌ dihydroxyacetone phosphate + glyceraldehyde 3-phosphate	Aldolase
5	Dihydroxyacetone phosphate ⇌ glyceraldehyde 3-phosphate	Triose phosphate isomerase
6	Glyceraldehyde 3-phosphate + Pi + NAD$^+$ ⇌ 1,3-bisphosphoglycerate + NADH + H$^+$	Glyceraldehyde 3-phosphate dehydrogenase
7	1,3-Bisphosphoglycerate + ADP ⇌ 3-phosphoglycerate + ATP	Phosphoglycerate kinase
8	3-Phosphoglycerate ⇌ 2-phosphoglycerate	Phosphoglycerate mutase
9	2-Phosphoglycerate ⇌ phosphoenolpyruvate + H$_2$O	Enolase
10	Phosphoenolpyruvate + ADP + H$^+$ → pyruvate + ATP	Pyruvate kinase

The more reactions required to form ATP, the longer the process takes and the less force the muscle cell can produce as a result. When stored ATP splits, it produces 100% force capacity because all the energy is immediately available. Because CP must donate a phosphate to ADP to re-synthesize ATP before it can be split for energy, the yield force capacity drops to 95-97%. And, when the ten-step glycolytic process takes over ATP production, maximal power output suffers an even greater decline. The energy released from ATP produced from glycolytic means is less than the energy provided by the immediate phosphagen sources. This explains why a person can lift more weight for three repetitions than he or she can for eight repetitions. The energy system employed composes a key element in maximal force output during a given activity.

The breakdown of CHOs, like most reactions, employs water as an assistive catalyst, along with enzymes, to fracture glucose into its respective parts outside of the mitochondria. Anaerobic glycolysis is unique in that glucose is the only carbon-fuel nutrient that yields energy without the use of oxygen. Fats and proteins cannot be employed anaerobically. However, fat, protein, and glucose can all be tapped to produce energy via aerobic metabolism, inside the mitochondria. In this instance, the hydrogen ions are essentially pulled off the different carbon fuels and transferred to molecular oxygen (O$_2$) to make water (H$_2$O). The anaerobic breakdown of glucose through glycolysis occurs without oxygen and, therefore, does not produce water. Consequently, the liberated hydrogen ions (which are very acidic) remain free in solution, increasing the acidity of the surrounding environment. From a practical perspective, this can be understood when considering discomfort: more H+ ions create a more acidic environment inside the body. A casual jog creates no discomfort as oxygen fuels aerobic metabolism, and there is not a significant increase in hydrogen ion concentration. The low force output of this activity does not require the use of phosphagen or anaerobic glycolysis to support it. On the other hand, weight lifting becomes uncomfortable because of the primarily anaerobic energy systems employed. When taxed, the anaerobic system rapidly increases the hydrogen concentration in the cell. The hydrogen promotes an acidic internal environment, which signals the need for oxygen. This causes **ischemic** stress and discomfort. Additionally, as the hydrogen concentration in the cell builds, the resultant pH changes inhibit the metabolic reactions and cause fatigue. Acids generally slow down metabolic activity by inhibiting the catalyst that helps facilitate the enzymatic reactions. This explains why aerobic activities can be performed for a long time, whereas anaerobic actions requiring high force cannot.

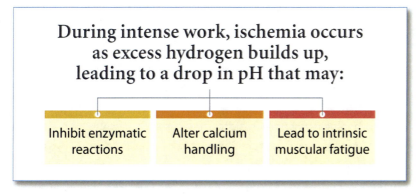

Most of the energy generated through glycolysis does not suffice to form high-bond ATP, and the body loses it as heat during each step in the process. The products of glycolysis include two molecules of ATP and two energy substrates: **lactic acid** (lactate) or **pyruvate**, depending on the work being done. When oxygen is available, pyruvate is the byproduct and is shuttled to an aerobic pathway to be further broken down to produce more energy. But when oxygen is limited, as during high-intensity work, the body converts pyruvate into lactate to support the anaerobic work. Although the process efficiency is only about 33%, significant energy can be derived from anaerobic glycolysis due to high glycolytic enzyme concentrations present in the muscle tissue as well as the speed of the associated reactions [7, 24, 84]. The ATP derived from this system is the major contributor to prolonged activities of maximal effort lasting up to 90 seconds [5, 7]. Therefore, anaerobic glycolysis is the primary energy system to fuel the average weight lifting set and the energy needs between burst actions in most sports like soccer and basketball.

When fueled by sugar, anaerobic metabolism commonly produces a burning sensation in active tissue. The discomfort and pain mentioned earlier result from insufficient oxygen, not lactic acid as many people think. Lactic acid is the buffer for the hydrogen by-product produced during intense work. It represents the internal cellular condition when oxygen supply cannot meet the oxygen demand [80]. Muscle ischemia causes pain, similar to the pain experienced if you placed a rubber band on the end of your finger to occlude blood flow or that associated with a myocardial infarction. During moderate levels of activity, the cellular pH stays in balance as the rate of energy re-synthesis matches energy utilization. However, this balance cannot be maintained during intense work. As the excess hydrogen builds up it promotes an ischemic environment [115, 116]. This (acidic-ischemic) environment leads to a drop in pH which may inhibit enzymatic reactions, alter calcium management, and lead to intrinsic localized muscular fatigue [115, 116]. Importantly, however, lactic acid is not the enemy that many have claimed it to be: on the contrary, it is essentially a sugar "part" that can be passed to a neighboring cell with adequate oxygen and turned back to pyruvate to yield additional energy [15, 80]. Lactate can also be transported in the blood to other skeletal muscles, the liver, the kidneys, the brain, or to the heart, where it can be efficiently metabolized. Although this can occur during exercise, lactic acid utilization commonly features importantly in the recovery phase.

DEFINITIONS

Ischemic (ischemia) –

A low oxygen state usually due to obstruction of arterial blood supply or inadequate blood flow leading to tissue hypoxia.

Lactic acid (lactate) –

Energy substrate produced as an end-product of glycolysis that can be used by various tissues of the body as fuel to continue ongoing work (e.g., aerobic cells, heart); it serves as a buffer for hydrogen ions created by sugar metabolism.

Pyruvate –

An energy substrate that results as an end-product of sugar metabolism during glycolysis in the presence of oxygen.

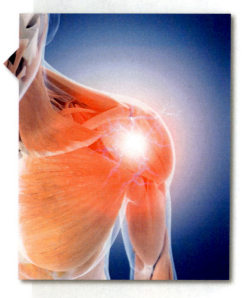

DEFINITIONS

Gluconeogenesis –

The creation of new glucose in the liver from other organic molecules, such as pyruvate, lactate, glycerol, and amino acids.

Cori cycle –

Name given to the process of lactate and pyruvate recycling in the liver to produce new glucose.

QUICK INSIGHT

Lactic acid (lactate) has been misrepresented as a detrimental byproduct of glycolysis, but this view is short-sighted and antiquated [15]. Ongoing exercise requires large amounts of ATP from metabolic sources to sustain work production. The body has contingency plans for all the substrate byproducts from metabolism. In this way, the body has potential energy stores ready to be converted to kinetic energy as dictated by exercise duration and intensity. Very little ATP results from glycolysis, and CHO substrates pyruvate and lactate are left over from the glycolytic process; the body can utilize this potential chemical energy by converting the carbon skeletons back to glucose in the liver [7]. Lactate and pyruvate enter a biochemical process of **gluconeogenesis** called the **Cori cycle**. In this process, the body can utilize the lactic acid produced from high-intensity activities to help preserve blood glucose levels. Blood glucose levels are crucial to physiological function, particularly in the brain, which, despite making up approximately 2% of the body's mass, represents 20% of blood glucose utilization [15, 70]. The remanufactured glucose from exercise byproducts can also be used to replenish liver and muscle glycogen stores [88], which suggests the important benefit of lactate.

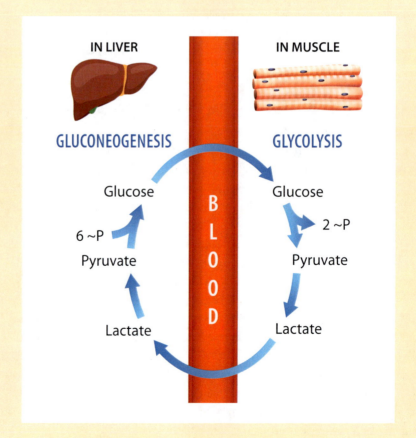

◆ Energy System Transition

The body maintains ATP levels through metabolic processes that take place either in the **cytosol** of the cell or in the mitochondria. Anaerobic processes occur in the cytosol and use fuel from phosphocreatine, glucose, glycogen, glycerol, and **deaminated** amino acids. These processes can contribute to maximal biological work lasting approximately three minutes. For activities lasting beyond three minutes, ATP re-synthesis occurs primarily through cellular oxidation via the **aerobic system**. This refers to the mitochondrial oxidation of fatty acids (fats), pyruvate from glucose (CHOs), and some deaminated amino acids (protein). Cellular oxidation in the human body reverses the process of photosynthesis: plants take CO_2 and H_2O to produce O_2 and glucose, lipids, and protein; the human body does the exact opposite.

QUICK INSIGHT

Transitioning Through the Energy Systems

A person rowing on an ergometer as fast as he or she can will travel through the energy pathways, experiencing a decline in force output as the weaker, more complex energy systems activate. The ATP-CP used in the first 10 seconds corresponds with the highest force output. As the body transitions from energy derived primarily from the phosphagen system to the glycolytic pathway, the rate of hydrogen ion accumulation begins to dramatically increase. Force production now declines relative to the rower's conditioning, as the acidity created from the H+ begins to slow down the glycolytic process. A well-trained rower will maintain a relatively high force output for 90-180 seconds, but, at some point, the activity speed will deteriorate due to the buildup of energy byproducts. The decline in anaerobic energy availability, muscle and liver glycogen, is met by an equal increase in energy production from aerobic sources. The rate of movement declines linearly with the decreasing anaerobic energy contribution due to consequential reduction in contractile force associated with aerobic metabolism.

DEFINITIONS

Cytosol –

The cytoplasmic fluid which surrounds all organelles within a cell.

Deaminate –

The process by which the liver breaks down a protein by removing an amino group for use as potential fuel; glutamate is also deaminated in the kidneys.

Aerobic system –

Metabolic pathway wherein the mitochondrion utilizes fats, pyruvate from carbohydrates, and amino acids from protein to produce ATP in the presence of oxygen.

Metabolic equivalent (MET) –

A measurement of energy use expressed as multiples of the resting metabolic rate; one MET equals an oxygen uptake rate of 3.5 ml of O_2 per kg of body weight per min of work (3.5 ml·kg-1·min-1).

At rest, the body uses the aerobic pathway, because its physical intensity is at the lowest waking level, 1 metabolic equivalent. A **metabolic equivalent**, or MET, represents a measurable quantity of oxygen used by the body. When a person goes from a state of rest (1 MET) to jogging on a treadmill (6-8 METS), the body's demand for oxygen changes significantly. So, at the onset of exercise, oxygen consumption undergoes a transitional phase to attempt to meet the new demand, and this creates an oxygen deficit. Physiological actions transpire to equalize the difference between the oxygen requirement of the activity and the oxygen available at the cell. The adrenal glands secrete hormones in recognition of the new stress, which triggers a response to promote oxygen delivery; this explains why the heart rate (HR) increases.

Consider this example. Measured by force production,

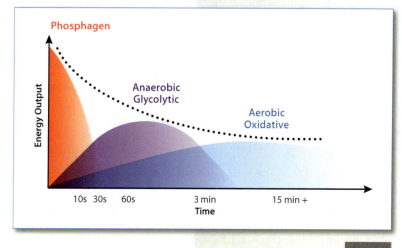

> **DEFINITIONS**
>
> **Anaerobic system –**
>
> *One of two major metabolic pathways, the ATP-PC phosphagen system or anaerobic glycolysis, that produces energy without the presence of oxygen. Anaerobic systems provide the energy for high power, high intensity activities.*
>
> **Steady state –**
>
> *A condition within the human body which indicates that the current level of oxygen utilization matches demand, signified by a leveling off or steady heart rate; it allows for minimal variance in heart rate (+/- 5 bpm) and other cardiovascular measures if the workload is not changed.*
>
> **Oxygen deficit –**
>
> *The difference between total oxygen consumed during the transition to steady state and the actual amount of oxygen required by the working tissues; it must be paid back after work is discontinued, resulting in an elevation in oxygen consumption (e.g., being out of breath after a sprint).*
>
> **Excess post-exercise oxygen consumption (EPOC) –**
>
> *A measurable increase in the rate of oxygen consumption following strenuous activity due to a deficit created by the work; it increases metabolism for hours after the bout as dictated by the duration, type, and intensity of the exercise.*

jogging is a low-intensity exercise, so the body does not necessarily need the **anaerobic system** to support the action. The body can manage the low force demands through aerobic metabolism independently. However, the body cannot just turn systems on and off. At the onset of exercise, the body must make cardiorespiratory adjustments to deal with the increased oxygen demands of the activity, which takes a few minutes. In the first three minutes of the exercise, the body deals with the abrupt change in intensity using energy from the anaerobic system. As time passes, these adjustments allow the aerobic system to come on-line, and oxygen is used to manage the stress of the exercise. When the utilization of oxygen matches the demand, the body is said to have reached metabolic **steady state**: HR and oxygen utilization level off and are maintained with minimal variance (+/- 5 bpm).

During the transition to steady state, the borrowed energy from anaerobic sources creates an **oxygen deficit**. This term quantitatively expresses the difference between the total oxygen consumed during the transition to steady state and the actual amount of oxygen required by the cells. When exercise stops, the body again

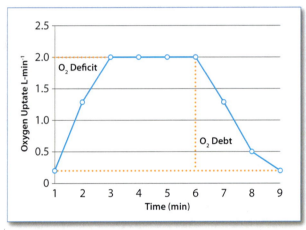

experiences a temporary state of disruption. **Excess post-exercise oxygen consumption (EPOC)**, historically referred to as oxygen debt, persists after exercise, representing the excess oxygen consumption needed to recover from the physical activity and to return the body to resting homeostasis. During short aerobic bouts of exercise at a mild intensity, about 50% of the oxygen recovery will occur within 30 seconds following exercise completion. This is termed the "fast component" and is used primarily to re-synthesize high-energy phosphates and replenish oxygen in the body fluids and muscle stores (myoglobin). Intense exercise and exercise of long duration cause an additional, longer-lasting phase of excess post-exercise oxygen consumption, termed the "slow component", which can last up to 24 hours following exercise [60, 98].

EPOC is attributed to:

- An elevated body temperature persisting post-exercise
- Ion-leakage across cell membranes, leading to greater reliance on active ionic transport across the membrane to preserve homeostasis
- Mitochondrial calcium uptake during exercise, reducing aerobic efficiency
- Increased levels of thermogenic hormones existing post-exercise
- The re-synthesis of glycogen in the liver from lactate
- The oxidation of the lactate in the mitochondria

All of the above processes require oxygen and burn additional calories. Transient bouts of high intensity exercise, such as interval training and weight lifting, can produce recovery oxygen periods lasting greater than an hour [61, 106, 111].

QUICK INSIGHT

While the body has the ability to manage most circumstances, it is the familiarity with a situation that leads to improved efficiency. Individuals who repeatedly train at higher intensities experience adaptations that allow the body to handle all levels of training much more proficiently than would an untrained individual. Trained persons experience significantly faster metabolic transition periods: from resting homeostasis to high level actions and back to rest. It is important to understand that exercise does not entail switching on and off different energy systems, but rather is a smooth blending and overlap of energy transfer from one pathway to another. All three systems interact constantly to manage homeostasis, but certain activities require greater contributions from particular systems. No system ever shuts off completely. With exercise training, the process of energy transfer among pathways becomes smoother, allowing trained individuals to reach exercise homeostasis sooner, a common marker of improved performance. In trained individuals, the complementary relationship between the energy systems increases metabolic harmony. The aerobic system cooperatively buffers the anaerobic system, while the anaerobic system more efficiently supports the aerobic system processes.

DEFINITIONS

Krebs cycle –

A series of enzymatic reactions that occur in the mitochondria involving aerobic metabolism of acetyl compounds which produce ATP for cellular energy; it is also known as citric acid cycle or the tricarboxylic acid (TCA) cycle.

Oxidative phosphorylation –

The formation of ATP energy created by the aerobic breakdown of various substrates, especially the organic compounds involved in the Krebs cycle.

Aerobic Metabolism

The previous section identified that the body transitions smoothly from one energy system to another. The shift from anaerobic metabolism to aerobic metabolism is initiated with the pyruvate molecules left over from the 10th step in glycolysis. The pyruvate is mobilized into the mitochondria, the organelle that houses enzymes and substrates used to make cellular fuel. The mitochondria functions like an organic blender, mixing oxygen and organic material freed by enzymes to feed the cell. When the pyruvate enters the mitochondria, it sparks the reaction called the citric acid cycle, tricarboxylic acid (TCA) cycle, or **Krebs cycle**. The Krebs cycle refers to the process in which energy or ATP is formed using oxygen and energy substrates called **oxidative phosphorylation**. Inside the organelle, glucose, oxygen, metabolic intermediates, and enzymes interact through 8 reactions to produce water, carbon dioxide, heat, and ATP.

The mitochondrial concentration within the muscle cell directly relates to the amount of energy that can be produced through aerobic means. In aerobic exercise, the three largest determinants of efficiency are the number and size of mitochondria, the concentration of enzymes inside them, and the amount of oxygen-rich blood which can be delivered to the cell. These factors also relate to the adaptations to muscle tissue when aerobic exercise is routinely employed. The metabolic pathway is characterized by the release of hydrogen ions from the metabolic intermediates NADH and FADH2 and the release of carbon dioxide as the CHO and oxygen molecules are transformed through the metabolic process.

The same process can be performed using **lipids** (fats) and proteins after they have been broken down into usable parts. When the body rests or functions at lower work intensities, lipids

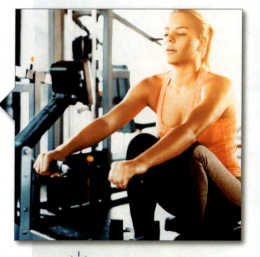

DEFINITIONS

Lipids –

Various classes of organic compounds composed of fatty acids or their derivatives; dietary sources include oils, fats, waxes, and cholesterol, while endogenous (internal) sources include free fatty acids, triglycerides, lipoproteins, and phospholipids.

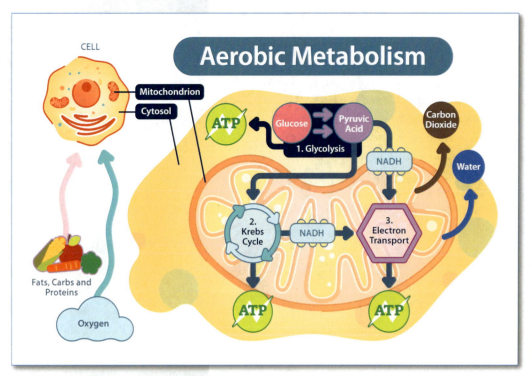

become the primary source of energy through aerobic metabolism. **FatMax** refers to the optimal work intensity for lipid metabolism, the highest intensity at which the body can work and maximize the aerobic oxidation of lipids. It usually lies between 40-70% of VO_2 max [47] and 60-80% HRmax. While training increases this value, most people reach FatMax at 60-65% of VO_2 max [16]. Interestingly, most people exercise to burn fat, but fat is actually the predominant fuel used for resting metabolism. For instance, when a person sits on the couch to watch TV or sits at his or her desk at work, approximately 70% of the aerobic energy is derived from lipid metabolism. This proportionately high value increases to roughly 80% during sleep. This may cause one to think increasing rest or sleep would increase fat metabolism, which is arguably true; however, at rest, the human body burns very few calories per hour compared to the metabolic costs of physical activity for the same duration. This fact limits the contribution of resting metabolism to weight loss and also contributes to the misconception that exercise for weight loss should be performed in the **fat-burning zone**. Though low intensity exercise (<60% of maximal aerobic output) utilizes fat as the preferred fuel, the low caloric expenditure reduces its benefits for weight loss unless durations are prolonged to 90 minutes. During low to moderate exercise, it takes approximately 10 minutes of continuous movement for lipids to significantly contribute to aerobic energy, so longer durations of exercise actually increase FatMax, a benefit for endurance.

In part, raising lipid use during activity takes substantial time because it requires significant processing to break it down into usable parts. **Triglycerides** represent 90% of the fat the body

DEFINITIONS

FatMax –

Is the highest intensity of work that can be performed where fat is the primary fuel for energy; it is also known as the aerobic limit.

Fat-burning zone –

Lower-intensity training (<65% of VO_2max) where the predominant fuel source is fat, as aerobic pathways can maintain the workload; not necessarily an optimal weight loss method as the relative quantity of total calories burned remains low compared to higher intensities.

Triglycerides –

Consist of a glycerol and three fatty acids bound together in a single large molecule; they serve as an important energy source and form much of the body's stored fat.

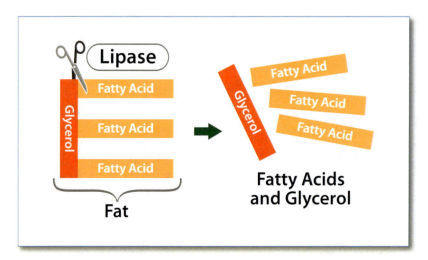

stores in **adipose tissue**. The enzyme, **lipase**, in the presence of water, splits triglycerides into a glycerol molecule and three fatty acids through **lipolysis**. The fatty acids hold most of the energy to be used by the muscle cell. These bind to plasma **albumin** to form **free fatty acids** (FFA) in the blood stream, where they can be transported to working tissue. Lipids can also be delivered by **lipoproteins** and freed to be used as fuel. The more oxygen-rich blood flow to the tissue, the greater the propensity for fat to be burned for energy. Individuals who routinely engage in aerobic exercise enhance their ability to use lipids for fuel because they have more mitochondria and capillaries. These adaptations improve CHO-sparing and increase exercise capacity, as fat can be utilized more efficiently. Additionally, exercise mediates lipid mobilization via the hormones epinephrine, growth hormone (GH), and glucagon. Hormone augmentation factors importantly in training adaptation. Many endurance athletes use long slow distance (LSD) training to improve these and other mechanisms of lipid metabolism [10].

When the lipids reach the cell, they have two pathways into oxidative phosphorylation. The glycerol molecule enters the same way glucose does by first forming pyruvate. Remember, all these molecules are essentially carbon chains of hydrogen and oxygen, so they can simply donate or accept ions to become something else. The fatty acids cannot enter this cycle in their current form: they first must go through a process in the mitochondria called **beta oxidation** via the protein complex that houses the **electron transport chain** (ETC). Here, the fatty acid molecules are reduced to **acetyl CoA**, a much smaller component that makes it easier to enter the Krebs cycle. Beta oxidation continues until the entire fatty acid molecule has been broken down and used. Through this process, a single triglyceride molecule can yield 460 ATP, which is more than 10 times more energy than a glucose molecule (30-36ATP) can provide. The glycerol backbone contributes to 19 ATP, while the three fatty acids provide 441 ATP. This clearly illustrates why lipids represent a valuable source of energy for the body and why it requires a lot of physical activity to reduce excess fat stores on the body.

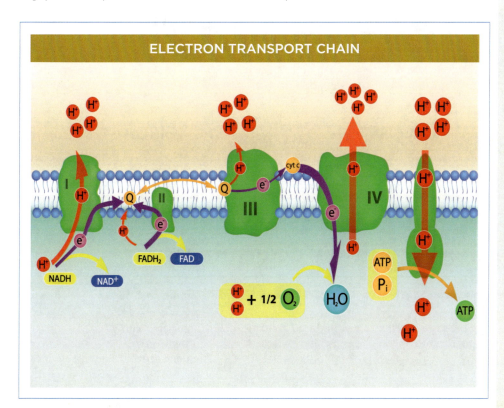

DEFINITIONS

Adipose tissue –
The storage form of fat tissue in the human body, which can be broken down for the liberation of necessary energy.

Lipase –
A specific enzyme capable of breaking down lipid molecules (fat stores) in the body.

Free fatty acids –
Liberated lipid molecules found in blood plasma that represent ~10% of fat in the body; due to the insolubility of fat, FFA must be bound and transported through the blood by the protein albumin

Lipolysis –
The breakdown of triglycerides from fat storage in the body for potential liberation into circulation to serve energy needs.

Albumin –
A blood protein produced in the liver that functions as a transporter for various molecules including FFA, hormones, and calcium.

Lipoproteins –
Protein-based compounds that transport various forms of lipids, such as cholesterol, in the bloodstream; there are high and low-density lipoproteins which serve various functions and have different implications related to the risk for heart disease.

Beta oxidation –
The process by which fats are oxidized, or broken down, in the mitochondria to produce acetyl CoA.

Electron transport chain –
A group of compounds which expedite a series of oxidation-reduction reactions for eventual aerobic production of ATP within the mitochondria.

Acetyl CoA –
Compound that functions as a co-enzyme in various biological reactions and is formed as an intermediate for the metabolism of carbohydrates, fats, or proteins in the mitochondria; it is critical in the first step of the Krebs Cycle.

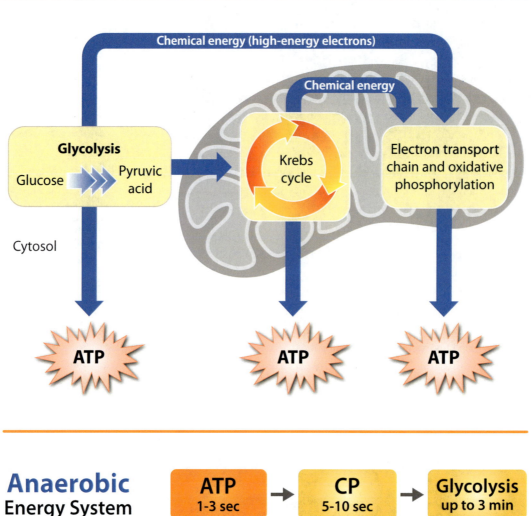

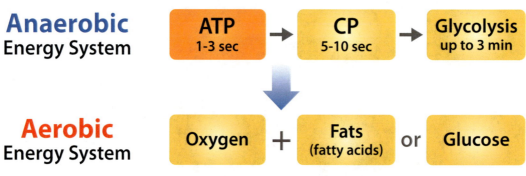

◆ Anaerobic Work to Increase Aerobic Capacity

If the work rate increases, the body again shifts to a greater reliance on glucose metabolism through both anaerobic and aerobic pathways. Metabolizing CHOs over fats proceeds much faster and provides a powerful energy source to support elevated force requirements, though the total amount of ATP that can be produced is only a fraction of that possible via lipid metabolism. A person on a Stairmaster™ who performs high-intensity intervals will notice the change in energy system contribution: he or she will experience an increase in ventilation and peripheral leg-muscle discomfort due to the increasing presence of hydrogen ions from glucose metabolism. For improvements in maximum aerobic capacity, CHOs are a necessary fuel, as they allow for training at higher intensities compared to lipid metabolism. High intensities create significant stress on the body, which allows for greater adaptations. Limited physiological adaptations occur at low intensities because the level of work stays below the threshold for a new perceived stress. Once adaptations to a stress occur, no new improvements will result unless the exercise demands increase.

When the body experiences prolonged energy demands, it can also elicit assistance from **amino acids** freed from protein sources [33, 79]. Cortisol released during exercise provides energy to working tissue by removing proteins from lean tissue. The **branched chain amino acids (BCAAs)** are particularly sensitive to catabolism, and, once liberated from muscle protein, they are transported to the liver and deaminated into keto-acidic carbon skeletons [3, 107]. These deaminated keto-acid skeletons can now enter the metabolic process as precursors to glucose or Krebs cycle intermediates. This ability to strip the nitrogen from the amino acid molecule also exists in the muscle itself in a process called **transamination**. Specific enzymes which break down muscle protein or amino acids in the cell increase as an adaptive response to endurance training. This partially explains total body weight loss (lean and fat mass) with endurance training, as the nitrogen removed from the amino acid is secreted through the kidneys via urea, highlighting the importance of adequate fluid intake. Muscle loss is associated with high-volume endurance training, particularly when exogenous CHO and/or protein intake are inadequate to support the volume of exercise [107, 122]. Depending on the type of protein and subsequent amino acids released, the route to entry into the Krebs cycle proceeds through several mechanisms [6, 113]. Amino acids can be turned into pyruvate, acetyl CoA, or enter through hydrogen ion exchange called electron transport. During prolonged exercise, using pyruvate is the preferred method. It should be noted that protein preservation during extended exercise requires adequate CHO consumption and storage.

DEFINITIONS

Amino acids –

Organic molecules consisting of hydrogen, carbon, oxygen, and nitrogen that combine to form the basic elements of proteins.

Branched chain amino acids (BCAAs) –

Includes leucine, isoleucine and valine; they serve as a potential fuel source during long-duration exercise bouts, have a nitrogen-sparing effect, and can bypass the liver and become available for uptake by muscle directly from circulation.

Transamination –

A reversible process involved in both anabolism and catabolism by which excess amino acids are diverted toward energy production as an amino group is transferred from one molecule to another.

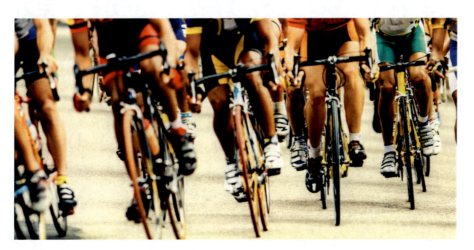

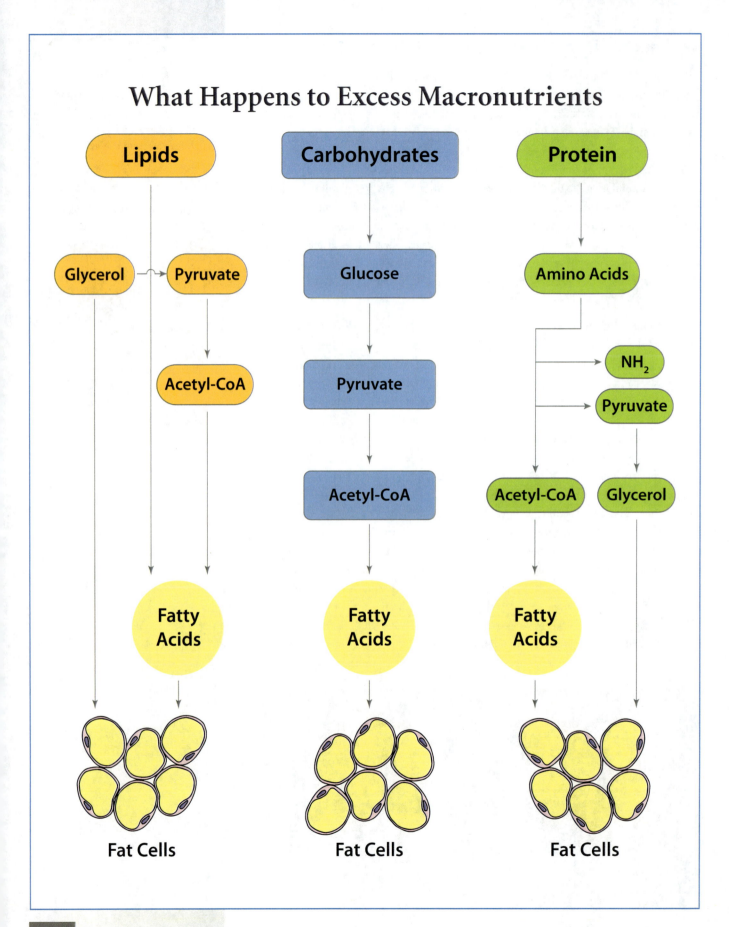

Muscular Fatigue

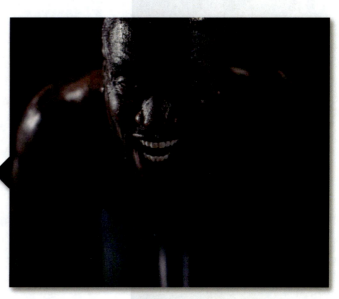

Lipid metabolism sustains low exercise intensity so that glycogen reserves may be spared. When the intensity elevates to moderately-high exercise or intermittent, high-intensity bouts, energy reserves deplete with increasing exercise duration [6]. The depletion rate of energy in particular fiber types is specific to the exercise intensity. Shorter duration bouts demanding high force output, such as one-minute sprints or heavy weight training, tend to deplete energy stores of fast-twitch fibers. In contrast, the slow twitch fibers become depleted during continuous low or repetitive bouts of moderately-high intensity. As would be expected, energy depletion is a factor of total muscle recruitment and time under tension.

Fatigue sets in when the body experiences significant decline in muscle and liver glycogen stores along with elevated byproduct concentration within the muscle cell. Energy depletion is related to intensity because it forecasts the demand for fuel and the rate of byproduct production. Since fats and proteins cannot support anaerobic exercise when sugars are gone, performance capabilities at higher intensities are lost. This pertains not only to maximal periods of exercise but to submaximal aerobic exercise as well. Even at levels where oxygen and lipids adequately meet the intensity demands of the work, the lack of CHOs in the body causes significant fatigue [13]. Endurance sports participants refer to this phenomenon as hitting the wall or "bonking." System inefficiency results from several sources: the necessity for glucose to support nervous system functions, the slow rate of lipid metabolism, and the consequent need for pyruvate to initiate oxidative phosphorylation [69, 74]. Untrained individuals experience an even higher rate of fatigue due to high levels of inefficiency and increased production of the rate-limiting enzymes at the same relative intensities [76]. Regardless, insufficient CHO intake leads to early decline in performance among both trained and untrained exercisers [76].

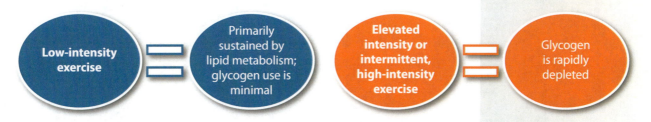

When inadequate CHO consumption occurs for an extended period of time, muscle and liver glycogen stores cannot be sustained at an adequate level to support activity, and the metabolic systems become dysfunctional. As mentioned earlier, a lack of CHO means a reduced quantity of pyruvate production in the mitochondria [21]. This lack of pyruvate consequently affects the quantity of **oxaloacetate** (byproduct of pyruvate metabolism) and its availability to bind with acetyl CoA to enter the Krebs cycle. This underscores the importance of adequate CHO intake to support lipolysis, as fatty acid metabolism will only occur when sufficient oxaloacetate is available for acetyl CoA produced through beta-oxidation [20]. This presents two problems: first, lipid metabolism yields only about half the power as that of CHOs; second, when CHOs are not available, the rate of lipid metabolism falls. Because CHO availability is lacking,

DEFINITIONS

Oxaloacetate –

An intermediate of the Krebs cycle that binds with acetyl-CoA to form citrate; it helps facilitate aerobic energy production.

the body requires lipids as the source for aerobic ATP formation. In this metabolic environment, **central fatigue** (via global neural mechanisms) and **general peripheral fatigue** (via local muscular mechanisms) inhibit performance [35].

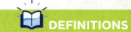

DEFINITIONS

Central fatigue –

Occurs with insufficient or systemic depletion of CHOs, resulting in reduced motor unit recruitment and firing rate; reflects a conscious and subconscious decision to reduce the intensity of exercise until energy replenishment and/or recovery have provided fuel for the re-initiation of work.

General peripheral fatigue –

Occurs with a lack of energy in working tissues due to low pre-exercise stores or localized depletion of anaerobic energy stores; acute rest intervals will not help, as muscular energy provisions are too low.

QUICK INSIGHT

Buffering That Muscular Burn

The body employs natural buffers that counteract the shift in pH associated with the glycolytic pathways during exercise performance. As liberated hydrogen ions rise, pH levels decline, adversely affecting enzyme activity and triggering an inhibitory response to muscle contractility. In lower-intensity activities, lactate moves to the liver to reformulate glucose through a process called gluconeogenesis. When production of lactic acid is met by equal buffering mechanisms (appearance = clearance), an exercise homeostasis is established. Due to the pH equilibrium, there are no metabolic consequences or disruptions. With increasing intensities, the tissue produces more acid (lactate and H+) than can be buffered by normal means. If the body is unable to compensate, the quantity of acid in the blood can reach high levels, dropping pH down to 6.8 from its comfortable 7.4. This generally is the point of physical exhaustion. Individuals will suffer nausea, headaches, vomiting, cramps, and even disorientation due to the total body acidity [87]. At this point, the body shuts down to allow the acid to be buffered in a process to regain homeostasis.

To prevent this from occurring, the body will increase its buffering capabilities through chemical, renal, and ventilatory adjustments. Chemical buffering is enhanced by an increase in bicarbonate formation and phosphate buffers [67, 68]. Renal buffering occurs via a shift in the rate of reabsorption of buffering agents with a concurrent increase in the number of hydrogen ions released into urine. Ventilation can also serve to buffer the blood by increasing the rate of carbon dioxide released by the body, consequently reducing carbonic acid concentrations and increasing fluid alkalinity [67].

Some theorize that buffering adaptations may occur in response to near maximal or maximal training efforts lasting 1-2 minutes, but increased buffering adaptations in the untrained can be seen with almost any level of increased activity. To assist with buffering, sodium bicarbonate and sodium citrate solutions can be consumed prior to events or training that are prolonged and primarily dependent on the glycolytic pathway and before 1-2-minute, all-out exercise bouts. These scenarios have been tested in experiments, showing positive effects. More research is needed, but the solutions seem to have a positive effect on hydrogen efflux (removal of acid) from the cells. No benefit has been shown in events lasting less than one minute, so it has little implication for traditional strength training.

When the anaerobic system is considered, fatigue again relates specifically to the intensity and duration of the training and the levels of pre-exercise energy storage. Depletion of stored ATP and CP during short, intense bouts of exercise is similar in untrained and trained individuals, with the differences lying in the trained individuals' increased ability to resynthesize CP during subsequent repetitions. In **acute peripheral fatigue**, increased lactic acid formation creates a temporary acidic environment that inhibits enzymatic reactions vital to the anaerobic pathway [54]. The increasing acidity negatively affects cellular activity because enzymes function at specific pH levels [55]. The low pH inactivates enzymes for energy metabolism and negatively effects contractility, causing the muscles' force output to decline [10]. Note that this specific type of acute fatigue does not result from energy depletion but rather from a temporary internal environment. Training that emphasizes the glycolytic pathway exposes the body to higher levels of lactate on a routine basis, enabling a higher lactate tolerance. With acute peripheral fatigue, the system needs time to utilize oxygen and buffer some of the acid, removing the inhibiting factors that contributed to the drop in pH. Once the pH rises, the exercise can be repeated. Peripheral fatigue is not temporary, as it is associated with depletion of energy provisions. Again, the rate of decline is linked with the intensity and time-under-tension. As mentioned, intense exercise causes high rates of glucose usage, whereas low intensity spares glucose. Performance decline, whether referring to speed, strength, or power, is directly related and linear to the decline of muscle glycogen [34]. When different muscles are used, as seen in a resistance training session, the rate of fatigue is inversely related to the total amount of tissue used for work. Dispersing the work over many muscle areas, as opposed to single tissues, avoids rapid depletion in individual muscle groups. Isolated muscle group activity, such as repeated sprint training or lower body plyometrics, can only be performed at high intensity for short training bouts due to the localized energy depletion of the lower extremities.

DEFINITIONS

Acute peripheral fatigue –

Occurs when cells experience dysfunction due to a metabolic reduction in pH; acid limits enzyme activity, requiring buffering compounds before work can be re-initiated.

Rest period –

The period of rest in between sets or structured periods of activity within a single exercise bout; the length of these intervals is dictated by the energy systems involved during the sets of work.

Recovery period –

The period of time in between separate exercise bouts so adaptations may occur.

◆ Recovery

Periods of recovery enable working tissue to avoid fatigue for longer periods of time. In highly intense, short burst activity, the muscles perform at peak or near peak levels, which leads to rapid fatigue. When the action stops for a time, the muscle fiber attempts to return to pre-exertion levels. The period of time between repeated actions, such as a sprint or squat performance, is called the **rest period** or rest interval. During this period of time, the muscle cell's recovery depends upon the return of intracellular energy supply, circulatory-based cellular by-product removal (reperfusion), and the delivery of oxygen. When the exercise bout halts completely, the cell has a much longer period of time to manage the disruption caused by the activity. This is referred to as the **recovery period**. During recovery from exercise, muscle fibers can rebuild their energy reserves to normal pre-exertion levels and fix any damage resulting from the production of force. The duration of the recovery period required to return the cell back to normal depends upon the degree and duration of the muscle fiber use [17, 28]. In cases of sustained high-level output, full recovery may take as long as one week [4]. To maximize safe and efficient training, recovery between exercise bouts must be an important consideration in the exercise prescription.

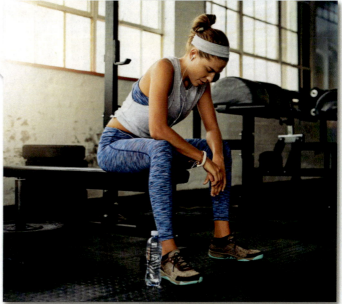

Central and Peripheral Fatigue Responses to Exercise and Recovery [18]

Acute Peripheral Fatigue	General Peripheral Fatigue	Central Fatigue
\multicolumn{3}{Characteristics of Fatigue via Exercise Intensity, Duration, and Recovery Characteristics}

Characteristics of Fatigue via Exercise Intensity, Duration, and Recovery Characteristics

Exercise Intensity and Recovery

Intensity: High Intensity (Sprints or Near Maximal Muscle Contraction)
- All muscle fibers recruited
- Metabolite accumulation occurs

Recovery: Recovery time is fast (<30s) after cessation and return of blood flow to the muscles, allowing for by-product buffering

Low Intensity (low force/endurance activities) – Fatigue threshold is low, and recovery is dependent upon the total duration of the low intensity activity

Exercise Intensity and Recovery

Intensity: High Intensity (Sprints or Near Maximal Muscle Contraction)
- Decreased voluntary muscle activation as the exercise is continued
- Decreasing responsiveness of recruitment MNs (motor neurons) throughout the activity

Recovery: Can be as short as 90 sec, with longer sustained, high intensity contraction requiring up to 3-5 minutes for full recovery

Note: when eccentric exercise occurs at high intensity, muscle activation may be decreased for 24+ hours

Low Intensity (low force/ endurance activities) – a decrease may be seen in the muscle activation due to decreased motor neuron excitability for as little as 1 min after activity up to 30 mins depending on the duration of the activity.

Causes and Effects of Fatigue

Accumulation of metabolic by-products which contribute to a decrease in action potentials across the sarcolemma, a slower muscle relaxation time, and/or a lowering of cellular pH, which contributes to slower chemical reactions and reduced ability to produce ATP. Examples of metabolites associated with acute peripheral fatigue:

- Potassium
- Calcium
- Anaerobic by-products (ADP, Pi, MG [magnesium], ROS [reactive oxygen species], Lactate, and H+) leading to a decrease in cellular pH

Decreased anaerobic fuel sources

Phosphagens: ATP and CP

(ATP, CP, Muscle Glycogen, Blood Glucose)

Causes and Effects of Fatigue

Decreased neural drive from the CNS resulting in subsequent decreases in muscle activation

Sites Affected

Peripherally
Alpha Motor Neuron
Neuromuscular Junction
Local Active Muscle cells

Centrally
CNS (i.e., Brain and Spinal Cord)

Sites of Central and Peripheral Fatigue

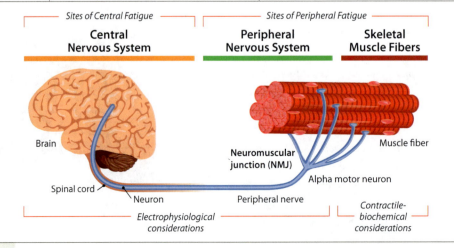

The importance of glucose and the body's reliance upon it cannot be overstated. When an intense activity demands the use of the body's endogenous CHO stores, the body attempts to refuel the depleted muscle tissue by releasing **glucagon**. This strong pancreatic hormone liberates glycogen (sugar) from the liver into the blood to aid in blood glucose homeostasis for the CNS and to fuel working tissues. Muscle tissues not being used in exercise will continue to maintain their glycogen reserves because the cells cannot donate energy to working tissues the way the liver can. Skeletal muscle cells do not contain the necessary enzymes to release glucose into the blood (glucose-6-phosphatase), as it is only found in the liver. When excessive sugars are being used, the body will attempt to reserve some glucose for the central nervous system to protect the brain via a glycogen-sparing mechanism controlled by hormones [70,76]. Therefore, the decline in performance stems not only from glycogen depletion caused by exercise, but also from the body's efforts to reserve glucose by reducing its availability through endocrine mediators. When muscle and liver glycogen depletion make glucose unavailable to serve all the actions of exercise, central fatigue will be compounded by peripheral fatigue [69]. Central fatigue signals depleted substrates and is more commonly associated with prolonged endurance training, whereas anaerobic fatigue (acute and peripheral) is mainly associated with limiting metabolites (pCr, pH).

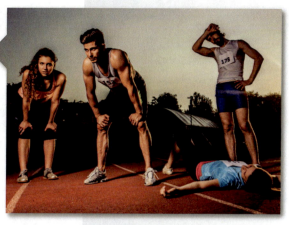

The most important component to maximizing exercise performance is the fuel available in the body. A high CHO, low fat meal consumed three hours before an event aids in available energy, but to promote maximal glycogen storage for subsequent training or events, it is more important for exercisers and athletes to consume adequate energy post-exercise [1,13]. The physiological environment created by depleted glycogen stores in the muscle and liver tissues cause a notable increase in energy substrate uptake immediately post-exercise. Scientists suggest that increased **cellular permeability** and heightened hormone sensitivity allows for increased storage capacity of glucose and protein in the four-hour period post-exercise [14]. Early literature in this area suggested that high amounts of CHOs (up to 500 g) should be consumed in 3-4 post-exercise meals [9,45]. Higher glycemic foods were recommended to allow for immediate glucose availability within the metabolic window following exercise.

 DEFINITIONS

Glucagon –

Hormone released from the pancreas to promote the breakdown of glycogen to glucose in the liver to aid in blood sugar homeostasis.

Cellular permeability –

The ability of nutrients and other substances to pass through the cellular wall: the greater the permeability, the greater the transfer of nutrients and other compounds.

The latest findings suggest that post-exercise muscle glycogen storage can be further enhanced with a CHO and protein meal (or supplement) over that of protein alone. This effect results due to the convergent interactions of CHO and protein on insulin secretion [8,71]. Studies analyzing CHO-protein recovery mixtures found that increases in both CHO and protein uptake occurring above that of the CHO-only solutions [46,125]. Additional research indicates that the rate of recovery couples with the rate of muscle glycogen replenishment, and suggests exercisers consume recovery supplements to optimize muscle glycogen synthesis and replace fluid post-exercise [89,121]. Importantly, in post-exercise replenishment, the quantity of calories should reflect the intensity and duration of the activity [8]. Low to moderate efforts do not significantly deplete glycogen stores, so increasing post-exercise consumption of calories may not be warranted. In heavy resistance training and intense endurance bouts, energy and fluid replenishment are critical for subsequent training efforts. The importance of glucose to the body's systems has been stated earlier, and the need to replenish liver and muscle glycogen stores post-exercise further emphasizes this point. A common fallacy is the importance of consuming protein when one's goal is the hypertrophy of muscle tissues. By now, it should be clear that glycogen replenishment is the primary goal of the body during and post exercise and will be prioritized over other functions and adaptations such as protein synthesis. If the goal is to build lean tissue, adequate CHO and protein intake are essential.

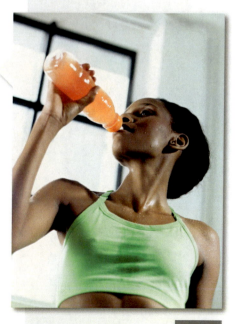

DEFINITIONS

Delayed onset muscle soreness (DOMS) –

Muscle soreness expedited by an inflammatory response to cellular damage, ischemia, and tonic spasms which presents 24-72 hours following an intense bout of exercise; common causes include performing new (unaccustomed) exercises, heavy eccentric work, and high work volume.

QUICK INSIGHT

Lactate is Not Your Enemy

Lactic acid (lactate) has been blamed for **delayed onset muscle soreness (DOMS)**, cramping, and inhibiting recovery from exercise. It is often considered to be a negative waste product from high intensity work. The reality is that none of these statements is true. Lactic acid results when glucose is metabolized during fast glycolysis. The breakdown leaves lactate and hydrogen ions as by-products. The hydrogen ions may build up under high intensity conditions that demand rapid metabolism and increase the acidity of the environment. This situation may interfere with the electrical signals from motor neurons, slow enzymatic reactions, and impair muscle contractility. With respect to lactate, however, it is a treasured fuel that is rapidly produced and easily used by metabolic tissues in the body [15]. The heart, slow twitch muscle fibers, and postural muscles thrive on lactate for energy because it is easily shuttled into the cell without insulin [81]. Lactate rapidly moves across the cell membrane through a process called facilitated transport, which enables the body to use the lactate without the detrimental effects of insulin in the blood [67, 81].

Lactate is produced in greater quantities when exercise intensity exceeds 50% of VO_2max. This production rises linearly with intensity as fast twitch fibers preferentially rely on carbohydrates for fuel. As the lactate is produced, the working muscle uses it, or the body transports it to other tissues via general circulation. The increased blood flow of exercise effectively mobilizes the lactate for use by different tissues. Liver glycogen storage is maintained in part by the gluconeogenic activity to create glycogen from the circulating lactate. Equally important, lactate in the blood maintains available energy for working tissues [87]. Recall that, unlike the liver, muscle tissue cannot free up glycogen stores and release glucose into the blood to aid other working tissues due to a missing enzyme (G-6-P). However, lactate steps in and provides the needed assistance via circulatory delivery to muscles that need energy. The transport and use of lactate coincides with what is often considered the "second wind" because more energy becomes available [81].

If exercise intensity becomes too elevated for an extended duration, the hydrogen ions produced inhibit muscle contractions via the mechanisms discussed previously. With a timely recovery interval, the production removal balance can be restored and training can continue. Training in the presence of lactic acid improves performance, as the body learns to become more efficient with lactate management and hydrogen removal [15]. Intense resistance conditioning – plyometrics, ballistics, sprints, intervals, stair running, and hill climbs – produces large quantities of lactic acid and stimulates the body to produce enzymes that increase the rate of lactic acid utilization.

Lactic acid is not to blame for cramps, DOMS, or inhibited recovery. Cramps are not caused by a sugar metabolite, but, more likely, the over-excitation of nerves from fatigue tonic disruption and intra/extracellular electrolyte imbalance. DOMS is an inflammatory response to cellular damage, ischemia, and tonic spasm, not from leftover lactic acid, which is completely removed from the system within hours of training cessation. Likewise, total system recovery is not inhibited by lactate [19]. The body has already used the leftover lactic acid for fuel before the next bout of exercise has even occurred. Lactate is a friend of intensity. If there is a foe, it's the hydrogen ion, and even that has been shown to be important for energy metabolism.

Cardiac Physiology

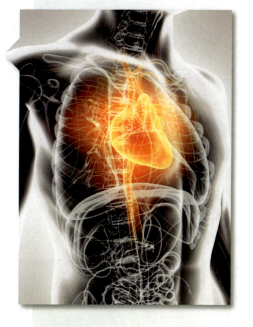

Several systems must harmoniously integrate to provide energy and keep cells alive. The cardiopulmonary system includes the lungs and right half of the heart, representing the start and end components of gas exchange. The cardiovascular system is made up of all the blood vessels and the left half of the heart. This system delivers oxygen to the body's cells via arteries and returns gases back to the heart and lungs via the veins. These systems collectively embody the oxygen delivery portion of VO_2. VO_2 is simply the abbreviation for volume of oxygen that the body can use in all capacities at a given moment. Absolute VO_2 reflects overall O_2 consumption and is expressed in liters per minute (L/min). Relative VO_2 considers the individual, so it represents the amount of O_2 consumption in one minute per kilogram (kg) of body weight of the person being assessed, with oxygen expressed in milliliters (ml/kg/min). When the volume of oxygen consumption by cells reaches the maximal limit, the individual is said to have reached VO_2max.

PRACTICAL INSIGHT

It should be noted that the definition of VO_2max has recently become controversial, as evidence postulates questions of test validity for the determination of this value. Scientists have reservations about whether the tests actually represent a true maximal value. Several recent findings provide evidence that the traditional **graded exercise tests** (GXT), used for decades to determine VO_2max, actually produce submaximal values. A variety of novel testing protocols have consistently elicited supramaximal (higher) VO_2 values than these GXTs when peak test criteria is applied. Possible explanations have been offered for these higher observed values; however, the mechanisms behind these findings remain unclear. While scientists have acknowledged the relevance of these supramaximal VO_2max values, they theorize that the actual implications may be minimal. More research is needed in the area, and the following information will help explain how VO_2max, no matter what is eventually determined, got its name in the first place.

VO_2 is a product of: the oxygen pumped from the heart as measured per minute, called **cardiac output** (CO) and the amount of that oxygen that is used by all bodily cells at a given time, called **(a-v) O_2 difference**. The equation is CO × (a-v) O_2 difference, the first part of the calculation, represents the maximal potential of "oxygen delivery" and is determined by multiplying the number of heart beats per minute by the **stroke volume** (ml) of the heart. Stroke volume represents the amount of blood expelled per beat from the left ventricle of the heart. The second half of the VO_2 equation denotes the amount of oxygen used by the cells, referred to as "oxygen extraction." Oxygen extraction represents the volume of oxygen present in the arteries (a) minus the amount of oxygen left in the veins (v) after the tissues have extracted all that they can use; this part of the equation demonstrates how much oxygen the working tissues consumed. All body tissues have the capacity to produce energy through aerobic metabolism by using the oxygen

DEFINITIONS

Graded exercise test (GXT) –

An exercise test which uses progressive stages to measure/estimate maximal oxygen consumption capacity; this type of test is often used to assess cardiovascular fitness.

Cardiac output (CO) –

The total volume of blood available for use by all bodily tissues, dictated by heart rate and stroke volume.

A-V O_2 difference –

The difference in oxygen saturation when comparing the arteries and veins (blood leaving and returning to the heart); it indicates the level of oxygen uptake efficiency of working muscles and other tissues.

Stroke volume –

The volume of blood expelled (to body tissues) per contraction from the left ventricle during each heartbeat.

diffused across the capillaries. So, two sides of the equation must be accounted for when considering exercise and the adaptations that can improve an individual's cardiorespiratory health and fitness: those that improve the rate and volume of oxygen delivery and those that increase oxygen extraction. Both will be further reviewed in the following text.

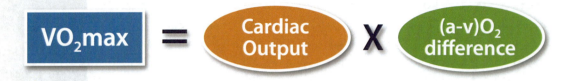

◆ The Heart

The heart is the body's most important muscle because it unites two systems which function to keep all cells alive: the cardiopulmonary and cardiovascular systems, together referred to as the cardiorespiratory system. To serve both systems, the heart is divided into two distinct sides, each responsible for different tasks. The right side of the heart receives deoxygenated blood from the working muscles and pumps it to the lungs (cardiopulmonary); the left side of the heart receives the newly oxygenated blood from the lungs and pumps it to the rest of the body through the arterial vessels (cardiovascular). The heart accomplishes both responsibilities by functioning with a dual pump action. By performing synchronized contractions balanced at both sides of the organ, the heart works continuously to deliver oxygen-rich blood and nutrients to tissues in the body. Each side of the heart has two distinct chambers separated by unidirectional valves to prevent any backflow of blood. The top chambers are called the **atria**, and the bottom chambers are the **ventricles**. The blood flows through each chamber as it is pushed by the force of the contracting cardiac tissue.

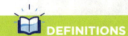 **DEFINITIONS**

Atria –

The two upper chambers in the heart that receive blood from the veins and push it into the ventricles; the left atrium receives oxygenated blood from the lungs while the right atrium receives deoxygenated blood from venous circulation.

Ventricles –

The two lower chambers of the heart. The right ventricle receives blood from the right atrium and pumps it into the lungs via the pulmonary artery, and the left ventricle receives blood from the left atrium and pumps the blood to the rest of the body via the aorta.

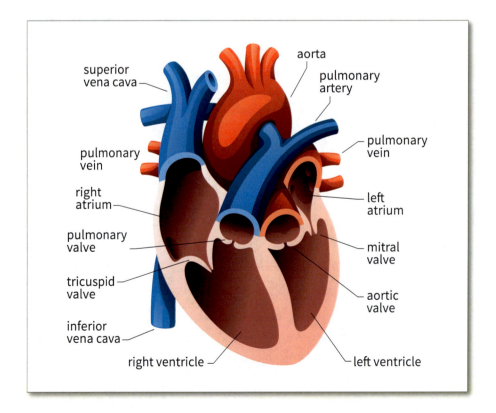

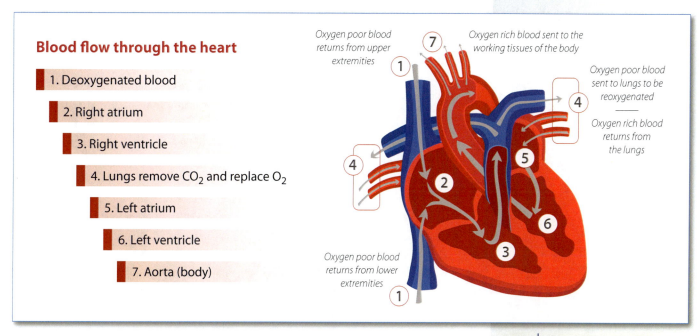

Descriptions of blood flow through the heart normally start with the right side, where the venous system delivers oxygen depleted blood to the right atrium through the superior and inferior vena cava. Earlier, it was stated that the heart is actually two pumps, which function in a synchronized manner. Between each heartbeat, a relaxation phase takes place, allowing both the right and left atria to fill with blood. This relaxed state is referred to as the diastolic phase or **diastole**. Once the atria fill, the heart contracts, driving blood into the large chambered ventricles. The contracted state of the heart is referred to as the systolic phase or **systole**. When the right atrium contracts, it mobilizes the blood through the tricuspid valve to the right ventricle. This interaction between the chambers and their corresponding one-way valves ensures that blood flows in only one direction, towards the ventricles. The familiar "lub-dub" sound of a heart beating is actually the sound that the valves make when they close. Upon filling, the right ventricle then contracts, pushing the blood into the pulmonary artery, which runs to the lungs. There, carbon dioxide (CO_2) is exchanged for oxygen (O_2). The oxygen diffuses into the blood across the lungs' **alveoli** and binds to **hemoglobin**. Hemoglobin is the iron containing component of **red blood cells** (RBCs) that serves as oxygen's transporter throughout circulation. Oxygen depleted dark blood turns bright red in the process of oxygenation and flows back to the heart via the pulmonary vein, reentering through the left atrium. Just as it was pumped out to the lungs, the now oxygen-rich blood is pushed through the bicuspid valve (mitral valve), which separates the left atrium from the left ventricle. Contraction of the left ventricle pushes the blood back against the bicuspid valve, closing it, while, at the same time, forcing the volume of blood through the aortic valve to the **aorta**. The aorta is the principal artery responsible for central distribution of blood to the rest of the body. Because the left ventricle powers blood delivery to the entire body, it is, not surprisingly, the largest of all the chambers and most susceptible to training improvements, especially endurance training.

DEFINITIONS

Diastole –

The heart's relaxation phase in which the atrial chambers fill with blood (diastolic phase).

Systole –

The contraction phase of the heart ventricles by which blood is pumped out to the body (systolic phase).

Alveoli –

The tiny, thin-walled, capillary-rich sacs found in the lungs where the exchange of oxygen and carbon dioxide takes place.

Hemoglobin –

A protein found in red blood cells that helps to transport oxygen to tissues.

Red Blood Cells (RBCs) –

The most common type of blood cell and the primary means of delivering oxygen to the tissues: also called erythrocytes.

Aorta –

The main artery of the body, supplying oxygenated blood from the left ventricle to the circulatory system.

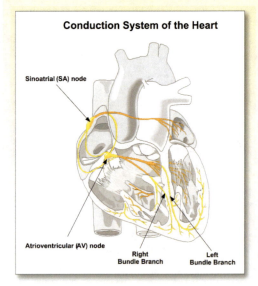

Conduction System of the Heart

PRACTICAL INSIGHT

The heart has its own conduction system to manage the dual pump mechanism. Alternating waves of depolarization and repolarization smoothly move blood through the respective chambers via simultaneous and synchronized contractions and relaxations. The heart uses nodes to dictate its pace based on the body's oxygen demands. The sinoatrial (SA) node, the natural pacemaker of the heart, and the atrioventricular (AV) node are modified cardiac muscle cells that connect to a conducting bundle. The nodes send electrical impulses that run down the connecting right and left bundle branches to the Purkinje fibers, which relay the electrical signal to the chambers of the heart. The signals from the SA and AV nodes dictate the contractile element of the heart, communicating to the atria and ventricles when to contract. This eloquent system of conduction allows the atria and ventricles to contract in harmony so that the forward flow of blood continues without interruption.

 DEFINITIONS

Myocardium –

The muscular tissue of the heart that is specialized to allow for continuous contractions; enhanced sarcoplasmic reticulum and calcium delivery systems allow this tissue to manage rapid and non-stop neural impulses: also called cardiac muscle.

◆ Cardiac Muscle Tissue

The heart muscle, also called the **myocardium**, exhibits similarities to skeletal muscle but is more specialized for its purpose of repeated, measured contractions. Cardiac muscle tissue, like that of skeletal muscle, has a sarcoplasmic reticulum for calcium storage and T-tubules to manage action potentials. It also possesses organized sarcomeres, which contain actin and myosin contractile proteins. However, distinct differences exist between cardiac and skeletal muscle due mainly to the continuous action of the heart. These differences allow the heart to function constantly, rather than serving the intermittent, voluntary actions common to skeletal muscle.

Cardiac tissue, like all tissue, relies on energy (ATP) for fuel. The heart requires a constant supply of ATP and oxygen, so it will not fatigue. This is crucial, as under conditions of high stress, oxygen would no longer be able to reach vital organs, causing a systematic failure and subsequent death. The versatile cardiac tissue utilizes substrates like fatty acids, glucose, amino acids, lactate, and ketone bodies to synthesize ATP; however, it relies heavily on the ATP produced from lipids. Lipid metabolism is crucial for the heart because it can produce large

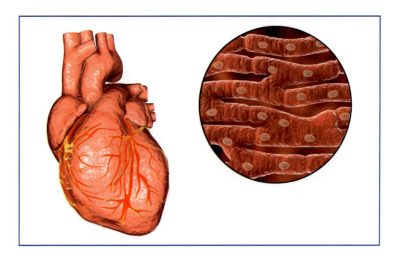

quantities of ATP aerobically compared to the other energy systems. This makes fat the ideal fuel, as the cardiac muscle almost exclusively employs oxidative metabolism to satisfy its energy demands. Oxidative phosphorylation supplies more than 95% of the heart's ATP consumption [54, 104]. To maximize the aerobic system's efficiency, cardiac muscle is densely packed with mitochondria and contains such an extensive network of **capillaries** that it actually has one capillary per cardiac-muscle fiber. This arrangement provides the mitochondria with a constant flow of oxygen-rich blood for ATP production via these small blood vessels. Consistent with skeletal muscle, cardiac muscle must utilize CHOs to fuel the higher force outputs required during intense exercise [104]. However, unlike skeletal muscle, the heart cannot allow hydrogen ions from glycolysis to build up as they might inhibit enzyme activity and contractility. To prevent this situation, myocardial tissues possess a greater capacity to utilize oxygen and blood to increase the rate of lactate conversion, effectively preventing fatigue. Remember, the heart is one of the main tissues that metabolizes and uses lactate for energy. Cardiac muscle extracts approximately 75% of the available oxygen, whereas skeletal muscle can only extract approximately 25% of the oxygen delivered.

DEFINITIONS

Capillaries –

The smallest vascular structures with the thinnest walls, which allow for oxygen and nutrient transport as well as waste product removal from muscles, organs, and other tissues.

◆ Cardiac Output

Training can generate an adaptation to the heart resulting in an increase in stroke volume (SV). Heart contraction strength and left ventricle blood volume collectively determine SV. Individuals who engage in endurance training increase the capacity of the heart to pump more blood to the tissues through specific adaptations that make the left ventricle cavity larger allows for greater filling capacity and enhances the force of the ventricular contraction [63, 78, 94, 95]. SV progresses relative to the intensity of the work being performed, up to a maximal point that occurs at roughly 50% of VO_2max among average people, but can be higher among trained athletes. When the volume of blood expelled per beat peaks, HR then becomes the body's mechanism to increase oxygen delivery. HR is always indicated by the number of beats per minute (bpm), expressing the quantity of oxygen used by the body. Therefore, when beats per minute (HR) is multiplied by the amount of blood expelled per beat (SV) at a given time, the total volume of blood available per minute (CO) can be determined. CO factors importantly in the body's ability to sustain physical activity and represents a key half of the VO_2 equation relating to adaptation [12].

Interestingly, as a person improves cardio-respiratory fitness, HRs decrease when measured, at all exercise intensities, including resting and maximal levels. Most people are initially surprised by the adaptation of the latter, but, logically, as the heart becomes more efficient, it does not need to work as hard: it needs less to do more. Remember, the body will adapt to the stress it experiences, and the heart is no different. The reduction in maximal HR among elite endurance athletes occurs because oxygen delivery is not the limiting factor to work capacity and oxygen consumption. At maximal levels, highly trained endurance runners already maintain more

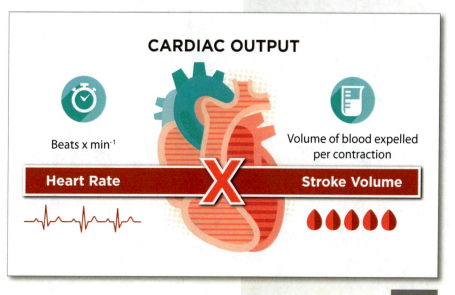

oxygen in circulation than can be extracted at the cellular level, so the heart does not benefit from additional beats[49]. At rest, the heart also gets a break because the stroke volume and conduction improvements account for a reduced need for beats. This accounts for the low resting heart rates (RHR) observed in trained individuals. Well-trained athletes have resting stroke volumes of 90-110 ml/beat compared to the 50-70 ml/beat of an average person. This explains resting HR measures of 30-40 bpm, which are not uncommon among very well-trained endurance athletes. These values are more than half of those found among same-age, sedentary individuals, who consistently have RHR values of >60 bpm. Further adaptations, such as **angiogenesis** and cellular mitochondria proliferation, increase the potential of the muscle to extract oxygen, adding to performance improvements and reducing cardiac stress.

> **DEFINITIONS**
>
> **Angiogenesis –**
>
> *The development of new blood vessels as an adaptation-specific response to aerobic training, resulting in greater capillary density and improved oxygen-extraction capacity.*

Resting Heart Rate in Men and Women (beats/min)										
	MEN					WOMEN				
%	20-29 y	30-39 y	40-49 y	50-59 y	60+ y	20-29 y	30-39 y	40-49 y	50-59 y	60+ y
90	50	50	50	50	52	55	55	55	55	52
80	54	55	54	55	55	59	58	60	60	57
70	58	58	58	58	58	60	62	62	61	60
60	60	60	60	60	60	63	65	64	64	62
50	63	63	62	63	62	65	68	66	67	64
40	66	65	65	65	65	70	70	70	69	66
30	70	68	69	68	68	72	74	72	72	72
20	72	72	72	72	72	75	76	76	75	74
10	80	77	78	77	77	84	82	80	83	79

> **DEFINITIONS**
>
> **Baroreceptors –**
>
> *Specialized receptors that detect changes in blood pressure and blood flow in order to inform the CNS to either decrease or increase blood pressure or heart rate. Baroreceptors are located in the aorta and carotid arteries.*
>
> **Blood pressure –**
>
> *A measure of the force or lateral pressure exerted by the circulating blood against the arterial walls; it is modulated in response to activity, nutrition, and health status: defined as cardiac output (CO) x total peripheral resistance (TPR).*
>
> **Vasodilation –**
>
> *The dilation or widening of a vascular structure, which decreases blood pressure and allows for increased blood flow and the potential for improved oxygen and nutrient delivery.*

◆ Blood Pressure

Blood leaving the heart through the left ventricle pushes through the resistance created from the periphery. It then enters into peripheral circulation via aortic distribution through the arteries. When this oxygen rich blood reaches the tissues, it engages in gas exchange, suppling oxygen and nutrients while removing cellular waste and by-products. To ensure that the flow of blood to the tissues remains at appropriate levels, the circulatory system's regulatory mechanisms control the pressure exerted throughout the arterial vessels. **Baroreceptors**, located in the heart's aorta and the carotid arteries in the neck's cervical area, manage **blood pressure (BP)**, measured during the heart's systolic and diastolic phases. When the body requires oxygen for working tissue, the pressure in the blood vessels adjusts to meet the demand through modulative constriction or dilation. Areas of the body which require more oxygenated blood experience expansion in their respective vessels' diameter as arteries relax (termed **vasodilation**), while areas requiring less oxygenated blood experience a narrowing of the vessels through arterial smooth muscle contraction that **vasoconstrict's** the vessels. By changing the diameter of the vessels, BP can be increased or decreased according to the body's relative demands at a given moment.

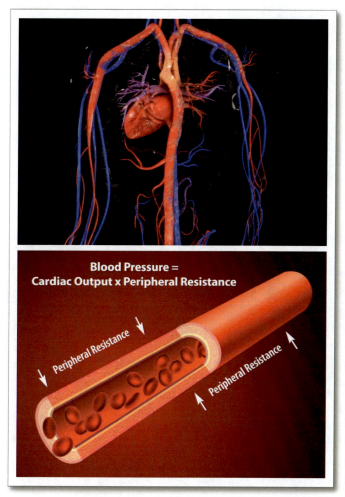

BP is determined by multiplying the CO of the heart by the **total peripheral resistance** (TPR) applied by the vessels and the rest of the body. When the body is at rest, CO is low, and the main determinant of BP is peripheral resistance. Peripheral resistance reflects the difficulty with which the blood passes through the vast network of vessels. Constricted, contracted, compressed, or arterial vessels that have plaque built up along the walls make it more difficult for the blood to pass because the diameter of the artery is acutely or chronically compromised. When blood experiences difficulty passing through a vessel, pressure increases, similar to blocking the flow of a water hose with one's thumb. This inhibition causes pressure behind the blockage to rise and become turbulent. This phenomenon is commonly observed among individuals who are obese or diabetic, older adults, and those who smoke [100, 119]. In small arteries and vessels like capillaries, the turbulent distress can lead to arterial disease, as the high pressure causes tears in the vessel wall. Large vessels do not present the same risk, partially based on the sheer size and diameter of these arteries: even when plaque buildup is observed, it provides little resistance to blood flow. Besides being able to contract and relax, arteries also have elastic properties and other mechanisms to further attenuate the high pressure in the vessels.

During exercise or high stress situations, HR increases, consequently increasing CO. The increase in CO forces blood through the circulatory system at a faster rate. The blood's high-speed circulation pushes out against the walls of the arteries as it flows past, creating a shear stress with increasing pressure. When this pressure is added to the peripheral resistance of the vessels, it equals the body's net BP. Due to elevations in HR during exercise, BP will be higher during activity than when the body is at rest. At rest, **mean arterial pressure** (MAP) in

> **DEFINITIONS**
>
> **Vasoconstriction –**
>
> *The constriction or narrowing of a vascular structure due to contraction of the muscular wall, which increases blood pressure and reduces blood flow; it is the opposite of vasodilation.*
>
> **Total peripheral resistance (TPR) –**
>
> *The resistance to blood flow experienced within peripheral vasculature which can be modulated by various internal/external factors; also referred to as systemic vascular resistance (SVR).*
>
> **Mean arterial pressure (MAP) –**
>
> *The average arterial pressure during one cardiac cycle.*

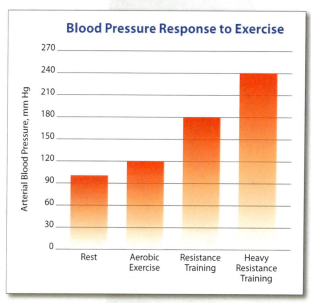

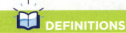

DEFINITIONS

Hypertension –

High blood pressure: a condition that has a negative impact on the cardiovascular system due to excessive pressure exerted upon arterial walls that causes damage over time.

Blood viscosity –

A measure of the thickness and stickiness of blood caused by variable quantities of various blood constituents; elevated viscosity measures can serve as a strong predictor for cardiovascular events.

Orthostatic hypotension –

A state of low blood pressure commonly caused by rapid changes in position from lying or seated to standing; it can also be caused by other internal factors.

Arteries –

The large, muscular-walled blood vessel structures that transport oxygenated blood away from the heart to the tissues.

Arterioles –

The smaller, thinner-walled arteries that serve as the connecting structures to capillaries.

the large arteries is about 100 mmHg. During aerobic exercise, the MAP will jump to 115-120 mmHg, and during heavy resistance training, that number can increase to values surpassing 200 mmHg. When selecting or prescribing exercise modalities for clients, personal trainers should consider BP response to ensure exercises are appropriate for the individual's current vascular health. Increasing BP in elderly clients or those with **hypertension** can dramatically increase the risk of vessel wall damage and may exacerbate tissue lesions and arteriosclerosis [37].

In some cases, BP is associated with acute internal conditions. BP is sensitive to blood volume and **blood viscosity**. Dehydration and electrolyte imbalances will cause an increase in BP. In the case of dehydration, HR increases due to the decrease in blood plasma, subsequently affecting BP [37]. This occurs in both resting and active states. Drinking alcohol and certain medications also can negatively affect BP response and, in some cases, cause temporary hypertension or **orthostatic hypotension**.

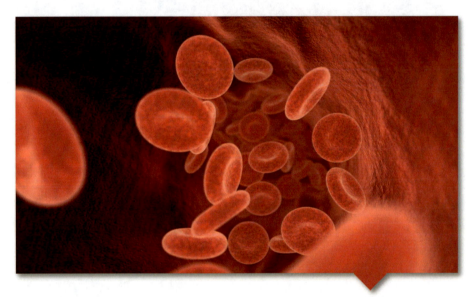

◆ Circulatory System

Vessel characteristics relate specifically to their role, size, and location. The large **arteries** with the greatest diameter maintain lower amounts of smooth muscle tissue when compared to smaller vessels, in part due to their role in delivery and their respective proximity to the heart. In the vascular (circulatory) system, they function primarily to deliver large quantities of blood to the main body segments. This is why they are referred to as the conducting arteries. Large arteries give way to medium size arteries, which turn into smaller branch arteries, then **arterioles**, and finally, capillaries. As artery diameter narrows, the amount of elastic tissue they contain lessens and is replaced by larger amounts of smooth muscle tissue. Medium-size arteries are called distributor arteries; they regulate what tissue areas get the most blood flow by governing vasodilation and vasoconstriction. During exercise, the medium arteries that supply blood to the gastrointestinal organs (stomach and intestines) constrict to decrease blood flow to these areas; concomitant vasodilation takes place in the medium vessels of the working tissue, rapidly increasing blood delivery. This process effectively shunts a larger amount of blood to the muscles, providing the needed oxygen to manage increased activity levels. The small arteries further control the flow of blood through a similar process.

Peripheral Circulatory System

An intricate network of varying-sized vessels provides blood to the body's working tissues. In the same fashion that a tree divides into limbs that further split into smaller branches, large vessels from the heart separate into smaller vessels that reach throughout the body. Blood leaving the heart enters into large arteries, following a path to smaller arteries and ending in even smaller capillaries. In the case of the ascending aorta, it leaves the heart and leads into large arteries that deliver blood to the brain: the carotid arteries in the neck and the brachiocephalic artery, which extends to arteries of the upper extremity, with a branch that includes the brachial artery. The descending aorta travels down the trunk to form the iliac artery, which eventually runs into the large femoral arteries. These arteries deliver blood to the lower limbs. The ascending aorta, like the trunk of the tree, is extensive, and along the way, has conduits that extend to the organs and tissues of the trunk.

Capillaries, the smallest blood vessels, directly supply the cells with oxygen and nutrients. Because these vessels do not have a muscle layer, the nutrients in the blood can diffuse across the capillary walls into the **interstitial spaces** for cellular use. The capillaries connect to the arterial system via arterioles. The smallest of the arteries, arterioles have only a couple of layers of smooth muscle surrounding the **endothelium**, and they do not have an elastic layer like their larger counterparts. Like the other vessels surrounded by smooth muscle, arterioles can constrict or dilate as needed to assist in blood flow management.

Once oxygen diffuses into the cells and carbon dioxide is absorbed into the blood, the blood travels from the capillaries to the venous side of the circulatory path, starting with the venules, which widen into small **veins**. Venules, like their microcirculatory counterparts, capillaries, enable nutrient transport across their walls; however, as those walls thicken in the transformation into small veins, the smooth muscle cells inhibit the exchange. The deoxygenated blood travels from these small veins to medium-sized veins back towards the heart. The vessels of the venous system resemble those of the arterial system in size and distribution but differ in makeup: arteries have more smooth muscle tissue, while veins hold significantly more blood. Arteries and

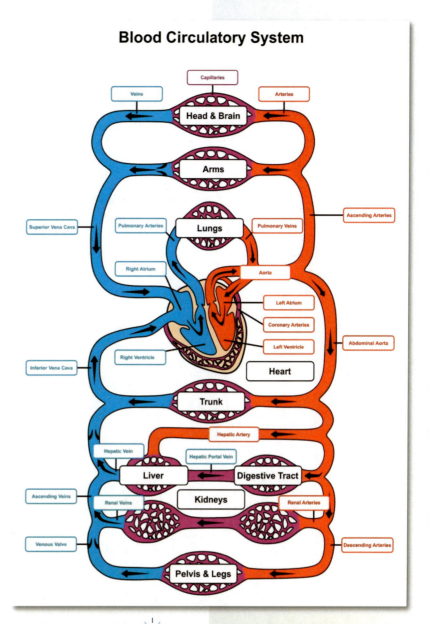

DEFINITIONS

Interstitial spaces –

Fluid-filled spaces between tissues that allow for the transfer of oxygen, nutrients, waste products, hormones, neurotransmitters, and other compounds.

Endothelium –

A thin layer of flat epithelial cells that line blood vessels. These cells allow for the diffusion of oxygen and waste products; the lining of blood vessels, when damaged, is associated with plaque build-up.

Veins –

Any of the blood vessels that are part of the circulatory system and transport deoxygenated blood back to the heart/ lungs; they are less muscular than arteries, and are often closer to the skin.

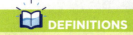

DEFINITIONS

Autonomic nervous system (ANS) –

A component of the nervous system responsible for bodily functions that are not consciously controlled, such as breathing, heart function, and digestive processes.

Diabetes –

A group of metabolic diseases (type 1 and 2) that involve insulin and glucose mismanagement; this results in a chronic state of excess sugar in the bloodstream, which causes numerous physical issues affecting the nervous system, vascular structures, and various organs.

veins run parallel to each other throughout the body, which is clearly illustrated by red (oxygenated blood) and blue (deoxygenated blood) color distinctions.

The major difference between veins and arteries is the amount of oxygen within the respective vessels and the way the fluid moves through circulation. A pulse can be felt in the arteries because blood flow is pushed by the rhythmic contractions of the heart. Each pump of the heart thrusts blood through the arterial system, and the pressure exerted on the walls of vessels can be felt and heard as the pulse. These contractile forces dissipate by the time blood arrives in the venous system; therefore, the vessels must use a skeletal pump mechanism. This effectively milks the blood through the veins' system via smooth muscle contractions and one-way valves that prevent any back flow. Veins larger than 2 mm contain valves that occlude the vessel when the blood attempts to reverse direction. Signals from the **autonomic nervous system (ANS)** stimulate the smooth muscle to contract so that blood returns and fills the right atrium of the heart, eventually moving to the lungs to be re-oxygenated. Greater venous return to the heart allows the chambers of the heart to be filled and stretched leading to a larger SV, due to Frank-Starling's Law.

QUICK INSIGHT

Blood Pooling and the Cool Down

When muscle tissue engages in work, the body floods the area with blood to satisfy the activity's oxygen demands. The mechanisms that precipitate the increased oxygen delivery continue until the activity stops. After exercise demands engorge the large muscles of the lower body with blood, they require a cool down of lighter rhythmic activities to effectively employ the muscle pump mechanism. When cool downs are neglected, blood remains in the tissue, and the vein's smooth muscles alone cannot complete bloods return [48]. This situation can cause blood to build up around the one-way valves called "blood pooling". This fluid is deoxygenated and high in bicarbonate and other byproducts of exercise metabolism. Because approximately 64% of all circulatory blood is located in the systemic veins, transitioning the body from heavy work to immediate rest may impede blood flow back to the heart [23, 48, 67]. Blood pooling prevents the necessary blood from returning to the heart, which can cause acute ischemia in the tissue and reduce cardiac output. Leg heaviness and discomfort signify blood pooling and can cause prolonged symptoms that can often make sleeping difficult.

Exercisers can avoid blood pooling if they routinely engage in activities that contract the muscles that were called upon to do work. Light aerobic exercise increases the flow of blood back to the heart due to the venous mobilization caused by rhythmic muscular contractions (skeletal pump mechanism). This begins to restore the body to its homeostatic, pre-exercise condition. The post-exercise activity increases by-product waste removal and conversion, including that of lactic acid, and sets up the tissue for more successful recovery. Elderly individuals or those with peripheral vascular problems, including those with **diabetes** and hypertension, should make use of longer warm-ups and cool downs to better regulate blood flow: older or damaged veins have a reduced capacity to return blood to the heart on their own, and an immediate cessation of activity can have negative effects on the vascular system.

◆ Assessing Pulse

A rhythmical pulse can be palpated at locations where large arteries lie close to the skin. This is caused by the pressure exerted on the arteries when the heart contracts. Several locations exist – at the arms, legs, head, and neck – where the heart's beat can be physically sensed. In the head and neck, the superficial temporal artery, facial artery, and common carotid artery can all be palpated. The carotid arteries are often easily identified by a strong pulse, as they ascend from the aorta and are the closest to the heart. They can be palpated on either side of the larynx just below the jaw. In the upper extremity, the radial artery's pulse is the most recognized and is often palpated for exercise pulse rate. In the upper arm, both the axillary artery and brachial artery can be felt with moderately light finger pressure. Although not commonly used for pulse assessment, the leg's femoral artery, popliteal artery, and dorsalis pedis artery all have a measurable pulse as well. During exercise, the blood flow volume increases through the arteries, making it easy to identify palpation sites.

Primary Pulse Assessment Locations

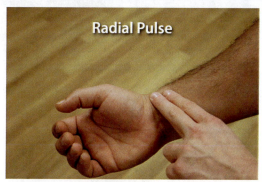
Radial Pulse

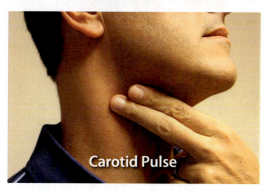
Carotid Pulse

The body maintains the tendency for vessels to match pressure with flow volume, a phenomenon called compliance. Compliance refers to a vessels ability to stretch in response to an increase in pressure. As pressures increase against the endothelium, mechanisms in place mediate the elastic vessels' expansion in compliance to accommodate an increase in blood flow, thereby reducing the pressure. Even small increases in pressure translate into large plasma volume shifts by compliant tissues. The veins have significantly more compliance to variations in BP than arteries. In fact, veins are almost 25x more compliant than arteries, which explains why veins contribute more to blood storage. Veins retain almost two-thirds of the body's blood supply at any given time; however, the venous system's ability to hold blood is sometimes detrimental because of blood pooling, which can constrain CO due to decreased levels of venous return. Low CO can increase cardiac event risk for certain individuals post-exercise and can also slow the recovery process: this underscores the need for cool down activities post exercise.

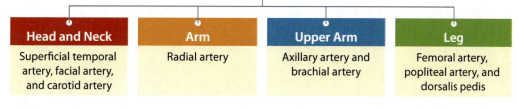

When palpating the areas where large arteries are close to the skin, one will feel a rhythmic pulse caused by the pressure exerted on the arteries when the heart contracts

Head and Neck	Arm	Upper Arm	Leg
Superficial temporal artery, facial artery, and carotid artery	Radial artery	Axillary artery and brachial artery	Femoral artery, popliteal artery, and dorsalis pedis

◆ Aging & Vessel Health

Similar to other tissues, the aging effect plays a role in vessel decline. The elastic properties of the arteries suffer degenerative changes, causing them to harden, losing pliability and compliance like an old rubber band.

The elastic properties of arteries suffer degenerative changes, causing increases in BP via: → Loss of pliability → Loss of compliance → Hardening of the vessel

DEFINITIONS

Arteriosclerosis –

A thickening and hardening of the arterial walls from chronic conditions such as high blood pressure, old age, or negative behaviors, such as smoking.

Atherosclerosis –

Refers to the deposit and buildup of fats, cholesterol, and other substances (known as plaque) in and on arterial walls, which can restrict blood flow and lead to heart attack or stroke.

Coronary artery disease (CAD) –

A disease of the coronary arteries often due to atherosclerosis; it leads to an obstruction of coronary circulation, potentially resulting in a dangerous cardiovascular event; it is also known as atherosclerotic heart disease or ischemic heart disease.

Varicose veins –

Veins that have become enlarged and twisted; as one ages, vascular structures lose elasticity. Some of the valves may also become weak or dysfunctional, increasing their hyper-dilated appearance.

This process of the hardening of the arteries is **arteriosclerosis**. Layers of the vessel thicken and experience chemical changes in elastic properties with a corresponding increase in mineral deposits. In between the elastic and collagenous fibers, fatty deposits build up over time, decreasing the diameter of the vessels. This state begins to impede blood flow as the wall thickens. The cholesterol-based materials further harden as calcium deposits and fibrous material progressively occlude blood flow. This process of plaque buildup and smooth muscle cell proliferation represents a specific type of arteriosclerosis, called **atherosclerosis**. This vessel dysfunction can dramatically reduce and even stop the flow of blood to tissues, leading to cellular death. Obesity, smoking, high cholesterol, physical inactivity, diabetes, and hypertension all relate to increased risk for arteriosclerosis and atherosclerosis, leading to diagnosed **coronary artery disease** (CAD).

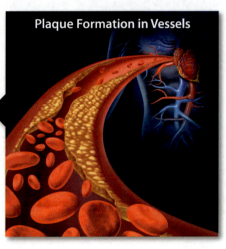

Plaque Formation in Vessels

Vascular degeneration reduces the circulatory system's capacity to respond to exercise's demands. Personal trainers should be cautious when working with hypertensive clients and elderly populations due to vascular system compromises, which reduce the vessels' efficiency at regulating pressures. Rapid changes in body position, particularly from supine to upright posture, can cause orthostatic hypotension or a drop in BP [31]. Caution is warranted when these exercisers perform activities with intense loads, as BP can skyrocket. Individuals with hypertension or reduced vascular compliance should not engage in heavy resistance training and should avoid machines that cause body compression: the leg press, for instance, will immediately increase BP as the body attempts to manage these loads. For these individuals, less than 70% of 1RM is recommended, often prescribed in rhythmic circuits.

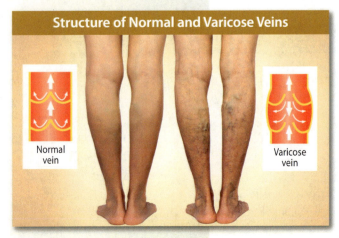

Structure of Normal and Varicose Veins

Normal vein / Varicose vein

If the veins experience tortuous lengthening or overstretching, the integrity of the valve system may be compromised. When this occurs, the one-way valves become progressively dysfunctional, decreasing their ability to perform their primary operation of preventing backflow. Compromised valves cause the vein to become abnormally dilated in response to back flow pressure, which induces localized swelling. The outcome is a vascular bulge of the blue-green superficial vessels, most often observed in the legs. Hyper-dilated, superficial veins are known as **varicose veins**. While most varicose veins are mainly a cosmetic concern and do not present a serious medical problem, some can lead to complications. Exercisers with pronounced varicose veins should avoid heavy resistance training [75]. Excessive pressure can increase back flow force, exacerbating the condition and causing pain. Aerobic or rhythmic physical activity is recommended because dynamic muscle contractions increase the blood's propensity to flow back to the heart. Phlebitis, or inflammation of the deep veins, poses more of a threat because it may lead to cellular ischemia and gangrenous tissue [42]. If it is deemed that they may pose a risk, surgery may be required to remove damaged vessels. Additionally, clot formation may occur when the vessel's blood flow becomes stagnant. These clots can lead to **deep vein thrombosis** (DVT), which poses the greatest risk for health complications. While blood clots in superficial veins rarely travel to the heart or lungs, deep vein clots can cause serious blockages and death from pulmonary embolism.

> **DEFINITIONS**
>
> **Deep vein thrombosis (DVT) –**
>
> *Deep vein blood clots that can cause serious circulation blockage and potential death from pulmonary embolism (blockage of pulmonary arteries).*

◆ The Role of Blood

During both rest and exercise, the circulatory system's dynamics depend upon the physics of blood flow and the vessels' tissue anatomy. Because they must satisfy blood flow demands for all body tissues, it makes sense that approximately 84% of the blood circulates systemically in the arteries and veins. The other 16% is being oxygenated in the pulmonary vessels or in the heart itself. Blood flows quickly through large arteries, with the rate of blood flow decreasing as the size of the vessels diminishes. The pressure also drops as the flow moves from large to small vessels. The average aortic pressure is 100 mmHg, which corresponds to the body's highest rates of blood flow. The pressure in the capillaries averages about 20 mmHg, the slowest rate of blood flow. This lower capillary pressure allows the cellular nutrients and waste products to be exchanged between the arterial entrance and the venous exit.

As mentioned earlier, capillaries allow fluids containing oxygen and nutrients to diffuse across the vessel walls. This is possible because capillaries have less smooth muscle compared to veins and arteries. The combination of interstitial pressure and BP drives this exchange. To facilitate this exchange, the BP pushes nutrients from the capillaries into surrounding tissues, while the interstitial pressure of the tissues drives metabolic waste from the tissue into the blood of the micro vessels. BP at the beginning (the arterial side) of the capillary-tissue exchange location is higher than the pressure on the venous side. This lends

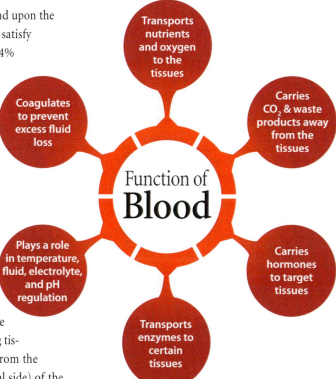

QUICK INSIGHT

Hemoglobin

Hemoglobin is a molecule made of proteins that require iron to carry oxygen in the body. Approximately 66% of the four grams of iron contained in humans is found attached to hemoglobin in the blood. Anytime blood is lost, hemoglobin and iron decrease as a consequence. This is a particular cause for consideration, as females lose iron through menstruation. The loss increases the need for dietary iron above the requirements of males. With insufficient iron availability, blood hemoglobin levels decrease, leading to a condition known as iron-deficiency anemia. Consequently, the body's ability to transport oxygen in the blood lessens. Additionally, cigarette smoking affects oxygen transport with hemoglobin. Cigarette smoke produces carbon monoxide, which bonds to hemoglobin, inhibiting oxygen transport in the blood. In its transport form with hemoglobin, 5-15% of blood may be composed of carbon monoxide, impeding physical capacity during activity due to decreased oxygen delivery to working tissue [44].

DEFINITIONS

Hematocrit –

The percentage of blood that consists of red blood cells; the most commonly used erythrocyte test.

Plasma –

The clear, liquid portion of blood that contains salts, glucose, amino acids, vitamins, urea, proteins and fats; it is extracted from circulation during dehydration as sweat.

White blood cells (WBC) –

A group of immunological cells in the bloodstream which serve various protective functions, such as protection from invasive pathogens.

Platelets –

Tiny cells responsible for blood coagulation (blood clotting) and the repair of damaged blood vessels.

itself to the regulatory mechanisms of exchange. Essentially, cellular nutrients leave the blood vessel at the beginning of the capillary as it approaches the tissue; waste enters the blood vessel at the end as it returns to the heart. Exercise increases the cellular demand for oxygen and nutrients and facilitates the removal of metabolic waste; as a result, the body responds by adding capillaries in an adaptive response called angiogenesis. Increasing the number of capillaries, or capillary density, within muscle tissue occurs mainly in response to endurance activities. This allows for increased oxygen and nutrient delivery to the muscle cells during exercise, consequently improving performance outcomes.

Whereas vessels represent the highway, blood functions as the delivery vehicle that connects tissues. The blood's ability to deliver nutrients and remove waste comes from its transport mechanisms and constitution. Of the normal 4-5 liters of blood in total circulation, part is comprised of cells and cell fragments called the formed element (44-54%) or **hematocrit**. The rest is composed of a fluid matrix (46-56%) called **plasma**. Approximately 95% of the hematocrit is red blood cells (RBCs). The remaining 5% is **white blood cells** (WBCs) and **platelets**. Males have nearly 14% more hematocrit than females, which represents an advantage in performance: the quantity of RBCs enables greater oxygen transport. Plasma is comprised of mostly water, interspersed with some dissolved or suspended molecules. Due to its high-water volume, plasma is often extracted from the blood during periods of dehydration. This is one mechanism by which dehydration causes body dysfunction: without exogenous hydration, the body pulls water from its only available source, the blood, causing an increase in blood viscosity. When the body dehydrates, the plasma volume decreases, increasing the formed element's proportion of the blood. During periods of dehydration, HR and BP responsively increase as the heart is forced to pump harder to maintain oxygen delivery to tissue, due to a decrease in the total blood volume.

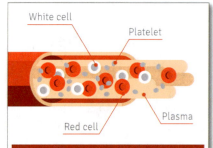

Major blood constituents:

Red blood cells (RBCs)
– transport oxygen and CO_2 to and from the tissues

White blood cells
– essential for a properly-functioning immune system

Platelets
– responsible for blood coagulation and for the repair of damaged blood vessels

Plasma
– clear, fluid portion of blood in which cells are suspended; extracted during dehydration

At any given time, numerous compounds constitute the blood. Each compound has a specific function and may vary based on internal and external conditions. During exercise, for instance, concentrations of dissolved components – ions, enzymes, hormones, nutrients, and metabolic by-products – increase in response to work demands. Concurrently, an increase in the concentration of RBCs corresponds to an increase in oxygen and carbon dioxide transport. RBCs also contain an enzyme, carbonic anhydrous, that catalyzes the reaction between carbon dioxide and water to form carbonic acid. This compound acts as buffer that ionizes the acidic hydrogen ions to form bicarbonate ions, increasing the blood's alkalinity. Bicarbonate ions diffuse into blood plasma, which represents the primary method of carbon dioxide transport to the lungs, and are then exhaled. Because bicarbonate buffers the waste products of sugar metabolism, it helps maintain blood pH as well.

PRACTICAL INSIGHT

When lifting or exerting high force, many exercisers hold their breath. This action, referred to as the **valsalva maneuver**, increases intra-abdominal pressure, allowing the diaphragm to forcefully contract against the viscera to support the spine. This process, however, dramatically increases blood pressure. Exercisers consciously exhale during concentric contractions and inhale during eccentric contractions to reduce the blood pressure response during exercise. This is especially important for hypertensive individuals.

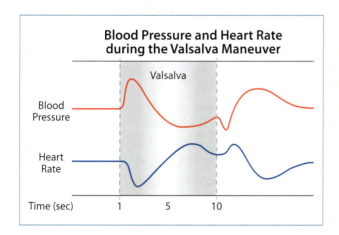

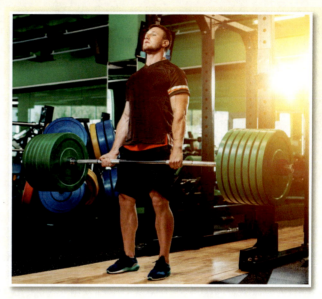

◆ Circulation During Activity

When the body performs activities involving elevated intensities, the circulatory system increases its capacity to deliver blood to the working tissues. At rest, only 20%-25% of the skeletal muscle's capillaries are open, and the heart rate is at its lowest working level. When the body begins engaging in activity, the circulatory system receives signals from the brain that prepare it to manage and respond to the increased oxygen demands. In anticipation of activity, HR increases before a person even picks up a weight or turns on the treadmill due to neural innervations and hormonal signaling. Concurrently, capillary beds open to provide oxygen to the tissues they feed. During exercise, 100% of the capillaries in active skeletal muscle respond to support the metabolic demands.

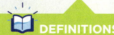
DEFINITIONS

Valsalva maneuver –

A strain against a closed airway, combined with muscle tightening; it occurs when a person holds his or her breath and tries to move a heavy object; it is contraindicated for those with hypertension, as it creates an immense increase in blood pressure.

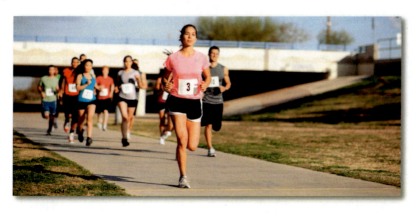

Three primary mechanisms related to the regulation of blood flow among tissues:

- Individual tissues can control blood flow based on metabolic need via humoral (immunological) reponses

- The nervous system can adjust sympathetic and parasympathetic signals to control MAP and shunt or distribute blood from one area of the body to another

- Hormonal communications can influence MAP and chemical release by tissues

Blood flow generally changes in proportion to the tissue's metabolic needs. Therefore, organs that are not needed during exercise, such as those of the digestive tract, have their blood redirected to active skeletal muscle tissue or metabolic organs. During times of activity, blood flow to skeletal muscles increases 15-20 fold. To accommodate the cell's increased oxygen need, the blood vessels react to vasodilators released into circulation in response to exercise. Lactic acid and carbon dioxide, as well as hydrogen and potassium ions, are key vasodilators. Their presence signals the body to an increased metabolic turnover and greater demand for oxygen in the active tissues. The nervous system interprets these metabolic messages and tells the less metabolically active tissues and non-working muscles to vasoconstrict, resulting in shunting and a redirection of blood flow to the dilated arteries of active tissues. Initially, the body responds to exercise by reducing blood flow to the skin. As body temperature begins to rise, however, nervous signals conduct more quickly and redirect the blood flow back to the skin to release the heat created from the metabolic activities.

The heart must work harder to accommodate the tissues' demand for blood. Sympathetic nervous system stimulation of the heart increases both HR and stroke volume, resulting in greater CO and increased BP of approximately 20-60 mmHg. At the same time, veins constrict, cooperating with the skeletal muscles to increase blood flow back to the heart for gaseous turnover in the lungs. Recall that the BP response in the vessels is a factor of CO and TPR; thus, the harder the body works, the more that pressure in blood vessels will increase. During activities of a rhythmic nature, such as running, swimming, or biking, the blood flows constantly and consistently back to the heart. Vasoconstriction efficiently manages venous return through coordinated smooth muscle action. Due to the relatively low forces produced by muscles during aerobic activities and rhythmic breathing rates, **diastolic blood pressure** (**DBP**) remains low. On the other hand, mean **systolic blood pressure** (**SBP**) and ventilation rates increase linearly with oxygen consumption and carbon dioxide production due to increases in CO and metabolic activity. When assessing exercise BP during aerobic steady-state work, exercise professionals should expect to see a rise in SBP consistent with the work rate but only a slight change in DBP compared to rest. This is important, as a continued increase in DBP during steady state exercise negatively associates with increased cardiac event risk.

Peripheral resistance increases when activities require greater intra-abdominal pressure for spinal stability and large muscle contractions mechanically compress arteries. Both DBP and SBP will increase linearly with the intensity of the effort during anaerobic exercise. The mag-

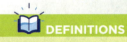
DEFINITIONS

Diastolic blood pressure –

The pressure within arteries in between heart beats when the ventricles are relaxed and filling with blood; it presents as the second value within blood pressure measurements (120/80 mmHg).

Systolic blood pressure –

The pressure within arteries during heart beats via contraction of the left ventricle; it presents as the first value within blood pressure measurements (120/80 mmHg).

nitude of the response is specific to the amount of muscle tissue employed and the intensity of the resistive load. BP increases further when internal compressive forces and external compressive forces combine. Exercises such as the back squat and leg press involve significant compressive forces from the external load, causing BP to increase dramatically. For this reason, hypertensive clients should avoid heavy lifting exercises, particularly those which apply compression to the body. Although factors that affect exercise BP can work independently, they usually work together to cause an additive effect.

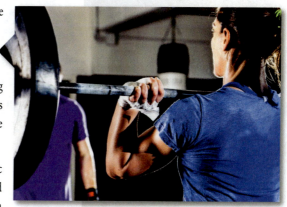

Exercise is crucial to promote a properly-functioning circulatory system. Aerobic exercise improves the body's BP response acutely and immediately following a period of exercise. When performed routinely, aerobic exercise has been shown to induce a chronic response at rest. It is suggested that alterations in the sympathetic nervous system reduce peripheral resistance, with increased renal secretion of sodium collectively accounting for the normal 8-11 mmHg reduction in BP following aerobic endurance training [39]. The chronic effects of resistance training do not yield the same results, but may provide slight improvement in resting measures. Measured BP response during resistance training has been shown to decrease with regular participation.

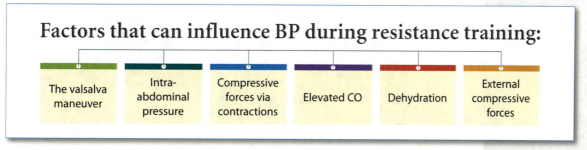

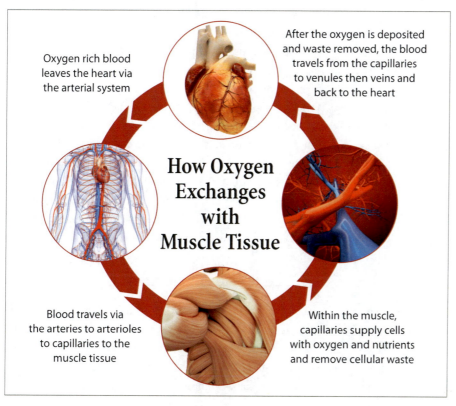

◆ Coronary Circulation

Like any other muscle, the heart's heightened action during physical activity increases its oxygen demand. However, the heart cannot pull oxygen from the blood in its atria or ventricles, as there are no circulatory channels inside the chambers. The coronary blood supply leaves the aorta through the main coronary arteries and enters an extensive network of myocardial blood vessels. This is termed coronary circulation. The myocardium is densely packed with capillaries and mitochondria, allowing for efficient extraction and utilization of oxygen. At rest, between 70-80% of oxygen is extracted from the 200-250 ml of coronary blood flow every minute. During activity, that value can jump 5-6 times if the activity is performed at a vigorous level [86]. The demand of work must be met by proportionate increases in coronary blood flow to maintain CO. As the myocardial tissue increases in metabolic function, the subsequent by-products' increasing concentration stimulates vasodilation, consequently increasing the flow of blood to the cardiac tissue. To estimate the oxygen demand of the heart, SBP is multiplied by the HR. The product, or myocardial oxygen demand, is called the **rate pressure product**.

> **DEFINITIONS**
>
> **Rate pressure product –**
>
> *An estimate of myocardial oxygen demand and cardiovascular disease risk; it is calculated as systolic blood pressure x heart rate.*
>
> **Myocardial infarction –**
>
> *The medical term for heart attack; it refers to the process by which one or more regions of the heart experience severe or prolonged ischemia due to a blockage of a coronary artery, resulting in the death of the affected cardiac tissue.*

PRACTICAL INSIGHT

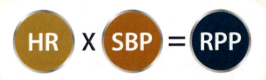

Rate Pressure Product (RPP)

Rate-pressure product (HR x SBP) is a little-known phenomenon with significant implications for health. An inability to supply oxygen to the myocardium when demand is high appears to contribute to several cardiovascular (CV) events: transient myocardial ischemia, acute **myocardial infarction**, and sudden death. The cardiac tissue's oxygen demand is a factor of activity; the more active the heart, the greater its oxygen demand. Ironically, as a person improves aerobic efficiency, the rate pressure product decreases at rest and during exercise. Sedentary individuals experience the opposite effect, which is one reason why a new exercise program causes discomfort. A high RPP at submaximal work means the cardiopulmonary system must labor harder relative to the activity. This further contributes to a heightened rate of perceived exertion (RPE). From a health perspective, RPP indicates CV risk when it exceeds 10,000 at rest, and this risk jumps as it passes 12,000. A person with a high BP of 160/90 mmHg and RHR of 80 bpm would have an RPP of 12800. To reduce cardiac event risk, RPP should be lowered to below 12,000 at rest using aerobic exercise; however, in many cases, physicians will also recommend pharmaceutical intervention due to the high level of hypertension.

As previously stated, cardiac muscle tissue is dense with mitochondria because it derives its energy almost exclusively from aerobic metabolism. Consequently, cardiac muscle is highly adapted for ATP production using lipid metabolism. In fact, the clear majority of the ATP the heart uses during rest comes from the metabolism of lipids. However, to accomplish increasingly intense exercise, energy metabolism comes from several sources: glucose, fatty acids, and lactate freed from skeletal muscle metabolism. During intense exercise, the heart is mainly fueled by aerobic metabolism of the lactate made available from CHO metabolism. When exercise is performed using a prolonged steady-state pace, heart tissue reverts to lipid metabolism to spare CHOs. When work is hard and CHOs are used as fuel, trained and untrained individuals are comparable in myocardial metabolic pathways. When work is moderate, trained individuals rely more on myocardial lipid metabolism when compared to their untrained counterparts, explaining lower relative RPE. Again, the differences reflect CHO-sparing in trained individuals.

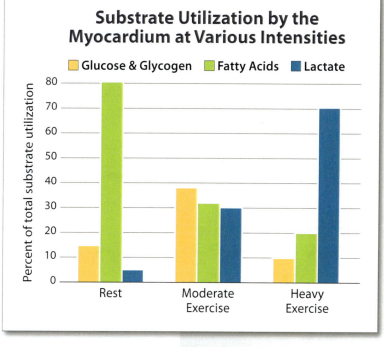

◆ Ventilation

During exercise, ventilation rates increase to meet the more active heart's oxygen demand. HR alone does not regulate the ventilation response. If it did, breathing rates would noticeably rise when the body experiences psychological nervousness or the presence of stimulants. Physiological control of respiration is multifaceted, based upon chemical, humoral, and neural mediation. At rest, pulmonary ventilation is largely controlled by factors that affect the chemical state of the blood: temperature, arterial gas concentrations, and pH. During the onset of exercise or work, body movement stimulates the brain's medulla through neurogenic means to increase respiration rates rapidly. This abrupt increase then levels and begins to reflect the intensity of the exercise more closely. Neurons in the brain and peripheral chemoreceptors in the vessels dictate ventilation rates to ensure adequate oxygen is available in the blood.

During exercise, ongoing ventilation will be controlled by chemoreceptor modulation based on concentrations of blood metabolites, temperature of the blood, and variations in gas exchange and blood pH. When the exercise is continuous and the body reaches steady-state, the ventilation rates are linear with respect to oxygen uptake. With intense exercise, the minute ventilation increases disproportionately to the oxygen uptake [108]. A dramatic upswing in breathing rate corresponds with a heightened rate of glycolysis. The by-products lactate, hydrogen ions, and carbon dioxide accumulation in the blood – trigger a signaling effect to restore blood homeostasis. In intense prolonged exercise that requires the highest levels of glycolytic activity, the onset of blood lactate accumulation (OBLA) progresses to **lactate threshold**. These markers promotes further increases in ventilation rates as the body attempts to make more oxygen available to the tissue and buffer the energy system's acidic by-products. Heavy resistance exercise performed

DEFINITIONS

Lactate threshold –

Reflects the maximal intensity at which steady state can be maintained: the intensity at which lactate accumulation begins to exceed lactate removal; muscle and blood lactate concentrations begin to increase exponentially; it is proposed as the best and most consistent predictor of endurance performance.

in short bouts also dramatically increases both heart and ventilation rates due to significant increases in blood lactate (51). This explains rapid post-lift respiration rates in exercises like the squat and deadlift but also in short distance sprinting.

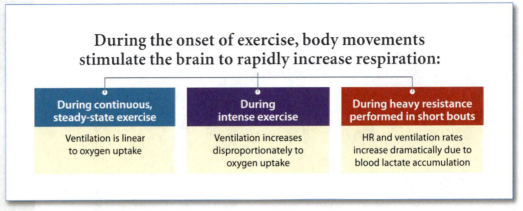

During the onset of exercise, body movements stimulate the brain to rapidly increase respiration:

During continuous, steady-state exercise	During intense exercise	During heavy resistance performed in short bouts
Ventilation is linear to oxygen uptake	Ventilation increases disproportionately to oxygen uptake	HR and ventilation rates increase dramatically due to blood lactate accumulation

Like cardiovascular adaptations, respiratory adaptations occur with specific training. In maximal measures, ventilation rates correspond to increases in oxygen consumption to match the greater oxygen levels required by the tissues. The increased turnover of oxygen to carbon dioxide triggers an increased ventilation rate to remove the CO_2 and infuse oxygen back into the blood. Over time, the body adapts to the stress, explaining why trained individuals expire about 3-4% less oxygen compared to untrained individuals at the same relative intensity. This results as the tissues use more oxygen, leading to less disruption and, consequently, lower respiration rates compared to untrained individuals. An improved rate of blood oxygen extraction by working tissues occurs in response to endurance adaptations, accounting for the differences between trained and untrained individuals.

The Endocrine System

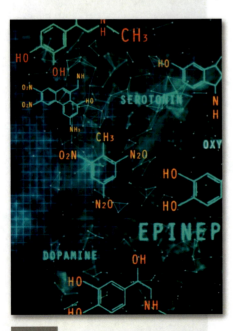

The endocrine system is a complex network of integrated organs that communicate directives to help regulate all other body systems. These effectively manage internal activities and maintain systemic homeostasis. Within the body, fine balances exist, with seemingly unlimited cause and effect patterns that occur in response to internal and external variations of environment. Although the systems of the body are often viewed independently, they are intimately integrated and do not function autonomously. The muscular and nervous systems' relationship illustrates one of many examples of interacting, networked systems. In essence, nerves serve as the brains behind all muscle activity, as a muscle cannot operate without neural communication. Additionally, the musculoskeletal system's function depends on the gastrointestinal system to supply it with nutrients for energy; and, of course, the cardiopulmonary system must work cooperatively with the cardiovascular system to deliver nutrients and oxygen while simultaneously eliminating the waste products of cellular metabolism. A less obvious relationship also exists between the muscular and endocrine systems. Most fitness professionals maintain a very limited knowledge of this relationship beyond being aware that it exists, with most attention directed towards the effects of anabolic hormones. Since exercise adaptations hinge upon this interactive relationship, exercise professionals must understand what stimulates the systems to adaptation in order to optimize health improvements and maximize performance.

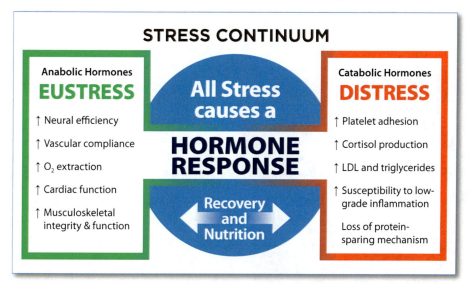

The endocrine system helps integrate and control operations needed to manage varying activities of the body. It provides internal balance to almost all aspects of human function. A group of small endocrine glands maintains homeostasis in every situation the body endures. This system's functions directly impact reproduction, growth, tissue maintenance and repair, and energy metabolism. In addition, it contributes importantly to the physiological actions that manage **eustress** and **distress**.

The endocrine system's main components include the pituitary, thyroid, adrenal, pineal, and thymus glands. Some hormonal providers include other functions in addition to their endocrine role, such as the **hypothalamus**, **pancreas**, and gonads (testicles and ovaries). In addition, certain other organs that aid in metabolic control further support this system: at least eight other hormones are produced in the stomach, duodenum, kidneys, heart, and plasma membranes of different bodily cells. However, this text will focus specifically on hormones and tissues most relevant to physical activity and the adaptations that most directly relate to participation in varying types of exercise.

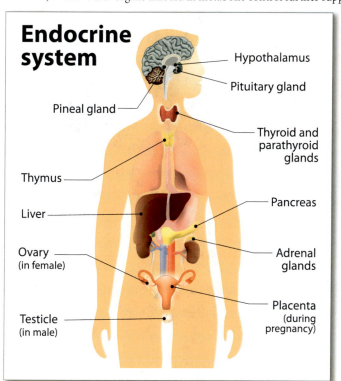

DEFINITIONS

Eustress –

A positive, desirable form of stress that influences physiological or psychological health; sources can include events such as exercise or working towards obtainable goals within one's occupation.

Distress –

A negative form of stress that influences physiological or psychological health; it can be caused by excessive stress of any type or forms of stress which are not associated with improving one's well-being, such as anxiety or lack of sleep.

Hypothalamus –

A region of the forebrain that coordinates the autonomic nervous system and governs the endocrine system via the pituitary gland; it directs homeostatic maintenance activities such as eating, drinking, body temperature regulation, sleep, and emotional responses.

Pancreas –

A relatively large gland that secretes digestive enzymes into the small intestines for macronutrient breakdown; it also produces the hormones insulin and glucagon for blood glucose regulation.

◆ Hormones

When endocrine glands produce and release hormones, they do so to communicate, directing the actions of other tissues via chemical messaging. Hormones fall into two classes: **steroids** (lipid based) and **polypeptides** (protein based). The type and structural basis of the hormone most often relates to its message and the tissue designed to receive it. During and following physical activity, hormones regulate electrolyte activity and acid/base balance and manage energy for biological work and recovery.

When a hormone is released, it travels through the body until it is picked up by the appropriate receptor on target cells. Cellular hormone receptors are small proteins on the outside of cells that bind to hormones and subsequently transmit the information into the cell to regulate the cells' behaviors. These receptors are generally specific to a single hormone, and not all cell types have every type of receptor. The concentration and location of hormone receptors depend upon the specific responsibility of the hormone. This efficient system ensures that only the tissue designated to receive the information gets it. This internal policy of communication is called target cell specificity. The messaging vehicle method used by e-mail provides an easy analogy to hormones and their receptors. When a person sends an e-mail, it travels through the internet, which is accessed by millions of people at any given time; however, only the designated recipients receive the information contained in it. Similarly, hormones travel past millions of cells but only interact with those cells that possess specific receptors with an affinity for that particular hormone.

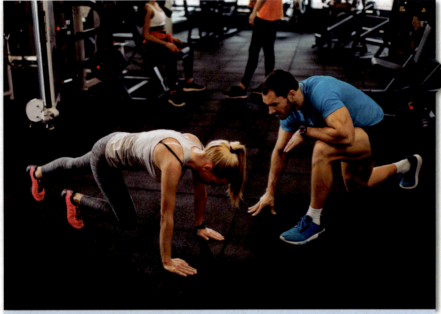

During and following exercise, hormones regulate electrolyte activity, acid/base balance and energy production for biological work and recovery.

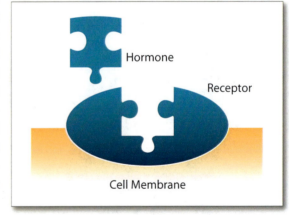

> **DEFINITIONS**
>
> **Steroid hormones –**
>
> *Organic, cholesterol-based hormone compounds that serve various functions related, but not limited to, sexual development, reproduction, tissue synthesis, inflammation regulation, and metabolism: examples include cortisol, aldosterone, estrogen, progesterone, and testosterone.*
>
> **Polypeptide hormones –**
>
> *A chain of amino acids synthesized on the ribosomes of the endoplasmic reticulum of endocrine cells; they attach to membrane receptors in order to activate second messenger systems: examples include insulin and glucagon.*

The specific activity each hormone regulates is often rather sophisticated because the signaling information is subject to variables. For instance, a hormone may relay information between itself and another hormone, but this message may be complicated by the internal environmental conditions. Factors such as the type of tissue the hormone binds to, what other hormones are binding to that tissue at that particular time, and the cellular environment occurring at the binding site all may compound the difficulty of relaying the correct information. Exercise of varied intensity challenges the endocrine system to ensure all metabolic factors are accounted for during the activity, as well as throughout the period that follows once the activity ceases. The process of returning the body back to its normal homeostatic condition requires a coordinated effort of hormone interactions across several systems.

Hormones are not produced at a constant rate but, rather, surge in response to variations in physiological and psychological demand; therefore, exercise and related stress have a notable effect on hormone activity [25, 38, 53, 93, 102, 109, 112]. Most endocrine glands do not store a large hormone reserve, and the hormones synthesized by the respective gland tend to equal the concentration of the hormone released. Rapid adjustments in production and excretion must occur to regulate the body's internal conditions when the environment changes from rest to activity. Generally, hormonal balance is consistent with maintaining a chemical uptake of hormone in reference to the rate of removal by the liver and kidneys. It seems the body constantly attempts to control concentration levels to maintain equilibrium so that hormones are only available to target tissues when needed.

Most of the controls that regulate hormone release and circulating concentrations are managed through a network of relational axes. This includes the hypothalamic-pituitary axis, GH-insulin-like growth factor (IGF) axis, and thyroid axis to name a few. The hypothalamus can be considered the coordinating center of the endocrine system. It consolidates signals derived from internal pathways and peripheral endocrine feedback, and responds to environmental cues such as light and temperature. Efficient data processing responds to perceived stress and allows the hypothalamus to deliver precise signals to the pituitary gland to release the appropriate hormones that influence most endocrine systems in the body. This is relevant to managing the stress from exercise, as the hypothalamic-pituitary axis directly affects the functions of the thyroid gland, the adrenal gland, and the gonads, as well as influencing growth and water balance. The homeostatic disruption of exercise causes different responses in each of the hormone axes. While the responses to exercise vary, it appears that immune and inflammatory responses and mediations may provide adaptive and regenerative response through the hormones of each respective axis [29, 32, 57, 77, 101]. This underscores the fact that signaling and resultant adaptations are training (stress) specific.

> **DEFINITIONS**
>
> **Anabolic hormones –**
>
> *Compounds involved in stimulating protein synthesis and tissue growth (muscle, organs, connective tissue); anabolism is associated with building tissues in general.*
>
> **Growth hormone (GH) –**
>
> *Promotes cell division and proliferation by facilitating protein synthesis; it protects glycogen reserves and limits carbohydrate metabolism by mobilizing lipids for fuel during exercise and plays a role in recovery.*
>
> **Testosterone –**
>
> *An anabolic hormone produced in the gonadal glands of both men and women. Men possess significantly (10x) greater quantities; it stimulates development of male secondary sexual characteristics.*
>
> **Insulin-like growth factor 1 (IGF-1) –**
>
> *Considered to be a central signaling hormone released from the liver that initiates muscle growth following resistance training.*

◆ Pituitary Hormones

Probably the most notable and easily-recognized hormones to those familiar with exercise are the **anabolic hormones**. Primary examples include **growth hormone (GH)**, **testosterone**, **insulin-like growth factor-1 (IGF-1)**: insulin and thyroid hormones produced from exercise [56, 57]. GH, formally called *somatotropin*, is excreted by the anterior pituitary gland and is one of the most relevant hormones in the body, having extensive responsibilities related to physiological activity [57, 117]. It promotes cell division and proliferation throughout the IGFs, as well as insulin. Each facilitates protein synthesis in muscle remodeling and aids in the adaptations of the body [12, 117]. It accomplishes this by increasing amino acid transport through plasma membranes, stimulating RNA formation, and activating cellular ribosomes [12]. GH also protects glycogen reserves and CHO breakdown by encouraging the mobilization and utilization of lipids for fuel during exercise, effectively decreasing the body's reliance on glucose for energy.

The hypothalamus constantly measures bodily stress. When stress increases, as with elevations in exercise intensity, the hypothalamus sends GH releasing-factor (GH-RF) hormones to the pituitary gland, stimulating pituitary secretion of GH. Since GH is released in proportion to intensity, the more intense the exercise, the greater the secretion and subsequent blood concentration of GH [56]. Factors that influence the release of GH-RF from the hypothalamus

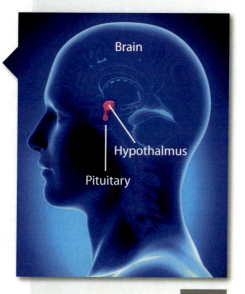

include low blood glucose, increased levels of certain amino acids, and stress, all of which occur during intense exercise. The elevation in GH during acute exercise benefits the active tissue and positively mediates energy metabolism [35, 50]. This action allows for prolonged work: the body relies on lipids for fuel while sparing CHOs [35]. Under certain exercise conditions, GH release does not appear to be dependent on training status, as untrained and trained individuals show similar levels of GH release when engaging in exercise to exhaustion. However, untrained individuals do show greater concentrations post exercise, which is likely due to the systems' inability to efficiently recover [90]. Likewise, during acute submaximal bouts, untrained individuals, when compared to conditioned individuals, show higher levels of GH [90]. These findings suggest that the perceived demand on the body determines the quantity of the GH production in response to exercise intensity [35].

DEFINITIONS

Myostatin –

A protein found primarily in skeletal muscle that functions to restrain the growth of muscular tissue; if myostatin were not restrained, muscle growth could theoretically have no limit, creating significant anatomical issues over time.

Androgenic hormone –

A generic term used to describe any natural or synthetic steroid-based hormone that controls the development and maintenance of masculine characteristics (e.g., facial hair, deepening of the voice).

The anabolic effect GH has on muscle mass, cartilage formation, and bone often occurs in conjunction and seems to be dependent upon another hormone, IGF-1 (35). By itself, GH does not have a profound effect on muscle mass. Rather, the interaction of IGF polypeptides and GH seems to be the main reason muscle fibers adapt by increasing the magnitude of their protein structures [35]. This occurs because IGF-1 plays a role in activating a key signaling pathway (Akt/mTOR-pathway) for muscle hypertrophy. The liver secretes IGF as dictated by the GH stimulation of liver cell DNA. The IGF binds to proteins, which transport and supervise the physiological mechanisms of the hormones [19]. A novel explanation of why IGF factors so importantly in hypertrophy is its effect on **myostatin**'s antagonist follistatin [62]. Because two crucial skeletal muscle growth factors, IGF-1 and IGF-2, are induced by myostatin inhibition, the stimulation of follistatin is needed to influence the IGF-IR/Akt/mTOR pathway, which promotes hypertrophy [62, 92]. Another important hormone, insulin, also affects follistatin-induced muscle hypertrophy. When either insulin or IGF-I is missing, anabolic adaptations can be maintained, but when both are deficient, as in the case of diabetics, follistatin fails to stimulate muscle growth [92]. It can be argued that a pro-diabetic environment inhibits muscle hypertrophic adaptations through this mechanism.

Testosterone has often been implicated as the premier anabolic hormone (probably due to the notability and effect of steroids), but it seems that the direct effect testosterone has on fiber hypertrophy is not as significant as that of IGF-signaling pathway [56]. It is important to understand that signaling dictates hypertrophy, not any one independent hormone. This explains why different types of training all have some hypertrophic effect. IGF directly increases protein synthesis activity when properly initiated through the GH signaling pathway, whereas **test**osterone's direct path depends heavily on androgen receptor affinity. While testosterone can have a marked effect on muscle mass, testosterone's main contribution to muscle hypertrophy stems more likely from its effect on increasing the quantity of GH released from the pituitary gland and the synergistic augmentation of GH response on target tissues, rather than through its direct effect on muscle cell DNA activity [56, 57].

◆ Gonadal Hormones - Testosterone

Testosterone is produced in the gonadal glands of men and women and is the primary **androgenic hormone** for secondary male characteristics. It is also the primary hormone responsible the visual and quantifiable differences between men and women. Testosterone, though, is not a male or female hormone; however, distinct differences exist in

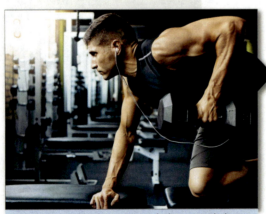

Testosterone's contribution to anabolic activity helps characterize the differences in lean mass and strength found between men and women.

the hormone's concentration within the respective sexes, as well as the specific androgen receptor density and affinity. Males demonstrate much higher concentrations of androgen receptors and circulating testosterone than do women.

Gender	Normal levels of testosterone
Men	270-1070 ng/dL (9-38 nmol/L)
Women	15-70 ng/dL (0.52-2.4 nmol/L)
Children	2-20 ng/dL (0.07-0.7 nmol/L)

Testosterone's contribution to anabolic activity helps characterize the differences in lean mass and strength found between men and women. Although the concentration of testosterone in women is ten times less than that in men, concentrations will increase in response to exercise in both genders[58]. Similar to testosterone, **estrogen** is not a gender-specific hormone. Testosterone is converted into estrogen (estradiol) in men and aids in the maintenance of bone throughout a male's lifespan. Estrogen is a key hormone in bone maintenance in both men and women. When men inject testosterone or take supplemental testosterone precursors such as dehydroepiandrosterone (DHEA), androstenediol, or androstenedione, the body may perceive excessively high concentrations and attempt to re-establish hormonal balance. It accomplishes this by converting the excess testosterone to estradiol through a process called **aromatization**[11]. This explains why male steroid users may develop breast tissue called **gynecomastia** and experience testicular **atrophy**.

When testosterone interacts with muscle tissue, it does so through direct and indirect mechanisms. Testosterone increases pituitary gland activity, causing the release of GH, which, in this case, would be an indirect influence on protein synthesis in the tissue[56]. As mentioned earlier, testosterone does directly communicate via signaling pathways (PI3K/Akt), which can control skeletal muscle mass through mTOR regulation of protein synthesis. These physiological signals are modulated through the interaction of testosterone with the intracellular androgen receptor. This relationship identifies the direct pathway testosterone takes to encourage increased protein synthesis, which depends heavily upon androgen receptor affinity, again demonstrating differences between the sexes. Testosterone also interacts with the nervous system to enhance force capacity and the physiological cross-sectional area via direct influence on neurons and structural protein changes. Increases in testosterone concentrations are attributed to participation in higher intensity exercises that utilize large amounts of muscle tissue.

◆ Pancreatic Hormones

CHOs are broken down primarily into simple sugars, so they can be absorbed by the blood stream. The most common outcome is glucose. When glucose enters the blood stream, the pancreatic receptors assesses the concentration level as blood flows through the pancreatic tissue. These receptors indicate the concentration of insulin to be released into the blood stream based on the blood glucose content. The greater the glucose concentration, the more insulin produced and secreted from the pancreatic beta cells in the islet of Langerhans. The pancreas attempts to maintain a homeostatic-state of blood glucose by modulating **insulin** concentrations to offset

> **DEFINITIONS**
>
> **Estrogen –**
>
> A steroid hormone that promotes the development and maintenance of female secondary characteristics (e.g., breast tissue).
>
> **Aromatization –**
>
> Chemical reaction process by which excess testosterone is converted to estrogen in order to maintain a homeostatic environment.
>
> **Gynecomastia –**
>
> An overdevelopment of the mammary glands among males (male breast tissue) due to hormonal imbalance; it is often cited as a side-effect of anabolic-androgenic steroid abuse.
>
> **Atrophy –**
>
> The wasting away of an organ, muscle, or other bodily tissue; it is often associated with the loss of muscle mass due to inactivity.
>
> **Insulin –**
>
> A hormone produced by the pancreas that serves various functions including blood glucose control and tissue growth; insulin dysfunction is related to diabetes.

The pancreas has two main functions:

The production of digestive enzymes to break down fat, carbohydrates, and protein for absorption via the lining of the small intestine	The regulation of blood sugar levels by the release of insulin and glucagon

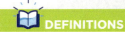

DEFINITIONS

Hyperglycemia –

An abnormally high blood glucose level; it is a hallmark sign of diabetes, which can potentially damage bodily tissues, including vascular structures.

Hypoglycemia –

A low blood sugar level that occurs when glucose concentrations drop below a critical concentration in the blood; where the metabolic demands of the brain and central nervous system cannot be met.

Catecholamines –

Potent neurotransmitters that help the body respond to stress or elicit "fight-or-flight" reactions: e.g., dopamine, epinephrine, norepinephrine.

changes associated with physical activity, eating, and drinking. After a meal when the blood sugar rises, the consequent release of insulin drives glucose, to be stored as glycogen, into the muscle and liver cells via the insulin regulated glucose sensor GLUT4 [43]. Through the GLUT4 receptor, insulin also pushes some of the excess sugar into adipocytes, where the imported glucose is converted into triglycerides (TG). This process helps lower blood glucose back to resting homeostatic levels. When insulin is appropriately regulated, CHO levels in the blood do not surpass the apparent glucose concentration threshold, which reduces the propensity of insulin to facilitate fat cell uptake of sugar [91]. Insulin's presence in circulation inhibits lipolysis because the body attempts to clear high levels of glucose, as chronic **hyperglycemia** damages vessel walls. To the contrary, in the absence of insulin, fat cells release fatty acids to fuel energy demands. Therefore, lowering glycemic loads upon the metabolic system will control insulin levels. Clearly, dietary intake of excess calories, simple sugars, and processed CHOs should be controlled to optimize fat utilization and reduce the risk of fat storage caused by high blood glucose concentrations [91].

Conversely, low blood glucose levels cause a condition called **hypoglycemia**. When this occurs, the alpha cells in the pancreas are stimulated to release glucagon. Glucagon shares a reciprocal relationship with insulin in terms of role and release rates. Glucagon quickly travels to the liver to stimulate the release of stored glucose from glycogen through a process called **glycogenolysis**. The freed glucose can now enter circulation to raise and stabilize the blood glucose concentration back to a steady-state. Regular exercise enables the body to manage blood glucose dynamics much more efficiently. Exercise increases the presence of **catecholamines**, which have an inhibitory effect on beta cells in the pancreas. Consequently, this inhibition reduces circulating insulin levels [103]. The drop in insulin during exercise is then matched by an enhancement in muscle cell permeability to energy substrates to balance the cells' need. Concurrently, liver cells become more sensitive to glucagon and epinephrine to raise (and sustain) glucose levels to meet the physical activity's demands [103]. As exercise duration increases, so does the contribution of fatty acids. The energy shift is necessary to account for the reduction in available glycogen from muscles and the liver. These are all positive adaptations. They not only reduce risk for diabetes and metabolic syndrome but can also reverse the process, particularly for those in a pre-diabetic state.

It is important to understand the anabolic nature of insulin. It is true that insulin's major function is to regulate glucose metabolism in the tissues through facilitated diffusion; however, insulin is more anabolically dynamic than many people realize [2]. As mentioned before, GLUT4 located in the cell membrane transports glucose into the cell in the presence of insulin. Without insulin, only trace quantities of glucose can enter the cell via muscular contractions. This fact explains why individuals with type 1 diabetes, who cannot produce insulin in the pancreas, must inject insulin for proper cellular function. Additionally, insulin's presence in the muscle cells increases enzyme activity via signaling mechanisms that facilitate heightened protein synthesis. Ipso facto, insulin is anabolic both in its effect on glucose's uptake in lipid and muscle cells, and also through the promotion of protein synthesis [107].

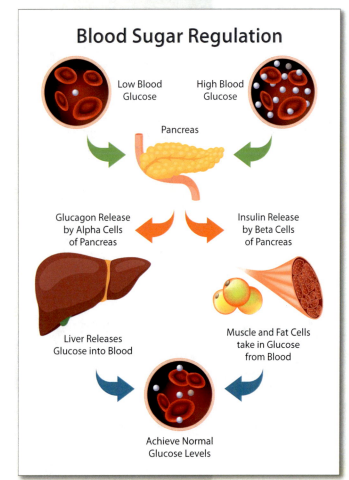

◆ Thyroid Hormones

The **thyroid** manages human metabolism through the action of its hormones thyroxine (T4) and tri-iodothyroxine (T3), which it makes by extracting iodine from the blood. T3 is the active form of thyroid hormone and increases the metabolic rate of all cells [1]. In fact, every cell depends on the thyroid to manage its metabolism.

Thyroid action is regulated via the hypothalamus-pituitary-thyroid axis. The hypothalamus senses low levels of thyroid hormone and, in response, releases thyrotropin-releasing hormone (TRH) which stimulates the pituitary to release thyroid-stimulating hormone (TSH). TSH then prompts the thyroid to secrete the pro-hormone thyroxin (T4) and, to a lesser extent, receptor-active T3 [72, 124]. The majority of circulating T3 comes from peripheral conversion of T4 by intracellular enzymes. Thyroid hormones have profound effects on growth and metabolism, and while not necessary for life, thyroid hormone deficiency does have consequences on normal health. Thyroid hormone is important for normal child development, and in adults is thought to serve a permissive role in lean mass maintenance and development. It does so by facilitating the actions of anabolic hormones and stimulating an increased secretion of GH in the pituitary gland and IGF-1 by the liver. During heavy exercise, thyroxine (T4) increases by about 35% [20]. This elevation possibly contributes to immediate short-term excess post-exercise oxygen consumption (EPOC) through an increase in temperature and metabolic rate of cells. The heightened metabolic activity purportedly benefits weight management due to an increased use of fatty acids for fuel [52, 97].

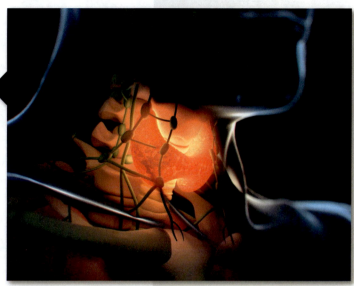

Individuals suffering from "slow metabolism" may actually be experiencing **hypothyroidism**. This condition occurs when the body lacks sufficient levels of thyroid hormones. While estimates vary, it is suggested that ~10 million Americans have this issue. Females may be more susceptible, as it is estimated that as many as 10% of women may have some degree of thyroid hormone deficiency. Hashimoto's thyroiditis is the common form of thyroid inflammation caused by one's own immune system. The disorder damages the thyroid and reduces its capacity to form and secrete hormones.

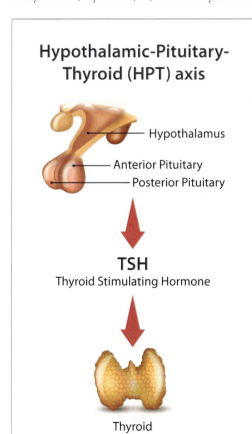

> **DEFINITIONS**
>
> **Thyroid** –
>
> *A gland which serves as the primary regulator for growth and development via the rate of metabolism within the body.*
>
> **Hypothyroidism** –
>
> *An abnormally low activity of the thyroid gland which results in "slow metabolism" and usually weight gain; it can result in retardation of growth and mental development.*

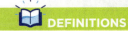

DEFINITIONS

Adrenal cortex –

The outer portion of the adrenal glands that secretes steroidal hormones such as cortisol and aldosterone.

Cortisol –

Regulates numerous metabolic and cardiovascular functions and helps to manage blood pressure; it is released in response to exercise stress and low blood glucose concentrations; a chronic elevation in cortisol levels is associated with overtraining.

Adrenal medulla –

The inner portion of the adrenal glands that converts the amino acid tyrosine into the catecholamines for release into the bloodstream.

Epinephrine –

A catecholamine hormone, also known as adrenaline, that is secreted by the adrenal glands during conditions of stress to increase blood circulation, ventilation, and carbohydrate metabolism to prepare skeletal muscles for exertion.

Norepinephrine –

A catecholamine hormone secreted from the adrenal glands in response to stress by increasing blood pressure and blood glucose levels; it has an affinity for different tissue receptors than epinephrine but facilitates similar responses.

◆ Adrenal Hormones

The adrenal glands produce two categories of hormones: steroidal and neural. Steroidal hormones are essential hormones secreted from the **adrenal cortex**. They include two main groups of corticosteroid hormones: glucocorticoids and mineralcorticoids. The hypothalamus triggers the pituitary gland to excrete adrenocorticotropin (ACTH) through the hypothalamus-pituitary-adrenal axis, which stimulates the adrenal cortex to secrete the glucocorticoid hydrocortisone, commonly known as **cortisol**, as well as corticosterone. Cortisol regulates metabolic and cardiovascular functions and helps to manage BP. Corticosterone works with cortisol to regulate immune response and suppress inflammatory reactions. Mineralcorticoids are mediated by signals triggered by the kidneys. The principle mineralcorticoid is aldosterone,

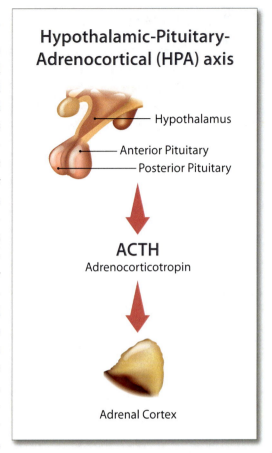

which functions to maintain the body's sodium and fluid balance and aids in BP regulation. The adrenal cortex also releases androgens, but their concentrations tend to be overshadowed by the quantities produced by the sexual glands.

The neural hormones originate in the **adrenal medulla** and are commonly referred to as catecholamines. Neural pathways stimulate the adrenal medulla, which provides a rapid release of the catecholamines **epinephrine** (adrenaline) and **norepinephrine** (noradrenaline). These

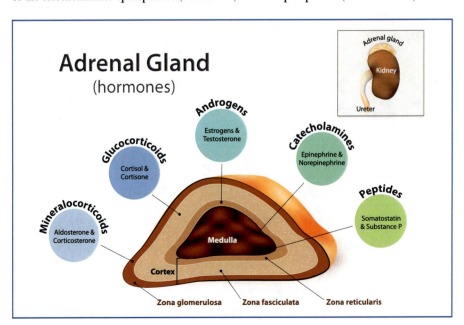

bind to adrenergic receptors on target cells where they induce the same effects as direct sympathetic nervous system stimulation. The adrenal medulla augments neural effects in response to varied levels of stress. When stress is perceived, the adrenal hormones increase energy provisions and oxygen to tissues by increasing CO, blood flow, and energy metabolism: this is commonly referred to as the **fight-or-flight response**. The release of catecholamines is based on the acute stress experienced by the body. As with the other adrenal hormones, prolonged stress leads to oversaturation of the receptors and decreased sensitivity, both of which contribute to poor recovery and other detrimental outcomes. The adrenal gland links very tightly to all components of training and recovery, including immuno-related activity [34]. This suggests that training needs to be dose-appropriate and balanced with other perceived stresses in the body to insure positive adaptive outcomes. Both sympathetic and parasympathetic overtraining syndromes may potentially have adrenal hormone implications.

All adrenal hormones relate very importantly to exercise: they are specifically designed to manage the internal responses of stress [65]. Epinephrine stimulates the cardiovascular system and releases energy into circulation. Aldosterone plays a key role in regulating electrolyte concentration via ion activity and water balance as it reabsorbs or excretes sodium. It also helps maintain proper mineral balance, which assists nerve transmission and subsequent motor function. Cortisol contributes to ongoing physical activity through glucose metabolism and the preservation of the body's sugar reserves [65]. During long duration exercise, cortisol acts as an insulin antagonist, catabolizing protein for sugar and inhibiting CHO uptake and oxidation in the body [22].

While stress hormones are not necessarily problematic, they can lead to health problems when chronically present. In particular, cortisol can present challenges for those suffering from high psychological stress because the body reacts to stress uniformly and does not distinguish between psychological and physical stresses. The chronic presence of cortisol leads to significant protein breakdown, thereby promoting muscle wasting and a negative **nitrogen balance**. It does so by increasing **proteolytic enzymes**, converting amino acids to glucose, and inhibiting protein synthesis in a process to provide energy and spare glucose. It also promotes visceral fat storage and inflammation during periods of chronic exposure to stress, which are compounded by obesity [64, 82, 118]. Additionally, sustained high levels of cortisol and corticosterone can suppress immune function, making the body more susceptible to infection [21]. This explains, in part, how psychological stress can play a role in inhibiting immune function [73]. Fortunately, the body does possess a natural defense against the catabolic effects of cortisol. Testosterone can block the genetic element in DNA from cortisol, or insulin can bind in greater numbers to receptors, trumping cortisol's effects on the protein [22, 109]. The hormones that are more prevalent and dominate the anabolic/catabolic balance determine what occurs in the tissue. This clearly accentuates the concept that stress must be controlled and balanced, as too much can be detrimental.

> **DEFINITIONS**
>
> **Fight-or-flight response –**
>
> *An acute increase in adrenal hormone activity which expedites enhancements in cardiac output, blood flow, and energy metabolism to rapidly deal with a perceived stress.*
>
> **Nitrogen balance –**
>
> *A comparison of nitrogen input and nitrogen output; it is widely used to determine recommended dietary intake for protein, as protein is almost the exclusive source of nitrogen to the body.*
>
> **Proteolytic enzymes –**
>
> *Function to break down protein compounds and eventually amino acids for energy use or protein recycling.*

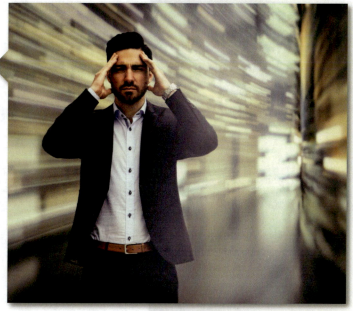

Endocrine Gland	Hormone	Action
Anterior Pituitary	Growth Hormone	Stimulates IGF, protein synthesis, growth and metabolism
Thyroid	Thyroxine	Stimulates metabolic rate, regulates cell growth and activity
Adrenal Cortex	Cortisol	Promotes use of fatty acids and protein catabolism; conserves sugar; maintains blood glucose level
Adrenal Cortex	Aldosterone	Promotes sodium, potassium metabolism and water retention
Adrenal Medulla	Epinephrine	Increases cardiac output; increases glycogen catabolism and fatty acid release
Adrenal Medulla	Norepinephrine	Has properties of epinephrine and constricts blood vessels
Pancreas	Insulin	Promotes glucose uptake by the cell, stores glycogen; aids in protein synthesis
Pancreas	Glucagon	Releases sugar from the liver into circulation
Liver	Insulin-like Growth Factors	Increases protein synthesis
Ovaries	Estrogen	Stimulates bone remodeling activity; female sex hormone
Testes	Testosterone	Stimulates growth; increases protein anabolism; reduces body fat; male sex hormone

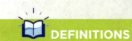

DEFINITIONS

Afferent stimuli –

Sensory information carried inward toward the brain and spinal cord from sensory and motor nerves throughout the body, as opposed to efferent stimuli, which carry information from the brain to the peripheral nerves.

◆ Hormone Considerations for Training

While at rest, sensory organs function through several mechanisms to ensure adequate homeostatic control. The coordinated secretions of several hormones regulate the daily operations for energy delivery and tissue health. When the motor neurons activate for exercise, sport, or self-preservation, the **afferent stimuli** to the brain cause a reactive communication to the endocrine system; this system then responsively secretes the appropriate hormones to manage the situation. As previously mentioned, acute hormonal, neural, and immune messengers are stimulated from physiological or psychological stress and from cellular disruption resulting from stress; these communicators direct hormonal activity specific to the type of stress the body experiences [56, 77]. Molecular mechanisms controlling muscle function and fiber type relate to the specific mode of muscle activation [26, 83, 114]. While a continuum exists, hormone responses to exercise can be distinguished by the force requirements and duration of tension applied. This simply categorizes modalities as low-force activities and high-force activities. Ergo, the responses one experiences from anaerobic endurance training are different from that elicited by muscular power and strength training. In turn, these differ from those of aerobic training. Each type of stress and the way that stress is applied triggers specific communications via the body's systems that manage the internal environment during and after an exercise session. The neural patterns activate hormonal patterns, shaping the adaptive response. Because the internal physiological environment is consistent in its response to the stress of a particular nature, outcomes are very predictive; thus, they depend upon the exercise-type, intensity, rest interval, and duration.

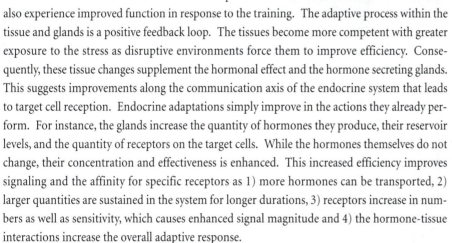

As the training regimen's intensity increases, the changes in both the muscular system, nervous system, and endocrine system become more apparent [56, 83, 109]. A great deal of attention is paid to the cellular activities of the target tissue; however, it is important to note that the hormones that most often dictate the adaptations also experience improved function in response to the training. The adaptive process within the tissue and glands is a positive feedback loop. The tissues become more competent with greater exposure to the stress as disruptive environments force them to improve efficiency. Consequently, these tissue changes supplement the hormonal effect and the hormone secreting glands. This suggests improvements along the communication axis of the endocrine system that leads to target cell reception. Endocrine adaptations simply improve in the actions they already perform. For instance, the glands increase the quantity of hormones they produce, their reservoir levels, and the quantity of receptors on the target cells. While the hormones themselves do not change, their concentration and effectiveness is enhanced. This increased efficiency improves signaling and the affinity for specific receptors as 1) more hormones can be transported, 2) larger quantities are sustained in the system for longer durations, 3) receptors increase in numbers as well as sensitivity, which causes enhanced signal magnitude and 4) the hormone-tissue interactions increase the overall adaptive response.

 ## Anaerobic Training Response

The positive adaptation that occurs in muscle protein is called muscle restructuring or remodeling. When the tissue experiences significant physiological stress, the consequent disruption and damage to the muscle cell stimulates an inflammatory response [27]. The nature of the physiological disruption determines the extent of remodeling from neural, hormonal, and immune system influences [27, 96]. The hormonal interaction of GH, testosterone, IGF, T3, and insulin causes the cell to synthesize new protein structures along the sarcomere [96]. Starting at the genetic level, cellular stimulation via the interaction of hormones initiates the action by which the muscle cells lay down new proteins [56]. The contractile proteins (actin and myosin) and the structural non-contractile proteins all experience enhancements, leading to greater tissue size and strength. The magnitude and specificity of the adaptations depend on fiber type. Fast-twitch fibers experience a far more dramatic effect in protein synthesis within the myofilaments than do slow-twitch fibers. This fact explains why they are most often targeted for muscle hypertrophy. However, the abundance of slow-twitch fibers distributed throughout the muscular system still plays a key role in muscle mass augmentation. Although limited protein synthesis occurs, slow-twitch fibers experience reduced degradation from hormone mediation. This combination of protein synthesis and reduced protein metabolism leads to noticeable gains in muscle tissue over time.

Resistance programs traditionally designed for strength training typically utilize heavy resistance, lower repetitions, and near maximal recovery periods (2-5 minutes) between sets in efforts to maximize force output. This formula makes the hormone activity very predictable. The training causes an increase in the presence of anabolic hormones. Early studies showed that this was explained by acute increases in testosterone without the more notable increases in GH-IGF signaling pathway. Highlighted earlier, IGF-1 affects protein synthesis via intramuscular anabolic signaling through the mTORC1 pathway. Some studies have previously shown that testosterone and neural factors contribute to increased force output in traditional high intensity strength training. In these findings, less protein synthesis seemed to occur due to reduced mTOR-mediated signaling; however, more recent studies show that this may not be the case. When the endocrine responses to traditional high-intensity strength training were compared to high volume strength training, some of the previous responses seemed to hold true: GH, cortisol, and insulin concentrations were higher following the traditional hypertrophy high volume training. However, IGF-1 and testosterone seemed to have a similar response to both training conditions. Though the different training protocols elicited different markers of muscle damage and different endocrine responses, intramuscular anabolic signaling and mTORC1 were similarly increased and activated [36].

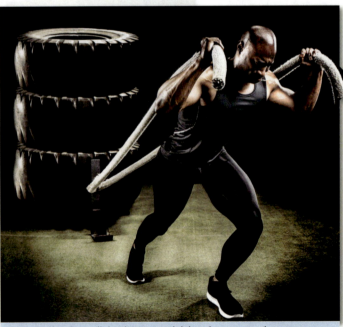

The early idea that cellular damage and delayed-onset muscle soreness (DOMS) is the only way to promote hypertrophy seemed to be overhyped with the thought of "break it down, to build up" - as many studies have shown that this is not necessary for muscle cell hypertrophy.

To increase lean mass, training can be modified to promote hypertrophic signaling using a variety of methods. Occlusion training using 20-30% 1RM indicates that mass can be gained at relatively low loads. This occurs due to the metabolic stress the muscle cells experience in the significant ischemic environment resulting from all-out efforts [99, 123]. Similarly, mass development can be triggered at moderately low intensities (50-75% 1RM), when rest is limited, relative to the intensity and volume employed. Significant increases in lean mass have also been associated with moderately high intensities as well: 75-90% 1RM and longer rest intervals allow sufficient recovery, so the repetitions at these higher intensities can be accomplished. Though the exact mechanisms behind the increase in lean mass seen throughout these protocols remain unclear, the literature does seem to lean towards a few commonly accepted ideas. One mechanism supported by occlusion training studies is that the tissue experiences a significant inflammatory effect due to metabolic stress caused by the hydrogen-induced ischemia of the cell.

The early idea was that cell damage and the related delayed-onset muscle soreness (DOMS) promoted hypertrophy. This theory was overhyped by the mainstream media: many studies have subsequently shown that this "break it down, to build it up" idea is unnecessary for muscle cell hypertrophy. Muscle activation due to mechanical load stress offers another mechanism that may explain the hypertrophic response of the high-intensity protocols: this process seems to increase intramuscular anabolic signaling and mTORC1 activation. Based on this information and other data, a variety of protocols seem available that all elicit muscle growth. A common theme across each mechanism is adequate volume. For optimal results, the same muscle group across 30-40 sets per bout should be used constantly to maximize activation and appropriate time-under-tension. Traditional approaches have consistently tested positively using multiple sets (3-5) of moderately heavy resistance (70-85% of 1RM) performed at maximal time under tension (6-12 repetitions) with short rest periods (30-90 seconds have demonstrated to be effective at dramatically raising serum concentrations of GH and IGF-1 signaling and intracellular phosphorylation [36, 56, 57]. Classically considered the recipe for bodybuilding, the previously mentioned collective activity utilizes all the appropriate reactive stimuli for muscle growth.

Notable factors to consider with hypertrophy training are the total volume of training and its effect on cellular ischemia; this method effects blood lactate, glucose, IGF, mTORC1 activation, and cortisol levels. Although the presence and products of stress hormones are often considered detrimental, a definite link exists between the stress that causes their presence and the response of the pituitary gland. Compared to other stress stimuli, it is suggested that the body manages cortisol activity differently in high-demand resistance-stress environments by blunting its catabolic effects via testosterone or insulin [105]. Ischemia and low blood pH are associated with concurrent cortisol release by the adrenal glands, which respond to high intensity, extended time-under-tension exercise. This is thought to be the environmental signaling path to the GH-IGF axis [35, 56, 57]. High-volume and short-rest periods stimulate both cortisol release and higher concentrations of GH and blood lactate, while heavy resistance training and long rest periods do not. This would explain why heavy strength training provides limited impact on hypertrophy compared to the bodybuilding approach. The most common errors in bodybuilding or activities aimed at hypertrophy are the following: lifting too light; not properly applying high enough volume of isolative overload via too few repetitions in relation to the resistance used; and/or resting too long between sets and exercises. These programmatic factors consequently reduce the magnitude of the hormonal response.

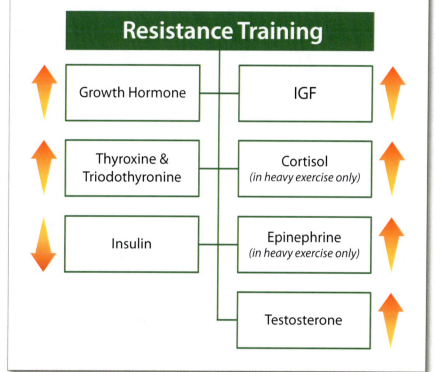

◆ Effects on Aerobic Fitness

Hormone signaling is different in response to endurance training compared to resistance training [109]. This occurs, in part, due to the activity's lower force requirements and the common employment of steady-state exercise that utilizes the repeated action of certain muscle groups. Hormone activity seems to be sensitive to variations of intensity, so when the intensity is sustained, a lower hormone response is observed [21, 109, 110]. Similar to resistance training, GH released in response to endurance activities depends upon the intensity [53, 57]. High-intensity training, particularly that done above one's lactate threshold, shows a greater increase in GH compared to that employing lower intensity [57]. On the other hand, testosterone seems to be suppressed during high-intensity aerobic activities, though plasma levels will increase modestly during lower levels of endurance training [21]. In sum, testosterone production during aerobic activities lags when compared to anaerobic exercise at similar rates of perceived exertion. Insulin sensitivity is heightened and glucagon levels will increase slightly as exercise becomes more prolonged [85]. During steady-state exercise, catecholamines seem to remain relatively stable throughout the bout, but cortisol will increase with ongoing work. In long endurance bouts, such as running a marathon, cortisol production will increase more dramatically to promote CHO sparing and help maintain energy stores [41]. Activities using aerobic metabolism do not stimulate the GH-IGF pathways, explaining why hypertrophy does not occur as a common adaptation. In fact, while moderate aerobic exercise has minimal effect on muscle mass, high-volume endurance training has a propensity to decrease lean mass [55].

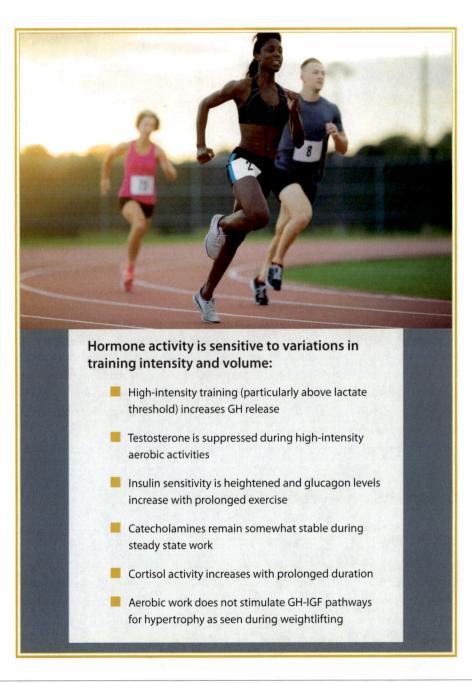

Hormone activity is sensitive to variations in training intensity and volume:

- High-intensity training (particularly above lactate threshold) increases GH release

- Testosterone is suppressed during high-intensity aerobic activities

- Insulin sensitivity is heightened and glucagon levels increase with prolonged exercise

- Catecholamines remain somewhat stable during steady state work

- Cortisol activity increases with prolonged duration

- Aerobic work does not stimulate GH-IGF pathways for hypertrophy as seen during weightlifting

REFERENCES:

1. Adamo K, Tarnopolsky M, and Graham T. Dietary carbohydrate and postexercise synthesis of proglycogen and macroglycogen in human skeletal muscle. *American Journal of Physiology-Endocrinology And Metabolism* 275: E229-E234, 1998.

2. Alessi DR, Andjelkovic M, Caudwell B, Cron P, Morrice N, Cohen P, and Hemmings B. Mechanism of activation of protein kinase B by insulin and IGF-1. *The EMBO journal* 15: 6541, 1996.

3. Anderson T, Lane AR, and Hackney AC. Cortisol and testosterone dynamics following exhaustive endurance exercise. *European journal of applied physiology* 116: 1503-1509, 2016.

4. Angeli A, Minetto M, Dovio A, and Paccotti P. The overtraining syndrome in athletes: a stress-related disorder. *J Endocrinol Invest* 27: 603-612, 2004.

5. Baker JS, McCormick MC, and Robergs RA. Interaction among Skeletal Muscle Metabolic Energy Systems during Intense Exercise. *J Nutr Metab* 2010: 905612, 2010.

6. Baker JS, McCormick MC, and Robergs RA. Interaction among skeletal muscle metabolic energy systems during intense exercise. *Journal of nutrition and metabolism* 2010, 2010.

7. Barclay CJ. Energy demand and supply in human skeletal muscle. *J Muscle Res Cell Motil*, 2017.

8. Berardi JM, Price TB, Noreen EE, and Lemon PW. Postexercise muscle glycogen recovery enhanced with a carbohydrate-protein supplement. *Medicine & Science in Sports & Exercise* 38: 1106-1113, 2006.

9. Blom P, Høstmark AT, Vaage O, Kardel KR, and MæHLUM S. Effect of different post-exercise sugar diets on the rate of muscle glycogen synthesis. *Medicine and Science in Sports and Exercise* 19: 491-496, 1987.

10. Borer KT. *Exercise endocrinology*: Human Kinetics, 2003.

11. Broeder C, Quindry J, Brittingham K, Panton L, Thomson J, Appakondu S, Breuel K, Byrd R, Douglas J, and Earnest C. The Andro Project: physiological and hormonal influences of androstenedione supplementation in men 35 to 65 years old participating in a high-intensity resistance training program. *Archives of Internal Medicine* 160: 3093-3104, 2000.

12. Brooks AJ and Waters MJ. The growth hormone receptor: mechanism of activation and clinical implications. *Nature Reviews Endocrinology* 6: 515-525, 2010.

13. Burke LM, Hawley JA, Wong SHS, and Jeukendrup AE. Carbohydrates for training and competition. *Journal of Sports Sciences* 29: S17-S27, 2011.

14. Burke LM, van Loon LJ, and Hawley JA. Postexercise muscle glycogen resynthesis in humans. *Journal of Applied Physiology* 122: 1055-1067, 2017.

15. Cairns SP. Lactic acid and exercise performance. *Sports Medicine* 36: 279-291, 2006.

16. Carey DG. Quantifying differences in the "fat burning" zone and the aerobic zone: implications for training. *J Strength Cond Res* 23: 2090-2095, 2009.

17. Carroll TJ, Taylor JL, and Gandevia SC. Recovery of central and peripheral neuromuscular fatigue after exercise. *J Appl Physiol (1985)* 122: 1068-1076, 2017.

18. Carroll TJ, Taylor JL, and Gandevia SC. Recovery of central and peripheral neuromuscular fatigue after exercise. *Journal of Applied Physiology* 122: 1068-1076, 2017.

19. Cheung K, Hume PA, and Maxwell L. Delayed Onset Muscle Soreness. *Sports Medicine* 33: 145-164, 2003.

20. Ciloglu F, Peker I, Pehlivan A, Karacabey K, Ihan N, Saygin O, and Ozmerdivenli R. Exercise intensity and its effects on thyroid hormones. *Neuroendocrinology letters* 26: 830-834, 2005.

21. Consitt LA, Copeland JL, and Tremblay MS. Endogenous anabolic hormone responses to endurance versus resistance exercise and training in women. *Sports Medicine* 32: 1-22, 2002.

22. Daly W, Seegers C, Rubin D, Dobridge J, and Hackney A. Relationship between stress hormones and testosterone with prolonged endurance exercise. *European journal of applied physiology* 93: 375-380, 2005.

23. de Chantemèle EB, Pascaud L, Custaud MA, Capri A, Louisy F, Ferretti G, Gharib C, and Arbeille P. Calf venous volume during stand test after a 90 day bed rest study with or without exercise countermeasure. *The Journal of physiology* 561: 611-622, 2004.

24. De Feo P, Di Loreto C, Lucidi P, Murdolo G, Parlanti N, De Cicco A, Piccioni F, and Santeusanio F. Metabolic response to exercise. *J Endocrinol Invest* 26: 851-854, 2003.

25. Douglas JA, Deighton K, Atkinson JM, Sari-Sarraf V, Stensel DJ, and Atkinson G. Acute exercise and appetite-regulating hormones in overweight and obese individuals: A meta-analysis. *Journal of obesity* 2016, 2016.

26. Drake JC, Wilson RJ, and Yan Z. Molecular mechanisms for mitochondrial adaptation to exercise training in skeletal muscle. *The FASEB Journal* 30: 13-22, 2016.

27. Egan B and Zierath JR. Exercise metabolism and the molecular regulation of skeletal muscle adaptation. *Cell metabolism* 17: 162-184, 2013.

28. Enoka RM and Duchateau J. Translating Fatigue to Human Performance. *Med Sci Sports Exerc* 48: 2228-2238, 2016.

29. Fragala MS, Kraemer WJ, Denegar CR, Maresh CM, Mastro AM, and Volek JS. Neuroendocrine-immune interactions and responses to exercise. *Sports Medicine* 41: 621-639, 2011.

30. Franchini E, Takito MY, and Kiss MAPDM. Performance and energy systems contributions during upper-body sprint interval exercise. *Journal of exercise rehabilitation* 12: 535, 2016.

31. Freeman R, Wieling W, Axelrod FB, Benditt DG, Benarroch E, Biaggioni I, Cheshire WP, Chelimsky T, Cortelli P, and Gibbons CH. Consensus statement on the definition of orthostatic hypotension, neurally mediated syncope and the postural tachycardia syndrome. *Clinical Autonomic Research* 21: 69-72, 2011.

32. Freidenreich DJ and Volek JS. Immune responses to resistance exercise. *Exercise immunology review* 18, 2012.

33. Friedman J and Lemon P. Effect of chronic endurance exercise on retention of dietary protein. *International journal of sports medicine* 10: 118-123, 1989.

34. Fry AC and Kraemer WJ. Resistance exercise overtraining and overreaching. *Sports medicine* 23: 106-129, 1997.

35. Gibney J, Healy M-L, and Sonksen PH. The growth hormone/insulin-like growth factor-I axis in exercise and sport. *Endocrine reviews* 28: 603-624, 2007.

36. Gonzalez AM, Hoffman JR, Townsend JR, Jajtner AR, Boone CH, Beyer KS, Baker KM, Wells AJ, Mangine GT, and Robinson EH. Intramuscular anabolic signaling and endocrine response following high volume and high intensity resistance exercise protocols in trained men. *Physiological reports* 3: e12466, 2015.

37. Guyenet PG. The sympathetic control of blood pressure. *Nature reviews Neuroscience* 7: 335, 2006.

38. Hackney AC, Anderson T, and Dobridge J. Exercise and Male Hypogonadism: Testosterone, the Hypothalamic-Pituitary-Testicular Axis, and Exercise Training. In: *Male Hypogonadism:* Springer, 2017, p. 257-280.

39. Halliwill JR. Mechanisms and clinical implications of post-exercise hypotension in humans. *Exercise and sport sciences reviews* 29: 65-70, 2001.

40. Haseler LJ, Hogan MC, and Richardson RS. Skeletal muscle phosphocreatine recovery in exercise-trained humans is dependent on O_2 availability. *J Appl Physiol* (1985) 86: 2013-2018, 1999.

41. Hill E, Zack E, Battaglini C, Viru M, Viru A, and Hackney A. Exercise and circulating cortisol levels: the intensity threshold effect. *Journal of endocrinological investigation* 31: 587-591, 2008.

42. Hingorani A and Ascher E. Superficial thrombophlebitis. In: *Essentials of Vascular Surgery for the General Surgeon:* Springer, 2015, p. 151-156.

43. Huang S and Czech MP. The GLUT4 glucose transporter. *Cell metabolism* 5: 237-252, 2007.

44. Huang Y-CT, O'Brien SR, Vredenburgh J, Folz RJ, and MacIntyre NR. Intrabreath analysis of carbon monoxide uptake during exercise in patients at risk for lung injury. *Respiratory medicine* 100: 1226-1233, 2006.

45. Ivy JL, Katz A, Cutler C, Sherman W, and Coyle E. Muscle glycogen synthesis after exercise: effect of time of carbohydrate ingestion. *Journal of Applied Physiology* 64: 1480-1485, 1988.

46. Jentjens R and Jeukendrup AE. Determinants of post-exercise glycogen synthesis during short-term recovery. *Sports Medicine* 33: 117-144, 2003.

47. Jeukendrup AE and Achten J. Fatmax: A New Concept to Optimize Fat Oxidation During Exercise? *European Journal of Sport Science* 1: 1, 2001.

48. Joyner MJ and Casey DP. Regulation of Increased Blood Flow (Hyperemia) to Muscles During Exercise: A Hierarchy of Competing Physiological Needs. *Physiological Reviews* 95: 549-601, 2015.

49. Kalliokoski KK, Oikonen V, Takala TO, Sipilä H, Knuuti J, and Nuutila P. Enhanced oxygen extraction and reduced flow heterogeneity in exercising muscle in endurance-trained men. *American Journal of Physiology-Endocrinology And Metabolism* 280: E1015-E1021, 2001.

50. Kanaley JA, Dall R, Møller N, Nielsen SC, Christiansen JS, Jensen MD, and Jørgensen JOL. Acute exposure to GH during exercise stimulates the turnover of free fatty acids in GH-deficient men. *Journal of Applied Physiology* 96: 747-753, 2004.

51. Kato T, Tsukanaka A, Harada T, Kosaka M, and Matsui N. Effect of hypercapnia on changes in blood pH, plasma lactate and ammonia due to exercise. *European journal of applied physiology* 95: 400-408, 2005.

52. Kilic M. Effect of fatiguing bicycle exercise on thyroid hormone and testosterone levels in sedentary males supplemented with oral zinc. *Neuro endocrinology letters* 28: 681-685, 2007.

53. Kindermann W, Schnabel A, Schmitt W, Biro G, Cassens J, and Weber F. Catecholamines, growth hormone, cortisol, insulin, and sex hormones in anaerobic and aerobic exercise. *European journal of applied physiology and occupational physiology* 49: 389-399, 1982.

54. Kolwicz SC, Purohit S, and Tian R. Cardiac metabolism and its interactions with contraction, growth, and survival of cardiomyocytes. *Circulation research* 113: 603-616, 2013.

55. Kraemer WJ, Patton JF, Gordon SE, Harman EA, Deschenes MR, Reynolds K, Newton RU, Triplett NT, and Dziados JE. Compatibility of high-intensity strength and endurance training on hormonal and skeletal muscle adaptations. *Journal of applied physiology* 78: 976-989, 1995.

56. Kraemer WJ and Ratamess NA. Hormonal responses and adaptations to resistance exercise and training. *Sports medicine* 35: 339-361, 2005.

57. Kraemer WJ, Ratamess NA, and Nindl BC. Recovery responses of testosterone, growth hormone, and IGF-1 after resistance exercise. *Journal of Applied Physiology* 122: 549-558, 2017.

58. Kraemer WJ, Staron RS, Hagerman FC, Hikida RS, Fry AC, Gordon SE, Nindl BC, Gothshalk LA, Volek JS, and Marx JO. The effects of short-term resistance training on endocrine function in men and women. *European journal of applied physiology and occupational physiology* 78: 69-76, 1998.

59. Krustrup P, Ferguson RA, Kjaer M, and Bangsbo J. ATP and heat production in human skeletal muscle during dynamic exercise: higher efficiency of anaerobic than aerobic ATP resynthesis. *J Physiol* 549: 255-269, 2003.

60. LaForgia J, Withers RT, and Gore CJ. Effects of exercise intensity and duration on the excess post-exercise oxygen consumption. *J Sports Sci* 24: 1247-1264, 2006.

61. Laforgia J, Withers RT, and Gore CJ. Effects of exercise intensity and duration on the excess post-exercise oxygen consumption. *Journal of sports sciences* 24: 1247-1264, 2006.

62. Lee S-J, Lee Y-S, Zimmers TA, Soleimani A, Matzuk MM, Tsuchida K, Cohn RD, and Barton ER. Regulation of muscle mass by follistatin and activins. *Molecular endocrinology* 24: 1998-2008, 2010.

63. Levine BD, Lane LD, Buckey JC, Friedman DB, and Blomqvist CG. Left ventricular pressure-volume and Frank-Starling relations in endurance athletes. Implications for orthostatic tolerance and exercise performance. *Circulation* 84: 1016-1023, 1991.

64. Martocchia A, Stefanelli M, Falaschi GM, Toussan L, Ferri C, and Falaschi P. Recent advances in the role of cortisol and metabolic syndrome in age-related degenerative diseases. *Aging clinical and experimental research* 28: 17-23, 2016.

65. Mastorakos G and Pavlatou M. Exercise as a stress model and the interplay between the hypothalamus-pituitary-adrenal and the hypothalamus-pituitary-thyroid axes. *Hormone and Metabolic Research* 37: 577-584, 2005.

66. McMahon S and Jenkins D. Factors affecting the rate of phosphocreatine resynthesis following intense exercise. *Sports Med* 32: 761-784, 2002.

67. McNaughton LR, Gough L, Deb S, Bentley D, and Sparks SA. Recent developments in the use of sodium bicarbonate as an ergogenic aid. *Current sports medicine reports* 15: 233-244, 2016.

68. McNaughton LR, Siegler J, and Midgley A. Ergogenic effects of sodium bicarbonate. *Current sports medicine reports* 7: 230-236, 2008.
69. Meeusen R, Watson P, Hasegawa H, Roelands B, and Piacentini MF. Central fatigue. *Sports Medicine* 36: 881-909, 2006.
70. Mergenthaler P, Lindauer U, Dienel GA, and Meisel A. Sugar for the brain: the role of glucose in physiological and pathological brain function. *Trends Neurosci* 36: 587-597, 2013.
71. Millard-Stafford M, Childers WL, Conger SA, Kampfer AJ, and Rahnert JA. Recovery nutrition: timing and composition after endurance exercise. *Current sports medicine reports* 7: 193-201, 2008.
72. Mullur R, Liu Y-Y, and Brent GA. Thyroid hormone regulation of metabolism. *Physiological reviews* 94: 355-382, 2014.
73. Nagaraja AS, Sadaoui NC, Dorniak PL, Lutgendorf SK, and Sood AK. SnapShot: stress and disease. *Cell metabolism* 23: 388-388. e381, 2016.
74. Nybo L and Nielsen B. Hyperthermia and central fatigue during prolonged exercise in humans. *Journal of applied physiology* 91: 1055-1060, 2001.
75. O'Flynn N, Vaughan M, and Kelley K. Diagnosis and management of varicose veins in the legs: NICE guideline. *Br J Gen Pract* 64: 314-315, 2014.
76. Ørtenblad N, Westerblad H, and Nielsen J. Muscle glycogen stores and fatigue. *The Journal of physiology* 591: 4405-4413, 2013.
77. Pedersen BK and Hoffman-Goetz L. Exercise and the immune system: regulation, integration, and adaptation. *Physiological reviews* 80: 1055-1081, 2000.
78. Pelliccia A, Culasso F, Di Paolo FM, and Maron BJ. Physiologic left ventricular cavity dilatation in elite athletes. *Annals of internal medicine* 130: 23-31, 1999.
79. Phillips SM and Van Loon LJ. Dietary protein for athletes: from requirements to optimum adaptation. *Journal of sports sciences* 29: S29-S38, 2011.
80. Philp A, Macdonald AL, and Watt PW. Lactate – a signal coordinating cell and systemic function. *J Exp Biol* 208: 4561-4575, 2005.
81. Philp A, Macdonald AL, and Watt PW. Lactate–a signal coordinating cell and systemic function. *Journal of Experimental Biology* 208: 4561-4575, 2005.
82. Purnell JQ, Kahn SE, Samuels MH, Brandon D, Loriaux DL, and Brunzell JD. Enhanced cortisol production rates, free cortisol, and 11 -HSD-1 expression correlate with visceral fat and insulin resistance in men: effect of weight loss. *American Journal of Physiology-Endocrinology and Metabolism* 296: E351-E357, 2009.
83. Qaisar R, Bhaskaran S, and Van Remmen H. Muscle fiber type diversification during exercise and regeneration. *Free Radical Biology and Medicine* 98: 56-67, 2016.
84. Racinais S and Perrey S. Energy Production Pathways During Exercise. In: *IOC Manual of Sports Cardiology*: John Wiley & Sons, Ltd, 2016, p. 21-31.
85. Richter EA and Hargreaves M. Exercise, GLUT4, and skeletal muscle glucose uptake. *Physiological reviews* 93: 993-1017, 2013.
86. Rigo F. Coronary flow reserve in stress-echo lab. From pathophysiologic toy to diagnostic tool. *Cardiovascular ultrasound* 3: 8, 2005.
87. Robergs RA, Ghiasvand F, and Parker D. Biochemistry of exercise-induced metabolic acidosis. *American Journal of Physiology-Regulatory, Integrative and Comparative Physiology* 287: R502-R516, 2004.
88. Robergs RA, Ghiasvand F, and Parker D. Biochemistry of exercise-induced metabolic acidosis. *Am J Physiol Regul Integr Comp Physiol* 287: R502-516, 2004.
89. Roberts PA, Fox J, Peirce N, Jones SW, Casey A, and Greenhaff PL. Creatine ingestion augments dietary carbohydrate mediated muscle glycogen supercompensation during the initial 24 h of recovery following prolonged exhaustive exercise in humans. *Amino acids* 48: 1831-1842, 2016.
90. Rubin MR, Kraemer WJ, Maresh CM, Volek JS, Ratamess NA, Vanheest JL, Silvestre R, French DN, Sharman MJ, and Judelson DA. High-affinity growth hormone binding protein and acute heavy resistance exercise. *Medicine & Science in Sports & Exercise* 37: 395-403, 2005.
91. Saltiel AR and Kahn CR. Insulin signalling and the regulation of glucose and lipid metabolism. *Nature* 414: 799-806, 2001.
92. Sandri M. Signaling in muscle atrophy and hypertrophy. *Physiology* 23: 160-170, 2008.
93. Sato K and Iemitsu M. Exercise and sex steroid hormones in skeletal muscle. *The Journal of steroid biochemistry and molecular biology* 145: 200-205, 2015.
94. Scharhag J, Schneider G, Urhausen A, Rochette V, Kramann B, and Kindermann W. Athlete's heart: right and left ventricular mass and function in male endurance athletes and untrained individuals determined by magnetic resonance imaging. *Journal of the American College of Cardiology* 40: 1856-1863, 2002.
95. Sequeira V and van der Velden J. Historical perspective on heart function: the Frank–Starling Law. *Biophysical reviews* 7: 421-447, 2015.
96. Sheffield-Moore M and Urban RJ. An overview of the endocrinology of skeletal muscle. *Trends in Endocrinology & Metabolism* 15: 110-115, 2004.
97. Silva JE. Thyroid hormone control of thermogenesis and energy balance. *Thyroid* 5: 481-492, 1995.
98. Skelly LE, Andrews PC, Gillen JB, Martin BJ, Percival ME, and Gibala MJ. High-intensity interval exercise induces 24-h energy expenditure similar to traditional endurance exercise despite reduced time commitment. *Applied Physiology, Nutrition, and Metabolism* 39: 845-848, 2014.
99. Slysz J, Stultz J, and Burr JF. The efficacy of blood flow restricted exercise: A systematic review & meta-analysis. *Journal of Science and Medicine in Sport* 19: 669-675, 2016.
100. Sun Z. Aging, arterial stiffness, and hypertension. *Hypertension* 65: 252-256, 2015.
101. Suzuki K, Nakaji S, Yamada M, Totsuka M, Sato K, and Sugawara K. Systemic inflammatory response to exhaustive exercise. Cytokine kinetics. *Exercise immunology review* 8: 6-48, 2002.
102. Suzuki K, Totsuka M, Nakaji S, Yamada M, Kudoh S, Liu Q, Sugawara K, Yamaya K, and Sato K. Endurance exercise causes interaction among stress hormones, cytokines, neutrophil dynamics, and muscle damage. *Journal of Applied Physiology* 87: 1360-1367, 1999.
103. Sylow L, Kleinert M, Richter EA, and Jensen TE. Exercise-stimulated glucose uptake [mdash] regulation and implications for glycaemic control. *Nature Reviews Endocrinology* 13: 133-148, 2017.

104. Taegtmeyer H, Young ME, Lopaschuk GD, Abel ED, Brunengraber H, Darley-Usmar V, Des Rosiers C, Gerszten R, Glatz JF, and Griffin JL. Assessing Cardiac Metabolism. *Circulation research*: RES. 0000000000000097, 2016.

105. Tarpenning KM, Wiswell RA, Hawkins SA, and Marcell TJ. Influence of weight training exercise and modification of hormonal response on skeletal muscle growth. *Journal of Science and Medicine in Sport* 4: 431-446, 2001.

106. Thornton MK and Potteiger JA. Effects of resistance exercise bouts of different intensities but equal work on EPOC. *Med Sci Sports Exerc* 34: 715-722, 2002.

107. Tipton KD and Wolfe RR. Exercise, protein metabolism, and muscle growth. *International journal of sport nutrition and exercise metabolism* 11: 109-132, 2001.

108. Tipton MJ, Harper A, Paton JF, and Costello JT. The human ventilatory response to stress: rate or depth? *The Journal of Physiology*, 2017.

109. Tremblay MS, Copeland JL, and Van Helder W. Effect of training status and exercise mode on endogenous steroid hormones in men. *Journal of Applied Physiology* 96: 531-539, 2004.

110. Tremblay MS, Copeland JL, and Van Helder W. Influence of exercise duration on post-exercise steroid hormone responses in trained males. *European journal of applied physiology* 94: 505-513, 2005.

111. Tucker WJ, Angadi SS, and Gaesser GA. Excess Postexercise Oxygen Consumption After High-Intensity and Sprint Interval Exercise, and Continuous Steady-State Exercise. *J Strength Cond Res* 30: 3090-3097, 2016.

112. Viru A. Plasma hormones and physical exercise. *International journal of sports medicine* 13: 201-209, 1992.

113. Wagenmakers AJ. 11 Muscle Amino Acid Metabolism at Rest and During Exercise: Role in Human Physiology and Metabolism. *Exercise and sport sciences reviews* 26: 287-314, 1998.

114. Wang Y-X, Zhang C-L, Ruth TY, Cho HK, Nelson MC, Bayuga-Ocampo CR, Ham J, Kang H, and Evans RM. Regulation of muscle fiber type and running endurance by PPAR. *PLoS biology* 2: e294, 2004.

115. Wasserman K, Beaver WL, Sun XG, and Stringer WW. Arterial H+ regulation during exercise in humans. *Respir Physiol Neurobiol* 178: 191-195, 2011.

116. Wasserman K, Cox TA, and Sietsema KE. Ventilatory regulation of arterial H(+) (pH) during exercise. *Respir Physiol Neurobiol* 190: 142-148, 2014.

117. Waters MJ. The growth hormone receptor. *Growth Hormone & IGF Research* 28: 6-10, 2016.

118. Weber-Hamann B, Hentschel F, Kniest A, Deuschle M, Colla M, Lederbogen F, and Heuser I. Hypercortisolemic depression is associated with increased intra-abdominal fat. *Psychosomatic Medicine* 64: 274-277, 2002.

119. Weisbrod RM, Shiang T, Al Sayah L, Fry JL, Bajpai S, Reinhart-King CA, Lob HE, Santhanam L, Mitchell G, and Cohen RA. Arterial stiffening precedes systolic hypertension in diet-induced obesity. *Hypertension*: HYPERTENSIONAHA. 113.01744, 2013.

120. Willardson JM. A brief review: factors affecting the length of the rest interval between resistance exercise sets. *J Strength Cond Res* 20: 978-984, 2006.

121. Williams MB, Raven PB, Fogt DL, and Ivy JL. Effects of recovery beverages on glycogen restoration and endurance exercise performance. *The Journal of Strength & Conditioning Research* 17: 12-19, 2003.

122. Wolfe RR. Control of muscle protein breakdown: effects of activity and nutritional states. *International journal of sport nutrition and exercise metabolism* 11: S164-S169, 2001.

123. Yasuda T, Loenneke JP, Thiebaud RS, and Abe T. Effects of blood flow restricted low-intensity concentric or eccentric training on muscle size and strength. *Plos one* 7: e52843, 2012.

124. Yen PM. Physiological and molecular basis of thyroid hormone action. *Physiological reviews* 81: 1097-1142, 2001.

125. Zawadzki K, Yaspelkis B, and Ivy J. Carbohydrate-protein complex increases the rate of muscle glycogen storage after exercise. *Journal of Applied Physiology* 72: 1854-1859, 1992.

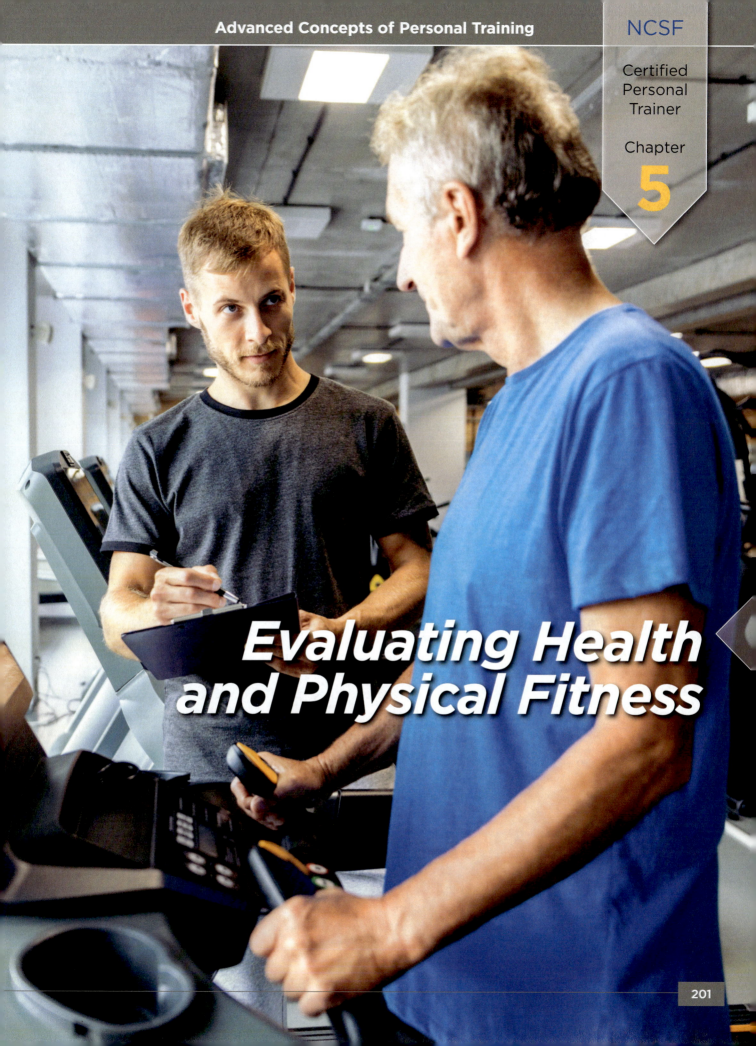

Factors that Affect Fitness

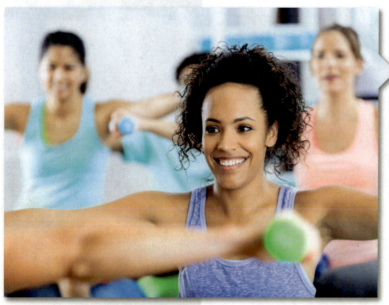

Baseline measures of fitness are heavily influenced by genetics, environment, and the stress the body experiences on a day-to-day basis. For a completely **sedentary** person, the strongest independent factor of health and fitness, other than the lack of activity, will be **genetic predisposition**; however, genetics alone do not fully account for a person's physical fitness. While the DNA blueprint begins as the foundation for all internal controls, environmental and eugenic factors can modulate genetic expression and activity. External environmental factors will all have implications for what occurs within the body: temperature, altitude, nutrition sufficiency, voluntary/involuntary stress, prenatal nutrition, and diet can all have an impact. Additionally, individual interests, education, and socio-economic factors all affect a person's physical fitness [1, 3, 6].

Genetics contribute to the measurable aspects of physical fitness at any given time during a person's lifespan and ultimately determine the body's potential capabilities. A person's genetics are estimated to account for at least 40%, and up to 66%, of uncontrolled, hereditable factors that affect physical health and performance components of fitness [8, 9, 18, 20]. With this being said, that leaves approximately 40-60% of controllable (or somewhat-controllable) factors that can be manipulated for improvement. Regardless of genetic makeup, virtually everyone can improve his or her health or performance by engaging in activities and behaviors that impact the body positively.

Numerous environmental factors affect physical fitness, with each primary factor carrying a subset of co-factors. These factors may be socially driven, such as those derived from one's family and friends, or from work-setting environments inclusive of influences of colleagues and supervisors. This implies a range of values, attitudes, financial means, and societal opportunities that impact the individual. Other factors may be physical, such as climate, altitude, exposure to pollutants, and access to resources. Early learned behaviors yield very powerful influences on the lifestyles of adults. Individuals born into families that place little value on healthy behaviors often

> **DEFINITIONS**
>
> **Sedentary –**
>
> *Describes a lifestyle behavioral pattern that includes very little physical activity.*
>
> **Genetic predisposition –**
>
> *Increased propensity towards a conditioning or outcome based on one's inherited genes.*

Behaviors vs. Genetics
Controllable vs. Uncontrollable Factors Affecting Physical Fitness

- 40% Estimated Uncontrollable Factors
- 60% Estimated Controllable Factors

do not have the habits or background knowledge to support positive choices. On the contrary, families that recognize the importance of health, emphasize it through routine health promotion and have the means to fulfill the financial requirements of total wellness are much more likely to engage in positive health behaviors. Many people who do not meet the guidelines for physical activity simply do not have the means to support proper nutrition and suffer greater risk of exposure to negative influences, which they often transfer to their children. Therefore, formative attitudes and behaviors from childhood to adulthood serve as a major consideration, since the behaviors established during one's youth potentially exert the strongest influences on what one does as an adult. During adulthood however, social environments are suggested to play a greater impact than family influences.

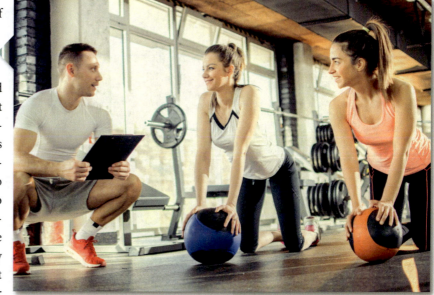

Interest also plays a key role in the types of behaviors in which people partake. Individual use of discretionary time is often connected with personal responsibility and enjoyment. Few people will voluntarily engage in activities that they find unpleasant. Individuals often preferentially select enjoyable activities over those without positive emotional associations. Exposure to a variety of activities during youth allows individuals to evaluate their interests and make decisions about adopting them into their lifestyle habits. In some cases, knowledge as to the benefits of certain activities or behaviors influences participation even when certain activities are perceived as less pleasurable. A sense of responsibility for one's health may cause people to exercise or eat right, even though they might prefer to make other decisions in the absence of consequences. Education factors importantly in this decision-making process. Individuals who understand that quality of life (QOL) outcomes closely link to one's health, participate more readily in healthy behaviors. For example, a person looking to have an active retirement may begin to emphasize healthy behaviors as they age in order to accomplish active retirement goals. Likewise, knowledge is paramount: understanding what benefits the body and what impacts health negatively profoundly informs the decision-making process associated

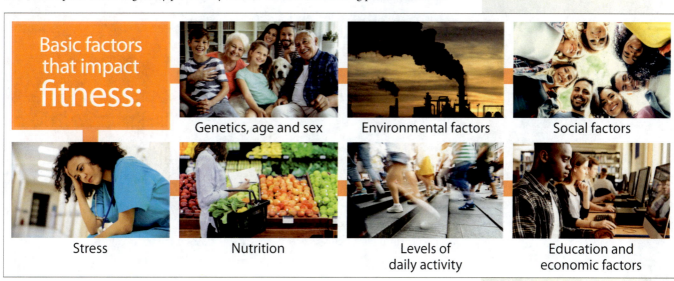

with physical activity participation. Even with the vast amounts of information available today, many people simply do not know how to implement healthy routines and habits. Granted, people know they should eat right and exercise, but what does that actually mean without reliable knowledge of what's truly healthy? Implementation of positive behaviors requires knowledge of the "whats and how-tos." Therefore, leadership in consumer education represents an important aspect of the fitness professional's job.

◆ Physical Activity & Life Quality

The World Health Organization has acknowledged health-related quality of life (HRQL) as an important outcome from wellness behaviors. In 1982, Kaplan and Bush coined this multidimensional concept that acknowledges the influences that health status has on tangible and perceived measures of life quality [13]. Clinical data has shown that physical activity has significant potential to positively influence a person's HRQL [7, 26, 33]. The areas that seem most directly affected include physical and psychological well-being, perceived physical function, and stress reduction. Additionally, a positive association exists between physical activity and self-efficacy in people of all ages [26].

The perception of improved physical function in activities of daily living (ADLs) is one important effect of physical activity. Although most people can perform daily tasks, the ease or proficiency of accomplishing physical work seems to improve with regular physical activity. Individuals suffering from maladies, such as heart disease and arthritis, who participate in physical activity report the highest rate of perceived improvement in daily functional capabilities [2, 14, 32]. In clinical trials, self-reported outcomes identified improvements in physical function and health in subjects who engaged in aerobic physical activity compared to sedentary controls [7]. Again, the individuals diagnosed with disease presented the greatest magnitude of positive improvement in both physical and psychological measures: understanding, of course, that they also had the most room to improve. This information is relevant from two perspectives: first, that routine engagement in exercise profoundly affects life quality and disease prevention, and secondly, that those with disease not only benefit but experience exponential improvements. The concept that exercise and physical activity can be used for

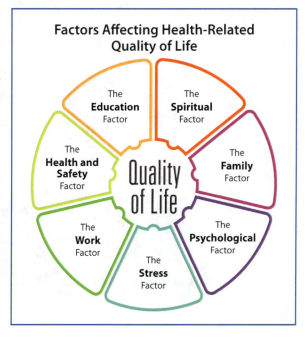

Factors Affecting Health-Related Quality of Life

- The Education Factor
- The Spiritual Factor
- The Health and Safety Factor
- The Family Factor
- The Work Factor
- The Psychological Factor
- The Stress Factor

Quality of Life

medicine is rapidly gaining momentum across the world. According to the World Health Organization, in highly developed countries, the predominant causes of **premature mortality** and overall **mortality** are controllable diseases [24]. Essentially, we are our own worst enemies, but concurrently also hold the solution to our potential health problems.

◆ Physical Activity & Risk for Injury

Exercise can help most people improve their QOL [7, 14], which holds true for apparently healthy individuals and also those diagnosed with disease. Exercise though, also offers the potential for negative outcomes if performed incorrectly, too aggressively, or too often. Training volume represents the combination of participation time and exercise intensity. Athletes are consistently at risk for injury simply due to their large quantity of daily activity. Individuals who increase physical activity should be familiar with the inherent risk of injury. Several types of common injuries are associated with exercise and sports participation. New exercisers are at particular risk for soft tissue strains, tears, and even stress fractures from inappropriately applied stress and repetitive motions that occur without proper acclimation to these increased demands. Progressing intensity levels too aggressively associates with greater risk for multiple-cause injuries. This represents one of the most common errors in new training programs, often resulting from a lack of knowledge, combined with a newly inspired motivation. Lower extremity injuries seem to be reported most commonly: in particular, at the articulation sites of the ankle, knee, and foot [28, 29]. Too much exercise implemented too quickly and/or too often will cause the onset of acute overuse injuries. Likewise, attempting a routine without the requisite training or education can also lead to a less than positive outcome. Special consideration for body acclimation should be made for new exercisers and those returning after an extended period of cessation.

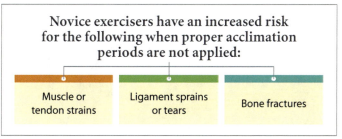

Novice exercisers have an increased risk for the following when proper acclimation periods are not applied:
- Muscle or tendon strains
- Ligament sprains or tears
- Bone fractures

Exercise participation also includes the possibility of metabolic injury. This injury, although rare, is mainly associated with prolonged duration, a pre-existing exercise condition, and/or environmental influences. Thermoregulatory dysfunction and abnormal metabolite concentration can be life threatening. Conditions such as **hyperthermia**, **hypothermia**, hypoglycemia, **rhabdomyolysis**, **hyponatremia**, and other electrolyte imbalances all may present acute life-threatening emergencies. Appropriate dietary considerations and fluid consumption, acclimation to stress, prudent decision making, and pre-exercise screening can help prevent incidences related to these issues. When exercise is implemented in a logical manner and considerations are made for

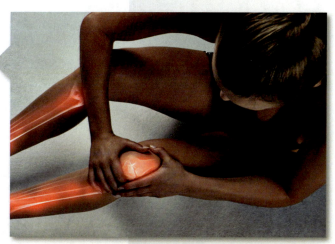

DEFINITIONS

Premature mortality –

A measure of unfilled life expectancy or death before age 75, usually caused by preventable factors.

Mortality –

Refers to death that occurs in a population or other group. It is often utilized as a term in research studies that examine rate of death due to a specific disease or ailment.

DEFINITIONS

Hyperthermia –

A potentially dangerous increase in body temperature above normal levels which can lead to heat-related illnesses, such as heat cramps, exhaustion, or stroke.

Hypothermia –

A potentially dangerous decrease in body temperature below normal levels which can lead to diminished neuromuscular control, frostbite, or death: body temperature below 95.0 °F (35.0 °C).

Rhabdomyolysis –

A potentially life-threatening condition resulting from the destruction of muscle tissue and subsequent release of muscle fiber content into the blood stream which may cause failure of major organs.

Hyponatremia –

Refers to a below-normal plasma sodium concentration (<135 mmol/L); it can be caused by excessive water consumption and is most commonly seen during endurance training in the heat.

environmental stress and safety, the risks for injury are very low. Exercise professionals must create conditions that present the safest situation for their clients, and to avoid any problems or risks, this should include pre-exercise screening for potential conditions and pre-exercise checklists for acute disorders.

Common Activities and Associated Injuries	
Jogging/Running	Torn cartilage, tendonitis, plantar fasciitis, shin splints
Bicycling	Ulnar nerve palsies, ischial bursitis, Achilles tendonitis, lower back pain
Swimming	Shoulder pain, shoulder impingement syndrome
Aerobic Dance	Shin splints, plantar fasciitis
Tennis	Epicondylitis, tendonitis

Considerations for Pre-Exercise Screening

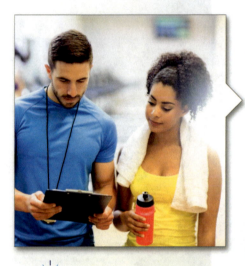

DEFINITIONS

Arrhythmia –

A potentially-dangerous abnormal heart rhythm which can be caused by physical exertion or without activity in cases where there is an issue with the cardiovascular system or presence of disease.

Acute angina –

A short-term chest pain caused by reduced blood flow to the heart. It is often precipitated by exertion and associated with cardiovascular disease.

Type 2 diabetes mellitus (T2DM) –

A metabolic disorder characterized by high blood sugar, insulin resistance, and relative lack of insulin production; it primarily occurs as a result of obesity and lack of physical activity.

Pre-exercise screening can pave the way for appropriate program modification that can help reduce the risk of many conditions affecting individuals during physical activity participation, particularly those known to cause death. For some individuals suffering from cardiovascular pathology, exercise may cause more harm than good. Individuals at risk may incite abnormal heart rates or rhythms due to a compromise to their coronary circulation during exertional stress. **Arrhythmias**, **acute angina**, and myocardial infarction may be precipitated by physical exertion in the presence of heart disease. Sudden death is not common but a definite possibility for high risk exercisers who participate without prior evaluation. It is important to recognize that these risks occur both during participation in the activity and also immediately following exercise. However, from a risk vs. benefit perspective, regular activity for medically-cleared participants yields more protective effects from disease than the risk for injury from an exercise-related cardiovascular event. Those designated as high risk are expected to exercise under expert supervision in specific cardiac care environments for optimal safety.

Another condition increasingly present among the United States population is **type 2 diabetes mellitus (T2DM)**. This metabolic condition is multi-factored and presents additional concerns during exercise. Clearly, the root to solving the population rise in T2DM lies in routine physical activity in conjunction with structured diet and exercise. Lipid infiltration into cells, desensitized endocrine receptors, and autoimmune dysfunction collectively create a metabolic setting that presents ongoing difficulty for sugar management. Diabetics cannot control their blood glucose properly under natural conditions, however exercise and physical activity play a large role in the ability to manage the phenomena. The problem and benefit lies in the tissues' metabolic response. Exercise invigorates cells and glucose receptors to better manage blood glucose; however, if the diabetic condition is not controlled, the activity may cause hypoglycemia, leading to a diabetic coma. Diabetics also must contend with hyperglycemia; however, due to the blood sugar used by muscle contractions during exercise, it does not present the same risk during physical activity. Exercise professionals should be aware that T2DM damages the vascular system due to chronic hyperglycemia, so getting oxygen to tissues may be compromised in those with later stage disease. This is particularly concerning for the heart, so diabetics should be thoroughly pre-screened for heart disease prior to the initiation of an exercise program.

Other health concerns related to exercise may warrant attention as well. Overtraining increases risk for infection from immuno-suppression and can cause stress-related injuries [10]. Likewise, pre-existing conditions, including asthma, tachycardia, abnormal heart murmurs, musculoskeletal injury, osteoporosis, hypertension, sickle cell anemia, and arthritis, all call for specific special considerations, as these can lead to additional problems during exercise participation. Studies show that previous injury and existing conditions strongly predict subsequent physical activity related injury [5, 12]. Although a myriad of adverse events can be associated with physical activity, the benefits of participation still far outweigh the problems inherent to a sedentary lifestyle.

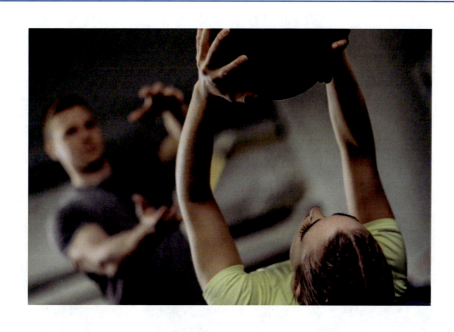

Contribute to a reduced risk and consequence of physical activity-related injuries:
- Identify risk factors and high-risk environments
- Thoroughly screen participants
- Provide structured acclimation to physical stress
- Prescribe exercise within individual capabilities
- Avoid activity when injured or when risk is elevated
- Have an emergency plan

Pre-Exercise Screening

A significant quantity of evidence supports daily physical activity as a vital part of healthy aging. Data suggests that the absence of routine exercise constitutes far more danger to health than the inherent risks of physical activity [25, 27]. Although this may be true, cautious steps can and should be taken by exercise professionals when encouraging exercise participation. Pre-exercise health screening comprises an important part of health management services and is a defined task requirement for personal trainers. The primary purpose for screening a client before activity participation is to identify possible factors that may increase the risk of injury when performing exercise or a particular activity. Factors may include physical limitations, medical conditions, or behaviors that may put the client at risk for a negative outcome from exercise testing or physical activity participation. Failure to appropriately screen a client that leads to an untoward event places significant liability on the personal trainer and place of employment. Age appropriate health screening is always a necessary part of fulfilling the duty of care owed to anyone paying for professional fitness or health services.

Pre-exercise screening provides additional benefits beyond simply attempting to identify and reduce risks for injury associated with participation. Secondary purposes for screening clients before activity are listed here.

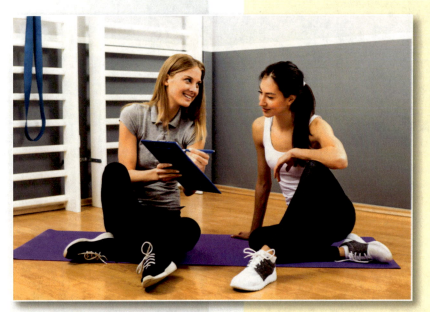

Benefits of Client Screening

1. Educating the client about relative health risks associated with their lifestyle, behaviors, and history.

2. Identifying current health status compared to recommended ranges.

3. Providing data that will be used to create a needs analysis as the basis for the exercise prescription.

4. Establishing starting points and predictions of performance.

5. Identifying particular interests, aptitudes, or possible limitations.

Screening for exercise participation has several advantages: it provides valuable information for creating an exercise prescription; it identifies client aptitude and interests in different types of activities; finally, it reveals short and long-term goals the client wishes to accomplish via training and health services. It is important to pinpoint the data most relevant to the purpose and goals identified through the screening process. This step allows the prescribed exercise program to start with a high likelihood for success and allows the client to participate with very low inherent risk. Note that part of the screening process involves an evaluation of psycho-emotional interest in physical activity. This allows one to gain insight into the motivation behind the decision to initiate exercise as well as an indication of the participant's potential exercise tolerance. This awareness is all very helpful in guiding decisions concerning starting points and potential motivators. The concept of "exercise tolerance" represents a relative consideration of how hard a person will work before perceiving the activity to be undesirable from a cost-benefit perspective and quitting. Many individuals do not like moderate-to-high exercise intensities, preferring health-related activities such as walking instead. This creates a conundrum for many exercise professionals: all indications point towards using specific intensities for desired physical adaptations; however, the client will not comply because he or she objects to the perceived discomfort of the activity level and believes it not worth the effort. This scenario manifests commonly among those who start exercise programs due to physicians' recommendations. Exercise professionals need to understand, in this case, the value of compromise. While an exercise professional should want to provide optimal conditions to promote health and fitness, it may be better to accommodate the client's sensitivities to exercise. Simply put, a client may not be interested in exercising at the optimal levels to promote beneficial adaptations; regardless, it is always better to have someone engage in some physical activity compared to none at all. In these cases, the exercise professional's ethical duty is to explain that fitness cannot be attained at subthreshold training levels and provide adequate support to encourage routine compliance at the highest tolerable level. Forcing a resistant person to perform exercise intensities beyond their comfort level will simply end in attrition.

In the recent past, some have criticized requiring testing and evaluation for clearing individuals for an unrestricted exercise program [4, 19]. Stringent screening protocols required men (>45 years) and women (>55 years) to undergo cardiac stress tests, cardiopulmonary tests, and in some cases, the completion of blood chemistry tests before being cleared for participation. The primary goal of this evaluation process is to identify those individuals who pose a risk for a cardiac event during exercise participation. Although this type of screening generates a thorough evaluation, the requirements are excessive and costly for participating in activities aimed at improving health. In addition, they may deter anyone already skeptical about initiating an exercise program [4]. Furthermore, cardiovascular events are not only rare and unpredictable, but cardiac stress tests and self-reported screening documents only effectively identify a small subset of individuals at risk [15-17, 22].

DEFINITIONS

Liability –

The state of being responsible for something, especially by law; a personal trainer maintains a fiduciary responsibility to function in the best interest of the client.

Professional negligence –

Failure to take proper care during standard protocol or to use reasonable care, potentially resulting in damage or injury to another person: doing something a reasonable person would not do or the omission of something that a reasonable person would do.

From a **liability** perspective, different screening level guidelines exist relative to the activity intensity and the individual; ignoring these may constitute a case of **professional negligence**. Exercise screening should not be an obstacle to participation or an unnecessary burden to initiating an exercise program but should serve a protective role. The screening protocols and depth of evaluation should always reflect the individual's needs. Whereas pre-exercise stress tests identify risk of participation in vigorous exercise, the reality is that most individuals engaging in activity do so at a moderate level of intensity. Novice and new exercisers, outside of those involved in fitness fads, rarely perform vigorous activity, and many people who exercise routinely never attain the interest or aptitude to participate in high-intensity exercise. The discomfort and the time it takes to acclimate to high-intensity training (HIT) or high intensity interval training (HIIT) deter this group. For this reason, comprehensive

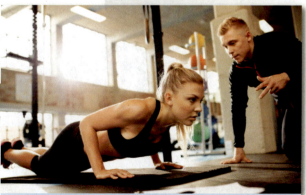

Exercise screening should not be an obstacle to participation or an unnecessary burden to initiating an exercise program - but should serve a relative protective role.

cardiovascular screening is not necessary unless indicated by a physician. A caveat to this discussion is the popularity of HIIT and similar protocols that make use of intense (typically grouped) activities accompanied with short rest intervals. Pre-exercise screening should always be specific to the individual and participation level of training. The goals of pre-screening are to safely get people to participate in physical activity and identify those individuals who truly need appropriate medical evaluation and clearance.

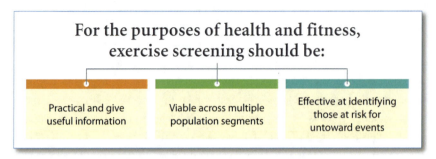

For the purposes of health and fitness, exercise screening should be:
- Practical and give useful information
- Viable across multiple population segments
- Effective at identifying those at risk for untoward events

Exercise professionals should individualize the screening process as much as possible for two reasons: health problems and risks for potential problems are identified from the beginning, and the specific findings can be analyzed to create an exercise program that is result-based and tailored to the individual. Several documents are available and can be employed in conjunction with industry guidelines to help the screening process become more efficient and effective. Common forms often employed include: Informed Consent, ParQ+, Health Risk Appraisal, Health Status Questionnaire (HSQ), Behavior Questionnaire, and Medical History Questionnaire. In general, the minimum requirement of an appropriate pre-screening process should include a health and medical history that identifies pre-exercise risk factors: a previous injury, any medications being taken and the reason the client is being medicated, and any other conditions warranting further investigation.

◆ Informed Consent

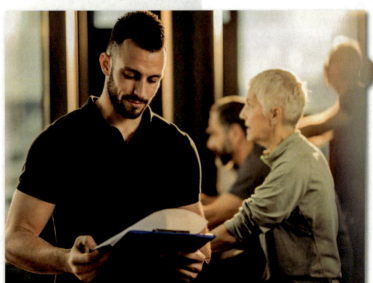

The informed consent is not necessarily a screening form but a waiver of sorts that requests voluntary permission or consent for health screening, fitness evaluations, and/or exercise participation. It represents a knowing and willful consent by an individual or guardian for testing procedures or participation in physical activity after being properly advised of the relevant facts and risks involved. An informed consent is a valuable document for personal training services: it provides powerful legal defense against claims that suggest a client was not informed about the protocols and the inherent risks associated with the activities they were instructed to perform. By law, clients who are exposed to or may be subject to possible physical or psychological injury must give informed consent prior to participation in the activities this document describes [11, 21, 30].

For the document to provide maximal protection for the exercise professional, company, or premises, it must include the following: a clear explanation of the contents; specific details related to the program and/or testing activities; risks and benefits that come from participation in said activities. In order for the informed consent to provide maximal defense during litigation, the document should be administered and explained in easily understood terms in front of a witness, so that, without doubt, the client fully understands the written language of the form before signing. Initials by each paragraph or section identify that the client was properly informed of the information contained in all of the document's subsections. Additionally, in order to realize full disclosure and informed consent requirements, the reading level of the consent form must be comprehensible by the client. Thus, the educational level of the individual being serviced must be taken into account. Finally, the form should be provided in the client's spoken language to ensure he or she fully understands the described content [23, 30, 31, 35].

The informed consent can serve, in part, as a liability waiver when implemented properly, using the appropriate language, and signed in the presence of a witness. Because of its legal implications, exercise professionals should use an agreement that has been reviewed and approved by an attorney to ensure the document's ability to serve its intended role. However, a signed informed consent does not prevent the client from taking legal action nor does it protect the exercise professional against negligence. It does, however, provide legal defensibility when the procedures in question have been correctly performed by a diligent, qualified practitioner. The informed consent should be the first document that is explained, signed, and added to a client's file. It serves as permission to move ahead with the personal training services, as it suggests the client is privy to the described procedures and expected outcomes. Once completed, the screening protocols can then be initiated.

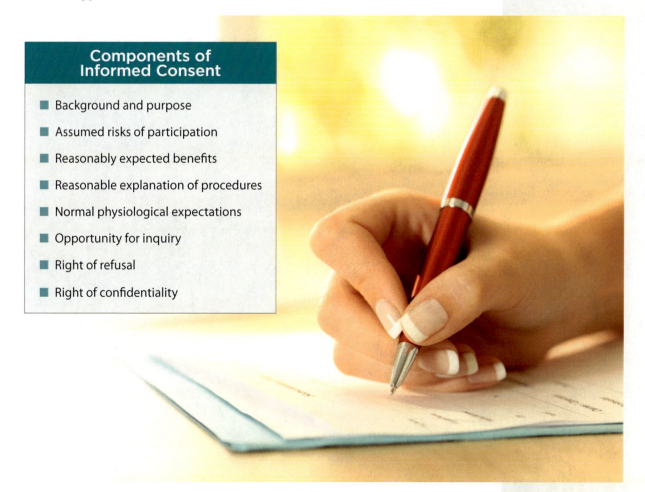

Components of Informed Consent

- Background and purpose
- Assumed risks of participation
- Reasonably expected benefits
- Reasonable explanation of procedures
- Normal physiological expectations
- Opportunity for inquiry
- Right of refusal
- Right of confidentiality

INFORMED CONSENT

Purpose and Explanation of Service

I understand that the purpose of the exercise program is to develop and maintain cardiorespiratory fitness, body composition, flexibility, muscular strength and endurance. A specific exercise plan will be given to me, based on my needs and abilities. All exercise prescription components will comply with proper exercise program protocols. The programs include, but are not limited to, aerobic exercise, flexibility training, and strength training. All programs are designed to place a gradually increasing workload on the body in order to improve overall fitness.

Risks

I understand, and have been informed, that there exists the possibility of adverse changes when engaging in a physical activity program. I have been informed that these changes could include abnormal blood pressure, fainting, disorders of heart rhythm, stroke and very rare instances of heart attack or even death. I have been told that every effort will be made to minimize these occurrences by proper screening and by precautions and observations taken during the exercise session. I understand that there is a risk of injury, heart attack, or even death as a result of my participation in an exercise program, but knowing those risks, it is my desire to partake in the recommended activities.

Benefits

I understand that participation in an exercise program has many health-related benefits. These may include improvements in body composition, range of motion, musculoskeletal strength and endurance, and cardiorespiratory efficiency. Furthermore, regular exercise can improve blood pressure and lipid profile, metabolic function, and decrease the risk of cardiovascular disease.

Physiological Experience

I have been informed that during my participation in the exercise program I will be asked to complete physical activities that may elicit physiological responses/symptoms that include, but are not limited to, the following: elevated heart rate, elevated blood pressure, sweating, fatigue, increased respiration, muscle soreness, cramping, and nausea.

Confidentiality and Use of Information

I have been informed that the information obtained in this exercise program will be treated as privileged and confidential and will consequently not be released or revealed to any person without my express written consent. Any other information obtained, however, will be used only by the program staff to evaluate my exercise status as needed.

Inquiries and Freedom of Consent

I have been given an opportunity to ask questions about the exercise program. I further understand that there are also other remote health risks. Despite the fact that a complete accounting of all these remote risks has not been provided to me, I still desire to proceed with the exercise program. I acknowledge that I have read this document in its entirety or that it has been read to me if I was unable to read. I consent to the rendition of all services and procedures as explained herein by all program personnel.

_____

Date

_____

Participant's Signature

_____

Witness's Signature

_____

Trainer's Signature

◆ PAR-Q+

PAR-Q+ stands for physical activity readiness questionnaire for everyone, with the plus representing the recent updates[34]. The original PAR-Q was designed to be used with the Canadian Fitness Testing program. It served as a seven-question assessment of self-reported health information to determine if one should see a physician before beginning or resuming an exercise program. Its primary objective was to identify those individuals at risk for a cardiac event. More recently, a collaboration of international authorities and regional health and fitness organizations sought to reduce barriers for low-to-moderate intensity physical activity participation, with a goal of specifically identifying those persons who might require additional screening prior to becoming more physically active. The collaboration's overall aim was to create an instrument to simplify physical activity participation clearance and expedite the involvement of physicians, allied health care professionals, and/or qualified exercise professionals. The new PAR-Q+ includes seven questions which serve as "red flag" indicators to identify individuals who require medical clearance before participating in any physical testing or exercise program. Essentially, a "yes" answer to any of the questions dictates medical clearance requirements. This basic screening instrument is practical for large numbers of individuals and requires little time or expertise to implement. It is limited to evaluating risk for low to moderate exercise but should not be used as clearance for vigorous activities. Additionally, the collaborative efforts also generated a second, more expansive tool. This includes questions regarding potential relative contraindications to unrestricted exercise, including those categorized as special populations by specific diagnosis. The electronic Physical Activity Readiness Medical Examination (ePARmed-X+) builds upon the PAR-Q+, with additional questions that direct the participant to a physical activity recommendation and/or a qualified health professional[34]. The tool addresses all of the common medical conditions found on health risk appraisal documents.

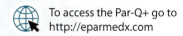
To access the Par-Q+ go to http://eparmedx.com

For the personal trainer, the Par-Q+ offers limited value beyond medical referral identification, and, in many cases, the ePARmed-X+ refers participants to exercise professionals for further evaluation. Investigative instruments including the Health Status Questionnaire, Behavior Questionnaire, comprehensive Health Risk Appraisal, and Medical History Questionnaire can provide additional data to identify individuals at risk of injury from a variety of possible events. Additionally, these screening tools further help identify those clients requiring medical clearance, while also being useful for specific program participation and exercise decision making. The assessment of a person's overall health profile provides coronary risk analysis, disease risk classification, lifestyle evaluation, general physical activity information, and behavior risk stratification. Additionally, the implementation process can help facilitate improved client-trainer rapport and help the client realize important health markers. Of added value, it helps participants become more educated about their current conditions. As a final note, in most court cases, prosecutors ask for documentation of medical and health history that the fitness professional formally employed before providing services, which pertain directly to liability.

◆ Health Status Questionnaire (HSQ)

The HSQ is divided into sections:
- General client information
- Current medical information
- Self-reported health status
- Self-reported physical fitness
- Psychological considerations

Traditionally, HSQs are generally split into the following sections: general client information, self-reported health and physical fitness status, current medical information, medical history, and self-reported psychological considerations. Numerous questionnaires are available for pre-exercise screening. These vary by format, number of questions, degree of thoroughness, and complexity level of each question.

The exercise professional should be present and actively assist the client with the completion of the document rather than having them fill it out off-site. Taking the time to administer the questionnaire orally is very effective for collecting the data and serves as yet again another opportunity to connect personally with the client. It helps initiate trust and confidence in the client-trainer relationship, enables the use of probing questions to expand on the questionnaire items, and helps to ensure that the client understands all of the questions so that the responses represent the appropriate and most complete answer regarding the questions' intentions. Likewise, administering the questionnaire verbally provides the opportunity for client education: the trainer can explain the relevance of the questions' subject matter and explain the information's value. Trainers should pay particular attention to key risk areas: family history of cardiovascular and metabolic disease, smoking history, sedentary lifestyle, obesity, high blood pressure, current medications, previous injuries or surgeries, undesirable blood lipid profiles, and impaired glucose tolerance. These areas are most likely associated with heightened disease risk, health complications, and potential cardiovascular events.

Key Risk Areas

- Family history of cardiovascular and metabolic disease
- Smoking history
- Sedentary lifestyle
- Obesity
- High blood pressure
- Current medications
- Previous injuries or surgeries
- Undesirable blood lipid profiles
- Impaired glucose tolerance

The highest quality health screening evaluations include a specific section for identifying diagnosed diseases, such as hypertension or diabetes, that warrant medical clearance. They also incorporate a separate section for symptoms that may represent undiagnosed diseases or conditions that require medical evaluation prior to exercise participation. Examples of symptoms that are warning signs include the following: chronic pain, dizziness, breathlessness, heart palpitations, edema, unusual fatigue, constipation, frequent thirst, and/or frequent urination or inability to urinate. Note that the role of an exercise professional is not to diagnose a disease or condition, but to identify those clients who require either medical referral or clearance prior to an exercise program's initiation. In addition, the exercise professional should note the frequency with which a potential client pursues medical exams. Many people do not get annual physical exams and rarely use a physician due to the real and perceived hassles and costs. Thus, a person may potentially have a disease for an extended period of time without knowledge of it, so documenting the date of his or her last examination is relevant, particularly among **geriatric** populations.

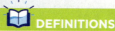

DEFINITIONS

Geriatric –

Used as a reference term for older populations or people, especially with regard to their health care or special needs.

HEALTH STATUS QUESTIONNAIRE

SECTION ONE – GENERAL INFORMATION

1. Date: _____

2. Name: _____

3. Mailing Address: _____ Phone (H): _____

   _____ Phone (W): _____

   Email: _____

4. EI Personal Physician: _____ Phone: _____

   Physician Address: _____ Fax: _____

5. EI Person to contact in case of Emergency: _____ Phone: _____

6. Gender (circle one):   Female   RF Male

7. RF Date of Birth: _____

8. Height: _____   Weight: _____

9. Number of hours worked per week: Less than 20   20-40   41-50   over 50

10. SLA More than 25% of the time at your job is spent *(circle all that apply)*:

    Sitting at desk   Lifting loads   Standing   Walking   Driving

HEALTH STATUS QUESTIONNAIRE

SECTION TWO – CURRENT MEDICAL INFORMATION

11. Date of last medical physical exam: _____

12. Circle all medicine taken or prescribed within the last 6 months:

    Blood thinner MC   Epilepsy medication SEP   Nitroglycerin MC

    Diabetic MC   Heart rhythm medication MC   Other: _____

    Digitalis MC   High blood pressure medication MC

    Diuretic MC   Insulin MC

13. Please list any orthopedic conditions. Include any injuries in the last six months.
    _____

14. Any of these health symptoms that occur frequently *(two or more times/month)* require medical attention. *Please check any that apply.*

    a. ___ Cough up blood MC   g. ___ Swollen joints MC
    b. ___ Abdominal pain MC   h. ___ Feel faint MC
    c. ___ Low-back pain MC   i. ___ Dizziness MC
    d. ___ Leg pain MC   j. ___ Breathlessness with slight exertion MC
    e. ___ Arm or shoulder pain MC   k. ___ Palpitation or fast heart beat MC
    f. ___ Chest pain RF MC   l. ___ Unusual fatigue with normal activity MC

    Other: _____

SECTION THREE – MEDICAL HISTORY

15. Please circle any of the following for which you have been diagnosed or treated by a physician or health professional:

    Alcoholism SEP   Diabetes SEP   Kidney problem MC
    Anemia, sickle cell SEP   Emphysema SEP   Mental illness SEP
    Anemia, other SEP   Epilepsy SEP   Neck strain SLA
    Asthma SEP   Eye problems SLA   Obesity RF
    Back strain SLA   Gout SLA   Phlebitis MC
    Bleeding trait SEP   Hearing loss SLA   Rheumatoid arthritis SLA
    Bronchitis, chronic SEP   Heart problems MC   Stress RF
    Stroke MC   Cancer SEP   High blood pressure SLA
    Thyroid problem SEP   Cirrhosis MC   HIV SEP
    Ulcer SEP   Concussion MC   Hypoglycemia SEP
    Congenital defect SEP   Hyperlipidemia RF   Other: _____

HEALTH STATUS QUESTIONNAIRE

SECTION THREE – *MEDICAL HISTORY (Continued)*

16. Circle any operations that you have had:

    Back *SLA*   Heart *MC*   Kidneys *SLA*   Eyes *SLA*   Joints *SLA*   Neck *SLA*

    Ears *SLA*   Hernia *SLA*   Lungs *SLA*   Other: _____

17. *RF* Circle any of the following who died of heart attack before age 55:

    Father   Brother   Son

18. *RF* Circle any of the following who died of heart attack before age 65:

    Mother   Sister   Daughter

SECTION FOUR – *HEALTH-RELATED BEHAVIORS*

19. *RF* Do you currently smoke?   Yes   No

20. *RF* If you are a smoker, indicate the number smoked per day:

    Cigarettes: 40 or more   20-39   10-19   1-9

    Cigars or pipes only: 5 or more or any inhaled less than 5

21. Have you ever smoked?   Yes   No

22. *RF* Do you exercise regularly?   Yes   No

23. Last physical fitness test: _____

24. How many days a week do you accumulate 30 minutes of moderate activity?

    0   1   2   3   4   5   6   7

25. How many days per week do you normally spend at least 20 minutes in vigorous exercise?

    0   1   2   3   4   5   6   7

26. What activities do you engage in a least once per week? _____

27. Weight now: _____   One year ago: _____   Age 21: _____

SECTION FIVE – *HEALTH-RELATED ATTITUDES*

28. These are traits that have been associated with coronary-prone behavior. *Circle the number that corresponds to how you feel toward the following statement:*

    I am an impatient, time-conscious, hard-driving individual.

    6 = Strongly agree   3 = Slightly disagree

    5 = Moderately agree   2 = Moderately disagree

    4 = Slightly agree   1 = Strongly disagree

HEALTH STATUS QUESTIONNAIRE

SECTION FIVE – HEALTH-RELATED ATTITUDES (Continued)

29. How often do you experience "negative" stress from each of the following?

	RF Always	*RF* Usually	*RF* Frequently	Rarely	Never
Work:	____	____	____	____	____
Home or family:	____	____	____	____	____
Financial pressure:	____	____	____	____	____
Social pressure:	____	____	____	____	____
Personal health:	____	____	____	____	____

30. List everything not included on this questionnaire that may cause you problems in a fitness test or fitness program.

_____
_____
_____
_____
_____
_____
_____

Action Codes

EI = Emergency Information - must be readily available.

MC = Medical Clearance needed - do not allow exercise without physician's permission.

SEP = Special Emergency Procedures needed - do not let participant exercise alone; make sure the person's exercise partner knows what to do in case of an emergency.

RF = Risk Factor of CHD (educational materials and workshops needed).

SLA = Special or Limited Activities may be needed - you may need to include or exclude specific exercises.

Other (not marked) = Personal information that may be helpful for files or research.

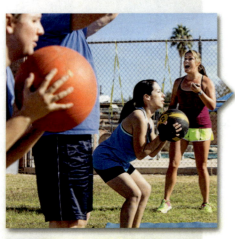

◆ Behavior Questionnaire

In a comprehensive screening process, the HSQ should be followed by a Behavior Questionnaire. The Behavior Questionnaire provides details about routine lifestyle habits, common behavior trends, and dietary practices. It can also help identify personal preferences and learned behavior traits. The behavior questionnaire can be very useful for several reasons, including:

1. Identifying obstacles to the program goals and needed improvements in health status.

2. Identifying factors correlating to current health status.

3. Providing the opportunity to educate clients about how their behaviors impact their health.

4. Identifying appropriate behavior management strategies.

Unhealthy behaviors can significantly impact a person's physical and mental condition. If unaccounted for, these behavior can impede program goal attainment, even with a properly constructed and implemented exercise prescription. Of the 168 total hours in a week, exercise professionals usually have 2-3 hours of control over the client's environment and behaviors. The other 165 hours remain at the client's discretion. If the client makes poor eating and drinking decisions, engages in sedentary living, or places him or herself in high stress environments, much of the work accomplished during the personal training sessions will be counteracted by these negative behaviors. This is most relevant if the behaviors exacerbate a current health condition. Individuals with disease, or at risk for diseases – such as diabetes, hypertension, **dyslipidemia**, coronary artery disease (CAD), **metabolic syndrome**, and obesity – must comply with the recommendations for managing their conditions. Of particular concern, are unchecked dietary habits (unhealthy eating and drinking), smoking, high alcohol consumption, and sedentary living, as these are clear markers for increased disease risk.

> **DEFINITIONS**
>
> **Dyslipidemia –**
>
> *A term used to indicate poor blood lipid profile measurements: elevated low-density cholesterol, low levels of high-density cholesterol, elevated total cholesterol levels or sub-optimal cholesterol ratio; it is a risk factor for cardiovascular disease and stroke.*
>
> **Metabolic syndrome –**
>
> *Recognized as a cluster of interrelated conditions--high blood pressure, poor glucose management, excess body fat (especially around the waist), systemic inflammation, and abnormal cholesterol levels--that significantly increases one's risk for heart disease, stroke, and diabetes.*

BEHAVIOR QUESTIONNAIRE

1. How many servings of fruits and vegetables do you eat per day?
       0   1   2   3+

2. How many caffeinated drinks (coffee, tea, cocoa, soft drinks) do you drink per day?
       0   1-2   3-4   5+

3. How many glasses (8 ounces) of water do you drink per day?
       0-3   4-5   6-7   8+

4. How many meals do you consume per day?
       1-2   3-4   5-6   7+

5. I cook with and eat fats:
   - ___ Nearly always cook/eat high fat foods (fried foods, shortening, butter, creams)
   - ___ Cook/eat mostly high fat
   - ___ Cook/eat both high and low fat foods
   - ___ Cook/eat mostly low fat
   - ___ Cook/eat only low fat

6. My bread/grain eating habit is:
   - ___ Nearly always eat refined (white bread, grains, rolls, crackers, cereal)
   - ___ Eat mostly refined grain products
   - ___ Eat a mixture of refined and whole grain products
   - ___ Eat primarily whole grain products
   - ___ Eat only whole grain products

7. How often do you eat out?
   - ___ I eat out nearly every day
   - ___ I eat out several times each week
   - ___ I eat out a few times each month
   - ___ I seldom or never eat out

BEHAVIOR QUESTIONNAIRE

8. My salty food habit is: (check all that apply)
   ___ I rarely eat salty foods (chips, pickles, soups, added salt)
   ___ Occasionally I eat salty foods
   ___ I regularly eat salty food
   ___ I add salt to the foods I eat

9. During the past 30 days, did you diet to lose weight or to keep from gaining weight?
             Yes   No
   If Yes Explain: _____

10. My high fat snack eating habit is:
    ___ I eat high fat snack foods (potato chips) 3 or more times daily
    ___ I eat high fat snacks once or twice daily
    ___ I eat high fat snacks a few times each week
    ___ I rarely or never eat high fat snacks

11. How often do you eat red meat?
    ___ I eat red meat nearly every day
    ___ I eat red meat several times each week
    ___ I eat red meat a few times each month
    ___ I seldom or never eat red meat

12. How often do you eat cookies, cakes, sweets?
    ___ I eat cookies, cakes, sweets nearly every day
    ___ I eat cookies, cakes, sweets several times each week
    ___ I eat cookies, cakes, sweets a few times each month
    ___ I seldom or never eat cookies, cakes, sweets

13. How many alcoholic beverages do you consume per week?
        0-3   4-5   6-7   8+

14. On average, I sleep ____ hours a night.
        3-4   5-6   7-8   8+

15. Outside of work, what physical and/or social activities do you engage in?
    _____
    _____

---

1. *Identified obstacles to program goals:*
   _____
   _____

2. *Needed improvements in health status:*
   _____
   _____

3. *Identified behavioral factors correlating to current health status:*
   _____
   _____

4. *Appropriate behavior management strategies:*
   _____
   _____

Compiling the Data

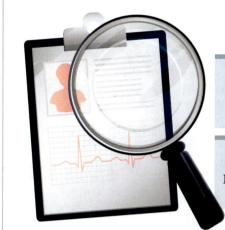

The health behavior questionnaire should complement the HSQ and be used in an attempt to correlate findings. For instance, if a client has been diagnosed with hypertension and his or her diet consists of high salt and fatty foods, these current lifestyle habits clearly promote the disease. Therefore, appropriate control strategies are needed to work to prevent negative health impact. Furthermore, if a client's weight measurements over time indicate a propensity for **creeping obesity**, and his or her normal lifestyle habits show a preference for nonphysical activities, these issues should be identified and explained that they are creating barriers to improved health and increasing susceptibility to additional weight gain. Most behavior questionnaires provide supportive evidence for the problems found on the HSQ. Rarely will someone live a very healthy lifestyle and suffer the consequences of diseases prevalent in the western world.

DEFINITIONS

Creeping obesity –

Obesity resulting from incremental weight gain over a period of time; usually attributed to sustained caloric intake coupled with a decrease in physical activity.

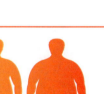

Creeping Obesity
One Pound Fat Mass = 3,500 kcals
Daily Caloric Need = 2,200 kcals
Daily Caloric Expenditure = 2,100 kcals
Positive 100 kcal/day
100 kcal/day x 365 days/year = 36,500 kcals per year
36,500 kcals per year ÷ 3,500 kcals per lb of fat =
10.4 lbs of fat per year

CREATE A NEEDS ANALYSIS

Health Needs
- Hypertension
- Pre-diabetes risk
- High body fat

Health Remedies
- Aerobic conditioning/weight loss (daily)
- Total body resistance training (<70% 1RM)
- Caloric control/expenditure (>1,000 kcal/wk)

Fitness Needs
- Flexibility
- Cardiovascular
- Strength imbalances

Fitness Remedies
- ROM activities (dynamic, static)
- Threshold aerobic training (33 ml/kg/min)
- Planned resistance exercises

Behavioral Needs
- High stress
- Poor diet

Health Remedies
- Educational assistance
- Educational assistance

Document findings by *Order of Importance*

DEFINITIONS

Needs analysis –

The identification, organization, and prioritization of physiological needs applicable to improving an individual's health and fitness measurements: a list of what the client needs to improve in his or her health and fitness.

Upon review of the HSQ and behavior questionnaire, personal trainers should attempt to identify and create a **needs analysis** that lists all the health problems and risks associated with the collected client's information. Once a list has been constructed, it should be ranked by order of health risk significance. Immediate and primary risks should be listed first. These risks can cause direct damage to a person's health and include smoking, inflammatory obesity, CVD, metabolic disease, and other major health problems: for example, asthma, leg pain, peripheral edema, chronic low back pain, and orthopedic injuries. The next group of risks should include those factors that compound these conditions or increase their potential adverse effects. Some examples are high fat diet, unmanaged stress, excessive alcohol consumption, poor sleeping habits, low fiber, and high sugar intake. These risks and any important information should be evaluated for relevance and used to correlate related factors. This model will allow for a more complete strategy to address the conditions appropriately. Jointly employed, these two forms can provide relevant details for effective risk stratification and program decision making.

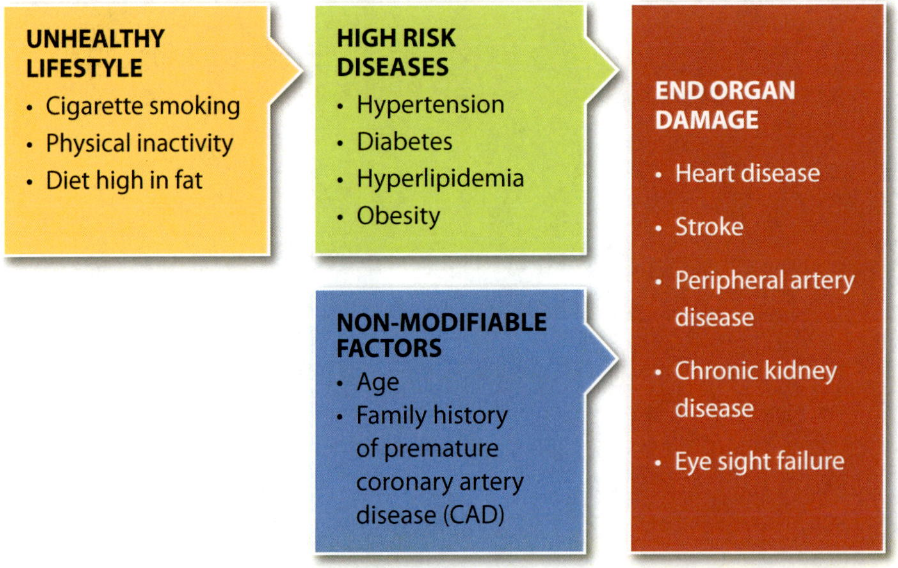

UNHEALTHY LIFESTYLE
- Cigarette smoking
- Physical inactivity
- Diet high in fat

HIGH RISK DISEASES
- Hypertension
- Diabetes
- Hyperlipidemia
- Obesity

NON-MODIFIABLE FACTORS
- Age
- Family history of premature coronary artery disease (CAD)

END ORGAN DAMAGE
- Heart disease
- Stroke
- Peripheral artery disease
- Chronic kidney disease
- Eye sight failure

Evaluating Health and Physical Fitness

REFERENCES:

1. Adler NE, Boyce T, Chesney MA, Cohen S, Folkman S, Kahn RL, and Syme SL. Socioeconomic status and health: The challenge of the gradient. *American psychologist* 49: 15, 1994.

2. Andenæs R, Bentsen SB, Hvinden K, Fagermoen MS, and Lerdal A. The relationships of self-efficacy, physical activity, and paid work to health-related quality of life among patients with chronic obstructive pulmonary disease (COPD). *Journal of multidisciplinary healthcare* 7: 239, 2014.

3. Barnekow Bergkvist M, Hedberg G, Janlert U, and Jansson E. Physical activity pattern in men and women at the ages of 16 and 34 and development of physical activity from adolescence to adulthood. *Scandinavian journal of medicine & science in sports* 6: 359-370, 1996.

4. Best TM. The preparticipation evaluation: an opportunity for change and consensus: LWW, 2004.

5. Brockett CL, Morgan DL, and Proske U. Predicting hamstring strain injury in elite athletes. *Medicine & Science in Sports & Exercise* 36: 379-387, 2004.

6. Brodersen NH, Steptoe A, Boniface DR, and Wardle J. Trends in physical activity and sedentary behaviour in adolescence: ethnic and socioeconomic differences. *British journal of sports medicine* 41: 140-144, 2007.

7. Brown DR, Carroll DD, Workman LM, Carlson SA, and Brown DW. Physical activity and health-related quality of life: US adults with and without limitations. *Quality of life research* 23: 2673-2680, 2014.

8. De Geus EJ and De Moor MH. Genes, exercise, and psychological factors. In: *Genetic and molecular aspects of sports performance:* Blackwell Publishing, Oxford, 2011, p. 294-305.

9. De Moor MH, Spector TD, Cherkas LF, Falchi M, Hottenga JJ, Boomsma DI, and De Geus EJ. Genome-wide linkage scan for athlete status in 700 British female DZ twin pairs. *Twin Research and Human Genetics* 10: 812-820, 2007.

10. Gomes EC and Florida-James G. Exercise and the Immune System. In: *Environmental Influences on the Immune System:* Springer, 2016, p. 127-152.

11. Grady C. Enduring and emerging challenges of informed consent. *New England Journal of Medicine* 372: 855-862, 2015.

12. Hootman JM, Macera CA, Ainsworth BE, Martin M, Addy CL, and Blair SN. Predictors of Lower Extremity Injury Among Recreationally Active Adults. *Clinical Journal of Sport Medicine* 12: 99-106, 2002.

13. Kaplan RM and Bush JW. Health-related quality of life measurement for evaluation research and policy analysis. *Health psychology* 1: 61, 1982.

14. Krops LA, Jaarsma EA, Dijkstra PU, Geertzen JH, and Dekker R. Health Related Quality of Life in a Dutch Rehabilitation Population: Reference Values and the Effect of Physical Activity. *PloS one* 12: e0169169, 2017.

15. Kwok Y, Kim C, Grady D, Segal M, and Redberg R. Meta-analysis of exercise testing to detect coronary artery disease in women. *The American journal of cardiology* 83: 660-666, 1999.

16. Ladapo JA, Blecker S, and Douglas PS. Physician Decision Making and Trends in the Use of Cardiac Stress Testing in the United StatesAn Analysis of Repeated Cross-sectional DataPhysician Decision Making and Trends in the Use of Cardiac Stress Testing. *Annals of internal medicine* 161: 482-490, 2014.

17. Ladapo JA, Blecker S, Elashoff MR, Federspiel JJ, Vieira DL, Sharma G, Monane M, Rosenberg S, Phelps CE, and Douglas PS. Clinical implications of referral bias in the diagnostic performance of exercise testing for coronary artery disease. *Journal of the American Heart Association* 2: e000505, 2013.

18. Lin X, Eaton CB, Manson JE, and Liu S. The Genetics of Physical Activity. *Current Cardiology Reports* 19: 119, 2017.

19. Lombardo JA and Badolato SK. The preparticipation physical examination. *Clinical cornerstone* 3: 10-22, 2001.

20. MacArthur DG and North KN. Genes and human elite athletic performance. *Human genetics* 116: 331-339, 2005.

21. McNeely E. Prescreening for the personal trainer. *Strength & Conditioning Journal* 30: 68-69, 2008.

22. Nandalur KR, Dwamena BA, Choudhri AF, Nandalur MR, and Carlos RC. Diagnostic performance of stress cardiac magnetic resonance imaging in the detection of coronary artery disease: a meta-analysis. *Journal of the American College of Cardiology* 50: 1343-1353, 2007.

23. Nishimura A, Carey J, McCormick JB, Tilburt JC, Murad MH, and Erwin PJ. Improving understanding in the research informed consent process: a systematic review of 54 interventions tested in randomized control trials. *BMC medical ethics* 14: 28, 2013.

24. Organization WH. Noncommunicable diseases country profiles 2014. 2014.

25. Pratt M, Norris J, Lobelo F, Roux L, and Wang G. The cost of physical inactivity: moving into the 21st century. *Br J Sports Med* 48: 171-173, 2014.

26. Rejeski WJ and Mihalko SL. Physical activity and quality of life in older adults. The Journals of Gerontology Series A: *Biological sciences and medical sciences* 56: 23-35, 2001.

27. Rowlands AV. Physical Activity, Inactivity, and health during youth. *Pediatric exercise science* 28: 19-22, 2016.

28. Schneider S, Seither B, Tönges S, and Schmitt H. Sports injuries: population based representative data on incidence, diagnosis, sequelae, and high risk groups. *British journal of sports medicine* 40: 334-339, 2006.

29. Schwebel DC and Brezausek CM. Child development and pediatric sport and recreational injuries by age. *Journal of athletic training* 49: 780-785, 2014.

30. Sekendiz B. Implementation and perception of risk management practices in health/fitness facilities. *International Journal of Business Continuity and Risk Management* 27 5: 165-183, 2014.

31. Sekendiz B, Ammon R, and Connaughton DP. An Examination of Waiver Usage and Injury-Related Liability Claims in Health/Fitness Facilities in Australia. *Journal of Legal Aspects of Sport* 26: 144-161, 2016.

32. Stubbs B, Eggermont L, Soundy A, Probst M, Vandenbulcke M, and Vancampfort D. What are the factors associated with physical activity (PA) participation in community dwelling adults with dementia? A systematic review of PA correlates. *Archives of gerontology and geriatrics* 59: 195-203, 2014.

33. Vagetti GC, Barbosa Filho VC, Moreira NB, Oliveira Vd, Mazzardo O, and Campos Wd. Association between physical activity and quality of life in the elderly: a systematic review, 2000-2012. *Revista Brasileira de Psiquiatria* 36: 76-88, 2014.

34. Warburton D, Jamnik VK, Bredin SS, and Gledhill N. The 2014 physical activity readiness questionnaire for everyone (PAR-Q+) and electronic physical activity readiness medical examination (ePARmed-X+). *Health & Fitness Journal of Canada* 7: 80, 2014.

35. Whitney SN. Consent in Biomedical Research. In: *Balanced Ethics Review:* Springer, 2016, p. 47-56.

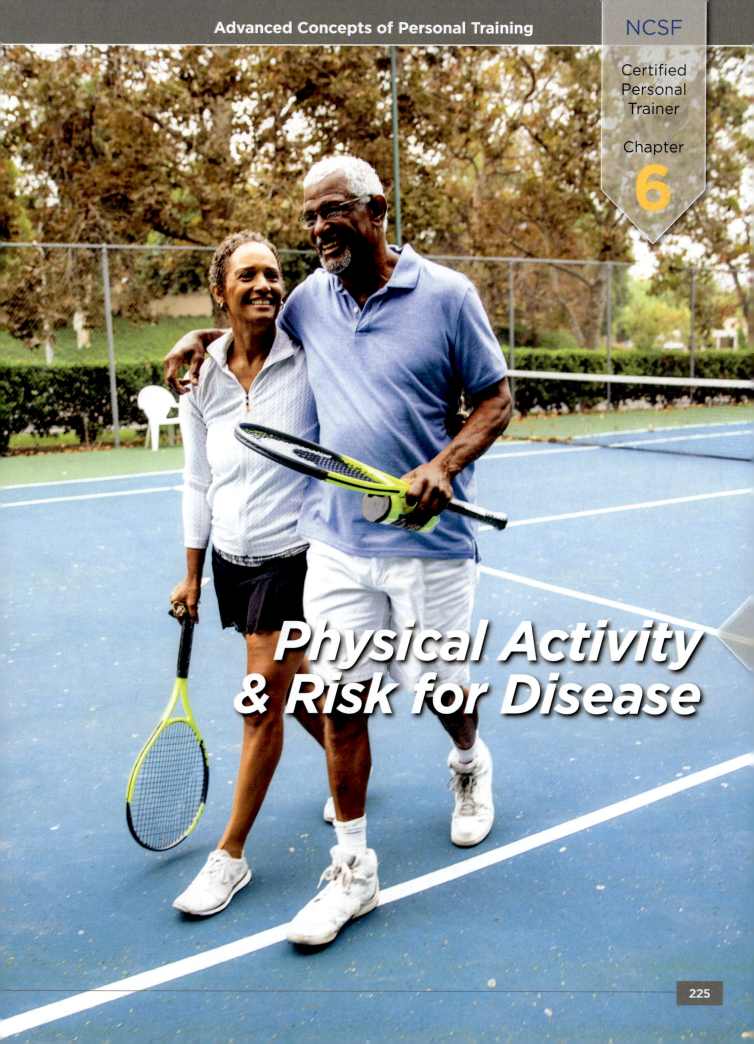

Advanced Concepts of Personal Training

NCSF Certified Personal Trainer

Chapter 6

Physical Activity & Risk for Disease

Physical Activity & Risk for Disease

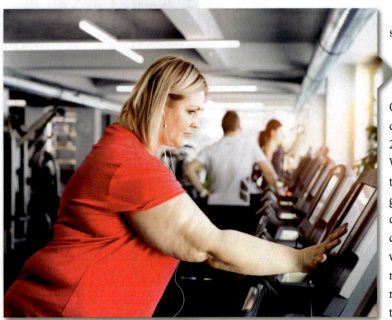

The rate of inactivity in the United States constitutes a significant societal health burden. The lack of participation in daily physical activity and the increase in access to calorically dense, processed food is partly to blame for the elevated incidence of controllable disease across the country. The Centers for Disease Control (CDC) estimates the number of deaths associated with physical inactivity to be approximately 200,000 annually when viewed as an independent risk factor. When linked with poor diet, that estimate jumps to 300,000 in the United States. Physical inactivity also contributes to a global pandemic responsible for approximately 5 million deaths per year [38, 80, 88]. It is likely that other risk factors associated with a sedentary lifestyle also contribute to these values, which speaks to the relevance of overall health accountability, rather than an emphasis on any single factor [38]. Simply removing a solitary consequential factor may not benefit mortality risk when it coincides with other negative risk factors.

The importance of physical activity cannot be overstated, as it is associated with a reduction in risk of all-cause mortality, coronary artery disease (CAD), hypertension, some cancers, non-insulin dependent diabetes mellitus, and mortality from all cardiovascular disease (CVD) combined [7, 25, 41, 104, 140]. The total global annual cost of physical inactivity is estimated at $67 billion [36, 37]. According to the World Health Organization (WHO), if the level of physical inactivity in the overall population of the world decreased by 10%, it could reduce the number of premature deaths by 533,000 annually. If the level of inactivity decreased by 25%, about 1.3 million premature deaths would be avoided globally every year. Research presented in this chapter identifies the relationship of physical activity and cardiorespiratory fitness (CRF) to a variety of health consequences. Epidemiological studies have identified the association of physical inactivity and health problems, the respective magnitude of such relationships, and the biological mechanisms for the onset of the diseases in question. Accounting for these relationships through behavioral modifications that increase the frequency and intensity of physical activity significantly improves life quality and prevents premature disability and death.

It is well known that individuals who regularly engage in physical activity and those with high levels of CRF have a lower mortality rate than those individuals who maintain low CRF, including individuals classified as sedentary [140]. The cited risk for dying from all-cause mortality is more than 2x higher for those classified as sedentary individuals and those with low CRF than those who are physically active. In this case, "physically active" includes not only exercise activities but also leisure-time physical activity, walking for transportation, and other non-exercise physical activity, as each activity type contributes to a reduced risk of all-cause and CVD mortality. In addition to a reduction in death rates associated with activity participation, a correlation exists between lifespan and the level of physical fitness [41, 104]. Individuals who engage in activities of longer duration and higher intensity tend to live longer regardless of the age at which they begin participation [6, 85, 87]. This correlation exists with limitations, however: individuals who overexert themselves routinely may actually harm their health and reduce overall lifespan due to associated chronic physical stress. This scenario again underscores the need for a healthy balance. To sum up, research demonstrates the profound effect of leisure-time physical activity (LTPA) on mortality but notes that it does further improve when performed at excessive levels.

◆ Physical Activity Relationship to Mortality Risk

Studies show that changes from low-level fitness to moderate-level fitness yield the greatest impact on death rates [60, 78, 105]. Essentially, exchanging a sedentary lifestyle for one which includes moderate physical activity will maximally impact risk for disease and yield a positive change in mortality. Improving one's fitness benefits any individual but not to the same extent as converting from a physically inactive to active state. In **longitudinal studies**, improvement from low CRF to moderate levels was related to a 44% lower death rate compared to those who remained at low fitness levels. After adjusting for other factors, that difference jumped to a 64% reduction in risk compared to those that remained sedentary [126]. This information adds to the mountain of literature that suggests individuals who engage in physical activity reduce their risk for all-cause mortality. Regular physical activity strongly indicates overall mortality rates and shows a significant dose-response relationship [126]. Individuals should adjust lifestyle habits to include daily physical activity to take control of their health and risk for death. Beyond this baseline level, increasing one's level of fitness decreases mortality risk when training at higher intensities and/or for longer durations and accounting for all other health-related components of fitness [41, 122].

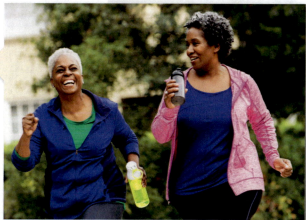

Exchanging a sedentary lifestyle for one which includes moderate physical activity will reduce the risk for disease as well as premature mortality.

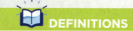
DEFINITIONS

Longitudinal studies –

A form of observational research in which data is gathered for a given sample of a population over a period of time to examine long-term effects or relationships; these studies can last years or even decades.

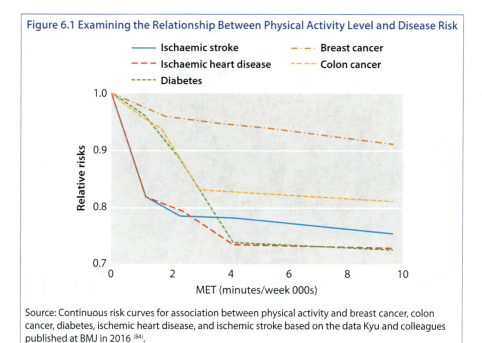

Figure 6.1 Examining the Relationship Between Physical Activity Level and Disease Risk

Source: Continuous risk curves for association between physical activity and breast cancer, colon cancer, diabetes, ischemic heart disease, and ischemic stroke based on the data Kyu and colleagues published at BMJ in 2016 [84].

Physical Activity & Cardiovascular Disease

The CDC identifies heart disease and stroke as the most common CVDs, representing the first and fifth leading causes of death in the United States, respectively [98]. According to the American Heart Association's Heart Disease and Stroke Statistics, CVD deaths were around 836,536 in 2018 [98]. Research suggests that these diseases account for almost 30% of all annual deaths, equating to one death every 40 seconds from CVD [98]. Although these largely preventable diseases occur more commonly in older individuals, the risk of sudden death has increased alarmingly in individuals less than 35 years of age [53]. The annual incidence of sudden cardiac death is estimated between 300,000 and 350,000 cases in the USA, which accounts for almost half of all cardiovascular deaths [83]. In the form of CAD, CVD is also the leading cause of premature, permanent disability among United States workers [160]. According to the CDC, every year about 735,000 Americans have a heart attack. Of these, 525,000 suffer a first heart attack and 210,000 experience a repeat heart attack. Additionally, over 1 million Americans become disabled from stroke alone. Collectively, CVD forces the hospitalization of over 6 million Americans [160]. Estimates suggest that more than 83.6 million Americans currently live with some form of heart disease, and the estimated direct and indirect cost of CVD for 2010 is $315.4 billion [98].

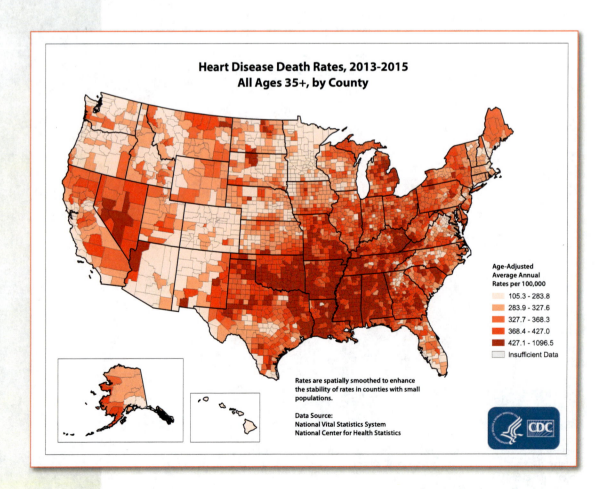

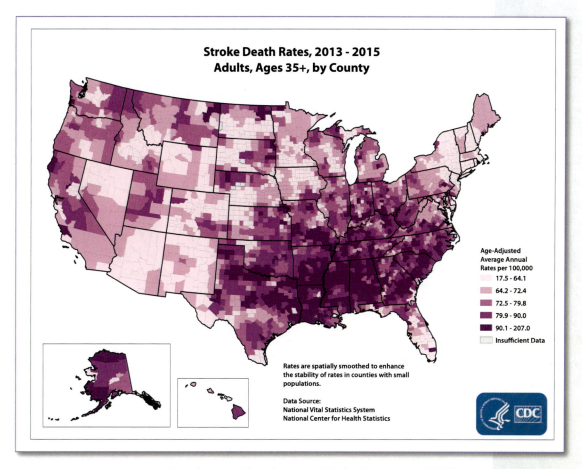

As mentioned, physical activity dramatically reduces the risk for developing CVD [78]. Several studies have shown that a dose-response gradient exists, further supporting the need for regular physical activity [84]. These research studies emphasize that some activity is better than none, and more activity is even better for mitigating CHD risk. As stated, lower CRF increases risk for mortality, which is consistent with its relationship with CVD-related death. Individuals with the highest fitness levels show the greatest reduction of risk [78, 104, 105]. The dose-response relationship suggests that benefits begin at moderate levels and increase consistently with activity intensity and duration. Therefore, physical activity demonstrates a strong inverse relationship with CVD risk [41, 60]. Numerous studies have analyzed the impact of physical activity on risk for specific forms of CVD [60, 87, 140]. The following text provides supportive evidence from **epidemiological studies** that analyze varied intensity and duration on measured outcomes of specific disorders.

DEFINITIONS

Epidemiological studies –

A form of research that focuses on the patterns, causes, and effects of health and disease conditions within specific populations (e.g., age groups, racial/ethnic groups, sexes).

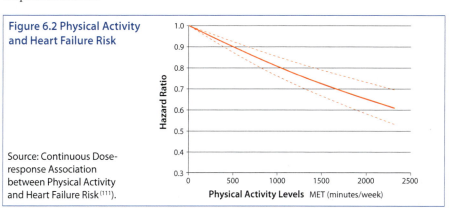

Figure 6.2 Physical Activity and Heart Failure Risk

Source: Continuous Dose-response Association between Physical Activity and Heart Failure Risk [111].

> **DEFINITIONS**
>
> **Comorbidities –**
>
> *Refers to the simultaneous presence of two or more chronic diseases in a patient; for example, obese individuals often have multiple concurrent comorbidities, such as diabetes, hypertension, and/or dyslipidemia.*
>
> **Thrombosis –**
>
> *The formation of a dangerous blood clot in a major blood vessel, heart, lungs or other body tissue which can cause various life-threatening issues, such as a stroke or pulmonary embolism.*
>
> **Cytokines –**
>
> *Various substances secreted by components of the immune system to modulate tissue functions or have an impact on other cells; these can serve as signalers, growth factors, or facilitators of inflammatory actions.*
>
> **Autoimmune disorders –**
>
> *A type of disease in which the body produces antibodies to attack its own tissues, leading to the deterioration and potential death of cells, glands, or organs; examples include lupus, multiple sclerosis, rheumatoid arthritis, etc.*

◆ Coronary Heart Disease (CHD)

There exists a transient risk of an acute coronary event when those with advanced coronary pathology participate in exercise but the inverse relationship between physical activity and CHD is so strong that exercise is even recommended for those with disease [101, 129]. For those without diagnosed disease it is simply safer to be physically active than not. Clearly, active people have a significantly lower risk for coronary events compared to sedentary persons or those with low CRF [108]. Participation in moderate-to-high intensity (60-80% VO_2max) aerobic exercise has been shown to improve CRF and dramatically reduce CHD risk [142]. Appropriate diet and lifestyle habits that reduce negative blood-content profiles and overall stress enhance this benefit.

Blood Lipid Profile Numbers to Know – *Based on Relative CVD Risk*

- **High-risk goals:** LDL < 100 mg/dL, non-HDL < 130 mg/dL, apoB < 90 mg/dL (apoB – protein involved in lipid metabolism and main constituent of LDL as well as VLDL)
    - Two or more risk factors and 10-year risk 10%-20%
    - Diabetes or Chronic Kidney Disease stages 3/4 with no other risk factors
- **Moderate-risk goals:** Same goals as high risk
    - Two or more risk factors and 10-year risk < 10%
- **Low-risk goals:** LDL < 130 mg/dL, non-HDL < 160 mg/dL, apoB not relevant
    - 0 risk factors

LDL – low-density lipoproteins, HDL – high-density lipoproteins, VLDL – very low-density lipoproteins

---

Most people assume high blood pressure and high cholesterol are adult-onset disorders, but CHD actually starts in childhood. In fact, nearly 1 in 250 children have high cholesterol levels that are beginning to promote plaque in their arteries, and those children who are obese, have diabetes or related **comorbidities**, experience additional risk [33]. Although a diagnosis for CHD is rare in children, sufficient evidence exists linking low levels of physical inactivity during childhood to risk for adult CHD [110]. The presence of CHD in adulthood is linked to coronary level plaque, and data shows atherosclerosis begins during childhood [123]. Of particular relevance, the childhood behaviors linked to the initial development of coronary plaque tend to persist into adulthood. Likewise, physical inactivity is linked to contributing factors for heart disease in all ages, including obesity, diabetes, hypertension, metabolic syndrome, and hyperlipidemia [151].

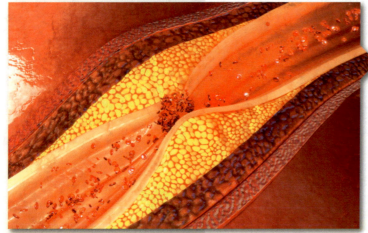

The reduction in risk for CHD associated with aerobic activity and CRF is likely attained through several physiological mechanisms. These include reductions in body fat, blood pressure, myocardial ischemia, **thrombosis**, and heart rhythm disturbances, as well as improvements in plasma lipid profiles and reduction in systemic inflammation [13, 22, 75, 76, 79, 91]. The latter is a relevant subject, as systemic inflammatory disorders are associated with numerous harmful **cytokines** and have been linked to **autoimmune disorders**.

CHD is caused by coronary artery occlusion due to vascular wall damage, which leads to atherosclerosis. Atherosclerosis has been described as a chronic inflammatory state characterized by the accumulation of cholesterol and immune cells within the artery wall which contributes to arteriosclerosis, hardening of the arteries. Atherosclerosis is a progressive disorder which starts in the cell wall of blood vessels. The accumulation of coronary plaque occurs when the arterial walls are injured from turbulent blood flow and high total vascular pressure. The harsh conditions applied to the vessel walls cause tears. The resultant lesions allow cholesterol fatty deposits to build up in the artery's lining. Circulating **low-density lipoproteins (LDL)** deliver cholesterol into the artery wall at the area of the initial insult, which promotes the negative association of LDL and **very low-density lipoproteins (VLDL)** in circulation. The large **high-density lipoproteins (HDL)** have been shown to be inversely related to risk for CVD, with some studies suggesting that HDLs provide a protection against **atherogenic** effects [82, 148]. When the vessel is exposed to foreign bodies, such as lipids, an inflammatory reaction occurs, similar to getting a splinter or a small cut. This inflammatory response attracts white blood cells, macrophages, or immune cells, which accumulate in the cell wall, where they ingest the fatty deposits. This event causes a proliferation of smooth muscle cells around the area, which are eventually replaced with hard collagen. A protective fibrous cap then forms between the fatty deposits and the artery lining. This process is commonly referred to as arteriosclerosis. At this point, the **lumen** of the artery is not narrowed. However, over the course of years, the plaque can form an **aneurism** (an abnormal dilation) of the vessel inner wall, which can rupture. When an aneurism of the plaque occurs in the wall, a clot can form, which can narrow or even occlude the artery so that little to no blood passes through. The inner wall damage is subject to additional build-up of fatty deposits, platelets, and other circulatory debris. With the decrease in blood flow through the artery, the tissue being fed by the vessel becomes ischemic and can die from lack of oxygen, essentially suffocating.

Factors Shown to Lower the Risk for Heart Disease

- Lower your blood pressure and cholesterol if elevated
- Consume a diet low in salt, refined sugars, total fat, saturated fat, and cholesterol
- Consume a diet rich in fiber via fresh fruits and vegetables and heart-healthy fats
- Exercise regularly (at least 150 minutes a week)
- Avoid excessive intake of alcohol and do not smoke
- Ensure safe use of medications and any over-the-counter drugs
- Educate oneself on appropriate stress management
- Lose weight and body fat if overweight

DEFINITIONS

Low-density lipoproteins (LDL) –

A complex of lipids and proteins that functions as a transporter for circulating cholesterol from the liver to various body tissues; LDLs were previously associated with a direct risk for cardiovascular disease as an explicit cause when found in elevated quantities within circulation due to its potential role in plaque accumulation as "bad cholesterol"; however, current research points to more complex synergistic considerations, such as carrier protein and total particle counts as well as cholesterol ratios.

High-density lipoproteins (HDL) –

A complex of lipids and proteins that functions to transport/remove cholesterol and lipids from circulation to the liver. HDLs have classically been associated with a reduced risk for atherosclerosis and heart disease ("good cholesterol"); however, contemporary research points toward HDL particle size and the impact of its carrier protein (apolipoprotein A-1) on inflammatory and oxidation dynamics as more integral to disease risk reduction than simply considering overall HDL concentration.

Very-low density lipoproteins (VLDL) –

Similar in structure, function, and circulatory impact to low-density lipoproteins, which aid in transporting cholesterol, triglycerides, and other lipids throughout the body; VLDLs were classically considered a component of "bad cholesterol," but contemporary research shows disease risk association is more complicated than originally thought.

Atherogenic –

A term used to describe dynamics which promote the formation of fatty plaques in vascular structures (arteries).

Lumen –

When referring to an artery or vascular structure, this term describes the inside open space of the tubular structure.

Aneurism –

An excessive localized enlargement of an artery (or abnormal dilation) caused by the weakening of an arterial wall due to issues such as hypertension and atherosclerosis or genetics; this bulge can rupture and cause life-threatening situations or sudden death when occurring within the brain or other integral organs.

◆ Exercise & Atherosclerosis

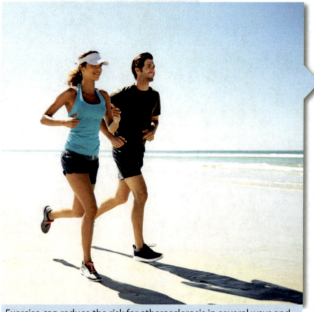

Exercise can reduce the risk for atherosclerosis in several ways and even reverse current vascular damage.

Exercise and physical activity reduce the risk of atherosclerosis via several concurrent mechanisms, presenting an opportunity for reversal of the damage. It has been shown that preventative exercise therapies can halt and even cause anti-atherogenic effects or reverse the atherosclerotic process [141, 153].

A key element in the process is managing the integrity of the vessel wall, called the endothelium. This inner lining can become stronger with consistent aerobic exercise. The vessels compliance increases due to the blood flow and pressure changes required to get blood from the heart to the skeletal muscles. Recall the importance of compliance, as it refers to the walls' ability to respond by either expanding (dilating) or contracting (constricting) in response to the demands of changing pressure and blood flow. When the vessel wall becomes healthier, it contributes to reducing blood pressure via dilation, therefore attenuating the primary instigator for damage. Concurrently, aerobic exercise reduces circulating LDL cholesterol (LDL-C) over time, addressing another potential factor in plaque formation. Extensive review has also shown that HDL cholesterol (HDL-C) increases via liver production in response to aerobic exercise [54, 153]. This increase is thought to promote reduced risk via a process involving structural and circulating LDL-C via a scavenger function. Historically, it was presumed high HDL-C was cardioprotective independently. In recent years, however, the importance of HDL-C levels and HDL particles (HDL-P) in atherosclerosis has been questioned [82, 148]. An increase in HDL-C levels has led to conflicting results regarding cardiovascular risk. Simply increasing the concentration of HDL-C via any mechanism does not demonstrate the expected protective impact that was once presumed. It seems the characteristics of the HDL-specific particles impact the outcome the molecules have on CVD risk. HDL particle number (HDL-P) concentrations seem to be superior as a reciprocated predictor of CHD compared to circulating levels of HDL-C. Pharmacological methods have focused on **statins** and niacin, but outcomes related to exercise-induced changes seem to be most beneficial. This may be due to systemic shifts rather than the independent alterations of HDL-C and LDL-C. Researchers are now analyzing anti-inflammatory functions of **monocytes** as well as specific components of HDL-C and their respective ability for reverse cholesterol transport. Further research is underway do help define the differences.

Regardless of the specific mechanism of improvement, exercise demonstrates a dose-response relationship between the amount of regular physical activity and the plasma levels of protective cholesterol components [114, 128]. Endurance-trained athletes have demonstrated 20% to 30% more circulating HDL-C than same- aged, sedentary, but otherwise healthy subjects [124]. Moderate-intensity aerobic activity seems to yield a similar benefit in HDL production compared to high-intensity exercise as long as one reaches a similar weekly energy expenditure value (1200-1600 kcal/week) [138]. In addition to elevations in HDL-C, routine exercise provides further benefit to blood profiles by reducing markers of low grade inflammation and circulating triglycerides while increasing lipoprotein lipase, the enzyme responsible for removing fatty acids and LDL-C from the blood [46]. The dose–response relationship between the lipid profile and energy expenditure seems to exist regardless of the exercise mode. Increases in caloric expenditure via intensity and/or duration through aerobic activity have been shown to positively influence lipoprotein lipase activity, HDL-C levels, and the lipid profile [112]. Resistance training

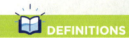

DEFINITIONS

Statins –

A group of drugs that function to reduce cholesterol and lipid levels in circulation to help lessen the impact and progression of cardiovascular disease, such as atherosclerosis.

Monocytes –

Large phagocytic (cells which can ingest other cells) white blood cells released from the immune system to deal with invading pathogens such as bacteria, viruses, and fungi; these cells are transported to sites throughout the body in response to inflammation.

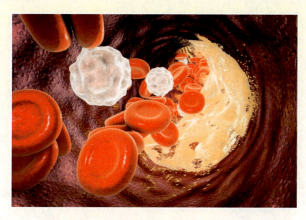

RESEARCH UPDATE: HDL-P

Recent landmark studies explored and tested markers to see if there were consistent ways to test HDL correlation with CVD. These studies showed that the body's ability to remove cholesterol in blood plasma, or efflux capacity, was a better predictor of CVD status than overall HDL-C concentration. It was also suggested that the measure of HDL particles or HDL-P was preferable to assess the contribution of HDL to CVD risk [5, 158]. Newer research suggests HDL components, such as HDL-P and mean HDL particle size, are more crucial contributors to the role that increased HDL-C plays in protecting the vascular system. These studies showed that **apolipoprotein A-I (apoA-I)**, the principle protein component of HDL, modulates cellular inflammation and oxidation. Additionally, ApoA-I, carried by HDL, plays a central role in the process of reverse cholesterol transport: the atheroprotective transfer of peripheral tissue cholesterol by HDL to the liver for excretion. Simply measuring plasma HDL-C does not give information on the number of HDL particles, HDL size distribution, or free versus ester cholesterol composition. Scientists now deem these latter factors to be more important to the role of HDL than the historical conception of HDL-C. Seemingly, these specific HDL components remove cholesterol from peripheral structures through reserve cholesterol transport. In conjunction with other beneficial mechanisms, they are the protective effect's source. According to researchers, the number and complexity of biochemical pathways that contribute to plasma HDL-C concentration make the current measure of assessing risk outdated. HDL-P seems to be the biomarker of choice when predicting risk for CHD, as it has been shown to provide superior predictability when compared to the previously suggested markers of HDL-C and apoA-I [116, 117, 121, 147]. Although reverse cholesterol transport is an important process, additional quantitative descriptors of endothelial and immune cell function are necessary before individual risk can be assessed. Further research is required to identify the specific action of particular atheroprotective markers and whether internal environments, such as those created by cardiovascular exercise, are needed to optimize reduction of CHD risk and to develop more effective pharmacological options.

> **DEFINITIONS**
>
> **Apolipoprotein A-I (ApoA-I) –**
>
> *The primary protein component of high-density lipoproteins (HDL); it plays specific roles in the metabolism of cholesterol and lipids; ApoA-I can impact cellular inflammation and oxidation actions within circulation, having an effect on vascular structures.*

also promotes positive changes in blood lipids when higher volumes of training are employed. Unlike aerobic exercise, high-intensity work does not present a greater effect [138]. Load-bearing work seems to impact the lipid profile more heavily when total volume of movement is increased via sets and/or repetitions compared to an increase in loads lifted [92, 95]. Both routine exercise and circuit training have demonstrated positive effects with loads less than 80% 1RM, and these benefits are potentially greater when combined with aerobic activity.

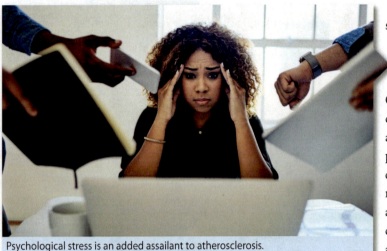

Psychological stress is an added assailant to atherosclerosis.

Psychological stress represents an accomplice to atherosclerosis. The hypothalamus-pituitary-adrenal (HPA) axis attempts to manage stress in non-physical environments, which promotes a negative metabolic effect. Stress directly promotes fat in the blood and platelet adhesion [50]. Combined with elevated blood pressure and pro-inflammatory cytokines, this state creates a dangerous scenario that promotes arterial plaque accumulation. Aerobic exercise mitigates platelet adhesion by attenuating the stress response and decreases circulating lipids, as previously detailed. Complementing the reduction in hazardous circulatory lipids and adhesive cells, exercise concurrently reduces stress-induced cytokines and staves off the effects of inflammation. As alluded to earlier, systemic low-grade inflammation is associated with the onset of cardio-metabolic syndrome and is a known contributor to atherosclerosis and metabolic disease. It is evident that aerobic exercise offers both a protective and healing effect against chronic inflammation. Whereas stress markers and inflammatory chemicals have been linked to atherosclerosis, researchers have found distinct gene alterations with exercise that likely direct monocytes in an anti-inflammatory, protective pathway, rather than promoting vessel wall mass [43, 51, 61, 118]. This suggests that, although exercise promotes an acute inflammation response, the adaptations are positive rather than negative. This seems to be an organism-wide trend, as many stress biomarkers are similar in exercise and non-exercise induced stress, and they present with different outcomes. The cause of the stress indicates the specific signaling effect or message expressed by the chemical and demonstrates that it may not be as simple as designating an individual circulating chemical marker as good or bad. To provide further clarity, a blood analysis following an intense bout of exercise would provide similar blood markers and cytokines when compared to a blood sample of a chronically stressed, inactive person. The exercise, however, provides positive adaptations, whereas the chronic stress promotes increased risk for disease and death. Clearly, there is more to the signaling process than simply the release of a particular chemical.

RESEARCH UPDATE: STRESS AND ATHEROSCLEROSIS

Psychological stress is associated with increased atherosclerosis. This response is mainly mediated by altered immune reactions through hormone-regulated mechanisms. Stress response activates or depresses the feedback mechanisms of the HPA axis. The HPA axis encompasses the interaction of three endocrine glands. The signaling effect of the HPA axis controls reactions to stress and regulates many body processes, including digestion and the immune system, as well as energy storage and expenditure. Its role in immune function affects vascular health via its influence on both the vascular endothelial function and the recruitment of circulating monocytes. Endothelial dysfunction and foam cell proliferation occur in response to chronic stress. Although the detailed mechanisms behind these processes are not well understood, it has been assumed that stress hormones' expression of pro- and anti-inflammatory cytokines, such as catecholamines and corticosteroids, may be involved [136]. It is presumed that prolonged psychological stress causes vascular low-grade inflammation which promotes atherosclerosis.

◆ Myocardial Ischemia

When the heart requires an amount of oxygen that cannot be met via purposeful mechanisms, it becomes ischemic. Ischemia describes the state when oxygen supply does not meet demand. When this occurs repeatedly over time, the condition becomes symptomatic, as in the case of **myocardial ischemia**. Exertion and consequential ischemia causes angina pectoris or chest pains and may cause irregularities in heart rhythm, previously referred to as arrhythmias. Endurance activities have been shown to cause adaptations in coronary circulation that can reduce ischemia [144]. Routine aerobic exercise leads to improved coronary blood flow and increased ventricular volume, allowing for more blood throughout the heart and also promotes increased oxygen utilization by the cardiac tissue. Adaptations to exercise that account for the improved efficiency seem to occur at the micro-RNA level: here, the stage is set for improved blood flow dynamics, the promotion of oxygen transfer, and remodeling of the vascular structures that augment oxygen delivery. Aerobic exercise, specifically, has demonstrated three important benefits: decreasing **cardiac fibrosis** and collagen inhibition (preventing vessel wall hardening), increasing angiogenesis (forming new vascular pathways), and modulating the **renin-angiotensin system** (reducing stress). The vascular structures increase in diameter, allowing more blood to pass, while new capillaries and arterioles form to enhance the myocardial vascular network. Furthermore, enhanced vascular reactivity and the subsequent distribution that manifests with increased vascular compliance combine to improve blood flow. Together, these adaptations to aerobic-based training cause a relative reduction in total peripheral resistance, thereby reducing the oxygen demand of the myocardium by lowering its workload [28].

Cardiac events related to CHD are often triggered by heart arrhythmias or thrombosis. Recall that arrhythmias are heart rhythm disturbances, which often occur in the presence of heart disease. These may appear in healthy individuals from an artery spasm, electrolyte imbalances, a response to certain medications or drugs, and/or a state of dehydration; however, they express more commonly in individuals with myocardial ischemia. The largest threat from arrhythmias occurs with **ventricular fibrillation**, where blockage causes the heart conduction system to malfunction. With ventricular fibrillation, the heart's electrical activity becomes disordered, and the signaling effect causes asynchronous contractions. When this happens, the heart's lower chambers contract in a rapid, unsynchronized manner, and the heart pumps little or no blood. If the heart is not defibrillated, the person will die from the phenomenon, known as sudden death from heart attack. Exercise reduces the risk of cardiac arrhythmias by increasing blood flow to the tissue, thereby better satisfying the myocardial oxygen demand while concomitantly suppressing sympathetic nervous system (SNS) activity. This combined effect reduces the risk of sudden death in both healthy persons and those diagnosed with disease by mediating the two primary triggers, ischemia and neural stimulus. The combination of dehydration and central nervous system stimulants, such as caffeine and intense exercise, all increase the risk of heart rhythm dysfunction and should be avoided.

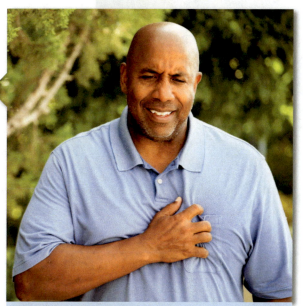

Myocardial ischemia can cause notable chest pain as a major red flag that insufficient oxygen is being delivered to the myocardium to meet baseline demands.

DEFINITIONS

Myocardial ischemia –

A symptomatic or asymptomatic condition where oxygen supply to the heart muscle does not meet demand; it can occur due to reduced blood flow through the coronary arteries as a result of progressive heart disease and plaque accumulation; a sudden, severe blockage can lead to a heart attack.

Cardiac fibrosis –

Refers to an abnormal thickening and stiffening of the heart valves (primarily tricuspid) and/or heart muscle walls, which can indicate a progression towards heart failure.

Renin-angiotensin system –

The hormone system which functions to regulate blood pressure and fluid balance throughout the body; improved function of this system can reduce daily workload and stress on the heart.

Ventricular fibrillation –

The most serious form of cardiac rhythm disturbance, where the ventricles essentially quiver or perform erratic mini-contractions; the heart is unable to pump any blood, resulting in cardiac arrest.

> **Common Cardiovascular Disease Medications**
>
> **Diuretics** – Act on the kidneys to prevent re-absorption of water.
>
> **Beta-Blockers** – Reduce myocardial vigor by inhibiting the nerve impulse to the heart and blood vessels.
>
> **Angiostensin Converting Enzyme (ACE) Inhibitors** – Cause blood vessels to relax by preventing the formation of the hormone angiotensin II, which causes constriction.
>
> **Angiostensin Antagonists** – Block angiostensin II, resulting in the prevention of vasoconstriction.
>
> **Calcium Channel Blockers** – Prevent calcium from entering the myocardium, reducing contraction.
>
> **Nervous System Inhibitors** – Relax blood vessels by controlling nerve impulses.
>
> **Vasodilators** – Directly open the blood vessels by relaxing the muscle in the vessel walls.

◆ Thrombosis

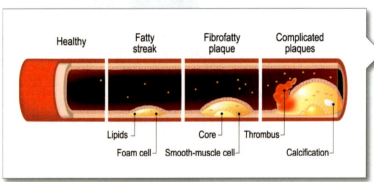

A thrombus, or blood clot, may also occlude a coronary artery, triggering a heart attack which, in turn, cuts off oxygen supply to a heart section. An acute thrombotic event often starts with a disruption or rupture of an atherosclerotic plaque site in the vascular system, tearing the inner wall of the vessel. Platelets then accumulate at the injury site, causing the aforementioned process of obstruction. The formation of a clot, or thrombosis, around the injury site is an expected immune response, but when it occurs in the artery, it can create a major obstruction to blood flow. Even without full occlusion, the ischemic catalyst can cause lethal disturbances in the heart rhythm, resulting in a myocardial infarction: heart attack.

Note that this process does not occur as rapidly as it may sound. It generally follows the slow progression of atherosclerosis, but the thrombosis is the acute precipitating occurrence that sets the catastrophic event in motion. The progression of the blockage signals the transition between silent CAD, where the lumen of the vessel is not disrupted and the condition is often asymptomatic, to significant occlusion and onset of symptoms. At this point, the individual may experience recurring chest pains called unstable angina, cardiac arrhythmias, acute myocardial infarction, or sudden death. Aerobic training not only promotes greater arterial diameter to help reduce the occurrence of blockage but also reduces the threat of thrombosis by enhancing the enzymatic activity at the site. The enzymes endurance training produces break down the blood clots and decrease platelet adhesion and aggregation, helping to reduce and prevent clot formation [79].

Deep vein thrombosis (DVT) occurs when a blood clot forms in the deep veins of the body, most often in the legs. Numerous factors exist that increase one's risk for developing DVT, and multiple factors compound risk. If a clot develops and is released into circulation, it may travel to the lungs and cause a **pulmonary embolism** (obstruction of an artery within the lungs). A

> **DEFINITIONS**
>
> **Pulmonary embolism –**
>
> *A serious, life-threatening type of blood clot that occurs in the pulmonary arteries which oxygenate the lungs themselves; it causes respiratory arrest and sudden death if the clot is big enough, while smaller clots may simply reduce blood flow and damage lung tissue.*

pulmonary embolism can be fatal; individuals that present with a high risk should watch for the following warning signs:

- Unexplained sudden onset of shortness of breath
- Chest pain or discomfort that worsens when you take a deep breath or when you cough
- Feeling lightheaded or dizzy, or fainting
- Rapid pulse
- Coughing up blood

Following a DVT, some individuals may develop a condition known as **postphlebitic syndrome**. This syndrome describes an inflammation within the walls of a vein, manifesting as a collection of signs and symptoms, including swelling and pain in the legs, skin color changes, and/or sores on the skin. This syndrome is caused by damage to the veins due to the prior blood clot. The damage reduces localized blood flow and can cause discomfort. Individuals with previously diagnosed DVT should consult a physician if these symptoms present at rest or at the onset of exercise.

DEFINITIONS

Postphlebitic syndrome –

Also known as post-thrombotic syndrome or venous stress disorder, it involves inflammation within the walls of a vein(s) which manifests as a collection of signs and symptoms: swelling and pain in the legs, skin color changes, and/or sores on the skin; it is caused by damage to venous structures due to a prior blood clot which reduces localized blood flow and can cause discomfort.

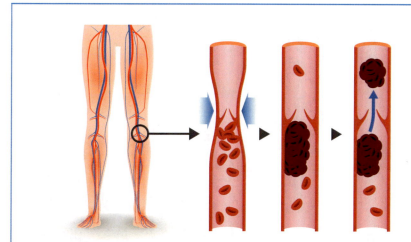

Common Risk Factors for DVT

- Inheriting a blood-clotting disorder
- Prolonged bed rest and lack of movement
- Injury or surgery
- Pregnancy
- Birth control pills or hormone replacement therapy
- Malignant varicose veins
- Being overweight or obese
- Smoking
- Heart failure
- Inflammatory bowel disease
- A personal or family history
- Age over 60

Stroke & Physical Activity

Stroke stands as the fifth leading cause of death and contributes significantly to disability, making it a major problem in developed countries like the United States [102]. Similar to a heart attack, a stroke occurs when a lack of oxygen causes the sudden death of an area of brain cells. The primary sources are vascular blockage, which impairs blood flow to the tissue (**ischemic stroke**), or an artery rupture (**hemorrhagic stroke**), which initiates bleeding within the brain. Ischemic stroke accounts for 80% of all stroke cases [102]. In ischemic stroke, interruption of the blood supply to the brain results in tissue **hypo-perfusion**, **hypoxia**, and eventual cell death. The main mechanisms involved in the development of ischemic strokes are associated with **atherothrombosis** and **embolic disease**.

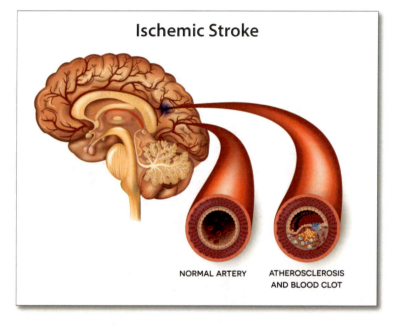

In atherothrombotic disease, the pathophysiology resembles CAD in the heart. Lipid deposits within the vascular system lead to the formation of plaque, which narrows the lumen of the vessel and results in turbulent blood flow through the area of **stenosis** (narrowed area of the vessel). The flow's turbulence and the resultant alterations in fluid movement velocities lead to vessel wall disruption or plaque rupture, both of which activate a clotting cascade. This process causes platelets to become activated and stick to the plaque surface, where they eventually form a fibrin clot. As the lumen of the vessel becomes more occluded, ischemia develops distally to the obstruction and can eventually lead to tissue infarction (cell death) as the tissue that relies on the parent vessel for oxygen delivery is starved. Embolic stroke occurs when dislodged thrombi travel distally and occlude vessels downstream. One-half of all embolic strokes are caused by atrial fibrillation (an abnormal

DEFINITIONS

Ischemic stroke –

Occurs as a result of an obstruction within a blood vessel that supplies oxygenated blood to the brain; this blockage type accounts for the vast majority of stroke cases.

Hemorrhagic stroke –

Occurs as a result of a weakened blood vessel rupture (aneurysm) in or on the surface of the brain; it is most commonly caused by prolonged and uncontrolled high blood pressure.

Hypoperfusion –

Essentially a shock response in a given tissue due to inadequate oxygen and nutrient supply which can quickly result in cellular death.

Hypoxia –

A state of oxygen deficiency in a given tissue, muscle or organ; this condition can be caused by intense work or a myriad of pathophysiological issues, such as cardiovascular disease.

Atherothrombotic disease –

Describes disease characterized by atherosclerotic lesion disruption which results in a dangerous blood clot(s) and occlusion of vascular structures; this condition is the major cause of acute coronary distress (i.e., heart attack) and the leading cause of mortality among industrialized nations.

Embolic disease –

Describes diseases where an embolus (blockage-causing material such as blood clots, lipids, or even air bubbles) inside vascular structures causes occlusion at some point in the body resulting in ischemia and potential cellular death (e.g., deep vein thrombosis, pulmonary embolism).

Stenosis –

Refers to the abnormal narrowing of a passage in the body, such as a vascular structure.

rhythm of the heart atria), while the rest are attributable to a variety of causes: among them, left ventricular dysfunction secondary to acute myocardial infarction (severe **congestive heart failure**), and **atheroemboli**. These latter emboli often arise from atherosclerotic lesions in the aortic arch, carotid arteries, and vertebral arteries, which break off and travel to the brain. Two of the most common risk factors for stroke include cigarette smoking and high blood pressure. This should offer no surprise, as these are two of the leading factors of arteriosclerosis [102].

Hemorrhagic stroke, as indicated above, is caused by an intracerebral hemorrhage, the rupture of a vessel within the brain tissue. The primary cause of these ruptures is hypertension. Hypertension can cause an aneurism (an abnormal ballooning of a vessel) to form in a brain artery. This aneurysm can burst, causing bleeding into the brain. Lifestyle variables play an important role in the reduction of stroke risk. The positive factors include physical activity, not smoking, and a dietary pattern including foods with low inflammatory potential [111]. Meta-analysis of 36 studies suggested previously sedentary individuals who achieve the recommended physical activity levels of moderate-intensity aerobic exercise experienced lower risk of CVD mortality by 23% and reduced CVD (including stroke) incidence by 17% after adjustment for body weight [150]. Large population studies identified elevated risk to be most associated with hypertension, atrial fibrillation, dyslipidemia, lack of physical exercise, and a previous stroke. Physical activity is implicated as effective treatment for both stroke prevention programs and as a therapy for stroke sufferers [76, 84].

> **DEFINITIONS**
>
> **Congestive heart failure –**
>
> *Characterized by an enlargement of the left ventricle and central portion of the heart in response to coronary heart disease and strain against vascular peripheral resistance (high blood pressure); the hypertrophic adaptations cause reduced blood flow through the heart, reduced valve function and a significant reduction in stroke volume that significantly limits oxygen availability and work capacity.*
>
> **Atheroemboli –**
>
> *Also known as a cholesterol embolism or blue toe, this condition occurs when cholesterol is released from an atherosclerotic plaque, travels as an embolus in the bloodstream, and ends up lodging (as a clot) in a specific area causing dangerous obstruction.*

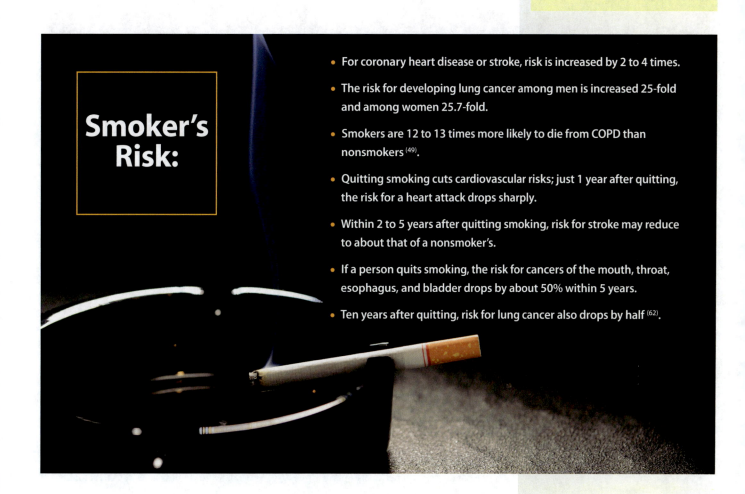

Smoker's Risk:

- For coronary heart disease or stroke, risk is increased by 2 to 4 times.
- The risk for developing lung cancer among men is increased 25-fold and among women 25.7-fold.
- Smokers are 12 to 13 times more likely to die from COPD than nonsmokers [49].
- Quitting smoking cuts cardiovascular risks; just 1 year after quitting, the risk for a heart attack drops sharply.
- Within 2 to 5 years after quitting smoking, risk for stroke may reduce to about that of a nonsmoker's.
- If a person quits smoking, the risk for cancers of the mouth, throat, esophagus, and bladder drops by about 50% within 5 years.
- Ten years after quitting, risk for lung cancer also drops by half [62].

Hypertension & Physical Activity

2017 High Blood Pressure Clinical Practice Guidelines[156].

Blood Pressure Category	SYSTOLIC mm Hg (Upper Number)		DIASTOLIC mm Hg (Lower Number)
NORMAL	Less than 120	and	Less than 80
ELEVATED	120 - 129	and	Less than 80
HIGH BLOOD PRESSURE (Hypertension) Stage 1	130 - 139	or	80 - 89
HIGH BLOOD PRESSURE (Hypertension) Stage 2	140 or Higher	or	90 or Higher
HYPERTENSIVE CRISIS Consult Your Doctor Immediately	Higher than 180	and/or	Higher than 120

High blood pressure has been implicated as a major underlying contributor to cardiovascular pathology. It is linked with cardiovascular complications and mortality. Currently, about one in every three persons in the United States is classifiably hypertensive (Systolic >130mmHg or Diastolic >80 mmHg)[156]. Of those individuals with hypertension, only half have the condition under control. Several large cohort studies have identified a relationship between physical activity and risk for hypertension. Epidemiological cohort studies have consistently demonstrated that sedentary, unfit persons have a 20% to 50% higher prospective risk of hypertension, as compared to physically-fit, active persons. After controlling for age, sex, baseline blood pressure, and body mass index (BMI), low CRF was identified as an independent risk factor for the development of hypertension. Low CRF was linked to a 72% higher risk of developing hypertension compared to individuals with the highest exercise capacity[81]. Consistent with other studies, a dose-response relationship exists between the amount of activity and the degree of protection from hypertension. Individuals who are the least active were shown to have a 30% increase in risk compared to those who were highly active. It should be noted that none of these studies analyzed higher-risk minorities, who present greater susceptibility in population studies. Reportedly, however, CRF does not depend on physical activity habits alone, as genetics also plays a role[122]. As it relates to demographics, CRF is higher in men than women, though it decreases with age, and non-Hispanic blacks have been reported to have lower levels of CRF than non-Hispanic whites. In these cases, socioeconomic influences cannot be overlooked, as the findings of many studies support this environmental influence.

Health Problems and Complications Related to Hypertension

Organ damage
Congestive heart failure
Hemorrhagic stroke
Aortic aneurysms and dissection
Renal failure
Retinopathy

Atherosclerosis Complications of Hypertension

Coronary heart disease
Ischemic stroke
Peripheral vascular disease

Conclusions of several meta-analyses suggest that aerobic exercise significantly affects both diastolic (DBP) and systolic blood pressure (SBP) response [122]. Participation in aerobic training 30-60 minutes a day, 3-4 days per week, at intensity ranges of 60-70% VO_2max caused a consistent decrease of approximately 4 to 10 mmHg in systolic and 3 to 8 mmHg in diastolic measures [81]. Different studies, lasting between 10 and 36 weeks, analyzed the aerobic exercise's intensity to determine the dose-response implications of the training. Both high and moderate intensity exercise training have been shown to reduce blood pressure; however, the reductions observed in response to low-intensity endurance training (<40% heart rate reserve or <55% heart rate maximum) were smaller compared to high and moderate-intensity exercise training [24, 29]. When comorbidities exist, aerobic exercise's impact seems to become more evident. After tracking blood pressure for 6 weeks to establish a baseline for medications, exercise was added to individuals with hypertension and those presenting with both diabetes and hypertension. In only 12 exercise sessions, SBP decreased by an average 16 points for those with diabetes and hypertensives and 17 points for those with only hypertension. Importantly, diastolic blood pressure decreased by 9 in participants with diabetes and hypertension and 6 mmHg in those with hypertension alone.

Blood pressure is the product of cardiac output and peripheral resistance in the blood vessels. From this basic equation, it follows that there are two potential aspects by which blood pressure can be manipulated: changes within the heart and changes within the vessels. Reducing relative heart rates and improving vessel compliance and responsiveness lower blood pressure. Exercise can contribute to this improvement, as it has been shown to relax vascular wall resistance acutely and chronically [28]. The acute response by the body to a bout of aerobic exercise causes an immediate and temporary reduction in vascular resistance through peripheral blood vessel dilation. This response has been measured several hours after a session of exercise. With repeated and appropriate exercise stress, peripheral resistance is lowered via attenuation of SNS activity. Routine aerobic exercise may

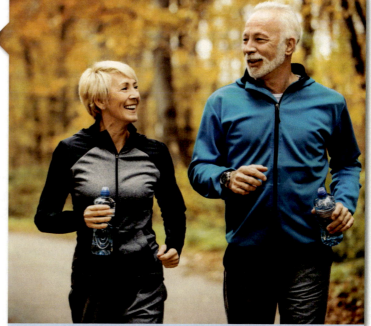

Exercise can help reduce high blood pressure by improving blood vessel compliance and enhancing cardiovascular efficiency.

Table 6.1 Prevalence of High Blood Pressure in Adults by Sex [102]

Age	Men (%)	Women (%)
20-34	8.6	6.2
35-44	22.6	18.3
45-54	36.8	32.7
55-64	54.6	53.7
65-74	62.0	67.8
75 and older	76.4	79.9
All	33.5	31.7

cause a reduction in renin-angiotensin system activity, arterial vasodilation, and baroreceptor adjustment [28]. Additionally, aerobic training allows for further enhanced management of blood pressure due to its positive effect on circulating insulin levels, as it decreases insulin-mediated re-absorption of sodium by the kidneys [42].

Both women and men are likely to develop high blood pressure during their lifetimes. However, for people under 45 years old, the condition appears more frequently in men, with the difference commonly attributed to the protective effects of estrogen in premenopausal women (Table 6.2). Interestingly, at older ages (>65 years), high blood pressure affects more women than men [102].

In addition to varying with age, blood pressure measures differ by race and ethnicity. Non-Hispanic Blacks are not only more susceptible to hypertension in general but also exhibit the condition at earlier ages than Hispanics and Non-Hispanic Whites. Interestingly, within certain ethic groups, more women than men have high blood pressure [102]. Individuals working with these higher risk populations should ensure programs reflect these concerns.

Table 6.2 Prevalence of High Blood Pressure by Population [102]

Race or Ethnic Group	Men (%)	Women (%)
African Americans	44.9	46.1
Mexican Americans	29.6	29.9
Whites	32.9	30.1
All	33.5	31.7

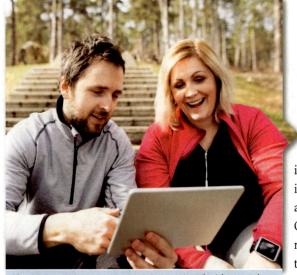

Obesity is a serious concern as it is associated with mental health issues, reduced quality of life, and an increased risk of early death due to diabetes, heart disease, stroke, and some types of cancer.

Obesity & Physical Activity

Obesity is a major health and economic issue facing the American population at this time. It is a complex problem to address due to the disease's multi-factorial nature. Genetics and medications play a role, but behaviors initially seem to be the largest problem. Behavioral contributions and influences include dietary patterns, physical activity, alcohol use, sleep, and stress. Additional influences come from socio-economic conditions, including financial well-being, access to education, community resources, and family-derived thoughts and values. Obesity is a serious concern: not only is it associated with mental health issues and reduced quality of life, but it also represents one of the leading causes of death in the U.S. and worldwide, due to diabetes, heart disease, stroke, and some types of cancer [134]. Documented increases in bodyweight have occurred substantially since the 1980s in all races and gender groups and have led to a health epidemic. The prevalence of obesity is about 40% in the United States [57]. In these individuals, commonly, poor food choices, high-calorie diets, and low levels of physical activity combine to create the metabolic disturbance that leads to progressive weight gain. This weight increase is most pronounced between the fourth and sixth decade of life; however, weight gain has been identified across all populations in the United States, and no significant difference exists in the prevalence of obesity between men and women overall or by age group [57, 107]. Recently, childhood obesity has also mushroomed, occurring in 17% of children and adolescents. Current surveys by the CDC suggest certain populations exhibit greater risk, as the prevalence among children and adolescents was higher among Hispanics (21.9%) and non-Hispanic blacks (19.5%) than among non-Hispanic whites (14.7%) [107].

Reductions in total activity and poor diet have made children fatter than ever before, leaving them susceptible to adult disorders such as diabetes and sleep apnea. Childhood obesity directly links to adult obesity, and overweight children present an elevated risk for adult diseases later in life, including hypertension, diabetes, and CVD [57]. Furthermore, the medical community has expressed rising concern because unhealthy body fat levels relate to emotional disorders and the mental health and development of obese children during puberty. In addition to the metabolic risk factors, substantial support exists that identifies obesity's association with internalizing disorders, **attention-deficit / hyperactivity disorder (ADHD)**, decreased- health-related quality of life, and low self-concept, self-efficacy, and self-esteem as products of obesity in childhood [30, 106]. Some medications used to manage these psycho-emotional conditions, including antidepressants and antipsychotics, have also been associated with additional weight gain.

DEFINITIONS

Attention-deficit/hyperactivity disorder –

A chronic condition marked by persistent inattention, hyperactivity, and potential impulsivity; often begins in childhood and progresses into adulthood.

Classifying Obesity

- **Body fat** = males <20% for fit-healthy; females <26% for fit-healthy
- **Stage 1 Obesity** = males ≥25% body fat; females ≥32% body fat; >38% old age
- **Stage 2 Obesity** = males ≥30% body fat; females ≥40% body fat
- **Stage 3 Obesity** = males ≥35% body fat; females ≥45% body fat
- **High risk** = males ≥40 inch waist circumference; females ≥35 inch (signifies significant visceral adiposity)
- **High risk** = BMI >30 obesity >35 morbid obesity males or females (must consider body fat)

In 2013, obesity was named a chronic disease by the American Medical Association (AMA). But obesity is much more dynamic than can be captured by the single definition of being "too fat". Paradoxical terms such as "healthy obese" and "skinny fat" have been used to describe overweight/overfat individuals who otherwise score well in the health-related components of fitness without any other risk factors for disease. Obesity from a disease perspective, describes its quantifiable negative effects on other bodily systems. A common theme that links many diseases and chronic illness, including obesity, is uncontrolled cellular inflammation. It factors in diseases including CVD, diabetes, a growing number of cancers, arthritis, and many autoimmune-related conditions. Obesity was added to this group of diseases as it was discovered to present a chronic low-grade inflammatory response within many of the body's tissues and was linked to the development of cardiovascular and metabolic disease [68]. It is well-known that being overweight is detrimental to one's health, but until recently, the harmful mechanisms were unclear. Scientists over the last decade have started to unravel the mystery and have begun to discover why obesity leads to premature death.

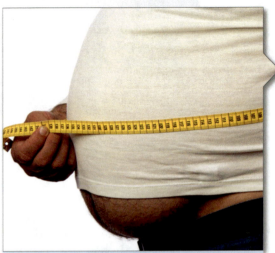

Visceral fat plays a major role in instigating metabolic dysfunction via hormonal influences and the promotion of systemic low-grade inflammation.

DEFINITIONS

Visceral fat –

Fat which directly surrounds the internal organs in the abdominal cavity; high quantities are associated with an increased risk for a number of health problems, including type 2 diabetes mellitus and low-grade systemic inflammation.

Adipokines –

A special type of cytokine released by adipose (fat) tissue to communicate energy needs and other information to various organs, including the brain, liver, immune system, and skeletal muscle; dysregulation of these signalers has been implicated in obesity, type 2 diabetes mellitus, and cardiovascular disease.

Hyperinsulinemia –

A condition in which excess levels of insulin are found in circulation relative to blood glucose; it often indicates progressive insulin resistance as a precursor to diabetes.

Leptin –

A type of cytokine released from adipose tissue that serves a role in fat storage regulation in the body; leptin dysfunction is associated with obesity and metabolic issues, giving it the common nickname of "obesity hormone."

Incretin –

A group of metabolic hormones that stimulate a decrease in blood glucose levels; they are released after eating and augment the secretion of insulin emitted from pancreatic beta cells of the islets of Langerhans.

Inflammation is, by design, a protective response used to repair tissue. When inflammation becomes chronic, as is the case with obesity, chemical mediators derived from different cellular activities change their signaling, which causes a progressive deterioration. Fat cells are dynamic immune organs that secrete numerous immune modulating chemicals [93]. **Visceral fat**, in particular, is associated with low-grade inflammation, which seems to be a contributing pathological feature for metabolic disease; this occurs via insulin resistance and the promotion of atherosclerotic build-up in circulatory vessels [45]. When high levels of visceral fat are combined with physical inactivity, over-nutrition, and aging, the effect becomes even more pronounced. Visceral fat is highly metabolic and contributes to cytokine hyperactivity [45]. **Adipokines** secreted from fat tissue influence the metabolic process and contribute to proper function [3,55,73]. The chronic low-grade inflammation associated with obesity disturbs adipokine secretion and function. Research has identified changes in specific adipokines including adiponectin, visfatin, **leptin**, and resistin that exhibit harmful internal effects in obese individuals and consequently, increase the risk for cardiometabolic disorders [73]. Adipokine dysfunction is further influenced by free fatty acids (FFAs) liberated directly into the liver from visceral fat tissue [73]. Visceral fat releases chemicals and fatty acids into the portal system, where they act on the connecting organs. The portal circulation system is a specialized network of blood vessels that connect the visceral organs to the liver. The excess fat in portal circulation has detrimental effects on insulin action, which obesity worsens. Obesity promotes beta-cell hypersecretion and reduced insulin clearance, resulting in **hyperinsulinemia** and leading to early stage diabetes [86]. Additionally, obesity promotes lipid deposits in the pancreas and other metabolic organs, further impairing **incretin** effects and promoting the onset of T2DM [39,66].

In normal conditions, adipokines promote health. Adiponectin for instance, is an anti-atherogenic or atheroprotective agent, meaning it helps prevent the development of atherosclerotic plaque in blood vessels and slows the progression of atherosclerosis in coronary vessels. It does this by acting directly upon the vessel wall, inhibiting adhesive molecules from contributing to plaque formation while acting as a blocking agent to foam cell formation. In skeletal muscle and the liver, adiponectin promotes insulin sensitivity and a positive blood lipid profile [155]. Visceral adiposity, however, reduces adiponectin concentrations, lessening the cardioprotective effect and leading to increased cardiovascular risk [11,143]. Another important adipokine is leptin, which regulates energy metabolism and balance in conjunction with the brain's hypothalamus. Leptin is currently being touted as having cardioprotective benefits among its other roles in metabolism. Early research demonstrated equivocal results; however, more recent studies have shown that leptin can decrease the size of atherosclerotic lesions and induce atheroprotective effects indirectly via upregulating adiponectin concentrations and reducing circulating cholesterol levels [65,133]. Leptin concentrations adjust negatively in response to obesity and contribute to insulin resistance, and these changes in leptin concentration have also been recognized as a risk factor for CHD. Similarly, increased resistin and visfatin concentrations correlate with obesity-related inflammation. Whereas resistin seems associated with the initiation and progression of atherosclerotic lesions, visfatin concentrations directly correlate to whole system inflammation. Due to its insulin mimetic effects, visfatin has been dubbed the fat cell's insulin and is a clinical marker for CVD [120]. Evaluating the adipokines as a whole suggests that a transition point exists where levels of leptin, visfatin, and resistin trigger a metamorphic shift in cell function. This seems to occur during early-stage obesity. Researchers have found that changes in the production of inflammatory biomolecules precede negative mRNA changes and coincide with immune cell changes in visceral adipose tissue. These changes are associated with serum resistin, visfatin, and leptin, each playing specific roles in the regulation of these cells and have been documented in persons with modest obesity and early metabolic dysfunction; this suggests it is vital to prevent the onset of obesity, as early stages begin the inflammatory-mediated changes that cause disease [55, 73, 139]. When persons with modest obesity were compared to those with severe obesity, the inflammatory chemical difference was far less than expected. Consequently, it follows that physical activity may function as a potent medicine for any stage of obesity due to the pronounced effect exercise has on mediating inflammatory chemicals.

Exercise provides some protection against the onset of obesity-related inflammation via heightened caloric expenditure, which attenuates some of the side effects. Obese individuals who engage in physical activity are more likely to experience a lower incidence of obesity-related health problems, compared to sedentary persons. Though more research is needed to fully support these widely accepted beliefs, exercise clearly helps decrease levels of white adipose tissue and lessens the obesity-induced dysregulation of circulating adipokines [125]. Although an active lifestyle alone cannot compensate for all potential health issues associated with obesity, most studies suggest that physical activity yields positive effects independently, even with limited changes in body weight. When diet is factored in, the results become more favorable. The combination of caloric control and physical activity appears to yield substantially more benefits than either diet or physical activity alone. Weight gain is associated with many more factors than simply energy balance: timing, type, quality, and quantity of food and drink consumed, as well as other factors. However, when energy intake exceeds caloric expenditure, weight gain often results. Increasing physical activity contributes to greater caloric expenditure via upregulated metabolic processes which improves weight management. Exercise yields positive results for the maintenance of metabolic rate, whereas diet alone does not have the same effect. Additionally, physical activity reduces the prevalence of central adiposity, which is important for lowering metabolic disease risk. Increased levels of visceral fat are directly related to metabolic diseases.

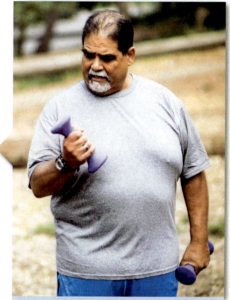

Exercise provides some protection against the onset of obesity-related inflammation via heightened caloric expenditure and the attenuation of some of the side effects.

Diabetes & Physical Activity

Diabetes mellitus, a chronic disease, involves abnormalities in the body's ability to manage glucose. In healthy individuals, the pancreas secretes the hormone insulin when carbohydrates are consumed and absorbed into the blood stream through normal digestion. As blood glucose rises, insulin is released, which signals muscle and other body cells to take up the glucose to regulate circulating levels. The glucose acquired by cells is then used for metabolism, stored as glycogen, or converted into fat for later use. Diabetes is diagnosed when the body either has an inability to make insulin – type 1 diabetes mellitus (T1DM) – or the cells have an inability to act in response to insulin (insulin resistance) – type II diabetes mellitus (T2DM).

Diagnosing Diabetes

- **Prediabetes:** *(for all tests, risk is continuous, extending below the lower limit of a range and becomes disproportionately greater at higher ends of the range)*
  - Fasting Plasma Glucose 100–125 mg/dL (5.6–6.9 mmol/L): Impaired Fasting Glycemia (IFG) Test
  - OR 2-hour Plasma Glucose 140–199 mg/dL (7.8–11.0 mmol/L): Impaired Glucose Test (IGT)
  - OR Hemoglobin A1c Test 5.7–6.4%

- **Diabetes:**
  - Fasting Plasma Glucose ≥126 mg/dL (7.0 mmol/L) on two separate occasions
  - OR 2-hour plasma glucose ≥200 mg/dL (11.1 mmol/L) during an Oral Glucose Tolerance Test (OGTT)
  - OR Hemoglobin A1c Test ≥6.5%
  - OR Classic diabetes symptoms + random plasma glucose ≥200 mg/dL (11.1 mmol/L)

*The Hemoglobin A1c Test indicates the average level of blood sugar over the past 2 to 3 months.

Type 2 diabetes represents one of the largest threats to US population health with an overall prevalence of 14.3% [99]. Approximately 3% of deaths are directly attributed to diabetes [63]. According to a recent study by the CDC, the lifetime risk of a 20-year-old developing diabetes has increased 20% for men and 13% for women, respectively, based on data collected from 1985-2011. For men, the likelihood of developing diabetes was 40.2% and for women 39.6%. With percentages over 50, Hispanic men and women and non-Hispanic black women present the highest risk of developing diabetes [56]. Not only are more people being diagnosed with disease, but those who are diagnosed are living longer, putting a greater strain on the health care system. Of the estimated 29 million Americans with diabetes, only 75% have been diagnosed. In addition, although diabetes is directly attributable as the 7th leading cause of death, this statistic greatly underestimates the role diabetes plays in premature death and disability among Americans. When diabetes is analyzed as a secondary cause (the disease that precipitated the event) the number of deaths associated with the disease doubles and is many times underrepresented [99]. Diabetes usually kills through CVD, including stroke, CHD, peripheral vascular disease, and congestive heart failure. Studies have shown that as much as 40% of the diabetics who have died do not have diabetes listed anywhere on the death certificate. In 2007, it was estimated that diabetes-related illness, treatment, or injury would cost the country $176 billion in direct medical costs: the actual costs determined in 2012 exceeded this number by 41%, coming in at $245 billion. This illustration highlights the heavy and ever rising burden the disease places on society [9]. Currently, close to 90 million Americans are living with pre-diabetes. Further, reported data suggests that by age 45, the remaining lifetime risk for developing diabetes is 48.9%, prediabetes 31.3%, and 9.1% for dependence on insulin use [90].

Diabetes is classified into groups based on the cause. T1DM was previously referred to as insulin-dependent diabetes mellitus (IDDM), or juvenile diabetes, as it was thought to be caused by a genetic autoimmune disorder that occurs in children. T1DM is characterized by atrophy and dysfunction of the pancreas. The beta cells are compromised by the immune system, which leads to a deficiency of circulating insulin. T2DM was previously called non-insulin dependent diabetes mellitus (NIDDM), or adult-onset diabetes, because the peak age of onset occurred much later than type 1 diabetes. T2DM results mainly from insulin insensitivity of muscle cells due to hyperinsulinemia, a reduction of insulin due to impaired secretion or a combination of both [149]. Diabetes may also occur during pregnancy due to metabolic disruption that occurs during the fetal development process, referred to as **gestational diabetes mellitus**.

DEFINITIONS

Gestational diabetes mellitus –

Defined as any degree of glucose intolerance with the onset of or during a pregnancy; the condition is caused by metabolic disruption due to weight gain and hormonal actions facilitated by the placenta that cause release of compounds that counteract insulin.

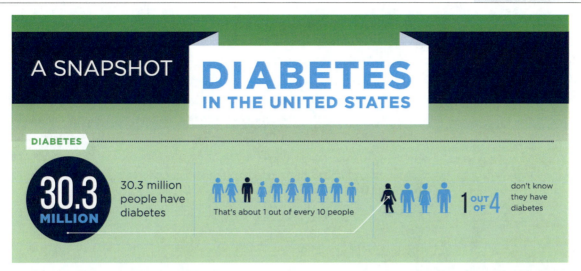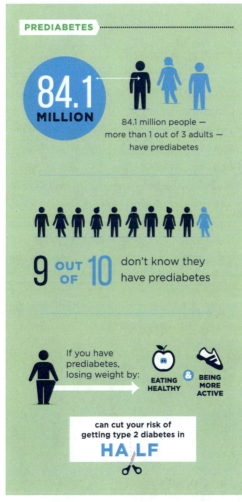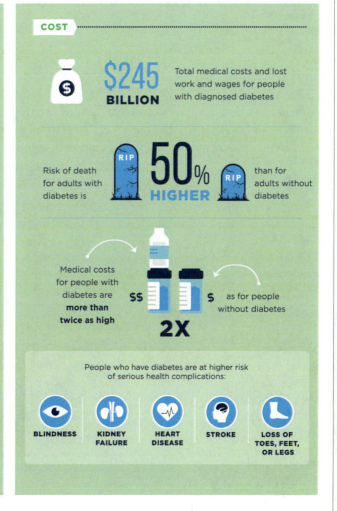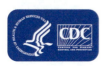

DEFINITIONS

Retinopathy –

A small blood vessel disease of the retina in the eye that can result in impairment or loss of vision, often as a result of diabetes; those with this condition should avoid heavy, compressive exercises (e.g., leg press) as well as activities that lower the head below the waist or jar the head.

Nephropathy –

A small blood vessel disease of the kidneys which causes damage to the organs, often as a result of diabetes; those with this condition should avoid heavy weightlifting or holding the breath during exercise and should maintain proper hydration.

Neuropathy –

A disease that impacts peripheral nerve tissue (often hands or feet) and can result in weakness, numbness, and/or pain; sufferers should avoid exercise that causes repetitive impact stress to the hands or feet and should wear proper footwear during exercise.

Cerebrovascular disease –

A collective term referring to diseases that impact the brain and its blood vessels: includes stroke, aneurysms, and vascular malformations.

Free radicals –

Charged and highly-reactive molecules with an odd (unpaired) number of electrons which form when oxygen interacts with certain molecules; oxygen consumption during activity causes free radical production within the body, which is linked to cellular aging and damaging oxidative stress; however, vitamin, mineral, and enzyme-related antioxidants serve to mediate their potential damage. Free radicals are also produced internally in response to various factors, such as pollution, cigarette smoke, excessive sunlight, heavy metal exposure, etc.

T2DM is the most common form of diabetes, representing 90-95% of all diagnosed cases. Although the most prevalent form of diabetes, T2DM is also the most preventable. Even though strong genetic factors exist, and the disease is more common in older age, the primary causes of T2DM are highly modifiable. Physical inactivity, obesity, and poor diet lead to the development of insulin resistance, glucose intolerance, and hyperinsulinemia (excessive secretion of insulin). When circulating glucose is not managed and remains elevated, it damages large and small vessels of the vascular system. Diabetic damage to blood vessels causes chronic complications and accounts for the significant morbidity and mortality related to the disease. As indicated above, these can be divided into large vessel (macrovascular) disorders – CAD, stroke, and peripheral vascular disease, which are the main causes of death and small vessel (microvascular) disorders – **retinopathy** (blindness/eye problems), **nephropathy** (kidney disease or damage), erectile dysfunction, **cerebrovascular disease**, and **neuropathy** (nerve damage), which are the main causes of morbidity. Diabetic macrovascular disease occurs due to the acceleration of atherogenesis, leading to cerebrovascular diseases: the leading cause of death in individuals with diabetes.

RESEARCH INSIGHT

Though a comprehensive understanding of the mechanisms responsible for hyperglycemic, small vessel disease is not clearly defined, mechanisms that have been reported to cause vascular disease in diabetics include the following: pathologic effects of advanced glycation-end-product accumulation, nitric oxide inhibition, mediated decreased vasodilation response, chronic systemic inflammation, dysfunction in the vascular muscle tissue, overproduction and exposure of endothelial growth factors, hemodynamic dysregulation, impaired ability to reduce blood clots, and enhanced platelet aggregation [21]. The oxidation of glucose releases **free radicals**, which may account for a number of cellular dysfunctions. Unfortunately, in recent human trials, the promise of antioxidants (such as vitamin C and vitamin E) in reducing diabetic complications has not materialized. But glycemic control with blood pressure and lipid-lowering therapy shows benefits in reducing the incidence and progression of small vessel disease.

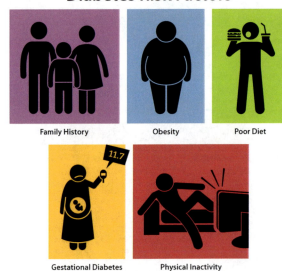

Diabetes Risk Factors: Family History, Obesity, Poor Diet, Gestational Diabetes, Physical Inactivity

Inactive lifestyles are linked with the development of T2D, as considerable evidence reveals that being sedentary is a prominent risk factor for T2DM [48, 132]. Physical activity, to the contrary, has shown to both protect against and have a pronounced effect on T2DM by reducing circulating glucose in a process that promoted insulin sensitivity in the cells. Physically inactive women ages 55-69 were found to have twice the risk for T2DM as their physically active counterparts [31]. On the other hand, obese physically inactive men had 17x the risk of developing diabetes, and obese physically active men had 13x the risk compared to physically active men with a healthy weight. Physical activity, regardless of weight, reduced the risk of developing T2DM [64]. Prospective cohort studies identified that physical activity provides a protective effect and is inversely related to the incidence of the disease [64, 132]. Researchers found that the intensity of physical activity was strongly correlated with decreased incidence of diabetes. Walking at a brisk pace, and/or striding, provided greater benefits when compared with walking at a leisurely pace and not walking at all. It is suggested that for each additional 500 kcal of expenditure per week from physical activity, risk for T2DM is reduced 6% [154]. Additionally, more vigorous activities were associated with the greatest benefit. A study of 34-59 year old women who reported engaging in vigorous physical activity at least once a week experienced a reduction in risk by 16% compared to women who did not participate in vigorous activities at all [96].

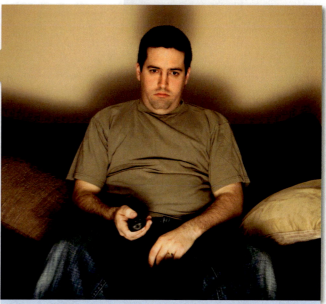
Sedentary lifestyles are directly linked to the development of T2DM.

Exercise has demonstrated an improvement in carbohydrate metabolism and glucose tolerance by enhancing the cellular uptake of sugar. Contracting muscle tissue causes a synergistic effect between insulin and cellular sensitivity, increasing glucose transport into the cell. Single, prolonged bouts of exercise increase cellular permeability for 24 hours, enabling better glucose management as skeletal muscle and hepatic cells replenish the lost glycogen stores. The increased sensitivity to insulin prevents hyperinsulinemia and improves glucose tolerance, providing a protective effect from the onset of the disease [69]. Both endurance and resistance training have been shown to provide benefits. Endurance athletes have demonstrated greater insulin sensitivity, allowing for lower insulin levels at relative blood glucose concentrations compared to sedentary subjects [1, 26]. Likewise, resistance-trained individuals seem to experience similar glucose/insulin dynamics as those who are aerobically trained [115, 131]. Physical activity has been shown to improve glucose management through muscle cell changes and fat cell response. Physical activity also leads to indirect benefits, including weight management, reduced visceral fat storage, and metabolic efficiency.

The combination of diet and exercise is recommended to prevent and treat diabetes. Individuals with mild disease who are not taking medication seem to experience the most benefit from the exercise therapy. Individuals with advanced T2DM may experience complications with excessive physical activity, including **ketosis**, an abnormality of the body's metabolic process resulting in increased ketones in the blood, hyperglycemia (high blood sugar), and a hypoglycemic (low blood sugar) response to vigorous exercise. Additionally, foot wounds, cardiovascular complications, and eye damage due to retinopathy are potential problems. Proper medical evaluation and screening can help identify individuals at greater risk and determine proper precautions.

DEFINITIONS

Ketosis –

A normal but potentially dangerous metabolic process when it progresses to severe ketoacidosis; ketosis occurs when the body does not have enough glucose for energy and burns stored fats instead. This results in circulating acid build-up caused by ketones. This condition can be caused by dietary measures, such as a low-carb diet, or diseases like diabetes.

Osteoarthritis & Physical Activity

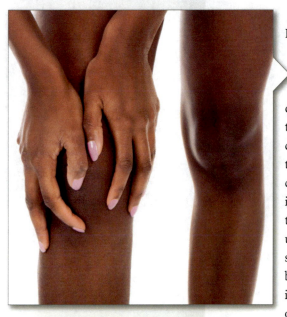

Osteoarthritis is the most common form of arthritis, but it is not a single disease. Rather, it is the end result of a variety of disorders leading to the structural or functional failure of one or more joints in the body. Osteoarthritis involves and affects the entire joint, including the nearby muscles, underlying bone, ligaments, joint lining, and the joint capsule. It is characterized by an advancing joint cartilage de**ge**neration. As the cartilage attempts to repair itself, the bone begins to remodel, the underlying (subchondral) bone hardens, which leads to the formation of bone cysts and **osteophytes** (bone spurs). Age is a key risk factor for osteoarthritis, with the greatest prevalence occurring in older adults. Cellular senescence describes the condition when cells lose the ability to divide due to age-associated deterioration and is the major factor contributing to age-related changes in cartilage homeostasis, function, and response to injury. The underlying mechanisms of this process are not fully understood, but like other age-related conditions, are associated with **telomere** erosion, DNA damage, oxidative stress, and inflammation. Osteoarthritis is credited with being the leading cause of activity limitation among many older adults. Previous joint injury, obesity, and occupational activity significantly correlate with an increased risk of knee and hip osteoarthritis [119]. It seems to be more common in individuals who play or participated in competitive sports or engage in high-intensity activity. Competitive running, football, soccer, and weightlifting are all associated with increased risk for the development of the disease [103, 146]. Osteoarthritis seems to occur more frequently in joints used repetitively and excessively, such as the pollex (thumb), hallux (big toe), knees, spinal column, and the hips. In a meta-analysis that assessed the relationship between sport participation and osteoarthritis, an increased osteoarthritis risk in elite athletes was observed in 19 out of the 24 studies [146].

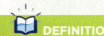

DEFINITIONS

Osteoarthritis –

The most common form of arthritis. It involves the degeneration of joint cartilage and the underlying bone, commonly associated with previous injury, but starting during middle age; the condition causes pain and stiffness, especially in the hip, knee, and thumb joints, when bones begin to run directly against each other (a.k.a. degenerative joint disease).

Osteophytes –

Also known as bone spurs or cysts that form as a result of bone remodeling in response to bone friction during progressive osteoarthritis; the condition includes a bone outgrowth deformity that can cause pain responses in the surrounding tissues (nerves, muscle, and other connective tissues).

Telomere –

A compound structure at the ends of a chromosome which serves as a protective cap that limits deterioration of DNA in all cells; telomeres have been associated with potential lifespan and longevity.

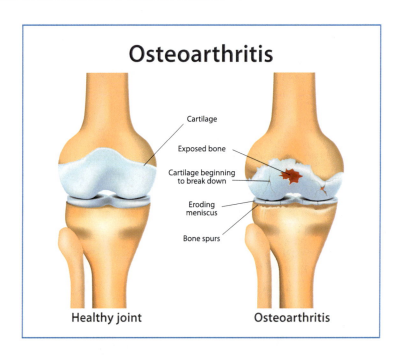

Osteoarthritis is strongly linked with injury in sedentary and active persons alike. Researchers suggest that osteoarthritis may be more prevalent in athletes than non-athletes because of the high incidence of injury reported in competitive sports [146]. When injury does not exist the incidence of osteoarthritis related to physical activity is reduced. For instance, high level soccer players who did not experience injury during competition demonstrated no greater incidence of arthritis than sedentary controls [40]. It appears that physical activity is not the sole impetus for osteoarthritis but increases one's risk of injury, which is seemingly the underlying cause of the degenerative process. **Post-traumatic arthritis (PTA)** develops acutely in response to direct trauma to a joint. PTA causes about 12% of all osteoarthritis cases and may increase risk of chronic conditions, particularly among those with inflammatory arthritis [103]. Common symptoms include edema, synovial effusion (joint swelling), pain, and, sometimes, intra-articular bleeding. The pathological mechanism seems to be the activation of inflammatory responses during the PTA acute phase, which appears to play a critical role in the chronic disease state's onset. Human studies have revealed that a series of inflammatory mediators are released in synovial fluid following acute joint trauma, increasing the risk of osteoarthritis.

Regular noncompetitive physical activity that is dose appropriate does not appear to be harmful to joints that have not been injured [146]. Physical activity that employs non-impact resistance and aerobic modalities, when performed at moderate levels, can improve function, reduce joint swelling, and relieve symptoms with both osteo- and **rheumatoid arthritis**. Increased levels of activity have been demonstrated to improve status in physical, psychosocial, and functional measures, particularly when longer warm-ups are used [109, 119]. In addition, self-reports by subjects with osteoarthritis suggest moderate intensity activity improves pain threshold, energy levels, and self-efficacy [137]. Moderate intensity exercise's benefits are likely related to the mechanisms that naturally keep joints healthy [67, 97]. Joints require movement to receive nourishment. Nutrients diffuse through the cartilage matrix via pressure gradients that cause fluid to flow when compressed. When the joints are appropriately loaded through normal functional range of motion, the **chondrocytes** amplify proteoglycan synthesis, increasing the cushioning effect. On the contrary, repeated high-impact, high-intensity loading disrupts this process, inhibiting cartilage matrix function. Inactivity also affects the cartilage matrix by reducing proteoglycan synthesis and cartilage integrity. Physical inactivity, particularly immobility, causes cartilage decline and makes the joint more susceptible to injury. Prolonged disuse associates with fibrous replacement and decline in function. When comparing injured versus non-injured joints, running had a positive effect on healthy joint water content and proteoglycan synthesis but had negative outcomes on injured joints, ultimately leading to the development of osteoarthritis [20]. However, the benefits of exercise, whether land based or water based, have been shown to be an appropriate treatment modality for those with knee osteoarthritis. Also of note, as little as 30 minutes of running with an intensity between approximately 6.5-9 miles per hour, decreases knee intra-articular, pro-inflammatory cytokine concentration, expressing benefits that go against the age-old thought process that "running is bad for your knees" [97]. But more is not additionally beneficial as excessive running volumes do not demonstrate the health equivalent.

>
> ### DEFINITIONS
>
> **Post-traumatic arthritis (PTA) –**
>
> *A type of arthritis where symptoms present acutely in response to a physical injury to a given joint; it can also include the wearing out/overuse of any joint which has had a previous injury, which places it at risk for inflammatory disorder and premature degradation.*
>
> **Rheumatoid arthritis –**
>
> *A chronic, progressive autoimmune disease that causes notable joint inflammation and results in painful deformities and/or significant immobility over time, especially in the fingers, wrists, feet, and ankles; this condition could be considered the most severe type of arthritis and can create the greatest limits to a client's exercise prescription.*
>
> **Chondrocytes –**
>
> *The only cells found within healthy cartilage which produce and maintain the cartilage's matrix integrity; they assist in amplifying the cushioning effect of cartilage during impact forces placed upon joints.*

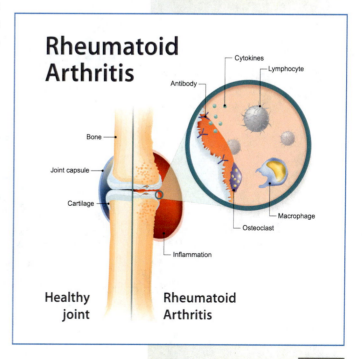

Osteoporosis & Physical Activity

Osteoporosis, a progressive bone disease, occurs due to a loss of bone mass and structural deterioration of the bone tissue. The disease's development is linked to three compounding factors: deficient peak bone mass, bone mass reduction after age thirty, and further loss of bone after age fifty. Each of these issues significantly contributes to the risk for disease. Osteoporosis makes the bone frail and brittle, creating conditions where the bone may fracture. The forearm, humerus, hip, and spine suffer the greatest risk of injury from the disease. Vertebral fractures are usually asymptomatic and lead to structural changes that often present as kyphotic disorders of the spine. Recall that kyphosis is an exaggerated rounding of the spine; when left untreated, it can progress toward a Dowager's hump (humpback), which is associated with significant functional decline, gastrointestinal and abdominal problems, and chronic back pain [19].

Injuries associated with hip fractures usually occur from falls. According to the International Osteoporosis Foundation, approximately 1.6 million hip fractures occur worldwide each year; by 2050, estimates predict that this number could reach between 4.5 million and 6.3 million [27, 70]. Death or disabilities are expected outcomes from hip fractures related to osteoporosis, with up to 20% of sufferers dying within 12 months of the injury [70, 89]. Following an osteoporotic hip fracture, the on-going mortality risk exists for five (5) years. Osteoporosis is more common in women than men due to lower peak bone mass, post-menopausal bone loss, and the simple fact that women live longer than men.

Bone stress from load-bearing activity is likely to be the most important factor in bone remodeling, and helps thwart the progression of osteoporosis.

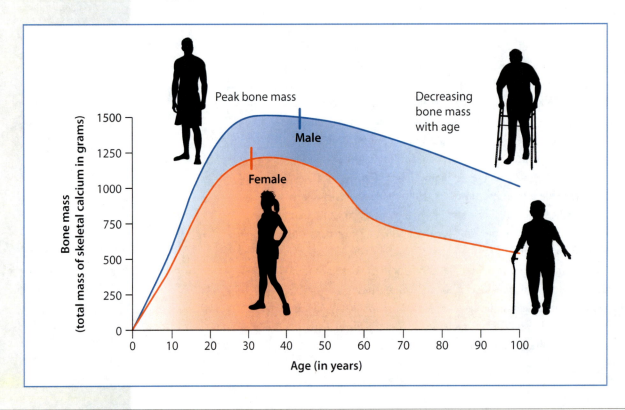

Physical activity is a vital part of bone health. Regular physical activity increases peak bone mass during youth and maintains this mass into adulthood. Active young adults demonstrate greater bone mass than their sedentary counterparts. The strength of the attached musculature, amount and intensity of physical activity performed, and level of aerobic fitness correlate with the bone mineral density (BMD). This suggests that activities promoting the greatest bone stress benefit bone mass the most. Repeated actions that encourage higher force outputs, such as resistance training, plyometrics, and weight-bearing endurance events have the greatest impact on bone maintenance. To maintain appropriate bone health, all persons should engage in routine weight-bearing physical activity consistent with the aforementioned guidelines. This is particularly true for postmenopausal women due to the estrogen production shift experienced during menopause and increased risk associated with age after 50. Evidence suggests that osteoporotic women may be able to reduce bone loss and facilitate improved BMD with exercise. This is even more important considering resistance exercise among elderly women who presented with osteopenia and osteoporosis has multiple benefits: it not only attenuates the loss of bone mass but actually improves bone BMD, inflammatory markers, insulin levels post-exercise, and physical fitness [2]. Emphasizing health-related components of fitness in programs aimed at older adults is paramount, especially for older females diagnosed with osteoporosis, as women who have a high fat mass relative to their BMI have been shown to have a lower BMD [159]. The use of resistance circuit training and weight bearing cardiovascular exercise combines benefits for overweight/obese older adults at risk for osteoporosis and comorbidities [152]. The degree of bone stress most likely determines the outcome. Resistance exercise seems to have a more pronounced effect when compared with endurance exercise; this effect occurs because resistance training employs more muscle mass and features higher mechanical stress. Bone stress, particularly in the axial skeleton, prompts adaptation and aids in prevention. Estrogen levels in both men and women seem to also be an important contributor to bone improvement. In postmenopausal women, greater BMD enhancements have been demonstrated with the use of estrogen replacement therapy [145].

Bone stress from load-bearing activity is likely the most important factor in bone remodeling. Bone cell formation occurs in response to mechanical loading, which improves structural balance and density. The effects of the load placed upon the bone are mediated by glucose-6-phosphate, prostaglandins, and nitric oxide, all of which enhance the adaptive response. Without appropriately applied stress, bone mass is compromised. Early astronauts actually developed osteoporosis in a matter of weeks due to the lack of gravity in space, which reduced the habitual impact levels commonly associated with physical activity [59]. In addition to mechanical factors, nutrition, medications, hormone concentrations, and age each have a relative contribution to bone health. Proper nutrition (in the form of adequate calcium and vitamin D) and physical activity are necessary throughout a person's lifespan to reduce the risk of osteoporosis.

In addition to the improvements and maintenance of bone that protect against osteoporosis, physical activity reduces the risk of fractures from falls. As previously mentioned, osteoporotic hip fractures account for a higher risk for premature death and disability than all other fractures combined. Studies analyzing physical activity and hip fracture occurrence found a lower risk among more active adults. Resistance exercise programs have not only proved beneficial in improving BMD in women with osteoporosis but also showed improvement in single leg stance; this suggests that, along with the increase in strength, enhance-

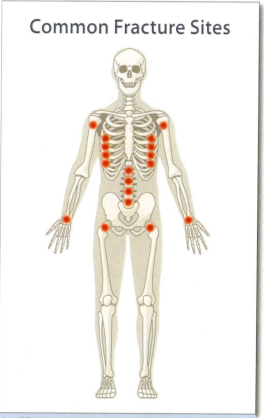

In addition to the maintenance of bone that protects against osteoporosis, physical activity also reduces the risk of fractures from falls.

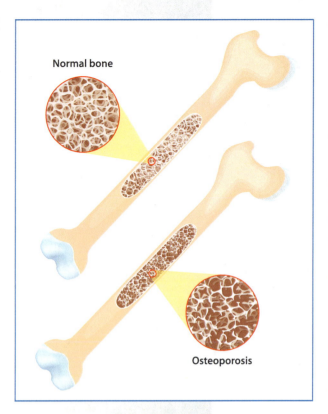

ments in body control and balance also occurred [2, 17, 152]. Although low-intensity, weight-bearing aerobic exercise exhibits protective effects, the greatest benefits seem to be related to higher intensity activity. It is likely the magnitude of the stress promotes structural bone adaptations consistent with the forces experienced during the activity. Low-to-medium impact forces have not produced the same positive associations with lower-limb bone size and strength compared to high-impact forces [59].

To further support the importance of progressive loading among older adults, a person's fall risk is inversely related to fitness performance scores and measures of functional task efficiency [16]. Compromised **gait**, balance, reaction time, strength, and range of motion, as well as impaired vision, all affect fall risk. Exercise profoundly reduces risk by enhancing strength and balance. Additionally, improvements in functional capacity, gait efficiency, speed, and reaction time may also positively impact those at risk. In measures of stair-climbing power, movement gait, and other functional tasks, frail elderly subjects suffering from chronic disease demonstrated improvements and reduced incidence of falls with weight training programs [16]. Individuals at high risk for falls should be encouraged to perform resistance and flexibility training activities aimed at improving strength and balance to reduce risk of injury and hip fractures [74].

DEFINITIONS

Gait –

The set of characteristics observed when a person walks or locomotes in other fashions; gait can include factors such as stride length, stride frequency, and various compensatory movements.

Cancer –

An abnormal growth of cells which tend to multiply in an uncontrolled way and sometimes spread (metastasize) to other tissues; the term cancer does not refer to a single pathology but rather includes more than 100 distinctive diseases that can involve any tissue of the body and may present as many different forms in each specific body area.

Cancer & Physical Activity

Cancer is reportedly the most feared of all diseases and is the second leading cause of death in the US, accounting for one-third of all deaths [130]. According to the American Cancer Society, cancer mortality has declined 25% in in the past two decades, with estimates of newly diagnosed cases around 1.7 million per year and nearly 600,000 deaths per year [130]. To put those numbers in perspective, that is over 4,600 new cases and 1,650 cancer deaths per day. World Cancer Research Fund estimates that about one-quarter to one-third of the new cancer cases expected to occur in the US will be related to being overweight or obese, physically inactive, and poorly nourished, and thus, could also be prevented. Cancer is actually a number of different diseases, characterized by an uncontrolled growth and spread of abnormal carcinogenic cells which have numerous forms and origins. It has been estimated that genetic disorders contribute to only 5-10% of cancer cases, whereas the remaining 90-95% of all cancer cases are related to lifestyle and environmental factors. These factors include the following: smoking, diet (processed foods, fried foods, and red meat), alcohol, environmental pollutants, radiation, sun exposure, stress, physical inactivity, sexually transmitted diseases, obesity and/or being overweight. As a result, many studies have provided evidence regarding cancer prevention as it relates to controllable factors: increasing physical activity levels and exercise, eating more fruits and vegetables, limiting caloric intake, moderating alcohol use, ceasing smoking, reducing meat consumption, avoiding direct exposure to sunlight, and scheduling regular check-ups to control or prevent infections and sicknesses [4]. At least one third of the most common cancers are related to lifestyle

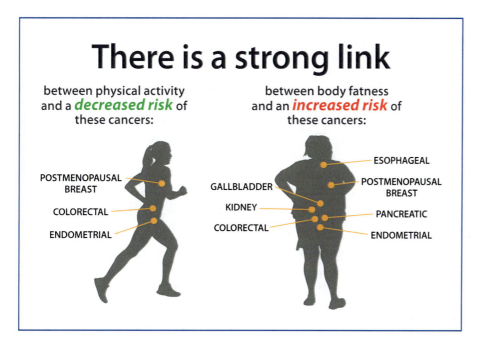

behaviors and controllable choices.

For individuals with early stage cancer, exercise training interventions have demonstrated efficacy for improving life quality, fatigue, and well-being [15, 127, 157]. Several published studies have included patients in the early stage of disease, and more recently, research has investigated populations of patients with advanced tumors of the breast, rectum, and lung who are undergoing therapy [8, 12, 71, 100]. While sample sizes in the study were small, exercise demonstrated improvements in both cardiopulmonary function and measures of muscular fitness. Cancer-related fatigue is the most limiting symptom in advanced stages of cancer, leading to significant decline in mobility and independence. In early stage cancers, physical activity and exercise should be used to promote health and the maintenance of lean body mass. Due to the side effects of treatment, an emphasis on overall well-being is important and should emphasize quality nutrition and individual-appropriate activity.

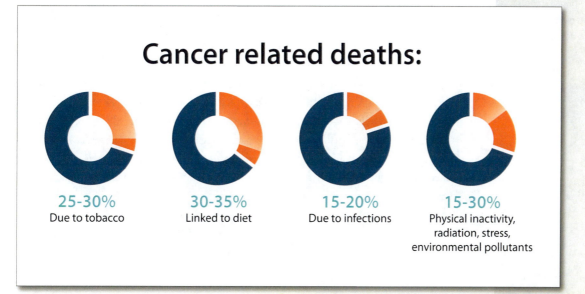

Mental Health & Physical Activity

Depression, anxiety disorders, and subjective feelings of self-worth affect psychological well-being. These disorders affect millions of people and are linked to suicide, currently the nation's 10th leading cause of death [136]. Statistical reports suggest 1 in 5 adults suffer from some type of mental illness in a given year, and approximately 1 in every 25 adults in the U.S. lives with a serious mental illness [125]. One study found 25% of people ages 15-54 reported mental disorders during the previous year [1]. Mental health and psychological well-being relate to mood, personality, cognition, and perception. Consequently, these factors are linked to physical health and perceived quality of life [153]. Exercise has been shown to be just as effective as antidepressants for those suffering from mild to moderate depression, and it has been recommended as a complementary therapy for those suffering from schizophrenia and/or mild and moderate depression [44,72,77]. Due to this association, physical activity can improve mood, self-esteem, self-efficacy, and cognitive function.

Epidemiologic research demonstrates an association between physical activity and the alleviation of symptoms of depression, clinical depression, and anxiety, as well as improvements in positive affect (disposition) and general well-being [113]. These trials suggest that improvements associated with physical activity occur in persons with diagnosed mental disorders and those reporting mood disturbances. Studies using aerobic training have demonstrated an acute temporary change in mental state based solely on a single episode of physical activity [113]. Subjects reported reduced anxiety, reduced muscle tension, and improvements in transient mood that lasted 2-6 hours post-exercise, consistent with the metabolic recovery period. In children, physical activity interventions had positive effects on externalizing problems, internalizing problems, self-concept, and academic achievement.

Although people with depression tend to be less physically active than non-depressed individuals, physical activity has been shown to significantly reduce depressive symptoms. Whereas the mechanism by which exercise inhibits depression symptoms is not clearly understood, many recent studies suggest that even low levels of frequent physical activity, such as walking <150 minutes/week, can be preventative [94]. Interestingly, people with depression have higher high rates of cardio-metabolic disorders and CVD and related premature death. Exercise appears to be a superior combatant when compared to pharmacological approaches for these populations [58]. Anxiety symptoms and panic disorder also improve with regular exercise, and the beneficial effects appear equal to other non-pharmacological treatments. The severity of anxiety disorders seems to be a major factor in exercise treatment plans. Acute anxiety responds better to exercise than chronic anxiety; similarly, low to moderate depression responds better than severe depression. For exercise to be optimally effective, participation should be routine and frequent. Increasing frequency of physical activity has demonstrated a pronounced effect on depression as an independent variable. It is not known if regular participation causes actual trait adjustments or simply results in "carry-over effect" of the transient changes associated with

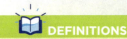

Exercise has been shown to be just as effective as anti-depressant medications for those suffering from mild-to-moderate depression.

DEFINITIONS

Depression –

A mood disorder that causes a persistent feeling of sadness and loss of interest; it can impact how a person feels, thinks, and behaves and can lead to a variety of emotional and physical problems.

the exercise bout. Adults who engaged in routine physical activity from exercise or sport experienced reduced symptoms of depression and anxiety compared to individuals reporting no physical activity [58]. In a **cross-sectional study** involving over 46,000 individuals, physical activity was associated with improved mood and general well-being and fewer symptoms of anxiety and depression [52]. On the contrary, studies analyzing the effects of physical inactivity on mental health found that both sedentary viewing time (seated television watching) and engagement in little or no recreational physical activity associated independently with greater incidence of depressive symptoms.

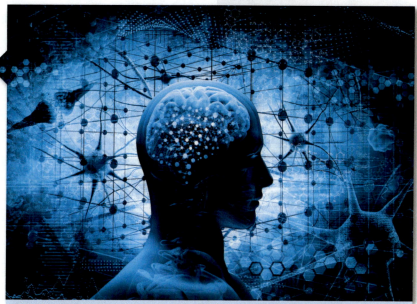

The biological mechanisms for improved mental health with exercise relates to concentrations of brain neurotransmitters and neuroreceptors (such as dopamine and serotonin) as well as psychosocial elements.

The activity engaged in and frequency of participation also seem to play a role in the mental shifts associated with physical activity. Women reported improvements in positive affect when the activity was recreational but did not show the same outcome when housework, measured via energy expenditure, contributed to the physical activity [18, 135]. Men reported a 27% lower incidence of depression when engaged in activity three or more days per week [135]. Additionally, individuals who expended 1,000-2,499 kcal per week showed a 17% reduction in risk, while those who exceeded 2500 kcal per week experienced a 28% reduction [35]. In a similar study, an inverse dose-response relationship was found between energy expended and depression incidence. Greater participation in activity seems to reduce risk for depression, consistent with the frequency and amount of work performed, up to a certain point. Notably, when individuals engage in strenuous or excessive activity, subjects reported negative mental health effects. No threshold of intensity or duration has been identified nor has an optimal volume been demonstrated; however, endurance athletes performing exorbitant quantities of vigorous exercise have reported negative effects on mental health [47]. These included mood disturbances, increased fatigue, anxiety, and symptoms of depression. These negative effects are consistent with some of the symptoms identified in overtraining syndrome. It would seem that the deleterious effects from strenuous, high-volume exercise correlate with overtraining, as mood improved when excessive work was tapered back.

The suggested biological mechanism for improved mental state with exercise relates to the concentration of brain neurotransmitters and neuroreceptors. Dopamine, norepinephrine, and **serotonin**, as well as **endorphins**, have been proposed components in the mood adjustments associated with activity. Additionally, the temperature changes and physiological adaptations associated with increased core temperature possibly explain the reduction in tension reported by subjects. It is also likely that some of the positive effects from exercise are psychosocial. Many people experience social interaction, healthy competitiveness, a positive body image, and social support in environments associated with physical activity, which may augment self-esteem, self-perception, self-efficacy, and relief of daily stressors. No matter what the particular impetus for improvement in mental health and well-being, physical activity performed at moderate levels throughout the week seems to positively effect one's mental health.

 DEFINITIONS

Cross-sectional study –

A type of observational study that analyzes data collected from a specific population or populations at a specific point in time to obtain "cross-sectional" data for comparisons; often examine the relationship between disease and other variables of interest that exist in a defined population.

Serotonin –

A hormone-based neurotransmitter which serves various roles, such as regulation of blood pressure, pain perception, the sleep-wake cycle, and even mood; it is released in response to exercise and other stimuli.

Endorphins –

A group of hormones secreted from the brain and central nervous system. They have a number of physiological functions and effects on the body and are released in relatively high quantities following exercise, activating opiate receptors that cause analgesic and pleasurable sensations.

Alzheimer's Disease

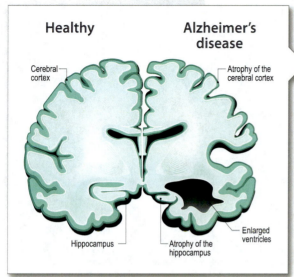

Age-related neurodegenerative disorders, like **Alzheimer's** or **Parkinson's disease**, are becoming a major issue in public health care. Alzheimer's and other **dementias** currently cost the American health care system approximately $236 billion dollars, with each family caregiver spending more than $5,000 per year to provide for an Alzheimer's sufferer. Alzheimer's is now the 6th leading cause of death in America and the 5th leading cause of death in those over 65 years of age. It kills more people than breast and prostate cancer combined [10]. Lifestyle factors appear to reduce the risk for Alzheimer's disease and dementia: specifically, novelties that provide intellectual stimulation, cognitive and social engagement, nutrition, and various types of exercise. Physical capacity and neurodegenerative brain decline seem to be linked. An example of this link is seen with the deterioration of walking speed, which is associated with negative performance in tests assessing psychomotor speed and verbal fluency among elderly individuals. Increases in physical activity and fitness training influence a wide range of cognitive processes, with the largest positive impact occurring at the frontal lobe. Frontal-lobe atrophy is associated with aging, neuro-physical impairments, loss of executive function, and overall cognitive decline [14]. Studies show that various types of exercise can improve additional cognitive functions; for instance, tasks mediated by the hippocampus and other neurological organs. The exercise-induced adaptations are multi-faceted, but brain tissue hypertrophy of key structures aids in slowing the aging process. Exercise-induced growth factors' production, such as the **brain-derived neurotrophic factor** (BDNF), has been shown to not only enhance neurogenesis (regeneration of brain tissue) but also plays a key role in positive cognitive effects. Several trials with elderly patients suffering from neurodegenerative diseases report exercise induced cognitive improvements and positive changes on these trophic factor levels including BDNF among others. Additional chemical messengers impacted by exercise, like the anabolic agent insulin-like growth factor (IGF-1), may mediate the exercise-induced response on BDNF, neurogenesis, and cognitive performance [23, 31, 32, 34]. Physical activity and interventions aimed at enhancing the effects of exercise likely significantly delay and attenuate neurodegenerative disorders.

Despite exercise's beneficial effects – preventing Alzheimer's disease and prolonging the survival rates of sufferers – adults at risk for the disease tend to engage in more sedentary behavior and less physical activity than those not in danger. Results indicated that, compared to controls, participants with neurodegenerative disease averaged 21% less activity. Due to the fact that most adults are not physically active to begin with, this presents additional, compound challenges. Researchers have identified several factors that enhance compliance with exercise among those with a family history of degenerative disorders; these include the opportunity to join an instructor-led exercise program, the perception of benefits from exercise, and social support. Participants reported high levels of extrinsic (fitness-related) and intrinsic (interest/enjoyment) motivation. Strategies that include these elements should be used for programs aimed at increasing physical activity participation and adherence among those at risk for neurodegenerative dementias.

DEFINITIONS

Alzheimer's disease –

A neurodegenerative disorder, or type of dementia, often occurring during older age, that causes progressive irreversible mental deterioration, memory loss, diminished cognition, and eventual loss of independence due to generalized degeneration of the brain.

Parkinson's disease –

A progressive neurodegenerative disease characterized by tremor, muscular rigidity, and slow, imprecise movement capabilities that primarily impacts middle-aged and elderly people; it is associated with degeneration of the basal ganglia of the brain and a deficiency of the neurotransmitter dopamine.

Dementia –

A chronic disorder of various mental processes caused by brain disease or injury that is characterized by memory disorders, personality changes, and impaired reasoning; the term is often used for a decline in mental ability severe enough to limit performance of daily living activities.

Brain-derived neurotrophic factor (BDNF) –

A protein-based compound released by nerves or brain support cells, such as astrocytes, that binds to a receptor on a nearby nerve cell to promote brain neuron survival by facilitating growth, maturation, and maintenance of these cells.

REFERENCES:

1. Aguiar EJ, Morgan PJ, Collins CE, Plotnikoff RC, and Callister R. Efficacy of interventions that include diet, aerobic and resistance training components for type 2 diabetes prevention: a systematic review with meta-analysis. *International Journal of Behavioral Nutrition and Physical Activity* 11: 2, 2014.

2. Ahn N and Kim K. Effects of 12-week exercise training on osteocalcin, high-sensitivity C-reactive protein concentrations, and insulin resistance in elderly females with osteoporosis. *Journal of physical therapy science* 28: 2227-2231, 2016.

3. Amato MC, Pizzolanti G, Torregrossa V, Misiano G, Milano S, and Giordano C. Visceral adiposity index (VAI) is predictive of an altered adipokine profile in patients with type 2 diabetes. *PLoS One* 9: e91969, 2014.

4. Anand P, Kunnumakara AB, Sundaram C, Harikumar KB, Tharakan ST, Lai OS, Sung B, and Aggarwal BB. Cancer is a preventable disease that requires major lifestyle changes. *Pharmaceutical research* 25: 2097-2116, 2008.

5. Anastasius M, Kockx M, Jessup W, Sullivan D, Rye K-A, and Kritharides L. Cholesterol efflux capacity: An introduction for clinicians. *American heart journal* 180: 54-63, 2016.

6. Arem H, Moore SC, Patel A, Hartge P, De Gonzalez AB, Visvanathan K, Campbell PT, Freedman M, Weiderpass E, and Adami HO. Leisure time physical activity and mortality: a detailed pooled analysis of the dose-response relationship. *JAMA internal medicine* 175: 959-967, 2015.

7. Arena R, McNeil A, Sagner M, and Hills AP. The Current Global State of Key Lifestyle Characteristics: Health and Economic Implications. *Prog Cardiovasc Dis* 59: 422-429, 2017.

8. Ashcraft KA, Peace RM, Betof AS, Dewhirst MW, and Jones LW. Efficacy and mechanisms of aerobic exercise on cancer initiation, progression, and metastasis: a critical systematic review of in vivo preclinical data. *Cancer research*, 2016.

9. Association AD. Economic costs of diabetes in the US in 2012. *Diabetes care* 36: 1033-1046, 2013.

10. Association As. 2017 Alzheimer's disease facts and figures. *Alzheimer's & Dementia* 13: 325-373, 2017.

11. Bastien M, Poirier P, Lemieux I, and Després J-P. Overview of epidemiology and contribution of obesity to cardiovascular disease. *Progress in cardiovascular diseases* 56: 369-381, 2014.

12. Battaglini CL, Mills RC, Phillips BL, Lee JT, Story CE, Nascimento MG, and Hackney AC. Twenty-five years of research on the effects of exercise training in breast cancer survivors: a systematic review of the literature. *World journal of clinical oncology* 5: 177, 2014.

13. Beavers KM, Brinkley TE, and Nicklas BJ. Effect of exercise training on chronic inflammation. *Clinica chimica acta* 411: 785-793, 2010.

14. Benedict RH, Bakshi R, Simon JH, Priore R, Miller C, and Munschauer F. Frontal cortex atrophy predicts cognitive impairment in multiple sclerosis. *The Journal of neuropsychiatry and clinical neurosciences* 14: 44-51, 2002.

15. Blaney J, Lowe-Strong A, Rankin J, Campbell A, Allen J, and Gracey J. The cancer rehabilitation journey: barriers to and facilitators of exercise among patients with cancer-related fatigue. *Physical therapy* 90: 1135-1147, 2016.

16. Bonder BR and Dal Bello-Haas V. *Functional performance in older adults*: FA Davis, 2017.

17. Borer KT. Physical activity in the prevention and amelioration of osteoporosis in women. *Sports medicine* 35: 779-830, 2005.

18. Brooks AG, Withers RT, Gore CJ, Vogler AJ, Plummer J, and Cormack J. Measurement and prediction of METs during household activities in 35- to 45-year-old females. *European journal of applied physiology* 91: 638-648, 2004.

19. Broy SB. The vertebral fracture cascade: etiology and clinical implications. *Journal of Clinical Densitometry* 19: 29-34, 2016.

20. Buckwalter JA and Martin JA. Sports and osteoarthritis. *Current opinion in rheumatology* 16: 634-639, 2004.

21. Cade WT. Diabetes-related microvascular and macrovascular diseases in the physical therapy setting. *Physical therapy* 88: 1322-1335, 2008.

22. Cai M and Zou Z. Effect of aerobic exercise on blood lipid and glucose in obese or overweight adults: a meta-analysis of randomised controlled trials. *Obesity research & clinical practice* 10: 589-602, 2016.

23. Cassilhas RC, Tufik S, and de Mello MT. Physical exercise, neuroplasticity, spatial learning and memory. *Cellular and molecular life sciences* 73: 975-983, 2016.

24. Ciolac EG, Bocchi EA, Bortolotto LA, Carvalho VO, Greve JM, and Guimarães GV. Effects of high-intensity aerobic interval training vs. moderate exercise on hemodynamic, metabolic and neuro-humoral abnormalities of young normotensive women at high familial risk for hypertension. *Hypertension Research* 33: 836-843, 2010.

25. Colberg SR, Sigal RJ, Yardley JE, Riddell MC, Dunstan DW, Dempsey PC, Horton ES, Castorino K, and Tate DF. Physical activity/exercise and diabetes: a position statement of the American Diabetes Association. *Diabetes Care* 39: 2065-2079, 2016.

26. Conn VS, Koopman RJ, Ruppar TM, Phillips LJ, Mehr DR, and Hafdahl AR. Insulin sensitivity following exercise interventions: systematic review and meta-analysis of outcomes among healthy adults. *Journal of primary care & community health* 5: 211-222, 2014.

27. Cooper C, Campion G, and Melton Lr. Hip fractures in the elderly: a world-wide projection. *Osteoporosis international* 2: 285-289, 1992.

28. Cornelissen VA and Fagard RH. Effects of endurance training on blood pressure, blood pressure–regulating mechanisms, and cardiovascular risk factors. *Hypertension* 46: 667-675, 2005.

29. Cornelissen VA and Smart NA. Exercise training for blood pressure: a systematic review and meta-analysis. *Journal of the American Heart Association* 2: e004473, 2013.

30. Cortese S, Moreira-Maia CR, St. Fleur D, Morcillo-Peñalver C, Rohde LA, and Faraone SV. Association between ADHD and obesity: a systematic review and meta-analysis. *American Journal of Psychiatry* 173: 34-43, 2015.

31. Cotman CW and Berchtold NC. Exercise: a behavioral intervention to enhance brain health and plasticity. *Trends in neurosciences* 25: 295-301, 2002.

32. Cotman CW, Berchtold NC, and Christie L-A. Exercise builds brain health: key roles of growth factor cascades and inflammation. *Trends in neurosciences* 30: 464-472, 2007.

33. De Ferranti SD, Rodday AM, Mendelson MM, Wong JB, Leslie LK, and Sheldrick RC. Prevalence of familial hypercholesterolemia in the 1999 to 2012 United States National Health and Nutrition Examination Surveys (NHANES). *Circulation* 133: 1067-1072, 2016.

34. de Melo Coelho FG, Gobbi S, Andreatto CAA, Corazza DI, Pedroso RV, and Santos-Galduróz RF. Physical exercise modulates peripheral levels of brain-derived neurotrophic factor (BDNF): a systematic review of experimental studies in the elderly. *Archives of gerontology and geriatrics* 56: 10-15, 2013.

35. De Moor M, Beem A, Stubbe J, Boomsma D, and De Geus E. Regular exercise, anxiety, depression and personality: a population-based study. *Preventive medicine* 42: 273-279, 2006.

36. Ding D, Kolbe-Alexander T, Nguyen B, Katzmarzyk PT, Pratt M, and Lawson KD. The economic burden of physical inactivity: a systematic review and critical appraisal. *Br J Sports Med* 51: 1392-1409, 2017.

37. Ding D, Lawson KD, Kolbe-Alexander TL, Finkelstein EA, Katzmarzyk PT, van Mechelen W, Pratt M, and Lancet Physical Activity Series 2 Executive C. The economic burden of physical inactivity: a global analysis of major non-communicable diseases. *Lancet* 388: 1311-1324, 2016.

38. Dishman R, Heath G, and Lee I-M. Physical activity epidemiology 2nd edition: *Human Kinetics*, 2012.

39. Drucker DJ and Nauck MA. The incretin system: glucagon-like peptide-1 receptor agonists and dipeptidyl peptidase-4 inhibitors in type 2 diabetes. *The Lancet* 368: 1696-1705, 2006.

40. Elleuch M, Guermazi M, Mezghanni M, Ghroubi S, Fki H, Mefteh S, Baklouti S, and Sellami S. Knee osteoarthritis in 50 former top-level footballers: a comparative (control group) study. Annales de réadaptation et de médecine physique. *Elsevier*, 2008, p. 174-178.

41. Erikssen G. Physical fitness and changes in mortality. *Sports medicine* 31: 571-576, 2001.

42. Evans EM, Racette SB, Peterson LR, Villareal DT, Greiwe JS, and Holloszy JO. Aerobic power and insulin action improve in response to endurance exercise training in healthy 77–87 yr olds. *Journal of Applied Physiology*, 2005.

43. Fernandes T, Baraúna VG, Negrão CE, Phillips MI, and Oliveira EM. Aerobic exercise training promotes physiological cardiac remodeling involving a set of microRNAs. *American Journal of Physiology-Heart and Circulatory Physiology* 309: H543-H552, 2015.

44. Firth J, Cotter J, Elliott R, French P, and Yung A. A systematic review and meta-analysis of exercise interventions in schizophrenia patients. *Psychological medicine* 45: 1343-1361, 2015.

45. Fontana L, Eagon JC, Trujillo ME, Scherer PE, and Klein S. Visceral fat adipokine secretion is associated with systemic inflammation in obese humans. *Diabetes* 56: 1010-1013, 2007.

46. Franklin BA, Durstine JL, Roberts CK, and Barnard RJ. Impact of diet and exercise on lipid management in the modern era. *Best Practice & Research Clinical Endocrinology & Metabolism* 28: 405-421, 2014.

47. Galper DI, Trivedi MH, Barlow CE, Dunn AL, and Kampert JB. Inverse association between physical inactivity and mental health in men and women. *Medicine & Science in Sports & Exercise* 38: 173-178, 2006.

48. Garber AJ, Abrahamson MJ, Barzilay JI, Blonde L, Bloomgarden ZT, Bush MA, Dagogo-Jack S, DeFronzo RA, Einhorn D, and Fonseca VA. Consensus statement by the American Association of Clinical Endocrinologists and American College of Endocrinology on the comprehensive type 2 diabetes management algorithm–2016 executive summary. *Endocrine Practice* 22: 84-113, 2016.

49. General S. The health consequences of smoking—50 years of progress: a report of the surgeon general. *US Department of Health and Human Services*. Citeseer, 2014.

50. Giannarelli C, Rodriguez DT, Zafar MU, Christoffel D, Vialou V, Peña C, Badimon A, Hodes GF, Mury P, and Rabkin J. Susceptibility to chronic social stress increases plaque progression, vulnerability and platelet activation. *Thrombosis and haemostasis* 117: 816-818, 2017.

51. Gondim OS, de Camargo VTN, Gutierrez FA, de Oliveira Martins PF, Passos MEP, Momesso CM, Santos VC, Gorjão R, Pithon-Curi TC, and Cury-Boaventura MF. Benefits of regular exercise on inflammatory and cardiovascular risk markers in normal weight, overweight and obese adults. *PLoS One* 10: e0140596, 2015.

52. Goodwin RD. Association between physical activity and mental disorders among adults in the United States. *Preventive medicine* 36: 698-703, 2003.

53. Goraya TY, Jacobsen SJ, Kottke TE, Frye RL, Weston SA, and Roger VL. Coronary heart disease death and sudden cardiac death: a 20-year population-based study. *American journal of epidemiology* 157: 763-770, 2003.

54. Gordon B, Chen S, and Durstine JL. The effects of exercise training on the traditional lipid profile and beyond. *Current sports medicine reports* 13: 253-259, 2014.

55. Graßmann S, Wirsching J, Eichelmann F, and Aleksandrova K. Association Between Peripheral Adipokines and Inflammation Markers: A Systematic Review and Meta Analysis. *Obesity* 25: 1776-1785, 2017.

56. Gregg EW, Zhuo X, Cheng YJ, Albright AL, Narayan KV, and Thompson TJ. Trends in lifetime risk and years of life lost due to diabetes in the USA, 1985–2011: a modelling study. *The lancet Diabetes & endocrinology* 2: 867-874, 2014.

57. Hales CM, Carroll MD, Fryar CD, and Ogden CL. Prevalence of obesity among adults and youth: United States, 2015–2016. *NCHS data brief*: 1-8, 2017.

58. Hallgren M, Stubbs B, Vancampfort D, Lundin A, Jääkallio P, and Forsell Y. Treatment guidelines for depression: Greater emphasis on physical activity is needed. *European Psychiatry* 40: 1-3, 2017.

59. Hannam K, Deere K, Hartley A, Al-Sari U, Clark E, Fraser W, and Tobias J. Habitual levels of higher, but not medium or low, impact physical activity are positively related to lower limb bone strength in older women: findings from a population-based study using accelerometers to classify impact magnitude. *Osteoporosis International* 28: 2813-2822, 2017.

60. Harber MP, Kaminsky LA, Arena R, Blair SN, Franklin BA, Myers J, and Ross R. Impact of cardiorespiratory fitness on all-cause and disease-specific mortality: Advances since 2009. *Progress in Cardiovascular Diseases*, 2017.

61. Hayashino Y, Jackson JL, Hirata T, Fukumori N, Nakamura F, Fukuhara S, Tsujii S, and Ishii H. Effects of exercise on C-reactive protein, inflammatory cytokine and adipokine in patients with type 2 diabetes: a meta-analysis of randomized controlled trials. *Metabolism* 63: 431-440, 2014.

62. Health UDo and Services H. How Tobacco Smoke Causes Disease: What It Means to You. US Department of Health and Human Services, Centers for Disease Control and Prevention. *National Center for Chronic Disease Prevention and Health Promotion, Office on Smoking and Health*: Atlanta, 2010.

63. Heron MP. Deaths: leading causes for 2012. 2015.

64. Hjerkind KV, Stenehjem JS, and Nilsen TI. Adiposity, physical activity and risk of diabetes mellitus: prospective data from the population-based HUNT study, Norway. *BMJ open* 7: e013142, 2017.

65. Hoffmann A, Ebert T, Klöting N, Dokas J, Jeromin F, Jessnitzer B, Burkhardt R, Fasshauer M, and Kralisch S. Leptin dose-dependently decreases atherosclerosis by attenuation of hypercholesterolemia and induction of adiponectin. *Biochimica et Biophysica Acta (BBA)-Molecular Basis of Disease* 1862: 113-120, 2016.

66. Holst JJ, Vilsbøll T, and Deacon CF. The incretin system and its role in type 2 diabetes mellitus. *Molecular and cellular endocrinology* 297: 127-136, 2009.

67. Hyldahl RD, Evans A, Kwon S, Ridge ST, Robinson E, Hopkins JT, and Seeley MK. Running decreases knee intra-articular cytokine and cartilage oligomeric matrix concentrations: a pilot study. *European journal of applied physiology* 116: 2305-2314, 2016.

68. Jarris PE. Obesity as disease: an opportunity for integrating public health and clinical medicine. *Journal of Public Health Management and Practice* 19: 610-612, 2013.

69. Jelleyman C, Yates T, O'Donovan G, Gray LJ, King JA, Khunti K, and Davies MJ. The effects of high intensity interval training on glucose regulation and insulin resistance: a meta analysis. *Obesity reviews* 16: 942-961, 2015.

70. Johnell O and Kanis J. An estimate of the worldwide prevalence and disability associated with osteoporotic fractures. *Osteoporosis international* 17: 1726-1733, 2006.

71. Jones LW, Kwan ML, Weltzien EK, Chandarlapaty S, Sternfeld B, Sweeney C, Bernard PS, Castillo AL, Habel LA, and Kroenke CH. Exercise and prognosis on the basis of clinicopathologic and molecular features in early stage breast cancer: the LACE and Pathways studies. *Cancer research*: canres. 3307.2015, 2016.

72. Josefsson T, Lindwall M, and Archer T. Physical exercise intervention in depressive disorders: Meta analysis and systematic review. *Scandinavian journal of medicine & science in sports* 24: 259-272, 2014.

73. Jung UJ and Choi M-S. Obesity and its metabolic complications: the role of adipokines and the relationship between obesity, inflammation, insulin resistance, dyslipidemia and nonalcoholic fatty liver disease. *International journal of molecular sciences* 15: 6184-6223, 2014.

74. Kannus P, Sievänen H, Palvanen M, Järvinen T, and Parkkari J. Prevention of falls and consequent injuries in elderly people. *The Lancet* 366: 1885-1893, 2005.

75. Kelley GA and Kelley KS. Effects of aerobic exercise on C-reactive protein, body composition, and maximum oxygen consumption in adults: a meta-analysis of randomized controlled trials. *Metabolism* 55: 1500-1507, 2006.

76. Kernan WN, Ovbiagele B, Black HR, Bravata DM, Chimowitz MI, Ezekowitz MD, Fang MC, Fisher M, Furie KL, and Heck DV. Guidelines for the prevention of stroke in patients with stroke and transient ischemic attack. *Stroke*: STR. 0000000000000024, 2014.

77. Knapen J, Vancampfort D, Moriën Y, and Marchal Y. Exercise therapy improves both mental and physical health in patients with major depression. *Disability and rehabilitation* 37: 1490-1495, 2015.

78. Kodama S, Saito K, Tanaka S, Maki M, Yachi Y, Asumi M, Sugawara A, Totsuka K, Shimano H, and Ohashi Y. Cardiorespiratory fitness as a quantitative predictor of all-cause mortality and cardiovascular events in healthy men and women: a meta-analysis. *Jama* 301: 2024-2035, 2009.

79. Koenig W and Ernst E. Exercise and thrombosis. *Coronary artery disease* 11: 123-127, 2000.

80. Kohl HW, Craig CL, Lambert EV, Inoue S, Alkandari JR, Leetongin G, Kahlmeier S, and Group LPASW. The pandemic of physical inactivity: global action for public health. *The Lancet* 380: 294-305, 2012.

81. Kokkinos P. Cardiorespiratory fitness, exercise, and blood pressure. *Hypertension* 64: 1160-1164, 2014.

82. Kontush A. HDL particle number and size as predictors of cardiovascular disease. *Frontiers in pharmacology* 6, 2015.

83. Kumar P and Mounsey JP. Sudden Cardiac Death. In: *Cardiomyopathies*: InTech, 2013.

84. Kyu HH, Bachman VF, Alexander LT, Mumford JE, Afshin A, Estep K, Veerman JL, Delwiche K, Iannarone ML, and Moyer ML. Physical activity and risk of breast cancer, colon cancer, diabetes, ischemic heart disease, and ischemic stroke events: systematic review and dose-response meta-analysis for the Global Burden of Disease Study 2013. *bmj* 354: i3857, 2016.

85. Lavie CJ, O'Keefe JH, and Sallis RE. Exercise and the heart—the harm of too little and too much. *Current sports medicine reports* 14: 104-109, 2015.

86. Lazar MA. How obesity causes diabetes: not a tall tale. *Science* 307: 373-375, 2005.

87. Lee I-M and Paffenbarger Jr RS. Associations of light, moderate, and vigorous intensity physical activity with longevity: the Harvard Alumni Health Study. *American journal of epidemiology* 151: 293-299, 2000.

88. Lee I-M, Shiroma EJ, Lobelo F, Puska P, Blair SN, Katzmarzyk PT, and Group LPASW. Effect of physical inactivity on major non-communicable diseases worldwide: an analysis of burden of disease and life expectancy. *The lancet* 380: 219-229, 2012.

89. Leibson CL, Tosteson AN, Gabriel SE, Ransom JE, and Melton LJ. Mortality, disability, and nursing home use for persons with and without hip fracture: a population based study. *Journal of the American Geriatrics Society* 50: 1644-1650, 2002.

90. Ligthart S, van Herpt TT, Leening MJ, Kavousi M, Hofman A, Stricker BH, van Hoek M, Sijbrands EJ, Franco OH, and Dehghan A. Lifetime risk of developing impaired glucose metabolism and eventual progression from prediabetes to type 2 diabetes: a prospective cohort study. *The lancet Diabetes & endocrinology* 4: 44-51, 2016.

91. Lin X, Zhang X, Guo J, Roberts CK, McKenzie S, Wu WC, Liu S, and Song Y. Effects of exercise training on cardiorespiratory fitness and biomarkers of cardiometabolic health: a systematic review and meta analysis of randomized controlled trials. *Journal of the American Heart Association* 4: e002014, 2015.

92. Lira FS, Yamashita AS, Uchida MC, Zanchi NE, Gualano B, Martins E, Caperuto EC, and Seelaender M. Low and moderate, rather than high intensity strength exercise induces benefit regarding plasma lipid profile. *Diabetology & metabolic syndrome* 2: 31, 2010.

93. Lyon CJ, Law RE, and Hsueh WA. Minireview: adiposity, inflammation, and atherogenesis. *Endocrinology* 144: 2195-2200, 2003.

94. Mammen G and Faulkner G. Physical activity and the prevention of depression: a systematic review of prospective studies. *American journal of preventive medicine* 45: 649-657, 2013.

95. Mann S, Beedie C, and Jimenez A. Differential effects of aerobic exercise, resistance training and combined exercise modalities on cholesterol and the lipid profile: review, synthesis and recommendations. *Sports Medicine* 44: 211-221, 2014.

96. Manson JE, Stampfer M, Colditz G, Willett W, Rosner B, Hennekens C, Speizer F, Rimm E, and Krolewski A. Physical activity and incidence of non-insulin-dependent diabetes mellitus in women. *The Lancet* 338: 774-778, 1991.

97. McAlindon TE, Bannuru RR, Sullivan M, Arden N, Berenbaum F, Bierma-Zeinstra S, Hawker G, Henrotin Y, Hunter D, and Kawaguchi H. OARSI guidelines for the non-surgical management of knee osteoarthritis. *Osteoarthritis and cartilage* 22: 363-388, 2014.

98. MEMBERS WG, Go AS, Mozaffarian D, Roger VL, Benjamin EJ, Berry JD, Blaha MJ, Dai S, Ford ES, and Fox CS. Heart disease and stroke statistics – 2014 update: a report from the American Heart Association. *circulation* 129: e28, 2014.

99. Menke A, Casagrande S, Geiss L, and Cowie CC. Prevalence of and trends in diabetes among adults in the United States, 1988-2012. *Jama* 314: 1021-1029, 2015.

100. Michaels C. The importance of exercise in lung cancer treatment. *Translational lung cancer research* 5: 235, 2016.

101. Mons U, Hahmann H, and Brenner H. A reverse J-shaped association of leisure time physical activity with prognosis in patients with stable coronary heart disease: evidence from a large cohort with repeated measurements. *Heart*: heartjnl-2013-305242, 2014.

102. Mozaffarian D, Benjamin EJ, Go AS, Arnett DK, Blaha MJ, Cushman M, Das SR, de Ferranti S, Després J-P, and Fullerton HJ. Heart disease and stroke statistics – 2016 update. *Circulation* 133: e38-e360, 2016.

103. Musumeci G, Aiello FC, Szychlinska MA, Di Rosa M, Castrogiovanni P, and Mobasheri A. Osteoarthritis in the XXIst century: risk factors and behaviours that influence disease onset and progression. *International journal of molecular sciences* 16: 6093-6112, 2015.

104. Myers J, McAuley P, Lavie CJ, Despres J-P, Arena R, and Kokkinos P. Physical activity and cardiorespiratory fitness as major markers of cardiovascular risk: their independent and interwoven importance to health status. *Progress in cardiovascular diseases* 57: 306-314, 2015.

105. Nauman J, Nes BM, Lavie CJ, Jackson AS, Sui X, Coombes JS, Blair SN, and Wisløff U. Prediction of cardiovascular mortality by estimated cardiorespiratory fitness independent of traditional risk factors: the HUNT study. *Mayo Clinic Proceedings*. Elsevier, 2017, p. 218-227.

106. Nigg JT, Johnstone JM, Musser ED, Long HG, Willoughby MT, and Shannon J. Attention-deficit/hyperactivity disorder (ADHD) and being overweight/obesity: new data and meta-analysis. *Clinical psychology review* 43: 67-79, 2016.

107. Ogden CL, Carroll MD, Fryar CD, and Flegal KM. *Prevalence of obesity among adults and youth: United States*, 2011-2014: US Department of Health and Human Services, Centers for Disease Control and Prevention, National Center for Health Statistics, 2015.

108. Okura T, Nakata Y, and Tanaka K. Effects of exercise intensity on physical fitness and risk factors for coronary heart disease. *Obesity* 11: 1131-1139, 2003.

109. Palmieri-Smith RM, Cameron KL, DiStefano LJ, Driban JB, Pietrosimone B, Thomas AC, Tourville TW, and Consortium ATO. The Role of Athletic Trainers in Preventing and Managing Posttraumatic Osteoarthritis in Physically Active Populations: a Consensus Statement of the Athletic Trainers' Osteoarthritis Consortium. *Journal of Athletic Training* 52: 610-623, 2017.

110. Pälve KS, Pahkala K, Magnussen CG, Koivistoinen T, Juonala M, Kähönen M, Lehtimäki T, Rönnemaa T, Viikari JS, and Raitakari OT. Association of physical activity in childhood and early adulthood with carotid artery elasticity 21 years later: the cardiovascular risk in Young Finns Study. *Journal of the American Heart Association* 3: e000594, 2014.

111. Pandey A, Garg S, Khunger M, Darden D, Ayers C, Kumbhani DJ, Mayo HG, de Lemos JA, and Berry JD. Dose response relationship between physical activity and risk of heart failure: a meta-analysis. *Circulation*: CIRCULATIONAHA. 115.015853, 2015.

112. Park Y-MM, Sui X, Liu J, Zhou H, Kokkinos PF, Lavie CJ, Hardin JW, and Blair SN. The effect of cardiorespiratory fitness on age-related lipids and lipoproteins. *Journal of the American College of Cardiology* 65: 2091-2100, 2015.

113. Penedo FJ and Dahn JR. Exercise and well-being: a review of mental and physical health benefits associated with physical activity. *Current opinion in psychiatry* 18: 189-193, 2005.

114. Pinto PR, Rocco DDFM, Okuda LS, Machado-Lima A, Castilho G, da Silva KS, Gomes DJ, de Souza Pinto R, Iborra RT, and da Silva Ferreira G. Aerobic exercise training enhances the in vivo cholesterol trafficking from macrophages to the liver independently of changes in the expression of genes involved in lipid flux in macrophages and aorta. *Lipids in health and disease* 14: 109, 2015.

115. Poehlman ET, Dvorak RV, DeNino WF, Brochu M, and Ades PA. Effects of resistance training and endurance training on insulin sensitivity in nonobese, young women: a controlled randomized trial. *The Journal of Clinical Endocrinology & Metabolism* 85: 2463-2468, 2000.

116. Qiu C, Zhou Q, Zhao X, and Zhang Z. High-density lipoprotein cholesterol efflux capacity is inversely associated with cardiovascular risk: a systematic review and meta-analysis. *Lipids in health and disease* 16: 212, 2017.

117. Rader DJ. Beyond high-density lipoprotein cholesterol levels. *Journal of the American College of Cardiology* 51: 2199-2211, 2008.

118. Radom-Aizik S, Zaldivar FP, Haddad F, and Cooper DM. Impact of brief exercise on circulating monocyte gene and microRNA expression: implications for atherosclerotic vascular disease. *Brain, behavior, and immunity* 39: 121-129, 2014.

119. Richmond SA, Fukuchi RK, Ezzat A, Schneider K, Schneider G, and Emery CA. Are joint injury, sport activity, physical activity, obesity, or occupational activities predictors for osteoarthritis? A systematic review. *journal of orthopaedic & sports physical therapy* 43: 515-B519, 2013.

120. Romacho T, Sánchez-Ferrer CF, and Peiró C. Visfatin/Nampt: an adipokine with cardiovascular impact. *Mediators of inflammation* 2013, 2013.

121. Rosenson RS, Brewer HB, Chapman MJ, Fazio S, Hussain MM, Kontush A, Krauss RM, Otvos JD, Remaley AT, and Schaefer EJ. HDL measures, particle heterogeneity, proposed nomenclature, and relation to atherosclerotic cardiovascular events. *Clinical chemistry* 57: 392-410, 2011.

122. Ross R, Blair SN, Arena R, Church TS, Després J-P, Franklin BA, Haskell WL, Kaminsky LA, Levine BD, and Lavie CJ. Importance of assessing cardiorespiratory fitness in clinical practice: a case for fitness as a clinical vital sign: a scientific statement from the American Heart Association. *Circulation*: CIR. 0000000000000461, 2016.

123. Sääkslahti A, Numminen P, Varstala V, Helenius H, Tammi A, Viikari J, and Välimäki I. Physical activity as a preventive measure for coronary heart disease risk factors in early childhood. *Scandinavian journal of medicine & science in sports* 14: 143-149, 2004.

124. Sagiv M and Goldbourt U. Influence of physical work on high density lipoprotein cholesterol: implications for the risk of coronary heart disease. *International journal of sports medicine* 15: 261-266, 1994.

125. Sakurai T, Ogasawara J, Shirato K, Izawa T, Oh-ishi S, Ishibashi Y, Radák Z, Ohno H, and Kizaki T. Exercise Training Attenuates the Dysregulated Expression of Adipokines and Oxidative Stress in White Adipose Tissue. *Oxidative medicine and cellular longevity* 2017, 2017.

126. Samitz G. Physical activity for decreasing cardiovascular mortality and total mortality. A public health perspective. *Wiener klinische Wochenschrift* 110: 589-596, 1998.

127. Santa Mina D, Alibhai S, Matthew A, Guglietti C, Steele J, Trachtenberg J, and Ritvo P. Exercise in clinical cancer care: a call to action and program development description. *Current Oncology* 19: e136, 2012.

128. Sattelmair J, Pertman J, Ding EL, Kohl HW, Haskell W, and Lee I-M. Dose response between physical activity and risk of coronary heart disease. *Circulation*: CIRCULATIONAHA. 110.010710, 2011.

129. Schnohr P, O'keefe JH, Lange P, Jensen GB, and Marott JL. Impact of persistence and non-persistence in leisure time physical activity on coronary heart disease and all-cause mortality: The Copenhagen City Heart Study. *European Journal of Preventive Cardiology* 24: 1615-1623, 2017.

130. Siegiel R, Miller K, and Jemal A. Cancer Statistics, 2017. *CA Cancer J Clin* 67: 7-30, 2017.

131. Sigal RJ, Kenny GP, Boulé NG, Wells GA, Prud'homme D, Fortier M, Reid RD, Tulloch H, Coyle D, and Phillips P. Effects of Aerobic Training, Resistance Training, or Both on Glycemic Control in Type 2 DiabetesA Randomized TrialEffects of Aerobic and Resistance Training on Glycemic Control in Type 2 Diabetes. *Annals of internal medicine* 147: 357-369, 2007.

132. Sigal RJ, Kenny GP, Wasserman DH, Castaneda-Sceppa C, and White RD. Physical activity/exercise and type 2 diabetes. *Diabetes care* 29: 1433-1438, 2006.

133. Smith CC, Dixon RA, Wynne AM, Theodorou L, Ong S-G, Subrayan S, Davidson SM, Hausenloy DJ, and Yellon DM. Leptin-induced cardioprotection involves JAK/STAT signaling that may be linked to the mitochondrial permeability transition pore. *American Journal of Physiology-Heart and Circulatory Physiology* 299: H1265-H1270, 2010.

134. Smith KB and Smith MS. Obesity statistics. *Primary Care: Clinics in office practice* 43: 121-135, 2016.

135. Stephens T. Physical activity and mental health in the United States and Canada: evidence from four population surveys. *Preventive medicine* 17: 35-47, 1988.

136. Strahler J, Rohleder N, and Wolf JM. Acute psychosocial stress induces differential short-term changes in catecholamine sensitivity of stimulated inflammatory cytokine production. *Brain, behavior, and immunity* 43: 139-148, 2015.

137. Sutton A, Muir K, Mockett S, and Fentem P. A case-control study to investigate the relation between low and moderate levels of physical activity and osteoarthritis of the knee using data collected as part of the Allied Dunbar National Fitness Survey. *Annals of the rheumatic diseases* 60: 756-764, 2001.

138. Swain DP and Franklin BA. Comparison of cardioprotective benefits of vigorous versus moderate intensity aerobic exercise. *The American journal of cardiology* 97: 141-147, 2006.

139. Sweeney G. Cardiovascular effects of leptin. *Nature Reviews Cardiology* 7: 22-29, 2010.

140. Swift DL, Lavie CJ, Johannsen NM, Arena R, Earnest CP, O'Keefe JH, Milani RV, Blair SN, and Church TS. Physical activity, cardiorespiratory fitness, and exercise training in primary and secondary coronary prevention. *Circulation Journal* 77: 281-292, 2013.

141. Szostak J and Laurant P. The forgotten face of regular physical exercise: a 'natural' anti-atherogenic activity. *Clinical Science* 121: 91-106, 2011.

142. Tanasescu M, Leitzmann MF, Rimm EB, Willett WC, Stampfer MJ, and Hu FB. Exercise type and intensity in relation to coronary heart disease in men. *Jama* 288: 1994-2000, 2002.

143. Tchernof A and Després J-P. Pathophysiology of human visceral obesity: an update. *Physiological reviews* 93: 359-404, 2013.

144. Thompson PD, Buchner D, Piña IL, Balady GJ, Williams MA, Marcus BH, Berra K, Blair SN, Costa F, and Franklin B. Exercise and physical activity in the prevention and treatment of atherosclerotic cardiovascular disease. *Circulation* 107: 3109-3116, 2003.

145. Torgerson DJ and Bell-Syer SE. Hormone replacement therapy and prevention of nonvertebral fractures: a meta-analysis of randomized trials. *Jama* 285: 2891-2897, 2001.

146. Tran G, Smith TO, Grice A, Kingsbury SR, McCrory P, and Conaghan PG. Does sports participation (including level of performance and previous injury) increase risk of osteoarthritis? A systematic review and meta-analysis. *Br J Sports Med* 50: 1459-1466, 2016.

147. van der Steeg WA, Holme I, Boekholdt SM, Larsen ML, Lindahl C, Stroes ES, Tikkanen MJ, Wareham NJ, Faergeman O, and Olsson AG. High-density lipoprotein cholesterol, high-density lipoprotein particle size, and apolipoprotein AI: significance for cardiovascular risk: the IDEAL and EPIC-Norfolk studies. *Journal of the American College of Cardiology* 51: 634-642, 2008.

148. Vergeer M, Holleboom AG, Kastelein JJ, and Kuivenhoven JA. The HDL hypothesis: does high-density lipoprotein protect from atherosclerosis? *Journal of lipid research* 51: 2058-2073, 2010.

149. Vijan S. Type 2 diabetes. *Annals of internal medicine* 152: ITC3-1-1, 2010.

150. Wahid A, Manek N, Nichols M, Kelly P, Foster C, Webster P, Kaur A, Smith CF, Wilkins E, and Rayner M. Quantifying the Association Between Physical Activity and Cardiovascular Disease and Diabetes: A Systematic Review and Meta Analysis. *Journal of the American Heart Association* 5: e002495, 2016.

151. Warburton DE, Nicol CW, and Bredin SS. Health benefits of physical activity: the evidence. *Canadian medical association journal* 174: 801-809, 2006.

152. Watson S, Weeks B, Weis L, Horan S, and Beck B. Heavy resistance training is safe and improves bone, function, and stature in postmenopausal women with low to very low bone mass: novel early findings from the LIFTMOR trial. *Osteoporosis International* 26: 2889-2894, 2015.

153. Wei C, Penumetcha M, Santanam N, Liu Y-G, Garelnabi M, and Parthasarathy S. Exercise might favor reverse cholesterol transport and lipoprotein clearance: potential mechanism for its anti-atherosclerotic effects. *Biochimica et Biophysica Acta (BBA)-General Subjects* 1723: 124-127, 2005.

154. Wei M, Schwertner HA, and Blair SN. The association between physical activity, physical fitness, and type 2 diabetes mellitus. *Comprehensive therapy* 26: 176-182, 2000.

155. Weyer C, Funahashi T, Tanaka S, Hotta K, Matsuzawa Y, Pratley RE, and Tataranni PA. Hypoadiponectinemia in obesity and type 2 diabetes: close association with insulin resistance and hyperinsulinemia. *The Journal of Clinical Endocrinology & Metabolism* 86: 1930-1935, 2001.

156. Whelton PK, Carey RM, Aronow WS, Casey DE, Collins KJ, Himmelfarb CD, DePalma SM, Gidding S, Jamerson KA, and Jones DW. 2017 ACC/AHA/AAPA/ABC/ACPM/AGS/ APhA/ASH/ASPC/NMA/PCNA Guideline for the Prevention, Detection, Evaluation, and Management of High Blood Pressure in Adults: A Report of the American College of Cardiology/American Heart Association Task Force on Clinical Practice Guidelines. *Journal of the American College of Cardiology*, 2017.

157. Wiskemann J and Huber G. Physical exercise as adjuvant therapy for patients undergoing hematopoietic stem cell transplantation. *Bone marrow transplantation* 41: 321-329, 2008.

158. Zhang J, Xu J, Wang J, Wu C, Xu Y, Wang Y, Deng F, Wang Z, Chen X, and Wu M. Prognostic usefulness of serum cholesterol efflux capacity in patients with coronary artery disease. *The American journal of cardiology* 117: 508-514, 2016.

159. Zhu K, Hunter M, James A, Lim E, Cooke B, and Walsh J. Discordance between fat mass index and body mass index is associated with reduced bone mineral density in women but not in men: the Busselton healthy ageing study. *Osteoporosis International* 28: 259-268, 2017.

160. Zipes DP, Camm AJ, Borggrefe M, Buxton AE, Chaitman B, Fromer M, Gregoratos G, Klein G, Moss AJ, and Myerburg RJ. ACC/AHA/ESC 2006 guidelines for management of patients with ventricular arrhythmias and the prevention of sudden cardiac death: a report of the American College of Cardiology/American Heart Association Task Force and the European Society of Cardiology Committee for Practice Guidelines (Writing Committee to Develop guidelines for management of patients with ventricular arrhythmias and the prevention of sudden cardiac death) developed in collaboration with the European Heart Rhythm Association and the Heart Rhythm Society. *Europace* 8: 746-837, 2006.

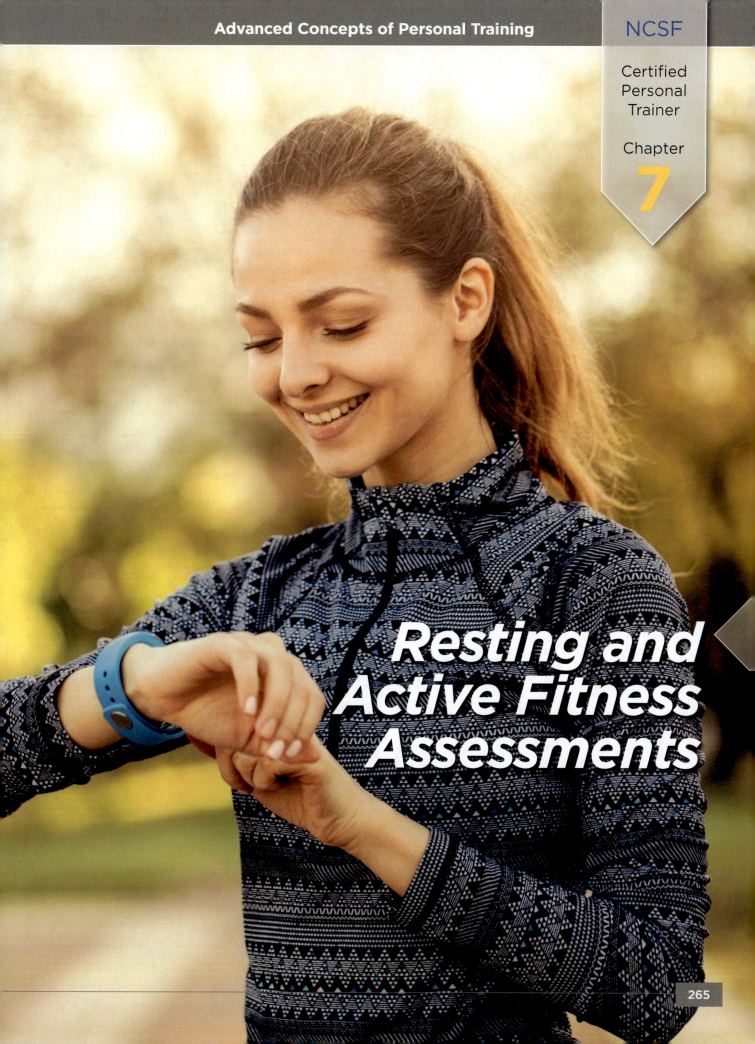

Resting Cardiovascular Tests

A comprehensive pre-exercise physical evaluation should be conducted in order to safely clear clients for fitness testing. These evaluations do not require physical activity and therefore, can be safely used to help establish participation status. Resting measurements are considered part of the laboratory process for pre-exercise screening. This collection of data provides physical information about the body's current condition at rest. The resting battery's purpose is to establish physical measures that can predict potential risk. These measurements include resting heart rate (RHR), blood pressure, body composition, height, weight, waist girth, body mass index (BMI), and standing posture. In addition, it may be worthwhile to evaluate blood chemistry to aid in the decision-making process and subsequent program development.

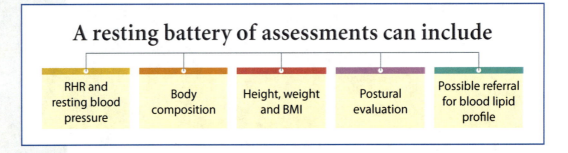

◆ Measurement Discrimination and Organization

Controllable factors that can affect the resting physical state should be accounted for and mitigated to ensure an efficient and effective assessment process. In some cases, external and internal variables can cause alterations within the body, so evaluators must recognize what conditions may adversely affect the outcome measures. Pretest readiness information and clear instructions enhance assessment accuracy. In addition, sleep, hydration, medications, and stimulants, like caffeine, are often controlled prior to testing, as they may reduce measurement legitimacy. The environment in which the measures are taken, the calibration of equipment, the technician's experience level, and the test subject's knowledge and understanding of the procedures also affect the testing outcomes. Accurate testing also requires knowledge, precision, organization, and experience, and a high level of discrimination: in other words, the level of rigor applied to measurement technique, consistency, adherence to protocol, and overall attention to detail during evaluation. The more discriminating a tester is, the more likely the test is to be valid and provide reliable results. Planning in advance, practicing the test, explaining the instructions to test subjects, and ensuring all equipment is available and operating properly all contribute to improved test performance and discrimination.

◆ Resting Heart Rate

RHR provides an indication of the heart's performance under non-stressed conditions. Numerous factors can alter heart rate from normal RHR measures, including lack of sleep, dehydration, medications, drugs or stimulants, alcohol, previous exercise, and real or perceived stress. Heart rate increases in response to catecholamines and stress hormones, which may be released due to both physical and psychological stimuli. Controlling external and internal influences enables proper measurement of heart efficiency. Heart rate is a factor of blood output and oxygen extraction, so when the heart expels appropriate amounts of oxygen-rich blood and the tissues can proficiently extract the oxygen, the heart functions well, causing a low RHR. It does not take much work for the heart to run a healthy and lean body. Measures of RHR among elite endurance athletes suggest that a very efficient heart will require only around 30-40 bpm at rest.

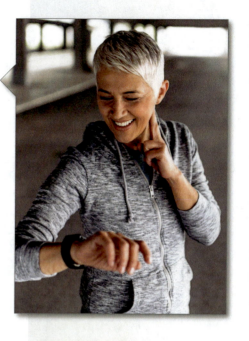

The combination of the following can allow the heart to run at reduced workloads:

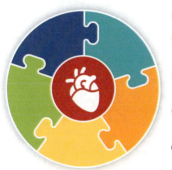

- High stroke volume
- Competent oxygen extraction capabilities *(expressed as A-V O$_2$ difference)*
- Adequate hydration to ensure proper hematocrit levels
- Adequate electrolyte intake to ensure proper ionic balance
- A low body mass *(the lighter the body is, the less energy it requires)*

When the heart is detrained, as in the sedentary population, it becomes inefficient and must function at higher rates, even when oxygen demand remains the same. Low stroke volume, poor oxygen extraction capability, increased fat mass, lower hemoglobin levels, reduced blood plasma, and unregulated stress hormones can cause elevations in RHR. Deconditioned individuals often have RHR in the 80s. Interestingly, factors that cause an elevated RHR eventually lead to its dysfunction. By contrast, aerobic exercise, weight management, proper hydration, and physical activity reduce RHR measures and consequently, lead to a healthier, more efficient cardiac muscle.

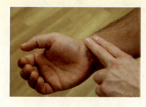

Assessing the Radial Pulse

1. Assessing resting heart rates requires a calm and relaxed physiological enviromnent. Any stimulus, perceived stress, or anxiety will cause the heart rate to accelerate beyond its resting requirements.
2. Personal trainers should instruct clients to avoid stimulants, such as caffeine and tobacco products, prior to assessing the pulse.
3. During the assessment, the client should not talk, as this can also elevate the heart rate. Have clients sit or lie down and place the arm to be assessed on a supportive structure. Have them maintain the position for two to five minutes to ease the postural shift and talk to them to reduce the anxiety of being tested.
4. Next, identify the site for measurement. Keep the arm supported at approximately heart height and palpate the radial pulse using the index and middle fingers.
5. For resting heart rate, the assessment should be for 60 seconds. Exercise heart rate can use a 15 second pulse count multiplied by four. Multiple recordings on subsequent visits will help predict an average waking resting heart rate.
6. If the value is consistently above 100 beats · min^{-1} the client should be referred to a physician before engaging in any physical testing or activity above walking.

◆ Blood Pressure

Another cardiovascular measure, blood pressure, illustrates the body's internal environment during resting metabolism. It has been well-documented that high blood pressure leads to numerous deleterious consequences for the body[22]. Vascular damage, stroke, kidney damage, and congestive heart failure all can occur in the presence of chronic hypertension. The latest recommendations are presented in the table below:

Blood Pressure Category	SYSTOLIC mm Hg (Upper Number)		DIASTOLIC mm Hg (Lower Number)
NORMAL	Less than 120	and	Less than 80
ELEVATED	120 - 129	and	Less than 80
HIGH BLOOD PRESSURE (Hypertension) Stage 1	130 - 139	or	80 - 89
HIGH BLOOD PRESSURE (Hypertension) Stage 2	140 or Higher	or	90 or Higher
HYPERTENSIVE CRISIS Consult Your Doctor Immediately	Higher than 180	and/or	Higher than 120

Blood pressure measurements above acceptable levels should be taken seriously and addressed as a key component in the exercise prescription and also incorporated into the behavior management strategy. It is important to inform clients about the threat of high blood pressure and the damage it causes to the vessels. Worldwide prevalence of high blood pressure

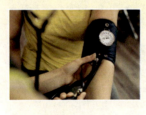

Assessing Blood Pressure

1. Have the subject sit in a chair with feet flat on the floor and arm supported by a desk or table.
2. Place the appropriate sized cuff around the right arm so that the bottom of the cuff is two fingers from the flexion crease of the elbow.
3. The arm used for the assessment should be at the same elevation as the heart. If using an electronic device, be sure the sensor is over the brachial artery.
4. A cuff that is too small will falsely increase the reading, whereas a cuff that is too large will have the opposite effect.
5. Inflate the cuff to 165 mmHg for females and 185 mmHg for males or 20 mmHg above the previous systolic reading. Let the client know you will take the measurement twice to validate the initial measure. This will prevent anxiety if the client suspects the second measure is being taken because something was wrong with the first reading.

Note: Hypertension cannot be diagnosed by a personal trainer even though it seems obvious given elevated measures on 3 different days. Clients with a systolic blood pressure ≥130 and/or a diastolic pressure ≥80 mmHg should be referred to their physician for proper diagnosis. If the measures are above 100 mmHg diastolic or 160 mmHg systolic, medical referral should be required before any activity participation.

is 1.3 billion, and approximately 103 million Americans are hypertensive, with 46% of adults over age 20 presenting with the disease [4, 22]. This statistic suggests that nearly half of all adults could benefit from hiring an exercise professional.

◆ Lipid Screening

Only a qualified health care professional can perform a blood lipid and chemistry profile. Information gained from a complete blood analysis helps in making program and behavioral modifications based on physician recommendations. Fasting blood glucose and blood lipid profiles are of particular importance, as they can identify certain diseases [2]. These blood values should reflect positive adaptations with regular exercise participation. Therefore, elevated measures should not be viewed as an impediment to aerobic exercise participation but as a risk factor that warrants physician review. For adults over 20 years of age, the National Cholesterol Education Program recommends that blood lipid profiles be evaluated every five years. While less-commonly followed, the National Heart, Lung, and Blood Institute recommends a cholesterol screening test between the ages of 9 and 11, and another cholesterol screening test between the ages of 17 and 21. Obesity and high blood pressure compound issues related to certain blood profiles, so individuals with comorbidities should consult with a physician for a management plan which includes timely re-evaluations.

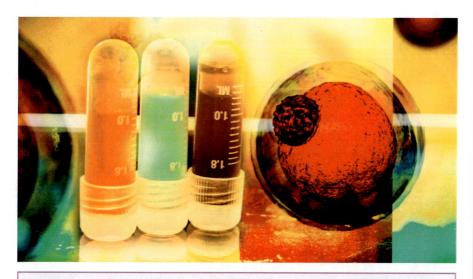

Classification of Cholesterol and Triglyceride Levels in mg/dL

Non-HDL-C*
<130	Desirable
130-159	Above desirable
160-189	Borderline high
190-219	High
≥220	Very High

LDL-C
<100	Desirable
100-129	Above desirable
130-159	Borderline high
160-189	High
≥190	Very High

HDL-C
<40 (men)	Low
<50 (women)	Low

Triglycerides
<150	Normal
150-199	Borderline high
200-499	High
≥500	Very high†

Potential medical referral values: Cholesterol ratio >5, total cholesterol >240 mg/dl, total triglycerides >200 mg/dl

HDL-C, high-density lipoprotein cholesterol; LDL-C, low-density lipoprotein cholesterol.

*Non-HDL-C = total cholesterol minus HDL-C.

†Severe hypertriglyceridemia is another term used for very high triglycerides in pharmaceutical product labeling.

National Lipid Association recommendations for patient-centered management of dyslipidemia: part 1 – full report. [7]

Treatment Goals for Cholesterol and Apo B – Based on Relative CVD Risk

Risk category	Treatment goal		
	Non-HDL-C	LDL-C	Apo B*
Low	<130	<100	<90
Moderate	<130	<100	<90
High	<130	<100	<90
Very high	<100	<70	<80

Apo, apolipoprotein; LDL-C, low-density lipoprotein cholesterol; Non-HDL-C, non-high-density lipoprotein cholesterol.

*Apo B is a secondary, optional target of treatment.

National Lipid Association recommendations for patient-centered management of dyslipidemia: part 1 – full report. [7]

QUICK INSIGHT

While an annual physical examination is often recommended as part of an ongoing prevention plan, physical examinations by a physician are not required prior to exercise participation for the majority of clients. Exercise professionals should encourage their clients to comply with physician recommendations for physicals and checkups. This is particularly important as people get older. When physiological problems are identified early, it makes them easier to manage, and in most cases, the consequential effects can be minimized. Individuals who go long periods of time without any physical assessment may place themselves at an unnecessarily high risk for disease or related complications. Pre-disease states respond more positively to proactive and early intervention compared to when they reach diagnostic criteria levels.

Body Composition and Anthropometrics

Obesity is a well-known comorbid disorder that places its sufferers at a heightened risk for developing many health problems: type 2 diabetes mellitus (T2DM), hypertension, dyslipidemia, cardiovascular disease (CVD), stroke, **sleep apnea**, **gout**, osteoarthritis, colorectal and prostate cancer in men, and, in women, endometrial (uterine) cancer, breast, and gall bladder cancer [13]. At one time, it was only classified as a comorbidity and a risk factor for other diseases; however, it is now recognized as an independent disease by the American Medical Association [10]. Individuals who become obese dramatically increase their risk for other diseases due to the chronic inflammatory response associated with excess body fat, a state that also promotes deleterious orthopedic problems. Measuring relative body fat is important, as body fat compositions above specific values are associated with higher rates of other diseases. Individuals with measured body fat compositions above 25% (males) and 32% (females) present an elevated risk for having or developing the comorbid diseases listed above. Individuals who reach measures of 30% (males) and 40% (females) respectively, are classified as morbidly-obese. Due to the likelihood of chronic comorbidities associated with morbid obesity, individuals who fall into this category require a physician's referral before exercise testing or

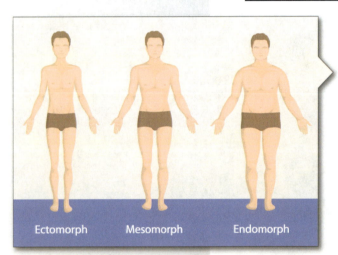

Ectomorph · Mesomorph · Endomorph

DEFINITIONS

Sleep apnea –

A potentially dangerous sleep disorder where the sufferer repeatedly stops breathing for short periods of time during sleep; the airway is intermittently blocked which often results in loud snoring or choking noises – usually waking the person for a quick moment before falling back asleep.

Gout –

A type of inflammatory arthritis that promotes joint redness, swelling, and pain; there are various nutritional triggers such as dehydration, sugary beverages, alcohol, red meat or seafood and it may also be instigated by surgery; if left untreated it can cause irreversible joint and/or kidney damage.

Classifying Obesity

- **Body fat** = males <20% for fit-healthy; females <26% for fit-healthy
- **Stage 1 Obesity** = males ≥25% body fat; females ≥32% body fat; >38% old age
- **Stage 2 Obesity** = males ≥30% body fat; females ≥40% body fat
- **Stage 3 Obesity** = males ≥35% body fat; females ≥45% body fat
- **High risk** = males ≥40 inch waist circumference; females ≥35 inch (signifies significant visceral adiposity)

participation. BMI and stature-weight index scores are most commonly used for obesity classification purposes. In addition to the role they serve in obesity classification, height and weight measurements should also be recorded for tracking and computing purposes.

BMI is the current metric used by physicians worldwide to determine risk associated with body fat. A value of 25 is the initial risk indicator; values above 27 are considered high risk, and a value of 30 or more indicates a diagnosis of obesity. Keep in mind that BMI-risk predictions are less meaningful among leaner, muscular individuals. For these subjects, waist circumference and body composition analysis serve as better risk predictors.

BMI Metric and English Calculations

Measurement Units	Formula and Calculation
Kilograms and meters (or centimeters)	Formula: weight (kg) / [height (m)]^2 With the metric system, the formula for BMI is weight in kilograms divided by height in meters squared. Because height is commonly measured in centimeters, divide height in centimeters by 100 to obtain height in meters. Example: Weight = 68 kg, Height = 165 cm (1.65 m) Calculation: 68 ÷ (1.65)^2 = 24.98
Pounds and inches	Formula: weight (lbs.) / [height (in)]^2 x 703 Calculate BMI by dividing weight in pounds (lbs.) by height in inches (in) squared and multiplying by a conversion factor of 703. Example: Weight = 150 lbs., Height = 5'5" (65") Calculation: [150 ÷ (65)^2] x 703 = 24.96

Classification of Overweight and Obesity by BMI, Waist Circumference, and Associated Disease Risk

	BMI (kg/m2)	Obesity Class	Disease Risk* (Relative to Normal Weight and Waist Circumference)	
			Men ≤40 in (≤102 cm) Women ≤35 in (≤88 cm)	>40 in (>102 cm) >35 in (>88 cm)
Underweight	<18.5		–	–
Normal†	18.5 - 24.9		–	–
Overweight	25.0 - 29.9		Increased	Increased
Obesity	30.0 - 34.9	I	High	High
	35.0 - 39.9	II	Very High	Very High
Extreme Obesity	≥40	III	Extremely High	Extremely High

*Disease risk for type 2 diabetes, hypertension, and CVD.
†Increased waist circumference can also be a marker for increased risk even in persons of normal weight.
2013 AHA/ACC/TOS Guidelines for the Management of Overweight and Obesity in Adults [8].

The formula for BMI is identical for both adults and children; however, it is interpreted differently in children. BMI measurements of children and adolescents should be age and gender specific due to the compositional changes that occur during development in boys and girls. The Centers for Disease Control (CDC) produces BMI-for-age growth charts, which take these differences into account and present them as a percentile ranking. Obesity among 2 to 19-year-olds is defined as a BMI at or above the 95th percentile of children of the same age and sex.

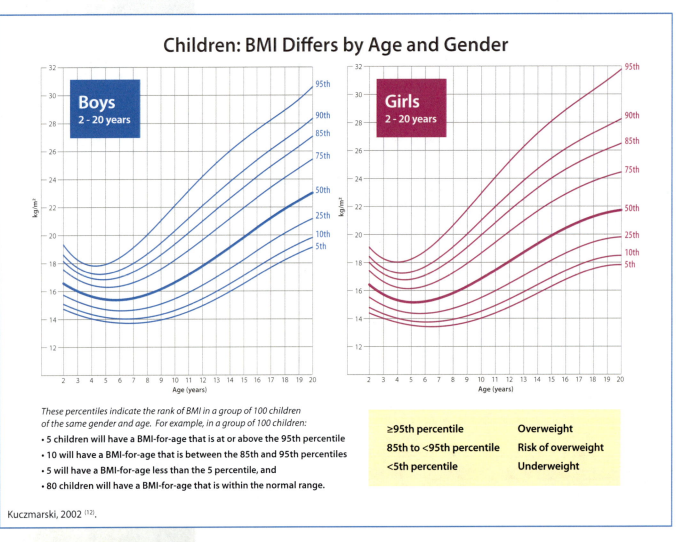

Children: BMI Differs by Age and Gender

These percentiles indicate the rank of BMI in a group of 100 children of the same gender and age. For example, in a group of 100 children:

- 5 children will have a BMI-for-age that is at or above the 95th percentile
- 10 will have a BMI-for-age that is between the 85th and 95th percentiles
- 5 will have a BMI-for-age less than the 5 percentile, and
- 80 children will have a BMI-for-age that is within the normal range.

≥95th percentile	Overweight
85th to <95th percentile	Risk of overweight
<5th percentile	Underweight

Kuczmarski, 2002 [12].

DEFINITIONS

Air displacement plethysmography –

A scientifically-validated method to measure human body composition that predicts body density based on volume and weight.

BMI should be used advisedly, as obesity diagnosis seems to suffer from a relatively high degree of misclassification compared with direct body fat measures (BF%). In a study of 6,123 Caucasian subjects aged 18 – 80 years (31% males and 69% females, respectively), researchers found flaws relating to classification by BMI: 29% of subjects designated as lean, and 80% of individuals categorized as overweight by BMI standards had a body-fat percentage that actually classified them as obese using **air-displacement plethysmography** [5]. Individuals with normal-weight obesity and metabolically healthy obesity are presumed to represent between 8-10% of the population, suggesting the number of obese individuals in the US is likely underestimated by more than 30 million [19]. This situation speaks to both health and financial concerns, as these individuals are not factored in to the 37.5% of the adult population in the United States who are considered obese.

◆ Girth/Circumference Values

Waist circumference also strongly predicts risk for developing metabolic and cardiovascular disease. It is a preferred measurement for disease prediction in individuals with BMI > 35 [18]. Waist girth helps identify central storage of both subcutaneous and visceral fat. Individuals with high BMI values and large centralized girth present with a notably elevated risk of disease, compared to those with low measures in both [3, 18]. Males exceeding 40 inches and females exceeding 35 inches in waist circumference are considered to be at high risk. Some arguments suggest these values should be lowered for physically inactive individuals and certain ethnic groups. Additionally, when all body-size measures (waist and hip circumference and body-mass index) are high, individuals experience an increased risk for cardiometabolic disease and venous thrombosis [16]. Regardless, when both BMI and central girth are high, exercise professionals should recommend clients see a physician for blood lipid profiling, hypertension-risk monitoring, and fasting glucose measures to ensure they do not already suffer from hyperlipidemia, hypertension, or glucose intolerance. Other areas with predictive circumference values are the neck, forearm, and calf, as they tend to be non-fat storage areas: ideal locations for a reference measurement. When the neck is used as an independent variable to predict disease among nonathletic populations, risk increased with size [2, 23]. Optimal neck circumference "cut-off points" to predict metabolic syndrome are suggested at >38 cm (~15") for men and >34 cm (13.5") for women respectively [17]. The calf and forearm represent novel circumference sites linked with risk prediction among older adults. Interestingly, the association of low measures predicts increased risk of premature mortality in the elderly.

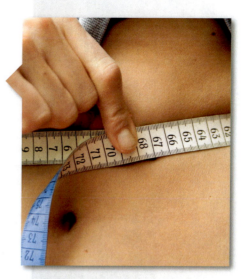

2-3 GIRTH BODY FAT ESTIMATION

The 2-3 girth method of body fat estimation can also be a viable option to predict body fat, particularly when working with the obese population and accurate caliper readings cannot be made. The advantage of the 2-3 girth measurement is the assessment utilizes two circumference values for men and 3 circumference values for women to estimate body fat. This may reduce the standard estimation of error (SEE) compared to other assessments when determining body composition. The standard estimation of error is about 3.5%.

Calculating your 2-3 girth measurement requires the use of Tables A and B on the following pages. The percent body fat can be found by using the derived circumference value (inches) and identifying the percent fat score that corresponds to the calculated value from the circumference measurements.

Step #1   Measure the appropriate anatomical positions.

Men:	Abdominal girth circumference	_____ in.
	Neck circumference	_____ in.
Women:	Upper abdominal circumference	_____ in.
	Hip circumference	_____ in.
	Neck circumference	_____ in.

Step #2   Find the derived circumference value (CV)

Men: (_____ Abdominal – _____ Neck) = _____ CV

Women: (_____ Upper abdominal + _____ Hip) = _____ – _____ Neck = _____ CV

Enter your derived Circumference Value (CV) here   _____

Step #3   Use the following tables (**Table A for Men** and **Table B for Women**) to find the estimated body fat % by matching the derived circumference value in the left hand column with your height in inches across the top.

Enter your 2-3 Girth body fat estimation here   _____ %

GIRTH/CIRCUMFERENCE MEASUREMENTS

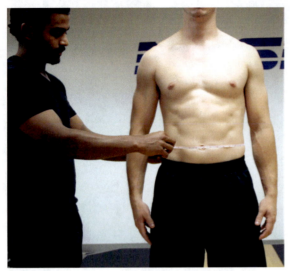

Abdominal
Across the umbilicus

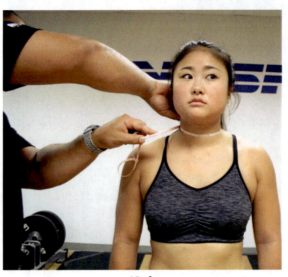

Neck
Across the center of the neck

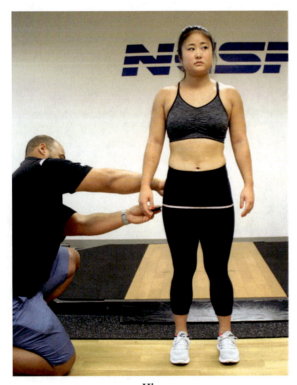

Hip
Across the thickest point of the hip
Feet should be inside the shoulders or together

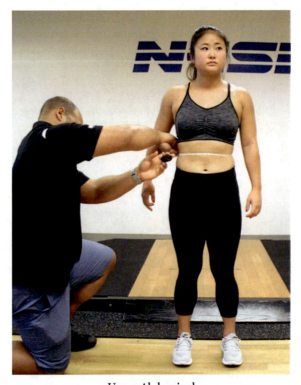

Upper Abdominal
Half way between the umbilicus and xyphoid process

TABLE A Men's BF % 2-3 Girth

Circumference value (in)	HEIGHT (IN)									
	60.0	60.5	61	61.5	62	62.5	63	63.5	64	64.5
11	3	2	2	2	2	1	1	1	1	1
11.5	4	4	4	3	3	3	3	2	2	2
12	6	5	5	5	5	4	4	4	4	3
12.5	7	7	6	6	6	6	6	5	5	5
13	8	8	8	8	7	7	7	7	6	6
13.5	10	9	9	9	9	8	8	8	8	8
14	11	11	10	10	10	10	10	9	9	9
14.5	12	12	12	11	11	11	11	11	10	10
15	13	13	13	13	12	12	12	12	12	11
15.5	15	14	14	14	14	13	13	13	13	12
16	16	15	15	15	15	15	14	14	14	14
16.5	17	17	16	16	16	16	15	15	15	15
17	18	18	17	17	17	17	16	16	16	16
17.5	19	19	19	18	18	18	18	17	17	17
18	20	20	20	19	19	19	19	18	18	18
18.5	21	21	21	20	20	20	20	19	19	19
19	22	22	22	21	21	21	21	20	20	20
19.5	23	23	23	22	22	22	22	21	21	21
20	24	24	23	23	23	23	22	22	22	22
20.5	25	25	24	24	24	24	23	23	23	23
21	26	26	25	25	25	25	24	24	24	24
21.5	27	26	26	26	26	25	25	25	25	24
22	28	27	27	27	27	26	26	26	26	25
22.5	28	28	28	28	27	27	27	27	26	26
23	29	29	29	29	28	28	28	28	27	27
23.5	30	30	30	29	29	29	29	28	28	28
24	31	31	30	30	30	30	29	29	29	29
24.5	32	31	31	31	31	30	30	30	30	29
25	33	32	32	32	31	31	31	31	30	30
25.5	33	33	33	33	32	32	32	31	31	31
26	34	34	34	33	33	33	32	32	32	32
26.5	35	35	34	34	34	33	33	33	33	32
27	36	35	35	35	34	34	34	34	33	33
27.5	36	36	36	35	35	35	35	34	34	34
28	37	37	36	36	36	36	35	35	35	35
28.5	38	37	37	37	37	36	36	36	36	35
29	38	38	38	38	37	37	37	37	36	36
29.5	39	39	39	38	38	38	37	37	37	37
30	40	39	39	39	39	38	38	38	38	37
30.5	-	-	40	40	39	39	39	39	38	38
31	-	-	-	-	40	40	39	39	39	39
31.5	-	-	-	-	-	-	-	40	40	39
32.0-35.0	-	-	-	-	-	-	-	-	-	40

TABLE A Men's BF % 2-3 Girth

Circumference value (in)	HEIGHT (IN)									
	65	65.5	66	66.5	67	67.5	68	68.5	69	69.5
11	0	0	-	-	-	-	-	-	-	-
11.5	2	2	1	1	1	1	1	0	0	-
12	3	3	3	3	2	2	2	2	2	1
12.5	5	4	4	4	4	4	3	3	3	3
13	6	6	6	5	5	5	5	5	4	4
13.5	7	7	7	7	6	6	6	6	6	5
14	9	8	8	8	8	8	7	7	7	7
14.5	10	10	9	9	9	9	9	8	8	8
15	11	11	11	10	10	10	10	10	9	9
15.5	12	12	12	12	11	11	11	11	11	10
16	13	13	13	13	12	12	12	12	12	11
16.5	14	14	14	14	14	13	13	13	13	13
17	16	15	15	15	15	14	14	14	14	14
17.5	17	16	16	16	16	16	15	15	15	15
18	18	17	17	17	17	17	16	16	16	16
18.5	19	18	18	18	18	18	17	17	17	17
19	20	19	19	19	19	19	18	18	18	18
19.5	21	20	20	20	20	19	19	19	19	19
20	22	21	21	21	21	20	20	20	20	20
20.5	22	22	22	22	22	21	21	21	21	20
21	23	23	23	23	22	22	22	22	22	21
21.5	24	24	24	24	23	23	23	23	22	22
22	25	25	25	24	24	24	24	24	23	23
22.5	26	26	25	25	25	25	25	24	24	24
23	27	27	26	26	26	26	25	25	25	25
23.5	28	27	27	27	27	26	26	26	26	26
24	28	28	28	28	27	27	27	27	27	26
24.5	29	29	29	29	28	28	28	28	27	27
25	30	30	30	29	29	29	29	28	28	28
25.5	31	31	30	30	30	30	29	29	29	29
26	32	31	31	31	31	30	30	30	30	29
26.5	32	32	32	32	31	31	31	31	30	30
27	33	33	32	32	32	32	32	31	31	31
27.5	34	33	33	33	33	33	32	32	32	32
28	34	34	34	34	33	33	33	33	33	32
28.5	35	35	35	34	34	34	34	33	33	33
29	36	36	35	35	35	35	34	34	34	34
29.5	36	36	36	36	35	35	35	35	35	34
30	37	37	37	36	36	36	36	35	35	35
30.5	38	38	37	37	37	37	36	36	36	36
31	38	38	38	38	37	37	37	37	37	36
31.5	39	39	39	38	38	38	38	37	37	37
32	40	39	39	39	39	38	38	38	38	38
32.5	-	-	40	40	39	39	39	39	38	38
33	-	-	-	-	40	40	39	39	39	39
33.5	-	-	-	-	-	-	-	40	40	39
34	-	-	-	-	-	-	-	-	-	40
34.5	-	-	-	-	-	-	-	-	-	-
35.0	-	-	-	-	-	-	-	-	-	-

TABLE A Men's BF % 2-3 Girth

Circumference value (in)	HEIGHT (IN)									
	70	70.5	71	71.5	72	72.5	73	73.5	74	74.5
11	-	-	-	-	-	-	-	-	-	-
11.5	-	-	-	-	-	-	-	-	-	-
12	1	1	1	1	0	0	0	-	-	-
12.5	3	2	2	2	2	2	1	1	1	1
13	4	4	4	3	3	3	3	3	2	2
13.5	5	5	5	5	4	4	4	4	4	4
14	7	6	6	6	6	6	5	5	5	5
14.5	8	8	7	7	7	7	7	6	6	6
15	9	9	9	8	8	8	8	8	7	7
15.5	10	10	10	9	9	9	9	9	9	8
16	11	11	11	11	10	10	10	10	10	9
16.5	12	12	12	12	12	11	11	11	11	11
17	13	13	13	13	13	12	12	12	12	12
17.5	14	14	14	14	14	13	13	13	13	13
18	15	15	15	15	15	14	14	14	14	14
18.5	16	16	16	16	16	15	15	15	15	15
19	17	17	17	17	17	16	16	16	16	16
19.5	18	18	18	18	18	17	17	17	17	17
20	19	19	19	19	18	18	18	18	18	17
20.5	20	20	20	20	19	19	19	19	19	18
21	21	21	21	20	20	20	20	20	19	19
21.5	22	22	22	21	21	21	21	21	20	20
22	23	23	22	22	22	22	22	21	21	21
22.5	24	23	23	23	23	23	22	22	22	22
23	25	24	24	24	24	23	23	23	23	23
23.5	25	25	25	25	24	24	24	24	24	23
24	26	26	26	25	25	25	25	25	24	24
24.5	27	27	26	26	26	26	26	25	25	25
25	28	27	27	27	27	27	26	26	26	26
25.5	28	28	28	28	28	27	27	27	27	27
26	29	29	29	29	28	28	28	28	27	27
26.5	30	30	29	29	29	29	29	28	28	28
27	31	30	30	30	30	30	29	29	29	29
27.5	31	31	31	31	30	30	30	30	30	29
28	32	32	32	31	31	31	31	31	30	30
28.5	33	33	32	32	32	32	31	31	31	31
29	33	33	33	33	33	32	32	32	32	31
29.5	34	34	34	33	33	33	33	33	32	32
30	35	35	34	34	34	34	33	33	33	33
30.5	35	35	35	35	35	34	34	34	34	33
31	36	36	36	35	35	35	35	34	34	34
31.5	37	36	36	36	36	36	35	35	35	35
32	37	37	37	37	36	36	36	36	36	35
32.5	38	38	37	37	37	37	37	36	36	36
33	39	38	38	38	38	37	37	37	37	37
33.5	39	39	39	38	38	38	38	38	37	37
34	40	39	39	39	39	39	38	38	38	38
34.5	-	-	40	40	39	39	39	39	39	38
35.0	-	-	-	-	40	40	40	39	39	39

TABLE A Men's BF % 2-3 Girth

Circumference value (in)	HEIGHT (IN)									
	75	75.5	76	76.5	77	77.5	78	78.5	79	79.5
11	-	-	-	-	-	-	-	-	-	-
11.5	-	-	-	-	-	-	-	-	-	-
12	-	-	-	-	-	-	-	-	-	-
12.5	1	1	0	0	-	-	-	-	-	-
13	2	2	2	1	1	1	1	1	1	0
13.5	3	3	3	3	3	2	2	2	2	2
14	5	4	4	4	4	4	3	3	3	3
14.5	6	6	5	5	5	5	5	5	4	4
15	7	7	7	6	6	6	6	6	6	5
15.5	8	8	8	8	7	7	7	7	7	6
16	9	9	9	9	8	8	8	8	8	8
16.5	10	10	10	10	10	9	9	9	9	9
17	11	11	11	11	11	10	10	10	10	10
17.5	12	12	12	12	12	11	11	11	11	11
18	13	13	13	13	13	12	12	12	12	12
18.5	14	14	14	14	14	13	13	13	13	13
19	15	15	15	15	15	14	14	14	14	14
19.5	16	16	16	16	16	15	15	15	15	15
20	17	17	17	17	16	16	16	16	16	16
20.5	18	18	18	18	17	17	17	17	17	16
21	19	19	19	18	18	18	18	18	18	17
21.5	20	20	20	19	19	19	19	19	18	18
22	21	21	20	20	20	20	20	19	19	19
22.5	22	21	21	21	21	21	20	20	20	20
23	22	22	22	22	22	21	21	21	21	21
23.5	23	23	23	23	22	22	22	22	22	21
24	24	24	24	23	23	23	23	23	22	22
24.5	25	25	24	24	24	24	24	23	23	23
25	26	25	25	25	25	25	24	24	24	24
25.5	26	26	26	26	26	25	25	25	25	25
26	27	27	27	26	26	26	26	26	25	25
26.5	28	28	27	27	27	27	27	26	26	26
27	28	28	28	28	28	27	27	27	27	27
27.5	29	29	29	29	28	28	28	28	28	27
28	30	30	29	29	29	29	29	28	28	28
28.5	31	30	30	30	30	30	29	29	29	29
29	31	31	31	31	30	30	30	30	30	29
29.5	32	32	31	31	31	31	31	30	30	30
30	33	32	32	32	32	32	31	31	31	31
30.5	33	33	33	33	32	32	32	32	32	31
31	34	34	33	33	33	33	33	32	32	32
31.5	34	34	34	34	34	33	33	33	33	33
32	35	35	35	34	34	34	34	34	33	33
32.5	36	35	35	35	35	35	34	34	34	34
33	36	36	36	36	35	35	35	35	35	34
33.5	37	37	36	36	36	36	36	35	35	35
34	37	37	37	37	37	36	36	36	36	36
34.5	38	38	38	37	37	37	37	37	36	36
35.0	39	38	38	38	38	38	37	37	37	37
35.5	39	39	39	39	38	38	38	38	38	37
36	40	40	39	39	39	39	39	38	38	38
36.5	-	-	40	40	39	39	39	39	39	38
37	-	-	-	-	-	40	40	39	39	39
37.5	-	-	-	-	-	-	-	40	40	40
38	-	-	-	-	-	-	-	-	-	-
38.5	-	-	-	-	-	-	-	-	-	-

TABLE B Women's BF % 2-3 Girth

Circumference value (in)	HEIGHT (IN)									
	58	58.5	59	59.5	60	60.5	61	61.5	62	62.5
34.5	1	0	-	-	-	-	-	-	-	-
35	2	1	1	1	0	-	-	-	-	-
35.5	3	2	2	2	1	1	0	0	-	-
36	4	3	3	3	2	2	1	1	1	0
36.5	5	4	4	4	3	3	2	2	2	1
37	6	5	5	4	4	4	3	3	3	2
37.5	7	6	6	5	5	5	4	4	4	3
38	7	7	7	6	6	6	5	5	5	4
38.5	8	8	8	7	7	7	6	6	5	5
39	9	9	9	8	8	7	7	7	6	6
39.5	10	10	9	9	9	8	8	8	7	7
40	11	11	10	10	10	9	9	8	8	8
40.5	12	12	11	11	10	10	10	9	9	9
41	13	12	12	12	11	11	11	10	10	10
41.5	14	13	13	13	12	12	11	11	11	10
42	14	14	14	13	13	13	12	12	12	11
42.5	15	15	15	14	14	13	13	13	12	12
43	16	16	15	15	15	14	14	14	13	13
43.5	17	17	16	16	15	15	15	14	14	14
44	18	17	17	17	16	16	16	15	15	14
44.5	19	18	18	17	17	17	16	16	16	15
45	19	19	19	18	18	17	17	17	16	16
45.5	20	20	19	19	19	18	18	18	17	17
46	21	20	20	20	19	19	19	18	18	18
46.5	22	21	21	20	20	20	19	19	19	18
47	22	22	22	21	21	20	20	20	19	19
47.5	23	23	22	22	22	21	21	21	20	20
48	24	23	23	23	22	22	22	21	21	21
48.5	25	24	24	23	23	23	22	22	22	21
49	25	25	25	24	24	23	23	23	22	22
49.5	26	26	25	25	24	24	24	23	23	23
50	27	26	26	26	25	25	24	24	24	23
50.5	27	27	27	26	26	26	25	25	24	24
51	28	28	27	27	27	26	26	25	25	25
51.5	29	28	28	28	27	27	27	26	26	25
52	29	29	29	28	28	28	27	27	27	26
52.5	30	30	29	29	29	28	28	28	27	27
53	31	30	30	30	29	29	29	28	28	27
53.5	31	31	31	30	30	30	29	29	28	28
54	32	32	31	31	31	30	30	30	29	29
54.5	33	32	32	32	31	31	31	30	30	29
55	33	33	33	32	32	32	31	31	30	30
55.5	34	34	33	33	33	32	32	31	31	31
56	35	34	34	33	33	33	32	32	32	31
56.5	35	35	34	34	34	33	33	33	32	32
57	36	35	35	35	34	34	34	33	33	33
57.5	36	36	36	35	35	35	34	34	34	33
58	37	37	36	36	36	35	35	35	34	34
58.5	38	37	37	37	36	36	35	35	35	34
59	38	38	38	37	37	36	36	36	35	35
59.5	39	38	38	38	37	37	37	36	36	36
60	39	39	39	38	38	38	37	37	37	36
60.5	40	40	39	39	39	38	38	37	37	37
61	41	40	40	39	39	39	38	38	38	37
61.5	41	41	40	40	40	39	39	39	38	38
62	42	41	41	41	40	40	40	39	39	38
62.5	42	42	42	41	41	40	40	40	39	39
63	43	42	42	42	41	41	41	40	40	40

TABLE B Women's BF % 2-3 Girth

Circumference value (in)	\multicolumn{10}{c}{HEIGHT (IN)}
	63	63.5	64	64.5	65	65.5	66	66.5	67	67.5
34.5	-	-	-	-	-	-	-	-	-	-
35	-	-	-	-	-	-	-	-	-	-
35.5	-	-	-	-	-	-	-	-	-	-
36	0	-	-	-	-	-	-	-	-	-
36.5	1	1	0	-	-	-	-	-	-	-
37	2	2	1	1	1	0	-	-	-	-
37.5	3	3	2	2	2	1	1	1	0	-
38	4	3	3	3	2	2	2	1	1	1
38.5	5	4	4	4	3	3	3	2	2	2
39	6	5	5	5	4	4	4	3	3	3
39.5	7	6	6	6	5	5	5	4	4	4
40	7	7	7	6	6	6	5	5	5	4
40.5	8	8	8	7	7	7	6	6	6	5
41	9	9	8	8	8	7	7	7	6	6
41.5	10	10	9	9	9	8	8	8	7	7
42	11	10	10	10	9	9	9	8	8	8
42.5	12	11	11	11	10	10	10	9	9	9
43	12	12	12	11	11	11	10	10	10	9
43.5	13	13	13	12	12	12	11	11	11	10
44	14	14	13	13	13	12	12	12	11	11
44.5	15	15	14	14	14	13	13	13	12	12
45	16	15	15	15	14	14	14	13	13	13
45.5	16	16	16	15	15	15	14	14	14	13
46	17	17	17	16	16	16	15	15	15	14
46.5	18	18	17	17	17	16	16	16	15	15
47	19	18	18	18	17	17	17	16	16	16
47.5	19	19	19	18	18	18	17	17	17	16
48	20	20	20	19	19	18	18	18	18	17
48.5	21	21	20	20	20	19	19	19	18	18
49	22	21	21	21	20	20	20	19	19	19
49.5	22	22	22	21	21	21	20	20	20	19
50	23	23	22	22	22	21	21	21	20	20
50.5	24	23	23	23	22	22	22	21	21	21
51	24	24	24	23	23	23	22	22	22	21
51.5	25	25	24	24	24	23	23	23	22	22
52	26	25	25	25	24	24	24	23	23	23
52.5	26	26	26	25	25	25	24	24	24	23
53	27	27	26	26	26	25	25	25	24	24
53.5	28	27	27	27	26	26	26	25	25	25
54	28	28	28	27	27	27	26	26	26	25
54.5	29	29	28	28	28	27	27	27	26	26
55	30	29	29	29	28	28	28	27	27	27
55.5	30	30	30	29	29	29	28	28	28	27
56	31	31	30	30	30	29	29	29	28	28
56.5	32	31	31	31	30	30	30	29	29	29
57	32	32	32	31	31	31	30	30	30	29
57.5	33	32	32	32	31	31	31	30	30	30
58	33	33	33	32	32	32	31	31	31	30
58.5	34	34	33	33	33	32	32	32	31	31
59	35	34	34	34	33	33	33	32	32	32
59.5	35	35	35	34	34	34	33	33	33	32
60	36	35	35	35	34	34	34	33	33	33
60.5	36	36	36	35	35	35	34	34	34	33
61	37	37	36	36	36	35	35	35	34	34
61.5	38	37	37	37	36	36	36	35	35	35
62	38	38	37	37	37	36	36	36	35	35
62.5	39	38	38	38	37	37	37	36	36	36
63	39	39	39	38	38	38	37	37	37	36

TABLE B Women's BF % 2-3 Girth

Circumference value (in)	HEIGHT (IN)									
	63	63.5	64	64.5	65	65.5	66	66.5	67	67.5
64	40	40	40	39	39	39	38	38	38	37
64.5	41	41	40	40	40	39	39	39	38	38
65	41	41	41	40	40	40	39	39	39	38
65.5	42	42	41	41	41	40	40	40	39	39
66	43	42	42	41	41	41	40	40	40	39
66.5	43	43	42	42	42	41	41	41	40	40
67	44	43	43	43	42	42	41	41	41	41
67.5	44	44	43	43	43	42	42	42	41	41
68	45	44	44	44	43	43	43	42	42	42
68.5	-	45	44	44	44	43	43	43	42	42
69	-	-	45	45	44	44	44	43	43	43
69.5	-	-	-	-	45	44	44	44	43	43
70	-	-	-	-	-	45	45	44	44	44
70.5	-	-	-	-	-	-	-	45	44	44
71.0-75.5	-	-	-	-	-	-	-	-	45	45

TABLE B Women's BF % 2-3 Girth

Circumference value (in)	HEIGHT (IN)									
	68	68.5	69	69.5	70	70.5	71	71.5	72	72.5
34.5	-	-	-	-	-	-	-	-	-	-
35	-	-	-	-	-	-	-	-	-	-
35.5	-	-	-	-	-	-	-	-	-	-
36	-	-	-	-	-	-	-	-	-	-
36.5	-	-	-	-	-	-	-	-	-	-
37	-	-	-	-	-	-	-	-	-	-
37.5	-	-	-	-	-	-	-	-	-	-
38	0	0	-	-	-	-	-	-	-	-
38.5	1	1	1	0	0	-	-	-	-	-
39	2	2	2	1	1	1	0	0	-	-
39.5	3	3	3	2	2	2	1	1	1	0
40	4	4	3	3	3	3	2	2	2	1
40.5	5	5	4	4	4	3	3	3	2	2
41	6	5	5	5	5	4	4	4	3	3
41.5	7	6	6	6	5	5	5	4	4	4
42	8	7	7	7	6	6	6	5	5	5
42.5	8	8	8	7	7	7	6	6	6	6
43	9	9	9	8	8	8	7	7	7	6
43.5	10	10	10	9	9	8	8	8	7	7
44	11	10	11	10	9	9	9	9	8	8
44.5	12	11	12	11	10	10	10	9	9	9
45	12	12	12	11	11	11	10	10	10	10
45.5	13	13	13	12	12	12	11	11	11	10
46	14	14	14	13	13	12	12	12	11	11
46.5	15	14	15	14	13	13	13	12	12	12
47	15	15	15	14	14	14	13	13	13	13
47.5	16	16	16	15	15	15	14	14	14	13
48	17	17	17	16	16	15	15	15	14	14
48.5	18	17	18	17	16	16	16	15	15	15
49	18	18	18	17	17	17	16	16	16	15
49.5	19	19	19	18	18	17	17	17	17	16
50	20	19	20	19	18	18	18	18	17	17
50.5	20	20	20	19	19	19	19	18	18	18
51	21	21	21	20	20	20	19	19	19	18
51.5	22	21	22	21	21	20	20	20	19	19
52	22	22	22	22	21	21	21	20	20	20

TABLE B Women's BF % 2-3 Girth

Circumference value (in)	HEIGHT (IN)									
	68	68.5	69	69.5	70	70.5	71	71.5	72	72.5
52.5	23	23	23	22	22	22	21	21	21	20
53	24	23	24	23	23	22	22	22	21	21
53.5	24	24	24	23	23	23	23	22	22	22
54	25	25	25	24	24	24	23	23	23	22
54.5	26	25	26	25	24	24	24	24	23	23
55	26	26	26	25	25	25	24	24	24	24
55.5	27	27	27	26	26	25	25	25	25	24
56	28	27	28	27	26	26	26	25	25	25
56.5	28	28	28	27	27	27	26	26	26	25
57	29	29	29	28	28	27	27	27	26	26
57.5	30	29	29	29	28	28	28	27	27	27
58	30	30	30	29	29	29	28	28	28	27
58.5	31	30	31	30	29	29	29	29	28	28
59	31	31	31	30	30	30	29	29	29	28
59.5	32	32	32	31	31	30	30	30	29	29
60	32	32	32	32	31	31	31	30	30	30
60.5	33	33	33	32	32	31	31	31	31	30
61	34	33	33	33	32	32	32	31	31	31
61.5	34	34	34	33	33	33	32	32	32	31
62	35	34	34	34	34	33	33	33	32	32
62.5	35	35	35	34	34	34	33	33	33	33
63	36	36	35	35	35	34	34	34	33	33
63.5	36	36	36	35	35	35	35	34	34	34
64	37	37	36	36	36	35	35	35	35	34
64.5	38	37	37	37	36	36	36	35	35	35
65	38	38	37	37	37	37	36	36	36	35
65.5	39	38	38	38	37	37	37	36	36	36
66	39	39	39	38	38	38	37	37	37	36
66.5	40	39	39	39	38	38	38	37	37	37
67	40	40	40	39	39	39	38	38	38	37
67.5	41	40	40	40	39	39	39	39	38	38
68	41	41	41	40	40	40	39	39	39	38
68.5	42	41	41	41	40	40	40	40	39	39
69	42	42	42	41	41	41	40	40	40	39
69.5	43	42	42	42	42	41	41	41	40	40
70	43	43	43	42	42	42	41	41	41	40
70.5	44	43	43	43	43	42	42	42	41	41
71	44	44	44	43	43	43	42	42	42	41
71.5	45	44	44	44	43	43	43	43	42	42
72	-	45	45	44	44	44	43	43	43	42
72.5	-	-	-	45	44	44	44	44	43	43
73	-	-	-	-	45	45	44	44	44	43
73.5	-	-	-	-	-	-	45	44	44	44
74	-	-	-	-	-	-	-	45	45	44
74.5	-	-	-	-	-	-	-	-	-	45

TABLE B Women's BF % 2-3 Girth

Circumference value (in)	HEIGHT (IN)									
	73	73.5	74	74.5	75	75.5	76	76.5	77	77.5
34.5-39.5	0	-	-	-	-	-	-	-	-	-
40	1	1	0	0	-	-	-	-	-	-
40.5	2	2	1	1	1	0	0	-	-	-
41	3	2	2	2	2	1	1	1	0	0
41.5	4	3	3	3	2	2	2	2	1	1
42	4	4	4	4	3	3	3	2	2	2

TABLE B Women's BF % 2-3 Girth

Circumference value (in)	HEIGHT (IN)									
	73	73.5	74	74.5	75	75.5	76	76.5	77	77.5
42.5	5	5	5	4	4	4	3	3	3	3
43	6	6	5	5	5	5	4	4	4	3
43.5	7	7	6	6	6	5	5	5	5	4
44	8	7	7	7	6	6	6	6	5	5
44.5	8	8	8	8	7	7	7	6	6	6
45	9	9	9	8	8	8	7	7	7	7
45.5	10	10	9	9	9	9	8	8	8	7
46	11	10	10	10	10	9	9	9	8	8
46.5	12	11	11	11	10	10	10	9	9	9
47	12	12	12	11	11	11	11	10	10	10
47.5	13	13	12	12	12	12	11	11	11	10
48	14	13	13	13	13	12	12	12	11	11
48.5	14	14	14	14	13	13	13	12	12	12
49	15	15	15	14	14	14	13	13	13	13
49.5	16	16	15	15	15	14	14	14	14	13
50	17	16	16	16	15	15	15	15	14	14
50.5	17	17	17	16	16	16	16	15	15	15
51	18	18	17	17	17	17	16	16	16	15
51.5	19	18	18	18	17	17	17	17	16	16
52	19	19	19	18	18	18	18	17	17	17
52.5	20	20	19	19	19	19	18	18	18	17
53	21	20	20	20	20	19	19	19	18	18
53.5	21	21	21	20	20	20	20	19	19	19
54	22	22	21	21	21	21	20	20	20	19
54.5	23	22	22	22	21	21	21	21	20	20
55	23	23	23	22	22	22	22	21	21	21
55.5	24	24	23	23	23	22	22	22	22	21
56	25	24	24	24	23	23	23	22	22	22
56.5	25	25	25	24	24	24	23	23	23	23
57	26	25	25	25	25	24	24	24	23	23
57.5	26	26	26	26	25	25	25	24	24	24
58	27	27	26	26	26	26	25	25	25	24
58.5	28	27	27	27	26	26	26	26	25	25
59	28	28	28	27	27	27	26	26	26	26
59.5	29	28	28	28	28	27	27	27	26	26
60	29	29	29	28	28	28	28	27	27	27
60.5	30	30	29	29	29	28	28	28	28	27
61	31	30	30	30	29	29	29	28	28	28
61.5	31	31	31	30	30	30	29	29	29	28
62	32	31	31	31	30	30	30	30	29	29
62.5	32	32	32	31	31	31	30	30	30	30
63	33	32	32	32	32	31	31	31	30	30
63.5	33	33	33	32	32	32	32	31	31	31
64	34	34	33	33	33	32	32	32	32	31
64.5	34	34	34	34	33	33	33	32	32	32
65	35	35	34	34	34	34	33	33	33	32
65.5	36	35	35	35	34	34	34	33	33	33
66	36	36	35	35	35	35	34	34	34	33
66.5	37	36	36	36	35	35	35	35	34	34
67	37	37	37	36	36	36	35	35	35	34
67.5	38	37	37	37	36	36	36	36	35	35
68	38	38	38	37	37	37	36	36	36	36
69	39	39	39	38	38	38	37	37	37	37
69.5	40	39	39	39	38	38	38	38	37	37
70	40	40	40	39	39	39	38	38	38	38
70.5	41	40	40	40	39	39	39	39	38	38
71	41	41	41	40	40	40	39	39	39	39
71.5	42	41	41	41	40	40	40	40	39	39

TABLE B	Women's BF % 2-3 Girth									
	HEIGHT (IN)									
Circumference value (in)	73	73.5	74	74.5	75	75.5	76	76.5	77	77.5
72	42	42	42	41	41	41	40	40	40	40
72.5	43	42	42	42	41	41	41	41	40	40
73	43	43	43	42	42	42	41	41	41	40
73.5	44	43	43	43	42	42	42	42	41	41
74	44	44	43	43	43	43	42	42	42	41
74.5	45	44	44	44	43	43	43	42	42	42
75	-	45	44	44	44	44	43	43	43	42
75.5	-	-	45	45	44	44	44	43	43	42

Adapted from Hodgdon and Beckett, 1984.

◆ Skinfold Assessments

The relative importance of body fat testing and commonly-used protocols has been described previously. This section focuses on reinforcing some key elements of the testing rationale and common areas of testing error. Consistent with other fitness tests, the subject is the central factor in the test selection for body composition analysis. Each specific assessment type used for body composition has advantages and disadvantages related to the test, and some have population limitations. The four biggest factors related to the decision of using one testing method over another are as follows: 1) test validity; 2) the subject population; 3) the tester's skill set; 4) the psychological impact the test presents to the client. Considering these factors and creating a value system for test selection may help in the decision to select one assessment option over another.

Increasing accuracy related to these four factors can be gained by increasing understanding and proficiency in the test protocols. Test validity can easily be ascertained by reviewing the documented research that supports the test and identifying the populations for whom the tests were designed. Matching the subject's population with tests that were devised for their characteristics will also help with validity. Testing accuracy is based on the tester's proficiency but also the standard estimation of error inherent in the test. In general, acceptable estimation error should not be higher than 4% because it may change the subject's fitness profile and affect appropriate decisions made for the program. The last factor to consider is the psychological impact the testing will have on the subject. Most people are cognizant of their level of fatness and may experience at least some body-image distress. Non-invasive techniques, like girth measurements or bioelectrical impedance, should be selected for individuals with obviously higher levels of body fatness.

As a rule of thumb, use skinfold assessments on lean individuals and girth measurements on everyone else. This limits the need for multi-protocol proficiency and caters to the advantages and disadvantages of both tests. Additionally, the standard estimation of error is about the same for both tests when competently administered and used for the appropriate population. Scans and air displacement technology can also be used. If it seems necessary to have a more accurate body composition measurement, then the subject should be tested clinically using hydrostatic weighing or dual-energy x-ray absorptiometry. In most cases, however, this will not be required.

Measurements related to body composition may also be used to identify risk related to disease. Recall that BMI measures above 27 are considered a high risk factor for disease, and a value of 30 or greater places the individual into the obese category, even if other non-direct measures of body fat have been taken. Waist circumference and waist-to-hip ratio may also be used to predict risk for disease, based on the charted findings. The identification of high central-adiposity levels correlates to elevated disease risk [18].

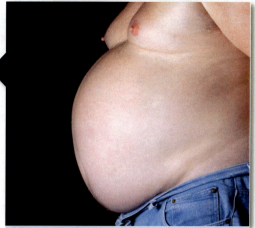

As a rule of thumb, use skinfold assessments on lean individuals and girth measurements on most other clients.

When exercise professionals explain findings from body composition tests, many individuals are surprised and convey feelings of disbelief because they have underestimated their body fat. Dealing with body fat results often requires a level of professional decorum and discretion so that the relevance of the information remains intact without causing the client to experience self-defeating emotions, such as acute depression and lack of self-worth. Emphasizing attainable change and adding a positive spin to the situation will help to keep the client focused on the important factors and can prevent feelings of apathy. Additionally, body composition changes take some time to alter; therefore, the trainer should avoid testing too frequently, as this may decrease motivation.

BODY COMPOSITION TEST: SKINFOLD

Equipment: Skinfold calipers
Pen (to mark sites)

Test: Prediction of body composition based on subcutaneous fat measures

Directions:

1) The test administrator should locate the correct sex-specific anatomical location(s). The following chart and illustrations provide a detailed description of the 3-site Jackson-Pollock model. The test administrator should refer to these when locating the proper skinfold location. Once the site has been identified, the test administrator should mark the site with an erasable marker so that the same location is used for subsequent measurements.

2) **Hand placement:** The test administrator should place the calipers in the right hand with the index finger in position to open the caliper. Slightly pronate the right hand so that the caliper can be easily read from above. Pronate the left hand so that the thumb of the left hand is pointing downward.

3) **Pinching of skinfold:** Using a pinch width of approximately two inches, firmly pinch the skinfold between the thumb and the first two fingers, lifting the subcutaneous fat and skin from the underlying muscle tissue.

4) **Placement of calipers:** Once the test administrator has successfully separated the subcutaneous fat and skin from the underlying muscle, the calipers should be placed on the fold. The pinchers of the caliper should be placed across the long axis of the skinfold at the designated site.

5) Using a 1 cm separation between the test administrator's fingers and the calipers should prevent the skinfold dimension from being affected by the finger pressure. The depth of the caliper placement is about half the distance between the base of the normal skin perimeter and the top of the skinfold.

6) Place the caliper jaws perpendicular to the skinfold site.

7) **Reading of calipers:** Calipers have a compression tension of $10g \cdot mm^2$. To get an accurate reading and prevent compression of the fat by the caliper, the test administrator must read the caliper to the closest half millimeter within two (2) seconds of releasing the caliper jaws on the fold.

8) The measurements should be recorded and the test repeated two times, allowing at least 15 seconds between subsequent measurements. If the measurements differ by more than two (2) millimeters, a third measurement should be taken and an average of the three measurements used.

9) In non-obese individuals, the skinfolds should not differ by more than two millimeters. The median values of the three trials are used for evaluation and prediction.

10) **Computation of results:** Once the data has been recorded, the test administrator should add the three skinfolds together to obtain the sum of the skinfolds in millimeters.

11) The sum of the skinfolds is then charted, or used in a body density equation, to determine the estimated body fat of the individual. The following charts contain the estimated, age-adjusted body composition computed by the Siri Equation. The test administrator can find the estimated body fat by referencing the following sex-specific table and matching the sum of the skinfolds in the left-hand column with the subject's age across the top row.

Male Three Sites

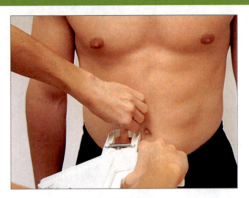

Abdominal Measurement:
Measure a vertical fold 2 cm from the midline of the umbilicus on the right side of the test subject. Be sure that neither the caliper nor the tester's fingers are in the umbilicus during the measurement.

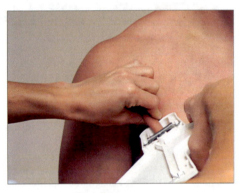

Chest Measurement:
The skinfold is a diagonal fold taken halfway between the anterior axillary line and the nipple. The right side is used for the pinch.

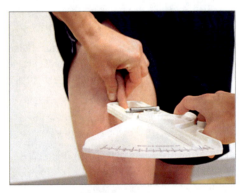

Thigh Measurement:
The measurement is a vertical fold taken over the quadriceps muscles on the midline of the right thigh. The measurement should be located halfway between the inguinal crease and the top of the patella.

Female Three Sites

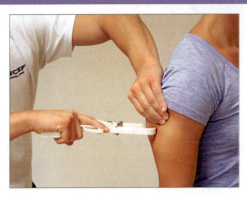

Triceps Measurement:
Measure the vertical fold over the center of the triceps muscle. Be sure the test subject relaxes the arm. The specific site is located on the posterior midline of the right triceps, halfway between the acromion and olecranon process.

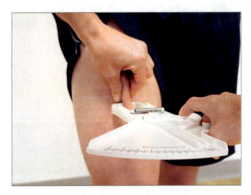

Thigh Measurement:
The measurement is a vertical fold taken over the quadriceps muscles on the midline of the right thigh. The measurement should be located halfway between the inguinal crease and the top of the patella.

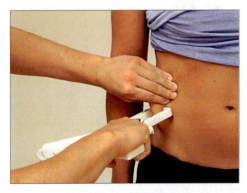

Suprailiac Measurement:
The skinfold is a diagonal fold measured in line with the natural angle of the iliac crest. The measurement should be taken along the anterior axillary line just above the iliac crest on the right side.

Percentage of Body Fat Estimation for Women From Age and Triceps, Suprailiac, and Thigh Folds

Sum of skinfolds (mm)	Under 22	23 to 27	28 to 32	33 to 37	38 to 42	43 to 47	48 to 52	53 to 57	Over 57
23-25	9.7	9.9	10.2	10.4	10.7	10.9	11.2	11.4	11.7
26-28	11.0	11.2	11.5	11.7	12.0	12.3	12.5	12.7	13.0
29-31	12.3	12.5	12.8	13.0	13.3	13.5	13.8	14.0	14.3
32-34	13.6	13.8	14.0	14.3	14.5	14.8	15.0	15.3	15.5
35-37	14.8	15.0	15.3	15.5	15.8	16.0	16.3	16.5	16.8
38-40	16.0	16.3	16.5	16.7	17.0	17.2	17.5	17.7	18.0
41-43	17.2	17.4	17.7	17.9	18.2	18.4	18.7	18.9	19.2
44-46	18.3	18.6	18.8	19.1	19.3	19.6	19.8	20.1	20.3
47-49	19.5	19.7	20.0	20.2	20.5	20.7	21.0	21.2	21.5
50-52	20.6	20.8	21.1	21.3	21.6	21.8	22.1	22.3	22.6
53-55	21.7	21.9	22.1	22.4	22.6	22.9	23.1	23.4	23.6
56-58	22.7	23.0	23.2	23.4	23.7	23.9	24.2	24.4	24.7
59-61	23.7	24.0	24.2	24.5	24.7	25.0	25.2	25.5	25.7
62-64	24.7	25.0	25.2	25.5	25.7	26.0	26.2	26.4	26.7
65-67	25.7	25.9	26.2	26.4	26.7	26.9	27.2	27.4	27.7
68-70	26.6	26.9	27.1	27.4	27.6	27.9	28.1	28.4	28.6
71-73	27.5	27.8	28.0	28.3	28.5	28.8	29.0	29.3	29.5
74-76	28.4	28.7	28.9	29.2	29.4	29.7	29.9	30.2	30.4
77-79	29.3	29.5	29.8	30.0	30.3	30.5	30.8	31.0	31.3
80-82	30.1	30.4	30.6	30.9	31.1	31.4	31.6	31.9	32.1
83-85	30.9	31.2	31.4	31.7	31.9	32.2	32.4	32.7	32.9
86-88	31.7	32.0	32.2	32.5	32.7	32.9	33.2	33.4	33.7
89-91	32.5	32.7	33.0	33.2	33.5	33.7	33.9	34.2	34.4
92-94	33.2	33.4	33.7	33.9	34.2	34.4	34.7	34.9	35.2
95-97	33.9	34.1	34.4	34.6	34.9	35.1	35.4	35.6	35.9
98-100	34.6	34.8	35.1	35.3	35.5	35.8	36.0	36.3	36.5
101-103	35.3	35.4	35.7	35.9	36.2	36.4	36.7	36.9	37.2
104-106	35.8	36.1	36.3	36.6	36.8	37.1	37.3	37.5	37.8
107-109	36.4	36.7	36.9	37.1	37.4	37.6	37.9	38.1	38.4
110-112	37.0	37.2	37.5	37.7	38.0	38.2	38.5	38.7	38.9
113-115	37.5	37.8	38.1	38.2	38.5	38.7	39.0	39.2	39.5
116-118	38.0	38.3	38.5	38.8	39.0	39.3	39.5	39.7	40.0
119-121	38.5	38.7	39.0	39.2	39.5	39.7	40.0	40.2	40.5
122-124	39.0	39.2	39.4	39.7	39.9	40.2	40.4	40.7	40.9
125-127	39.4	39.6	39.9	40.1	40.4	40.6	40.9	41.1	41.4
128-130	39.8	40.0	40.3	40.5	40.8	41.0	41.3	41.5	41.8

Percentage of Body Fat Estimation for Men From Age and Chest, Abdominal, and Thigh Folds

Sum of skinfolds (mm)	Under 22	23 to 27	28 to 32	33 to 37	38 to 42	43 to 47	48 to 52	53 to 57	Over 57
8-10	1.3	1.8	2.3	2.9	3.4	3.9	4.5	5.0	5.5
11-13	2.2	2.8	3.3	3.9	4.4	4.9	5.5	6.0	6.5
14-16	3.2	3.8	4.3	4.8	5.4	5.9	6.4	7.0	7.5
17-19	4.2	4.7	5.3	5.8	6.3	6.9	7.4	8.0	8.5
20-22	5.1	5.7	6.2	6.8	7.3	7.9	8.4	8.9	9.5
23-25	6.1	6.6	7.2	7.7	8.3	8.8	9.4	9.9	10.5
26-28	7.0	7.6	8.1	8.7	9.2	9.8	10.3	10.9	11.4
29-31	8.0	8.5	9.1	9.6	10.2	10.7	11.3	11.8	12.4
32-34	8.9	9.4	10.0	10.5	11.1	11.6	12.2	12.8	13.3
35-37	9.8	10.4	10.9	11.5	12.0	12.6	13.1	13.7	14.3
38-40	10.7	11.3	11.8	12.4	12.9	13.5	14.1	14.6	15.2
41-43	11.6	12.2	12.7	13.3	13.8	14.4	15.0	15.5	16.1
44-46	12.5	13.1	13.6	14.2	14.7	15.3	15.9	16.4	17.0
47-49	13.4	13.9	14.5	15.1	15.6	16.2	16.8	17.3	17.9
50-52	14.3	14.8	15.4	15.9	16.5	17.1	17.6	18.2	18.8
53-55	15.1	15.7	16.2	16.8	17.4	17.9	18.5	19.1	19.7
56-58	16.0	16.5	17.1	17.7	18.2	18.8	19.4	20.0	20.5
59-61	16.9	17.4	17.9	18.5	19.1	19.7	20.2	20.8	21.4
62-64	17.6	18.2	18.8	19.4	19.9	20.5	21.1	21.7	22.2
65-67	18.5	19.0	19.6	20.2	20.8	21.3	21.9	22.5	23.1
68-70	19.3	19.9	20.4	21.0	21.6	22.2	22.7	23.3	23.9
71-73	20.1	20.7	21.2	21.8	22.4	23.0	23.6	24.1	24.7
74-76	20.9	21.5	22.0	22.6	23.2	23.8	24.4	25.0	25.5
77-79	21.7	22.2	22.8	23.4	24.0	24.6	25.2	25.8	26.3
80-82	22.4	23.0	23.6	24.2	24.8	25.4	25.9	26.5	27.1
83-85	23.2	23.8	24.4	25.0	25.5	26.1	26.7	27.3	27.9
86-88	24.0	24.5	25.1	25.7	26.3	26.9	27.5	28.1	28.7
89-91	24.7	25.3	25.9	26.5	27.1	27.6	28.2	28.8	29.4
92-94	25.4	26.0	26.6	27.2	27.8	28.4	29.0	29.6	30.2
95-97	26.1	26.7	27.3	27.9	28.5	29.1	29.7	30.3	30.9
98-100	26.9	27.4	28.0	28.6	29.2	29.8	30.4	31.0	31.6
101-103	27.5	28.1	28.7	29.3	29.9	30.5	31.1	31.7	32.3
104-106	28.2	28.8	29.4	30.0	30.6	31.2	31.8	32.4	33.0
107-109	28.9	29.5	30.1	30.7	31.3	31.9	32.5	33.1	33.7
110-112	29.6	30.2	30.8	31.4	32.0	32.6	33.2	33.8	34.4
113-115	30.2	30.8	31.4	32.0	32.6	33.2	33.8	34.5	35.1
116-118	30.9	31.5	32.1	32.7	33.3	33.9	34.5	35.1	35.7
119-121	31.5	32.1	32.7	33.3	33.9	34.5	35.1	35.7	36.4
122-124	32.1	32.7	33.3	33.9	34.5	35.1	35.8	36.4	37.0

◆ Postural Assessment

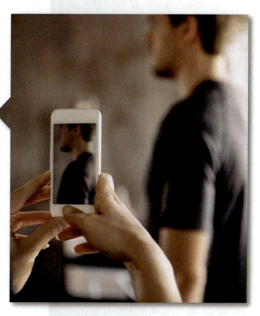

Postural assessments outside of clinical environments have gained popularity and can provide useful data to educated practitioners. Two categories of posture exist: **static** and **dynamic**. The first provides predictions for dynamic applications and aids as symptomatic and asymptomatic reference points. For instance, if a person in a static, standing position exhibits asymmetries between the left and right side that present as a dropped shoulder, clearly something is not right within or around the affected areas. There may be a tendency to favor one side, a pre-existing condition, a lower spine issue, a previous injury, or even a congenital abnormality. Earlier chapters implicated that changes in skeletal alignment can cause potential movement issues and, in some cases, pain-related pathologies. Complimenting static appraisals, dynamic postural assessments can identify what, if anything, is wrong with the biomechanical movement of the body through the different planes of motion during various joint actions. In many cases, a static postural assessment predicts faulty movement and muscular compensation patterns. In other words, it can help frame a risk analysis while also serving to provide details as to why a dysfunction occurs.

Common Postural Deviations Include:
(not an inclusive list)

- Forward head position
- Abducted scapulae
- Hyperlordotic lumbar spine
- Knee/ankle deviations
- Rounded shoulders
- Thoracic Kyphosis
- Lateral pelvic tilting

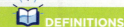

DEFINITIONS

Static posture –

Biomechanical alignment when standing motionless that is usually assessed via a plumb line; can provide predictions for issues during physical activity and the relative risk of injury or symptomatic conditions due to musculoskeletal malalignment.

Dynamic posture –

Biomechanical proficiency, or lack thereof, during movements of the body such as locomotion, stepping, jumping etc.; assessment allows for the detection of faulty movement patterns, strength imbalances and risk for injury during given activities.

Center of gravity –

A point within a given object such as the human body where the line of gravitational pull is equal in all directions; for example, the center of gravity for the body should be directly down the midline of the body in the frontal plane if the body is symmetrical on both sides.

Static postural assessments are surprisingly helpful at identifying skeletal deficiencies across a broad age range, but most significant dysfunction is found among the elderly. Conversely, children without genetic dysfunctions tend to demonstrate better posture than adults. Natural play and primal movements have historically accounted for postural health in children; however, the recent and increasing decline in physical activity among the nation's youth, increased reliance on technology, and even more so on handheld devices, have compounded the risks of developing poor posture, faulty biomechanics, and reduced joint function earlier in life [6, 21]. Increased risk of postural deficit occurs with physical inactivity and elevated sitting time per week [20, 21]. Likewise, poor posture has deleterious effects on overall health and well-being and is associated with premature loss of independence among the elderly [9, 15].

The ability to perform an accurate postural assessment requires an understanding of proper anatomical positioning. During proper upright posture, the line of gravity passes through the axis of each joint when the joint segments align vertically. The gravitational vector line is represented by a vertical line drawn through the body's **center of gravity**. Therefore, the closer a person's postural alignment lies to the center of all joint axes, the more efficient the position. During proper upright posture, less gravitational stress is placed on the soft tissue components of supporting systems due to the system's structural alignment or form closure. Muscle strength balance (proper strength ratios across joints) and resting length affect the joint actions, resting position, and range of motion (ROM). Force couples maintain the body position in three

> **DEFINITIONS**
>
> **Synergistic muscles –**
>
> *Muscles that work together at a given joint or body segment that regulate controlled rotation of the joint and total range of motion so that no compensatory actions occur; these muscles work together to effectively transfer force across the body.*

dimensions across all planes of motion. When balance is lost between force couples, it affects the joint segments' axes of rotation, often presenting as faulty joint motions. Notably, this may be seen in a variety of postural deformities, such as a kyphotic exaggeration or changes in pelvic angles (tilts). Under those circumstances, complications at peripheral sites can promote imbalances and loss of forces directed to the limbs. These postural faults provide information which can be used to identify alterations in tissue strength, length, and pliability. Although it is often concluded that imbalances represent one muscle group that is too tight while its antagonist is reciprocally relaxed, this is not always the case. **Synergistic muscles** around a joint may also affect the joint's function, based on strength, length, activation patterns, and inhibitory characteristics. Imbalances affecting the spine, scapula, and hip are particularly problematic, as they lead to undesirable joint positions. Poorly aligned articulations promote faults across the length of the kinetic chain. When the issues occur at spinal regions, they are particularly pervasive in promoting alignment problems in other joints, due to the architectural relationships. These faults may limit motion in soft tissues and often negatively affect activation patterns. Due to the alignment issues, these muscles tend to become lax and weak.

Standing Postural Assessment

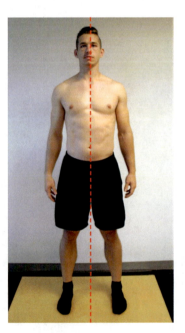
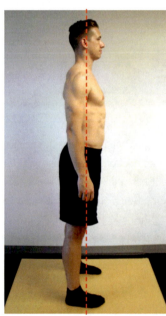
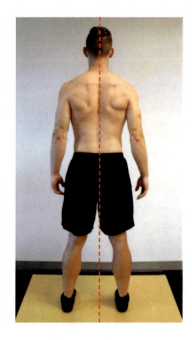

1. Prior to evaluation, an assessment of medical history, prior injuries, limb dominance (sports), and any symptoms should be performed.

2. Subject should dress in a manner (without shoes) that provides a clear view of all relevant anatomical landmarks used for reference.

3. Any subjects who use orthotics should be assessed with and without them to determine their effectiveness in correcting posture.

4. Subject should assume a comfortable and relaxed posture and be informed that, while the analysis is being performed, no conscious, voluntary muscle activation should take place (i.e, trying to assume "good posture" for the assessment).

Anterior View	Lateral View	Posterior View
Plumb line: The line bisects the head at the midline into equal halves.	*Plumb line:* The line falls through the ear lobe to the acromion process.	*Plumb line:* The midline bisects the head through the external occipital protuberance; head is usually positioned squarely over the shoulders so that eyes remain level.
Plumb line: A vertical line bisects the sternum and xiphoid process	*Plumb line:* It falls through the acromion process.	*Plumb line:* It runs midline of all cervical vertebrae and falls midway between the medial borders of the scapulae.
Plumb line: Line runs through the umbilicus.	*Plumb line:* The line falls midway between the abdomen and back and slightly anterior to the sacroiliac joint.	*Plumb line:* The line bisects the spinous process of the thoracic and lumbar vertebrae.
Plumb line: The line runs equidistant between the thighs.	*Plumb line:* The line falls slightly anterior to the sacroiliac joint and posterior to the hip joint, through the greater trochanter.	*Plumb line:* The line bisects the pelvis and the gluteal cleft, and the posterior superior iliac spines are on the same horizontal plane; the iliac crests, gluteal folds, and greater trochanters are level.
Plumb line: The line runs between the medial femoral condyles of the knees.	*Plumb line:* The line falls slightly anterior to the knee joint.	*Plumb line:* The plumb line lies equidistant between the knees.
Plumb line: The line runs between the medial malleoli.	*Plumb line:* The line lies slightly anterior to the lateral malleolus.	*Plumb line:* The line is equidistant from the malleoli.

A systematic static posture assessment employs three views using established reference lines. These lines bisect the body into equal side-by-side and front-and-back halves using the midline and the mid-axillary lines for reference. Postural analysis is most commonly performed by assessing the body's alignment from the lateral, posterior and anterior views using a **plumb line**. This provides data pertinent to alignment disruptions across all the joints. A number of factors affect the validity and reliability of postural analysis assessments as a tool for identifying skeletal issues.

In addition to evaluating static posture, dynamic everyday actions, such as walking (gait) and stepping, should also be viewed. Observing inefficient alignment of body segments while these movements are performed helps in detecting faulty muscle patterns and challenges to joint stability and mobility. Greater quality of movement and proper alignment of gravitational forces through joint axes lead to a more efficient motion sequence. When postural alignment improves so does joint proficiency.

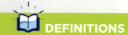

DEFINITIONS

Plumb line –

Linear testing tool used to assess posture and observe variations in anatomical positions.

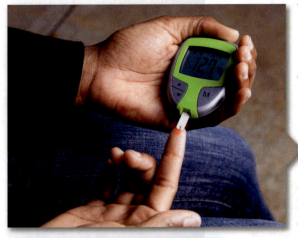

Exercise Participation Clearance

Findings from the resting evaluation battery should be added to the needs analysis and reviewed for added risk for activity participation. The data collected using the aforementioned screening tools should provide a clear picture as to a subject's potential risk for adverse events during physical activity. At this point, activity participation status must be determined before exercise testing can occur. Exercise professionals will classify the individual in one of the following four categories:

Signs and Symptoms of Disease

Cardiovascular
- High blood pressure
- Hypotension
- High resting heart rate
- Leg pain
- High lipid profile
- Chest or left arm pain
- **Dyspnea** on exertion
- Edema
- Heart palpitations

Metabolic
- Increased thirst
- Increased urination
- Glucose intolerance
- Obesity
- High or low blood glucose
- Increased or unexplained fatigue
- Unexplained weight loss
- Amenorrhea
- Blurred vision
- Insomnia
- Jaundice *(yellow colorization of skin and eyes)*
- Delayed wound healing

Pulmonary
- Labored breathing
- Breathlessness *(mild exertion)*
- Nocturnal dyspnea
- Frequent or chronic cough
- Exercise induced asthma
- Hemoptysis *(coughing up blood)*
- Wheezing

1. **Unrestricted exercise** – There is no evidence to support that exercise participation will harm the individual at any intensity. Program participation should reflect the individual's current fitness level.

2. **Modified exercise program** – The observed data stipulates that the individual is at a low risk, but certain indications suggest some activities can be modified to accommodate those concerns. Instructor recommended activities are ideal.

3. **Supervised program** – This individual demonstrates risks that may cause an adverse event or present an increased likelihood for a problem, such as stage 2 hypertension. Exercise instruction should be guided by a professional in small group or one-on-one instruction.

4. **Medically supervised program** – This individual requires medical clearance and/or was referred by a physician to initiate an exercise program specifically supervised in a medical facility or by a trained health-care professional. These individuals demonstrate a high risk for a cardiac or metabolic event and often include those with symptomatic inflammatory obesity, uncontrolled diabetes, heart failure, or similar conditions.

Individuals who do not present any significant risk are cleared for unrestricted activity and prepared for a full physical fitness evaluation. Individuals who possess a concerning number of risk factors or any signs and symptoms of disease, as indicated by health status coding, should obtain documented medical clearance from a physician before beginning any exercise program or test (see Health Status Questionnaire). An exercise professional may be considered negligent if he or she identifies criteria that necessitate a medical referral or medical clearance during the screening process yet allows the client to proceed without physician approval. In some cases, findings by a physician indicate an individual should begin in a medically supervised program, but these cases are rare among the general population. Most individuals with lower-level hypertension, controlled diabetes, and stabilized metabolic syndrome can participate in exercise in a public or private training facility when using a certified exercise professional qualified to manage these conditions.

 DEFINITIONS

Dyspnea –
Difficult or labored breathing; shortness of breath due to some inefficiency or disease.

Liability and Fiduciary Care

No one wants medical clearance to be a barrier to participation, particularly when partaking in exercise is likely to improve a client's condition. However, sticking with generally accepted protocols reduces liability risks. If a client has been to a physician in the past year, the standard method for efficiently clearing him or her for exercise is to attain a physician contact form or have the client fax the request to the general practitioner for clearance. The form indicates that the individual willingly requests to engage in activity and allows the physician to make recommendations and restrictions for participation. This process allows the client to simply fax, email, or even text a picture of the document to his or her physician and attain quick clearance without a complete physical examination. Exercise professionals should comply with any recommendations or restrictions, and in some cases, a physician may require a face-to-face visit. Due to the transfer of liability attained from the medical clearance document, exercise professionals must adhere to any requirements outlined by the physician.

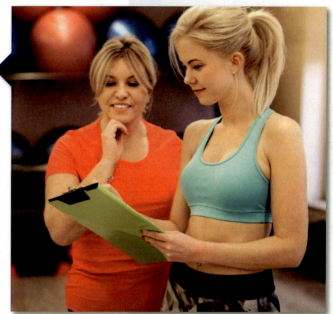

If a client needs to see his or her physician for clearance, the exercise professional should provide him or her with a release form. An acknowledgement of clearance without the supportive evidence of written documentation does not suffice for reducing professional liability. Exercise professionals must keep a written history of all activities, personal information, and clearance documentation to manage risk properly. In addition, this information assists the trainer in developing an exercise prescription and subsequently tracking health-related changes. Then, the documents can be easily digitized and placed into the client's file. This prevents clutter or the loss of important paperwork over time. It is important to note however, that personalized digital information should be held securely to prevent infringement of the client's privacy. A diligent and prudent health professional can minimize risk associated with personal data by ensuring only the appropriate personnel have access to client information.

Creating a client file is part of the first step to providing appropriate client services. Throughout the screening process, all documentation should be recorded and filed appropriately. Documents that are recommended for effective risk management include the informed consent, health status and behavior questionnaires, documentation of any resting battery assessments, any medical referral documents, physical testing records, and data, including pictures or videos, and all subsequent program documents. Exercise professionals should implement an organized filing and tracking system to ensure a consistent, ongoing paper trail of the client's history while receiving personal training services. Although this adds responsibilities to the job requirements, it is good business practice and enhances the quality of service. Taking the time to document and track services allows for insight into what works and what may require modification within the program, while simultaneously reducing the liability risk. Additionally, tracking and reviewing files can help to identify compliance with recommendations and to ascertain obstacles to goal attainment.

MEDICAL CLEARANCE FORM

Name of Patient _____   Date _____

Your patient wishes to take part in an exercise program and/or fitness assessment at or with _____.
After initial screening it has been determined that this individual requires physician consent prior to engaging in the exercise program and/or fitness assessments due to _____.

The participant will engage in the following exercise programming and/or fitness assessments:

Exercise Programming
- ___ Muscular Strength
- ___ Flexibility
- ___ Muscular Endurance
- ___ Cardiorespiratory Fitness
- ___ Other*

Fitness Assessments
- ___ Muscular Strength
- ___ Muscular Endurance
- ___ Flexibility
- ___ Body Composition
- ___ Cardiorespiratory Fitness

*Explain: _____
_____

Physician's Recommendations
Please indicate below for which of the following your patient is cleared to participate

Muscular Strength & Endurance Training and Assessment

___ Yes with no limitations   ___ Yes with limitations below   ___ No cannot participate

Limitations/ recommendations: _____
_____

Cardiorespiratory Fitness and Assessment

___ Yes with no limitations   ___ Yes with limitations below   ___ No cannot participate

Limitations/ recommendations: _____
_____

Flexibility Training and Assessment

___ Yes with no limitations   ___ Yes with limitations below   ___ No cannot participate

Limitations/ recommendations: _____
_____

_____   _____
Signature of Physician/Primary Care Provider   Date

_____   Please return this form to:
Printed Name of Physician/Medical Group

_____
Street Address

_____
City   State   Zip

Exercise Testing

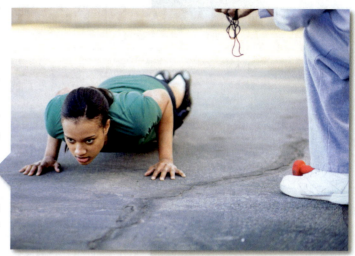

Fitness testing is a fundamental part of designing an exercise prescription and is most useful when the tests are valid, client appropriate, and specific to the program goals. This suggests no single testing protocol is perfect for all clients. Results, observations, and findings from physical fitness tests allow exercise professionals to create an individualized health and fitness profile of each client and provide the basis for making educated decisions that will most efficiently address the client's current condition(s).

Test Rationale

- Identifying baseline data of physical measures
- Identifying strengths and weaknesses
- Assessing capabilities
- Identifying starting points
- Determining readiness for training activities
- Establishing program and progress tracking criteria
- Determining goal setting data
- Evaluating psychological considerations
- Educating clients
- Establishing program activities and evaluating their effectiveness

Test Selection Criteria

- What is the purpose of the test?
- Is the test valid, reliable, and objective?
- What does the data provide and how will it be used?
- How will improvements in subsequent test measures affect the goals of the training?
- What does it predict?
- Does it match the goals of the training?
- Is it consistent with important program components?
- Is it appropriate for the specific individual being tested?
- Will the client be able to effectively perform the test?
- Is it safe for the client?
- Does the test present psychological barriers or anxiety?
- Is the client comfortable performing the test?

The rationale for testing is well justified and fairly extensive; that being said, each individual test should have a specific purpose, or it has no place in the testing battery. The decision to select certain exercise tests for each client should be thoughtful and thorough to ensure the client performs individually appropriate assessments. The tests need to be chosen based on specific criteria and should be in line with the client's age and abilities. A common error is asking a client to complete a test that requires actions he or she has never performed or which exceed the person's level of fitness and cannot be completed competently. All assessments must be practiced before the evaluation to ensure that both client and tester perform the test correctly by all measurable parameters. The **validity** and subsequent **reliability** of an assessment depends on the implementation method. Test proficiency and scoring discrimination are key elements that determine the value of the measurement and the subsequent data it provides.

Individualizing test selection for the client maximizes the testing effectiveness and experience and serves to ensure the best outcome for his or her well-being. The client's experience, capabilities, training status, age, and gender will be relevant factors when deciding on the most appropriate assessments. Personal trainers must remain conscious of any health risks or safety issues when selecting tests to avoid a negative experience or outcome associated with the testing

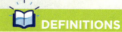

DEFINITIONS

Test validity –

The ability of a test to accurately measure what it is designed for; enhanced by maintaining proper protocol, tester and testee proficiency, strict scoring discrimination, etc.

Test reliability –

The ability of a test to allow for consistent reproduction of measures during retesting events; enhanced by duplicating testing conditions every time, using the same protocol every time, ensuring consistency in pretest factors, etc.

protocol or environment. In most cases, repeat practice of the test, in whole or in part, helps with the decision of whether the test should be used. Would it make sense to have a client perform a maximal repetition back squat test if the person was not proficient at squatting? Similarly, would it be valid to have a client perform a 1.5 mile run test if he or she had not practiced the distance and/or attained the capacity to set a proper pace? Many times, exercise professionals test clients before the person is proficient, which invalidates the results and increases the risk of a potential negative outcome. This scenario results in useless data and wasted time for everyone involved. When deciding on the test or protocol to be used, a trainer must evaluate each test's validity, reliability, objectivity, and the value of the data potentially provided. A test is considered valid when it accurately measures what it is designed to measure. The goal when designing a testing battery is to identify assessment protocols that have proven validity through appropriate research methodologies and will best match the client's characteristics. The tests provide better data when reliability is confirmed by clinical trials that are appropriately chosen for the tested population and implemented with the proper protocol. This necessitates understanding the assessment protocol and complying with the defined methodology in an appropriate environment.

Increasing Validity and Reliability of Tests

Validity

- Make sure the protocol is valid
- Make sure the tester is skillful and experienced in the test protocols
- Make sure the client is proficient in the test action
- Use strict discrimination in measurement
- Psychologically prepare the client for the event and properly motivate them
- Make sure the environment is safe and ideal for the test
- Make sure all the equipment functions properly and is calibrated
- Make sure the client has met pretest instructions
- Make sure no variable has entered the equation such as illness or high stress
- Clearly defined scoring system

Reliability

- Duplicate the conditions (time, environment, location, recovery)
- Strict adherence to the protocol
- Consistent pretest factors: warm-up and motivation
- Consistency with scoring system
- Emphasize tester consistency
- Use the same assessment instrument

To understand how validity can be gained or lost, consider the following scenarios:

Scenario 1

A personal trainer asks a previously sedentary 37-year old female to run a mile on a high school track. The trainer assumes that the track distance is 1,320 feet because when he ran the mile in high school, four laps was equal to a mile. The test takes place on the third meeting, but the trainer did not inform the client what exercises or evaluations she would be performing that day. The client has worn designer athletic shoes, but they are not ideal for running. In addition, it is a hot and humid summer day, and the client trains at lunch time.

Scenario 2

A personal trainer researches the distance of an indoor track before deciding to use it with her 28-year-old male client. He has routinely jogged between 6-9 miles per week for the past six months to stay fit; she has used the data he has provided to calculate his one mile pace. For the next training session, she asks him to bring his running shoes with him for a scheduled assessment of his performance in a maximal one-mile run. In their previous two meetings, she used the track for some pace training with the client to practice his laps at peak speed for the specific distance so that he would be familiar with the surface, pace, and running distance. She instructs him not to run any significant amount on his own for at least two days before the test and gives him a pretest checklist to follow to ensure he is optimally prepared for the assessment.

Clearly, the second situation would provide a much better experience for the client and would likely have a much higher testing validity for his actual cardiorespiratory fitness (CRF). The second trainer has selected a test that is consistent with the client's capabilities and experience. She has provided the client with appropriate details regarding the test, assessed the distance for accuracy, accounted for environmental factors, and properly planned the event. Conversely, scenario one may actually place the client at risk. The trainer did not select the appropriate test for the client, did not mentally or physically prepare her for the event, failed to account for environmental influences, and did not provide pretest information that would increase the assessment's accuracy. The personal trainer's job is to account for all the factors that may invalidate a test and confirm that they have been removed before implementation.

Methodology that deviates in any way from proper protocol damages assessment validity. This is commonly seen when subjects or test administrators incorrectly perform the techniques used in the assessment. Incorrect body position, poor biomechanics, incomplete ROM, and using momentum or other compensatory action for improved scoring all serve to invalidate the assessment. Validity may also be compromised when the testing equipment or the evaluation instrument performs poorly or is not properly calibrated. This can occur when using inferior, improperly calibrated equipment that is employed in unsuitable environments or which is not functioning properly for some reason: for example, having depleted batteries in the device.

When deciding on the test or protocol to be used for a client, evaluate each test's validity, reliability, objectivity, and the value of the data each test will provide.

When the proper steps have been taken to limit assessment errors, the measurement can provide high validity. Exercise professionals should document the testing environment (time of day, temperature, humidity, etc.), the specific details related to the client's preparation, and the protocol's implementation. In doing so, he or she can increase the opportunity for effective reliability in follow-up testing. Reliability suggests reproducibility: the test's ability to provide consistent measures in subsequent re-testing. Any change present in the testing activities or environment may decrease predictive reliability, consequently invalidating the data for comparative purposes, as reliability requires consistency. With multiple tests, conditions should remain the same in order to maximize the data's accuracy for comparison to previous trials. This means using the same measurer, methods, instruments, testing environment, and pretest protocols for each succeeding retest. Even though reproducibility of a test affects retest validity, the two are not synonymous. A test can be invalid and still be reproducible. For instance, the sit-and-reach test has been used for decades and has demonstrated consistently reproducible measures; however, a meta-analysis from 34 sit-and-reach criterion-validity studies showed that this test has a moderate mean criterion-related validity for estimating hamstring extensibility but a low mean for estimating lumbar extensibility [14].

Validity and reliability errors may be impossible to remove completely because test participants are human and, therefore, subject to innumerable physiological and psychological variables, any of which may affect a test outcome. Despite this obstacle, the test administrator can improve a test's validity and reliability, and when testers are highly trained and well-versed in testing protocols, the results will be more accurate. Applying meticulous detail to all the test factors and being organized will add to the success of any program developed from test data.

Testing Considerations

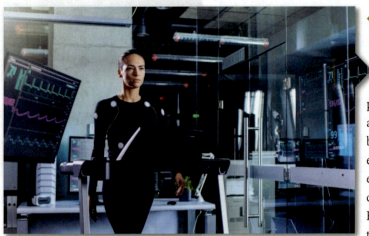

◆ Testing Environment

The testing environment can either add to or detract from validity and reliability. Obvious environmental factors include ambient air temperature, time of day, altitude, humidity, and pollution, including gases, noise, and toxins. However, most variables that affect the testing environment are not as obvious. While being mindful of the difficulty of accounting for the human factor, exercise professionals must also try to control for it. If the testing environment includes other users or bystanders, the client may be distracted and possibly self-conscious, thereby affecting the testing. For this reason, private testing may help the client to focus on the task, rather than experience environment-related test anxiety. Safety should also be thoroughly accounted for when creating the test environment. Tests should be performed in environments similar to those in which the client practiced the test. Equipment must be tested and deemed safe, and the client should be wearing the appropriate clothing and footwear prior to beginning any testing.

Environmental factors to consider:

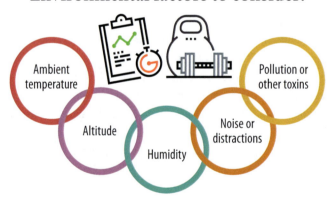

◆ Test Administration

Test administration factors crucially in client assessment outcomes. Properly organized and administered testing procedures provide quality data for the exercise program. Acquiring technical skills and mastering test protocols is vital to being a successful personal trainer. Just as clients should practice the test activities, administrators should also practice and have experience implementing the test protocol. A test administrator's proficiency conducting and managing the assessment improves greatly with his or her expertise in, and experience with, the specific protocols being employed. Performing the tests and practicing the protocols on others can help identify problems and circumstances that may reduce client testing accuracy. Test invalidation due to administrator error or incompetence related to the procedure can be avoided by diligent practice and use of a premeditated, organized plan. Making a checklist and complying with it will yield efficient test management. Likewise, preparing an **emergency plan** in case something goes wrong helps reduce negative outcomes and provides an invaluable addition to the protocol.

◆ Test Economy

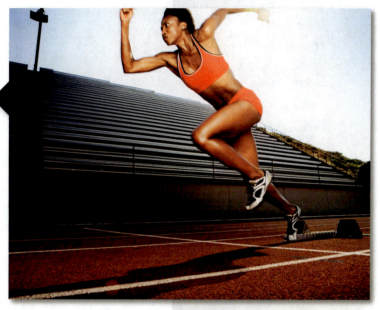

Test economy is another variable that often compromises test validity. Test economy describes the subject's proficiency in test performance, as well as his or her compliance with the instructions. When exercise professionals do not properly educate clients in test techniques or fail to point out pitfalls and common errors, the assessment is likely to provide poor and/or inaccurate data. Personal trainers should have clients practice techniques to allow for adequate skill acquisition before implementing the protocol. When the client attains proficiency in the test skills required, the validity increases dramatically. For example, a client performs a pull up test and achieves five (5) partial repetitions but fails to complete a single full repetition across the entire range of the motion, what is his or her score? In this case, a discriminating test administrator would give the client a score of zero: but is that mark accurate and useful? The answer, clearly, is no. Proactive communication concerning the standard for a full repetition and a practice session of the test would allowed for a more valid outcome.

To summarize, practicing the skills required of a specific test prior to the actual test implementation yields several benefits:

1) The tester will be able to predict the individual's capabilities and best align the method to the subject.
2) The test subject's confidence increases with exposure to the parameters.
3) The actions of the test will be understood, as will the discrimination of the scoring.

The psychological component of testing should not be underestimated. In addition to the physical requirements asked of a client, some psychological aspects related to testing are always present. People experience different levels of test anxiety. In some cases, the unease stems from pressure to perform well, internal questioning of one's ability to perform, or concerns that one may do poorly and suffer embarrassment. In other cases, the client may have had a negative experience or poor outcome on similar tests in the past. These subconscious feelings often surface when individuals are faced with a similar situation. Proper test preparation, checklists, and practice all help alleviate many of these misgivings. In this vein, two types of pretest checklists exist, one for the administrator and one for the client. For the test administrator, the checklist should include factors that will guide safe and efficient test performance. It will cover items that ensure correctly calibrated and functioning equipment appropriate to the tasks, as well as having the appropriate forms and a properly prepared environment. The client's pretest instructions will include test day preparations, such as appropriate clothing, adequate rest, and hydration,

DEFINITIONS

Emergency plan –

A comprehensive plan for dealing with emergency situations that may arise during exercise testing and performance. This plan should include a list of possible emergencies, consequences, required actions, written procedures and the resources available in a particular facility.

Test economy –

Used to describe the proficiency of the client in performing a given test and their compliance with the testing instructions; can be compromised by choosing an inappropriate test for a given client's fitness level, goal(s), sources of motivation, special needs or limitations.

and direct the client to avoid stimulants or other ingested items that may affect the test results. The best assessment administrators are organized and detail oriented. When everything is properly accounted for, the likelihood of success is very high. On the other hand, a lack of preparation significantly increases the chance for error.

Pretest Checklists

Client Pretest Instructions

___ I have read and understand any pretest procedures.

___ I am familiar with the tests I will perform.

___ I have acquired adequate rest the night before testing.

___ I have consumed adequate fluid.

___ I have consumed a moderate dietary intake.

___ I have abstained from tobacco, stimulants, and nonprescription medications.

___ I have the proper clothing and footwear for the activity.

___ I am not ill or injured.

Administrator Checklist for Testing

___ Client has been screened and signed an informed consent.

___ Equipment is available, in working condition, and calibrated.

___ All records and scoring sheets are prepared.

___ Protocol is clearly understood.

___ Subject has practiced the test.

___ Subject has been properly instructed for the test.

___ Testing environment has been defined and is prepared.

___ External conditions are appropriate for testing.

___ Determine the test termination criteria.

___ Warm-up and cool-down procedures are defined.

◆ Testing Format

When more than one test is to be administered on a given day, exercise professionals should establish a well-organized testing format considering the two primary components, time and accuracy. For example, some tests take more time than others to set up and administer. Others have minimal time requirements but can invalidate subsequent tests by causing fatigue within one of the body's systems. Identifying an appropriate sequence can help guarantee the test session's efficiency and accuracy. Attempting to perform all the tests in one day, for instance, may be desirable from a time perspective; however, if this act dilutes the data, then the time saved was of little value. Knowledge should drive proper decision making when determining the test sequence or what tests should be administered together. Tests that are demanding of the nervous system and/or the immediate energy systems should be performed first in a sequence of testing, following any resting battery. Tests that produce fatigue should be placed later in the test sequence. Such evaluations should mirror the physiological demand and energy system, so they may be ordered by time-intensity relationships. When deciding on a logical progression, categorize the tests into those lasting < 10 sec, 10-20 sec, up to 30 sec, up to 60 sec, up to 90 sec and >90 seconds. The following guidelines and examples can assist in the sequencing decision.

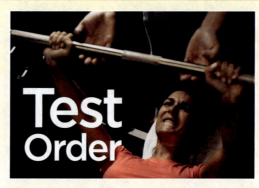

1. **Resting test or test of minimal fatigue:** Body composition, flexibility, and mobility

2. **Strength, power and speed tests:** Maximal repetition(s) tests (3RM) and anaerobic power tests (vertical jump)

3. **Anaerobic endurance tests:** Multi-rep bench press, pull-up, push-ups, and abdominal curl-ups

4. **Anaerobic capacity tests:** 30-60-90 jump test and 400m run

5. **Aerobic tests:** Yo-yo beep test, 12-min run or swim, 1.5-mile run, jog, walk, and step tests

For maximum effectiveness, tests should be split up and implemented on different days. Strength tests, **anaerobic capacity** tests, and aerobic tests are generally most valid when performed independently of other tests. If several tests are being performed on a single day, non-fatiguing tests may be employed between tests of more intense activity to provide a full recovery period for the client and still make good use of time. Specific decisions will be relative to the tests employed, the capabilities of the client, and other relevant factors. A good strategy when designing testing days is to implement a particular test and then use the rest of the training day to practice other physical fitness evaluations to be performed on subsequent test days.

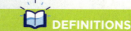

DEFINITIONS

Anaerobic capacity –

The total amount of energy for work obtained from anaerobic sources which is measured with an all-out effort; the capacity to run bodily systems without using oxygen.

PRACTICAL INSIGHT

Measures from training bouts can be used as tracking metrics in lieu of testing. Consider, for instance, a client able to perform six (6) repetitions with the heaviest resistance at 135 lbs. who uses a pyramid training set design for maximal strength improvements: his training performance can be converted to a predictive 1RM using the 3% formula (160 lbs.). Likewise, if anaerobic power-step repetitions performed at maximal speed are counted during a training bout for 15 seconds, the value can be used in future determinations of performance by either calculating watts (W) from the distance covered in 15 seconds, or by repetitions performed in 15 seconds. Repeat 30-second Wingate tests on a cycle ergometer can function similarly. Using performance data from ongoing training bouts adds value to testing information, particularly for predictions, but also has independent merit.

◆ Health and Safety Considerations

Safety must be a fundamental concern in the personal trainer's delivery of services. As with any trainer-supervised environment, the testing conditions must be controlled and managed in a way that ensures the best possible outcome for the client. Using the aforementioned strategies will certainly assist in helping to prevent negative incidents from occurring, but a premeditated safety and emergency plan should always be in place. Even though clients have gone through a proper screening process before being cleared for exercise testing, problems may still arise, as injury is an inherent, elemental risk of physical activity. In addition to establishing a safe environment and implementing a pretest checklist, trainers should explain stop-test protocols and communicate methods to help reduce injury during testing. They should visually survey the area before and during the test for external hazards and ensure the client is adequately prepared in mind and body for the assessment, while also being aware of the client's responses to the testing procedures. Likewise, trainers should be able to execute the emergency plan to efficiently address any situation that may arise. Some prudent considerations include having ice available (bagged in a portable cooler) in case of a musculoskeletal injury, having juice or sugar-based fluids to address a hypoglycemic reaction, and readying an EMS action plan in the event of a more serious situation. If a client has a medical condition, such as asthma, ensure the person has medication readily available in case of an emergency. In cases of medicated clients, such as those with controlled diabetes and hypertension, learning about how medications can affect exercise and what to expect will ensure the most positive outcome for the clients.

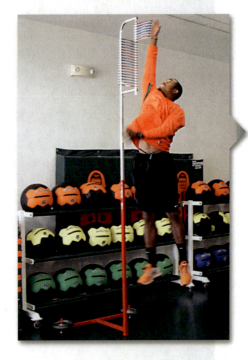

◆ Test Interpretation

Once the exercise testing data has been collected, the trainer must analyze and interpret it for the client. Clients often demonstrate high interest in their performance relative to others in their population group. To help them understand their level of fitness, trainers should compare the test scores to established age and gender norms. In some cases, the scoring system uses ranges that will encompass the client's scores in order to identify his or her current fitness level. Other test norms use percentile ranking to classify individual performance on a given test, compared to others within a homogenous group. Explaining scores and the respective classification in understandable terms and context helps clients recognize where they fall on the fitness continuum. In all cases, an effective personal training service should strive to maintain a positive outlook on the outcome. This is especially important when clients fall into categories that define their current fitness levels as low, which can lead to feelings of embarrassment and inadequacy. These counterproductive mindsets must be avoided as they can easily derail exercise motivation. To combat this potential problem, personal trainers should emphasize that these are starting points and that the training program is designed specifically to enhance the scores assessed. Avoid using negative terms, such as "poor" or "low," and apply action words instead that frame the results as a starting point for positive progress. Constructive terms would include "we will work" or "focus" on these areas. Letting the client know that the deficient result can be improved upon, providing a realistic timeline for the expected improvements, and revealing how it will be emphasized during the exercise program can help a great deal. Additionally, always convey to the client that many of their peers fall into these categories as well and that improvement in fitness is why he or she is working with a fitness professional in the first place.

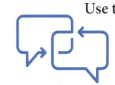

Use tact when explaining subpar test scores to clients:
- Emphasize that results are starting points and improvements will occur
- Avoid the use of negative or demeaning terms

◆ Motivational Strategies

When providing support and motivation, the focus should be on the end goal. Avoid overemphasizing current deficiencies. Most clients realize they are not in peak condition but need to know what they can achieve in a reasonable period of time. This information should be factual and provide for realistic activities and outcomes. Sugar coating the facts will simply lead to future disappointment. Focus on the steps to success, reinforcing confidence in your knowledge and the client's ability to achieve realistic outcomes. This time also provides the perfect opportunity to set interim and short-term goals. Let the client know that progress will be tracked, and that by complying with the program recommendations, improvement will come by the next evaluation. In this instance, **tracking** becomes a useful tool for motivation: demonstration of physical improvement is clear evidence the program is working.

When interpreting the recorded measures from the assessments for program decision-making purposes, exercise professionals should evaluate each area of fitness and then determine the greatest areas of individual need. Obviously, the lowest scores reflect the greatest room for

DEFINITIONS

Tracking –

The act of documenting all applicable testing and program data for a client which allows for an optimized understanding of how they are progressing towards their goals; allows the trainer to develop the best exercise prescription possible and make the most appropriate adjustments over time as the client improves, or fails to respond to training.

improvement, but certain attributes must become foundations for positive improvements. Many individuals will score low in multiple areas, and for these individuals, a plan toward securing function and endurance in aerobic and anaerobic pathways will provide for cross-adaptive benefit. CRF, mobility, and muscle-strength balance compose the initial emphasis, due to their respective roles in health and disease prevention. For those who are significantly overweight, the emphasis should be on consistency and limiting orthopedic limitations while improving endurance. Losing weight is a relatively slow process, so focusing on improvements in strength and mobility while tracking endurance gains will overshadow limited weight loss. Emphasize the most rapidly occurring adaptations to keep the client positive and motivated. In adults over 65, the focus shifts to strength, movement balance, and power training, as these closely correlate to independence and longevity. This does not suggest that the other areas should be overlooked, but that low levels of certain fitness parameters have specific consequences on other health and fitness measures, and therefore, should be given priority. All of the values ascertained from fitness testing should be added to the needs-analysis list, so they can be appropriately emphasized and accounted for in the exercise program. Each area will warrant appropriate attention, which will help to define the **program matrix**.

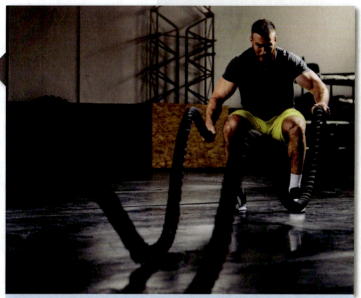

Tracking is useful for motivation because it clearly shows the client's improvements and gives evidence that the program is working.

DEFINITIONS

Program matrix –

Term used to describe all the necessary components to an exercise prescription which will allow the client to safely and effectively attain their training goals.

◆ Needs Analysis

The long list of data collected from the resting and exercise evaluations will lead to relevant findings and dictate the appropriate response via the exercise prescription. The needs analysis involves reviewing the collected information and identifying the specific issues that the exercise program needs to address. This process requires personal trainers to determine and prioritize the exercise prescription's goals, based on the data collected and the findings' relationship to positive and negative health outcomes. The initial review should single out the most negative influencing factors, as they pose the greatest risk for health consequences and may be barriers to improvements in health status. These negative factors should be evaluated and addressed with a specific strategy to generate plausible solutions to these problems. For instance, if flexibility scores are low, the limitations will affect the exercises a client can perform. The exercise professional should identify effective strategies that will improve upon the identified musculoskeletal limitations and simultaneously promote additional adaptations.

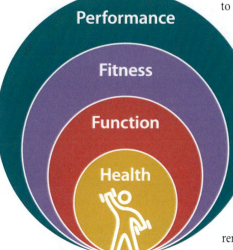

An easy way to create a needs analysis is using a two-column listing system, matching each need with one or more suitable remedies. The selected remedies serve the exercise professional by providing appropriate options to use within the exercise program. Additionally, evaluating the needs list based on the problems' severity and adaptation rate can be used to determine short and long-term goals. From an operational perspective, the order of importance works outward from those central deficiencies that present the greatest health risks, to improvements in function, to establishing adequate health-related fitness, and finally, to attain optimal fitness for performance. This structured system serves first to reduce the risk for premature death or disability, next to improve the body's systems to provide a solid base level of functional movement, and, in the end, leads to client-specific performance goals.

Category of Fitness	Measures	Issues	Recommendations
Posture	Slight anterior shoulder migration	Increased risk of impingement syndrome, scapular rhythm and shoulder complex dysfunction	Stretch pectoralis muscles Increase strength of posterior deltoids, rhomboids and mid/low trapezius Increase function of the rotator cuff
Flexibility mobility	Failed Apley back stretch test Failed Thomas test Failed trunk flexion test Failed straight-leg hip flexion test	Tight rotator cuff Tight latissimus dorsi Tight iliopsoas Tight low back Tight hamstrings	Dynamic mobility work (good morning, Bulgarian squat with overhead reach, forward lunge with cross reach) Active isolation stretches for latissimus dorsi, pectoralis, calf, hamstring, and low back
Strength balance	Imbalances in push to pull in frontal and sagittal plane Overall deconditioned	Poor back strength Limited work on overall muscle balance	Seated row, modified pull-ups, single-arm row, cable row, wide-grip overhead bar reach Emphasize total body agonist-antagonist training
Aerobic fitness	33 ml/kg/min	Low CRF (<10 METS)	Increase VO_2 by 20% Body weight metabolic circuits and intervals
Body composition	23% body fat	Body fat too high	Long term goal: decrease fat weight by 13 lbs. (18% body fat) Short term: lose 2% body fat
Additional notes	Intermittent low back discomfort	Poor flexibility in hamstrings and low back Weak core	Increase strength in abdominal and core muscles Stretch pelvic musculature

◆ Goal Setting

Nearly all new exercise professionals find goal setting initially difficult, as estimates of adaptation associated with effort and compliance are hard to ascertain. As such, typical errors frequently occur in this area. Fitness enthusiasts and professionals alike often set goals that do not align with the designated adaptation timeframe. This sets the client up for failure. When goals are not attained, clients lose momentum, and this disappointment negatively affects motivation and program compliance. When goals are set appropriately, they reinforce and promote adherence, compliance, and effort, often renewing motivation toward further improvements. The two most common errors made when defining goals are setting unrealistic targets and not creating an appropriate system of accountability and tracking to monitor objectives and short-term aims. To effectively set goals, exercise professionals should thoughtfully analyze the capabilities of the client and then determine a timeframe to reach the goals based on the actual quantity and quality of effort necessary to attain them. Effective goal setting starts with educating clients so that they understand what separates attainable goals from those that may be unrealistic or ineffective. Goals should reflect controllable behaviors, be specific, measurable, realistic, and rewarding to the client. They should have a designated time frame that matches the client's individual characteristics, motivations, and capabilities.

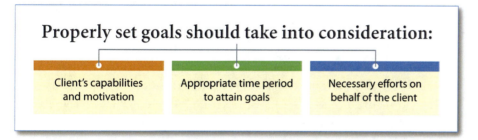

Goal setting entails outlining an action plan. In most cases, a reverse approach can effectively define the timeline, based on milestones towards the goal. Defining a timeline employs knowledge of adaptations as they relate to the actual volume of exercise to be used. Long-term personal training goals should be split into at least two categories: first, the ultimate goal to be achieved by the program, and second, a more modest goal that the client can accomplish in three to six months. Losing thirty pounds, for instance, would reflect an ultimate long-term goal, whereas losing twelve pounds would still be significant but could be attained within a reasonable timeframe. This objective would allow for a 12-week training cycle, progressively implemented and monitored using weekly and monthly milestones. Defining the terms of an action plan will ultimately proceed on a case-by-case basis due to relative physiological and psychological differences among individual clients and the numerous individual factors in play. A person new to exercise who is fairly deconditioned and previously sedentary may require more time to accomplish an ambition than a well-conditioned client. Likewise, an individual that works with an exercise professional 4x a week will likely get to the target faster than someone working with a trainer 2x a week. Psychological conditioning, often expressed as "mental attitude" or "mental toughness," is another factor that must be considered when determining a time frame with goals. Clients should understand that the proposed time line to achieve goals is based on approaching exercise with a certain intensity: if that intensity is not met, this sub-par effort can prevent or delay the timeline for goal completion.

Using the reverse model, the long-term goal helps to establish the short-term goals, based

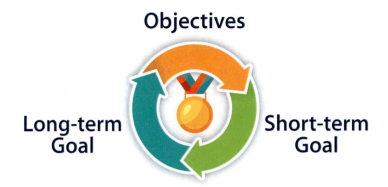

on the timeline. In the same example, a weight loss of twelve pounds in a twelve-week period suggests that the short-term goal would be one pound of weight loss a week, an average of at least four pounds of weight loss per month. Short-term goals are generally accomplishable in a month or less and can be broken down further into weekly goals. The short-term goals must be attainable because they foster motivation and pace the accomplishment of the longer-term goals. The weekly short-term targets can be further broken down into daily objectives. If the long-term aim is twelve pounds in three months and the short-term one is a pound a week of weight loss, then the daily objective would be a negative caloric balance of 500 calories (kcals). Here, the goal is to achieve a total caloric deficit of 500 kcals below the determined daily need, which will be accomplished through a regular effort of caloric restriction, combined with physical activity and exercise. If the client routinely achieves the daily objectives, he or she will reach the short-term goal of 1lb. per week, and the long-term goal becomes more attainable. Keeping the focus on daily objectives and weekly milestones provides the client with shorter, more manageable outcomes and a visible goal line. This approach has been proven to be more effective than just trying to accomplish one long term ambition, as it accounts for daily actions. Exercise professionals that intend to help people accomplish life-changing ambitions should implement short-term targets to ensure program adherence while motivating and supporting clients in efforts to attain a better lifestyle. The inability to attain goals can almost always be traced back to unrealistic expectations and false pretenses. Part of the problem is that meaningful behavioral change and physiological adaptations are fairly slow when compared to the rate of influence from negative behaviors. Attempting to force the rate of change beyond the typical human process may be sustained for a short period but will most often result in failure.

Exercise Testing

Cardiorespiratory Fitness

CRF is often considered the single most important measure of health-related fitness because it plays a role in physiological function and correlates strongly to disease and lifespan [1, 11]. Participation in cardiovascular activities positively affects the other health related components of fitness, including body composition and muscle endurance, making it a key component of any exercise program. Nonetheless, CRF alone does not suffice for optimal health measures, which include muscle strength, power, and flexibility. These attributes contribute importantly to aging well and maintaining independence. A robust evaluation of physical fitness components can be useful in discerning where to focus programmatic efforts.

Physical fitness evaluations should include periodic assessment of CRF to ensure appropriate levels of aerobic function are maintained throughout a person's life. When CRF tests are administered, they are intended to identify a person's VO_2max, or maximum oxygen uptake. VO_2max reflects the body's ability to intake, transport, and utilize oxygen. It measures the efficiency with which the lungs, heart, and blood supply oxygen to the muscles, and the ability of the muscles to extract and use the oxygen for energy metabolism and muscular contraction during exercise. Tests to measure oxygen consumption may be maximal, where an individual is required to perform an all-out effort at 100% intensity (VO_2max test), or submaximal, where heart rate is measured at lower intensities and extrapolated to predict the maximal oxygen uptake based on known relationships (sub-max VO_2 test).

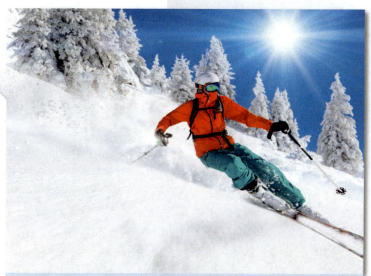

CRF is often considered the single most important measure of health-related fitness due to its role in physiological function and its relationship to disease and lifespan.

Submaximal VO_2 Tests vs Maximal Tests

Exercise professionals rarely employ maximal cardiorespiratory protocols due to the need for experience and practice in conducting them, risk of possible negative outcomes, increased resources required for accurate implementation, and the time and complexity of administration. On the other hand, submaximal testing is often easier to employ, requires minimal equipment, presents limited risk for injury or cardiovascular incident, and is well-tolerated by most people. These tests include walking and running protocols, stationary bike tests, step tests, and even swim tests, if warranted by the test population.

Most submaximal assessments require subjects to perform activities at a predetermined pace with a protocol-specific level of difficulty, although some tests do utilize gradually increasing submaximal workloads. The tests are performed for an assigned duration, until a designated distance is reached, or until steady-state heart rate has been attained at a selected intensity level. The specific test protocol determines the measuring system and termination criteria to be used. Once the test data has been collected, it is normally entered into a protocol-specific calculation or graphed to identify a predictive score or value. Note that submaximal protocols differ from maximal protocols in that they generate a prediction of an individual's VO_2max. They are less accurate due this indirect measurement of CRF, whereas maximal protocols represent a direct measurement.

Predicting Maximal Values

Predictive equations convert the measured performance unit into an expression of oxygen utilization. The predictive quantity of oxygen utilization is expressed in absolute terms: milliliters or liters of oxygen used per minute of activity ($ml \cdot min^{-1}$ or $L \cdot min^{-1}$), or in relative terms, milliliters of oxygen used per kilogram of body weight per minute of activity ($ml \cdot kg^{-1} \cdot min^{-1}$). The absolute terms represent the total quantity of oxygen consumed by the body per minute, whereas the relative expression represents the oxygen used by the subject's body mass per minute. If a large person and small person both have the same absolute measure of oxygen usage, the smaller person possesses a better oxygen utilization capacity per pound or kilogram of his or her respective weight. For this reason, relative expressions are more commonly used so that the measures display the subjects' individualized efficiency levels, and are, therefore, more useful for comparisons among individuals.

The predicted measure of oxygen utilization identified by the test will mean very little to a client if presented using scientific expression (ml · kg^{1-} · min^{1-}). The findings should be explained in easy to understand language and compared to norms consistent with the client's sex and age. Personal trainers should become familiar with what the scores mean for different population segments so that the exercise prescription is appropriately constructed to help meet the client's defined goals.

Each submaximal test of CRF will have specific protocols for proper implementation. Early text discussed the importance of matching the client to the appropriate test, based on his or her specific characteristics. For each of the following protocols, it should be assumed that the client has already signed an informed consent, has been successfully screened for risk factors, and has been cleared for exercise participation consistent with the level of testing being conducted. He or she should have complied with the pretest checklist and be appropriately prepared for testing. Additionally, each protocol has indicators to abort the test (**Stop Test Indicators**) that should be strictly adhered to, along with an emergency plan in the unlikely event of a problem.

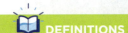

DEFINITIONS

Stop test indicators –

A list of absolute and relative signs that an exercise test should be terminated immediately.

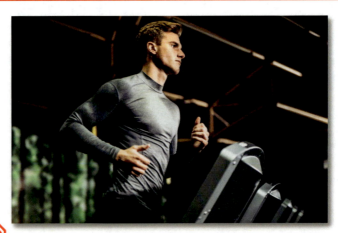

Indications for Test Termination

- Subject no longer feels comfortable doing the test.
- Subject's skin becomes pale.
- Subject fails to keep cadence for 20 seconds or more.
- Subject has an inability to focus attention.
- Subject experiences faintness, dizziness, or lightheadedness.
- Subject experiences upset stomach or vomiting symptoms.
- Subject experiences dysfunction in breathing.
- Subject experiences chest pain.
- Subject experiences side stitch, cramp, strain, fatigue.

FITNESS TEST PREPARATION CHECKLIST

Subject Preparation

1. Subject has completed the informed consent. _____
2. Subject has been screened and cleared for participation. _____
3. Subject has read and understands the test procedures. _____
4. Subject understands the starting and stopping procedures. _____
5. Subject knows the stop test indicators. _____
6. Subject understands what is expected for each stage of the test. _____
7. Subject has complied with all pre-test instructions concerning:
    A. Rest _____
    B. Food _____
    C. Beverage and hydration status _____
    D. Drugs – including prescription, stimulants, depressants, alcohol, and tobacco _____
    E. Appropriate attire _____
8. Subject does not have illness or injury. _____
9. Subject is not fatigued, stressed, or anxious. _____
10. Subject is not on any medication (prescription or non-prescription). _____
11. Subject has participated in the proper warm-up procedure. _____

Tester Preparation

1. Test to be administered has been determined. _____
2. The protocols for administration are understood. _____
3. Equipment has been tested, calibrated, and is in good working order. _____
4. All necessary equipment, supplies, and recording sheets are ready. _____
5. The test environment is within acceptable limits for:
    A. Cleanliness _____
    B. Temperature _____
    C. Humidity _____
    D. Noise _____
6. The timing and sequence of testing are set. _____
7. The starting and stopping instructions are clear. _____
8. The subject has been prepared appropriately and meets all guidelines for testing. _____
9. The test atmosphere and environment are controlled. _____
10. Post test activities and responsibilities are set. _____
11. Emergency procedures are determined and understood. _____

Chapter 7

CARDIORESPIRATORY FITNESS TEST: 1 MILE WALK TEST

Equipment

1 mile course
Stopwatch

Test

Walk as quickly as possible for 1 mile. Immediately record the HR at the culmination of the test if wearing a HR monitoring device, or measure 10 second heart rate immediately following completion of the mile distance.

Directions

1) **Test Preparation:** Subject should comply with pretest checklist requirements including all test instructions. He or she should have practiced the distance and been instructed on proper HR assessment.

2) **Test Start:** Have subject ready him or herself behind the beginning mark of the measured mile. Test administrator initiates the test, stating "Ready, Set, Go!" and starts the watch. The subject will then walk the measured mile distance as fast as possible.

3) **Test Finish:** At the end of the measured mile (4 laps on standard track), the tester identifies the subject's time as he or she crosses the measured mile marker and records the number below. **The heart rate at the end of the test should also be recorded.** If not using a HR monitor, immediately palpate and assess the subject's heart rate for 10 seconds. Record the 10-second heart rate, and calculate the subject's 60-second heart rate by multiplying by 6.

Time to Completion _____   **Heart Rate** _____

4) **Cool Down:** Have the subject perform an adequate cool down following the assessment.

5) **Organize Data:** To calculate the subject's fitness level you will need to have the following data: age, current body weight, and gender (this information should have already been gathered prior to any physical activity assessments). In addition, your recording sheet should have the subject's 1-mile walk time and 60-second pulse count from Steps 3 and 4.

6) **Calculating Fitness Level:** The following formula is used to calculate an estimated VO2max (ml · kg^{-1} · min^{-1}) for the 1-mile walk test from the recorded information. Using the equation template below, calculate the estimated VO_2max.

$$VO_2\text{max (ml} \cdot \text{kg}^{-1} \cdot \text{min}^{-1}) =$$
$$132.853 - 0.0769\text{ (weight)} - 0.3877\text{ (age)} + 6.315\text{ (gender)} - 3.2649\text{ (time)} - 0.1565\text{ (HR)}$$

- Weight is in pounds
- Age is in years
- Gender = 0 for females and 1 for males
- Time is in minutes and hundredths of a minute (ex. 13.06)
- Heart rate is in beats per minute

Aerobic Fitness Classification for the General Population ($ml \cdot kg^{-1} \cdot min^{-1}$)

MEN

Age (Years)	20-29	30-39	40-49	50-59	60+
Above Average	>46.8	>44.6	>41.8	>38.5	>35.3
Average	42.5 – 46.7	41.0 – 44.5	38.1 – 41.7	35.2 – 38.4	31.8 – 35.2
Below Average	<42.4	<40.9	<38	<35.1	<31.7

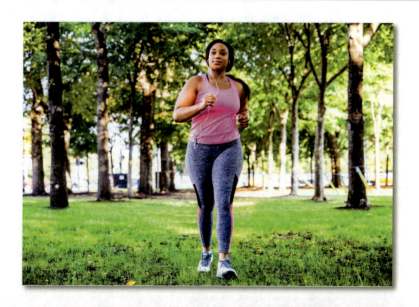

Aerobic Fitness Classification for the General Population ($ml \cdot kg^{-1} \cdot min^{-1}$)

WOMEN

Age (Years)	20-29	30-39	40-49	50-59	60+
Above Average	>38.1	>36.7	>33.8	>30.9	>29.4
Average	35.2 – 38	33.9 – 36.6	30.9 – 33.7	28.3 – 30.8	25.9 – 29.3
Below Average	<35.1	<33.8	<30.8	<28.2	<25.8

CARDIORESPIRATORY FITNESS TEST: 12 MINUTE RUN TEST

Equipment

Measured track
Stopwatch

Test

On a measured track, run as quickly as possible for 12 minutes. Periods of walking and jogging are acceptable if the overall exertion is maximal.

Directions

1) **Test Preparation:** Subject is checked for compliance with the pretest checklist and instructed in a proper warm-up activity.

2) **Test Start:** When ready to begin the test, the subject will line up at the starting line of the pre-measured track. The test administrator will say "Ready, Set, Go!" and the subject will begin the test.

3) The subject will (run, jog, and/or walk) for the designated time period (12 min) at the fastest tolerable pace.

4) The test administrator should supply motivational support and shout out the duration of time remaining following each lap.

5) **Test Finish:** Toward the end of the 12 minute duration, the test administrator should place himself or herself in close proximity to the subject to identify the specific location that the subject reached on the track at the end of 12 minutes period: the identified finishing spot should be within 10 yards of the true spot attained by the subject.

6) **The testing administrator should not have the subject stop for the sake of identifying the finishing spot; the subject should be allowed to continue moving through the end of the test.** This explains why the test administrator must position himself or herself appropriately as the time approaches the 12 minute limit.

7) Have the subject perform a cool down activity.

8) **Calculating Fitness Level:** The fitness level of the subject is determined by consulting the following table.

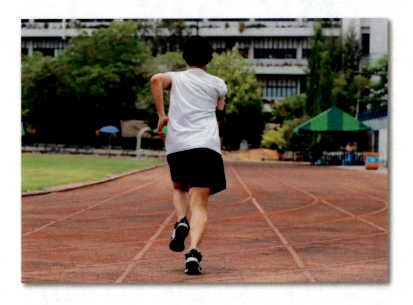

Fitness Level vs. 12-min Distance for Men and Women Ages 13-59 years

12 – Minute Distance (Miles)

Fitness Level	Age (Years)	13-19	20-29	30-39	40-49	50-59
Very Poor	Men	<1.30	<1.22	<1.18	<1.14	<1.03
	Women	<1.0	<0.96	<0.94	<0.88	<0.84
Below Average	Men	1.30 - 1.37	1.22 - 1.31	1.18 - 1.30	1.14 - 1.24	1.03 - 1.16
	Women	1.00 - 1.18	0.96 - 1.11	0.95 - 1.05	0.88 - 0.98	0.84 - 0.93
Fair	Men	1.38 - 1.56	1.32 - 1.49	1.31 - 1.45	1.25 - 1.39	1.17 - 1.30
	Women	1.19 - 1.29	1.12 - 1.22	1.06 - 1.18	0.99 - 1.11	0.94 - 1.05
Good	Men	1.57 - 1.72	1.50 - 1.64	1.46 - 1.56	1.40 - 1.53	1.31 - 1.44
	Women	1.30 - 1.43	1.23 - 1.34	1.19 - 1.29	1.12 - 1.24	1.06 - 1.18
Excellent	Men	1.73 - 1.86	1.65 - 1.76	1.57 - 1.69	1.54 - 1.65	1.45 - 1.58
	Women	1.44 - 1.51	1.35 - 1.45	1.30 - 1.39	1.25 - 1.34	1.19 - 1.30
Superior	Men	>1.87	>1.77	>1.70	>1.66	>1.59
	Women	>1.52	>1.46	>1.40	>1.35	>1.31

Maximal Oxygen Consumption (VO$_2$max) vs. 12-Minute Distance

12-Min Distance (miles)	VO$_2$max (ml · kg^{-1} · min^{-1})
<1.0	<25.0
1.0 - 1.24	25.0 - 33.7
1.25 - 1.49	33.8 - 42.5
1.50 - 1.74	42.6 - 51.5
1.75 - 2.0	51.6 - 60.2
>2.0	>60.2

CARDIORESPIRATORY FITNESS TEST: 1.5 MILE RUN

Equipment
Measured track
Stopwatch

Test
On a measured track, run as quickly as possible for 1.5 miles. Periods of walking and jogging are acceptable if the overall exertion is maximal.

Directions

1) **Test Preparation:** Check that the subject has complied with pretest checklist and have him or her perform an appropriate warm-up activity.

2) **Test Start:** Have subject get ready behind the beginning mark of the measured 1.5 miles. The test administrator initiates the test, stating "Ready, Set, Go!" and starts the watch as the subject begins running the 1.5 mile distance (6 laps on a standard track).

3) **Monitor:** As the subject passes the start/stop line, the trainer informs the subject of the lap number and the time. The test administrator should also look for signs of physical distress.

4) **Test Finish:** At the completion of lap 6, or 1.5 miles, the tester records the subject's time and has him or her perform a cool down activity.

5) **Review of Formula:** Calculating the fitness level (estimated VO_2max) from the subject's 1.5-mile run time involves the use of the following formula:

$$VO_2 = \text{horizontal velocity m·min}^{-1} \times \frac{0.2 \text{ ml} \cdot \text{kg}^{-1} \cdot \text{min}^{-1}}{\text{m} \cdot \text{min}^{-1}} + 3.5 \text{ ml} \cdot \text{kg}^{-1} \cdot \text{min}^{-1}$$

6) **Finding horizontal running velocity (m · min^{-1}):** The first factor that must be calculated is the average horizontal running velocity of the subject in meters per minute. To do this, convert the distance completed into meters, and divide it by the number of minutes the subject took to complete the run.

Example Meter Conversion

1.5 miles = 2,413.8 meters

2,413.8 must then be divided by the time it took to complete the run in minutes (use whole numbers).

Example (m · min^{-1}) conversion

If it took 12:00 minutes to complete the run, divide the 2,413 meters by 12 minutes.

2,413.8 m ÷ 12 min = 201.15 m · min^{-1} (horizontal velocity)

If it took 12:13 to complete the run, then the divisor would be 12.21.

12 min + (13 sec ÷ 60 sec)

Perform your conversion below:

2,413.8 meters ÷ _____ minutes = _____ m · min^{-1} (horizontal velocity)

7) **VO₂max conversion:** The last calculation that must be performed will provide you with the client's estimated VO₂max. Consider the previous example:

$$VO_2\,max = \text{horizontal velocity } m\cdot min^{-1} \times \frac{0.2\ ml\cdot kg^{-1}\cdot min^{-1}}{m\cdot min^{-1}} + 3.5\ ml\cdot kg^{-1}\cdot min^{-1}$$

$$VO_2 max = 201\ \cancel{m\cdot min^{-1}} \times \frac{0.2\ ml\cdot kg^{-1}\cdot min^{-1}}{\cancel{m\cdot min^{-1}}} + 3.5\ ml\cdot kg^{-1}\cdot min^{-1}$$

$$VO_2 max = 43.7\ ml\cdot kg^{-1}\cdot min^{-1}$$

The following chart can also be used as a quick reference:

1.5 Mile Time min:s	VO₂max ml·kg⁻¹·min⁻¹	1.5 Mile Time min:s	VO₂max ml·kg⁻¹·min⁻¹
<7:31	75	12:31 - 13:00	39
7:31 - 8:00	72	13:01 - 13:30	37
8:01 - 8:30	67	13:31 - 14:00	36
8:31 - 9:00	62	14:01 - 14:30	34
9:01 - 9:30	58	14:31 - 15:00	33
9:31 - 10:00	55	15:01 - 15:30	31
10:01 - 10:30	52	15:31 - 16:00	30
10:31 - 11:00	49	16:01 - 16:30	28
11:01 - 11:30	46	16:31 - 17:00	27
11:31 - 12:00	44	17:01 - 17:30	26
12:01 - 12:30	41	17:31 - 18:00	25

CARDIORESPIRATORY FITNESS TEST: 3 MINUTE STEP TEST

Equipment

Step or Box (16.25 inch)
Metronome
Stopwatch

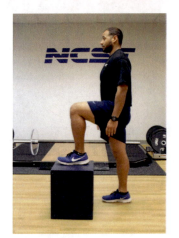

Test

This test requires subjects to step up and down on a 16.25-inch step at a set metronome pace for three minutes. A fifteen-second recovery heart rate is taken between five and twenty seconds following the test and converted to a predicted VO_2max.

Directions

1) **Test Preparation:** Ensure the subject has complied with the pretest checklist.

2) **Practice stepping:** Using a 16.25 in box or step, have the subject stand facing toward the box and practice stepping with each foot completely on and off the box. A metronome is set at 88 (women) or 96 (men) tones per minute, and the subject should practice stepping up and down using a four-count cadence.

"Up-one"	Foot #1 goes to the top of the step.
"Up-two"	The other foot (#2) follows to the top of the step.
"Down-one"	Foot #1 descends to the floor.
"Down-two"	Foot #2 descends to the floor.

   The subject should practice until he or she can establish cadence (ideally ambidextrously to avoid single leg fatigue).

   Once proficiency has been demonstrated, allow the subject a rest period for the duration of time it takes to return the pulse back to a resting state.

3) **Begin Assessment:** Following the rest interval, re-establish the metronome's pace – 96 tones per minute for men and 88 tones per minute for women – and ask the subject to take the starting position (facing the box). When the subject feels ready, he or she can begin stepping. As soon as the client takes the first step, the test administrator should begin timing the assessment.

4) **Test Performance:** Have the subject continue stepping on and off the box, keeping with the cadence, for 3 minutes.

5) **RPE:** The trainer should maintain visual assessment of the subject throughout the duration of the test to identify any signs and symptoms listed on the Stop Test Indicator check list. The trainer should also periodically ask the subject how he or she is feeling, based on their RPE. The RPE for this type of submaximal assessment should not exceed 7 on a 1 to 10 scale, or 16 on a 1 to 20 scale.

6) **Palpation Preparation:** When the stopwatch reaches 3:00, have the subject stop stepping. Be sure to keep the watch running, as it will be used to assess the subject's recovery heart rate. Immediately locate the subject's radial pulse as the clock continues to run. Marking the site before beginning the test may aid in rapid identification.

7) **Recovery Heart Rate Palpation:** Once the stopwatch reads 3:05, the test administrator begins counting the subject's recovery heart rate through the palpation of the radial artery.

8) Monitoring/counting of the subject's heart rate should start at the 3:05 mark and end at the 3:20 mark. This will provide the subject's heart rate in 15 seconds.

9) Record the 15-second recovery heart rate. Then have subject perform a cool down.

Recovery heart rate (15 seconds) _____ beats min^{-1}

Procedures for Estimating VO₂max:

10) **Calculate Fitness Level Score:** Using the 15-second recovery heart rate recorded in step #9, calculate the subject's predicted VO_2.

Maximal oxygen uptake in ml/kg/min is estimated per the following equations:

Men: Maximal oxygen uptake = 111.33 - (0.42 * recovery heart rate in bpm)
Women: Maximal oxygen uptake = 65.81 - (0.1847 * recovery heart rate in bpm)

Example: The recovery fifteen-second heart rate for a male subject following the three-minute step test is found to be 39 beats. Maximal oxygen uptake is estimated as follows:

Fifteen-second heart rate = 39 beats

Minute heart rate = 39 * 4 = 156 bpm

Maximal oxygen uptake = 111.33-(0.42*156) = 45.81 ml · kg⁻¹ · min⁻¹

Enter score here _____ (ml · kg⁻¹ · min⁻¹)

11) **Evaluating the Results:** To find out what fitness category the client falls into, refer to the table titled below.

Enter classification here _____

Sex	Age	Poor	Fair	Average	Good	Excellent
Men	<29	<25	25 - 33	34 - 42	43 - 52	53+
	30 - 39	<23	23 - 30	31 - 38	39 - 48	49+
	40 - 49	<20	20 - 26	27 - 35	36 - 44	45+
	50 - 59	<18	18 - 24	25 - 33	34 - 42	43+
	60 - 69	<16	16 - 22	23 - 30	31 - 40	41+
Women	<29	<24	24 - 30	31 - 37	38 - 48	49+
	30 - 39	<20	20 - 27	28 - 33	34 - 44	45+
	40 - 49	<17	17 - 23	24 - 30	31 - 41	42+
	50 - 59	<15	15 - 20	21 - 27	28 - 37	38+
	60 - 69	<13	13 - 17	18 - 23	24 - 34	35+

CARDIORESPIRATORY FITNESS TEST: YO-YO BEEP TEST

Equipment

Cones
Metronome
Stopwatch

Test

This test requires subjects to sprint to failure in 20m shuttle runs between cones at a set metronome pace. A ten-second recovery is used between shuttle attempts. The number of shuttles completed is converted to a predicted VO₂max.

Yo-Yo IR1 Protocol

1) **Test Preparation:** Ensure the subject has complied with the pretest checklist.
2. **Warm-up:** Have the subject perform a warm-up, emphasizing continuous movement for 5-10 minutes.
3. **Set up:** Place two cones in line 20m apart and a third recovery cone 5m from the start cone.

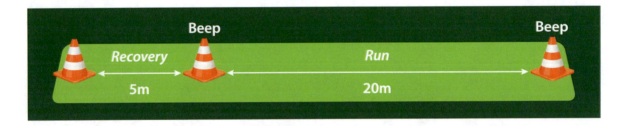

4. **Practice:** The subject must run 40m (shuttles) with intermittent 10-second active recovery periods that include 10 meters of jogging around a recovery cone.
5. Once the subject is familiar with the test, have him or her start at the first shuttle cone. On the "Ready, Go!" command, the subject must run to the second cone and back before the second beep sounds. They will decelerate around the recovery cone and reposition at the start within 10sec.
6. The test is terminated when the subject fails to finish 2 consecutive shuttles before the "beep" sounds.
7. The subject performs the first four shuttles at 10 km/h.
8. He or she then performs 7 shuttles at 13.5-14 km/h.
9. If the subject has not failed by the 11 shuttle, he or she will perform another 8 shuttles with the cadence speed increased by 0.5 km/h.
10. This is repeated until the subject fails.
11. VO₂max is obtained using the formula: **VO$_2$max = IR distance in meters x 0.0084 + 36.4.**

Estimated VO$_2$max: _____

Testing for Muscular Fitness

Testing for muscular fitness includes assessing a client's capacity for both **muscular strength** and **endurance**. Traditionally, these components of fitness have used specialized equipment: hand grip dynamometers, cable tensiometers, and isokinetic machines to predict body strength and endurance in clinical settings or 1RM dynamic resistance exercises for use with athletic populations. However, this testing method did not account for the fact that individual muscles vary in their ability to produce and sustain force. This is compounded by force variability in the direction of the force application. Using only one or two measures to assess the body's force production capabilities or the body's ability to sustain force output means that the outcome may not be valid for movements or exercises other than the ones used for the testing. For instance, a person may perform well on a bench-press test but not have the strength to perform a pull-up; he or she may be able to perform leg/knee extension using 150 lbs. but only produce 50 lbs. of force during knee flexion, placing him or her at an increased risk for muscle strains and joint injuries due to strength imbalances. For this reason, exercise professionals should evaluate different strength and endurance capabilities with an emphasis on agonist/antagonist strength balance across the joint.

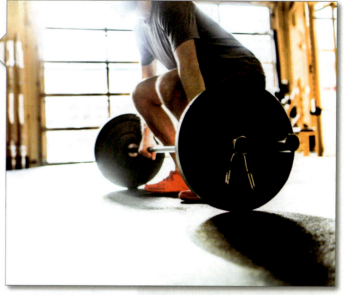

Muscle Balance Ratio Goals

Trunk Flexors: Extensors	1:1
Hip Flexors: Extensors	1:1
Shoulder Flexors: Extensors	2:3
Knee Flexors: Extensors	2:3
Shoulder Int. Rotators: Ext. Rotators	3:2
Elbow Extensors: Flexors	1:1
Ankle Plantar Flexors: Dorsiflexors	3:1

Adequate strength and endurance in all body muscles is a central goal for health. When measures such as the bench press or leg press are emphasized, the criteria for retest performance only apply to the muscle groups employed. A person may, in fact, perform well on those tests and receive a high ranking for muscle strength, but this should not be viewed as a true representation of the whole body. In the ideal situation, exercise professionals would be able to ascertain the strength and fitness of all the major muscle groups to identify deficiencies and imbalances. Normalized data can be used for traditional assessments where population norms have been established, while multi-repetition assessments and one-repetition predictive calculations can help provide information regarding movements that do not currently have defined comparable data.

As previously suggested, a balance of muscular strength between agonist and antagonist muscle groups aids proper joint stability and function. Muscles that cause joint movement maintain an opposing relationship across the joint. The nature of the joints' architectural efficiency and muscle attachment sites determine the force (balance) relationship of the opposing muscles, and attaining the appropriate ratio for each group should be a primary goal of any exercise program.

> **DEFINITIONS**
>
> **Muscular strength –**
>
> *The external force that can be generated by a specific muscle or muscle groups; it is commonly expressed in terms of resistance met or overcome.*
>
> **Endurance –**
>
> *The ability of a muscle group to execute repeated muscle actions over a period of time sufficient to cause muscular fatigue, or to maintain a specific percentage of the 1 Repetition Maximum (1RM) for a prolonged period of time.*

Muscular Strength Assessments

Strength assessments pose a level of risk for musculoskeletal injury due to mechanical strain, particularly in deconditioned clients. To reduce this risk, clients should be well-versed in the exercise movements and appropriately familiarized with the load and velocity the assessment requires. Of course, near maximal strength assessments are not the ideal time for practice or experimentation; test practice should be performed prior to actual testing in order to improve test validity and reliability. Since muscle strength is generally associated with 1-10 repetitions, selecting multi-repetition tests is recommended for the average healthy population. Lower repetition maximal tests can be performed safely with healthy populations, but inherent problems exist. Some of these problems include the following: increased risk associated with the testing; difficulty in identifying the correct maximal load to be lifted; changes to the movement mechanics due to the high load and stability requirements; questions of qualifying technique; performance ROM; and, finally, dramatic increases in pressure associated with the lifts. Outside of specific performance purposes, low-repetition, maximal-strength tests are generally not recommended.

Resistance exercises used for strength testing feature many variations. Some tests employ static resistance or isometric strength tests, while others use variable resistance or constant resistance machines. Still others utilize free-weight modalities. Although the decision to employ any test will be client specific, free-weight assessments feature advantages over exercise machines. In addition to assessing strength, free weight tests can identify relative joint stability during the movement performance. Since joint stabilizers always represent the weak link in the kinetic chain, free weights better identify true strength. Machine tests only measure linear or angular force and will not identify significant weaknesses associated with joint instability due to the fixed movement arms. Humans require balance, coordination, and stability during real world applications of energy transfer; therefore, it is logical to employ these factors when testing.

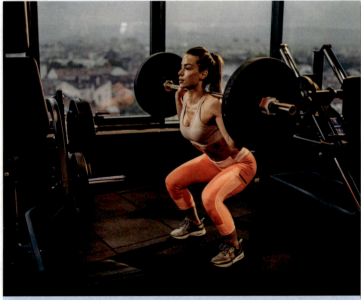

Strength assessments possess a level of risk for musculoskeletal injury due to mechanical strain, particularly in deconditioned clients. To reduce this risk, clients should be well-versed in the exercise movements and appropriately familiarized with the load and velocity being used in the assessment.

MUSCULAR STRENGTH TEST: MULTI-REP BENCH PRESS

Equipment

Flat bench, Olympic bar and weights

Test

Maximal repetition test to predict 1RM strength using a bench press.

Directions

1) **Starting Position:** Subject should begin in a supine position on a flat bench with feet flat on the floor. Subject should assume a neutral spine position and place hands just outside of shoulder width using a closed, pronated grip (thumps wrapped around the bar).

2) Perform three warm-up sets, progressing from estimated 50, 65, 75% resistance for up to 8 repetitions. Allow a two-minute recovery between sets and three minutes after the final warm-up set.

3) Place an estimated 85% 1RM or what the subject expects to lift for 5-7 repetitions on the bar.

4) The test administrator assists the subject in lifting the bar off the rack to a position over the subject's chest. The subject should maintain the bar position with fully extended arms. At this point, the test starts, and the subject performs as many repetitions as possible to failure.

5) **Downward Movement Phase:** The subject should lower the bar using a quick but controlled movement down toward the chest. As the descent is made, the body should remain fixed on the bench with no extraneous movement.

6) **Upward Movement Phase:** Once bar contact has been made with the chest, the subject will press the bar upward in the same plane of motion as employed during the descent phase.

7) The bar is pressed upward until the arms are fully extended but not locked. This is repeated to volitional failure.

8) **Spotting:** The test administrator should lift the bar off the rack to the start position only. During the test, the administrator should spot the lifter with his or her hands supinated under the bar (without making contact) inside the subject's grip position.

9) At the test's end, the test administrator should assist with re-racking the bar.

10) The predicted maximum can be calculated using the following formula:

3% Formula

[(0.03 x reps performed) + 1.0] x total weight weight used

[(0.03 x Reps _____) + 1.0] x weight used _____ lb.

(_____ + 1.0) x _____ lb.

Estimated Bench Press 1RM = _____ lb.

11) **Interpret Results.** The table below illustrates *Relative Bench Press Strength Norms* based on body weight in both males and females. To find your subject's strength classification, divide the subject's calculated 1RM by current body weight.

Weight Lifted ÷ Body Weight = Upper Body Strength Rating

Upper Body Strength Rating _____

Age (Years)	20-29		30-39		40-49		50-59		60 +	
Classification	M	F	M	F	M	F	M	F	M	F
Above Average	>1.17	>.72	>1.01	>.62	>.91	>.57	>.81	>.51	>.74	>.51
Average	.97 - 1.16	.59 - .71	.86 - 1.00	.53 - .61	.78 - .90	.48 - .56	.70 - .80	.43 - .50	.63 - .73	.41 - .50
Below Average	<.96	<.58	<.85	<.52	<.77	<.47	<.69	<.42	<.62	<.40

MUSCULAR STRENGTH TEST: 3-5 RM SQUAT

Equipment

Squat rack

Olympic bar and weights

Test

Maximal repetition test to predict 1RM strength using a Back Squat.

Directions

1) Prior to the test performance, the subject must demonstrate squatting efficiency using a barbell and should practice in the required depth for each repetition to be scored as valid. Ideally, the subject has a benchmark squat score (e.g., an estimated 10RM or heavier).

2) Calculate predicted max using benchmark squat performance.

$$[(0.03 \times \text{Reps performed}) + 1.0] \times \text{weight used} = \text{Predicted 1RM}$$

$$\text{Multiply Predicted 1 RM} \times 90\% = \text{Multi-rep weight}$$

3) **Starting Position:** the correct bar height must be set so that the subject can safely position the bar across the shoulders and step clear of the rack.

4) Once the bar is set at the correct height, the subject faces the bar and grasps it with a closed, pronated grip. The hands should be placed slightly wider than shoulder width apart.

5) The subject then steps under the bar and positions it across the superior aspect of the scapula on top of the trapezius. **DO NOT** place the bar across the cervical spine. The scapula should be retracted to help provide rigidity to the upper spine.

6) To attain the correct starting position, the subject must extend the knees to lift the bar off the rack. Once the weight is suspended and the client has established control under the load, he or she must slowly step backward (one-two foot clearance) to avoid coming in contact with the rack during the execution phase of the lift.

7) Once clear of the rack, the subject again places the feet shoulder width apart and positions the feet so that they are pointing forward and slightly outward. The degree of outward rotation will be consistent with the natural standing gait of the subject and is dictated by the degree of hip abduction.

8) Have the subject warm-up using 3 sets: 1 each of 10-8-6 repetitions, using 65%, 70%, and 80% of predicted or estimated 1RM. Allow for full recovery between sets.

9) Place an estimated 90% 1RM or what the subject expects to lift for 4-5 repetitions on the bar.

10) The test administrator assumes the spotting position as the subject lifts the bar off the rack to the start position. At this point, the test starts, and the subject must perform as many repetitions as possible to failure.

11) **Downward Movement Phase:** The subject initiates the controlled downward movement by simultaneously flexing the hips and knees. The trunk remains isometrically contracted, the head remains forward, and the chest elevated as the subject flexes the hips and knees to at least 90° of knee flexion. The ideal end-point ROM is exhibited when the top of the thigh is parallel with the floor. The knees should not break the anterior plane of the toes during the entire downward movement phase.

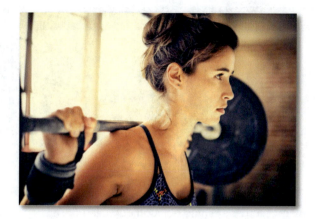

12) **Upward Movement Phase:** Once end-point ROM has been reached, the subject extends the knees and hips to return to the start position. This is repeated to failure.

13) The back should not round or move towards the floor on the ascent, and the legs should not adduct or abduct during any phase of the execution process.

14) Once the 3-5RM have been completed, re-rack the bar, checking to be sure the bar rests safely on the rack.

15) **Spotting:** The squat spotter should utilize an upper trunk hand placement technique. The hands of the spotter should be located outside of the anterior aspects of the rib cage. Spotters should immediately assume the position at the liftoff from the rack and walk the subject to the starting position.

16) The spotter should mirror the lifter's form and speed. This allows the hips to extend and move the subject safely into an upright position.

17) When the lift is complete, the spotter should walk the subject back to the rack and watch the bar to make sure it is racked correctly.

18) Calculate the predicted 1RM using the following formula.

Step One:

3 repetitions performed 1.09 x _____ weight used = _____ predicted 1RM

4 repetitions performed 1.12 x _____ weight used = _____ predicted 1RM

5 repetitions performed 1.15 x _____ weight used = _____ predicted 1RM

Step Two: _____ predicted 1RM / _____ body weight

Classification of Relative Squat Strength (1 RM/body mass)											
Age (Years)	20-29		30-39		40-49		50-59		60 +		
Classification	M	F	M	F	M	F	M	F	M	F	
Above Average	>1.84	>1.36	>1.21	>1.21	>1.57	>1.13	>1.47	>1.08	>1.37	>1.00	
Average	1.63 - 1.84	1.26 - 1.36	1.55 - 1.64	1.13 - 1.21	1.50 - 1.57	1.06 - 1.13	1.40 - 1.47	.86 - 1.08	1.31 - 1.37	.85 - 1.00	
Below Average	<1.63	<1.26	<1.55	<1.13	<1.50	<1.06	<1.40	<.86	<1.31	<.85	

MUSCULAR STRENGTH TEST: 10 RM LEG PRESS

Equipment

Leg press, adequate weight

Test

Maximal repetition test to predict 1RM strength using a leg press.

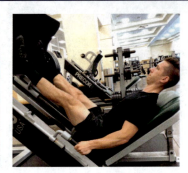

Directions

1) **Starting Position:** The subject assumes a seated position in the leg press machine.
2) The back is pressed flat against the back pad, and feet are placed flat on the footplate, approximately shoulder width apart.
3) The lumbar spine should be pressed firmly into the pad, and the knees should be slightly flexed in readiness to disengage the machine's support arms.
4) **Downward Movement Phase:** The subject extends the legs slowly and disengages the weight (usually by a rotating handle). With the back pressed firmly against the back pad, the weight is dropped in a controlled manner, causing the knees to flex in front of the subject's torso. As the weight descends, the lumbar spine and glutes must stay in contact with the back support and seat pad.
5) The weight is lowered until full, functional ROM has been reached with a neutral pelvic tilt. This will vary from person to person. Individual flexibility limitations of the glutes, low back, and hamstrings will dictate specific endpoint ROM. At no point should the glutes rise off the back pad to create a posterior pelvic tilt.
6) The subject's knees should not be flexed more than 90°, and at no point should the knees break the plane of the toes.
7) **Upward Movement Phase:** Once full, functional ROM has been attained or the knees have reached 90° of flexion, the subject returns the resistance to the start position. The knees are never placed into full extension or a "locked" position at any point during the execution, even during a break between repetitions.
8) Subjects should perform at least two warm-up sets before attempting the 10-repetition maximal lift.
9) Use the following formula to calculate the predicted 1RM from the subjects best ten-repetition performance.

Step One:

9 reps 1.27 x _____ weight used = _____ predicted 1RM

10 reps 1.3 x _____ weight used = _____ predicted 1RM

11 reps 1.33 x _____ weight used = _____ predicted 1RM

Step Two:

_____ predicted 1RM / _____ body weight

Classification of Relative Leg Press Strength (1 RM/body mass)											
Age (Years)	20-29		30-39		40-49		50-59		60 +		
Classification	M	F	M	F	M	F	M	F	M	F	
Above Average	>1.97	>1.42	>1.85	>1.47	>1.74	>1.35	>1.64	>1.24	>1.56	>1.18	
Average	1.91 - 1.97	1.32 - 1.42	1.71 - 1.85	1.26 - 1.47	1.62 - 1.74	1.19 - 1.35	1.52 - 1.64	1.09 - 1.24	1.43 - 1.56	1.08 - 1.18	
Below Average	<1.91	<1.32	<1.71	<1.26	<1.62	<1.19	<1.52	<1.09	<1.43	<1.08	

MUSCULAR STRENGTH TEST: PULL-UP

Equipment

Pull-up bar

Test

Measure of upper body pulling strength relative to body weight.

Directions

1) **Starting Position:** Following a proper warm-up, the subject should start by grasping a pull-up bar with hands in a pronated position approximately shoulder width apart and attain a straight-arm hanging position. Note: pull-up performance should be evaluated before the test for proper score discrimination and subject understanding of the ROM required per scored repetition.

2) **Upward Movement Phase:** From a complete (arm extended) hang position, the upward ascent requires the subject's chin to pass the top of the bar without ANY extraneous leg assistance.

3) **Downward Movement Phase:** After the chin has passed the top of the bar, the subject should initiate the downward phase of the movement to full arm extension.

4) Count the total number of repetitions completed. Score _____

5) Compare to the sex-appropriate table below.

Classification for Males (> 17 Y)		
Below Average	Average	Above Average
<7	8-10	>11

Classification for Females (> 17 Y)		
Below Average	Average	Above Average
0	1	>1

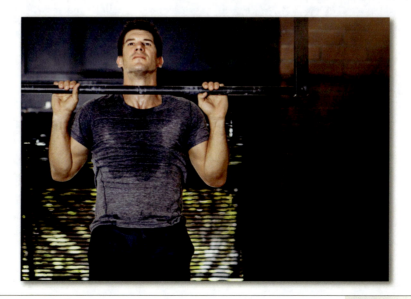

Muscular Endurance Assessments

Endurance tests require that the subject either sustains an isometric contraction for an extended period, performs a maximal number of repetitions in a designated time frame, or performs a particular movement to failure. Flexed-arm hangs used with elementary school children exemplify static contractile force assessed by time. Paced abdominal curl-ups represent a test in which the exerciser stays in cadence for a designated period or until the subject can no longer maintain the pace. Maximal repetition tests may have a time limitation, as seen with the one-minute body squat test, or allow the exerciser to reach failure, as is the case with the maximal push-up test or YMCA Bench Press test. Regardless of the test criteria, the goal is to ascertain the decline in a muscle's force production over time. The abdominal curl-up is likely the most common single assessment used for overall prediction because it focuses on the endurance capabilities of trunk postural muscles. However, this assumes that postural muscle endurance reflects other muscles' endurance, which is not always accurate. Local muscle endurance often depends upon the activity status of the individual and the movements or actions he or she performs on a routine basis. A person who rides a bike most days of the week will likely have better endurance in the muscles used for that activity compared to others. Although trunk postural muscle endurance is important, other muscles in the body also have endurance requirements.

Much like strength testing, it is equally appropriate to perform endurance movements for comparative scoring purposes. Although normative data is not available, the number of correctly performed movements with a certain resistance will provide details regarding the muscle's endurance and can be easily repeated for re-evaluation data. This will allow the exercise professional to track changes within an individual muscle group or movement despite the lack of normative data.

Successful completion of endurance testing requires adequate strength, so this is a key consideration. A person who performs three push-ups or one pull-up is not being assessed for endurance but, rather, strength. For local muscular endurance to be appropriately gauged, the number of repetitions should ideally reach double digits, or force production should reach at least 30 seconds. If a client cannot perform at least ten repetitions for a given assessment, then a different test should be selected to evaluate endurance. Modifications to the test can be made by reducing the resistance applied during the movement. Doing push-ups off a bench, for instance, is mechanically advantaged and may be appropriate for a client that cannot perform push-ups from the ground. This movement can be used as an alternative to the traditional exercise, even though no norms for scoring exist. Having comparative norms is helpful, but intake data is also valuable primarily for contributing to exercise program generation and providing a basis to identify improvement. If a person performs poorly in all strength and endurance tests, resistance training should be encouraged, with initial repetition ranges between 12 and 15. This will provide for client acclimation to resisted movements and still encourage both strength and endurance adaptations.

One key consideration for endurance testing is that successful completion requires adequate strength. A person who performs three push-ups or one pull-up is not being assessed for endurance but rather strength.

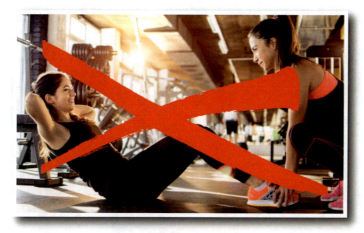

Testing Error

Estimation error is very common in tests used for muscular fitness. The error most commonly relates to four key measurement factors, which include:

1. Inadequate practice and the subject's lack of neuromuscular proficiency or familiarity in the tested movement.
2. Indiscriminate performance criteria used for scoring.
3. Lack of experience with the resistance loads used for the test.
4. Movement compensation and undefined ROM performance requirements.

Strategies to reduce error risk require identifying and accounting for likely pitfalls. Following the guidelines outlined in the previous text will aid in reducing organizational and administrative error and can also limit subject-related error. A trainer should employ strict testing and scoring protocol, ensure the subject is proficient in the movement and comfortable with the resistance used, and adequately practice the test prior to assessment to clarify scoring criteria for the client. All of these characterize quality procedures and will enhance test validity.

When using muscular tests to evaluate older adults, trainers should be mindful of additional considerations to ensure safety and a successful outcome. Standard protocols are often inappropriate/unsafe for older adults. Fortunately, a battery of functional tests has been created to predict independence and the ability to successfully complete **activities of daily living (ADLs)**. ADLs include tasks such as cooking and cleaning, getting in and out of vehicles, carrying and storing groceries, climbing stairs, dressing, and bathing. The most common tests are the grip strength, single arm-curl, 30-second chair stand, timed up-and-go, foot tapping, hand tapping, trunk rotation, functional reach, single-leg balance, and 2 and 6-minute walk tests. Trainers can implement these practical tests easily and acquire valid, reliable, normalized data for individuals between the ages of 60 and 94. Classifications of scores should be viewed along a continuum of function, keeping in mind that difficulty or failure to perform these tests correlates with disability and independence loss.

DEFINITIONS

Activities of Daily Living (ADLs) –

The fundamental skills typically needed to manage basic physical needs comprised of the following areas: grooming/personal hygiene, dressing, toileting/continence, transferring/ambulating and eating.

MUSCULAR ENDURANCE TEST: PUSH-UP

Equipment

Towel or foam roller

Test

Measure of upper body endurance relative to body weight.

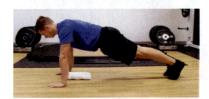
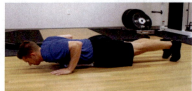
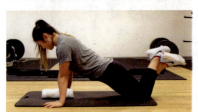
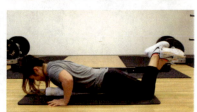

Directions

1) **Starting Position:** Subject starts in a prone position on the floor with body extended. Hands should be placed approximately shoulder-width apart with thumbs located directly under the shoulders with arms extended. The feet should be or no more than 6" apart.

2) Place a towel (rolled up to a thickness of approximately 3" in width) or a halved foam roller directly under the chest of the subject.

3) **Practice:** From the start position, the subject should descend in a rigid, straight position until the chest contacts the towel. The test subject should complete 3-5 practice reps to demonstrate compliance with the movement technique requirements.

4) **Begin Assessment:** When ready, the test administrator should give the "Ready, Go!" command and begin counting.

5) **Movement Repetition:** The subject should begin performing push-ups, contacting the towel with the chest and ensuring the body uniformly returns to the start position for each completed repetition. Resting is permitted in the "arms-extended" position only.

6) The subject should perform to failure or until proper technique is lost. The test administrator should count each correct repetition out loud.

7) **Note:** During the execution of the test, the trainer should ensure that the subject performs the movement through full ROM. Not uncommonly, individuals limit ROM to try to achieve a higher score. In addition, the subject must maintain a rigid, aligned body position. At no time should the pelvic angle change nor should the spine/torso be placed in a flexed or hyperextended position.

8) **Record:** Record the number of repetitions successfully performed on the Data Recording Sheet. Note: This test can be timed for one or two minutes, according to preference.

Number of Repetitions Completed _____

	Classifications for Push-up Test						
	Age (Years)	15-19	20-29	30-39	40-49	50-59	60-69
Men	Above Average	>28	>28	>21	>16	>12	>10
	Average	22-28	21-28	17-21	13-16	10-12	8-10
	Below Average	<22	<21	<17	<13	<10	<8
Women	Above Average	>24	>20	>19	>14	>11	>10
	Average	18-24	15-20	13-19	11-14	7-11	5-10
	Below Average	<18	<15	<13	<11	<7	<5

MUSCULAR ENDURANCE TEST: MODIFIED PULL-UP

Equipment

Smith machine or equivalent

Test

Measure of upper body endurance relative to body weight.

Directions

1) **Starting Position:** Using an overhand, pronated grip, the subject should walk the feet forward until they have established a 45° floor-to-body position while hanging from the bar. The subject's body should be straight with feet on the ground. He or she should perform 2-3 repetitions to ensure the pull places the bar just below the chest across the inferior portion of the xyphoid process.

2) **Start the Test:** Once the position has been established, the test administrator should give the "Ready, Go!" command to start the evaluation. The repetition is completed every time the bar touches the chest.

3) The subject should return to the starting position in a controlled manner, repeating the movement as many times as possible.

4) **Stop the Test:** Discontinue the test once proper form is compromised or the subject cannot perform any more repetitions.

5) Record: Document the results.

Number of Repetitions Completed _____

Classification for the Modified Pull-up (Adults 17+)		
	Male	Female
Above Average	>22	>9
Average	14-21	4-8
Below Average	<14	<4

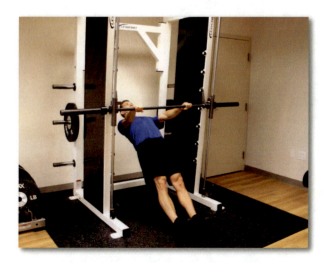
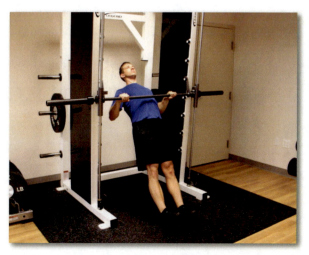

MUSCULAR ENDURANCE TEST: ABDOMINAL CURL-UP

Equipment

Mat, metronome

Test

Measure of trunk endurance relative to body weight.

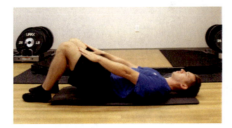 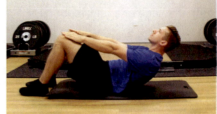

Directions

1) **Starting Position:** Have the subject assume a supine position with knees flexed and feet flat on the floor approximately 12" apart.

2) The subject should extend the arms with hands positioned palms down on the thighs and fingertips pointing at the knees.

3) **Practice the Assessment:** Set a metronome for a cadence of 40 beats · min^{-1} and ask the subject to practice the cadence for 4-5 reps.

4) On the "Ready, Go!" command, the subject flexes the trunk to perform curls-up in a controlled manner until the fingers reach the top of the knees as the cadence sounds.

5) Each beat represents a transitional change in the movement. The movements should be controlled and must remain on pace with the metronome through a full ROM.

6) **Movement Repetition:** After touching the knee tops, the client then returns to the starting position with the upper back in contact with ground. The movements should not be jerky or use momentum. This should be repeated until the client cannot perform any more repetitions or completes 75 repetitions.

7) **Data Collection:** The test administrator should count each correct repetition out loud.

8) **Stop the Test:** If the subject performs 75 repetitions, stop the test, and record the results.

9) Individuals stopping before the terminal score should have the score recorded at the test's end.

10) **Interpretation of Results:** The table below indicates the trunk flexion endurance ratings for both males and females. It is based on the number of completed curl-ups for each age category.

Number of Repetitions Completed _____

	Classification for Abdominal Curl-up Test					
	Age (Years)	20-29	30-39	40-49	50-59	60-69
Men	Above Average	>21	>18	>18	>17	>16
	Average	16 - 20	15 - 17	13 - 17	11 - 16	11 - 15
	Below Average	<16	<15	<13	<11	<11
Women	Above Average	>18	>19	>19	>19	>17
	Average	14 - 17	11 - 18	11 - 18	10 - 18	8 - 16
	Below Average	<14	<11	<11	<10	<8

Assessment of Anaerobic Power & Capacity

Muscular strength and endurance can contribute to a functional measure of anaerobic power and capacity. Note that neither strength and power nor muscular endurance and anaerobic capacity are synonymous. Each impacts and works in conjunction with the other, although specific physiological factors distinguish each independently. Rather than analyzing neurophysiological contractile factors such as recruitment, synchronicity, and firing rate, anaerobic power and capacity emphasizes biochemical measures, including energy system efficiency, fatigue rate, and the resultant total work over time.

Power is the amount of work performed in a given time and is a key component in functional health, especially for the ageing population. Individuals who lack adequate power have difficulty rising from bed, getting out of a chair, and often suffer significant decline in gait speed. Low power levels correlate to disability, loss of independence, and reduced quality of life (QOL). Therefore, low power measures require special attention in the exercise prescription, which should emphasize improving movement rate and body segment velocity to prevent functional decline. Whereas an older adult may be assessed using the chair sit-to-stand test, healthy individuals are more commonly tested by vertical jump or anaerobic power stepping.

Anaerobic capacity simply measures power-rate decline: the length of time that a muscle can perform an activity while utilizing the anaerobic glycolytic pathway to regenerate ATP until the onset of local metabolic fatigue. In other words, it represents the ability to perform sustained work at elevated intensity levels for extended periods of time. Most capacity tests last 15, 30, 60, or 90 seconds, depending on what component of capacity is being emphasized. The two components of anaerobic capacity are either the body's ability to sustain high intensity levels for a short duration of time (average peak power) or the ability to perform moderate intensity levels until fatigue (sustained power capacity). Performances lasting less than 30 seconds gauge the duration maximal output can be sustained. Tests lasting 60 to 90 seconds analyze the power rate of decline. Some tests can be used to identify both anaerobic power and capacity, including the Wingate bike test and anaerobic power step test, as both protocols use measures taken at different time segments throughout the test. A measure is done at 5 or 15 seconds and then again at 30 or 60 seconds, respectively. Each value is then placed in a predictive equation to calculate watts or joules (units of power). Anaerobic capacity tests most likely predict functional capability better than strength tests due to the number of physiological factors involved, but they may also be associated with an elevated degree of risk when employed with the wrong population. Individuals should be appropriately categorized by health and demonstrate suitable levels of fitness before engaging in these anaerobic capacity tests.

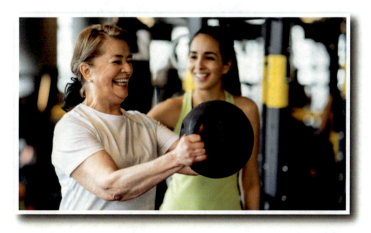

MUSCULAR POWER TESTS: NON-COUNTER MOVEMENT VERTICAL JUMP

Equipment

Tape measure, chalk, stopwatch

Test

Measure of lower body power relative to body weight.

Directions

1) **Test Set-up:** Secure a measuring tape against a sturdy surface at least 48 inches above the maximum reach point of the subject.
2) **Warm-up:** The subject should perform a 5 to 10-minute warm-up consisting of activities designed to increase muscle temperature and enhance nervous system excitation.
3) **Measure Reach:** The subject should stand erect, with both feet flat on the floor with the dominant side facing the wall or measuring surface.
4) The subject then extends the dominant arm straight up with the palm facing the measuring surface for a single-arm maximum-reach measurement. The highest point of the reach should be measured to the closest increment and recorded.
5) **Mark Reach Hand:** The subject should chalk his or her finger tips on the dominant hand (reach arm) prior to the initial trial, so the measurement can be marked and maximum jump height assessed accurately.
6) **Test Prep:** The subject then prepares to make the first attempt by assuming an isometric jumping position.
7) Once the subject has established the jumping position, the feet cannot move, nor may the body position change. If the subject uses any other preparatory counter-movement action, the jump should be discounted.
8) **Test:** The subject should then make the first attempt by jumping and reaching as high as possible, placing a mark on the measurement surface with the chalked fingers.
9) The test administrator should observe the reach mark and record the measurement. Test administrators should be on an elevated surface to get a more accurate reading at eye level.
10) **Trials:** Three attempts should be performed (resting up to 90 sec. between trials), with the best trial recorded.
11) **Record and Calculate Data:** Record the subject's results.
12) Subtract the initial reach height from the recorded height on the tape to calculate vertical jump distance.

Recorded Height _____

Vertical Jump Classification (inches)				
Age (Years)	21-25		26-30	
Classification	M	F	M	F
Above Average	>25.7	>16.6	>25.2	>16.4
Average	18.7 - 25.6	11.6 - 16.5	18.6 - 25.1	11.6 - 16.3
Below Average	<18.7	<11.6	<18.6	<11.6

Adapted from D. Patterson, D. Fred Peterson, 2004, "Vertical Jump and Leg Power Norms for Young Adults" Measurement in Physical Education and Exercise Science

MUSCULAR POWER TEST: 30-SECOND CHAIR STAND

Equipment

Stable chair, stopwatch

Test

Measure of lower body power relative to body weight among older adults.

Directions

1) For the Chair Stand Test, select a stable chair that will not move during the test. The height of the chair should be at a level that allows for approximately 90° of knee flexion at the starting position.

2) **Warm-up:** The subject should perform a 5 to 10-minute warm-up, consisting of activities that increase muscle temperature and enhance movement-specific readiness.

3) **Start Position:** The subject should sit in the middle of the chair with back straight, knees flexed, and feet flat on the floor at shoulder width.

4) Arms should be crossed across the chest.

5) **Test Start:** At the "Ready, Go!" the subject should attempt to stand to a full upright position and then back down to a full seated position in the chair. The subject should perform continuous repetitions for 30 seconds.

6) **Test Stop:** At the end of the 30-second period, the trainer should verbally indicate "Stop." The number of correctly completed chair stands should be recorded by the test administrator.

Number of Completed Chair Stands _____

30-Second Chair Stand (#. of Stands)														
Age (Years)	60-64		65-69		70-74		75-79		80-84		85-89		90-94	
Classification	M	F	M	F	M	F	M	F	M	F	M	F	M	F
Above Average	>19	>17	>18	>16	>17	>15	>17	>15	>15	>14	>14	>13	>12	>11
Average	14-19	12-17	12-18	11-16	12-17	10-15	11-17	10-15	10-15	9-14	8-14	8-13	7-12	4-11
Below Average	<14	<12	<12	<11	<12	<10	<11	<10	<10	<9	<8	<8	<7	<4

ANAEROBIC CAPACITY TEST: ANAEROBIC POWER STEP

Equipment

Step or box

Stopwatch

Test

Measure of lower body anaerobic capacity relative to body weight.

Directions

1) **Warm-up:** The subject should perform a 5 to 10-minute warm-up, consisting of activities designed to increase muscle temperature and to enhance movement-specific readiness.

2) **Start Position:** The subject should stand alongside a box or bench. The height of the step should be set so the knee is flexed at 90°.

3) **Practice:** The subject starts with the foot of the dominant leg (testing leg) centered on top of the box or bench with the support leg extended under the hip. The step foot will remain flat and in the same location throughout the duration of the test. Have the subject perform five (5) repetitions to demonstrate compliance with the execution technique and required ROM.

4) **Start Test:** On the "Ready, Go!" command, the test administrator starts the timer and the subject begins the step-up. On each step, the subject's legs and back should be straightened, with the arms remaining at the sides and used for balance only. The arms should not move for the purpose of added momentum.

5) The cadence for the test is a 1-2 count; the 1 count is up, and the 2 count is down.

6) **Scoring:** A step is counted each time the subject's step leg is straightened and then returned to the starting position. Steps are not counted if the client does not straighten the step leg or if the subject's hip is flexed.

7) The test administrator should call out the time remaining every 15 seconds. The total number of completed steps should be recorded for the 60 second period.

8) Tests should not be paced but performed at an all-out exertion for the entire duration (60 seconds).

9) **Stop Test:** At the end of the 60 second period, the test administrator should stop the test and record the number of step-ups completed.

Number of Steps Completed _____

10) Have the client perform a cool down to prevent blood from pooling in the action leg.

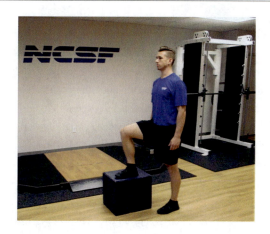
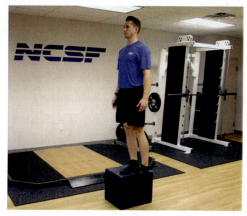

How to Calculate

Anaerobic Capacity (kgm · min⁻¹) = {_____ kg x [(0.4 m x _____ step score)/1]} x 1.33

= [_____ kg x (_____) m / 1] x 1.33

= _____ kg x _____ m · min⁻¹ x 1.33

= _____ (kgm · min⁻¹)

Watts = _____ (kgm · min-1) ÷ 6.12 W/ kgm · m⁻¹

Example

A 100 kg (220 lbs.) male completed 60 steps for the entire one-minute test duration.

Anaerobic Capacity (kgm · min⁻¹) = 100 x [(0.40 x 60)/1] x 1.33

= [100 x (24/1)] x1.33

= 100 x 24.0 x 1.33

= 3192 (kgm · min⁻¹)

Conversion to Watts (6.12 kgm · min⁻¹ = 1 W)

Watts = 3192 ÷ 6.12

= 521.6 W

Classification for Anaerobic Capacity		
	Male (W)	Female (W)
Above Average	>507	>339
Average	460 - 506	307 - 338
Below Average	<460	<307

Flexibility and Mobility Assessments

Often, fitness evaluations overlook or undervalue flexibility testing, and consequently, exercise prescriptions based on these limited or neglected assessments reflect this devaluation. This error may stem from time limits, lack of knowledge of effective stretches, or the fact that flexibility activities do not provide tangible changes in body composition. In any case, flexibility is the least employed health-related component of fitness. Interestingly, flexibility directly relates to functional independence in the elderly and represents a key factor in activity decline with age. A negative, self-perpetuating loop exists in which flexibility declines with reduced physical activity, and as flexibility declines, limited movement capacity reduces subsequent physical activity status. This further diminishes an individual's flexibility and leads to a significant decrease in physical activity throughout later stages of life. Poor flexibility can result in acute and chronic low-back pain and musculoskeletal injuries. For all of these reasons, exercise professionals should emphasize flexibility in exercise programming and use a battery of tests to ensure adequate levels are maintained throughout a person's lifespan. An additional benefit of flexibility is that it clearly contributes to sports-related performance. Aside from their contribution to normal function, flexibility exercises should be further emphasized for those individuals looking to increase performance in sports and competitive endurance activities.

In traditional health and fitness testing batteries, flexibility assessment has employed the modified sit-and-reach as the staple evaluation protocol. However, since flexibility is joint specific, the sit-and-reach test has obvious limitations as a suitable assessment for total body flexibility. Flexibility, like strength, is specific to a joint movement. This suggests that several assessments should be employed to identify the range of motion in all movement capabilities of the body. The need for multiple measures is further supported by common differences between bilateral joints. For lateralized joints like the shoulder, trainers should assess both the right and left sides, as discrepancies often exist based on the actions an individual may regularly perform. For example, a tennis player who holds the racquet in his or her right hand may have excellent right shoulder flexibility but limited left shoulder flexibility due to the usage difference.

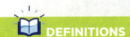

DEFINITIONS

Goniometer –

An instrument used to measure joint angles or range of motion of a specific joint.

Additionally, as seen with strength considerations, a similar agonist-antagonist relationship exists at each joint. Range of motion deficiencies on one side of a joint can lead to structural adjustments, as the tight side places an uneven pull on the components composing the articulation. Identifying areas of concern before they manifest in serious limitations or injuries should be a goal of any exercise program.

The difficulty with most flexibility assessments lies in the evaluation method and tester scoring. This is common of **goniometer** measurements, which measure the angle of a given joint during full attainable range of motion. The device works like a mathematical protractor. The pivot point, or axis of rotation, is placed over the joint, and the arms of the instrument are aligned with the joint's bones to determine the angle. A source of error, however, can occur when repeated placements of the goniometer are not done properly or consistently; similar to skinfold analysis, initial errors or inconsistent repetition in the test's execution affect validity and reliability. Electronic inclinometers and other specialized devices may

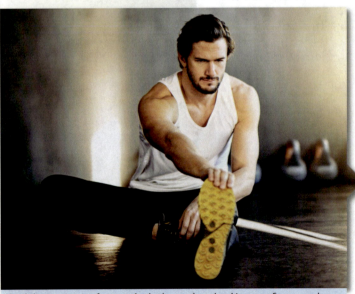

Flexibility testing is often overlooked or undervalued in many fitness evaluations, but this health-related component of fitness is critical to maintaining functional movement capacity, improving performance, and reducing the risk for injuries.

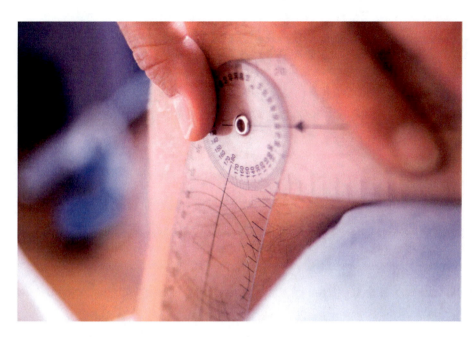

also be used for accurate assessment but require a higher level of expertise and may be cost prohibitive. Limited normative data exists for all flexibility tests, but again, the primary goal of the assessment is to identify baseline measures for exercise prescriptions and retesting of an individual client.

Another group of measuring devices used for quantifiable data are alignment posters or mats. These floor or wall mats use 360-degree or line patterns to identify the client's range of motion angle. They are relatively inexpensive, easy to use, and provide quality data for range determination and retest analysis. Any movement can be performed on or in front of the mat to assess the degree of range. To retain accurate data sets and to track progress, trainers should video or take still photographs of the start and finish positions.

If a measuring device is not used, visual assessments can still be useful. Predetermined angles related to function can be identified and used in the evaluation process. Taking still photographs of the start and end range of motion using a digital camera can provide excellent data for retest comparisons. Additionally, observed biomechanical adjustments that occur during the assessment should be recorded for analysis, and any pain associated with the movements should be documented. Keeping detailed and organized records helps streamline the program and aids in the decision-making process.

Once flexibility has been determined, mobility should be assessed to identify fascial-line limitations. People often use the terms flexibility and mobility interchangeably, but this is not accurate. Flexibility is range of motion attainable at a single joint in one plane. Mobility is the ability of the body to move through a range of motion while maintain proper joint biomechanics. Whereas flexibility looks at one muscle or group, mobility looks at the interaction of the fascia when more than one joint is involved. A very common assessment used for mobility is the overhead squat. Interestingly, the flexibility of the latissimus dorsi and trunk may be satisfactory during a flexibility assessment but categorically "fail" during the mobility assessment. This occurs because of aggravating forces that manifest when the joints of the spine and hip are added to the assessment. In many cases, flexibility assessments will predict the mobility outcomes.

FLEXIBILITY TESTS: APLEY BACK SCRATCH TEST/SHOULDER ROTATORS

Assessed Structures:

Shoulder Capsule, Subscapularis, Infraspinatus, Anterior Deltoid, Medial Deltoid, Teres Minor, Triceps, Latissimus Dorsi, Pectoralis Major.

Directions

1) Have the subject stand in an upright posture.
2) Have the subject reach one arm behind the back and maximally flex the elbow; the other arm should reach outward in the frontal plane and rise until it reaches 180° or terminal ROM. Next, flex the upper arm to a maximal position: both hands should be held in either an open palm or closed fist position.
3) The subject should attempt to overlap the fingers or touch the knuckles together (closed fist) with the humerus directed straight up and straight down.
4) Test administrators should then use the observation scale below or measure the distance between the knuckles; normal ROM is 2-3 inches of separation between the knuckles.
5) Be sure to repeat test contralaterally.
6) Flexibility evaluation is categorized as either good, borderline, or needs work (could differ from left to right shoulder rotator).

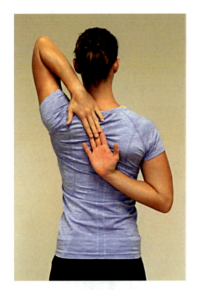

Observation	Score
Fingers are touching	1 - Good
Fingers are not touching but less than two inches apart	2 – Borderline
Fingertips are greater than two inches apart	3 – Needs work

Errors	Problem
Upper humerus rotates forward	Tight internal rotators/Tight latissimus dorsi
Lower humerus angles outward	Tight external rotators
Lower humeral head migrates forward	Tight internal rotators
Upper arm not fully flexed	Tight tricep-latissimus dorsi fascia
Lower arm shoulder drops	Tight joint capsule
Lower arm Scapula wings out	Tight external rotators

FLEXIBILITY TESTS: HIP EXTENSION (MODIFIED THOMAS TEST)

Assessed Structures:

Iliopsoas, Rectus Femoris, Hip Capsule Restrictions

Directions

1) Subject assumes a supine position on a table or bench with the edge aligned with the center of the hamstrings.

2) Instruct the subject to pull both legs to the chest (hands on hamstrings) attaining at least 120° without any negative change in pelvic angle. An excessive posterior tilt will cause a false positive.

   Note: When pelvic tilt is not controlled, the modified Thomas test displays poor criterion reference validity and, as per previous studies, poor reliability. However, when pelvic tilt is controlled, the modified Thomas test appears to be a valid test for evaluating peak hip extension angle.

3) Once the start position is attained, the subject releases one leg, extending the released leg off the edge of the table.

4) The hamstring of the released leg should come to rest on the table for normal ROM of the iliopsoas.

5) Assess both sides.

6) Next, repeat the test using a flexed, released leg. This will indicate limitations associated with the rectus femoris.

7) If the release leg externally rotates, note that this indicates IT band tightness.

8) Flexibility evaluation is categorized as either good, borderline, or needs work (note that the catergorization could differ from left to right hip flexor).

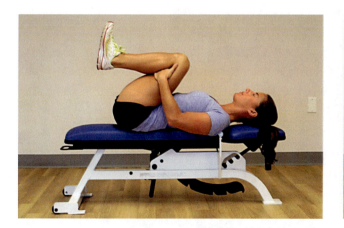
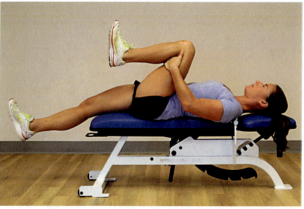

Observation	Score
Straight leg or flexed knee contact with bench	1 - Good
Hamstring <1 inch	2 – Borderline
Hamstring >1 inch	3 – Needs work

FLEXIBILITY TESTS: TRUNK EXTENSION

Assessed Structures:

Anterior Flexors (Hip Flexors, Abdominals)

Directions

1) Have the subject assume a prone position.

2) The subject should then place hands directly under the shoulders.

3) The subject should then fully extend the arms, while keeping the pelvis (hips) in contact with the mat or ground.

4) Measurement: note perpendicular distance from suprasternal notch (top of the sternum) to the floor.

5) If not measuring the distance, then note the height of the hips off the ground at terminal arm extension: it indicates whether or not the client has tight anterior flexors.

6) **If a client has a history of Low Back Pain (LBP), do not perform this assessment.**

7) Flexibility evaluation is categorized as either good, borderline, or needs work.

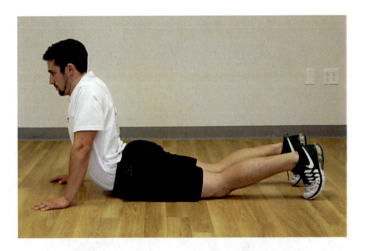

Scoring with suprasternal notch measurement	
Excellent	> 12 inches (30 cm)
Good	> 8 inches (20 cm)
Fair	> 4 inches (10 cm)
Scoring with Iliac crest measurement	
Good	Hips remain on the ground
Borderline	< 1 inch (2.54 cm)
Needs work	> 1 inch (2.54 cm)

FLEXIBILITY TESTS: TRUNK FLEXION

Assessed Structures:

Back Extensors

Directions

1) The subject should sit on a chair or box, and legs should be abducted to 45°.

2) Thighs should be parallel with the ground.

3) The subject then reaches down and backward between the legs, contracting the rectus abdominis.

4) Instruct the subject to move in a controlled manner and not to bounce while reaching as far as possible.

5) Normal ROM for this test occurs when the subject's glenohumeral joint reaches at least parallel with the acetabulum (hip capsule). Rounding of the back is acceptable for this test.

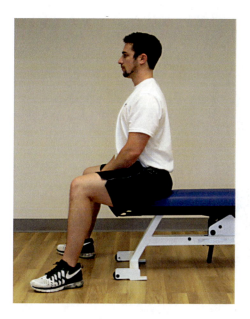
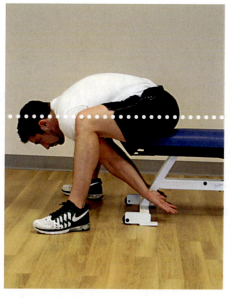

Scoring	
Good	Alignment of the centers of shoulder and hip capsules
Borderline	< 1-inch (2.54 cm) deviation between center of capsule
Needs work	> 1-inch (2.54 cm) deviation between center of capsule

FLEXIBILITY TESTS: UNILATERAL KNEE FLEXION

Assessed Structures:

Quadriceps

Directions

1) Have the subject assume a prone position with legs together.

2) Instruct the subject to flex the knee of one leg, bringing the heel to the gluteal of the same side.

3) The subject may grasp the ankle, using the ipsilateral hand and pulling the leg as close as possible to the gluteal.

4) For normal ROM, the heel should contact the gluteal, without hip flexion.

5) Assess both sides.

6) Flexibility evaluation is categorized as either good, borderline, or needs work (could differ from left to right quadriceps).

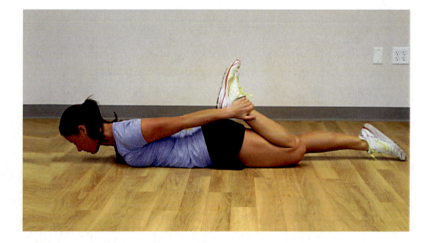

Scoring	
Good	Heel touches glute without hip flexion
Borderline	< 1 inch (2.54 cm) heel without hip flexion
Needs work	> 1 inch (2.54 cm) with* or without hip flexion
	*indicates significant tightness in rectus femoris

FLEXIBILITY TESTS: ACTIVE KNEE EXTENSION TEST

Assessed Structures:

Hamstrings

Directions

1) Have the subject assume a supine position with legs outstretched.

2) Instruct the subject to actively flex the hip and knee of one leg, bringing the knee toward the chest.

3) Then, instruct the subject to extend the flexed knee upwards by contracting the quadriceps, keeping the ankle neutral.

4) The down leg must maintain hamstring and calf contact with the ground (may not flex) or externally rotate.

5) The subject should be able to hold the fully extended leg at 90° of flexion from the hip joint, with the lower leg maintaining contact with the floor for normal ROM.

6) Assess both sides by measuring the horizontal distance between the lateral malleolus and the hip capsules.

7) Flexibility evaluation categorized as either: good, borderline, or needs work (could differ from left to right leg).

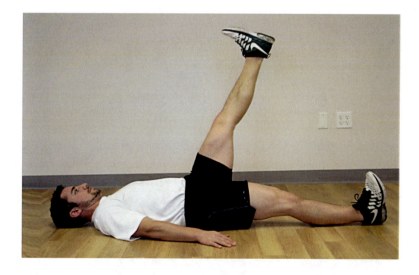

Scoring	
Good	Lateral malleolus and the hip capsules
Borderline	< 3 inches (7.5 cm) deviation between center of capsule
Needs work	> 3 inches (7.5 cm) deviation between center of capsule

FLEXIBILITY TESTS: OVERHEAD SQUAT TEST

Assessed Structures: Total Body Mobility

Directions

1) Instruct the subject to wear shorts and a short sleeve shirt and have him or her remove shoes. This will make it easier to identify faulty movement patterns of the foot and ankle.

2) Provide the subject with a dowel rod or similar object held at chest height with 90° of arm flexion. Have the subject then extend both arms and raise the dowel overhead.

3) Verbally instruct the subject to stand with feet shoulder width apart, with the inside of the feet aligned with the outside of the shoulders. Feet will align with the knee angle as determined by degree of hip abduction.

4) Then, instruct the subject to attain a neutral pelvic position to reduce the risk of pre-activation influence of the hip flexors and low back.

5) Have the subject practice squatting to at least 90° of knee flexion or functional ROM, as warranted.

6) Once the execution is understood, have the subject perform 4 repetitions in each of three views: anterior, lateral, posterior.

7) Anterior: view from the ground up, and focus on the foot, ankle, knee, hip, and shoulder positions.

8) Lateral: view top down, and focus on the elbow, shoulder, spine, hip, and knee (dorsiflexion) positions.

9) Posterior: focus on the middle down, looking for spine, hip, and femoral alignment and frontal plane deviation.

Note that learned behaviors may affect this assessment.

Common errors include the following:

1) Attempting the posterior movement of the hips, emulating a back squat. This will cause limitations in dorsiflexion and promote a "turn off" of the core visible as a posterior pelvic tilt at the bottom of the movement.

2) Obvious abduction of the hips, common of trunk weakness and tightness.

3) Excessive dorsiflexion; this occurs when the individual has tightness in the anterior aspects of the upper body and low back.

4) External shoulder rotation with arm flexion; this movement compensates for tightness in the upper posterior.

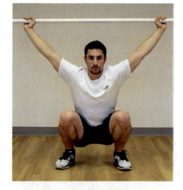

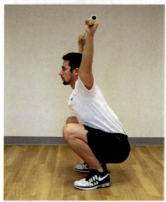

Overhead Squat Test
☐ No Dysfunctions Noted

L	**Front View**	R
☐	Foot Turns Out	☐
☐	Knee Shifts In	☐
☐	Knee Shifts Out	☐

Side View
☐ Heels Lift
☐ Excessive Forward Lean
☐ Low Back Arch
☐ Low Back Rounds
☐ Arms Fall Forward

L	**Rear View**	R
☐	Foot Flattens	☐
☐	Asymmetrical Weight Shift	☐

Common Observations	Potential Tightness	Potential Weakness
Feet externally rotate	Soleus, lateral gastrocnemius	Medial gastrocnemius, tibialis posterior
Feet flatten out	Peroneal complex	Tibialis posterior
Heel rises	Soleus	Anterior tibialis
Hip abducts	Piriformis, iliopsoas, sartorius, biceps femoris	Adductors, semitendinosis, semimembranosis
Hip adducts	Adductors, medial hamstrings	Gluteus maximus, gluteus medius
Hips internally rotate	Medial hamstrings, TFL, IT band, gluteus medius	Deep gluteal hip rotators
Lumbar hyperextension	Iliopsoas, lumbar erectors, latissimus dorsi, quadratus lumborum	Gluteals, rectus abdominis, obliques
Lumbar flexion	Obliques, hamstrings, rectus abdominis, adductor magnus	Iliopsoas, lumbar erectors, latissimus dorsi, quadratus lumborum
Protruded abdomen	Iliopsoas, lumbar erectors, quadratus lumborum	Rectus abdominis, obliques, gluteus maximus, transverse abdominis
Arms forward	Latissimus dorsi, pectorals, upper abdominals	Rhomboids, mid trapezius, thoracic extensors
Elbows bent	Pectoralis major, latissimus dorsi	Infraspinatus, teres minor, mid trapezius
Shoulder blade winging	Pectoralis major, serratus anterior	Mid trapezius, rhomboids

Resting and Active Fitness Assessments

REFERENCES:

1. Barry VW, Baruth M, Beets MW, Durstine JL, Liu J, and Blair SN. Fitness vs. fatness on all-cause mortality: a meta-analysis. 56: 382-390, 2014.

2. Borel A-L, Coumes S, Wion N, Reche F, Arvieux C, and Pépin J-L. Neck circumference is the best anthropometric marker for sleep apnoea and cardiometabolic risk in class II or III obese women: *Eur Respiratory Soc*, 2017.

3. Cerhan JR, Moore SC, Jacobs EJ, Kitahara CM, Rosenberg PS, Adami H-O, Ebbert JO, English DR, Gapstur SM, and Giles GG. A pooled analysis of waist circumference and mortality in 650,000 adults. *Mayo Clinic proceedings*. Elsevier, 2014, p. 335-345.

4. Collaboration NRF. Worldwide trends in blood pressure from 1975 to 2015: a pooled analysis of 1479 population-based measurement studies with 19· 1 million participants. *Lancet (London, England)* 389: 37, 2017.

5. Gómez-Ambrosi J, Silva C, Galofré J, Escalada J, Santos S, Millán D, Vila N, Ibañez P, Gil M, and Valentí V. Body mass index classification misses subjects with increased cardiometabolic risk factors related to elevated adiposity. *International journal of obesity* 36: 286, 2012.

6. Howie EK, Coenen P, Campbell AC, Ranelli S, and Straker LM. Head, trunk and arm posture amplitude and variation, muscle activity, sedentariness and physical activity of 3 to 5 year-old children during tablet computer use compared to television watching and toy play. *Applied ergonomics* 65: 41-50, 2017.

7. Jacobson TA, Ito MK, Maki KC, Orringer CE, Bays HE, Jones PH, McKenney JM, Grundy SM, Gill EA, and Wild RA. National Lipid Association recommendations for patient-centered management of dyslipidemia: part 1 – full report. *Journal of clinical lipidology* 9: 129-169, 2015.

8. Jensen MD, Ryan DH, Apovian CM, Ard JD, Comuzzie AG, Donato KA, Hu FB, Hubbard VS, Jakicic JM, and Kushner RF. 2013 AHA/ACC/TOS guideline for the management of overweight and obesity in adults: a report of the American College of Cardiology/American Heart Association Task Force on Practice Guidelines and The Obesity Society. *Journal of the American college of cardiology* 63: 2985-3023, 2014.

9. Kell RT, Bell G, and Quinney A. Musculoskeletal fitness, health outcomes and quality of life. *Sports Medicine* 31: 863-873, 2001.

10. Khaodhiar L, McCowen KC, and Blackburn GL. Obesity and its comorbid conditions. *Clinical cornerstone* 2: 17-31, 1999.

11. Kodama S, Saito K, Tanaka S, Maki M, Yachi Y, Asumi M, Sugawara A, Totsuka K, Shimano H, and Ohashi Y. Cardiorespiratory fitness as a quantitative predictor of all-cause mortality and cardiovascular events in healthy men and women: a meta-analysis. *Jama* 301: 2024-2035, 2009.

12. Kuczmarski RJ. 2000 CDC growth charts for the United States; methods and development. 2002.

13. Li Q, Blume SW, Huang JC, Hammer M, and Ganz ML. Prevalence and healthcare costs of obesity-related comorbidities: evidence from an electronic medical records system in the United States. *Journal of medical economics* 18: 1020-1028, 2015.

14. Mayorga-Vega D, Merino-Marban R, and Viciana J. Criterion-related validity of sit-and-reach tests for estimating hamstring and lumbar extensibility: A meta-analysis. *Journal of sports science & medicine* 13: 1, 2014.

15. Morais PCA, Mauricio TF, Moreira RP, Guedes NG, Rouberte ESC, Ferreira JDF, and de Lima PA. Nursing Diagnosis of Impaired Physical Mobility in Elderly People at Primary Health Care. *International Archives of Medicine* 10, 2017.

16. Nazare J-A, Smith J, Borel A-L, Aschner P, Barter P, Van Gaal L, Tan CE, Wittchen H-U, Matsuzawa Y, and Kadowaki T. Usefulness of measuring both body mass index and waist circumference for the estimation of visceral adiposity and related cardiometabolic risk profile (from the INSPIRE ME IAA study). *American Journal of Cardiology* 115: 307-315, 2015.

17. Onat A, Hergenç G, Yüksel H, Can G, Ayhan E, Kaya Z, and Dursuno lu D. Neck circumference as a measure of central obesity: associations with metabolic syndrome and obstructive sleep apnea syndrome beyond waist circumference. *Clinical nutrition* 28: 46-51, 2009.

18. Organization WH. Waist circumference and waist-hip ratio: report of a WHO expert consultation, Geneva, 8-11 December 2008. 2011.

19. Romero-Corral A, Somers VK, Sierra-Johnson J, Korenfeld Y, Boarin S, Korinek J, Jensen MD, Parati G, and Lopez-Jimenez F. Normal weight obesity: a risk factor for cardiometabolic dysregulation and cardiovascular mortality. *European heart journal* 31: 737-746, 2009.

20. Shan Z, Deng G, Li J, Li Y, Zhang Y, and Zhao Q. Correlational analysis of neck/shoulder pain and low back pain with the use of digital products, physical activity and psychological status among adolescents in Shanghai. *Plos one* 8: e78109, 2013.

21. Straker L, Harris C, Joosten J, and Howie EK. Mobile technology dominates school children's IT use in an advantaged school community and is associated with musculoskeletal and visual symptoms. *Ergonomics*: 1-12, 2017.

22. Whelton PK, Carey RM, Aronow WS, Casey DE, Collins KJ, Himmelfarb CD, DePalma SM, Gidding S, Jamerson KA, and Jones DW. 2017 ACC/AHA/AAPA/ABC/ACPM/AGS/APhA/ASH/ASPC/NMA/PCNA guideline for the prevention, detection, evaluation, and management of high blood pressure in adults: a report of the American College of Cardiology/American Heart Association Task Force on Clinical Practice Guidelines. *Journal of the American College of Cardiology*: 24430, 2017.

23. Zhou J-y, Ge H, Zhu M-f, Wang L-j, Chen L, Tan Y-z, Chen Y-m, and Zhu H-l. Neck circumference as an independent predictive contributor to cardio-metabolic syndrome. *Cardiovascular diabetology* 12: 76, 2013.

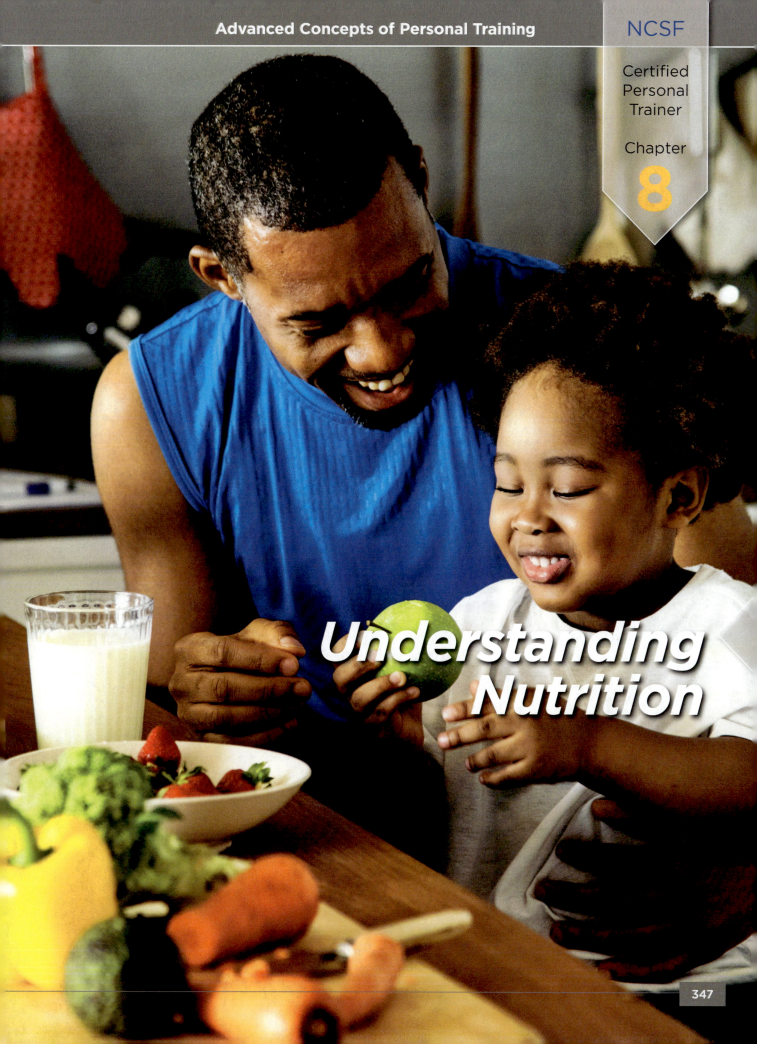

Energy Value of Food

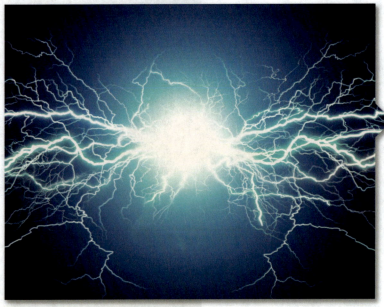

◆ Energy

The first scientific law of thermodynamics, known as the Law of Conservation of Energy, states that energy cannot be created nor destroyed. Instead, it is transferred from one form to another through a variety of mechanisms. Humans have the capacity to consume, store, and release energy. In most cases, human energy originates with plants, which derive this "power" from sunlight, water, and carbon dioxide (CO_2) in the process of photosynthesis. This energy is stored in the bonds that connect the molecules within the plant's structure. When humans eat plants, or animals that consume plants, the energy transfers from one organism to another. The energy conveyed through food represents a form of heat energy, measured by a unit called a **calorie**. A calorie represents the amount of heat required to raise the temperature of 1 g of water 1° Celsius. If calories were accurately used in the United States as the unit for food energy on nutritional labels, the energy value per gram of a nutrient would actually be expressed in the thousands. For this reason, the United States uses the kilocalorie. The kilocalorie (kcal) represents 1,000 calories, or the measurement of heat required to raise 1 kg (1L) of water 1° Celsius. To avoid consumer confusion, U.S. nutrition labels use the word calorie, but the value reflects units in kilocalories. The international unit of energy is the kilojoule (kJ), which is equal to 4.2 kilocalories.

> **DEFINITIONS**
>
> **Calorie –**
>
> *The basic unit of heat measurement, defined as the heat required to raise the temperature of 1 gram of water 1 degree Celsius.*
>
> **Energy-yielding nutrients –**
>
> *Macronutrients (carbohydrates, protein, fats) that provide the body with energy, measured in calories.*

◆ Energy Value of Food

The energy value of food derives from the respective combustion heat yielded when the product is burned. This suggests "energy potential" through its chemical structure. **Energy-yielding nutrients** contain carbon, hydrogen, and oxygen, and protein also contains nitrogen.

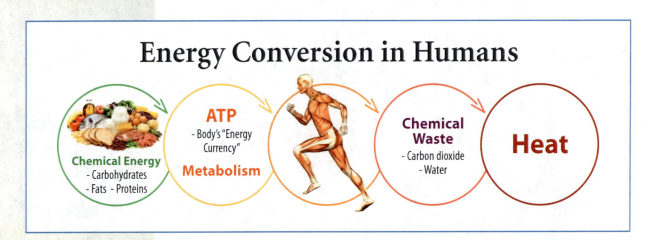

As mentioned, the energy is held in the bonds structured across the carbon chains. Water's chemical formula does not contain carbons, and as a result, does not provide energy. Since water, vitamins, and minerals do not provide any calories, they are referred to as **non-energy-yielding nutrients**. All foods contain both energy-yielding and non-energy-yielding components.

> **DEFINITIONS**
>
> **Non-energy-yielding nutrients –**
>
> *Micronutrients (vitamins, minerals) that provide the body with elements necessary for homeostasis.*

Slight variations exist in the heat created between foods composed of similar energy substrates. To account for these variations in a practical manner, a food's energy value is rounded to a whole number. For instance, fat values vary between animal lipids (mean = 9.5 kcal) and plant lipids (mean = 9.3 kcal), so food labels simply round down, listing any dietary fat as 9 kcal per gram. Similarly, the arrangement of atoms in different carbohydrates (CHO) causes variations in the net value of the food. Glucose has a very simple molecular structure, so it is valued at 3.74 kcal per gram; conversely, complex CHOs, such as glycogen and starch, are valued at 4.2 kcal per gram. Labels use the rough average of 4 kcal per gram for all CHO sources. Variations also exist in protein, where the energy values are based on the structure and nitrogen content that each protein contains. On average, protein yields 5.65 kcal of energy when burned. However, in the body, the nitrogen-containing amine group is cleaved off, stealing hydrogen in the process. This lowers the energy value to 4.6 kcals, which is further reduced to 4 kcal per gram when expressed on food labels.

PRACTICAL INSIGHT

Atwater general factors represent the value food is assigned for nutritional purposes. The average net value for protein and CHO is set at 4 kcal per gram, while fats are valued at 9 kcal per gram. Alcohol also contributes to energy intake when consumed but is not a nutrient. Pure alcohol is valued at 7 kcal per gram (ml). When the weight of each energy nutrient is known, the calories can be determined for a select food or meal. Food labels attempt to identify the energy value in foods clearly and are expressed in both weight (g) and energy (kcal).

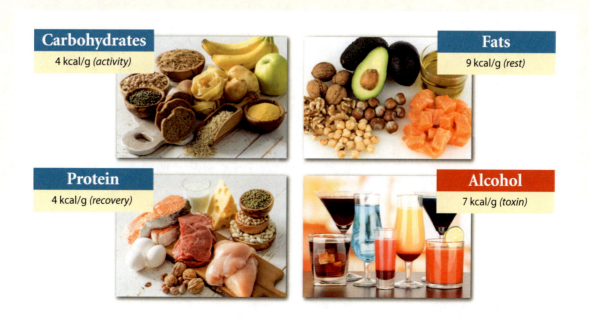

Carbohydrates 4 kcal/g *(activity)*

Fats 9 kcal/g *(rest)*

Protein 4 kcal/g *(recovery)*

Alcohol 7 kcal/g *(toxin)*

Understanding Nutrition

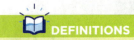

DEFINITIONS

Coefficient of digestibility –
The proportion of food that is digested compared to what is absorbed, expressed as a percentage.

The net energy of food is also affected by the digestion and absorption process, referred to as the **coefficient of digestibility**. The coefficient of digestibility reflects the total energy the body has available from the food it consumes. Certain components of food are indigestible and pass body absorption, adding to excrement. Fibrous foods affect this rate, reducing digestibility by as much as 5-10% [64]. The fiber cannot be broken down, which promotes increased mobility through the intestines, thus reducing absorption time. Plant proteins seem to yield the lowest digestibility coefficient, whereas animal products seem to yield the highest measured levels [25, 85]. In general, the body absorbs 97% of CHO, 95% of lipid, and 92% of protein energy for fuel.

PRACTICAL INSIGHT
Net Metabolizable Energy (NME)

Metabolizable energy calculations, derived from the Atwater general factors, make for easy interpretation of food values. They are widely used, even though they do not accurately measure the precise amount of energy entering the body. Traditional scaled energy values can actually be modified to further account for energy lost from different substrates via fermentation and energy that would not be available to fuel metabolism for ATP production. This results in the NME factors. The NME system employs a single factor for each energy-yielding compound. The energy sources are separated into CHOs, fiber, fats, protein, sugar alcohol, and alcohol. NME factors in the loss of energy through digestion, absorption, and urinary excretion [50]. This loss is most pronounced with the true energy content of protein, non-digestible, fermentable CHO sources (i.e., dietary fibers and other resistant starches), and alcohol. The NME factor for protein is 13 kJ/g (3.2 kcal/g); dietary fiber is 6 kJ/g (1.4 kcal/g); fermentable fiber is 8 kJ/g (2.0 kcal/g); alcohol is 26 kJ/g (6.3 kcal/g). The lower NME values for fermentable, non-digestible dietary fiber occur due to a higher assumed loss of energy through heat via the process of fermentation; protein loss occurs through metabolic inefficiency and thermogenesis, while rates for alcohol seem to be due to thermogenesis and pass-through waste with increased consumption. Diets high in protein and fiber present the greatest net loss from traditional energy predictions by some 25%, clearly denoting the pronounced effect these nutrients have on weight management.

◆ Dietary Nutrients

Factors that affect dietary sufficiency include:
- Food and nutrient timing
- Food quantity and type
- Variations in nutrient digestion, absorption, and assimilation
- Individual requirements for energy based on physical factors: age, sex, physical activity
- Other influences, such as dietary practices, preferences, and risk of food allergies

Nutrients are divided into two categories, each with three separate classes. The energy-yielding category includes CHOs, proteins, and lipids/dietary fats. The non-energy-yielding category includes vitamins, minerals, and water. Collectively, each plays a vital role in proper body function as it responds to varying physiological and environmental conditions. A healthy diet provides nutrient sufficiency in support of all normal biological functions, without excessive consumption or imbalance.

These factors further indicate that no universal diet for optimal nutrition exists [38, 65, 82]. However, careful evaluation of food consumption habits, coupled with complementary food-intake planning in accordance with sound nutritional guidelines, results in improvements in overall health, fitness, and performance.

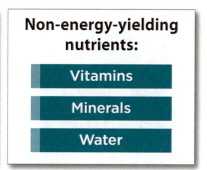

◆ Energy-Yielding Nutrients

Energy-yielding nutrients provide the body tissues with usable energy to form ATP. All energy-yielding nutrients contain the chemical element carbon. The carbon atoms bind together into carbon chains, often referred to as carbon skeletons. Carbon chains link with atoms of other elements to form lipids, CHOs, and proteins. When consumed, digestion breaks food down to its most basic energy form. In the small intestine, the nutrients are absorbed into the blood stream and are transported though the arteries to tissues, so they may perform their respective jobs throughout the body.

Once energy enters the blood stream, chemoreceptors within tissues identify each of the specific nutrients and subsequently determine the appropriate course of action based on the internal environment's current status. The body can either manipulate the energy to meet a particular demand, or store the energy for later use, as necessary. Metabolic organs determine the outcome of the energy consumed in the diet based on hormonal signaling. The liver is the primary metabolic organ used to manipulate the energy form based on the acute internal needs of the body. If needed, the liver can convert proteins into CHOs or excess proteins and CHOs into fatty acids (FA) and triglycerides (TG) by rearranging the carbon chains and elements to reflect the desired energy substrate. The body's ability to reformulate nutrients that are needed but lacking in the diet allows for energy needs to be met but also allows energy to be stored for later use.

| Fundamental steps involved in the use of **energy** by the body: | When energy-yielding nutrients are consumed, the process of digestion breaks the food down into its most basic form of energy | In the small intestine, the basic nutrient forms are absorbed into the blood and transported to tissues to perform their respective jobs | Metabolic organs determine the ultimate outcome of the energy consumed via hormonal regulation |

Carbohydrates

Although all nutrients are necessary for proper body function, CHOs are the most important nutrient related to physical activity and central nervous system (CNS) function because glucose fuels the brain. CHOs represent the primary fuel source for intense work and are necessary for the formation of ATP in the CNS, making the nutrient an indispensable part of a

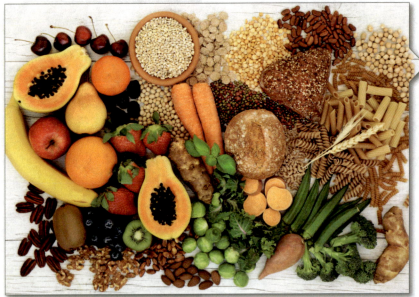

healthy diet. CHOs fall into three general categories, **mono**saccharides, **di**saccharides, and **poly**saccharides, based on their respective chain complexity. Monosaccharides are the most basic form of CHO, representing a single sugar component. Variations between monosaccharides are based on their carbon-to-hydrogen-to-oxygen sequence.

These differences in sequence determine a CHO's biochemical characteristics. For example, glucose and galactose are monosaccharides with the same number of carbon, hydrogen, and oxygen atoms; however, they are arranged differently, which causes them to behave and taste slightly differently. Disaccharides, as their name implies, are formed by the joining of two separate monosaccharides. Lactose, for instance, is a disaccharide which features a combined glucose and galactose molecule. Both monosaccharides and disaccharides are referred to as simple sugars because they are easily digestible and require little manipulation by the cell for energy use. Finally, polysaccharides are chains of monosaccharides linked together in sequences from as few as three sugars to as many as several thousand. As the chains of monosaccharide sugars increase in length and diversity, the nutrient complexity increases. Polysaccharides are more commonly referred to as complex CHOs and have chain linkages of tens to thousands of monosaccharide residues. These complex chains are classified as either plant or animal polysaccharides, depending on their source.

Glycogen and **starch** are two common forms of polysaccharides in our diets. Glycogen is the storage form of CHOs in animal tissue, while starch is the term used for the storage form of CHOs in plants. Starch is the larger component in seeds, corn, potatoes, beans, and the various grains that make up common foods like pasta, bread, and cereals. Plant starch remains the most important source of CHOs for most Americans, accounting for more than 50% of the total CHOs consumed. This number has decreased by 30% since the turn of the century, when starches comprised about 80% of CHO sources. This significant decline has been met by an equally significant increase in simple sugar consumption.

 DEFINITIONS

Monosaccharides –

The simplest form of carbohydrate: glucose, fructose, and galactose.

Disaccharides –

The carbohydrate formed when two monosaccharides bond to each other: sucrose, lactose, and maltose.

Polysaccharides –

Carbohydrate molecules composed of long chains of monosaccharides.

Starch –

Chains of sugars that can be digested and metabolized for energy.

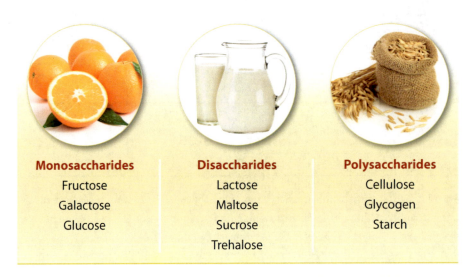

Monosaccharides	Disaccharides	Polysaccharides
Fructose	Lactose	Cellulose
Galactose	Maltose	Glycogen
Glucose	Sucrose	Starch
	Trehalose	

PRACTICAL INSIGHT

Nutraceuticals define a new category where food functions in place of drugs. As per its definition, a nutraceutical is "a food or part of a food that provides health benefits in addition to its nutritional content." Commonly, phytonutrient complexes extracted from plants function as active substances, useful in prevention and/or support for other therapies for diagnosed pathological conditions. Diet and lifestyle are essential to promote and maintain well-being, as well as to prevent the onset of many diseases with age. Plant-based nutrition is a key instrument in the battle against western disease states, particularly metabolic syndrome. Plant-based nutrition and nutraceuticals may prevent and treat the cascade of risk factors that lead to premature death, including obesity, insulin resistance, hypertension, and dyslipidemia. Based on the unsustainable costs of inflammatory obesity, diabetes, and heart disease, prevention is the best strategy as it functions as an effective and proactive medicine.

Fiber

Fiber is a non-starch polysaccharide classified as a CHO. Cellulose is its most common form in the diet, which represents the most abundant organic molecule found on earth. Cellulose resists enzymatic breakdown in the intestines, making it indigestible by humans, except for a small portion that can be fermented by intestinal/gut bacteria. Fiber is commonly categorized as either **soluble** or **insoluble**. The bacterial breakdown of fiber generally contributes <2 kcal per gram, making it an excellent addition to calorie-controlled diets, not only for its low caloric density but also for its positive effect on blood sugar regulation and metabolism. Its consumption is linked with lower occurrences of several "Western" diseases, including obesity, diabetes, hypertension, intestinal disorders, some cancers, and heart disease [25]. In fact, fiber is a key component to support plant-based diets for disease prevention and anti-inflammation. Most Americans consume about half (16 g) the recommended 20-35 grams of fiber per day, predisposing consumers to an elevated disease risk [31].

In less industrialized nations, the fiber content of the average diet is higher due to plant consumption, as protein is very expensive. Worldwide however, dietary intake is well below the recommended intake levels [37].

Additionally, the foods associated with a high fiber diet often support health by being lower in calories and more nutrient-rich, particularly with **phytochemicals** [5, 57]. For this reason, the source of the fiber is very important, and consideration should be given to fiber consumed through food sources rather than supplements. As addressed previously, whole grain products, fruits, legumes, and leafy green vegetables exemplify foods high in fiber.

Fiber:
- Enhances gastrointestinal (GI) function
- Reduces irritation to the intestinal wall
- Mobilizes harmful chemicals and compounds, inhibiting their activity
- Shortens the time for intestinal transport and excretion
- Decreases the length of time **carcinogenic** materials stay in the intestines
- Slows down the absorption rate of CHOs, which has a positive effect on blood-glucose dynamics

DEFINITIONS

Soluble fiber –

A fiber found in oat bran, barley, nuts, seeds, beans, and some fruits and vegetables; it attracts water and turns to gel during digestion, slowing the digestive process.

Insoluble fiber –

A fiber found in wheat bran, vegetables, and whole grains; it adds bulk to stool and helps food pass more quickly through the stomach and intestines.

Carcinogenic –

A substance having the potential to promote cancer formation in the body.

Phytochemicals –

Non-nutritive chemical compounds produced by plants that have various beneficial impacts on health.

Types of Fiber	Soluble or Insoluble	Sources	Health Benefits
Cellulose, some hemicellulose	Insoluble	Cellulose is the major cell wall component of plants; both are naturally found in nuts, whole wheat, cereal grains, bran, seeds, edible brown rice, and skins of produce.	"Nature's laxative": reduces constipation, lowers risk of diverticulitis, and can help with weight loss.
Resistant oligosaccharides (fructans, inulin, etc.)	Soluble	Found in numerous foods, including wheat, fruits, onions, garlic, asparagus, beets, lentils, and seeds; added to processed foods to boost fiber.	May increase "good" bacteria in the gut and enhance immune function.
Lignin	Insoluble	Found naturally in cereal grains and some vegetables, such as celery.	Good for heart health, weight management, and possibly immune function.
Mucilage, beta-glucans	Soluble	Naturally found in cereals such as barley (5-11% volume) and oats (3-7% volume), and in smaller amounts in rye, maize, wheat, and rice.	May help lower LDL cholesterol, reduce the risk of coronary artery disease (CAD), and type 2 diabetes mellitus; use caution with celiac disease or gluten intolerance.
Pectin and gums	Soluble (some pectins can be insoluble)	Naturally found in fruits, berries, and seeds; also extracted from citrus peel and other plants to boost fiber in processed foods.	Slows the passage of food through the intestinal tract and may help lower blood cholesterol.
Polydextrose	Soluble	Added to processed foods as a bulking agent and sugar substitute; made from dextrose, sorbitol, and citric acid.	Adds bulk to stools and helps prevent constipation; may cause bloating or gas.
Psyllium	Soluble	Extracted from seeds or husks of plantago ovata plant; used in supplements, fiber drinks, and added to foods.	Helps lower cholesterol and prevent constipation.
Resistant starch	Soluble	Starch in plant cell walls naturally found in un-ripened bananas, oatmeal, and legumes; also extracted and added to processed foods to boost fiber.	May help manage weight by increasing fullness and can help control blood sugar fluxes.
Wheat dextrin	Soluble	Extracted from wheat starch, and widely used to add fiber to processed foods.	May help lower cholesterol (LDL and total); may help lower blood sugar and reduce risk for CAD, but more research is needed; avoid with celiac disease or gluten intolerance.

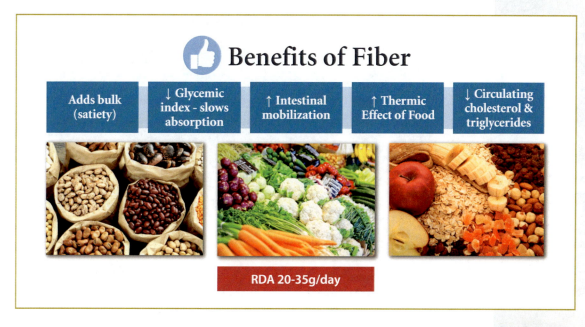

Sugars

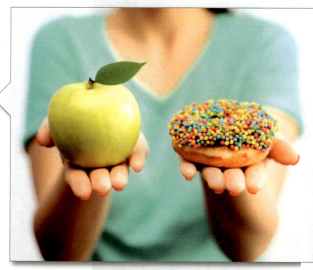

CHOs serve as the primary fuel source for physical activity and represent the largest portion of energy in the diet. The recommended dietary intake for CHOs is 55%-60% of total daily calories, with the majority being derived from polysaccharide (complex) sources. However, the average American consumes only about 40-50% of their total diet from CHO sources, with 50% of those calories being derived from monosaccharides and disaccharides (simple sugars). It has been estimated that at least 25% of the American diet is simple sugar, a trend that significantly contributes to an increased risk for obesity, diabetes, and heart disease. Most people consume more than 100 lbs. of sugar annually, mainly in the form of sucrose and high-fructose corn syrup [26].

Sugars fall into the categories of monosaccharides and disaccharides. They are similar in chemical formula but differ by specific carbon, hydrogen, and oxygen linkage. Glucose is the main monosaccharide used by the body. It can be split to form ATP, stored in muscle tissue or the liver for later use as glycogen, or converted into a lipid form following its absorption into the cells. Fructose is nature's fruit sugar. It is the sweetest of the sugars per gram. When ingested, it is converted into glucose by the liver. Another monosaccharide, galactose is an animal sugar found in dairy products.

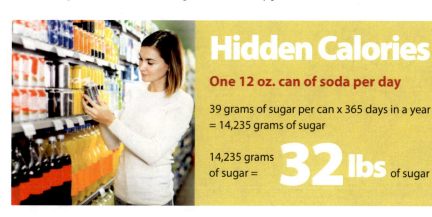

Hidden Calories
One 12 oz. can of soda per day

39 grams of sugar per can x 365 days in a year = 14,235 grams of sugar

14,235 grams of sugar = **32 lbs** of sugar

Understanding Nutrition

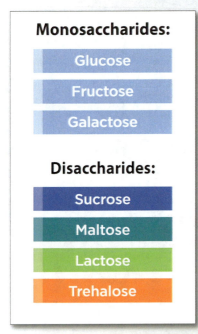

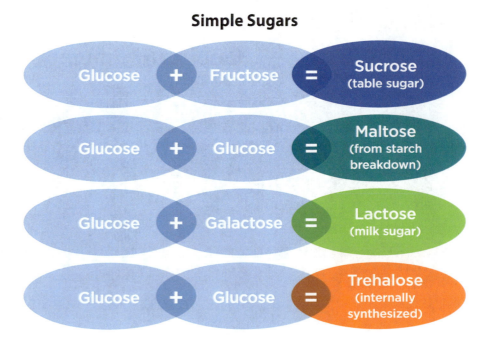

Sucrose is table sugar, the most commonly consumed sugar form. As mentioned, it can represent as much as 25% of American diets [26]. It is commonly consumed in baked goods but is also added to many foods for taste and preservation. Lactose, or dairy sugar, is formed from glucose and galactose. Individuals who lack sufficient enzymes to break down lactose, particularly the enzyme lactase, experience what is called lactose intolerance. When two glucose molecules are combined, they form maltose, which is present in cereals, germinating seeds, and beer.

◆ **Glycemic Response**

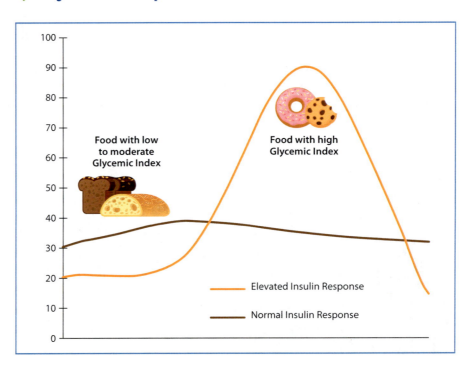

When sugars enter the blood, they immediately raise blood glucose levels. The specific response is based on the quantity (total amount) and type (simple vs complex) of sugar consumed. The elevation in blood glucose concentrations is quantified using a measurement system called glycemic indexing. The **glycemic index** describes the effect CHO sources have on circulating blood glucose levels by rate and concentration over a measured period of time. The rate at which the food increases blood glucose is called the **glycemic response**, whereas the amount of CHO in the meal multiplied by the glycemic index is referred to as the **glycemic load**.

> **QUICK INSIGHT**
>
> *Monosaccharides can be broken down to form derivatives which the body can use. Sugar acids, sugar alcohols, and amino sugars are all formed when monosaccharides break down and are metabolized. Amino sugars and sugar acids are present in connective tissue and assist in supporting the tissue's metabolic needs. Sugar alcohols have become a popular additive to supplements and foods to provide flavor with a decreased energy value (<4kcals/gram). Glycerol and sorbitol, among others, are used in energy bars and foods that attempt to reduce sugar content and glycemic spikes in the diet. They are often not counted under the total CHOs measured on food labels, or they are advertised as "non-impact carbs" for CHO-conscious consumers. They generally provide 1-3 calories and effect blood glucose dynamics less* [69, 98].

> **DEFINITIONS**
>
> **Glycemic index –**
>
> *A measure of the blood-glucose-raising potential of the carbohydrate content of a food. A value of 100 represents the standard or the equivalent of pure glucose.*
>
> **Glycemic response –**
>
> *The effect a food or meal has on blood glucose following consumption.*
>
> **Glycemic load –**
>
> *An index that simultaneously describes the blood-glucose-raising potential of the carbohydrate in a food and the quantity of carbohydrate in a food; it is calculated by multiplying the glycemic index by the amount of carbohydrate in grams provided by a food and dividing the total by 100.*

American diets contain much less fiber than just 50 years ago. Food manufacturing, which has put more focus on mass production, has denatured grain-based, complex CHOs into processed (partially digested or broken down) starches and simple sugars. In this "pre-digested" form, the complexity of the CHO is lost, and it can now enter the blood stream rapidly. The consequent increase in blood glucose causes the release (often over-release) of insulin, which can create a state of hyperinsulinemia [74, 75]. Consistently eating high-glycemic foods leads to overproduction of insulin, thereby decreasing muscle-insulin sensitivity in both sedentary children and adults [49]. The muscle's reduced insulin sensitivity causes the pancreas to release even higher amounts of insulin in response to elevations of blood sugar. This response, in conjunction with sedentary lifestyle habits and obesity (independently and cooperatively), is linked to the development of T2DM.

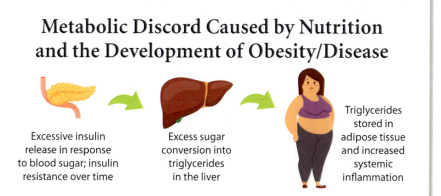

Metabolic Discord Caused by Nutrition and the Development of Obesity/Disease

Excessive insulin release in response to blood sugar; insulin resistance over time

Excess sugar conversion into triglycerides in the liver

Triglycerides stored in adipose tissue and increased systemic inflammation

As mentioned earlier, high amounts of insulin in the body facilitate the conversion of sugar into TGs in the liver, which are then stored as fat in adipose tissue. Diets high in sugar link directly to an increased risk for obesity and raise the potential for metabolic issues. On the contrary, diets high in fiber, digestion-resistant starch, and protein slow the absorption rate of sugars, attenuating surges of blood glucose. Similarly, combining fat with simple CHOs also reduces the glycemic effect [7, 95]. A reduction in the rate at which sugar enters the blood benefits the body by lowering the insulin response. This suggests that drinking sugary beverages or snacking on sugary foods presents greater metabolic mayhem than consuming sugar mixed with protein, fiber, digestion-resistant starch, and even fat. Consider a trail mix versus a candy bar. Both are high in calories, but the fiber, fat, and protein in the trail mix promote a moderated blood-glucose response. This also explains why healthy nuts are recommended as a snack for diabetics. Regular exercise also exerts a notably positive influence on the body's sensitivity to insulin, making regular physical activity a key component in the prevention and management of diabetes. The following identifies the glycemic-index values of select food products, which reflect consequent insulin responses.

Glycemic Index

Grain/Starches		Vegetables		Fruits		Dairy		Proteins	
Rice Bran	27	Asparagus	15	Grapefruit	25	Low-Fat Yogurt	14	Peanuts	21
Bran Cereal	42	Broccoli	15	Apple	38	Plain Yogurt	14	Beans, Dried	40
Spaghetti	42	Celery	15	Peach	42	Whole Milk	27	Lentils	41
Corn, sweet	54	Cucumber	15	Orange	44	Soy Milk	30	Kidney Beans	41
Wild Rice	57	Lettuce	15	Grape	46	Fat-Free Milk	32	Split Peas	45
Sweet Potatoes	61	Peppers	15	Banana	54	Skim Milk	32	Lima Beans	46
White Rice	64	Spinach	15	Mango	56	Chocolate Milk	35	Pinto Beans	55
Cous Cous	65	Tomatoes	15	Pineapple	66	Fruit Yogurt	36	Black-Eyed Peas	59
Whole Wheat Bread	71	Chickpeas	33	Watermelon	72	Ice Cream	61		
Muesli	80	Cooked Carrots	39						
Baked Potatoes	85								
Oatmeal	87								
White Bread	100								
Bagel, White	103								

Low GI (<55) • Medium GI (56-69) • High GI (>70)

The glycemic values in the table derive from data collected following the ingestion of 50 grams of the food source. The resultant blood-sugar level is tracked over a two-hour period and then compared to a standard for CHOs, which has an assigned value of 100. The corresponding value on the table expresses, as a percentage, the total area under the curve, set by the reference standard. Pure glucose is used as the standard and represents 100% of the curve; thus, if a food encompasses 45% of the total area, it would be assigned a glycemic index of 45. International values for glycemic index do exist and are most often based on glucose as the standard; with this said, when comparing specific trials, slight discrepancies will arise due to variations in the foods used.

◆ Processed Carbohydrates

Food manufacturing manipulates the biological integrity of many food sources, consequently affecting the glycemic response, as detailed previously. For example, whole grains are processed and broken down to create a more desirable consistency, as seen with enriched flour. The reduction from the original biochemical complexity to a simpler form increases the glycemic index of the food, thereby creating a more rapid surge in blood glucose levels. The complex chains are broken down to reflect a simplified food source. The end product from grain processing produces a CHO that is more easily digestible and more quickly absorbed into the blood. In some instances, such as after exercise or training events, this rapid rise in blood glucose may be beneficial to the internal environment for glycogen replenishment; however, for the average underactive person, this translates to excessive circulating blood sugars, leading to increased insulin levels and potential increases in fat storage.

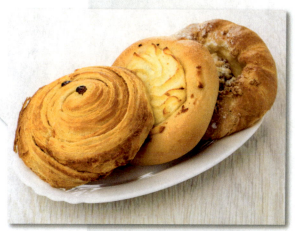

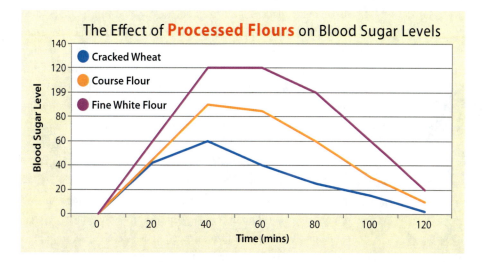

QUICK INSIGHT

Certain sugars, such as sucrose and high fructose corn syrup (HFCS), can wreak havoc on blood glucose stability. Naturally occurring fructose is touted as a more desirable sugar because of its sweetness and lower glycemic index. It is particularly favorable when consumed from non-juiced, whole-fruit sources that include the natural coupling fiber often found in the skin and internal structures of the fruit. Unlike naturally occurring fructose, commercially formulated HFCS absorbs quickly into the blood stream and causes a rapid rise in the body's blood glucose concentration. Research trials identified increased serum cholesterol and low-density-lipoprotein (LDL) concentrations in the blood when 20% of the dietary calories came from this monosaccharide. Additionally, researchers found that people who routinely consume sugary beverages containing HFCS produced dose-dependent increases in circulating lipid/lipoprotein risk factors for CVD, further explaining why cardiovascular mortality is positively associated with consuming higher amounts of added sugars. When excess quantities of simple sugars are consumed on a regular basis, the body works hard to remove the glucose from the blood, as it can cause damage to the vessels. Once liver and muscle glycogen stores have been replenished, the body may metabolize the sugar as fuel or convert it in the liver into TGs, which are then stored as fat in adipose cells. Insulin is lipogenic, meaning it increases fat storage. Thus, consistently elevating blood glucose leads to the release of insulin, causing an increased susceptibility to fat gain. This phenomenon contributes greatly to weight gain and the obesity epidemic in America.

Potentially associated with high dietary sugar intake:

- Obesity, cardiometabolic disease, and systemic inflammation
- T2DM or normal-weight diabetes and hepatic insulin resistance
- Elevated visceral fat storage
- Hyperlipidemia
- Increased (waking) cortisol levels
- Young age (premature) arthritis

It is estimated that a large portion of the American population routinely exceeds 20% of total dietary calories from sucrose and HFCS. This is compounded by a diet rich in processed grains but low in complex CHO. Excessive consumption of processed CHOs disrupts normal metabolic pathways, leading to endocrine fatigue, the onset of obesity, and pre-diabetes. To make this problem worse, excessive consumption of refined CHO often pairs with a concomitant reduction in dietary fiber, further promoting diabetes.

Beta- and alpha-cells in the pancreas regulate the metabolic hormones that control the level of circulating blood sugar. Elevated blood glucose causes the pancreas to release insulin in proportion to the rate and quantity of sugar absorption. Insulin signals the body's tissues to take up the glucose in the blood; conversely, low glucose levels are managed by the release of the hormone glucagon, which converts stored liver glycogen into glucose to be released in the blood to increase the waning glucose levels. So, insulin facilitates an uptake of the circulating blood sugar into skeletal muscle and the liver, where it is stored as glycogen, and glucagon promotes sugar release from the liver into circulation to sustain muscle work and energy for the CNS.

Ideally, the body keeps blood sugar concentrations within a consistent homeostatic range throughout the day, adjusting for times when blood glucose levels might dip too low (hypoglycemia), which can cause fatigue, or rise too high (hyperglycemia). However, a large number of Americans have significant, detrimental fluctuations in their blood glucose levels within a 24-hour period. If circulating blood glucose levels of the average American individual were plotted on a line graph, they would look somewhat erratic, with varied peaks and valleys. After meals, especially those high in simple sugars, blood glucose concentrations peak after a dramatic rise, often referred to as "spiking." These large fluctuations occur as most Americans consume the majority of their calories in two to four sittings. The body's blood glucose responses to a small number of large meals throughout the day exceed regulatory functions: the glycemic loading with each meal is too high and significant rebounding from hypoglycemic "valleys" occurs. As mentioned earlier, the pancreas releases insulin any time it senses high blood-sugar levels and, thus, increases glucose uptake by cells. Poor eating patterns cause the body to respond to polarized conditions: in this scenario, blood glucose level constantly fluctuates from one extreme to the other, resulting in higher concentrations of pancreatic hormones in circulation. Energy nutrients are utilized poorly in these conditions, changing the cellular use of glucose and promoting fat storage. To counter this pattern, some nutritionists have proposed eating small meals and lowering caloric intakes to create a better metabolic situation in humans.

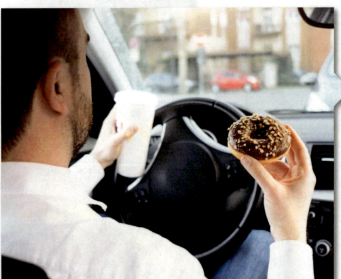

Many Americans have large, detrimental fluctuations in their blood glucose levels within a 24-hour period due to a hectic lifestyle and poor nutritional planning.

This can be accomplished by consuming smaller quantities of food in 90 to 120-minute intervals throughout the day. This suggests that the average portion of food consumed needs to be lower in calories than the traditional Western meal in order to maintain optimal blood glucose levels that do not deviate to hyper or hypoglycemic levels. Greater eating frequency seems to be related to reduced cardiovascular disease and diabetes risk [86]. Grazing and foraging animals such as deer and wild boar follow this eating pattern and maintain low levels of body fat, never developing T2DM or cardio-metabolic disease. Obviously, this occurs in part because their foods are high in fiber and low in calories, but stable (lower) blood glucose levels also play a role [32]. Although 7-9 meals may be unrealistic, "grazing" on small meals more frequently throughout the day may help avoid notable spikes in blood glucose.

Increasing the consumption frequency of necessary CHOs and consuming calories in smaller portions also works to thwart hunger. When chemical receptors in tissues identify reduced levels of blood glucose, the hypothalamus stimulates the physiologically controlled **hunger** mechanism to communicate the need for food. This makes sense, if one remembers that the brain's main fuel source is CHO. At the onset of hunger, the caloric intake required to meet the current energy needs is often low, equal to perhaps a couple hundred calories. If food is consumed at this time, the hunger mechanism is relieved and blood glucose levels are appropriately re-established. However, if the hunger response is not attended to, hunger soon turns into **appetite**. Appetite is a physio-psychological perception of caloric need. The brain's psychological discernment of need exceeds the physiological requirements for food and predisposes an individual to over-consume calories. Anyone who has ordered and consumed appetizers before the main course at a restaurant has probably realized he or she was not as hungry as originally thought by the time the main dish arrived. Addressing hunger when it presents itself to avoid appetite-related eating patterns is important and can prevent overeating habits [11].

DEFINITIONS

Hunger –

A biological need to eat in response to declining blood sugar.

Appetite –

A motivational drive to obtain food, often influenced by one's experiences and environment.

Thermic Effect of Food (TEF) –

The amount of energy expenditure above resting metabolic rate due to the cost of processing food for use as fuel or for storage.

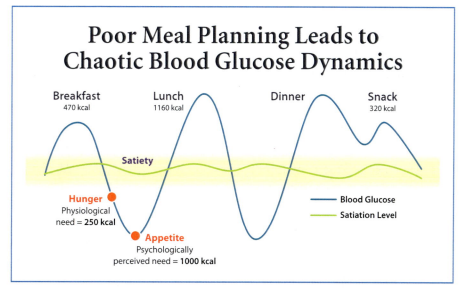

When appropriate CHO selections are made, they can effectively help reduce body weight and improve health. CHOs account for most of the **thermic effect of food** (**TEF**) (when they are 50-60% of total kcals consumed), which can represent up to 10% of daily caloric expenditure. As previously stated, complex CHOs are nutrient dense and can provide dietary fiber, which reduces the risk of digestive and bowel disorders. In addition, they tend to be low in calories when consumed from appropriate sources. Likewise, phytochemicals and other compounds found in whole grains can reduce the risk of certain severe ailments, including cancer and cardiovascular disease (CVD) [33, 88]. Compliance with the suggested guidelines for CHO consumption seems to be one of the problems with the American diet. The majority of CHO calories in the average daily intake comes from processed and sugar sources: of course, the health benefits from these foods are minimal, and the thermic effect associated with the average diet is low. Authors of diet books have recognized this pattern and recommend reducing total CHOs to control weight by decreasing the negative systemic effects of sugar and processed sources. Whereas lipids were once the primary focus for weight control and disease risk, CHOs can

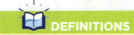

DEFINITIONS

Isocaloric –

Having similar caloric values.

Protein-sparing mechanism –

The process by which the body derives energy from fat and carbohydrate to avoid converting protein into energy.

clearly be much more influential when compared in **isocaloric** conditions. From an energy nutrient perspective, the type of CHO consumed, the quantity and timing of the consumption, and the level of physical activity one engages in have the greatest impact on resultant body composition, bodyweight, and disease risk.

The current trend toward reducing consumption of CHOs should emphasize reducing simple sugar and processed CHO intake, not uniformly cutting all sources of CHOs, as this would include removing fiber, dietary starches, and other complex CHOs from the diet. The common misconception that carbs are bad lies in the dissemination of information to the general public. In many cases, the popularized low-CHO diets cause weight loss, but much of the initial weight is water. Cutting CHOs reduces stored glycogen within the liver and muscles. Glucose bonds with three water molecules to form one molecule of glycogen in the cell. Reducing glycogen stores within the body diminishes the body's water content, thereby lowering total body weight. In addition, the body will significantly diminish its CHO stores in about 24 hours under an extended fast, which can also account for significant water loss [34]. This mechanism explains most of the initial weight loss in higher-protein, low-CHO diets, but unfortunately, the body's fat storage has not been significantly altered. Many see this reduction in water weight as a positive effect of the diet; in reality, however, the reduction in CHOs only contributed to water loss, which, in some cases, can deactivate the body's **protein-sparing mechanism**. This effect can lead not only to losing water but also lean mass without any positive alterations in body composition. Calorie control and exercise have been touted as the most effective way to lose weight and keep it off, which explains why most low CHO dieters gain the weight back soon after finishing the diet. In fact, attempting to lose weight by diet alone usually is only successful for approximately 2-5% of the population (15, 36). Most dieters gain the weight back within 6-9 months, with some even gaining rebound poundage, ultimately weighing more than when they started the diet. Additionally, low-CHO diets are contrary to the metabolic functions that promote activity. When glycogen stores are low, so is the body's capacity to work at prolonged, high intensities. In general, low-CHO diets should not be recommended for physically active people. With that said, it should be understood that controlling refined sugar and processed CHOs is not the same as a low-CHO diet.

◆ Carbohydrate Depletion

CHO availability affects more than energy output alone; it also affects metabolic biochemistry. When CHO consumption is reduced through any of the following means, the body reacts to compensate for the deficit:

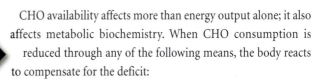

- **Poor food selections**
- **High-protein diets**
- **Reduced energy intake**
- **Starvation or fasting**
- **Intentional CHO restriction**

Reduced glycogen reserves and low plasma glucose concentrations trigger glucose synthesis through a process called gluconeogenesis (GNG) in the liver and, to a lesser extent, in the kidneys. The primary carbon skeletons used for GNG derive from

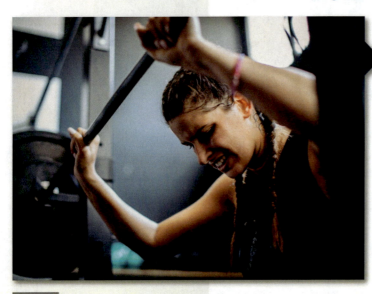

pyruvate, lactate, glycerol, and the amino acids alanine and glutamine. These molecules are rearranged to form sugar to fuel the body's need. The gluconeogenic conversion steals substrates from the blood that have been liberated from lean mass (broken down proteins from muscle tissues) and fat mass to augment CHO availability. Normally, the body has a natural protein-sparing mechanism, maintained by an adequate consumption of CHOs and calories, but restricting CHO availability alters this typical state.

Typically, the body does not want to use protein for fuel. Proteins and amino acids are the building blocks for all tissues. Even if a person consumes adequate protein to meet functional requirements, protein-sparing may not occur because this process is regulated by a neural and hormonal assessment of CHO stability. Without protein-sparing, muscles are broken down so that the amino acids can be liberated from lean mass, primarily skeletal muscle, and reformulated in the liver into CHOs, which will be used to sustain energy. Prolonged effects of lean-mass catabolism can lower the body's total metabolic rate and, over time, contribute to reduced force production capability. This problem is exacerbated by the fact that the body relies on CHOs as the primer for fat metabolism. As mentioned earlier, because the by-products of CHO breakdown are reduced, fat mobilization increases, and capacity for fat oxidation decreases. Under this state of insufficient CHO availability and lowered metabolism, more fat is mobilized than can be oxidized. This produces an incomplete breakdown of the fat and the build-up of acetone byproducts known as ketone bodies. For this reason, low-CHO diets are also referred to as ketogenic diets. Only adequate consumption of CHOs will prevent this phenomenon from occurring.

CHO consumption proves to be of even further significance due to the fact that the brain and CNS require CHOs for proper function. Under normal conditions, the brain uses blood glucose almost exclusively for fuel. When the body is deprived of CHOs, gluconeogenesis (using blood substrates to create glucose) and glycogenolysis (breaking down liver glycogen stores to create glucose) occur in order to maintain blood glucose concentrations for nerve-tissue metabolism and as a fuel for red blood cells. In a low CHO environment, blood glucose can drop to hypoglycemic levels: 70 milligrams per deciliter (mg/dL) or less. This condition can cause central fatigue, and, when sustained at very low levels, may trigger fainting or unconsciousness.

Ketone Build-up

	Ketone concentration in blood (mmol L^{-1})
Normal blood glucose	0.01
2 day depleted	2.9
7 day depleted	4.5

Issues related to loss of the protein-sparing mechanism:

- Prolonged periods of lean mass catabolism (amino acid use) can reduce metabolism
- Fat oxidation is reduced as the body relies on CHO (as a primer) for fat metabolism
- Incomplete breakdown of liberated triglycerides causes the buildup of ketone bodies, increasing risk for acidosis

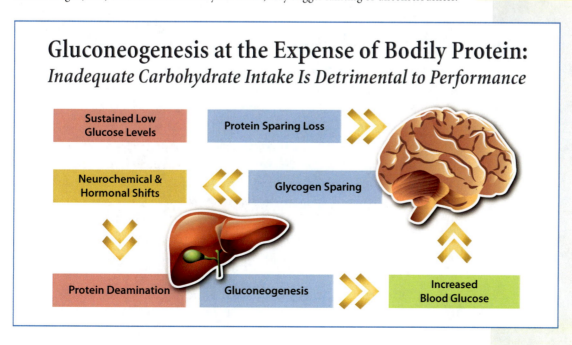

Gluconeogenesis at the Expense of Bodily Protein: *Inadequate Carbohydrate Intake Is Detrimental to Performance*

◆ Carbohydrate Need

When consuming a normal diet, the storage capacity for glycogen is between approximately 300-500 grams, or 1,200-2,000 kcal, of energy, of which about 75% is stored in the skeletal muscles [2]. CHOs fuel both high and moderate-intensity exercise via anaerobic-energy pathways and contribute substantial amounts of energy in higher-intensity aerobic training. Energy derived from the breakdown of absorbed glucose and glycogen, stored in the muscles and liver, powers the protein-contractile elements during muscle contractions and concurrent biological work in the tissues and organs. Glycogen stores rapidly deplete during intense or prolonged exercise. For physically active people, CHO intake should mirror the training volume on a daily or weekly basis. Low CHO consumption can lead to premature glycogen depletion, causing the storage volume to become too low to support higher-intensity activities. The following graphic illustrates the varying fuel-source contribution to glycogen storage and its role in prolonging steady-state exercise.

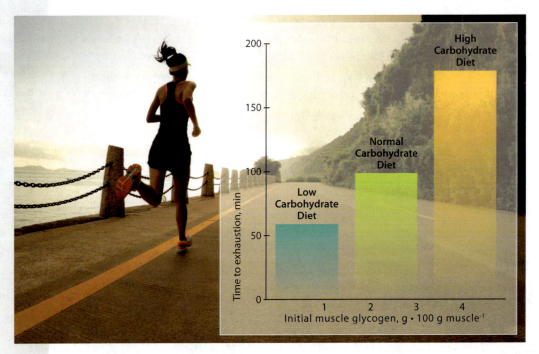

The consumption of CHOs is relative to specific need but has a definite lower limit. The exact quantity consumed depends on the amount and type of physical activity an individual engages in on a regular basis. In a sedentary person, acceptable CHO consumption may be as low as 45% of the total diet because the level of activity routinely performed is equally low. For individuals who exercise regularly, CHOs should comprise roughly 55-60% of the total diet [53, 58]. It is recommended that the majority of CHOs come from complex sources with no more than 10% derived from simple sugar. Total CHO intake recommendation jumps to 65-70% for individuals who engage in regular, moderate-to-high volume, intense training although few attain this level of CHO consumption [58]. Conceptually, "carb-loading," the intake of high amounts of CHOs prior to a race, optimizes glycogen reserves, much like topping off a car's fuel tank before a trip [29, 87]. Frequently, however, athletes attempting to "carbo-load" overeat the amount of CHOs required, not only consuming at inappropriate times to store CHOs optimally, but also promoting fat gain [10]. Additionally, diets that overemphasize protein often fail to meet the CHO needs of most physically active individuals.

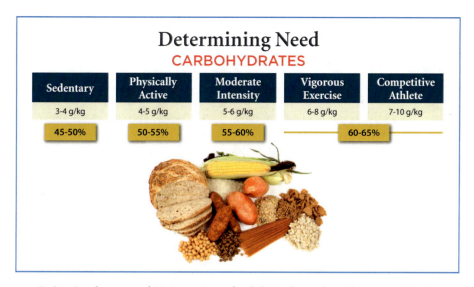

Estimating the grams of CHOs necessary for daily intake needs can be accomplished in two ways. One method entails calculating the value using a predicted daily need and subsequent percentage rate based on activity factors. The other method involves using recommended grams per kilogram of body weight (g/kg of BW), based on estimations or clinical measures of activity status, as seen in the previous figure. The two are similar in predictability when calculated correctly. This number can be a moving target because relative CHO needs change based on daily-activity status. If training volume and intensity fluctuate, the CHO intake should reflect the shifts in training. Additionally, the timing and specific nutrient types are key components of consideration to optimally effect glycogen management for sport and fitness training.

Method One

The following example demonstrates the amount of carbohydrates needed for a 35 year old 5' 5" male, weighing 75 kg, who participates in regular, moderate exercise most days of the week.

Daily Caloric Intake Requirement	2744 kcal
Recommended CHO Intake	60%

Step 1: 2744 × 60% = 1646 kcal CHO
Step 2: 1646 kcal CHO ÷ 4 kcal/g = 412 g
Step 3: 412 g ÷ 75 kg body weight = 5.5 g CHO per kg of body weight

Method Two

The following example demonstrates the amount of carbohydrates needed for a 35 year old 5' 5" male, weighing 75 kg, who participates in regular, moderate exercise most days of the week.

Daily Caloric Intake Requirement	2744 kcal
Recommended CHO Intake	60%

Body weight in kilograms × selected active status

Step 1: 75 kg × 5.5 g = 412 g
Step 2: 412 g × 4 kcal = 1648 kcal CHO

Population	Carbohydrate Requirements
Sedentary Individual	3-4 g/kg of body weight (BW)
Physically Active	4-5 g/kg of BW
Moderate Exercise	5-6 g/kg of BW
Vigorous Exercise	6-8 g/kg of BW

Understanding Nutrition

Fats

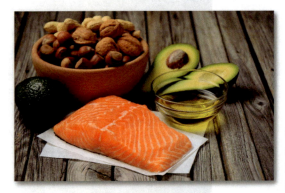

Fats are also known as dietary lipids. They represent the other primary source of energy the body uses to fuel biological work. Lipid molecules have the same structural elements as CHOs (carbon, oxygen, and hydrogen), but differ in the way the atoms are linked. This marked difference determines the way lipids are metabolized and stored in the body. Like CHOs, lipid classes are differentiated by chain length and molecular complexity. The three categories include **simple lipids**, **compound lipids**, and **derived lipids**. The following table identifies the specific characteristics related to each type of lipid.

DEFINITIONS

Simple lipids – *Formed primarily from fatty acids: waxes, fats, and oils.*

Compound lipids – *Lipids conjoined with other substances: phospholipids, glycolipids, sulpholipids, lipoproteins.*

Derived lipids – *Substances derived from simple and compound lipids by hydrolysis.*

Lipid Characteristics & Examples

Simple Lipids	Compound Lipids	Derived Lipids
Triglycerides	Phospholipids Glycolipids Lipoproteins	Fatty acids Steroids Hydrocarbons
Glycerol + 3 Fatty Acids		
Saturated Monounsaturated Polyunsaturated	Triglyceride + Phosphorus group + nitrogenous base Fatty acids + CHO + Nitrogen Protein + Triglycerides or Phospholipids	Rings of simple and compound lipids
		Cholesterol
98% of dietary lipids 90% of fat in the body	Lecithin Chylomicron High Density Lipoprotein Low Density Lipoprotein Very Low Density Lipoprotein	Produced in the body - 70% Consumed in diet - 30%
Play a major role in risk of disease Primary storage form of fat		Builds plasma membranes Vitamin D precursor Aid in formation of adrenal gland and sex hormones Component for bile Forms tissue, organ and body structures during fetal development
	Approximately 10% of body fat	
	Modulate fluid movement across the cell membrane Maintain cell structure integrity Play a role in blood clotting Protects nerve fibers Cholesterol transport Transport fat soluble vitamins	

Lipids perform many functions:

- Provision of energy
- Transportation of molecules in the blood
- Storage of nutrients and vitamins
- Service as conduction canals in the nervous system
- Formation of hormones
- Protection of organs
- Regulation of body temperature
- Communication of energy needs
- Formation of cell membranes

Most people view fat as a negative constituent of the diet because of the perceived link to being overweight and obese. This common misconception is unwarranted, as fat actually serves a multitude of crucial body functions. Lipids are required for a number of normal cellular activities and serve as necessary components to many of the body's tissues, including cell membranes.

The number of lipid-dependent functions in the body underscores the importance of adequate fat consumption in the diet. Problematic issues related to fat in the diet are associated with the source and quantity of the fat. At 9 kcal per gram, fat provides more than twice the energy of CHOs and proteins per gram, a characteristic that makes it easy for fats to contribute significantly to a positive caloric balance. Potential pitfalls exist, however, because dietary fats are more easily stored as adipose tissue throughout the body compared to CHOs or protein. Unlike CHOs, where endogenous stores are physiologically limited and oxidation rate occurs rapidly, the human body has an almost unlimited ability to store lipids. Additionally, biological mechanisms exist to protect the body in times of starvation, and these promote fat storage in situations where high amounts of calories are consumed. According to the NHANES data collected from 2009-2012, the average fat intake of American adults measures approximately 33% of total caloric intake [66]. About 34% of these dietary fats originated from non-animal sources, while the majority, 66%, came from animal sources. In addition, sixty percent of the US adult population were at or above the recommended levels of saturated fat consumption [66].

DEFINITIONS

Trans fat –

Also known as partially-hydrogenated oils, these fats are created by adding hydrogen molecules to vegetable oils. This process changes the chemical structure of the oil, turning it from liquid to semi-solid. Research has found these fats to significantly increase the risk of heart disease.

Monounsaturated fatty acids –

"Good" fat: molecules with one unsaturated carbon bond in the molecule.

Polyunsaturated fatty acids –

"Good" fat: molecules with more than one unsaturated carbon bond in the molecule.

Saturated fats –

Fats that have no double bonds between carbon molecules because they are saturated with hydrogen molecules.

Dietary fats are classified as saturated or unsaturated based on their fatty acid (FA) characteristics. While a food may contain different types of dietary fat, current food labels must only identify the total fat content and the quantity of saturated and **trans fat** included in a serving size. Because the type of fat consumed plays a role in health, consumers would benefit if the label identified the concentration of unsaturated fats as well. Unsaturated fats include **monounsaturated** and **polyunsaturated fatty acids** and are commonly found in plant-based sources of fat, such as avocados and nuts. Animal sources of fat often contain higher amounts of **saturated fats**, which are easily observed under the skin of fowl and in the white marbling present in red meat. It is generally recommended that 20-30% of an individual's total caloric consumption be derived from fat sources, with no more than 7-10% coming from saturated fat [66]. According to the 2013 dietary report card from the Center for Science in the Public Interest, Americans need to pay closer attention to their fat intake. The report suggests the average American eats 79 grams (>700 kcal) of dietary fat each day. This breaks down to 26 grams of saturated fat, 30 grams of monounsaturated fats, 16 grams of polyunsaturated fats, and 5.3 grams of trans fats [48]. These numbers represent the average, and there are clear distinctions between the fat intake of males and females. Teenage and adult males

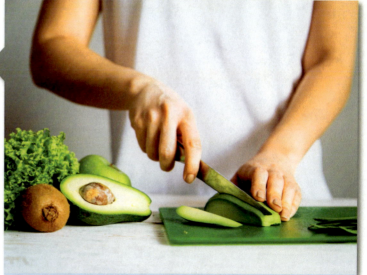

Although there are variances due to special needs, it is generally recommended that 20-30% of an individual's total caloric consumption be derived from fat sources, with no more than 7-10% coming from saturated fat.

consume between 80-90 grams of fat per day, whereas their female counterparts consume an average of 50-60 grams of fat a day. Based on these statistics, the average American consumes 20 pounds more fat per year than in 1970. Of even greater concern, approximately 19% of total calories that Americans consume everyday come from saturated and trans fat [48]. The top sources of solid fats in the American diet are grain-based desserts, pizza, and full-fat cheese. This is relevant, as a relationship exists between fat intake, specifically saturated fat intake, and coronary heart disease. Diets high in saturated fats lead to a pronounced change in the blood lipid profile, particularly in LDL cholesterol, whereas diets higher in monounsaturated fats have been linked to a lower risk of coronary heart disease [61, 83].

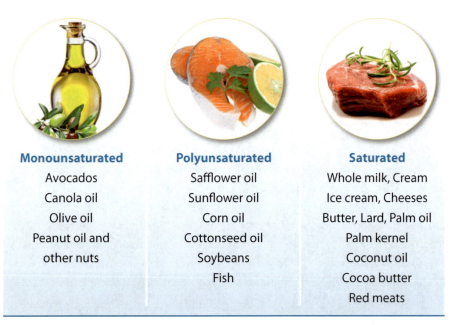

Monounsaturated	Polyunsaturated	Saturated
Avocados	Safflower oil	Whole milk, Cream
Canola oil	Sunflower oil	Ice cream, Cheeses
Olive oil	Corn oil	Butter, Lard, Palm oil
Peanut oil and other nuts	Cottonseed oil	Palm kernel
	Soybeans	Coconut oil
	Fish	Cocoa butter
		Red meats

Unsaturated and saturated fats differ according to their structural bonds and respective carbon element compositions. Saturated fatty acids do not have double bonds between the carbon atoms, which maximizes the number of attachment sites that hydrogen can bond to, "saturating" the FA. Monounsaturated fatty acids are characterized by a single double bond within the carbon chain, and polyunsaturated fatty acids have multiple double bonds, thereby reducing the number of hydrogen attachments. Additionally, the location of the double bond plays a role in the dynamics of the FA as well. For instance, when the first double bond is next to the sixth carbon, the FA is an omega-6, and when the first double bond is next to the third carbon, it is an omega-3 fatty acid, as is the same for omega-9 fatty acids. The quantity of hydrogen atoms and double bonds and the location of the double bonds play a role in how the FA reacts in the body. The following illustration demonstrates the chemical differences between saturated and unsaturated fats. Notice the differences in the bonds and hydrogen concentration.

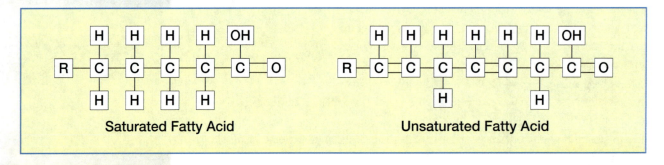

When FAs are consumed in the diet, they enter the blood stream in varying proportions, based on type and quantity. FAs enter circulation through the small intestine and are picked up by lipoproteins called chylomicrons. The circulating lipids are then transported and metabolized in the liver, where they are attached to very low-density lipoproteins (VLDL) and delivered to adipocytes, or fat cells, to be stored or utilized as fuel in the form of triglycerides. The VLDL gives up the transported lipids to form an LDL. Lipoprotein density refers to the protein to fat ratio, and VLDLs are 95% fat. LDL cholesterol circulates in the blood en route back to the liver where it can form bile. LDL is considered a hazardous cholesterol form because its small size enables it to seep into the lining of damaged arteries. This affinity for arterial wall cells increases risk of oxidation and proliferation of smooth muscle cells, thereby adding to arterial plaque, a condition known as atherosclerosis. On the other hand, High-density lipoprotein (HDL) has a cardioprotective role, inhibiting arterial plaque formation and making HDL the more desirable circulating cholesterol. This protective function seems to be associated with not only the HDL-C but also the HDL particles. Current data from clinical trials suggest that diminished HDL particle numbers can be superior to lower HDL levels in terms of cardiovascular risk prediction [44]. Thus, a broad spectrum of functional components in HDL seem to exist, as the particles contribute to a variety of athero-protective activities. This conclusion is supported by the results of large-scale clinical trials, which identify measurements of HDL, circulating concentrations of HDL particles, and HDL particle profiles. These findings have proven to be useful in improving clinical assessment of cardiovascular risk [44, 70].

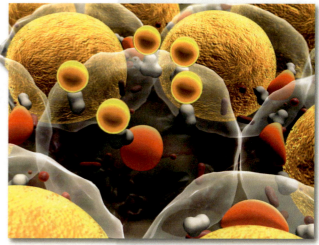

Cholesterol is not essential to the diet as the body produces about 70% of its daily need internally (~1000 mg); however, cholesterol is found in many food products. Recent guideline changes acknowledge that dietary cholesterol is not as hazardous as once believed and have led to the abandonment of the 300 mg/day limit. Healthy recommendations still suggest limiting intake as this substance is commonly found in foods higher in saturated fat, such as animal products. Cholesterol is necessary for the body to perform complex functions, including the formation of plasma membranes and hormones. It also works in digestive settings, as in the formation of bile, and serves as a precursor for vitamin D. Common cholesterol-rich foods include egg yolks, red and processed meats, dietary liver, shell fish, shrimp, and fast food products.

◆ Trans Fatty Acids

Identifying which fats to consume has become increasingly difficult due to the manipulation of fats in processed food. At room temperature, in a pure state, saturated fats are solid, whereas unsaturated fats are liquid. To elongate the shelf-life of food, however, scientists created ways to manipulate the dynamics of these FAs by manufacturing products with a synthetic, man-made, specialized fat that takes advantage of the desirable chemical components of both saturated and unsaturated fats. These trans-fatty acids have become an ever present component in many manufactured food compounds and are commonly found in fast foods, boxed foods, baked goods, and processed snacks. A key ingredient for many of these products is "partially hydrogenated oils," a form of trans-fatty acids commonly infused into foods. Through **hydrogenation**, food manufacturers create a preferable texture and consistency for foods like margarine, cookies, and ice cream. Consequently, this molecular alteration changes the way the

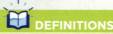

Hydrogenation –

Chemical reaction in which hydrogen reacts to an organic compound. In the context of food processing, it refers to the saturation of unsaturated liquid oils with hydrogen atoms.

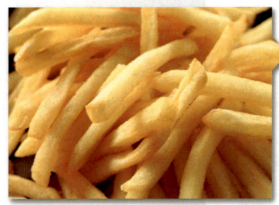

lipids act in the body. Trans-fatty acids have a profound effect on serum lipoproteins and can possibly contribute to compounded adverse health effects by increasing LDL cholesterol and triglycerides, while simultaneously reducing HDL cholesterol and promoting an increased risk of CHD [45-47]. Although trans fat exists naturally in some animal foods, trans-fatty acids do not occur in nature, and their intake may have other unknown detrimental effects. The CDC estimates that trans-fatty acids account for 30,000 deaths annually from heart disease. In 2013, the American Heart Association and CDC recommended that 0% of the diet come from trans-fat sources [22].

Not all lipids have the same capacity to increase CAD risk. Studies performed on Eskimos have shown a low incidence of coronary heart disease despite their high fat-consumption levels; however, no detrimental effects have been associated with the omega-3 fatty acids found in the high quantities of fish they consume. Theoretically, these polyunsaturated fatty acids found in cold-water fish oils reduce the formation of clots on the arterial wall and decrease plasma triglyceride levels: in conjunction, these properties lessen the risk for CHD [8, 97]. Monounsaturated fats have also been implicated as a healthier fat choice because they are benign to vessels. Mediterranean diets are often high in monounsaturated fat, like olive oil, which sometimes represents more than 50% of the dietary fat consumed. Even though the average person in Greece consumes at least 40% of his or her diet from fat, Greeks experience much lower incidences of heart disease due to the type of dietary fat consumed [16, 52]. Notably, a Mediterranean diet is low in animal products and high in vegetables, fruits, olives, and legumes. Scientists are not sure whether the Mediterranean diet as a whole contributes to reduced heart disease or if the elevated amounts of monounsaturated fat are an independent variable. Most safely conclude that the effect stems from the overall quality of the Mediterranean diet.

Trans fats have a profound effect on the blood lipid profile and health by:			
Increasing LDL cholesterol	Increasing serum triglycerides	Reducing HDL cholesterol	Increasing the risk for HD

The amount of trans fat can vary within food categories:

Food Category	Range of Trans Fat Per Serving
Margarine and spreads	0.0-3.0 g
Cookies	0.0-3.5 g
Frozen desserts	0.0-4.5 g
Frozen pizza	0.0-5.0 g
Savory snacks	0.0-7.0 g

As Reported by the CDC [21]

QUICK INSIGHT

The Mediterranean diet is associated with reduced risk of heart disease and is characterized by a high intake of olive oil, fruit, nuts, vegetables, and cereals with only a moderate intake of fish and poultry. The diet is low to very low in dairy products, red meat, processed meats, and sweets. Additionally, the primary alcohol consumed is red wine (in moderation) and notably, it is taken with meals. It has been observed that individuals that comply with the Mediterranean diet for prolonged periods consistently experience benefits with respect to cardiovascular risk. A systematic review published in the New England Journal of Medicine ranked the Mediterranean diet as ideal for the protection against coronary heart disease. The Mediterranean diet (unrestricted calories), supplemented with extra-virgin olive oil or with nuts, far outperformed a calorie controlled, low-fat diet in primary cardiovascular prevention [23].

Even with the beneficial effects some fats have on reducing coronary risk factors, these fats still need to be consumed in moderation due to their caloric content. Dietary fats can be converted to adipose tissue very efficiently when the diet is too lipid rich, no matter the lipid type. In addition, fat intake that exceeds 30% of the total diet increases the risk for developing many diseases, even when the diet is within recommended total caloric intake for the individual. On the contrary, cutting fats out of the diet is not a prudent decision either. Diets that drop dietary fat below 20% of the recommended intake can cause insufficient consumption of the essential FAs, **linolenic** and **linoleic acids**[12,72]. This is not uncommon in dieting, as most people prefer to reduce fat in the diet over practicing balanced caloric restriction. For the majority of the population, simply following the dietary guidelines will help reduce the risk of heart disease associated with the Western diet.

DEFINITIONS

Linolenic acids –

Essential polyunsaturated fatty acid (PUFA) belonging to the omega-3 fatty acids group. Highly concentrated in certain plant oils and has been reported to reduce inflammation and help prevent certain chronic diseases.

Linoleic acids –

Essential polyunsaturated fatty acid (PUFA) belonging to the omega-6 fatty acids group.

QUICK INSIGHT

When excess fat accumulates in the body, the risk for CVD dramatically increases. For this reason, manufacturers produce fat-replacers, such as sugar, which serve as tasty substitutes for the higher calorie lipids. These replacers have actually caused more problems in the American diet than they have solved. People seem to confuse fat-free foods with calorie-free foods and consume larger volumes of the food product than they would if real fat were an ingredient. This leads to excessive caloric intake and a positive caloric balance. Although the fat percentage in the diet has declined from just over 40% in the early eighties to approximately 33% today, the total amount of fat has increased because many diets are higher in calories. Additionally, higher sugar intake is common because sugar is used to improve the taste lost from the removal of the fat and serves as a quality preservative, further contributing to the problem. In most cases, moderation of fat and non-fat products will help reduce the chances of over eating calories.

◆ Dietary Fat and Disease

CVD is the number one killer in the United States. Although other factors contribute to heart disease, such as smoking and physical inactivity, dietary fat also claims some responsibility, as it has a strong, direct effect on blood lipid profiles. Additionally, dietary fat contributes to increases in fat mass and risk for obesity, which is linked to both heart and metabolic diseases. A high amount of saturated fat in the diet increases blood cholesterol dramatically, which can lead to CAD. This is further compounded by a Western diet rich in sugar, processed CHOs, processed meat, and trans fatty acids. Likewise, when high amounts of fat are consumed on a regular basis, body fat, particularly visceral fat, often increases, and the risk for disease tracks upward as well. For this reason, the recommendation is to con-

Determining Fat Intake

Daily caloric need × recommended percentage of fat in the diet = **Calories of fat in diet**

Calories of fat in diet ÷ 9 cal per gram = **Grams of fat in the diet**

Grams of fat in the diet ÷ Kilograms of body weight = **Grams of fat per kg of bodyweight**

Example

220 lb Male
2744 Calorie per day diet
30% Recommended calories from fat

2744 cal × 30% = 823 calories of fat in diet

823 ÷ 9 cal per gram = 91 Grams of fat in the diet

91 ÷ 100 Kilogram of body weight = .91 Grams of fat per kg bodyweight

sume ≤30% of total calories from fat. Categorizing fat intake is a useful step that can further serve dietary improvement. A healthy ratio of dietary fat intake contains >50% monounsaturated, ~30% polyunsaturated, and 5% or less from saturated sources [72]. Following this recommendation alone would drastically reduce many people's CAD risk.

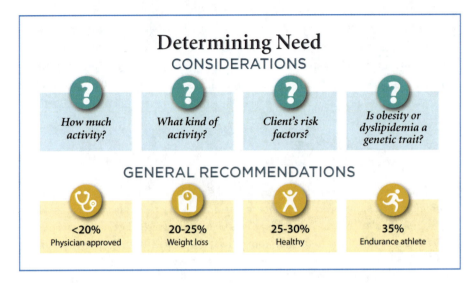

Protein

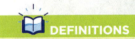

DEFINITIONS

Amino acids –

Organic compounds that combine to form proteins in the body.

Proteins represent the primary structural components of non-bony tissues and serve thousands of body functions. Proteins are made up of building blocks called **amino acids**. In the same way that many monosaccharides are chained together to form a complex CHO, multiple amino acids link together in a chain to form a protein. Like the other macronutrients, amino acids are composed of carbon, hydrogen, and oxygen; however, they are unique because they contain nitrogen, which forms an amine group (NH2). Amino acids also contain side chains, which provide each structure with an exclusive identity. Proteins are comprised of different amino acid sequences, making up approximately 50,000 different protein-containing compounds in the body. The configuration and number of the amino acids within a given protein determine its distinguishing properties. In fact, not many physiological reactions occur within the body that do not require a protein's presence at some point in the process. Twenty (20) different amino

QUICK INSIGHT

Hundreds of amino acids exist in nature, but until recently, only 20 were thought to function as protein building blocks. All of the other amino acids serve as metabolites, messengers, and regulators of biological processes. Some sources suggest that there are actually 22 amino acids, which include selenocysteine and pyrrolysine. But these amino acids are rare, unique, genetically-coded, incorporating into only certain proteins. Some texts will include selenocysteine and pyrrolysine as the 21st & 22nd amino acids, but the two additional amino acids are not generally accepted as key building blocks, pyrrolysine is limited to archea and bacteria and only selenocysteine is considered to be an addition to the 20 proteinogen amino acid groups.

acids serve as building blocks for protein, each differing from the side chains that attach to the amine group, carboxyl group, and associated carbon skeleton. The side chains dictate the biochemical affinity of the amino acid, which determines the role they serve. The body can combine elements to create amino acids, and link amino acids to form an almost infinite number of proteins. As the following picture makes clear, amino acids are carbon chains with different linkage options which ultimately determine the amino acid type and its specific characteristics.

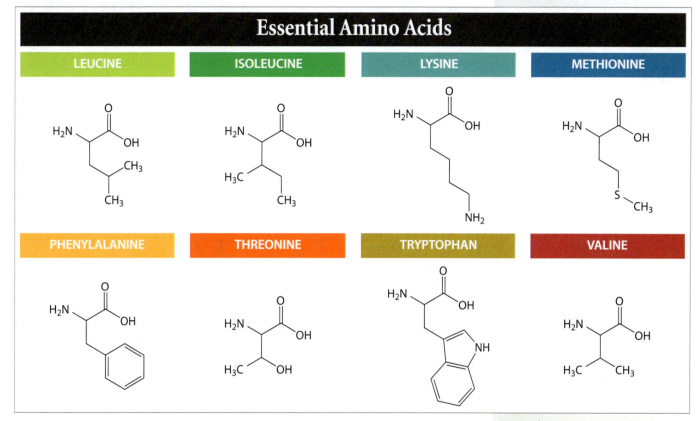

All body tissues can form amino acids, but the liver, and to a lesser extent the intestines, function as the primary organs for amino acid synthesis. Unlike bacteria and plants, which can synthesize all 20 types of amino acids, humans can only synthesize five (5) of them in sufficient quantities under any condition. These include alanine, asparagine, aspartate, glutamate, and serine, collectively referred to as **non-essential amino acids**. The amino acids that cannot be synthesized are termed **essential**, as they must be obtained from dietary sources. The nine (9) essential amino acids include histidine, isoleucine, leucine, lysine, methionine, phenylalanine, threonine, tryptophan, and valine (see following table). Older texts commonly list eight (8) essential amino acids, but histidine is now included due to the additional needs of developing infants and children. Infants cannot synthesize histidine, and children have been identified to have a reduced capacity to form histidine, as well as arginine, lysine, and cysteine[63]. The remaining six (6) amino acids were historically grouped as 'non-essential' but are now more commonly referred to as 'conditional' (semi-) essential amino acids due to challenges the body sometimes has in forming them. Conditionally essential amino acids include arginine, cysteine, glutamine, glycine, proline, and tyrosine (see following table). Though each of these amino acids can be synthesized within the body, supplementation is generally required from dietary sources under some conditions. Age, health, stress, and illness can all possibly affect amino acid synthesis and the dietary requirements needed to be able to form them.

> **DEFINITIONS**
>
> **Non-essential amino acids –**
>
> *Amino acids that are produced by the body.*
>
> **Essential amino acids –**
>
> *Nine (9) amino acids that cannot be produced by the body and must be consumed in the diet.*

Nonessential	Conditionally Essential*	Essential
Alanine	Arginine	Histidine
Asparagine	Cysteine	Isoleucine
Aspartate	Glutamine	Leucine
Glutamate	Glycine	Lysine
Serine	Proline	Methionine
	Tyrosine	Phenylalanine
		Threonine
		Tryptophan
		Valine

*Required to some degree in young, growing humans, and/or sometimes during illness.

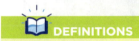

Complete protein –

A source of protein that contains an adequate proportion of all nine of the essential amino acids.

Incomplete protein –

A source of protein lacking in one or more of the essential amino acids.

Note that the groupings 'essential,' 'conditionally essential,' and 'non-essential' do not imply any difference in importance or priority. The body requires sufficient stores of all amino acids, regardless of grouping. Additionally, overall protein requirements differ from person to person, and the amount of conditionally essential and non-essential amino acids produced by the body depends on many different factors: age and mental and/or physical stress or distress situations. Environmental exposure and internal conditions also determine the various amino acid levels required by the body to remain healthy at any given time.

The source of the amino acid does not affect the body's ability to synthesize proteins, so the proteins can be consumed as animal or plant foods. A **complete protein** is considered to be of higher quality because it contains all of the essential amino acids in appropriate quantity and ratio for nitrogen balance, whereas an **incomplete protein** lacks one or more of the essential amino acids.

Animal sources generally receive the highest rating among dietary proteins. For the average American, animal proteins account for up to 70% of the total dietary protein consumed [66]. This represents an increase of 20% from the early 1900's. One problem associated with this increased animal protein intake is that they are often accompanied by higher amounts of saturated fats and cholesterol. Plant proteins, although often incomplete, can supply all essential amino acids when consumed through a variety of sources and are often accompanied with natural fiber and other beneficial nutrients. This suggests that vegetarians can get adequate protein from the foods they consume, as long as their diets maintain a variety of plant food sources that together appropriately provide all the essential amino acids. Dietary recommendations established by the Food and Nutrition Board of the National Research Council and National Academy of Science reflect the nutritional needs of the general population, not each individual's specific requirements. The protein recommendation of 0.8-0.9 grams per kilogram of bodyweight meets the protein needs and requirements of most individuals. Based on American averages, this adds up to around 56 grams for men and 46 grams for women per day, respectively, according to the Food and Nutrition Board at the Institute of Medicine. But the average American eats nearly twice that amount every day. According to *What We Eat in America*, a 2014 report published by the U.S. Department of Agriculture, men over the age of 20 consumed an average of 98.9 grams of protein a day, and their female counterparts consumed over 68 grams. In fact, the 2015 Nutritional Guidelines specifically recommended that teenage boys and men reduce animal-based protein intake.

Those who are more physically active may require a protein intake greater than the 0.8-0.9g recommendation. However, in most cases, the normal daily intakes of most Americans, especially males, already meet the added need. Additionally, higher protein consumption is often associated with extra calories consumed to meet the heightened energy needs for exercise, which further (over) satisfy any additional protein needs. Individuals who engage in high volume resistance programs or participate in endurance training programs often need more protein in order to meet the tissue re-synthesis requirements associated with recurring microtrauma or, in the case of the endurance athlete, protein loss associated with energy metabolism.

It is important to consider that protein consumption beyond 1.6 grams per kilogram of

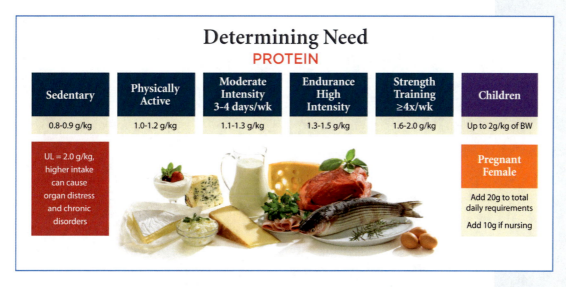

body weight has been associated with elevated saturated fat in the diet due to higher amounts of animal foods consumed. Protein consumed above and beyond need has also been linked to some cancers, osteoporosis, kidney disease, and kidney stones in the urinary tract, along with increasing renal and liver distress in certain individuals. Individual protein requirements are based on the frequency, duration, and intensity of activity or exercise. High-intensity endurance and resistance-training activities increase protein requirements significantly, especially when compared to sedentary and low-level physical activity participation. To calculate the estimated protein requirements of an individual, use the protein-intake chart presented earlier and the formula strategy presented in the following:

Determining Protein Needs

Body weight in lbs ÷ 2.2 lbs per kg = **Kilograms of body weight**

Kilograms of body weight × desired grams of protein per kilogram = **Daily protein requirement in grams**

Daily protein requirement in grams × 4 kcal per gram = **Total protein calorie requirement**

Example
220 lb Male
Population: Physically active

220 lbs ÷ 2.2 lbs per kg = 100 kg
100 kg × 1.1 grams per kg = 110 grams of protein
110 grams of protein × 4 kcal per gram = 440 kcal of protein

Protein intake above 2.0 g/kg of bodyweight, which is considered the upper limit (UL), often causes increased renal stress due to high quantities of nitrogen [54]. Protein consumption that exceeds requirements for anabolic processes can force the body into additional work, causing even more stress on the organs, as they now have to deal with the overflow. This occurs because protein is broken down into amino acids during digestion, and as mentioned earlier, deamination occurs in the liver where the amino acid loses its nitrogen group to form urea. When protein is needed in the body, the deaminated amino acids formulate into new amino acids. Excessive protein intakes can cause the deaminated amino acid to formulate and be stored as CHO or fat, depending on the physiological environment. When protein is overconsumed, the kidneys and liver must process the surplus and therefore, become stressed from additional biochemical reactions. Furthermore, the kidneys will require more water to create urine when the solute concentration of urea is high. This can lead to increased fluid loss and dehydration, creating a dangerous situation for those who do not compensate with increased fluid consumption. Clearly, excessive protein intake over an extended period of time can harm the body.

> 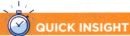 **QUICK INSIGHT**
>
> *Most people consume two times the protein needed for the day. If Americans complied with the recommended 10-15% of total calories coming from protein, they would most likely meet their nutritional needs. The American diet relies heavily on protein as a staple in most meals, making the diet rich in nitrogen. For most exercisers, additional protein is not warranted, based on their current consumption level and relative intensity of the activities they regularly complete. Many new exercisers want to buy protein supplements to encourage muscle gain. However, increasing protein alone will add no new benefits and is likely to contribute to weight gain from a positive caloric balance. Likewise, increasing protein intake requires an equal increase in water consumption to manage excess nitrogen. If protein supplements are deemed necessary to meet training demands, many experts recommend whey protein as a first choice.*
>
> *A 175-lb. male with 15% body fat, training four days a week and using moderate resistance training would have a recommended protein intake of approximately 110 grams and a total calorie requirement of 2912 kcal per day. His protein needs can easily be met by consuming 15% of his calories from protein.*
>
> *3000 calorie diet x 10-15% = 300-450 kcal or 75-113 g*

When manipulating protein intake for weight gain or weight loss, some key recommendations should be followed. As described earlier, a high-protein diet does not increase weight loss rate compared to balanced diets of similar calorie content. Most early weight loss associated with high protein diets comes from losses in cellular water, as glycogen and fluid stores decline. Though some protein diets have demonstrated fat loss, most weight reduction is attributed to caloric control and a reduction in sugar and processed CHOs. To ensure adequate protein is consumed during dietary restriction, protein should be consumed at approximately 15% of the total calories with additional adjustments made according to activity status.

If weight gain is intended, the additional calories can come from protein sources. In general, adding 30-50 grams (120-200 kcal) of protein is recommended for increases in lean mass, as long as the total amount reflects a value less than 2.0 grams per kilogram of body weight. Additional calories beyond a positive caloric balance of 200 kcal per day may lead many individuals to gain fat, as the body cannot process and absorb the protein, and must convert the excess proteins into CHOs and fat. If protein supplements are consumed to increase muscle-protein synthesis, the most appropriate times seem to be post-exercise, pre-sleep (casein), and every 3-4 hours, evenly spaced throughout the day [35, 41, 92]. In the presence of insulin cellular use of protein is heightened, as is cellular uptake of CHOs. This explains common recommendations for a CHO/protein mix immediately post-exercise. Up to 40g of protein can be consumed immediately after a workout to serve the goal of lean mass gain. The same amount of protein ingestion before bed has been shown to increase muscle

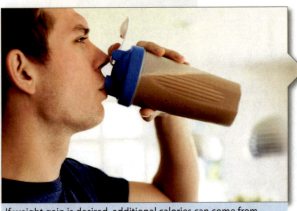

If weight gain is desired, additional calories can come from protein sources. In general, adding 30-50 grams (120-200 kcal) of protein is recommended as long as the total amount reflects a value less than 2.0 grams per kilogram of body weight.

protein synthesis [35, 92]. When selecting protein sources for post-exercise consumption, not all foods are considered equal. Animal proteins tend to be higher quality sources but have differing digestion rates due to the fat content. The efficient physical processing of whey protein and its high concentration of leucine make it an ideal post-exercise source to aid recovery. Casein, the other milk protein, can be used at night, as it digests slowly, adding to the amino acid pool, and promotes protein adequacy during the recovery state [35]. Protein consumption and lean mass changes are further reviewed in the supplement section of this text.

Protein Quality Rankings

Protein Type	Protein Efficiency Ratio	Biological Value	Net Protein Utilization	Protein Digestibility Corrected Amino Acid Score
Beef	2.9	80	73	0.92
Black Beans	NA	NA	NA	0.75
Casein	2.5	77	76	1.00
Egg	3.9	100	94	1.00
Milk	2.5	91	82	1.00
Peanuts	1.8	NA	NA	0.52
Soy Protein	2.2	74	61	1.00
Wheat Gluten	0.8	64	67	0.25
Whey Protein	3.2	104	92	1.00

Source: FAO 2013 Expert Consultation Report [47]

QUICK INSIGHT

Nitrogen balance occurs when the amount of nitrogen in consumed protein equals the amount of nitrogen the body excretes. When nitrogen balance is positive, the tissues utilize the largest amount of protein for anabolic processes, such as growth, maintenance, and repair. This is commonly seen during the stages of developmental growth, pregnancy, and illness and with resistance-trained individuals through protein synthesis. When the nitrogen balance becomes negative, the nitrogen output exceeds the intake, and protein is utilized by the body as a source of energy. Inadequate consumption of CHOs and fats can lead to, and sometimes force, a negative nitrogen balance, even in the presence of what would seem adequate protein intake. Low-CHO diets, inadequate nutrition, and excessive exercise have all been implicated in negative nitrogen balance and the consequential loss of lean mass proteins.

◆ Dietary Reference Intakes (DRI)

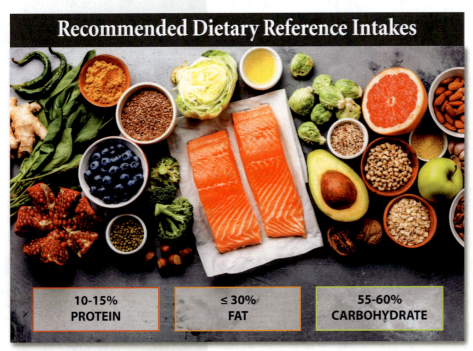

The American government funds the expert committee of the Food and Nutrition Board of the National Academy of Sciences' Institute of Medicine to establish recommendations and guidelines for nutrient intake. In 1995, a Standing Committee on the Scientific Evaluation of Dietary Reference Intakes was established to review scientific research on nutrients and recommend levels that would prevent deficiency and chronic diseases, as well as estimate intake levels that may be hazardous to health. Collectively, the values are called the **Dietary Reference Intakes (DRI)**.

The DRIs encompass four categorical sets of reference values, including the **Estimated Average Requirement (EAR)**, **Recommended Dietary Allowance (RDA)**, **Adequate Intakes (AI)**, and the **Tolerable Upper Intake Level (UL)**. Although not enough research exists to cover every nutrient in each category, significant information exists to provide values for the large majority of nutrients. The DRIs are based on the bioavailability of the nutrient, which considers the actual quantity that is absorbed by the intestines, not just the amount ingested. The nutrient recommendations establish a range that consumers can follow to meet their individual nutritional needs. Individuals who exercise or suffer from chronic illness have additional nutrient requirements above the sedentary population's needs. Therefore, nutritional experts may assign a consumption value near the tolerable upper intake level of particular nutrients for these individuals. On the contrary, individuals who do not engage in physical activity may only need to consume the nutrient quantities reflected by the RDA. The RDAs are evidence-based estimates of what intakes are necessary to support good health and lower risk for disease.

The concept of "more is better" does not often apply in nutrition. Physiological homeostasis depends upon several biochemical reactions, and adding more of a particular element or compound will not necessarily increase the level of the desired reaction. High vitamin intakes cause increased chemical concentrations once enzyme systems are saturated, and these additional circulating compounds impact system function. In fact, supplementing with excessive amounts of most nutrients can cause adverse effects. Mega-dosing vitamins can cause irreversible damage even if the vitamin is water soluble [4, 56]. Although a daily vitamin is often recommended to ensure adequate nutritional status, when combined with other supplements and normal dietary consumption, it may cause intake values to rise above the upper limit for safe consumption.

DEFINITIONS

Dietary Reference Intakes (DRI) –

An umbrella term encompassing specific standards for dietary intake; the quantity of each nutrient needed for proper function and health is defined in one of the DRIs.

Estimated Average Requirement (EAR) –

The average daily nutrient-intake level estimated to meet the requirement of half the healthy individuals in a particular group; this value is needed in order to set the RDA values.

Recommended Dietary Allowance (RDA) –

The average daily dietary-intake level sufficient to meet the nutrient requirement of nearly all (97-98%) healthy individuals in a particular group.

Adequate Intakes (AI) –

Formerly the Estimated Safe and Adequate Daily Dietary Intake, it is the recommended average daily-intake level, based on observed or experimentally-determined approximations or estimates of nutrient intake by a group or groups of apparently healthy people.

Tolerable Upper Intake Level (UL) –

The highest average daily nutrient-intake level that is likely to pose no risk of adverse health effects to almost all individuals in the general population.

Estimated Average Requirements (EAR)	Recommended Dietary Allowance (RDA)
The amount of each nutrient that meets the requirements of half of healthy people in a particular life-stage and gender group.	The amount of each nutrient that meets the needs of 97% of healthy people in a particular life-stage and gender group. The RDAs are determined using the EARs. Therefore, if an estimated average has not been determined for a nutrient, it will not be assigned a value in the RDAs.
Adequate Intakes (AI)	**Tolerable Upper Intake Level (UL)**
The average intake of each nutrient needed to sustain health, based on studies of people in a particular life-stage and gender group as determined by the DRI Committee. AIs are used when an RDA does not exist.	The highest level of daily nutrient intake that is likely to pose no risk of adverse health effects to almost all individuals in the general population. Exceeding the UL may lead to adverse health effects.

Vitamin Overdose Effects	
Vitamin C	Increases serum uric acid and may cause gout and kidney stones
Vitamin B6	May cause liver and nerve damage
Riboflavin (B2)	May impair vision
Niacin	May cause flushing of the skin, headache, fatigue, nausea, and possible liver dysfunction
Pyridoxine	May cause skin lesions and nerve damage
Vitamin E	May cause headache, fatigue, blurred vision, gastrointestinal disorders, muscular weakness, and low blood sugar
Vitamin A	May cause hair loss, dry skin, headache, bone and muscle pain, liver damage, bone abnormalities, nervous system toxicity, and possible death
Vitamin D	May cause nausea, elevated blood pressure, kidney damage, and failure

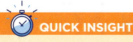

QUICK INSIGHT

Food manufacturers are aware of the nutrients in the foods they sell. When nutrients are lost during the manufacturing process, "enrichment" is utilized, a practice of replacing the lost nutrients to improve the food's nutritional quality. In some cases, the manufacturer will add nutrients that exist in small quantities or are not present in the food at all. Fortified foods have nutrients added into the product to improve the overall nutritional value. Common examples are Vitamin D-fortified milk or calcium-fortified orange juice.

Vitamins and Minerals

◆ Vitamins

Unlike CHOs, fats, and proteins, vitamins do not provide energy to the body. They function primarily as metabolic catalysts that release energy from food consumed and help maintain homeostasis within the body.

There are currently thirteen different vitamins classified as either water-soluble or fat-soluble:

- **Water-soluble vitamins** regulate metabolic reactions, control the process of tissue synthesis, aid in the protection of the cell's plasma membrane, and facilitate proper tissue function.

- **Fat-soluble vitamins** function to enhance tissue formation and integrity, prevent cell damage, and serve as constituents of certain compounds.

Vitamin requirements are generally met by the consumption of a well-balanced diet. Unlike CHOs and protein structures, the body cannot reassemble vitamins from other chemical compounds, with the exception of vitamin D, and therefore, these must be consumed in the diet. Some vitamins, such as A, D, niacin, and folic acid, require activation from an inactive precursor known as a pro-vitamin. A common example of a pro-vitamin is beta-carotene, the precursor for vitamin A.

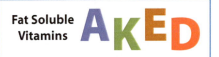

A well-balanced diet will usually meet most individuals' requirements regardless of age and physical activity level. For those who are highly active, a multi-vitamin may be warranted to provide any additional nutrient needs. This may be particularly important for individuals who do not consume enough vitamin C and folic acid (B_9). Additionally, B vitamins may provide added protection against heart disease [3]. They reduce high blood **homocysteine** levels that have been linked to coronary heart disease by converting it to cysteine (B_6) or methionine (B_{12}) [18; 30]. Other beneficial actions of certain vitamins include their roles as **antioxidants**. During both aerobic and anaerobic metabolism, **free radical** formation occurs, caused by electron leakage along the electron-transport chain. Under normal metabolic conditions, as much as 2-5% of oxygen used by the body forms oxygen-containing free radicals. These chemically-reactive molecules increase the potential for cellular damage and can increase the oxidation of LDL cholesterol, accelerating the process of atherosclerosis [68, 84, 94]. Free radical production is associated with cigarette smoke inhalation, environmental pollutants, and even exercise due to the high oxygen consumption. They have been linked with oxidative stress, leading to advanced aging, cancer, diabetes, heart disease, and a decline in the immune system. Food high in anti-oxidants, which include vitamins A, C, E, and the vitamin precursor beta-carotene, can serve a protective function against free radical activity, notably lowering risks of cancer and heart disease [68, 94].

DEFINITIONS

Water-soluble vitamins –

Vitamins that travel freely throughout the body, but are not necessarily stored in the body. Excess amounts are excreted by the kidneys and thus are not as likely to reach toxic levels as fat-soluble vitamins.

Fat-soluble vitamins –

Vitamins that are soluble in fat and predominantly stored in the body, primarily in the liver. Excess supplemental amounts can cause adverse health effects.

Homocysteine –

An amino acid that is produced by the body by chemically altering adenosine; it can be a marker of increased CVD risk.

Antioxidants –

Can be man-made or natural substances that may prevent or delay some types of cell damage; it is found in foods and available as dietary supplements.

Free radicals –

Highly unstable molecules, naturally formed during exercise or when the body converts food to energy; can cause oxidative stress, triggering cellular damage.

Vitamin	Adult RDA[a] Men	Adult RDA[a] Women	Functions	Sources	UL[o]
Thiamin (B1)	1.2 mg	1.1 mg	Part of a coenzyme used in energy metabolism, supports normal appetite and nervous system functions	Occurs in all nutritious foods in moderate amounts; pork, bacon, ham, whole grains, nuts, legumes	ND
Riboflavin (B2)	1.3 mg	1.1 mg	Part of a coenzyme used in energy metabolism, supports normal vision and skin health	Milk, yogurt, cottage cheese, meat, green leafy vegetables, and whole grains	ND
Niacin	16 mg	14 mg	Part of a coenzyme used in energy metabolism, supports health of skin, nervous system, and digestive system	Milk, eggs, meat, poultry, fish, whole-grain and enriched breads & cereals, nuts	35 mg
B6	1.3 mg	1.3 mg	Part of a coenzyme used in amino acid and fatty acid metabolism, helps convert tryptophan to niacin, helps make red blood cells	Green and leafy vegetables, meats, fish, poultry, shellfish, legumes, fruits, whole grains	100 mg
Pantothenic acid	5 mg*	5 mg*	Part of a coenzyme used in energy metabolism	Whole-grain cereals, bread, dark green vegetables	ND
Folic Acid	400 µg	400 µg	Functions as coenzyme in synthesis of nucleic acids and protein	Green vegetables, beans, whole-wheat products	1000 µg
B12	2.4 µg	2.4 µg	Part of a coenzyme used in new cell synthesis, red blood cell formation, helps maintain nerve cells	Animal products such as meat, fish, poultry, milk, cheese, eggs	ND
Biotin	30 µg	30 µg	Part of a coenzyme used in the synthesis of fatty acids and glycogen	Egg yolk, dark green vegetables	ND
C	90 mg	75 mg	Intracellular maintenance of bone, capillaries, and teeth	Citrus fruits, green peppers, tomatoes	2000 mg
A	900 µg	700 µg	Vision, skin health, bone and tooth growth, reproduction, hormone synthesis and regulation, immunity	Retinol: Fortified milk, cheese, carrots, butter, fortified margarine, eggs, liver	3000 µg
D	15 µg*	15 µg*	Mineralization of bones, calcium absorption	Fortified milk, margarine, butter, cereals, eggs	50 µg
E	15 mg	15 mg	Antioxidant, stabilization of cell membranes, regulation of oxidation reactions	Polyunsaturated plant oils, green and leafy vegetables, wheat germ, whole grain products, nuts, seeds	1000 mg
K	120 µg*	90 µg*	Synthesis in blood clotting proteins and a protein that binds calcium in the bones	Bacterial synthesis in the digestive tract, green leafy vegetables, cabbage-type vegetables, potatoes	ND

[a]Values are Recommended Daily Allowance (RDA) for adults 19 to 50 years of age, unless marked with an asterisk. The requirements may vary for children, older adults, and pregnant or lactating women.
*Values are Adequate Intakes (AI), indicating that sufficient data to set the RDA are unavailable.
[o]Tolerable Upper Intake Levels (UL) for adults 19 to 50 years of age. Intakes above the UL may lead to negative health consequences.
ND = not yet determined.

Source: 2015–2020 Dietary guidelines for Americans.[30]

Understanding Nutrition

PRACTICAL INSIGHT

According to the Centers for Disease Control and Prevention (CDC) in 2012, about 10% or less of the general population had nutritional deficiencies for selected vitamin and minerals. The rates of deficiency are shown below, along with some notable differences by age, gender, and race/ethnicity:

- **Vitamin A:** Less than 1%; however, 2% were at risk for excess vitamin A, with older adults most likely to be at-risk for excess vitamin A (4.8%)
- **Vitamin B6:** 10.5%
- **Vitamin B12:** 2%; older adults are the most likely to be deficient (4%)
- **Vitamin C:** 6%; men (7%) were more likely to be deficient than women (5%)
- **Vitamin D:** 8.1% (with deficiency defined as serum 25-hydroxyvitamin D level less than 12 ng/mL); an additional 24% were at-risk for *inadequacy* (level of 12 ng/mL to 20 ng/mL); non-Hispanic black (31%) and Mexican American (12%) people were more likely to be deficient than non-Hispanic white people (3%)
- **Vitamin E:** Less than 1%
- **Folate:** Less than 1%; deficiency has decreased since mandatory folic acid fortification of enriched cereal grain products in 1998, raising levels by about 50%

DEFINITIONS

Minerals –
Micronutrients that the body needs in small amounts that must be obtained through diet.

◆ Minerals

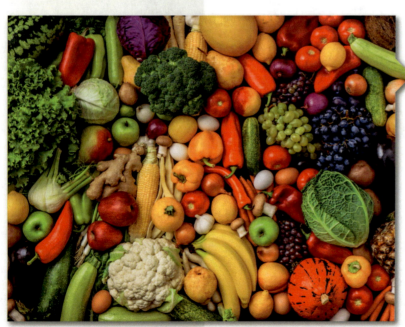

Minerals compose roughly 4% of total body mass. These inorganic compounds are mainly metallic elements that serve as constituents of enzymes, hormones, and vitamins. **Minerals** are often incorporated into structures and chemicals in the body. Their functions include:

- Providing components for bone and teeth.
- Regulation of cellular metabolism, actions of the heart, muscle, and nervous system.
- Maintenance of acid base balance.
- Regulation of cellular fluid balance.

Minerals play an extensive role in the catabolic and anabolic cell processes, activating the numerous reactions necessary to release energy from the breakdown of energy-yielding nutrients. Minerals also help assist with the synthesis of metabolic compounds, which enables the biological nutrient formation of glycogen, triglycerides, and protein from glucose, FAs, and amino acids. Minerals are fundamental parts of most activities of the body and, although they are consumed in small amounts, play a significant role in physiological homeostasis.

Mineral	Adult RDA[a] Men	Adult RDA[a] Women	Functions	Sources	UL[o]
Calcium	1000 mg*	1000 mg*	The principal mineral of bones and teeth. Normal muscle contraction and relaxation, nerve function, blood clotting, blood pressure, immune defenses	Milk and milk products, oysters, sardines, tofu (bean curd), greens, legumes	2500 mg
Chloride	2,600 mg	2,600 mg	Nerve and muscle function water balance (with sodium)	Table salt	ND
Magnesium	420 mg	320 mg	Bone mineralization, building of protein, enzyme action, normal muscular contraction, transmission of nerve impulses, and maintenance of teeth	Nuts, legumes, whole grains, dark green vegetables, seafood, chocolate, cocoa	350 mg^
Phosphorus	700 mg	700 mg	Important in cells' genetic material, in cell membranes as phospholipids, bones and teeth	All animal tissues	4000 mg
Potassium	4,700 mg	4,700 mg	Nerve and muscle function	All whole foods: meats, milk, fruits, vegetables, grains, legumes	ND
Sodium	500 mg*	500 mg*	Maintains cells' normal fluid balance and acid-base balance in the body; nerve impulse transmission	Salt, soy sauce, processed foods	ND
Chromium	35 µg*	25 µg*	Associated with insulin and required for the release of energy from glucose	Meat, unrefined foods, fats, vegetable oils	ND
Copper	900 µg	900 µg	Necessary for the absorption and use of iron in the formation of hemoglobin; part of several enzymes	Meat, nuts, seafood	10,000 µg
Fluoride	4 mg	3 mg	An element involved in the formation of bones and teeth; helps to make the teeth resistant to decay	Drinking water, tea, seafood	10 mg
Iodine	150 µg	150 µg	Thyroid hormone function	Iodized salt, seafood	1100 µg
Iron	8 mg	18 mg	Part of the proteins hemoglobin and myoglobin, necessary for the utilization of energy	Red meats, fish, poultry, shellfish, eggs, legumes, dried fruits	45 mg
Manganese	2.3 mg*	1.8 mg*	Enzyme function	Whole grains, nuts, fruits, vegetables	11 mg
Molybdenum	45 µg	45 µg	Energy metabolism in cells	Whole grains, organ meats, peas, beans	2000 µg
Selenium	55 µg	55 µg	Works with vitamin E	Meat, fish, whole grains, eggs	400 µg
Zinc	11 mg	8 mg	Part of the hormone insulin and many enzymes; involved in making genetic materials and proteins, immune reactions	Meats, fish, shellfish, poultry, grains, vegetables	40 mg

[a]Values are Recommended Daily Allowance (RDA) for adults 19 to 50 years of age, unless marked with an asterisk. The requirements may vary for children, older adults, and pregnant or lactating women.
*Minimum estimated daily intake requirement
[o]Tolerable Upper Intake Levels (UL) for adults 19 to 50 years of age. Intakes above the UL may lead to negative health consequences.
^This refers to pharmacological agents only, and not amounts contained in food and water. No evidence of ill effects from ingestion of naturally occurring amounts in food and water.
ND= not yet determined

Source: 2015–2020 Dietary guidelines for Americans.[30]

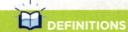

DEFINITIONS

Calcium –

The most abundant mineral in the body; it is required for vascular contraction and vasodilation, muscle function, and other body functions including bone rigidity.

Osteoclasts –

A cell responsible for dissolution and absorption of bone.

Osteoblasts –

A cell responsible for forming new bone.

The average American diet usually meets the nutritional requirements for every mineral except iron, and in some populations, calcium, most particularly deficient in female older adults, teenagers, minorities, and those of low income [66]. **Calcium** is the most abundant mineral in the body, carrying out numerous roles to support normal biological processes. It is involved in muscle contractions and the transmission of nerve impulses, serves as an activator for several enzymes, and helps transport fluids across cell membranes. Calcium combines with phosphorus in the body to form bone and teeth, which represents about 75% of the total mineral content found in humans. Due to its role in bone formation, calcium deficiencies significantly impact bone health.

A common misconception is that bones are static, when in fact, they are quite dynamic and are constantly undergoing modifications. Earlier chapters identified that bones are continuously being broken down and rebuilt in a process known as bone remodeling. Bone remodeling is controlled by two types of bone cells, **osteoclasts** and **osteoblasts**. This catabolic/anabolic relationship allows the bone to remain healthy and facilitates repair of damage. When the main construction material, calcium, is unavailable, the process of remodeling becomes impaired. Bones represent the largest storage pool of calcium in the body, so when inadequate amounts of calcium are supplied by the diet, the body pulls calcium from the bone and transfers it to the blood stream to maintain other biological processes that rely on calcium. When calcium is repurposed from bone, the restorative balance becomes disproportionate, leading to osteopenia and, eventually, osteoporosis. The average adult female consumes approximately half of the recommended 1,000-1,500 mg per day [66], which supports the current trend, where osteoporosis is reaching near-epidemic numbers. Estimates suggest that more than 30% of women over 50 and 77% of women over 80 develop the disease [99].

Life Stage Group		Calcium (mg)
Infants	0 - 6 mo	200
	6 - 12 mo	260
Children	1 - 3 y	700
	4 - 8 y	1,000
Males	9 - 13 y	1,300
	14 - 18 y	1,300
	19 - 30 y	1,000
	31 - 50 y	1,000
	51 - 70 y	1,000
	>70 y	1,200
Females	9 - 13 y	1,300
	14 - 18 y	1,300
	19 - 30 y	1,000
	31 - 50 y	1,000
	51 - 70 y	1,200
	>70 y	1,200
Pregnancy	14 - 18 y	1,300
	19 - 30 y	1,000
	31 - 50 y	1,000
Lactation	14 - 18 y	1,300
	19 - 30 y	1,000
	31 - 50 y	1,000

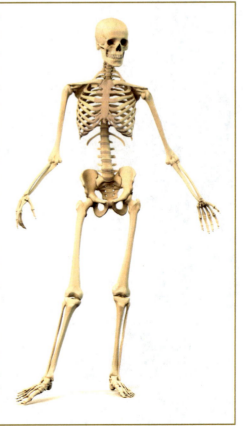

QUICK INSIGHT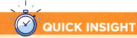

Osteopenia is characterized by a reduction in bone-mineral density. The disorder affects nearly 51% of adult women over the age of fifty [100]. Osteopenia is the precursor for the disease osteoporosis. Characterized by significant bone loss, the diagnostic criterion for osteoporosis is a loss of bone equivalent to 2.5 standard deviations below the average measured bone-mineral density for a given age range. Caucasian and Asian women suffer the highest incidence of osteoporosis. Osteoporosis increases risk for bone fracture and commonly afflicts the hip bones, vertebral column, and wrists. For optimal skeletal health, individuals should strive for >1000 mg calcium in the diet each day and a maintenance of serum 25(OH)D levels of 50 to <75 nmol/L. Of added importance, resistance training using weight-bearing exercise can significantly reduce the risk for developing the disease.

DEFINITIONS

Osteopenia –

A bone density that is lower than normal peak density but not low enough to be classified as osteoporosis.

Female athlete triad –

The interrelationship of menstrual dysfunction, low energy availability (with or without an eating disorder) and decreased bone mineral density; relatively common among young women participating in sports.

Without proper nutrition, bone mass can begin to decrease even before one turns 30 years of age; however, this can be significantly reduced with adequate consumption of calcium and load-bearing exercise, such as resistance training [18, 90]. Females may lose up to 1% of bone mineral density (BMD) a year after the age of 35. Menopause aggravates this loss because it is a time during which estrogen production drops dramatically and calcium absorption is also decreased. This change causes as much as a 3-6% loss of bone mass annually for the five years following menopause [45]. Estrogen is a vital hormone in calcium regulation. It facilitates intestinal absorption of calcium, reduces calcium excretion, and enhances calcium retention by the bone in both men and women. Despite the obstacles aging presents for men and women, adequate calcium, vitamin D, and exercise can reverse the developmental decline of osteoporosis [90].

Even without nutrient deficiency, research findings suggest that the relationship of inadequacy between both vitamin D and calcium perpetuates the risk of bone disease more than the individual consumption of either nutrient [90]. When both daily calcium intake and serum 25(hydroxy) vitamin D were insufficient, risk of osteopenia and osteoporosis significantly increased in both the hip and spine. Furthermore, among the elderly, an association between nutrient insufficiency and risk for osteoporosis was even more prominent when the subjects also suffered from sarcopenia. It is important for exercise professionals to convey the importance of calcium and vitamin D as well as resistance or body-weight exercise to maintain bone health.

QUICK INSIGHT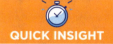

FEMALE TRIAD AND RELATIVE ENERGY DEFICIENCY IN SPORTS (RED-S)

The **female athlete triad** is a combination of disordered eating, amenorrhea, and osteoporosis. It is estimated that at least 25% of female athletes are at risk of suffering the consequences of estrogen imbalance due to insufficient caloric intake and excessive exercise stress. Body fat levels below essential requirements disrupt menstrual activity, causing a reduction in circulating estrogen concentrations [60]. The reduced level of estrogen causes calcium regulation to become dysfunctional. When combined with restricted diets that are low in calcium, the risk for osteoporosis is dramatically elevated [20]. While the term Female Athlete Triad may be the most commonly referenced aspect of energy-related risk, the concept of energy deficiency is not unique to women, as relative energy deficiency in sports is also found among male athletes in weight-regulated sports [59, 60].

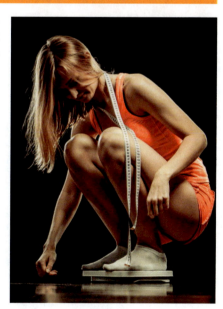

Common characteristics, signs, and symptoms of the female triad include:

- Young adult females
- Lean or low body mass
- Recurrent stress fractures
- Exercise fanatic
- Low self-esteem
- Self-critical
- Hard-driving personality
- Highly competitive
- Signs of depression
- Emotional highs and lows

◆ Iron

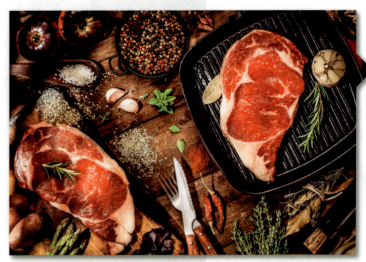

Iron deficiency is the most common nutrient deficiency in the world [51]. The mineral serves key functions in the formation of oxygen-carrying materials, including hemoglobin and myoglobin. In these molecules, iron is responsible for the binding of oxygen, so it can be transported to and also within cells. Iron is also an important component of many enzyme systems and physiological processes. The intestinal absorption of iron is consistent with the type of iron source consumed, but in general, is relatively low. Approximately 2-10% of the iron from plant-based foods (**non-heme iron**) is absorbed, compared to the 10-30% of the heme-iron found in animal products [27, 73]. In fact, well-known plant sources of iron, including spinach and soybeans, have absorption rates of only 2% and 7%, respectively. Foods high in vitamin C or in heme-iron can increase non-heme absorption rates when these sources are combined. Studies analyzing this relationship identified that as little as 65 mg of vitamin C can triple iron absorption. Foods including citrus, dark-green, leafy vegetables, melons, tomatoes, and strawberries, as well as beef, poultry, salmon, and pork, will all improve the absorption of non-heme iron. As with heme iron, foods rich in vitamin C must be eaten at the same time as foods high in non-heme iron to increase absorption. Additionally, it should be noted that calcium-rich foods like milk may inhibit iron absorption rates.

Inadequate iron consumption poses another problem for females. Iron loss during menstrual cycles can be as high as 45 mg (5-45 mg) [28, 101]. This loss is compounded by the fact that heme-iron consumption is often lower in females than in male populations. This problem leads to insufficient iron levels in approximately 30-50% of the adult female population [101]. Due to the role iron plays in the formation of hemoglobin, insufficient consumption reduces oxygen transport in the blood, consequently affecting oxygen delivery to cells. Iron-deficiency anemia occurs when iron or hemoglobin levels drop too low. Common signs and symptoms of iron-deficiency anemia include fatigue, loss of appetite, and reduced capacity to perform activity. Individuals with iron-deficiency anemia will suffer a noticeable decline in performance associated with a reduced capacity for oxygen transport. To avoid iron-deficiency anemia, those at the greatest risk should consume more iron-rich foods, particularly animal-source iron, to enhance absorption capabilities. While supplementation may help, eating animal meat increases iron status most effectively, even when supplements are consumed with vitamin C [91]. In addition to animal sources and vitamin C, exercise can also augment iron absorption when supported by proper nutrition [1].

DEFINITIONS

Non-heme iron –

Iron from plant-based foods like beans, fruits, vegetables and nuts. It is absorbed more effectively when eaten with meat, poultry and fish or with food that is high in vitamin C.

Population	Age	Iron (mg)
Children	1 - 3 y	7
	4 - 8 y	10
Males	9 - 13 y	8
	14 - 18 y	11
	19 - 30 y	8
	31 - 50 y	8
	51 - 70 y	8
	>70 y	8
Females	9 - 13 y	8
	14 - 18 y	15
	19 - 30 y	18
	31 - 50 y	18
	51 - 70 y	8
	>70 y	8
Pregnancy	> 16 y	27
Lactation	< 18 y	10
	> 18 y	9

Recommended Dietary Allowances For Iron Dietary Reference Intakes for Iron 2001, National Academy of Sciences, Institute of Medicine. Food and Nutrition Board.

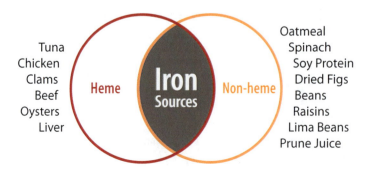

◆ Electrolytes

Some additional minerals are of particular interest for exercise professionals due to their role in fluid balance and cellular regularity. **Electrolytes** are electrically charged ions that come from the minerals sodium, potassium, chloride, calcium, magnesium, and phosphate. Sodium and chlorine combine to form sodium chloride, and together, these electrolytes represent the main minerals contained in blood plasma and extracellular fluid, while potassium mainly resides in the cell. Magnesium is needed for proper muscle, nerve, and enzyme function and aids in energy metabolism and cellular transport of sodium and potassium. Electrolytes modulate fluid exchange between the cell and the extracellular environment. This balance is maintained by well-regulated electrical and concentration gradients that enable all the cellular activities required for biological homeostasis to occur on an ongoing basis.

> *All of the following depend on the electrical balance control of electrolytes:*
> - Signals from the nervous system
> - Muscular contractions
> - Glandular function
> - Regulation of pH balance

> **DEFINITIONS**
>
> **Electrolytes –**
>
> *Minerals (sodium, calcium, potassium, chlorine, phosphate, magnesium) found in blood, urine, tissues and other bodily fluids that help balance the amount of water and pH level in the body based on osmolar relationships.*

Poor intake of electrolytes in the diet and unmanaged environmental stress leading to mineral deficits like hyponatremia can lead to imbalances and manifest into serious physiological problems. Of major concern is the thermoregulatory system, whose proper function depends upon the regulation of water balance. When the system becomes impaired, heat illness can result and increase the risk of permanent neurological injury or death. Excessive body fluid loss from sweat or illness will lower internal water and electrolyte levels. Proper diet and water consumption should be maintained to ensure adequate intake of electrolytes and proper hydration. Beverages containing electrolytes can be a viable re-hydration option following intense training, GI illness, or any situation in which the body loses high levels of fluid.

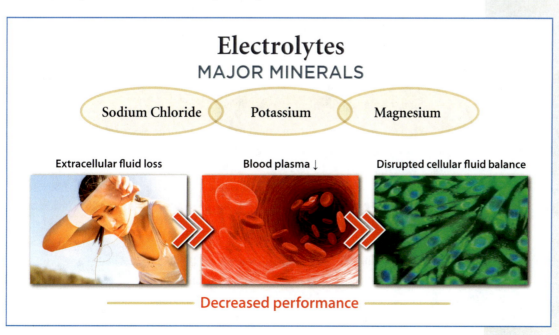

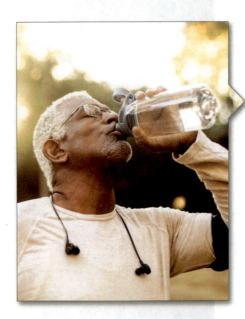

◆ Water

Water constitutes nearly 75% of muscle weight and approximately 50% of fat weight (76). It is the most abundant and important nutrient in the body. Without water, life can only be sustained for a limited number of days. It plays a role in almost all the functions of the body as a constituent of compounds, transporter, reactant, and principal of gaseous diffusion.

> *As a functional component, water:*
> - **Lubricates joints**
> - **Protects moving organs**
> - **Provides body volume and form**
> - **Serves in thermoregulation**
> - **Is used in chemical balance**
> - **Serves as an ingredient in cellular metabolism**

Water serves more roles than any other single nutrient in the body. If water consumption does not meet requirements and dehydration occurs, the body fails to function properly. An important relationship exists between water and minerals within the body, which makes proper daily consumption vital for health. Minerals need water to form electrolytes, and in turn, water needs minerals to maintain fluid balance via specific osmolality levels inside and outside the cell membrane. Body water is generally categorized into two divisions: intracellular and extracellular fluids. Most water is found inside of the cells as intracellular fluid, while approximately one-third of body water exists outside of the cell as extracellular fluid. Extracellular fluid includes blood plasma, the water found between the cells (interstitial fluid), lymph, saliva, fluid secreted by glands and organs, and the fluids that hydrate the spinal cord. Cells are permeable, so water moves relatively easily through the cellular membrane as dictated by the physiological environment. This mobility allows the body to maintain a system that prevents cells from losing too much fluid or becoming over saturated; minerals play an important role in facilitating this regulatory mechanism. When minerals dissolve in water, they become ions (or electrolytes). As stated earlier, the term electrolyte is given to these ions because they have an electrical charge and conduct electricity. When these electrical conductors are maintained in correct concentration within and outside of the cell, water balance is maintained. The electrolyte responsible for maintenance of intracellular fluid volume is potassium, while extracellular fluid is regulated by sodium and chlorine. Magnesium inside and outside of the cell also contributes to the action but is rarely identified with the other electrolytes [19].

When excess fluid loss disturbs the cellular environment, electrolyte imbalances occur. Individuals experiencing excessive fluid loss through exercise, heat, vomiting, or diarrhea can reach a hazardous state of dehydration [62]. When extracellular fluid is lost due to any of these physiological agitators, the reduction of extracellular fluid draws intracellular fluid from the cell as it attempts to restore balance. Electrolytes are also lost during this process, which changes the osmolarity, further exacerbating this problem. This creates a hazardous situation because the fluid regulatory mechanism is compromised, which in extreme cases, increases risk for kidney and heart failure [62]. Once balance is lost, immediate fluid replenishment is imperative to restore it; however, the content of the fluid consumed for rehydration is relevant. In severe cases of dehydration, intravenous (IV) therapy is used to increase fluid volumes using an electrolyte-balanced solution. In less severe cases, water and electrolyte solutions should be consumed orally due to their effect on extracellular fluid osmolality and volume [24]. The following charts illustrate normal fluid intake and fluid output pathways.

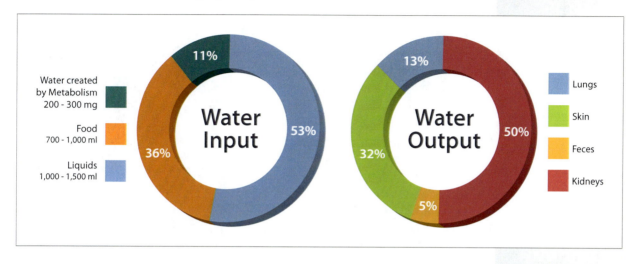

Daily Fluid Intake

Daily fluid intake prevents dehydration and heat illness, but most people do not consume enough water to meet their daily requirements, particularly when they are physically active. Fluid is gained and lost through a variety of mechanisms. A daily intake of 2.7 L of water for adult women and 3.7 liters of water for adult men will meet the daily needs for the majority of people [77]. When the environment is hot and the intensity and duration of activity increases, the physiological demand for water jumps dramatically. Fluid intake volumes may increase to 5 L or even 10 L under extreme physiological stress.

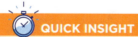 **QUICK INSIGHT**

*The **sodium-potassium relationship** is very important to maintain homeostasis. Together, the electrolyte ions regulate the fluid balance in tissues by establishing the proper electrical gradient across cell membranes. When excess salt is consumed in the diet, it increases the excretory function of the kidneys by decreasing aldosterone, the hormone that increases sodium re-absorption. In some cases, the excess sodium cannot be adequately regulated, causing too much sodium to remain in the body. The excess sodium pulls water into the blood, causing the blood to become hyper-hydrated, which increases blood pressure. Sodium-induced hypertension occurs in approximately 33% of the individuals who are diagnosed with hypertension [89]. The average American consumes twice the recommended intake of salt in the diet (>5000 mg) [66], but this high intake is not often met by an appropriate balance of potassium. Individuals who have an elevated risk for high blood pressure should reduce salt in their diets and consume adequate quantities of potassium. Tomatoes, avocados, potatoes, winter squash, bananas, coconut water, and meat are good potassium sources.*

 DEFINITIONS

Sodium-potassium relationship –

Electrolytes that control the distribution of fluids throughout the body; a higher potassium intake can cause the excretion of more sodium through urine which can help lower blood pressure.

QUICK INSIGHT

WATER LOSS

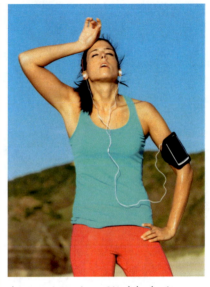

Dehydration is the adverse consequence of inadequate water intake. The symptoms of acute dehydration vary with the degree of water deficit [1]. For example, fluid loss of 1% of body weight impairs thermoregulation, triggering thirst. Thirst increases at 2%, with dry mouth appearing at approximately 3%. Vague discomfort and loss of appetite also appear at 2%. The threshold for impaired exercise thermoregulation occurs at a mere 1% dehydration, and at 4%, work capacity declines 20-30%. Difficulty concentrating, headache, and sleepiness are observed at 5%, and heat-illness risk increases significantly. Tingling and numbness of extremities can be seen at 6%, and collapse can occur at around 7% dehydration. A 10% loss of body water through dehydration is life-threatening [2]. While the vague discomfort that accompanies a 2% dehydration may not have a significant impact, the 20 – 30% reduction in work capacity seen at 4% can seriously impair productivity.

Three primary sources can satisfy daily fluid intake requirements: liquids consumed, foods consumed, and metabolic processes. Fluid consumption should attempt to focus on pure water or electrolyte containing beverages. It is argued that some of the hydration effects of soda, coffee, and tea are negated due to the diuretic effects of the caffeine contained in these beverages; however, recent research has shown that when the caffeine content is low there is no evidence of increased diuresis [42, 80]. Additionally, supplement drinks with diuretics, and some medicines may also negatively affect water balance. Healthy food sources, particularly fruits and vegetables, contain considerable amounts of water, whereas breads and sweets have relatively low water content. Metabolic water represents H_2O liberated from the breakdown of energy molecules such as glycogen. It provides about 25% of daily water requirements for a sedentary person. During physical activity, the breakdown of CHOs supplies additional systemic water as glycogen liberates the water that bonds it to glucose. Each gram of glycogen contains 2.7 grams of water, accounting for more than 1,000 grams of water maintained inside the body when glycogen stores are at full capacity.

Metabolic Water Produced From Energy Substrate Breakdown	
Energy Nutrient (100g)	**Metabolic Water (grams)**
Carbohydrates	55 g
Protein	100 g
Fats	107 g

◆ Fluid Loss

The body's water output proceeds relatively efficiently. The four primary pathways for fluid loss include urine, water loss through the skin, water loss as water vapor during respiration, and water lost in feces. Fluid loss through urine is determined by the re-absorption rate of the kidneys and the amount of solute that passes through the kidneys each day. The average re-absorption rate of water is about 99%, leaving roughly 1000-1500 ml of fluid to be excreted as urine each day [9; 32; 78]. This fluid loss is increased with alcohol consumption and when high quantities of protein are used as energy, which may accelerate the dehydration rate. The excretory function of removing fecal matter also requires water. To ensure the matter moves easily through the large intestine, water constitutes approximately 70% of the total volume of human excrement (100-200 ml of water). This becomes increasingly relevant when an individual suffers from diarrhea, which can cause a fluid loss between 1500-5000 ml [19].

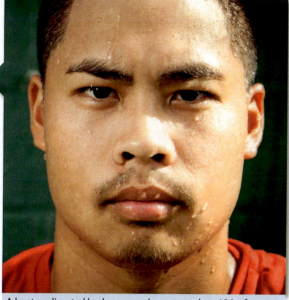

A heat-acclimated body can produce as much as 12 L of sweat in one day - at a rate of 1 L per hour (or more) during prolonged intense exercise.

Water lost from the skin and through respiration accounts for the rest of the fluid lost each day. Water vapor leaves the body with each breath, and accounts for about 250-300 ml of water lost each day through normal respiration. When under the stress of exercise, fluid loss increases due to increased ventilatory requirements and can equal approximately 2 to 5 ml per minute of vigorous exercise, depending on the environment [78, 96]. Interestingly, this rate is highest in colder climates and higher altitudes because the body must release water to moisten inspired air to help it move through the pulmonary airways.

The skin also experiences increased fluid loss during exercise and in heated environments. Under normal conditions, the skin will lose about 350 ml of fluid per day to "insensible perspiration." This perspiration occurs as water seeps from deeper tissues out to the skin and is evaporated before one feels the "sweat" on the skin. Water can also be excreted from sweat glands that lie beneath the skin's surface. Generally, the body will lose between 500-750 ml of water to normal daily sweating, which serves as a refrigeration mechanism to help cool the body. As the body produces sweat, it is evaporated from the skin, causing a cooling effect. This is the body's best defense against overheating. A heat-acclimated body can produce as much as 12 L of sweat in one day at a range of 0.5 to 2 with an average of 1.2 L per hour during prolonged intense exercise [9]. In addition to the aforementioned conditions and physiological functions of the body, fluid output can be affected by several other factors as well.

> **Factors increasing the need for additional water intake:**
> - Low-calorie diets
> - Pregnancy and lactation
> - Illness
> - High sodium consumption
> - Higher protein and fiber diets
> - The consumption of alcohol and caffeine [39]

Each factor requires a specific amount of water to compensate for the added fluid lost through one of the four fluid-loss mechanisms. Determining how much additional water is necessary requires understanding what facilitated the loss in the first place. Examining each mechanism and its relative mean fluid-loss value will help to determine how much more water must be ingested in order to meet daily need.

◆ Exercise and Fluid Loss

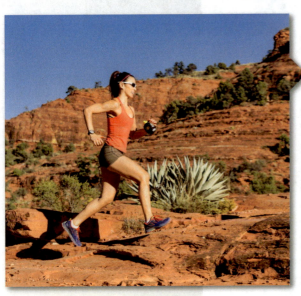

Exercise exacerbates the effects of water loss due to cardiovascular adjustments and evaporation. The dissipation of metabolically generated heat can cause excessive sweating, which may lead to an accompanying reduction of plasma volume, causing fluid shifts out of the intercellular and interstitial compartments. When the environmental climate includes high heat and humidity, the cardiovascular system is taxed by the physiological demands of heat management. During these conditions, the blood must transfer metabolic heat to the periphery for cooling. This requirement reduces the amount of available blood for oxygen delivery and is one reason why relative intensity is affected by hot conditions. In addition, exercising in the heat lowers absolute VO_2 because the reduced amount of available blood directly lowers stroke volume. As a result, heart rate increases to compensate for the decrease in stroke volume, and thereby produces higher heart rates at all submaximal exercise levels. At maximal aerobic capacity, in these types of environments, the heart rate cannot make up for the reduced stroke volume, causing a reduction in VO_2max.

During exercise, the body experiences rapid internal temperature changes. Heat generated by the active muscles will lead to an elevated **core temperature**. A modest rise in core temperature creates the optimal thermal environment for physiologic and metabolic function, as heat catalyzes reactions used by these systems. Although this response is normal, body thermodynamics still require a well-regulated, heat reduction response. The brain's hypothalamus contains the coordinating center for temperature control, making thermoregulatory adjustments in response to deviations in temperature. Heat regulating mechanisms activate via signals from thermal receptors in the skin and by the temperature of blood, both of which directly stimulate the thermoregulatory center. In response to this information, the body mobilizes fluid for a cooling effect. Evaporation provides the major physiological defense against overheating during rest and activity. When the body experiences environmental heat and internal heat activated by physical activity, the situation is handled primarily by increased perspiration. This results in a decrease of body fluid and leads to rapid dehydration.

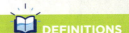

DEFINITIONS

Core temperature –

The operating temperature of an organism which is normally maintained within a narrow range; typically obtained most accurately through rectal measurement.

Dehydration –

Occurs when the body loses more fluid than is taken in; signs and symptoms include increased thirst, headache, dry skin, dizziness, increased heart rate and BP, decreased urine output and dry mouth.

◆ Dehydration

Thirst is the primary controller of hydration status. Unfortunately, the threshold for the initiation of thirst occurs at a point where a person may already be mildly dehydrated [40, 46]. For most people, basing water consumption on thirst will likely lead to inadequate water consumption. This is a particular concern for the elderly, as the thirst mechanism becomes impaired due to attenuation of central volume receptors that occurs with age [40, 46]. **Dehydration** occurs at a body weight deficit of 1.0% or more due to fluid loss and occurs when fluid output is greater than fluid intake. As indicated earlier, water is lost through multiple body functions, and all metabolic activity requires water in some capacity. On average, humans cycle through all the water in the body about once every 10-12 days. Athletes in heavy training generally replace all their water about once every six days. Whenever fluid dynamics become output dominated (>2% loss of body weight), body functions are impaired [78]. Moderate exercise can cause a fluid loss of 0.5 to 1.5 L • hour-1. This number significantly increases up to 3 L • hr-1 when conditions become more strenuous, either through increased physical exertion or environmental factors [78]. Fluid loss can reach life-threatening levels in a very short period, and accumulative fluid loss can be just as dangerous. Consistently losing water over an extended period without adequate replenishment can cause a normal bout of exercise to become a significant health hazard due to poor hydration status. The risk of heat-related illness, such as a stroke, greatly increases when the body is dehydrated. This same problem occurs with prolonged exercise.

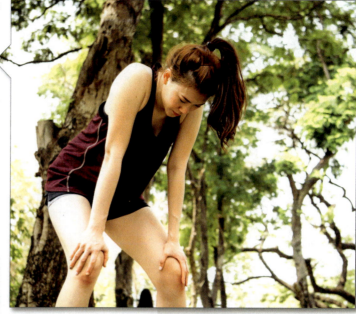

Early Signs of Dehydration
- Fatigue
- Headache
- Heat Intolerance
- Dry Mouth or Cough
- Flushed Skin
- Appetite Loss
- Sensation of Being Light-Headed
- Dark Urine with Strong Odor

Hypovolemia and sweat gland fatigue can occur once hydration status reaches a fluid loss greater than 5% of body mass [55]. Since most of the fluid lost from sweat is supplied by blood plasma, cardiovascular function is impaired due to a reduced availability of oxygen and a lower cardiac output. This reduction in cardiac output can cause kidney dysfunction, heart dysfunction, and possibly stroke. Additionally, the reduced blood plasma volume further compromises the body's thermoregulatory capacity [55]. These thermoregulatory and physiological functions experience decreased efficiency with almost any level of dehydration. The fact that dehydration can occur when swimming, exercising in colder environments, and at higher altitudes is often overlooked. Diuretic use also contributes to dehydration status by decreasing the amount of water recycled by the kidneys via an increased urine output. In addition, the fluid excreted through urine from diuretic consumption comes from blood plasma. As mentioned earlier, individuals who consistently consume diuretic-containing beverages instead of water may be impairing their hydration status. The same is true for alcohol consumption.

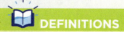

DEFINITIONS

Hypovolemia –

State of decreased blood volume that can result in multiple organ failure death due to inadequate circulating volume and subsequent inadequate perfusion.

PRACTICAL INSIGHT

To be well hydrated, the average sedentary, adult male should consume at least 3.7 liters of fluid per day, while the average sedentary, adult female should consume at least 2.7 liters of fluid per day [13]. The fluid should be in the form of non-caffeinated, non-alcoholic beverages, soups, and foods. Water in its pure form is the most readily used by the body. Drinking tea, coffee, and other soft drinks can over-stimulate the CNS, and at the same time, increase dehydration risk due to the strong diuretic action of caffeine on the kidneys, which causes increased urine production. In fact, persons who regularly drink coffee or soda without additional adequate water intake can cause mild dehydration without participating in any physical activity whatsoever.

Chronic dehydration has been linked to the development of numerous major health problems. It is generally thought that the prevalence of kidney stones increases in populations with low urinary volume. Decreased fluid intake leads to low urine volume and increased concentrations of all stone-forming salts. Recommendations for individuals at risk for urinary stone formation, as well as patients with stones, include the consumption of at least 250 ml of fluid with each meal, between meals, before bedtime, and upon waking [13,43,93]. This pattern ensures that fluid intake is spread throughout the day and that urine doesn't become concentrated. These measures decrease the chance for kidney stone development.

Chronic dehydration can result in debilitating conditions such as:

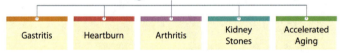

Gastritis | Heartburn | Arthritis | Kidney Stones | Accelerated Aging

Low fluid consumption may increase the incidence of certain cancers. A link seems to exist between patients with urinary tract cancer (bladder, kidney, prostate, and testicle) and low fluid consumption [2,5]. No association with specific fluid volumes has been found, but one study found that women who drank more than five glasses of water per day had a 45% decreased risk of colon cancer compared with those who drank two or fewer glasses. Among the men, there was a 32% decrease in risk with increased water consumption [1,4]. This effect probably stems from the fact that fecal mobility increases with proper fluid intake. It is thought that higher fecal mobility reduces the duration of time that carcinogenic toxins remain in the large intestine.

Water also plays a primary role in fat metabolism. One of the liver's many functions is to mobilize stored fat for energy utilization. Water is a key ingredient in this metabolic process. In times of water shortage, the kidneys cannot perform as required for waste removal. This results in the liver being called upon to aid the kidneys in their efforts, resulting in less efficient metabolism. Additionally, water serves to further aid in reducing dietary caloric content. Unlike juices and sodas, water is calorie-free. People who consume regular amounts of water experience feelings of satiety (fullness) by maintaining a higher gastric volume. With more contents in the stomach, there is a tendency to eat less. Adequate water intake can take the edge off hunger, reducing the caloric peaks and valleys that many people experience when eating large meals.

◆ Maintaining Proper Hydration

Fluid replacement is the key to maintaining healthy body dynamics. When proper hydration combines with adequate **acclimation** to the training and environment, the synergistic effect greatly reduces the risk for dehydration and heat-related illnesses.

For individuals with proper acclimation to training and environmental stress, several physiological adjustments can occur:

- Increased plasma volume
- Increased sweat sensitivity and earlier onset of sweating
- Increased sweat rate and distribution
- Lower core temperature
- Increased release of antidiuretic hormone (ADH) and aldosterone
- Improved cutaneous blood flow
- Lower RPE

> **DEFINITIONS**
>
> **Acclimation –**
> *A physiological adjustment by an organism in response to an environmental change such as altitude, temperature, humidity or systemic pH.*
>
> **Gastric emptying –**
> *The process of emptying food from the stomach; strongly influenced by the volume and composition of gastric contents.*

The effects of acclimatization must be complemented with regularly scheduled fluid consumption throughout the day and during activity. Ingesting fluids during exercise increases blood flow to the skin, causing a more effective cooling process through sweat evaporation. Strictly following an adequate fluid replacement schedule prevents dehydration and its consequences, particularly hyperthermia. Fitness professionals must remain diligent about keeping scheduled fluid intakes throughout their client's training regimens, especially in hot climates and environments with high humidity, as this prevents sweat evaporation from the skin, and limits the body's ability to cool itself. Most exercisers and athletes under-consume their recommended fluid intake when left to monitor their own hydration [17]. This is important, as a fully-hydrated individual will experience improvements in performance compared to efforts made in a state of compromised hydration.

◆ Pre-Exercise Hydration

Pre-exercise hydration can help provide added protection against heat stress delaying dehydration and increases in core temperature [77,79,93]. This consumption can start 24 hours before the exercise bout or competition and should continue up to 20 minutes before the training begins. Pre-exercise fluid consumption should be approximately 400-600 ml of water, which serves to increase stomach volume and optimizes **gastric emptying** [78]. This pre-exercise hydration can be very important for endurance activities and training in hot climates where it is difficult to balance intake with output.

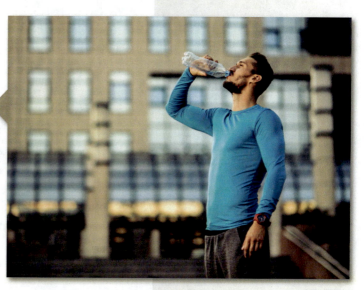

◆ Hydration During & Post-Exercise

To maintain proper hydration, fluid should be consumed throughout exercise. Fitness professionals can ensure that hydration status is optimized by tracking urine composition and bodyweight changes. In a well-hydrated individual, urine should typically be produced in large volumes, have a limited odor, and exhibit a light coloration. Urine that is dark and gives off noticeable odor suggests dehydration. Likewise, changes in pre and post-exercise bodyweight indicate fluid lost during the training bout. Charting training weight differences between pre and post exertion enables the exercise professional to gauge the normal fluid loss for each client. This provides clear data for fluid replacement quantities. On average, one pound of weight loss equates to 450 ml (15 oz) of water loss.

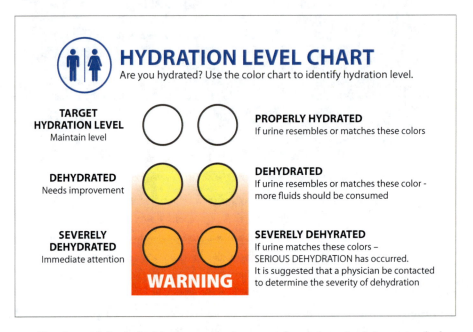

Time intervals for replenishment are also important factors in maintaining proper hydration status. For fluid loss of 1000 ml per hour, 250 ml of water should be consumed every 15 minutes. For fluid loss in excess of 1000 ml per hour, the same quantity should be consumed every 10 minutes [6, 24, 67, 81]. Identifying the actual amount of fluid lost is the first step to replacing the lost contents adequately. Rehydration fluid intake does not have to be limited to water. Palatable CHO-electrolyte solutions (4-8% CHO solution) can serve to facilitate more complete hydration than plain water alone [6]. This active and facilitated hydration can be used both during and following exercise and competition. Beverages containing 20-60 mmol/L have shown to increase recovery hydration and electrolyte balance post-exercise [6, 24]. Additionally, small amounts of potassium 2-5 mmol/L may enhance the retention of water in intracellular space and may diminish any extra potassium loss from sodium retention by the kidneys.

Immediately after exercise, pure water is quickly absorbed and dilutes the plasma-sodium concentration to the point that it decreases plasma osmolarity. This, in turn, increases urine production and inhibits the sodium-dependent stimulation process that initiates the brain's thirst mechanism. When fluids have the correct concentration of sodium, plasma-sodium concentrations remain elevated, which sustains the thirst sensation, promotes the retention of ingested fluid, and speeds up plasma-volume restoration during rehydration [6, 14, 24, 93]. CHO-electrolyte drinks contribute to the ideal solution for activity and recovery hydration. The

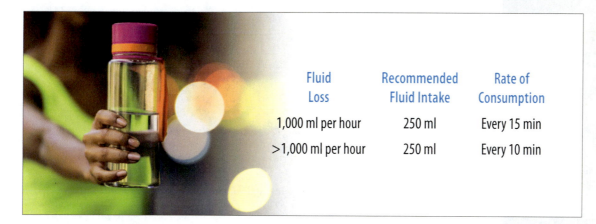

Fluid Loss	Recommended Fluid Intake	Rate of Consumption
1,000 ml per hour	250 ml	Every 15 min
>1,000 ml per hour	250 ml	Every 10 min

glucose solutions stimulate active absorption of both sodium and water in the intestines, and when combined with fructose, can take advantage of facilitated transport. CHO-electrolyte drinks have proven to be effective in aiding fluid replenishment [24]. However, when CHO concentrations are too high, gastric emptying and the rate of intestinal fluid absorption is negatively affected. Total gastric volume plays an important role in the rate of gastric emptying, as higher volumes increase this rate. Since many people experience discomfort when exercising with greater gastrointestinal contents, CHO concentration is very important if a sports drink is used for hydration. One caveat to CHO-replenishment drinks is that sport drinks are intended for individuals who exercise at levels that compromise water balance and glycogen stores. Many individuals do not reach the exercise intensities or durations that warrant CHO-electrolyte solutions. These glucose solutions usually contain 100+ calories in the form of sugar. Over-consuming replenishment drinks can contribute to a positive caloric balance and undesirable insulin response. Water alone does not have any calories and, therefore, will usually be adequate for most participants performing low-to-moderate exercise.

REFERENCES:

1. Abbaspour N, Hurrell R, and Kelishadi R. Review on iron and its importance for human health. *Journal of research in medical sciences: the official journal of Isfahan University of Medical Sciences* 19: 164, 2014.

2. Acheson K, Schutz Y, Bessard T, Anantharaman K, Flatt J, and Jequier E. Glycogen storage capacity and de novo lipogenesis during massive carbohydrate overfeeding in man. *The American journal of clinical nutrition* 48: 240-247, 1988.

3. Albert CM, Cook NR, Gaziano JM, Zaharris E, MacFadyen J, Danielson E, Buring JE, and Manson JE. Effect of folic acid and B vitamins on risk of cardiovascular events and total mortality among women at high risk for cardiovascular disease: a randomized trial. *Jama* 299: 2027-2036, 2008.

4. Alhadeff L, Gualtieri CT, and Upton M. Toxic effects of water soluble vitamins. *Nutrition Reviews* 42: 33-40, 1984.

5. Alissa EM and Ferns GA. Functional foods and nutraceuticals in the primary prevention of cardiovascular diseases. *Journal of nutrition and metabolism* 2012, 2012.

6. Armstrong LE, Casa DJ, Maresh CM, and Ganio MS. Caffeine, fluid-electrolyte balance, temperature regulation, and exercise-heat tolerance. *Exercise and sport sciences reviews* 35: 135-140, 2007.

7. Augustin LS, Kendall CW, Jenkins DJ, Willett WC, Astrup A, Barclay AW, Björck I, Brand-Miller JC, Brighenti F, and Buyken AE. Glycemic index, glycemic load and glycemic response: An international scientific consensus summit from the international carbohydrate quality consortium (ICQC). *Nutrition, Metabolism and Cardiovascular Diseases* 25: 795-815, 2015.

8. Bäck M. Omega-3 fatty acids in atherosclerosis and coronary artery disease. *Future science* OA 3: FSO236, 2017.

9. Baker LB. Sweating rate and sweat sodium concentration in athletes: a review of methodology and intra/Interindividual variability. *Sports Medicine* 47: 111-128, 2017.

10. Bartlett JD, Hawley JA, and Morton JP. Carbohydrate availability and exercise training adaptation: too much of a good thing? *European journal of sport science* 15: 3-12, 2015.

11. Berthoud HR. Homeostatic and non homeostatic pathways involved in the control of food intake and energy balance. *Obesity* 14, 2006.

12. Bhattacharya A, Banu J, Rahman M, Causey J, and Fernandes G. Biological effects of conjugated linoleic acids in health and disease. *The Journal of nutritional biochemistry* 17: 789-810, 2006.

13. Campbell S. Dietary Reference Intakes: Water, Potassium, Sodium, Chloride, and Sulfate. *Clinical Nutrition Insight* 30: 1&hyhen, 2004.

14. Casa DJ, Armstrong LE, Hillman SK, Montain SJ, Reiff RV, Rich BS, Roberts WO, and Stone JA. National Athletic Trainers' Association position statement: fluid replacement for athletes. *Journal of athletic training* 35: 212, 2000.

15. Christiansen T, Bruun JM, Madsen EL, and Richelsen B. Weight Loss Maintenance in Severely Obese Adults after an Intensive Lifestyle Intervention: 2 to 4 Year Follow Up. *Obesity* 15: 413-420, 2007.

16. Costacou T, Bamia C, Ferrari P, Riboli E, Trichopoulos D, and Trichopoulou A. Tracing the Mediterranean diet through principal components and cluster analyses in the Greek population. *European Journal of Clinical Nutrition* 57: 1378, 2003.

17. Coyle EF. Fluid and fuel intake during exercise. *Journal of sports sciences* 22: 39-55, 2004.

18. Dawson-Hughes B, Harris SS, Krall EA, and Dallal GE. Effect of calcium and vitamin D supplementation on bone density in men and women 65 years of age or older. *New England Journal of Medicine* 337: 670-676, 1997.

19. De Baaij JH, Hoenderop JG, and Bindels RJ. Magnesium in man: implications for health and disease. *Physiological reviews* 95: 1-46, 2015.

20. De Souza MJ, Nattiv A, Joy E, Misra M, Williams NI, Mallinson RJ, Gibbs JC, Olmsted M, Goolsby M, and Matheson G. 2014 Female Athlete Triad Coalition Consensus Statement on treatment and return to play of the female athlete triad: 1st International Conference held in San Francisco, California, May 2012 and 2nd International Conference held in Indianapolis, Indiana, May 2013. *Br J Sports Med* 48: 289-289, 2014.

21. Doell D, Folmer D, Lee H, Honigfort M, and Carberry S. Updated estimate of trans fat intake by the US population. *Food Additives & Contaminants: Part A* 29: 861-874, 2012.

22. Eckel RH, Jakicic JM, Ard JD, De Jesus JM, Miller NH, Hubbard VS, Lee I-M, Lichtenstein AH, Loria CM, and Millen BE. 2013 AHA/ACC guideline on lifestyle management to reduce cardiovascular risk: a report of the American College of Cardiology/American Heart Association Task Force on Practice Guidelines. *Journal of the American College of Cardiology* 63: 2960-2984, 2014.

23. Estruch R, Ros E, Salas-Salvadó J, Covas M-I, Corella D, Arós F, Gómez-Gracia E, Ruiz-Gutiérrez V, Fiol M, and Lapetra J. Primary prevention of cardiovascular disease with a Mediterranean diet. *New England Journal of Medicine* 368: 1279-1290, 2013.

24. Evans GH, James LJ, Shirreffs SM, and Maughan RJ. Optimizing the restoration and maintenance of fluid balance after exercise-induced dehydration. *Journal of Applied Physiology* 122: 945-951, 2017.

25. Fuller S, Beck E, Salman H, and Tapsell L. New Horizons for the Study of Dietary Fiber and Health: A Review. *Plant Foods for Human Nutrition* 71: 1-12, 2016.

26. Gaby AR. Adverse effects of dietary fructose. *Alternative medicine review* 10: 294, 2005.

27. Hallberg L and Hulthén L. Perspectives on iron absorption. *Blood Cells, Molecules, and Diseases* 29: 562-573, 2002.

28. Harvey LJ, Armah CN, Dainty JR, Foxall RJ, Lewis DJ, Langford NJ, and Fairweather-Tait SJ. Impact of menstrual blood loss and diet on iron deficiency among women in the UK. *British Journal of Nutrition* 94: 557-564, 2005.

29. Hawley JA, Schabort EJ, Noakes TD, and Dennis SC. Carbohydrate-loading and exercise performance. *Sports medicine* 24: 73-81, 1997.

30. Health UDo and Services H. 2015–2020 Dietary guidelines for Americans. *Washington (DC)*: USDA, 2015.

31. Health UDo and Services H. *Dietary Guidelines for Americans 2015-2020*: Skyhorse Publishing Inc., 2017.

32. Hoffman R, Kronfeld D, Cooper W, and Harris P. Glucose clearance in grazing mares is affected by diet, pregnancy, and lactation 1. *Journal of animal science* 81: 1764-1771, 2003.

33. Hooper L, Kroon PA, Rimm EB, Cohn JS, Harvey I, Le Cornu KA, Ryder JJ, Hall WL, and Cassidy A. Flavonoids, flavonoid-rich foods, and cardiovascular risk: a meta-analysis of randomized controlled trials. *The American journal of clinical nutrition* 88: 38-50, 2008.

34. Izumida Y, Yahagi N, Takeuchi Y, Nishi M, Shikama A, Takarada A, Masuda Y, Kubota M, Matsuzaka T, and Nakagawa Y. Glycogen shortage during fasting triggers liver–brain–adipose neurocircuitry to facilitate fat utilization. *Nature communications* 4: ncomms3316, 2013.

35. Jäger R, Kerksick CM, Campbell BI, Cribb PJ, Wells SD, Skwiat TM, Purpura M, Ziegenfuss TN, Ferrando AA, and Arent SM. International society of sports nutrition position stand: protein and exercise. *Journal of the International Society of Sports Nutrition* 14: 20, 2017.

36. Jehn M, Patt M, Appel L, and Miller Er. One year follow up of overweight and obese hypertensive adults following intensive lifestyle therapy. *Journal of human nutrition and dietetics* 19: 349-354, 2006.

37. Jones JM. CODEX-aligned dietary fiber definitions help to bridge the 'fiber gap'. *Nutrition journal* 13: 34, 2014.

38. Katz D and Meller S. Can we say what diet is best for health? *Annual review of public health* 35: 83-103, 2014.

39. Kavouras SA. Assessing hydration status. *Current Opinion in Clinical Nutrition & Metabolic Care* 5: 519-524, 2002.

40. Kenefick RW. Drinking Strategies: Planned Drinking Versus Drinking to Thirst. *Sports Medicine*: 1-7, 2018.

41. Kerksick CM, Arent S, Schoenfeld BJ, Stout JR, Campbell B, Wilborn CD, Taylor L, Kalman D, Smith-Ryan AE, and Kreider RB. International society of sports nutrition position stand: nutrient timing. *Journal of the International Society of Sports Nutrition* 14: 33, 2017.

42. Killer SC, Blannin AK, and Jeukendrup AE. No evidence of dehydration with moderate daily coffee intake: a counterbalanced cross-over study in a free-living population. *PloS one* 9: e84154, 2014.

43. Kleiner SM. Water: an essential but overlooked nutrient. *Journal of the American Dietetic Association* 99: 200-206, 1999.

44. Kontush A. HDL particle number and size as predictors of cardiovascular disease. *Frontiers in pharmacology* 6: 218, 2015.

45. Lane NE. Epidemiology, etiology, and diagnosis of osteoporosis. *American Journal of Obstetrics & Gynecology* 194: S3-S11, 2006.

46. Leib DE, Zimmerman CA, and Knight ZA. Thirst. *Current Biology* 26: R1260-R1265, 2016.

47. Leser S. The 2013 FAO report on dietary protein quality evaluation in human nutrition: Recommendations and implications. *Nutrition Bulletin* 38: 421-428, 2013.

48. Liebman B. Changing American Diet: A Report Card: Center For Science In The Public Interest, 2013.

49. Liese AD, Schulz M, Fang F, Wolever TM, D'Agostino RB, Sparks KC, and Mayer-Davis EJ. Dietary glycemic index and glycemic load, carbohydrate and fiber intake, and measures of insulin sensitivity, secretion, and adiposity in the Insulin Resistance Atherosclerosis Study. *Diabetes care* 28: 2832-2838, 2005.

50. Livesey G. Thermogenesis associated with fermentable carbohydrate in humans, validity of indirect calorimetry, and implications of dietary thermogenesis for energy requirements, food energy and body weight. *International journal of obesity* 26: 1553, 2002.

51. Lopez A, Cacoub P, Macdougall IC, and Peyrin-Biroulet L. Iron deficiency anaemia. *The Lancet* 387: 907-916, 2016.

52. Mackenbach JP. The Mediterranean diet story illustrates that "why" questions are as important as "how" questions in disease explanation. *Journal of clinical epidemiology* 60: 105-109, 2007.

53. Manore MM. Exercise and the Institute of Medicine recommendations for nutrition. *Current sports medicine reports* 4: 193-198, 2005.

54. Martin WF, Armstrong LE, and Rodriguez NR. Dietary protein intake and renal function. *Nutrition & metabolism* 2: 25, 2005.

55. McGee S, Abernethy III WB, and Simel DL. Is this patient hypovolemic? *Jama* 281: 1022-1029, 1999.

56. Meyers DG, Maloley PA, and Weeks D. Safety of antioxidant vitamins. *Archives of internal medicine* 156: 925-935, 1996.

57. Mirmiran P, Bahadoran Z, and Azizi F. Functional foods-based diet as a novel dietary approach for management of type 2 diabetes and its complications: A review. *World journal of diabetes* 5: 267, 2014.

58. Moore DR. Nutrition to support recovery from endurance exercise: optimal carbohydrate and protein replacement. *Current sports medicine reports* 14: 294-300, 2015.

59. Mountjoy M, Sundgot-Borgen J, Burke L, Carter S, Constantini N, Lebrun C, Meyer N, Sherman R, Steffen K, and Budgett R. Authors' 2015 additions to the IOC consensus statement: Relative Energy Deficiency in Sport (RED-S): BMJ Publishing Group Ltd and British Association of Sport and Exercise Medicine, 2015.

60. Mountjoy M, Sundgot-Borgen J, Burke L, Carter S, Constantini N, Lebrun C, Meyer N, Sherman R, Steffen K, and Budgett R. The IOC consensus statement: beyond the female athlete triad – Relative Energy Deficiency in Sport (RED-S). *Br J Sports Med* 48: 491-497, 2014.

61. Mozaffarian D, Micha R, and Wallace S. Effects on coronary heart disease of increasing polyunsaturated fat in place of saturated fat: a systematic review and meta-analysis of randomized controlled trials. *PLoS medicine* 7: e1000252, 2010.

62. Noakes TD. Dehydration during exercise: what are the real dangers? Clinical journal of sport medicine: *official journal of the Canadian Academy of Sport Medicine* 5: 123-128, 1995.

63. Organization WH and University UN. *Protein and amino acid requirements in human nutrition*: World Health Organization, 2007.

64. Ötles S and Ozgoz S. Health effects of dietary fiber. Acta scientiarum polonorum *Technologia alimentaria* 13: 191-202, 2014.

65. Pagoto SL and Appelhans BM. A call for an end to the diet debates. *Jama* 310: 687-688, 2013.

66. Rehm CD, Peñalvo JL, Afshin A, and Mozaffarian D. Dietary intake among US adults, 1999-2012. *Jama* 315: 2542-2553, 2016.

67. Rehrer NJ. Fluid and electrolyte balance in ultra-endurance sport. *Sports Medicine* 31: 701-715, 2001.

68. Riccioni G, Bucciarelli T, Mancini B, Di Ilio C, Capra V, and D'Orazio N. The role of the antioxidant vitamin supplementation in the prevention of cardiovascular diseases. *Expert Opinion on Investigational Drugs* 16: 25-32, 2007.

69. Robertson MD, Bickerton AS, Dennis AL, Vidal H, and Frayn KN. Insulin-sensitizing effects of dietary resistant starch and effects on skeletal muscle and adipose tissue metabolism–. *The American journal of clinical nutrition* 82: 559-567, 2005.

70. Rosenson RS, Brewer HB, Chapman MJ, Fazio S, Hussain MM, Kontush A, Krauss RM, Otvos JD, Remaley AT, and Schaefer EJ. HDL measures, particle heterogeneity, proposed nomenclature, and relation to atherosclerotic cardiovascular events. *Clinical chemistry* 57: 392-410, 2011.

71. Ross AC, Taylor CL, Yaktine AL, and Del Valle HB. Institute of medicine (US) committee to review dietary reference intakes for vitamin D and calcium. *Dietary Reference Intakes for Calcium and Vitamin D National Academies Press, Washington (DC)*, http://www/ ncbi nlm nih gov/books/NBK56056/(accessed 0201 16), 2011.

72. Sacks FM, Lichtenstein AH, Wu JH, Appel LJ, Creager MA, Kris-Etherton PM, Miller M, Rimm EB, Rudel LL, and Robinson JG. Dietary fats and cardiovascular disease: a presidential advisory from the American Heart Association. *Circulation* 136: e1-e23, 2017.

73. Saini RK, Nile SH, and Keum Y-S. Food science and technology for management of iron deficiency in humans: A review. *Trends in Food Science & Technology* 53: 13-22, 2016.

74. Samuel VT. Fructose induced lipogenesis: from sugar to fat to insulin resistance. *Trends in Endocrinology & Metabolism* 22: 60-65, 2011.

75. Samuel VT and Shulman GI. The pathogenesis of insulin resistance: integrating signaling pathways and substrate flux. *The Journal of clinical investigation* 126: 12-22, 2016.

76. Sarvazyan A, Tatarinov A, and Sarvazyan N. Ultrasonic assessment of tissue hydration status. *Ultrasonics* 43: 661-671, 2005.

77. Sawka MN, Cheuvront SN, and Carter R. Human water needs. *Nutrition reviews* 63, 2005.

78. Sawka MN, Cheuvront SN, and Kenefick RW. Hypohydration and human performance: impact of environment and physiological mechanisms. *Sports Medicine* 45: 51-60, 2015.

79. Sawka MN and Montain SJ. Fluid and electrolyte supplementation for exercise heat stress–. *The American journal of clinical nutrition* 72: 564S-572S, 2000.

80. Seal AD, Bardis CN, Gavrieli A, Grigorakis P, Adams J, Arnaoutis G, Yannakoulia M, and Kavouras SA. coffee with high but not low caffeine content augments Fluid and electrolyte excretion at rest. *Frontiers in nutrition* 4: 40, 2017.

81. Shirreffs SM and Maughan RJ. Rehydration and recovery of fluid balance after exercise. *Exercise and sport sciences reviews* 28: 27-32, 2000.

82. Simpson SJ, Le Couteur DG, and Raubenheimer D. Putting the balance back in diet. *Cell* 161: 18-23, 2015.

83. Siri-Tarino PW, Sun Q, Hu FB, and Krauss RM. Meta-analysis of prospective cohort studies evaluating the association of saturated fat with cardiovascular disease–. *The American journal of clinical nutrition* 91: 535-546, 2010.

84. Siti HN, Kamisah Y, and Kamsiah J. The role of oxidative stress, antioxidants and vascular inflammation in cardiovascular disease (a review). *Vascular pharmacology* 71: 40-56, 2015.

85. Slavin JL. Position of the American Dietetic Association: health implications of dietary fiber. *Journal of the American Dietetic Association* 108: 1716-1731, 2008.

86. St-Onge M-P, Ard J, Baskin ML, Chiuve SE, Johnson HM, Kris-Etherton P, and Varady K. Meal timing and frequency: implications for cardiovascular disease prevention: a scientific statement from the American Heart Association. *Circulation* 135: e96-e121, 2017.

87. Stellingwerff T and Cox GR. Systematic review: Carbohydrate supplementation on exercise performance or capacity of varying durations. *Applied Physiology, Nutrition, and Metabolism* 39: 998-1011, 2014.

88. Surh Y-J. Cancer chemoprevention with dietary phytochemicals. *Nature Reviews Cancer* 3: 768, 2003.

89. Takahashi H, Yoshika M, Komiyama Y, and Nishimura M. The central mechanism underlying hypertension: a review of the roles of sodium ions, epithelial sodium channels, the renin–angiotensin–aldosterone system, oxidative stress and endogenous digitalis in the brain. *Hypertension Research* 34: 1147, 2011.

90. Tang BM, Eslick GD, Nowson C, Smith C, and Bensoussan A. Use of calcium or calcium in combination with vitamin D supplementation to prevent fractures and bone loss in people aged 50 years and older: a meta-analysis. *The Lancet* 370: 657-666, 2007.

91. Teucher, Olivares, and Cori. Enhancers of iron absorption: ascorbic acid and other organic acids. *International journal for vitamin and nutrition research* 74: 403-419, 2004.

92. Thomas DT, Erdman KA, and Burke LM. Position of the academy of nutrition and dietetics, dietitians of canada, and the american college of sports medicine: Nutrition and athletic performance. *Journal of the Academy of Nutrition and Dietetics* 116: 501-528, 2016.

93. Trangmar SJ and González-Alonso J. New insights into the impact of dehydration on blood flow and metabolism during exercise. *Exercise and sport sciences reviews* 45: 146-153, 2017.

94. Varadharaj S, Kelly OJ, Khayat RN, Kumar PS, Ahmed N, and Zweier JL. Role of Dietary Antioxidants in the Preservation of Vascular Function and the Modulation of Health and Disease. *Frontiers in cardiovascular medicine* 4, 2017.

95. Venn B and Green T. Glycemic index and glycemic load: measurement issues and their effect on diet–disease relationships. *European journal of clinical nutrition* 61: S122, 2007.

96. Westerterp KR, Plasqui G, and Goris AH. Water loss as a function of energy intake, physical activity and season. *British journal of nutrition* 93: 199-203, 2005.

97. Wiktorowska-Owczarek A, Berezinska M, and Nowak JZ. PUFAs: structures, metabolism and functions. *Adv Clin Exp Med* 24: 931-941, 2015.

98. Wölnerhanssen BK, Cajacob L, Keller N, Doody A, Rehfeld JF, Drewe J, Peterli R, Beglinger C, and Meyer-Gerspach AC. Gut hormone secretion, gastric emptying, and glycemic responses to erythritol and xylitol in lean and obese subjects. *American Journal of Physiology-Endocrinology and Metabolism* 310: E1053-E1061, 2016.

99. Wright N, Saag K, Dawson-Hughes B, Khosla S, and Siris E. The impact of the new National Bone Health Alliance (NBHA) diagnostic criteria on the prevalence of osteoporosis in the USA. *Osteoporosis International* 28: 1225-1232, 2017.

100. Wright NC, Looker AC, Saag KG, Curtis JR, Delzell ES, Randall S, and Dawson Hughes B. The recent prevalence of osteoporosis and low bone mass in the United States based on bone mineral density at the femoral neck or lumbar spine. Journal of Bone and Mineral Research 29: 2520-2526, 2014.

101. Zimmermann MB and Hurrell RF. Nutritional iron deficiency. *The Lancet* 370: 511-520, 2007.

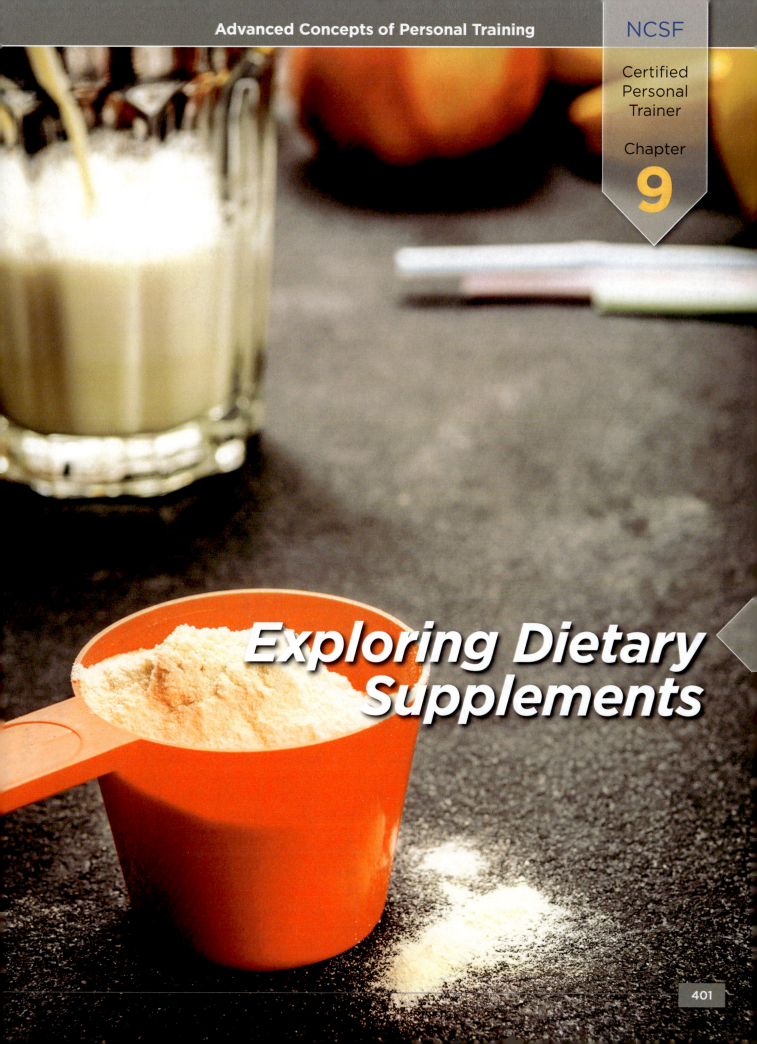

Advanced Concepts of Personal Training

NCSF Certified Personal Trainer

Chapter 9

Exploring Dietary Supplements

401

Introduction

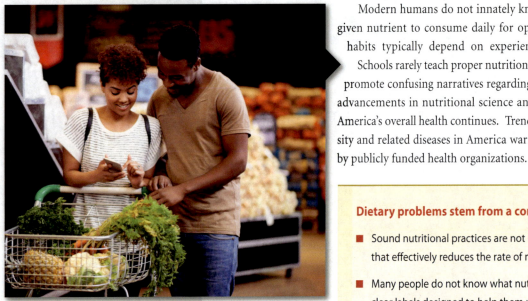

Modern humans do not innately know what and how much of any given nutrient to consume daily for optimal nutrition. Consumption habits typically depend on experience, culture, and convenience. Schools rarely teach proper nutrition, and marketing campaigns often promote confusing narratives regarding what is healthy to eat. Despite advancements in nutritional science and medicine, a steady decline in America's overall health continues. Trends toward increased rates of obesity and related diseases in America warrant the serious concerns raised by publicly funded health organizations.

Dietary problems stem from a combination of sources:

- Sound nutritional practices are not reaching the public in a way that effectively reduces the rate of negative, health-related issues.

- Many people do not know what nutrients are in foods, even with clear labels designed to help them understand food products.

- Americans cite time and pressure demands as excuses for poor nutritional choices.

- The amount of daily physical activity performed does not match the energy being consumed across all age levels.

- Manufacturers promote and endorse quick-fix solutions, creating numerous obstacles to a balanced diet by taking advantage of people's natural tendency to choose convenience.

- The media presents incomplete or incorrect information, and no regulatory body oversees what is being communicated to consumers from books and magazines.

The government provides outlets for quality information; however, many people find it challenging to implement the information effectively. Historically, the United States Department of Agriculture (USDA) has used initiatives like the Food Pyramid and MyPlate as easy tools to help provide Americans with a practical approach to good nutrition. The government programs' goals have been to provide simple guidelines for nutrient sources, as well as the recommended servings from defined categories, such as grains, meats, fruits, and vegetables. These programs were intended to meet the nutritional needs of approximately 90% of the population. As digital apps and other resources flood the market however, these projects may be discontinued. A case in point: June 30, 2018 marked the last day for Supertracker, the nutrient-tracking software associated with MyPlate, due to the number of private-company apps available free to consumers.

Reading a Food Label

◆ Food Labels

The government requires that producers and retailers display basic nutritional facts on the labels of pre-packaged food products. The information on food labels can be very helpful in managing a healthy diet. Therefore, learning how to read and interpret the information on a food label, such as discerning the difference between a portion and a serving size, is an integral part of being able to track dietary intake. Presenting clients with examples of appropriate serving sizes is an excellent method that can be used to help them realize the dietary-intake quantities that will fulfill, but not exceed, their relative need. The chart below describes what a typical serving size should look like from each category.

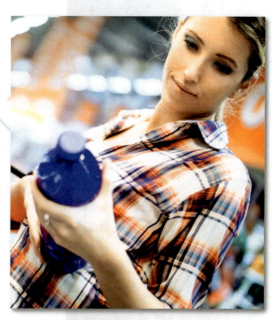

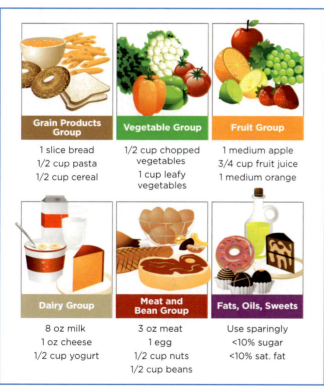

A food label provides specific information required by the Nutrition Education Labeling Act of 1990. This act requires a mandatory nutrient list and an ingredient list, which is in descending order by weight, to be on the label for pre-packaged foods. When consumers purchase foods in a prepared form, reading the labels on the container is necessary to identify contents, nutrients, and caloric breakdown of the product because there are several ingredients. The **Nutritional facts label** is also required and identifies the number of servings per container, reflecting the amount of food by weight or volume that constitutes a single serving. A serving size is the portion that contains the nutrient amounts listed on the label. In 2016, the US Food and Drug Administration (FDA) approved a new Nutrition Facts label for packaged foods to

> **DEFINITIONS**
>
> **Nutritional facts label –**
>
> *A label required on most packaged foods that was updated by the FDA in 2016 to reflect new scientific information, including the link between diet and chronic disease.*

reflect the newest scientific information, including the link between diet and chronic diseases, such as obesity and heart disease.

The following nutrient information is required of each label:

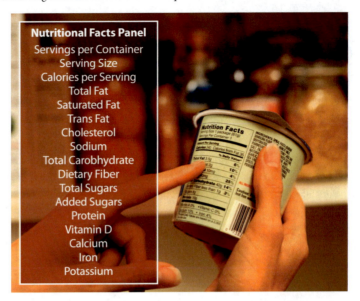

Sample Food Label

Nutrition Facts
8 servings per container
Serving size 2/3 cup (55g)

Amount per serving
Calories 232

	% Daily Value*
Total Fat 8g	10%
Saturated Fat 1g	5%
Trans Fat 0g	
Cholesterol 0mg	0%
Sodium 160mg	7%
Total Carbohydrate 37g	13%
Dietary Fiber 4g	14%
Total Sugars 12g	
Includes 10g Added Sugars	20%
Protein 3g	
Vitamin D 2mcg	10%
Calcium 260mg	20%
Iron 8mg	45%
Potassium 235mg	6%

* The % Daily Value (DV) tells you how much a nutrient in a serving of food contributes to a daily diet. 2,000 calories a day is used for general nutrition advice.

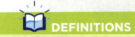

DEFINITIONS

Daily Values (DV) –

A nutrition-label guide to the nutrients in one serving of food, based on a 2,000-calorie diet for healthy adults.

The nutritional fact panel attempts to provide additional clarity by expressing the nutrient list through **Daily Values**. The Daily Values are represented by the nutritional content of one serving by weight as it applies to a 2,000-kcal diet. The product's total energy is listed next to each nutrient by percentages of the Daily Value. This is to assist consumers in meeting their energy and nutritional intake requirements according to the recommended percentage in the diet.

Using the percentage of calories from carbohydrates (CHO), fats, and proteins would seem to be a reasonable way to track energy nutrients; however, the actual work required to correctly track energy intake this way is very difficult. A person would have to know his or her actual total daily caloric intake and the specific intake in grams or calories for each nutrient to calculate the percentages. This would involve tracking the specific number of grams from each energy source, converting them to caloric value, totaling the calories consumed, and dividing total calories by the nutrient total calories to get the percentages. Knowing the exact serving size and caloric value of every food consumed and the nutrients therein would be required for true accuracy, illustrating why this is not a reasonable method for tracking dietary intake. The methodology is relevant for an exercise professional but impractical for the consumer, as it is much too difficult to employ. Below is the method used to convert energy nutrient weight into the percentage of dietary calories.

Converting Grams to Percentages

125 grams of fat consumed in a 2,700 kcal diet

125 ~~gram~~ x 9 kcal/~~gram~~ = 1,125 kcals from fat

1,125 kcals from fat ÷ 2,700 kcal diet = 41% fat

41% of the total calories in the diet come from fat

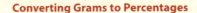

Food description terminology can also challenge consumers. For most individuals looking to eat better, boxes labeled 'light,' 'low-fat,' 'non-fat,' and 'reduced-calorie' all look very appealing, but very few people recognize what the terms actually mean. The government has made efforts to help by generating **nutrient content descriptors**: terms used to market foods based on improved consumer-health awareness. The FDA and Food Safety and Inspection Service of the USDA regulate the specific descriptive information found on food labels. The following terms are commonly found on many food product labels.

DEFINITIONS

Nutrient content descriptors –

Terms used to describe the relevant aspects of a food source, for example "free," "low," "high," "good source."

Food Descriptors

- **Free** – often associated with fat-free or sugar-free, means the product contains no amount of, or only trivial quantities of, the referred components. Less than 0.5 g per serving or less than 5 kcal per serving.
- **Low** – can be used if the foods can be consumed regularly without causing excessive intakes of its referred components.
- **Low-Calorie** – less than 40 kcal per serving.
- **Low-Fat** – less than 3g per serving.
- **Low-Cholesterol** – less than 20 mg per serving.
- **Low-Sodium** – less than 140 mg per serving.
- **Light** – has three possible meanings: 1) 1/3rd fewer calories or half the fat, 2) the sodium content of a low calorie, low fat food has been reduced by 50%, 3) the term describes the color, texture or other property as long as it explains intent e.g. "light brown sugar."
- **Reduced** – the contents contain at least 25% less of the component than the referenced product.
- **Lean** – less than 10g fat, 4.5g or less saturated fat, and less than 95 mg of cholesterol per serving and per 100 g.
- **Extra Lean** – less than 5 g of fat, less than 2 g of saturated fat, less than 95 mg of cholesterol per serving.
- **Good Source** – 10-19% of the Daily Value.
- **High In** – 20% or more of the Daily Value.
- **Extra** – at least 10% more than the Daily Value in the reference food.
- **Very Low Sodium** – 35 mg or less sodium.
- **Sodium Free** – less than 5 mg per serving.
- **High Fiber** – 5g or more per serving.

Consumers can rely on these descriptors because they are properly regulated, although some confusion still exists as to when they are appropriate. For instance, a jelly-bean package that advertises itself as 'fat-free' falls within the agency's regulations, but the food is a protein-based gum infused and covered in pure sugar. Certainly, the product does not contain any fat, and therefore is 'fat-free'; however, the fact is that jelly beans have never contained fat. The company makes the "fat-free" claim to confuse consumers into thinking it is a healthier food choice. Exercise professionals should educate clients on appropriate food-selection practices and help make them aware of the label descriptors.

Exploring Dietary Supplements

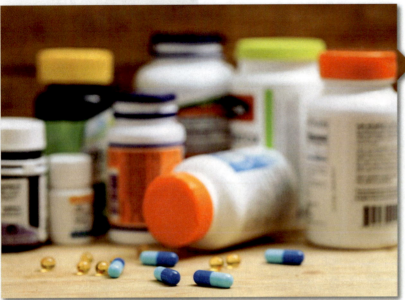

Every person's nutritional requirements differ in some capacity due to the broad number of factors that affect the individual's energy needs. When there is greater physiological and/or psychological stress placed upon the body, the supportive nutrient need increases in tandem. The specificity of the demand will dictate the change in nutritional needs. When the stress stimulus arises from physical activity, its modality, intensity, and duration become relevant factors in determining the appropriate nutritional makeup of the diet. For instance, heavy resistance training requires different nutritional adjustments than does long-distance endurance training. The amount of energy used during activity, the physiological recovery and repair mechanisms, and the goals of the training play a role in differentiating the proper nutrition for optimal outcomes.

◆ Post-Exercise Recovery Considerations

During high-volume, heavy resistance training, muscle glycogen provides the largest portion of calories available for work. For this reason, glycogen levels in muscle tissue should be maximized before engaging in intense resistance training. Research has shown that when muscle-glycogen levels are low, premature fatigue results, limiting intense exercise duration. Cellular glycogen saturation is best initiated immediately following an exercise bout. Physical exertion depletes glycogen at a rate consistent with intensity; depletion consequently signals the cells to absorb nutrients for glycogen resynthesis. During the four hours immediately post-exercise, cells have an increased permeability to nutrients and an increased sensitivity to anabolic hormones, including insulin. During this time, CHO should be consumed at 1 g/kg of body weight to optimize this systematic recovery process [22]. Consuming a mixture of protein and CHOs immediately post exercise increases both glycogen saturation and protein synthesis in the muscle tissue [8, 60, 121]. The quantity of CHOs consumed should reflect the energy needs of the next training or competition bout, as the pre-exercise levels of glycogen play an integral role in the tissues' capacity. Several studies suggest that, during intense training programs, the replenishment of total calories expended is the most important factor following exercise in order to mitigate subsequent performance detriments [44]. Some studies even suggest intakes of up to 10 g of CHO per kilogram of body weight consumed over the course of several hours following each exercise bout [19, 21, 31]. The key factors to glycogen replenishment are as follows: 1) the total energy utilized from CHOs versus other sources (i.e. fat, protein) during exercise; 2) how soon CHOs are consumed after exercise, with early ingestion showing substantial benefits over late ingestion [44]. When glycogen is significantly depleted, it becomes more difficult to fully refuel for the next event.

Immediately following an exercise bout, simple CHOs or high glycemic foods with a CHO component that is quickly absorbed into the blood stream are an ideal choice to replenish CHO [20]. The internal biological environment makes better use of the glucose, because in its simple form, it quickly enters circulation. The cellular availability of nutrients is very important to the post-exercise metabolic process, which explains why quickly digested and absorbed nutrients are ideal during this time (e.g., simple sugars and whey protein) [15]. This holds true for both stop-and-go anaerobic activities, which are typical of resistance training and repeat sprints, as well as sustained aerobic exercise events. Research trials consistently found that inadequate CHO consumption in the hours following exercise led to reduced performance in subsequent training bouts [44]. Based on these findings, many athletes and fitness enthusiasts who perform high-intensity exercise utilize post-exercise recovery drinks. CHO-electrolyte solutions can contribute to replenishment, but, when consumed alone, tend to be inadequate in terms of supplying sufficient calories to satisfy the recovery demands fully. Though immediate post-exercise energy replenishment represents an integral part of the recovery process, it is only the first step. Additional CHO sources should be consumed during the four-hour period following exercise and throughout the day to maintain adequate caloric intake relative to the training bout.

Recovery beverages or commercially blended meal-replacement drinks offer an alternative to regular food due to their digestibility and convenience. The actual energy breakdown of the beverages varies by manufacturer and the product's intention. Protein drinks consumed immediately after exercise can contribute to tissue recovery but are generally too low in CHOs to replenish glycogen stores. In addition, the protein content often exceeds the rate of protein-synthesis stimulation. Fluid energy mixtures that provide both CHOs and protein can be an ideal solution for post-exercise energy consumption when appropriate food sources are not available. Low-fat chocolate milk has enjoyed significant scientific support due to its 3.5:1 CHO to protein mixture [70, 110, 118, 131]. Possible benefits include increased digestibility and absorption rates compared to many whole food choices. In addition, beverages are convenient, providing a practical alternative to the labor and time requirements of meal preparation. As a rule of thumb for immediate post exercise nutrient consumption, most literature supports a 3-4:1 ratio of CHO to protein [72, 100]. Additionally, literature-backed recommendations suggest total energy from glucose should not exceed 60g per hour due to the 1g/min absorption rate and maximal protein consumption should not exceed 40g per serving for similar reasons [47, 66, 85]. Following sleep or any 8-12-hour period when eating does not occur, glycogen stores become reduced. One strategy that can be employed to help encourage glycogen storage is pre-exercise food consumption. Pre-activity fuel should be mainly in CHO form to ensure adequate energy stores for high intensity work. Consuming a meal high in protein or fat will not satisfy the energy needs of the working tissue during heavy or intense training. CHOs consumed approximately 3-4 hours before the exercise bout provide adequate time for digestion and absorption of the nutrients [53]. Adequate fluid should also be consumed during this period to prepare the body for activity participation.

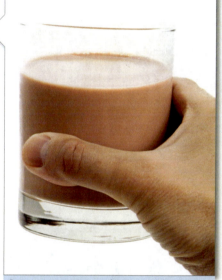

Consuming a mixture of protein and carbohydrates, immediately post exercise, increases both glycogen saturation and protein synthesis in the muscle tissue.

◆ Ergogenic Aids

To further enhance physical performance, many exercise enthusiasts and athletes supplement their dietary intake of nutrients. The term **supplement** implies enhancing consumption of nutrients required for proper nutrition, which may or may not have been attained by an

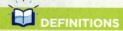

DEFINITIONS

Supplement –

Products that are intended to fulfill or complement the diet and may contain one or more ingredients, such as vitamins, herbs, amino acids, or their constituents.

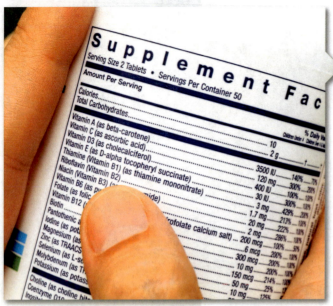

DEFINITIONS

Ergogenic aid –

Any product that offers a mental or physical edge while exercising or competing, also called performance enhancers.

individual through normal dietary intake. The most common dietary supplements consumed in the United States are multi-vitamin and mineral pills. They represent the largest portion of the dietary supplement industry and are estimated to cover 70-90% of all supplements marketed and sold [128]. Per the American Dietetic Association, more than 50% of adults have taken or currently take vitamin pills as a supplement to their diet. Many exercisers also believe that taking additional vitamins is necessary for improved performance and health [39, 40]. Supplements an individual takes above what is necessary for normal homeostasis are classified as **ergogenic aids**. Dietary ergogenic aids are supplemental nutrients or compounds that, when consumed, enhance one or more body functions.

For many people, the hardest concept to accept is that "more is not always better." If adequate nutrition is attained through the diet, then further intake through supplemental sources is unnecessary. Over 50 years of research concludes that additional supplementation above relative nutritional adequacy does not provide exercise-performance enhancement. Consuming an extra serving of protein or a single multi-vitamin will likely not be detrimental; however, caution should be used when consuming large quantities of any nutrient, especially when also consuming other supplements [17, 28]. The Tolerable Upper Intake Limit (UL) should provide the ceiling for prudent ingestion of any nutrient. A variety of food sources, particularly plant-based foods, should be used to meet the majority of the body's nutrient needs. That being said, numerous nutrients, compounds, herbs, and chemical agents purport to enhance performance-related physiological functions, which are generally categorized by the specific "claimed" effect the supplement is supposed to have on the body. The following list includes the most popular categories found in most nutrition stores.

Popular supplement/ergogenic aid categories:

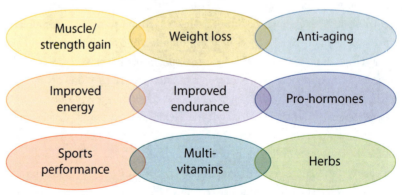

Hundreds of products fall within each of these categories. The contentious claims associated with dietary supplement consumption vary dramatically. Some products claim to offer numerous health benefits, while others advertise that consumption will improve a single body function. Given the seemingly endless products offered, combined with limited peer-reviewed literature supporting the alleged claims, only the most popular supplements are reviewed.

◆ Consumer Caution

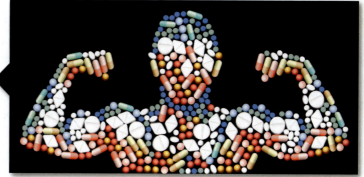

The supplement industry remains a "buyer beware" market. The FDA regulates dietary supplements under a different set of regulations than those covering "conventional" food and drug (prescription and over-the-counter) products. Under the Dietary Supplement Health and Education Act of 1994 (DSHEA), the dietary supplement manufacturer is responsible for ensuring that a dietary supplement is safe before it is marketed, and the FDA is only responsible for acting against any unsafe dietary supplement product after it reaches the market. Despite the fact that manufacturers must make sure that product label information is truthful and not misleading, they do not generally need to register their products with the FDA or get FDA approval before producing or selling dietary supplements.

The supplement industry's pseudo self-regulation has created an environment where, legally, almost anything goes, as long as the product label does not make a medical claim or suggest that the product can cure or prevent a disease. These loose reins on the multi-billion-dollar supplement industry have not only opened the gates but cleared the way for unethical "health hustling." Interestingly, only a limited number of supplements have been both reviewed by scientifically sound research trials and demonstrated efficacy in performance enhancement, including weight loss and hypertrophy.

The product labels are also a source of concern when buying supplements. Numerous well-controlled studies have found inconsistencies in both supplement potency and implied or listed concentrations of the active ingredients on supplement labels. This situation stems from the fact that companies manufacturing and selling supplements are not necessarily scrutinized for quality-control practices. If supplements are purchased, they should come only from reputable companies certified by NSF/ANSI and should be Good Manufacturing Practices (GMP) registered.

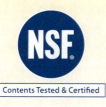

"Good Manufacturing Practices (GMPs) are guidelines that provide a system of processes, procedures and documentation to assure a product has the identity, strength, composition, quality and purity that appear on its label. These GMP requirements are listed in Section 8 of NSF/ANSI 173 which is the only accredited American National Standard in the dietary supplement industry developed in accordance with the FDA's 21 CFR part 111.

NSF International independently registers manufacturers as meeting GMP requirements. The program is open not just to manufacturers of dietary supplements but also to manufacturers of ingredients and raw materials, as well as distribution, warehousing and packaging companies, who want to demonstrate their commitment to public safety." NSF International 2018

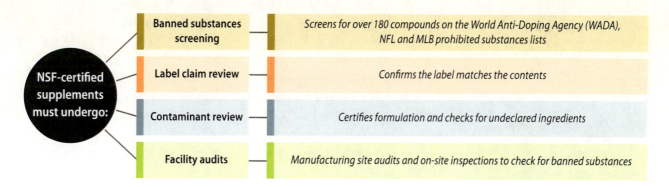

Exploring Dietary Supplements

All consumers should beware of advertising and marketing that uses:
- Testimonials
- "Independent research"
- Free trials
- Celebrity endorsements
- Guarantees of quick results
- "Secret" ingredients
- Proprietary blends

DEFINITIONS

Creatine monohydrate –

Used as a dietary supplement to improve muscle strength and athletic performance. Creatine is a naturally occurring chemical in the body and is commonly found in the diet via the consumption of red meat and seafood.

Branched-Chain Amino Acids (BCAAs) –

Essential nutrients (leucine, isoleucine, and valine) that the body obtains from proteins found in food, especially meat, dairy products, and legumes.

Glutamine –

The most abundant amino acid found naturally in the body; it is produced in the muscles and distributed by the blood to the organs that need it. Athletes supplement with glutamine for enhanced exercise performance.

Nitric oxide (NO) –

A signaling molecule in the body responsible for vasodilation. Athletes supplement with NO to support the flow of blood and oxygen to skeletal muscle.

Beta-hydroxy Beta-methylbutyrate (HMB) –

A metabolite of the essential amino acid leucine. As a dietary supplement, it is reported to enhance gains in strength and lean body mass associated with resistance training.

Other suspicious marketing buzzwords include "doctor recommended" or "physician approved with amazing results." Companies often make these labels appear pharmaceutical and may come as a free trial giveaway where "you just pay the shipping." Likewise, when the findings do not match the conventional wisdom of science or governmental recommendations, or the research is not published in peer-reviewed journals, buyers should become suspicious. Scientifically valid information is typically extremely welcome and exchanged amongst the top scientists and researchers. This raises the question of why supplement "research," if it is indeed valid, is done independent of these prestigious circles.

Mass and Strength Gains

When the training focus is on muscle hypertrophy, many exercisers and body builders ingest compounds to aid in the formation of new muscle mass. The most common ergogenic aids that fall within these categories include **creatine monohydrate**, supplemental protein, **branch chain amino acids (BCAAs)**, **glutamine**, **nitric oxide (NO)**, and **beta-hydroxy beta-methylbutyrate (HMB)**. The proposed mechanism for improving muscle mass is not the same for each of these dietary supplements, so bodybuilders may consume all of them, hoping to gain from potential synergistic effects.

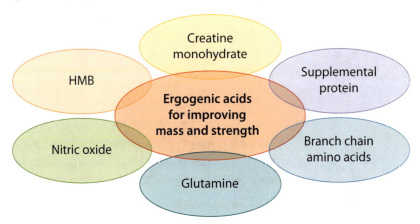

Creatine

A French scientist in the 1800's first identified creatine while he was studying the organic components of meat. Creatine is a naturally occuring amino acid, with the chemical name methyl guanidine-acetic acid, that can be converted into the phosphocreatine and used as an anaerobic source of immediate energy. Only about 5% of creatine in the body is stored outside of the skeletal muscle. Intramuscular stores of creatine are composed of two different forms: 1) free-form creatine, which accounts for approximately 40% of these stores; 2) phosphorylated creatine or creatine phosphate [9]. Creatine is also found in animal muscle and is often consumed through foods, such as meat, poultry, and fish, which provide natural dietary sources. These animal sourced foods contain approximately 4-5 grams of creatine per kilogram (2.2 lbs) of food.

In the human body, the liver, kidneys, and pancreas produce creatine from the non-essential amino acids arginine, glycine, and methionine. Creatine provides the primary immediate energy used for high-force-output exercise and is involved in acid buffering and glycolysis regulation. Due to the body's conservative nature, and the fact that creatine is a relatively heavy molecule, the body does not maintain large stores and only synthesizes about 1 to 2 grams of creatine per day. When the body needs more creatine, instead of relying on the stored quantities, the body prefers to re-phosphorylate the molecule into its active form in response to energy demands. Although fast-twitch fibers contain the greatest creatine concentrations, slow-twitch fibers more efficiently **re-phosphorylate** the molecule due to their aerobic capacity and communicable mitochondrial content. No significant differences exist in creatine storage pattern or needs between males and females.

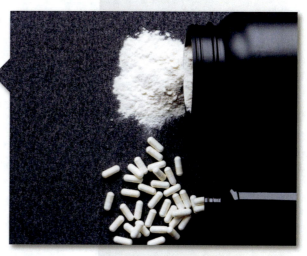

Proposed Mechanisms of How Creatine Enhances Performance

- Increased intramuscular creatine and phosphocreatine content
- Greater resynthesis of phosphocreatine
- Increased metabolic efficiency
- Enhanced adaptations with training

DEFINITIONS

Re-phosphorylate –

The phosphorylation (attachment of a phosphoryl group) of a compound that has been previously dephosphorylated.

Creatine monohydrate is one of the most popular supplements consumed for performance enhancements. Studies have shown that 20-25 g per day for 3-5 days increases intramuscular free creatine stores from 10-30% and phosphocreatine stores from 10-40% [64, 78]. The magnitude the storage gain correlates to initial levels of creatine in the body prior to supplementation. Those who consume plant-based diets or limited quantities of meat and fish display the greatest increases in creatine stores following supplementation. Increased concentrations are associated with improvements in short-burst performances of the highest intensities as well as in the rate of resynthesis during recovery [114, 117, 136]. In addition to improving immediate energy availability, creatine supplementation is also associated with body mass increases. This may be attributed to increases in fat-free mass and/or fluid retention [103]; however, no consensus exists as to the exact causes of the mass gains [103]. Though dietary creatine supplementation has undoubtedly been shown to increase intramuscular creatine stores and creatine phosphate resynthesis rates, no conclusive evidence suggests that creatine supplementation aids in long-duration aerobic-based activities, such as distance running [116]. Interestingly, certain individuals do not respond to creatine supplementation, which further complicates published findings. Creatine has shown efficacy when consumed using a loading phase consisting of 20 to 30g of creatine for five to six days, followed by a maintenance phase of 2 to 5 grams of creatine per day [116]. It has also been used effectively without the loading phase. Longer-term, low doses of 3 grams of creatine per day similarly increased total muscle creatine content [62, 101]. It appears that once a specific amount of creatine is stored, a physiological upper limit is reached, and any excess in the body is excreted in urine as creatinine.

Anecdotal reports of side effects associated with creatine supplementation have included abdominal cramping, muscle cramping, gastrointestinal distress, stiffness, and strains. These case study reports do not

Creatine has no clinically proven side effects, but anecdotal reports include:

- Abdominal and or muscle cramping
- Diarrhea
- Muscle stiffness
- Strains

Exploring Dietary Supplements

represent well-controlled trials, and since short-duration, high-intensity types of activities alone may result in these types of symptoms, no causal relationship between creatine and these side-effects has been established [11, 79, 97]. No long-term, empirical studies on humans have been conducted that prove that excessive amounts of creatine will have adverse effects on the liver, kidneys, or cardiac muscle in healthy individuals. New studies are looking at creatine supplementation as a means to combat other physiological and mental deficits, as prior studies have hinted at possible neuroprotective mechanisms of creatine [2, 3, 26]. It is imperative that individuals taking creatine be educated regarding proper dosages. Additionally, co-ingestion of caffeine with creatine has produced equivocal results in the research, with some studies reporting that caffeine negates creatine's ergogenic benefits, while others conclude that caffeine augments the ergogenic effects [56, 65, 81, 112, 124]. When ingesting creatine for enhancements in body composition via skeletal muscle hypertrophy, one should practice effective timing of the supplementation by consuming creatine before and/or after the training session [32].

> **QUICK INSIGHT**
>
> *Supplement timing seems to be important for optimal benefit. Research indicates that the consumption of supplements can be categorized into 5 specific times. These include pre-exercise (nitrate, caffeine, sodium bicarbonate, creatine, CHO, and protein), during exercise (CHO), post-exercise (creatine, CHO, protein), at meal time (β-alanine, creatine, sodium bicarbonate, nitrate, CHO, and protein), and before sleep (protein). In addition, the dose amounts may or may not be subject to body size. For instance, recommended dosing assignments for supplements such as nitrate and β-alanine are fixed irrespective of body weight, whereas dosing protocols for sodium bicarbonate, caffeine, and creatine supplements are related with corrected body weight (mg/kg of body weight). Additionally, some supplements function acutely, whereas others demonstrate effectiveness over time. The intake duration of creatine and β-alanine requires chronic exposure time < 2 weeks, while caffeine and sodium bicarbonate have acute responses (1-3 hours). Nitrate supplementation is both chronically < 28 days and acutely (2-2.5 h) relevant* [32, 93].

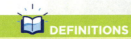

Muscle hypertrophy –
An increase in size of skeletal muscle.

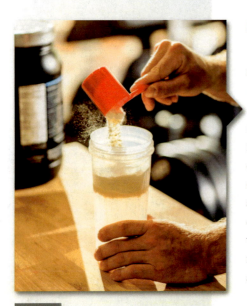

Protein

Protein is the key component in forming and repairing muscle tissue through its integral role in protein synthesis. In muscle tissue, amino acids interact with one another to form structural and contractile proteins that aid in muscles' capacity to produce force. These contractile proteins increase in size and number when appropriate stress is applied, creating a larger cross-sectional area (CSA) of the muscle, contributing to **muscle hypertrophy**. The Recommended Daily Allowance (RDA) for protein and amino acids is 0.8 gram of protein per kilogram of body weight in sedentary populations or 12-15 percent of the total calories consumed. Data collected by the National Health and Nutrition Examination Survey (NHANES) suggests the average American diet easily supplies this amount of protein, and on average, most people exceed their daily needs [96]. Activity levels seem to be the strongest determinant of protein need, with research suggesting individuals who engage in elevated intensities experience higher requirements for proteins than the RDA recommendation [83]. Studies suggest that the highest average recommended intake of protein is 2.0 g/kg of body weight [135]. This level of protein intake only appears beneficial for the recovery needs of competitive power lifters and body builders [92].

The consumption of excessive amounts of protein has not been shown to create additional muscle growth independently [92]. The effect of greater protein synthesis efficiency negates the increased protein recommendations derived from other research. Exercise has been shown to increase the efficiency by which the body utilizes protein, making it unnecessary to increase protein consumption above relative need for the maximal protein synthetic response [123]. Chronic high protein intake (>2 g per kg BW per day for adults) may result in digestive, renal, and vascular abnormalities and should be avoided [135].

Readily available protein is the key to protein synthesis. Inadequate protein availability promotes a **catabolic** environment, negatively affecting muscle size and strength. Research indicates that adding protein to the diet during periods of caloric insufficiency may be enough to attenuate muscle protein breakdown in active individuals [98, 111]. The timing of consumption is also important. Protein consumption prior to and post-exercise, as well as pre-sleep, has demonstrated optimal effect for muscle hypertrophy [85, 120]. Consuming adequate protein following a workout creates the best anabolic environment, promoting the greatest detected rates of protein synthesis when high quality protein (25-40g) is consumed [85].

DEFINITIONS

Catabolic –

A state in which the body is breaking down molecules in metabolism.

Training tenure –

The length of time an individual has actively participated in an activity or specific exercise program.

No evidence confirms the effectiveness of consuming dietary protein supplements over quality protein sources found in beef, fish, poultry, eggs, and milk when amino acid concentrations in the body are comparable. However, digestibility does matter as it relates to timing. Complete proteins derived from animal sources seem to be more effective than plant sources; though most whole food sources take too long to digest and absorb when immediate amino acid pools are depleted. Whey protein has been suggested to be a better form than other sources of protein due to its overall digestibility, absorption rate, and amino acid configuration [61]. In post-exercise trials, increased absorption occurs when whey protein mixes with high glycemic CHOs. This combination likely enhances nutrient uptake via hormonal mechanisms. Post-exercise insulin concentrations, stimulated by CHO intake, speed the movement of amino acids into muscle cells, thus promoting muscle hypertrophy or muscle repair [104]. This mix may be as simple as a glass of milk [43, 55].

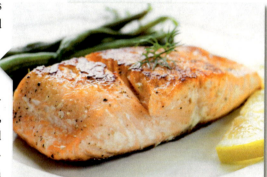

No concrete evidence confirms the effectiveness of consuming dietary protein supplements over quality protein sources found in whole foods.

QUICK INSIGHT

A balance between muscle protein synthesis and catabolism regulates skeletal muscle mass. In healthy humans, synthesis is 4-5x more sensitive to changes in protein consumption and muscle loading. Performing resistance exercise then consuming quality protein augments protein synthesis and (over time) will lead to muscle hypertrophy when all internal factors are appropriate. The magnitude of the exercise-induced increase in muscle protein synthesis is dictated by a variety of nutrition and loading factors including the following: the dose and source of protein, the distribution and timing of protein ingestion, the frequency of resistance training sessions, time under tension, total volume, and the **training tenure** *of the individual. Protein consumption timed around resistance training promotes muscle hypertrophy. Timely ingestion of protein provides indispensable amino acids, which trigger and support an increase in muscle protein synthesis, suppression of muscle protein breakdown, and net positive protein balance. Leucine is the primary amino acid responsible for inducing the rise in protein synthesis. Ingesting proteins with a high leucine content assists protein synthesis signaling. Research indicates that protein quality may have important ramifications for muscle adaptations made with resistance exercise as well as muscle remodeling [43]. Cheese, soybeans, and meat all have high leucine concentrations.*

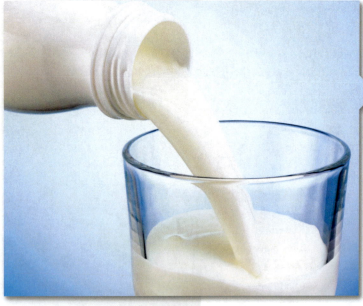

Milk Proteins

Cow's milk contains whey and casein protein. Whey is a high-quality protein with vast nutritional properties. Whey protein positively affects protein synthesis when consumed within an hour of resistance exercise due to the rapid absorption and cell membranes' increased permeability during this period. Whey also contains glutathione, a powerful antioxidant that boosts immune function. This may provide an additional benefit for strength training athletes, who may experience immune-system compromise due to repeated highly intense training bouts [90]. In its pure form, whey protein contains very little fat, cholesterol, or lactose, making it an excellent milk substitute for lactose-intolerant individuals. It is also reputed to suppress appetite, which makes it a popular protein supplement aimed at muscle maintenance and weight loss.

Casein composes a majority of the protein found in milk, which, like whey, is another high-quality protein. However, unlike the quick-digesting whey, casein releases amino acids slowly and is not ideal for rapid protein replacement following physical activity. Glutamine, an anti-catabolic amino acid, exists in high concentrations in casein. Due to the slow digestion rate of casein, it should be consumed before sleep to support recovery [119]. Casein does contain a small amount of lactose or milk sugar that could cause a problem for lactose intolerant individuals.

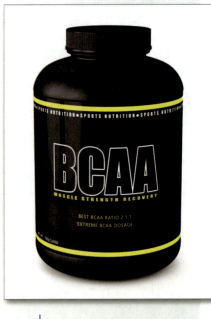

Branched Chain Amino Acids–Subunits of Proteins

In the nutrition section of this text, it was stated that amino acids are the building blocks of proteins and may form numerous subunits. Valine, isoleucine, and leucine make up the branched-chain amino acids (BCAA). BCAAs are essential amino acids that account for one third of the protein in muscle tissue. This significant contribution makes them important for muscle remodeling and the mechanistic functioning of the muscle cells. Importantly, BCAAs have been found not only to have anabolic effects but also anti-protein degradation effects on muscle, as they activate key enzymes for protein synthesis after exercise. These anabolic effects are mediated through key signaling pathways via activation of BCAAs in the recovery period following exercise [13]. BCAAs are easily attained in the diet. A 6oz. serving of chicken, beef, or fish will satisfy the daily need. Supplemental BCAAs are common amongst bodybuilders but do not add additional benefit when adequate quality protein is consumed [73]. BCAAs break down easily to spare other amino acids, and this process decreases the catabolic effect of tissue by sparing other proteins [99]. This function particularly benefits endurance athletes [30]. Trials conducted in both endurance running and cycling populations have found that BCAA supplementation can prevent catabolic effects in human muscle [13]. BCAAs also serve as precursors to other muscle-building amino acids, such as glutamine and **alanine** [37,59]. Glutamine is a non-essential amino acid that aids in muscle recovery and rebuilding and is an important fuel source for the immune system. Strength training depletes the concentrations of glutamine and alanine, but since these amino acids are of the non-essential variety, they are resynthesized within the body from the normal intake of BCAAs.

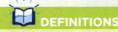

DEFINITIONS

Alanine –

A non-essential amino acid known for increasing immunity and providing energy for the brain, central nervous system, and muscles.

Glutamine

Glutamine is a non-essential, naturally occurring amino acid found within the muscle cell. As stated previously, during prolonged exercise, amino acids begin to be used as a fuel source via **gluconeogenesis** in the liver. Glutamine is released from muscle tissue into the blood stream and is extracted by the liver to form glucose for energy during stressful periods in which glucose levels are depleted.

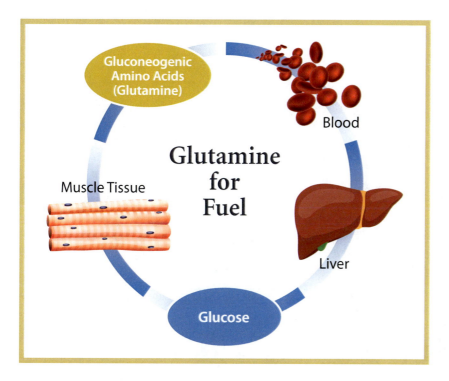

> **DEFINITIONS**
>
> **Gluconeogenesis –**
> *A metabolic pathway that leads to the production of glucose from sources such as pyruvate, lactate, glycerol, and certain amino acids in the liver.*

Supplementing glutamine is thought to increase post-exercise glycogen stores and recovery as well as to reduce the amount of protein degradation associated with stress hormones [33]. Other claims include enhanced protein sparing and increased buffering capacity of lactic acid, consequently increasing the time until fatigue. The premise behind glutamine supplementation is to reduce functional changes in muscle tissue and negative nitrogen metabolism [25, 138]. Though some data has shown that glutamine can counteract some levels of muscle atrophy, studies have not suggested that glutamine supplementation directly effects protein sparing and/or decreases muscle wasting in humans in response to normal exercise. It has shown some promise in helping those in excessive stress states, such as burn victims and immunosuppressed patients but not in normally trained individuals who consume adequate nutrients [38]. Even when glutamine supplementation was combined with a six-week resistance-training program, there was no difference in lean body mass or strength when compared to a placebo group [23].

Although glutamine seems to provide limited benefit when consumed by healthy individuals who meet their protein requirements, it may have merit when mixed with other amino acids or their derivatives. Glutamine supplementation combined with either whey protein or creatine seems to be effective in enhancing muscular strength [82]. This data suggests that a supplement containing glutamine and/or other key amino acids may contribute positively to an improvement in training efficiency through positive effects on protein sparing.

DEFINITIONS

L-arginine –

Essential amino acids obtained from the diet (found in red meat, poultry, fish, dairy); l-arginine changes into Nitric Oxide.

L-arginine

L-arginine (arginine) is a conditional amino acid produced naturally in the body that is purported to have numerous beneficial effects. The normal functions of arginine include:

- **Aiding in protein synthesis**
- **Increasing immune and nervous system function**
- **Increasing oxygen delivery to the heart**
- **Regulating growth hormone (GH) levels**

For athletes and body builders, the claim that arginine plays a role in GH stimulation holds particular interest. Increasing GH levels promotes strength, increases lean body mass, and reduces body fat. Laboratory results display a 100% increase in GH with very large doses of arginine while at rest. However, exercise alone can trigger a 300-500% increase in GH, and when L-arginine is combined with exercise, only a 200% increase occurs in GH compared to resting levels. This indicates a diminished GH response when L-arginine supplementation is combined with exercise [125]. Several studies have also have tested claims of increased strength, ability to breakdown fat, and development of lean mass. No positive findings were reported to support these statements; only equivocal evidence has been presented regarding muscle blood flow when it was examined in conjunction with arginine supplementation [69, 125].

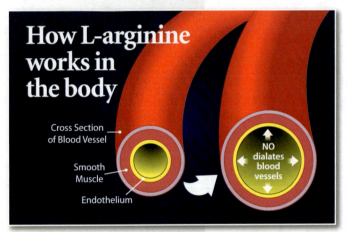

L-arginine serves as a precursor to Nitric Oxide (NO), which functions as a vasodilator, allowing for increased oxygen delivery to the heart muscles and reducing blood pressure. Arginine's positive effect on atherosclerotic properties via its stimulation of NO release seems to improve the exercise abilities of patients displaying coronary blood flow disruptions, such as those associated with coronary artery disease [1, 27, 51]. Ingestion of 6 g of arginine per day for 3 days has been shown to increase exercise tolerance due to increased coronary blood flow in patients with compromised coronary arteries [12]. A caveat here is to remember these are patients in a clinical setting with cardiovascular diseases and that no evidence supports increases in NO production in healthy individuals consuming adequate nutrients [4].

Arginine, a semi-essential amino acid, can be synthesized in sufficient amounts from the average diet. The recommended daily intake of arginine is 3.5 to 5 grams, and the average diet contains approximately 3-6 g of arginine. High amounts of arginine can be found in walnuts, peanuts, watermelon, and even chocolate, as well as in foods high in protein [29]. Arginine seems to cause no significant adverse effects when the source is whole food and the consumption level is under 25 g per day. However, diabetics should not consume high amounts of arginine due to its effect on insulin production [84].

Nitric Oxide

While NO is synthesized from L-arginine in almost all body cells, many dietary supplement manufacturers produce NO in supplemental form. NO is a strong vasodilator and has been shown to assist in the metabolic regulation of glucose, fatty acids, and amino acids. Its effect on smooth muscle promotes arterial dilation, which increases regional blood flow. The endothelium releases NO and related vasodilating substances in response to aerobic training to increase blood flow and oxygen delivery to muscle. Training improves the tissues' ability to secrete NO due to the shear stress of the blood flow against the endothelial walls: signs of a healthy blood vessel [57]. This training adaptation has also been shown to occur in cardiac patients with aerobic training, increasing their blood vessels' health and responsiveness [75, 77, 86]. Cardiac medications dependent upon nitrate, such as nitroglycerin, work on this principle of blood vessel dilation, with the goal of increasing blood flow to the heart's cardiac muscle tissue. Some fitness enthusiasts believe that ingesting supplemental NO will provide greater availability of oxygen and nutrients during the exercise bout by increasing blood flow, which will also enhance recovery immediately following exercise. These individuals will experience an acute "pump" during exercise due to an increased blood flow to active tissues. Currently, however, no conclusive evidence exists that NO increases performance in normal exercise bouts or augments post-exercise recovery.

Beta-hydroxy Beta-Methylbutyrate

HMB is a bioactive metabolite of leucine, the primary amino acid affecting muscle protein synthesis. HMB is thought to be anti-catabolic, decreasing the breakdown of protein resulting from intense exercise [76]. The body naturally produces small amounts of HMB depending on an individual's diet. The normal bodily synthesis is between 0.3-1.0 g per day. The recommended daily dosage for the supplement is a total of 3 g/day separated into three 1g quantities. Again, however, research concerning the benefits of HMB remains inconclusive [95, 130, 132]. A review of literature on the ergogenic effects of HMB showed minimal or zero benefit with supplementation [109, 133]. Some recent studies suggest supplementation may have an advantageous effect on aerobic capacity and may promote increased peak anaerobic power but with no effect on indices of anaerobic adaptations [102]. Other literature contradicts these findings [109, 133]. It has been suggested that creatine and HMB can increase lean body mass and strength and that the effects are additive [68]. Although not definitive, some study results suggest that creatine and HMB act by different mechanisms, which may complement each other. Again, more research is necessary to verify this conclusion.

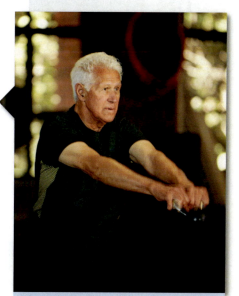

HMB may be useful for sedentary older adults, but the research is not conclusive.

The research on reduced protein breakdown in trained individuals is inconclusive. However, limited data supports a decrease in catabolism with supplementation in recreationally trained and untrained individuals as well as sedentary older adults [42, 102, 129]. Age and sex play a role in HMB concentration within the body. Findings suggested that mean plasma HMB drops significantly with increasing age, with children having the highest mean HMB concentration, followed by young adults and older adults. Females demonstrate lower levels across all age groups. A positive correlation between HMB concentration and appendicular lean mass and handgrip strength has been reported. However, a variety of studies demonstrate inconclusive evidence for any change in body composition or strength with HMB supplementation in trained individuals [42, 102, 129]. To date, there have been no adverse effects associated with HMB. Promising research suggests that a free acid (FA) form of HMB may provide greater bioavailability of the leucine metabolite and increase muscle anabolism [129]. Combinations with supplemental ATP have also shown promising effects on lean body mass and body composition by way of decreases in fat mass, strength, and anaerobic power output, with more studies needed to provide conclusive support [42, 102, 129].

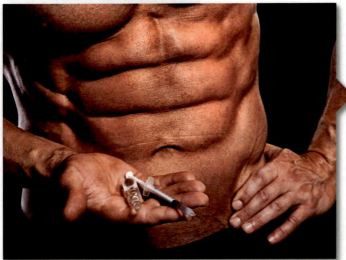

Androgenic-Anabolic Steroids

Androgenic-anabolic steroids (AAS) is an official definition for all male sex steroid hormones, their synthetic derivatives, and their active metabolites. Although AAS drugs have specific therapeutic purposes, they are more commonly used for aesthetically driven, non-therapeutic reasons by a large number of healthy individuals. AAS have reached the public spotlight due to their heavy presence in professional and Olympic sports. Athletes employ AAS to enhance performance and, even more importantly, to increase recovery from high volumes of physical exertion due to training, practice, and competition. The use of AAS is well documented in body building, weightlifting, and both anaerobic and aerobic sports. Following suit, recreational exercisers and fitness "athletes" have increased their AAS consumption. Unfortunately, steroid use in adolescent populations has also elevated significantly, with estimates climbing to millions of student users. Self-reported surveys suggest roughly 1:18 high school students use or have used AAS [58, 67, 91].

> **DEFINITIONS**
>
> **Androgenic-anabolic steroids (AAS) –**
>
> *Synthetically produced variants of the naturally occurring male sex hormones.*

Increases in mass, reductions in body fat, and notable amplifications of strength are all very desirable for athletes, those who emphasize vanity, and individuals who experience issues related to insecurity or low self-confidence. Dissatisfaction with one's body and poor self-esteem associate with the so-called "reverse anorexia syndrome," or body dysmorphia, a condition that sometimes predisposes individuals to use AAS. Early research trials suggested that AAS offered little benefit as an ergogenic aid, likely due to the low doses that were administered. But today, supra-physiologic dose administration shows conclusive evidence of AAS' effectiveness for increasing protein synthesis within cells. Scientific literature has documented that short-term administration can increase strength and bodyweight when used in conjunction with resistance training. Strength gains between 5-20% above starting value and lean mass gains of 2-5 kg have

Risks Associated with AAS Abuse

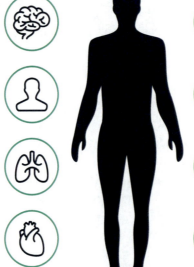

Mind
Extreme aggression, mood swings, anxiety, dizziness, drowsiness, psychotic depression, suicidal thoughts

Face and Hair
Swollen appearance, greasy skin, severe acne, mouth and tongue soreness, male-pattern hair loss, increased growth of face and body hair

Voice
Irreversible deepening of voice

Chest
In males, breathing difficulty, breast development
In females, breast atrophy

Heart
Heart disease, heart attack, stroke, hypertension, increased LDL, drastic reduction in HDL

Abdominal Organs
Nausea, vomiting, bloody stool, liver tumors, liver damage, kidney stones

Blood
Blood clots, high risk of blood poisoning, risk of contracting blood born pathogens

Reproductive System
In males, shrinkage of testes, prostate enlargement with increased risk of cancer, sexual dysfunction, loss of fertility
In females, loss of menstruation and fertility, permanent enlargement of external genitalia

Muscles, Bones, and Connective Tissue
Increased susceptibility to injury, cramps, tremors

been observed with moderate dosages. Increases in red blood cell counts and hemoglobin concentrations have been documented with anabolic steroid use as well. Although limited research exists due to the nature of human testing, it is strongly suggested that AAS yield dramatic improvements in recovery and subsequent performance in response to any event that stresses tissue to the point of micro-trauma. The exposure of AAS-using athletes from the cycling world has shown that AAS have found their place in all sports, regardless of the related metabolic energy system employed.

Anabolic steroid abuse can lead to various adverse effects, and the degree of the side effects seems to be dose related. High-level doses commonly used for body building, increases in strength, and athletic enhancement can result in serious and irreversible organ damage, primarily to the liver, heart, and cardiovascular system as a whole [54, 87]. These adverse effects stem from documented increased rates of hypertension and atherosclerosis, blood clotting, myocardial hypertrophy, decreased ventricular chamber size, jaundice, hepatic neoplasms and carcinoma, tendon damage, and also psychiatric and behavioral disorders [87]. The primary negative effects of short and long-term anabolic steroid abuse that is self-reported by males include the occurrence of **acne vulgaris**, increased body hair, **gynecomastia**, and anger and aggressive behavior [41]. Women and young adolescents may also experience masculinization [24]. The increased presence of blood testosterone inhibits the natural production of testosterone and gonadotrophins. This reduced or halted production of testosterone from gonad glands may persist for months, even after steroid use has stopped [115].

As indicated above, anabolic steroid use can cause harmful cardiovascular alterations, including elevation of blood pressure that can lead to **myocardial hypertrophy** and depression of serum high-density lipoprotein concentration (HDL) [94]. Anabolic steroid-induced arterial hypertension can cause increases in left ventricular hypertrophy and other **cardiomyopathies** [126]. Additionally, blood clotting and **fibrinolysis** are negatively affected, and several case studies of thrombus formation (blood clots that can cut off the blood supply to downstream organs) exist in young strength athletes using AAS. Sudden death is also a serious possibility with steroid abuse [36, 45, 126]. Cases exist of sudden cardiac events leading to death in seemingly healthy subjects. In fatal and non-fatal myocardial infarctions associated with steroid abuse, coronary arteries demonstrated significant atherosclerotic plaque [6].

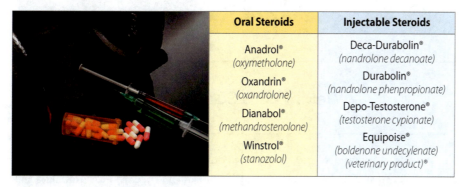

> **DEFINITIONS**
>
> **Acne vulgaris –**
>
> *A common, chronic skin disease involving blockage and/or inflammation of hair follicles and their accompanying sebaceous gland.*
>
> **Gynecomastia –**
>
> *A swelling of the breast tissue in boys or men caused by an imbalance of the hormones estrogen and testosterone.*
>
> **Myocardial hypertrophy –**
>
> *A disease in which the heart muscle becomes abnormally thick, making it harder for the heart to pump blood; often goes undiagnosed because many people have few, if any, symptoms.*
>
> **Cardiomyopathies –**
>
> *A disease of the heart muscle that makes it harder for the heart to pump blood to the rest of the body, which can lead to heart failure.*
>
> **Fibrinolysis –**
>
> *A process that occurs naturally inside the body to break down (fibrin) blood clots that can be induced by medications or occur as a result of stress or disease.*
>
> **Prohormones –**
>
> *An inactive compound that is converted by enzymes into a biologically active hormone.*

Individuals looking for the steroid effect without the direct risk often first turn to **prohormone** or steroid precursor supplements. Prior to a ban in the early 2000's, androstenedione pills were a popular and legal supplement used to increase blood testosterone levels to increase strength, lean body mass, and sexual performance. Research on androstenedione and its related compounds, including androstenediol and 19-norandrostenedione, has not shown evidence that prohormone supplementation works to increase strength or lean body mass in humans [88, 122].

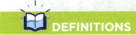

DEFINITIONS

Dehydroepiandrosterone (DHEA) –

A hormone produced by the adrenal glands that, in turn, helps produce other hormones, including testosterone and estrogen. Synthetic versions are available for supplementation and are reported to ward off chronic illness and improve physical performance.

Dehydroepiandrosterone (DHEA) has also been used in attempts to elevate testosterone levels to enhance muscle mass and strength. A weak androgen, DHEA, is purported to provide anti-aging effects, including improved libido, vitality, and immunity levels. Research demonstrates that DHEA supplementation does not increase serum testosterone, nor provide any of the touted effects. In fact, prohormones are often converted to estradiol, increasing male estrogen levels [7, 18].

QUICK INSIGHT

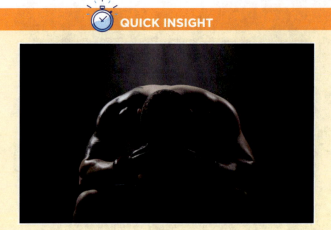

Psychological and personality adjustments are well documented with steroid abuse. AAS can cause aggression, hostility, and anger as well as depression. Mood disturbances are likely to be dose and drug dependent, as well as individually specific, with those already prone to aggression or depression more likely to experience larger responses. Other adverse effects include disturbances within the endocrine and immune systems, liver dysfunction and damage, as well as alterations of the urogenital tract and the skin's sebaceous system. It is likely that additional effects occur but are not documented or are underestimated because scientific studies using humans administer relatively low dosages. The mechanism of action is specific to the particular steroid molecule and its affinity to androgen receptors. Therefore, side effects can differ between each compound and combination of compounds.

Weight Loss Supplements

Weight-loss supplement sales generate well over one billion dollars annually. There are currently more than 50 individual dietary supplements and over 125 commercial formulas sold for weight-loss purposes. Weight-loss supplements appeal to consumers as a "quick fix" solution that obviates the labor of exercise or dieting. Although very few products report any level of effectiveness, few people investigate whether evidence-based efficacy exists beyond the manufacturer's claims. Weight-loss supplements have attained particular popularity due to the social stigma associated with obesity and the difficulties most people experience when attempting to lose weight through diet, exercise, or a combination of both. Weight-loss supplements are classed by their professed biological mechanism. The general categories of dietary weight-loss supplements contain chemicals or compounds that function in one of the five following ways:

- Increase energy expenditure
- Modulate CHO metabolism
- Suppress appetite
- Increase fat oxidation or reduce fat synthesis
- Block dietary fat absorption

Clinical data to support the effectiveness of most weight loss supplements is limited. Chemical agents that affect the sympathetic nervous system seem to be the only type of supplement that has shown any level of effectiveness in research. The two most investigated sympathetic agents are caffeine and ephedra, both commonly consumed in a mixture with other compounds. The sale of ephedra alkaloids was once banned by the FDA due to reports of adverse cardiovascular events associated with ingestion but has since been reapproved as a medicinal agent. It is commonly used in asthma medications and as an expectorant in cold medications. Caffeine is commercially available in many over the counter products and drinks, but is in fact a regulated chemical by many sporting bodies.

> **DEFINITIONS**
>
> **Caffeine –**
> *A central nervous-system stimulant.*

Caffeine

Caffeine occurs naturally and is widely consumed in a variety of forms. It is a common ingredient in coffee, tea, colas, chocolate, energy drinks, and nutritional supplements. Caffeine is also becoming popular as an additive, being combined with liquids, foods, and other ingestible products. It produces multiple physiologic and psychological effects throughout the body, which are likely mediated through actions at centrally located adenosine receptors. Caffeine's stimulant effects are frequently used for both weight loss and performance enhancement.

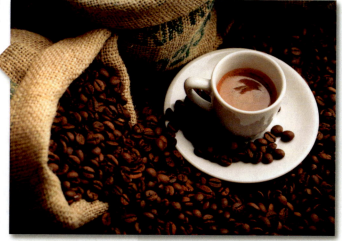

Caffeine ingestion has been shown to improve concentration, reduce fatigue, and enhance alertness. It has been well researched for its potential use as an ergogenic aid, with several studies demonstrating an improvement in exercise performance in submaximal endurance activities [18]. Its potential ergogenic effect in acute, high-intensity exercise is less clear. It is relatively safe and has no known negative performance effects when consumed within recommended dosages. Because of its potential use as an ergogenic aid, its use in sports is regulated by most sanctioning bodies. Pre-competition quantities are regulated and tested in athletes participating in International Olympic Committee (IOC) and National Collegiate Athletic Association (NCAA) sanctioned events [71,105].

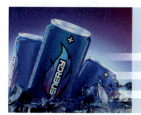

Shown to provide the following ergogenic benefits (250-700mg):
- Improved concentration and alertness
- Reduced fatigue
- Improved performance during sub-maximal endurance activities

Exploring Dietary Supplements

The level of caffeine necessary to produce an ergogenic effect is 250 to 700 mg [71]. By comparison, the drip method used to make a regular cup of coffee yields between 110 to 150 mg of caffeine. Anything above these levels could lead to disqualification from an NCAA or IOC event. It is important to note that not all the caffeine contained within a supplement will be accurately reported on the product. A research investigation revealed that, of more than 100 dietary supplements samples, 26.6% of the products contained more than 120% of the declared, specified content [35]. The daily intake of caffeine above the safe limit of 400 mg may lead to symptoms, such as sweating, nervousness, and an overall feeling of uneasiness, associated with anxiety. These side effects occur due to increases in heart rate, blood pressure, vasoconstriction, increased amounts of fatty acids in the blood, and increased production of gastric acid. Excessive consumption may cause an upset stomach and even vomiting. Due to these possible side effects, caffeine ingestion by children, teens, and pregnant females warrants caution. Additionally, routine caffeine consumption may lead to tolerance or dependence, and abrupt discontinuation produces irritability, mood shifts, headache, drowsiness, or fatigue [80].

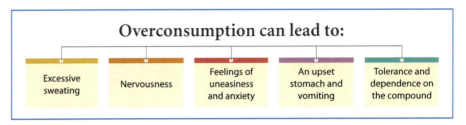

Ephedra - Alkaloids

Ephedra alkaloids are commonly used for weight loss or enhanced athletic performance. They come from a plant containing **sympathomimetic** compounds. Ephedra is sold commercially as a **bronchodilator** but is commonly used as a weight loss supplement among fitness enthusiasts and athletes. Individuals usually couple ephedra supplementation with caffeine or botanical caffeine from **guarana** due to the synergistic effect that results in appetite suppression. This combination often includes aspirin as well, referred to as an "ECA stack" [50]. The mixture is intended to cause stimulation of the sympathetic nervous system with subsequent vasodilation. Ephedra, like caffeine, is often referenced as an appetite suppressant, likely from the stimulant effects associated with its ingestion. Ephedra has successfully shown its efficacy as a fat loss aid due to its ability to increase internal temperature and promote availability of fatty acids for fuel [48]. Meta-analysis of research trials that used ephedra-containing substances showed a consistent weight loss of 0.9 kg per month compared to placebo [113]. Although its use for short-term weight loss seems to be efficacious, serious risks, including cardiac problems and stroke, are associated with its consumption among at risk populations, and long-term effects have not been studied.

Data collected from 50 trials of ephedra supplementation yielded estimates of 2.2 to 3.6-fold increases in the likelihood of psychiatric, autonomic, or gastrointestinal symptoms and heart palpitations [113]. It is estimated that consequential responses, the hazard rate for ephedra-only products, is 250 per 1000 exposures, while those containing ephedra plus additional ingredients is 267 per 1000 [134]. Reports of adverse events associated with the use of this non-prescription supplement raised concerns in the United States regulatory community [10]. A review of FDA-collected data of adverse effects from ephedra between 1997 and 1999 identified episodes of hypertension, arrhythmias, myocardial infarction, stroke, and seizures. Acute

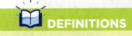

Sympathomimetic –

A drug that mimics the effects of sympathetic activation on the heart and circulation, causing vascular smooth-muscle contraction and vasoconstriction.

Bronchodilator –

A substance that dilates, or opens, the bronchi and bronchioles and decreases resistance in the respiratory airway, thereby increasing airflow to the lungs.

Guarana –

A substance derived from the seeds of a South American tree, which has among the highest caffeine concentration of any plant.

changes in blood pressure and insulin have been shown to subside with cessation [49, 137]. During those three years, at least ten deaths and thirteen permanent disabilities stemmed from these episodes, and 40% of the incidences occurred at the recommended dosages in persons without pre-existing cardiovascular conditions. Despite many studies reporting positive effects of fat loss without harm, the reported risks are sufficient to shift the risk-benefit ratio against ephedra, which should not be used unless prescribed by a physician [5].

Synephrine

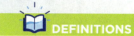

Since 2004, synephrine has been a substitute for ephedra and is marketed in products labeled as "ephedra-free." These supplements are presumed to promote the same desired effects, including energy enhancement, weight loss, and appetite suppression [108]. Citrus aurantium extract (Bitter Orange) contains the botanical **adrenergic** amines **synephrine** and **octopamine**. Synephrine is structurally similar to epinephrine, and, like ephedra, is a sympathomimetic alkaloid. Little evidence suggests products containing bitter orange effectively aid weight loss [63]. Some authorities question the likelihood of bitter orange working as an effective weight-loss supplement at all because synephrine has **lipolytic effects** in human fat cells only at high doses, and octopamine has not been shown to yield lipolytic effects in humans at all [46, 63]. No evidence suggests that bitter orange is any safer than ephedra, and it is a NCAA-banned substance for collegiate athletes due to its stimulatory effects.

> **DEFINITIONS**
>
> **Adrenergic –**
> Relates to nerve cells in which epinephrine or norepinephrine act as neurotransmitters.
>
> **Synephrine –**
> (Also called bitter orange) a plant in which the peel, flower, fruit and fruit juice are used to create medicinal products for treatment of skin infections, weight loss, chronic fatigue syndrome and many GI disorders.
>
> **Octopamine –**
> Biosynthesized sympathomimetic amine used to treat hypotension.
>
> **Lipolytic effects –**
> Causing lipolysis, the breakdown of lipids into glycerol and free fatty acids.

Conjugated Linoleic Acid (CLA)

Conjugated linoleic acid (CLA) is a naturally occurring fatty acid found in meat and dairy products. Early studies on animals suggested that CLA potentially provided numerous positive effects on health including [46]:

- Body fat reduction
- Weight loss maintenance
- Lean muscle mass retention
- Improved control of type 2 diabetes

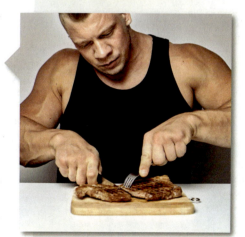

Although previous studies on humans did not lead to consistent results, the popularity of CLA as a weight loss product for overweight people and as a muscle-building substance for athletes remains high today. Proposed anti-obesity mechanisms of CLA include regulation of one or more of the following: adipogenesis, lipid metabolism, inflammation, adipocyte apoptosis, browning of adipose tissue, and energy metabolism [46]. Among the obese and those with certain disease states, some support exists to show that CLA provides a positive effect. Clinical trials have documented statistically significant decreases in body-fat mass among overweight humans, improved weight loss maintenance, and specific regional fat loss among overweight and obese adults [12].

Tea (Catechin Polyphenols)

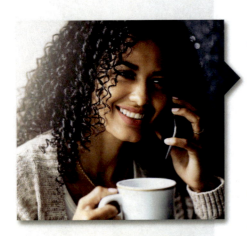

Dietary catechin polyphenols are found in green, black, and oolong tea [139]. Cellular studies suggest that proper doses of these dietary polyphenols can:

- Reduce the viability of adipocytes and proliferation of preadipocytes
- Suppress adipocyte differentiation and triglyceride accumulation
- Stimulate lipolysis and fatty acid β-oxidation
- Reduce inflammation

These polyphenols demonstrate positive effects through a variety of proposed mechanisms, including the modulating of signaling pathways that regulate adipogenesis and lipolysis, as well as antioxidant and anti-inflammatory responses. Recent animal studies strongly support polyphenols as having a pronounced effect on obesity. Studies using obese rats have demonstrated beneficial effects, including lower body weight, fat mass, and triglycerides through enhanced energy expenditure, fat utilization, and modulation of glucose hemostasis [127]. As with many supplements, a limited number of human studies exist, and there are inconsistencies in the anti-obesity impact of dietary polyphenols [89, 127]. This may be due to variation in study duration and design, variation among subjects (age, gender, ethnicity), chemical forms of the dietary polyphenols used, and confounding factors, such as other weight-reducing agents.

There is adequate support that tea polyphenols may present a level of efficacy against inflammatory obesity [14, 16]. However, the actual molecular mechanisms of how tea catechins modulate obesity and regulate fat metabolism, particularly in adipose tissue, remain poorly understood [106]. The current literature has been focused on a few major processes: [52]

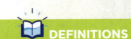

DEFINITIONS

Lipogenesis –

The process of fatty acid and triglyceride synthesis from glucose or other substances, stimulated by a diet high in carbohydrates.

- Inhibiting lipid and CHO digestion, absorption, and intake (reduced calorie intake)
- Promoting metabolism of fat by activating AMP-activated protein kinase to reduce **lipogenesis** and enhance lipolysis
- Decreasing lipid accumulation by inhibiting the differentiation and proliferation of preadipocytes
- Blocking the pathological processes of obesity and comorbidities of obesity by reducing oxidative stress

Larger human trials are needed to validate these mechanisms and the true benefits of tea consumption on obesity.

Weight-Loss Drugs

The prevalence of weight gain in America has caused physicians to turn to pharmacological therapy in order to manage cases of significant obesity. Prescribed weight loss drugs differ from over-the-counter (OTC) supplements in that they require a doctor's prescription to obtain for use. In most cases, a person must have a BMI above 30 (clinically obese), or greater than 27 (clinically overweight=25) and coronary risk factors to qualify for medication. Obesity medications primarily have three goals: weight loss, the maintenance of weight loss, and reductions in cardiovascular and metabolic disease risk. Drug interventions focus specifically on overall weight loss, with changes in body-fat composition and a reduction of health risks as secondary end points.

Several drugs and pharmacologic interventions have been used to fight obesity, including Orlistat, Belviq, Contrave, Saxenda, Phentermine, and Qsymia. The proposed mechanisms for the weight loss agents include decreased appetite, reduced absorption of fat, or increased energy expenditure [107]. Most pharmacotherapies have shown effectiveness at reducing body weight compared to placebo when used in conjunction with a calorie-controlled diet or lifestyle intervention in short-term trials [34, 107].

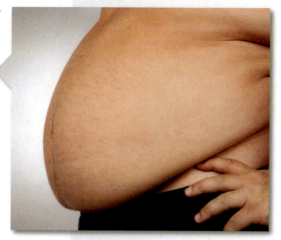

Name	How it works	Side Effects	Considerations
Orlistat (Xenical)	Blocks (30%) fat absorption	Abdominal cramping, passing gas, leaking oily stool, having more bowel movements, and not being able to control bowel movements	Non-prescription OTC is called ALLI (1/2 dosage Xenical) Temporarily makes it harder for your body to absorb vitamins A, D, E, and K
Belviq	Appetite suppression	Headache, dizziness, nausea, fatigue, dry mouth, and constipation Can cause hypoglycemia in diabetics	Women who are pregnant or planning to get pregnant shouldn't take Belviq
Contrave	Combines, naltrexone and bupropion, used to suppress addictive cravings	Nausea, constipation, headache, vomiting, dizziness, insomnia, dry mouth, and diarrhea	May increase blood pressure and heart rate Potential increase of suicide risk
Saxenda	It mimics an intestinal hormone that tells the brain that the stomach is full	Nausea, vomiting, diarrhea, constipation, low blood pressure, and increased appetite	Serious side effects include raised heart rate, pancreatitis, gallbladder disease, kidney problems, and suicidal thoughts
Phentermine	Appetite suppression	High blood pressure or heart palpitations, restlessness, dizziness, tremor, insomnia, shortness of breath, chest pain	Approved for short-term use (a few weeks) only A doctor must review current medical status
Qsymia	Increases satiation, making foods taste less appealing, and burns additional calories	Tingling hands and feet, dizziness, altered sense of taste, insomnia, constipation, and dry mouth	Combines low dose phentermine with the seizure/migraine drug topiramate

Conclusions and Relevance: Among overweight or obese adults, orlistat, lorcaserin, naltrexone-bupropion, phentermine-topiramate, and liraglutide, compared with placebo, were each associated with achieving at least 5% weight loss at 52 weeks. Phentermine-topiramate and liraglutide were associated with the highest odds of achieving at least 5% weight loss [74].

Weight-loss drugs are not a desirable choice as a first intervention to reduce body fat, simply due to the acute side effects of the drugs and the limited information associated with long-term use. For moderately to severely obese individuals, the drugs may be an effective assistive strategy in the journey to reduce body weight, subsequently reducing disease risk. The use of weight-loss medications should be closely monitored by a physician and should only be used in conjunction with a healthy diet and lifestyle. Due to the risk for injury, personal trainers should be familiar with the side effects of the medications their clients use and closely monitor their exercise participation.

PRACTICAL INSIGHT
BARIATRIC SURGERY

Bariatric surgery started in the 1950's and, at that time, was performed only for those at the highest risk for weight-associated mortality. Since that time, it has demonstrated successful achievement of significant and sustainable weight loss in a large number of individuals at varied age ranges. The surgeries have provided a number of benefits across several metabolic disorders, including type 2 diabetes mellitus and hyperlipidemia. It is considered fairly safe despite the high-risk nature of the individuals who undergo these procedures. In studies analyzing post-surgery patient efficacy, many individuals reported a motivation related to physical health and interest in positive health pursuits. Once cleared for exercise, bariatric patients can and should start an exercise program to aid in weight-loss maintenance.

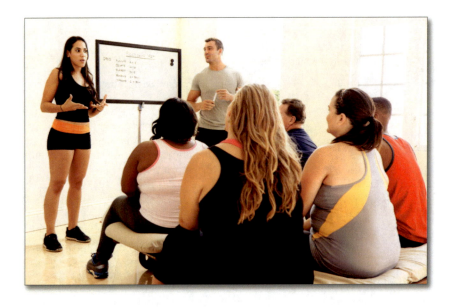

REFERENCES:

1. Adams MR, McCredie R, Jessup W, Robinson J, Sullivan D, and Celermajer DS. Oral L-arginine improves endothelium-dependent dilatation and reduces monocyte adhesion to endothelial cells in young men with coronary artery disease. *Atherosclerosis* 129: 261-269, 1997.

2. Ainsley Dean PJ, Arikan G, Opitz B, and Sterr A. Potential for use of creatine supplementation following mild traumatic brain injury. *Concussion* 2: CNC34, 2017.

3. Allen PJ. Creatine metabolism and psychiatric disorders: Does creatine supplementation have therapeutic value? *Neuroscience & Biobehavioral Reviews* 36: 1442-1462, 2012.

4. Alvares TS, Conte-Junior CA, Silva JT, and Paschoalin VMF. Acute L-Arginine supplementation does not increase nitric oxide production in healthy subjects. *Nutrition & metabolism* 9: 54, 2012.

5. Andraws R, Chawla P, and Brown DL. Cardiovascular effects of ephedra alkaloids: a comprehensive review. *Progress in cardiovascular diseases* 47: 217-225, 2005.

6. Baggish AL, Weiner RB, Kanayama G, Hudson JI, Lu MT, Hoffmann U, and Pope HG. Cardiovascular Toxicity of Illicit Anabolic-Androgenic Steroid Use Clinical Perspective. *Circulation* 135: 1991-2002, 2017.

7. Bahrke MS and Yesalis CE. Abuse of anabolic androgenic steroids and related substances in sport and exercise. *Current opinion in pharmacology* 4: 614-620, 2004.

8. Beelen M, Koopman R, Gijsen AP, Vandereyt H, Kies AK, Kuipers H, Saris WH, and van Loon LJ. Protein coingestion stimulates muscle protein synthesis during resistance-type exercise. *American Journal of Physiology-Endocrinology and Metabolism* 295: E70-E77, 2008.

9. Bemben MG and Lamont HS. Creatine supplementation and exercise performance. *Sports Medicine* 35: 107-125, 2005.

10. Bent S, Tiedt TN, Odden MC, and Shlipak MG. The relative safety of ephedra compared with other herbal products. *Annals of internal medicine* 138: 468-471, 2003.

11. Bizzarini E and De Angelis L. Is the use of oral creatine supplementation safe? *Journal of Sports Medicine and Physical Fitness* 44: 411, 2004.

12. Blankson H, Stakkestad JA, Fagertun H, Thom E, Wadstein J, and Gudmundsen O. Conjugated linoleic acid reduces body fat mass in overweight and obese humans. *The Journal of nutrition* 130: 2943-2948, 2000.

13. Blomstrand E, Eliasson J, Karlsson HK, and Köhnke R. Branched-chain amino acids activate key enzymes in protein synthesis after physical exercise. *The Journal of nutrition* 136: 269S-273S, 2006.

14. Bogdanski P, Suliburska J, Szulinska M, Stepien M, Pupek-Musialik D, and Jablecka A. Green tea extract reduces blood pressure, inflammatory biomarkers, and oxidative stress and improves parameters associated with insulin resistance in obese, hypertensive patients. *Nutrition research* 32: 421-427, 2012.

15. Boirie Y, Dangin M, Gachon P, Vasson M-P, Maubois J-L, and Beaufrère B. Slow and fast dietary proteins differently modulate postprandial protein accretion. *Proceedings of the National Academy of Sciences* 94: 14930-14935, 1997.

16. Bose M, Lambert JD, Ju J, Reuhl KR, Shapses SA, and Yang CS. The major green tea polyphenol,(-)-epigallocatechin-3-gallate, inhibits obesity, metabolic syndrome, and fatty liver disease in high-fat-fed mice. *The Journal of nutrition* 138: 1677-1683, 2008.

17. Brown AC. An overview of herb and dietary supplement efficacy, safety and government regulations in the United States with suggested improvements. Part 1 of 5 series. *Food and Chemical Toxicology* 107: 449-471, 2017.

18. Brown GA, Vukovich MD, Sharp RL, Reifenrath TA, Parsons KA, and King DS. Effect of oral DHEA on serum testosterone and adaptations to resistance training in young men. *Journal of Applied Physiology* 87: 2274-2283, 1999.

19. Burke LM, Collier GR, Davis PG, Fricker PA, Sanigorski AJ, and Hargreaves M. Muscle glycogen storage after prolonged exercise: effect of the frequency of carbohydrate feedings. *The American journal of clinical nutrition* 64: 115-119, 1996.

20. Burke LM, Collier GR, and Hargreaves M. Muscle glycogen storage after prolonged exercise: effect of the glycemic index of carbohydrate feedings. *Journal of applied physiology* (Bethesda, Md : 1985) 75: 1019-1023, 1993.

21. Burke LM, Loon LJCv, and Hawley JA. Postexercise muscle glycogen resynthesis in humans. *Journal of Applied Physiology* 122: 1055-1067, 2017.

22. Burke LM, van Loon LJ, and Hawley JA. Postexercise muscle glycogen resynthesis in humans. *Journal of applied physiology* 122: 1055-1067, 2017.

23. Candow DG, Chilibeck PD, Burke DG, Davison SK, and Smith-Palmer T. Effect of glutamine supplementation combined with resistance training in young adults. *European journal of applied physiology* 86: 142-149, 2001.

24. Casavant MJ, Blake K, Griffith J, Yates A, and Copley LM. Consequences of use of anabolic androgenic steroids. *Pediatric Clinics* 54: 677-690, 2007.

25. Cersosimo E, Williams P, Radosevich P, Hoxworth B, Lacy W, and Abumrad N. Role of glutamine in adaptations in nitrogen metabolism during fasting. *American Journal of Physiology-Endocrinology And Metabolism* 250: E622-E628, 1986.

26. Chamberlain KA. *The role of creatine in promoting oligodendrocyte survival and modulating axonal mitochondria in the CNS*: Georgetown University, 2017.

27. Clarkson P, Adams MR, Powe AJ, Donald AE, McCredie R, Robinson J, McCarthy SN, Keech A, Celermajer DS, and Deanfield JE. Oral L-arginine improves endothelium-dependent dilation in hypercholesterolemic young adults. *The Journal of clinical investigation* 97: 1989-1994, 1996.

28. Clemens R and Pressman P. Nutritional and Dietary Supplements: Code or Concern. In: *Preventive Nutrition: The Comprehensive Guide for Health Professionals*, edited by Bendich A and Deckelbaum RJ. Cham: Springer International Publishing, 2015, p. 47-62.

29. Collins JK, Wu G, Perkins-Veazie P, Spears K, Claypool PL, Baker RA, and Clevidence BA. Watermelon consumption increases plasma arginine concentrations in adults. *Nutrition* 23: 261-266, 2007.

30. Coombes J and McNaughton L. Effects of branched-chain amino acid supplementation on serum creatine kinase and lactate dehydrogenase after prolonged exercise. *Journal of sports medicine and physical fitness* 40: 240, 2000.

31. Coyle EF. Timing and method of increased carbohydrate intake to cope with heavy training, competition and recovery. *Journal of Sports Sciences* 9: 29-52, 1991.

32. Cribb PJ and Hayes A. Effects of supplement-timing and resistance exercise on skeletal muscle hypertrophy. *Medicine & Science in Sports & Exercise* 38: 1918-1925, 2006.

33. Cruzat VF, Krause M, and Newsholme P. Amino acid supplementation and impact on immune function in the context of exercise. *Journal of the International Society of Sports Nutrition* 11: 61, 2014.

34. Curry SA. Obesity epidemic: pharmaceutical weight loss. *RI Med J* 100: 18-20, 2017.

35. da Justa Neves DB and Caldas ED. Determination of caffeine and identification of undeclared substances in dietary supplements and caffeine dietary exposure assessment. *Food and Chemical Toxicology* 105: 194-202, 2017.

36. Darke S, Torok M, and Duflou J. Sudden or unnatural deaths involving anabolic androgenic steroids. *Journal of forensic sciences* 59: 1025-1028, 2014.

37. Darmaun D and Déchelotte P. Role of leucine as a precursor of glutamine alpha-amino nitrogen in vivo in humans. *American Journal of Physiology-Endocrinology And Metabolism* 260: E326-E329, 1991.

38. De-Souza DA and Greene LJ. Intestinal permeability and systemic infections in critically ill patients: effect of glutamine. *Critical care medicine* 33: 1125-1135, 2005.

39. Dickinson A, Blatman J, El-Dash N, and Franco JC. Consumer Usage and Reasons for Using Dietary Supplements: Report of a Series of Surveys. *Journal of the American College of Nutrition* 33: 176-182, 2014.

40. Dickinson A, MacKay D, and Wong A. Consumer attitudes about the role of multivitamins and other dietary supplements: report of a survey. *Nutrition Journal* 14: 66, 2015.

41. Duffy R and Kelly B. Steroids, psychosis and poly-substance abuse. *Irish Journal of Psychological Medicine* 32: 227-230, 2015.

42. Durkalec-Michalski K and Jeszka J. The effect of -hydroxy- -methylbutyrate on aerobic capacity and body composition in trained athletes. *The Journal of Strength & Conditioning Research* 30: 2617-2626, 2016.

43. Elliot TA, Cree MG, Sanford AP, Wolfe RR, and Tipton KD. Milk ingestion stimulates net muscle protein synthesis following resistance exercise. *Medicine & Science in Sports & Exercise* 38: 667-674, 2006.

44. Ferguson-Stegall L, McCleave EL, Ding Z, Doerner PG, 3rd, Wang B, Liao YH, Kammer L, Liu Y, Hwang J, Dessard BM, and Ivy JL. Postexercise carbohydrate-protein supplementation improves subsequent exercise performance and intracellular signaling for protein synthesis. *Journal of strength and conditioning research* 25: 1210-1224, 2011.

45. Frati P, P Busardo F, Cipolloni L, De Dominicis E, and Fineschi V. Anabolic androgenic steroid (AAS) related deaths: autoptic, histopathological and toxicological findings. *Current neuropharmacology* 13: 146-159, 2015.

46. Fugh-Berman A and Myers A. Citrus aurantium, an ingredient of dietary supplements marketed for weight loss: current status of clinical and basic research. *Experimental biology and medicine* 229: 698-704, 2004.

47. Gonzalez JT, Fuchs CJ, Betts JA, and van Loon LJC. Glucose Plus Fructose Ingestion for Post-Exercise Recovery—Greater than the Sum of Its Parts? *Nutrients* 9: 344, 2017.

48. Gutiérrez Hellín J and Del Coso J. Acute p synephrine ingestion increases fat oxidation rate during exercise. *British journal of clinical pharmacology* 82: 362-368, 2016.

49. Haller CA and Benowitz NL. Adverse cardiovascular and central nervous system events associated with dietary supplements containing ephedra alkaloids. *New England journal of medicine* 343: 1833-1838, 2000.

50. Haller CA, Duan M, Benowitz NL, and Jacob Iii P. Concentrations of ephedra alkaloids and caffeine in commercial dietary supplements. *Journal of analytical toxicology* 28: 145-151, 2004.

51. Hambrecht R, Hilbrich L, Erbs S, Gielen S, Fiehn E, Schoene N, and Schuler G. Correction of endothelial dysfunction in chronic heart failure: additional effects of exercise training and oral L-arginine supplementation. *Journal of the American College of Cardiology* 35: 706-713, 2000.

52. Hanhineva K, Törrönen R, Bondia-Pons I, Pekkinen J, Kolehmainen M, Mykkänen H, and Poutanen K. Impact of dietary polyphenols on carbohydrate metabolism. *International journal of molecular sciences* 11: 1365-1402, 2010.

53. Hargreaves M, Hawley JA, and Jeukendrup A. Pre-exercise carbohydrate and fat ingestion: effects on metabolism and performance. *Journal of sports sciences* 22: 31-38, 2004.

54. Hartgens F and Kuipers H. Effects of androgenic-anabolic steroids in athletes. *Sports medicine* 34: 513-554, 2004.

55. Hartman JW, Tang JE, Wilkinson SB, Tarnopolsky MA, Lawrence RL, Fullerton AV, and Phillips SM. Consumption of fat-free fluid milk after resistance exercise promotes greater lean mass accretion than does consumption of soy or carbohydrate in young, novice, male weightlifters. *The American journal of clinical nutrition* 86: 373-381, 2007.

56. Hespel P, Eijnde BOt, and Leemputte MV. Opposite actions of caffeine and creatine on muscle relaxation time in humans. *Journal of Applied Physiology* 92: 513-518, 2002.

57. Higashi Y, Sasaki S, Kurisu S, Yoshimizu A, Sasaki N, Matsuura H, Kajiyama G, and Oshima T. Regular Aerobic Exercise Augments Endothelium-Dependent Vascular Relaxation in Normotensive As Well As Hypertensive Subjects. *Role of Endothelium-Derived Nitric Oxide* 100: 1194-1202, 1999.

58. Hoffman JR, Faigenbaum AD, Ratamess NA, Ross R, Kang J, and Tenenbaum G. Nutritional supplementation and anabolic steroid use in adolescents. *Medicine & science in sports & exercise* 40: 15-24, 2008.

59. Hole M. Relation between glutamine, branched-chain amino acids, and protein metabolism 1. *Nutrition* 18: 130-133, 2002.

60. Howarth KR, Moreau NA, Phillips SM, and Gibala MJ. Coingestion of protein with carbohydrate during recovery from endurance exercise stimulates skeletal muscle protein synthesis in humans. *Journal of applied physiology* (Bethesda, Md : 1985) 106: 1394-1402, 2009.

61. Hulmi JJ, Lockwood CM, and Stout JR. Effect of protein/essential amino acids and resistance training on skeletal muscle hypertrophy: A case for whey protein. *Nutrition & Metabolism* 7: 51, 2010.

62. Hultman E, Soderlund K, Timmons J, Cederblad G, and Greenhaff P. Muscle creatine loading in men. *Journal of applied physiology* 81: 232-237, 1996.

63. Inchiosa MA. Experience (Mostly Negative) with the Use of Sympathomimetic Agents for Weight Loss. *Journal of Obesity* 2011: 764584, 2011.

64. Jagim AR, Oliver JM, Sanchez A, Galvan E, Fluckey J, Riechman S, Greenwood M, Kelly K, Meininger C, Rasmussen C, and Kreider RB. A buffered form of creatine does not promote greater changes in muscle creatine content, body composition, or training adaptations than creatine monohydrate. *Journal of the International Society of Sports Nutrition* 9: 43-43, 2012.

65. Jerônimo DP, Germano MD, Baccin F, Fiorante LB, da Silva Neto LV, de Souza RA, da Silva FF, and Carlos A. Caffeine Potentiates the Ergogenic Effects of Creatine. 2017.

66. Jeukendrup A. A Step Towards Personalized Sports Nutrition: Carbohydrate Intake During Exercise. *Sports Medicine* (Auckland, Nz) 44: 25-33, 2014.

67. Johnston LD, O'Malley PM, Bachman JG, Schulenberg JE, and Miech R. Monitoring the Future national survey results on drug use, 1975-2015: Volume II, college students and adults ages 19-55. 2016.

68. Jówko E, Ostaszewski P, Jank M, Sacharuk J, Zieniewicz A, Wilczak J, and Nissen S. Creatine and -hydroxy- -methylbutyrate (HMB) additively increase lean body mass and muscle strength during a weight-training program. *Nutrition* 17: 558-566, 2001.

69. Kanaley JA. Growth hormone, arginine and exercise. *Current Opinion in Clinical Nutrition & Metabolic Care* 11: 50-54, 2008.

70. Karp JR, Johnston JD, Tecklenburg S, Mickleborough TD, Fly AD, and Stager JM. Chocolate Milk as a Post-Exercise Recovery Aid. *International Journal of Sport Nutrition and Exercise Metabolism* 16: 78-91, 2006.

71. Keisler BD and Armsey TD. Caffeine as an ergogenic aid. *Current sports medicine reports* 5: 215-219, 2006.

72. Kerksick C, Harvey T, Stout J, Campbell B, Wilborn C, Kreider R, Kalman D, Ziegenfuss T, Lopez H, Landis J, Ivy JL, and Antonio J. International Society of Sports Nutrition position stand: Nutrient timing. *Journal of the International Society of Sports Nutrition* 5: 17-17, 2008.

73. Kerksick CM, Rasmussen CJ, Lancaster SL, and Magu B. The effects of protein and amino acid supplementation on performance and training adaptations during ten weeks of resistance training. *Journal of strength and conditioning research* 20: 643, 2006.

74. Khera R, Murad MH, Chandar AK, Dulai PS, Wang Z, Prokop LJ, Loomba R, Camilleri M, and Singh S. Association of pharmacological treatments for obesity with weight loss and adverse events: a systematic review and meta-analysis. *Jama* 315: 2424-2434, 2016.

75. Kingwell BA. Nitric oxide-mediated metabolic regulation during exercise: effects of training in health and cardiovascular disease. *The FASEB journal* 14: 1685-1696, 2000.

76. Knitter A, Panton L, Rathmacher J, Petersen A, and Sharp R. Effects of -hydroxy- -methylbutyrate on muscle damage after a prolonged run. *Journal of Applied Physiology* 89: 1340-1344, 2000.

77. Krause M, Rodrigues-Krause J, O'Hagan C, Medlow P, Davison G, Susta D, Boreham C, Newsholme P, O'Donnell M, and Murphy C. The effects of aerobic exercise training at two different intensities in obesity and type 2 diabetes: implications for oxidative stress, low-grade inflammation and nitric oxide production. *European journal of applied physiology* 114: 251-260, 2014.

78. Kreider RB. Effects of creatine supplementation on performance and training adaptations. *Molecular and cellular biochemistry* 244: 89-94, 2003.

79. Kreider RB, Ferreira M, Wilson M, Grindstaff P, Plisk S, Reinardy J, Cantler E, and Almada A. Effects of creatine supplementation on body composition, strength, and sprint performance. *Medicine and science in sports and exercise* 30: 73-82, 1998.

80. Kutlu FY and Dikec G. Problems Related to Substance and Alcohol Misuse. In: *European Psychiatric/Mental Health Nursing in the 21st Century:* Springer, 2018, p. 395-421.

81. Lee C-L, Lin J-C, and Cheng C-F. Effect of caffeine ingestion after creatine supplementation on intermittent high-intensity sprint performance. *European journal of applied physiology* 111: 1669-1677, 2011.

82. Lehmkuhl M, Malone M, Justice B, Trone G, Pistilli E, Vinci D, Haff EE, Kilgore JL, and Haff GG. The effects of 8 weeks of creatine monohydrate and glutamine supplementation on body composition and performance measures. *Journal of strength and conditioning research* 17: 425-438, 2003.

83. Lemon PWR. Beyond the Zone: Protein Needs of Active Individuals. *Journal of the American College of Nutrition* 19: 513S-521S, 2000.

84. Liu Z and Barrett EJ. Human protein metabolism: its measurement and regulation. *American Journal of Physiology-Endocrinology and Metabolism* 283: E1105-E1112, 2002.

85. Macnaughton LS, Wardle SL, Witard OC, McGlory C, Hamilton DL, Jeromson S, Lawrence CE, Wallis GA, and Tipton KD. The response of muscle protein synthesis following whole body resistance exercise is greater following 40 g than 20 g of ingested whey protein. *Physiological Reports* 4: e12893, 2016.

86. Maiorana A, O'Driscoll G, Cheetham C, Dembo L, Stanton K, Goodman C, Taylor R, and Green D. The effect of combined aerobic and resistance exercise training on vascular function in type 2 diabetes. *Journal of the American College of Cardiology* 38: 860-866, 2001.

87. Maravelias C, Dona A, Stefanidou M, and Spiliopoulou C. Adverse effects of anabolic steroids in athletes: a constant threat. *Toxicology letters* 158: 167-175, 2005.

88. Maughan RJ, King DS, and Lea T. Dietary supplements. *Journal of sports sciences* 22: 95-113, 2004.

89. Meydani M and Hasan ST. Dietary polyphenols and obesity. *Nutrients* 2: 737-751, 2010.

90. Micke P, Beeh K, Schlaak J, and Buhl R. Oral supplementation with whey proteins increases plasma glutathione levels of HIV infected patients. *European journal of clinical investigation* 31: 171-178, 2001.

91. Miech RA, Johnston LD, O'malley PM, Bachman JG, and Schulenberg JE. Monitoring the Future national survey results on drug use, 1975-2015: Volume I, Secondary school students. 2016.

92. Morton RW, Murphy KT, McKellar SR, Schoenfeld BJ, Henselmans M, Helms E, Aragon AA, Devries MC, Banfield L, Krieger JW, and Phillips SM. A systematic review, meta-analysis and meta-regression of the effect of protein supplementation on resistance training-induced gains in muscle mass and strength in healthy adults. *British Journal of Sports Medicine*, 2018.

93. Naderi A, de Oliveira EP, Ziegenfuss TN, and Willems ME. Timing, optimal dose and intake duration of dietary supplements with evidence-based use in sports nutrition. *Journal of exercise nutrition & biochemistry* 20: 1, 2016.

94. Nieminen MS, Rämö M, Viitasalo M, Heikkilä P, Karjalainen J, Mäntysaari M, and Heikkila J. Serious cardiovascular side effects of large doses of anabolic steroids in weight lifters. *European Heart Journal* 17: 1576-1583, 1996.

95. O'Connor D and Crowe M. Effects of [beta]-hydroxy-[beta]-methylbutyrate and creatine monohydrate supplementation on the aerobic and anaerobic capacity of highly trained athletes. *Journal of sports medicine and physical fitness* 43: 64, 2003.

96. on Diet C and Council NR. Dietary Intake and Nutritional Status: Trends and Assessment. 1989.

97. Ostojic SM and Ahmetovic Z. Gastrointestinal Distress After Creatine Supplementation in Athletes: Are Side Effects Dose Dependent? *Research in Sports Medicine* 16: 15-22, 2008.

98. Pasiakos SM, Margolis LM, and Orr JS. Optimized dietary strategies to protect skeletal muscle mass during periods of unavoidable energy deficit. *The FASEB Journal* 29: 1136-1142, 2015.

99. Platell C, Kong SE, McCauley R, and Hall JC. Branched chain amino acids. *Journal of gastroenterology and hepatology* 15: 706-717, 2000.

100. Poole C, Wilborn C, Taylor L, and Kerksick C. The Role of Post-Exercise Nutrient Administration on Muscle Protein Synthesis and Glycogen Synthesis. *Journal of Sports Science & Medicine* 9: 354-363, 2010.

101. Poortmans JR and Francaux M. Long-term oral creatine supplementation does not impair renal function in healthy athletes. *Medicine and science in sports and exercise* 31: 1108-1110, 1999.

102. Portal S, Zadik Z, Rabinowitz J, Pilz-Burstein R, Adler-Portal D, Meckel Y, Cooper DM, Eliakim A, and Nemet D. The effect of HMB supplementation on body composition, fitness, hormonal and inflammatory mediators in elite adolescent volleyball players: a prospective randomized, double-blind, placebo-controlled study. *European journal of applied physiology* 111: 2261-2269, 2011.

103. Powers ME, Arnold BL, Weltman AL, Perrin DH, Mistry D, Kahler DM, Kraemer W, and Volek J. Creatine Supplementation Increases Total Body Water Without Altering Fluid Distribution. *Journal of Athletic Training* 38: 44-50, 2003.

104. Rasmussen BB, Tipton KD, Miller SL, Wolf SE, and Wolfe RR. An oral essential amino acid-carbohydrate supplement enhances muscle protein anabolism after resistance exercise. *Journal of applied physiology* 88: 386-392, 2000.

105. Reardon CL and Factor RM. Considerations in the use of stimulants in sport. *Sports Medicine* 46: 611-617, 2016.

106. Rocha A, Bolin AP, Cardoso CAL, and Otton R. Green tea extract activates AMPK and ameliorates white adipose tissue metabolic dysfunction induced by obesity. *European journal of nutrition* 55: 2231-2244, 2016.

107. Rodríguez JE and Campbell KM. Past, present, and future of pharmacologic therapy in obesity. *Primary Care: Clinics in Office Practice* 43: 61-67, 2016.

108. Rossato LG, Costa VM, Limberger RP, de Lourdes Bastos M, and Remião F. Synephrine: from trace concentrations to massive consumption in weight-loss. *Food and chemical toxicology* 49: 8-16, 2011.

109. Rowlands DS and Thomson JS. Effects of -Hydroxy- -Methylbutyrate Supplementation During Resistance Training on Strength, Body Composition, and Muscle Damage in Trained and Untrained Young Men: A Meta-Analysis. *The Journal of Strength & Conditioning Research* 23: 836-846, 2009.

110. Roy BD. Milk: the new sports drink? A Review. *Journal of the International Society of Sports Nutrition* 5: 15, 2008.

111. Ryan TH, Stephen AM, Robert GM, Juan BOG, Jorge AC-B, Roland ND, Daren KH, Hoffer LJ, Frederick AM, Claudia RM, Douglas P-J, Jayshil JP, Stuart MP, Saúl JR, Menaka Sarav MD, Peter JMW, Jan W, Jill H-R, Craig JM, and Beth T. Summary Points and Consensus Recommendations From the International Protein Summit. *Nutrition in Clinical Practice* 32: 142S-151S, 2017.

112. Santana JO, de França E, Madureira D, Rodrigues B, and Caperuto EC. Combined effect of creatine monohydrate or creatine hydrochloride and caffeine supplementation in runners' performance and body composition. *RBPFEX-Revista Brasileira de Prescrição e Fisiologia do Exercício* 11: 844-854, 2018.

113. Shekelle PG, Hardy ML, Morton SC, and et al. Efficacy and safety of ephedra and ephedrine for weight loss and athletic performance: A meta-analysis. *JAMA* 289: 1537-1545, 2003.

114. Solis MY, Artioli GG, Otaduy MCG, da Costa Leite C, Arruda W, Veiga RR, and Gualano B. Effect of age, diet, and tissue type on PCr response to creatine supplementation. *Journal of Applied Physiology* 123: 407-414, 2017.

115. Strauss RH and Yesalis CE. Anabolic steroids in the athlete. *Annual review of medicine* 42: 449-457, 1991.

116. Terjung RL, Clarkson P, Eichner E, Greenhaff P, Hespel P, Israel R, Kraemer W, Meyer R, Spriet L, and Tarnopolsky M. American College of Sports Medicine roundtable. The physiological and health effects of oral creatine supplementation. *Medicine and Science in Sports and Exercise* 32: 706-717, 2000.

117. Theodorou AS, Paradisis G, Smpokos E, Chatzinikolaou A, Fatouros I, King R, and Cooke CB. The effect of combined supplementation of carbohydrates and creatine on anaerobic performance. *Biology of Sport* 34: 169-175, 2017.

118. Thomas K, Morris P, and Stevenson E. Improved endurance capacity following chocolate milk consumption compared with 2 commercially available sport drinks. *Applied Physiology, Nutrition, and Metabolism* 34: 78-82, 2009.

119. Trommelen J, Kouw IWK, Holwerda AM, Snijders T, Halson SL, Rollo I, Verdijk LB, and Loon LJCv. Pre-sleep dietary protein-derived amino acids are incorporated in myofibrillar protein during post-exercise overnight recovery. *American Journal of Physiology-Endocrinology and Metabolism* 0: ajpendo.00273.02016.

120. Trommelen J and Van Loon LJ. Pre-sleep protein ingestion to improve the skeletal muscle adaptive response to exercise training. *Nutrients* 8: 763, 2016.

121. Upshaw AU, Wong TS, Bandegan A, and Lemon PWR. Cycling Time Trial Performance 4 Hours After Glycogen-Lowering Exercise Is Similarly Enhanced by Recovery Nondairy Chocolate Beverages Versus Chocolate Milk. *International Journal of Sport Nutrition and Exercise Metabolism* 26: 65-70, 2016.

122. Van Gammeren D, Falk D, and Antonio J. Effects of norandrostenedione and norandrostenediol in resistance-trained men. *Nutrition* 18: 734-737.

123. van Loon LJ. Is there a need for protein ingestion during exercise? *Sports Medicine* 44: 105-111, 2014.

124. Vandenberghe K, Gillis N, Leemputte MV, Hecke PV, Vanstapel F, and Hespel P. Caffeine counteracts the ergogenic action of muscle creatine loading. *Journal of Applied Physiology* 80: 452-457, 1996.

125. Vieira Teixeira da Silva D, Adam Conte-Junior C, Margaret Flosi Paschoalin V, and da Silveira Alvares T. Hormonal response to L-arginine supplementation in physically active individuals. *Food & nutrition research* 58: 22569, 2014.

126. Vinereanu D, Florescu N, Sculthorpe N, Tweddel AC, Stephens MR, and Fraser AG. Differentiation between pathologic and physiologic left ventricular hypertrophy by tissue Doppler assessment of long-axis function in patients with hypertrophic cardiomyopathy or systemic hypertension and in athletes. *American Journal of Cardiology* 88: 53-58, 2001.

127. Wang S, Moustaid-Moussa N, Chen L, Mo H, Shastri A, Su R, Bapat P, Kwun I, and Shen C-L. Novel insights of dietary polyphenols and obesity. *The Journal of nutritional biochemistry* 25: 1-18, 2014.

128. Wheatley VM and Spink J. Defining the Public Health Threat of Dietary Supplement Fraud. *Comprehensive Reviews in Food Science and Food Safety* 12: 599-613, 2013.

129. Wilkinson D, Hossain T, Hill D, Phillips B, Crossland H, Williams J, Loughna P, Churchward Venne T, Breen L, and Phillips S. Effects of leucine and its metabolite hydroxy methylbutyrate on human skeletal muscle protein metabolism. *The Journal of physiology* 591: 2911-2923, 2013.

130. Wilkinson DJ, Hossain T, Hill DS, Phillips BE, Crossland H, Williams J, Loughna P, Churchward-Venne TA, Breen L, Phillips SM, Etheridge T, Rathmacher JA, Smith K, Szewczyk NJ, and Atherton PJ. Effects of leucine and its metabolite -hydroxy- -methylbutyrate on human skeletal muscle protein metabolism. *The Journal of Physiology* 591: 2911-2923, 2013.

131. Wilkinson SB, Tarnopolsky MA, MacDonald MJ, MacDonald JR, Armstrong D, and Phillips SM. Consumption of fluid skim milk promotes greater muscle protein accretion after resistance exercise than does consumption of an isonitrogenous and isoenergetic soy-protein beverage1–3. *The American Journal of Clinical Nutrition* 85: 1031-1040, 2007.

132. Wilson GJ, Wilson JM, and Manninen AH. Effects of beta-hydroxy-beta-methylbutyrate (HMB) on exercise performance and body composition across varying levels of age, sex, and training experience: A review. *Nutrition & Metabolism* 5: 1, 2008.

133. Wilson GJ, Wilson JM, and Manninen AH. Effects of beta-hydroxy-beta-methylbutyrate (HMB) on exercise performance and body composition across varying levels of age, sex, and training experience: A review. *Nutrition & Metabolism* 5: 1-1, 2008.

134. Woolf AD, Watson WA, Smolinske S, and Litovitz T. The severity of toxic reactions to ephedra: comparisons to other botanical products and national trends from 1993–2002. *Clinical Toxicology* 43: 347-355, 2005.

135. Wu G. Dietary protein intake and human health. *Food & function* 7: 1251-1265, 2016.

136. Yquel RJ, Arsac LM, Thiaudiere E, Canioni P, and Manier G. Effect of creatine supplementation on phosphocreatine resynthesis, inorganic phosphate accumulation and pH during intermittent maximal exercise. *Journal of Sports Sciences* 20: 427-437, 2002.

137. Zhang M, Schiffers P, Janssen G, Vrolijk M, Vangrieken P, and Haenen GR. The cardiovascular side effects of Ma Huang due to its use in isolation in the Western world. *European Journal of Integrative Medicine*, 2018.

138. Ziegler TR, Young LS, Benfell K, Scheltinga M, Hortos K, Bye R, Morrow FD, Jacobs DO, Smith RJ, and Antin JH. Clinical and metabolic efficacy of glutamine-supplemented parenteral nutrition after bone marrow transplantation: a randomized, double-blind, controlled study. *Annals of internal medicine* 116: 821-828, 1992.

139. Zuo Y, Chen H, and Deng Y. Simultaneous determination of catechins, caffeine and gallic acids in green, Oolong, black and pu-erh teas using HPLC with a photodiode array detector. *Talanta* 57: 307-316, 2002

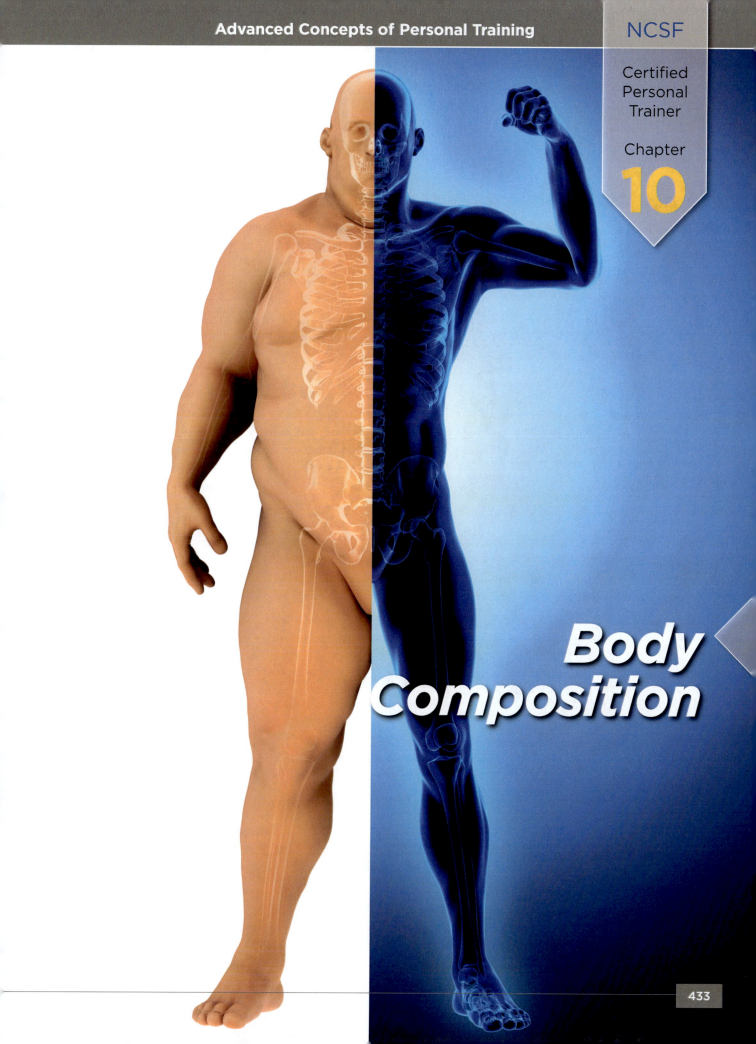

Obesity: A Worldwide Health Issue

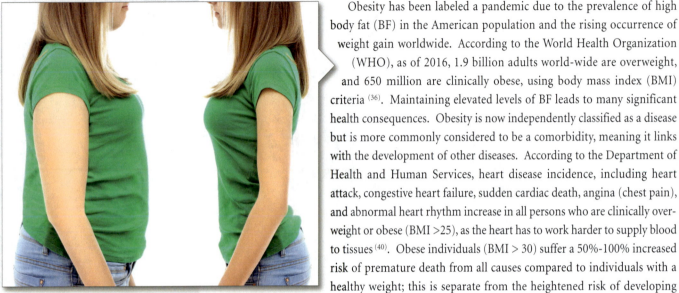

Obesity has been labeled a pandemic due to the prevalence of high body fat (BF) in the American population and the rising occurrence of weight gain worldwide. According to the World Health Organization (WHO), as of 2016, 1.9 billion adults world-wide are overweight, and 650 million are clinically obese, using body mass index (BMI) criteria [36]. Maintaining elevated levels of BF leads to many significant health consequences. Obesity is now independently classified as a disease but is more commonly considered to be a comorbidity, meaning it links with the development of other diseases. According to the Department of Health and Human Services, heart disease incidence, including heart attack, congestive heart failure, sudden cardiac death, angina (chest pain), and abnormal heart rhythm increase in all persons who are clinically overweight or obese (BMI >25), as the heart has to work harder to supply blood to tissues [40]. Obese individuals (BMI > 30) suffer a 50%-100% increased risk of premature death from all causes compared to individuals with a healthy weight; this is separate from the heightened risk of developing some cancers, musculoskeletal diseases such as osteoarthritis and degenerative joints, diabetes,

BODY FAT FACTS

High blood pressure is twice as common in adults who are obese than in those who are at a healthy weight.

Obesity is associated with elevated triglycerides (blood fat) and decreased HDL cholesterol ("good cholesterol").

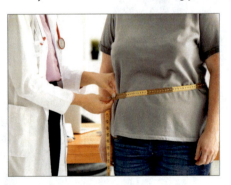

A weight gain of 11 to 18 pounds increases a person's risk of developing type 2 diabetes to twice that of individuals who have not gained weight.

Over 80% of people with diabetes are overweight or obese.

Overweight and obesity are associated with an increased risk for some types of cancer, including endometrial (cancer of the lining of the uterus), colon, gall bladder, prostate, kidney, and postmenopausal breast cancer.

Women gaining more than 20 pounds from age 18 to midlife double their risk of postmenopausal breast cancer, compared to women whose weight remains stable.

Sleep apnea (interrupted breathing while sleeping) is more common in obese persons.

Obesity is associated with a higher prevalence of asthma.

For every 2-pound increase in weight, the risk of developing arthritis increases by 9% to 13%.

Obesity during pregnancy is associated with increased risk of death in both the baby and the mother and increases the risk of maternal high blood pressure by a factor of 10.

In addition to many other complications, women who are obese during pregnancy are more likely to have gestational diabetes and problems with labor and delivery.

Obesity during pregnancy is associated with an increased risk of birth defects, particularly neural tube defects, such spina bifida.

and an increase in stroke risk [6, 15, 27, 28]. Obesity and overweight combine as the second leading cause of preventable deaths in the United States, with estimates of 300,000 associated deaths per year, a correlation which increases proportionately to fat mass gains. Moderate weight gain of even 10-20 lbs. increases the risk of death, particularly among adults aged 30 to 64 years [45]. Interestingly, all the world has gained weight, as there are more people who are obese than underweight in every area of the world, except parts of sub-Saharan Africa and Asia [36].

◆ Body Composition

As one of the five components of health-related fitness, body composition composes an important part of an individual's overall health profile. The body is composed of water, protein, minerals, and fat. Using a two-component model, it represents the ratio of fat mass to fat-free mass (FFM): two important variables when tracking changes in physical fitness. Body composition is most commonly expressed as the percentage of body weight composed of fat. For instance, a 200lb. man with a BF percentage of 20% would maintain 40lbs of fat mass on his body, meaning that 20% of his 200lb weight is fat. In and of itself, fat is not a risk factor for disease; however, the percentage of fat one carries can impact health risk due to metabolic changes associated with the ratio of fat to lean mass. Categorical risks associated with percentage of fat differ by sex and age due to the differing physiological needs that exist between males and females. Males, in general, require less total BF for normal physiological function than do females. This is due to hormonal receptor characteristics that dictate storage patterns, the body's natural developmental purposes related to childbirth, and the endocrine regulations of body functions.

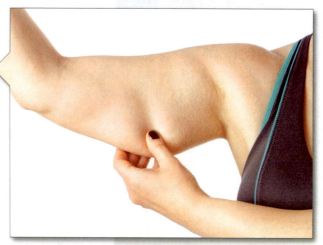

◆ Essential Body Fat Levels

Men and women have minimal values of BF required to facilitate normal, but important, physiological activities. The lowest level of BF for proper homeostasis is referred to as **essential body fat**. Essential levels are necessary for key body functions, such as promoting cell membrane health and formation, temperature regulation and maintaining myelin sheaths for nerve conduction.

The categorical levels of essential BF for males fall between 3% and 5%. When fat levels drop below these values, dysfunctions within the thermoregulatory and metabolic systems occur. Females have the same need as males to support basic human functions, and thus have similar essential values as men; however, females also have an additional BF need of 8-10%, called sex characteristic fat, which increases the total level of essential fat to between 11%-14%. Females require higher levels of essential fat content for hormone balance, as tracked by menstrual cycles. Endocrine disturbances associated with female BF percentages below the essential levels include **oligomenorrhea** and **amenorrhea** [5]. This reduction impairs homogenous estrogen levels and may cause an

Roles of Fat
- Transports and stores vitamins and lipids
- Forms cell membranes
- Provides insulation and protection
- Aids functions of the nervous system
- Assists formation of hormones

DEFINITIONS

Essential body fat –

Necessary fat present in nerve tissues, bone marrow, and organs. Loss of this fat compromises physiological function.

Oligomenorrhea –

A condition of infrequent menstruation, with menstrual periods occurring at intervals greater than 35 days.

Amenorrhea –

The absence of menstruation in a woman of childbearing age.

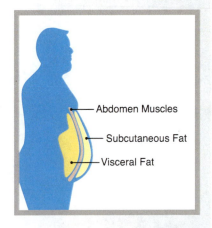

DEFINITIONS

Subcutaneous fat –

A layer of adipose tissue sitting beneath the skin, comprising the largest compartment of fat storage.

Intramuscular fat –

Lipid deposits stored within skeletal muscle fibers.

Visceral fat –

Central body fat stored within the abdominal cavity around internal organs.

TOFI (Thin-outside-fat-inside) –

Term used to describe lean individuals who carry a disproportionate amount of adipose tissue in the abdominal cavity.

Android storage –

Central (or apple shaped) fat pattern associated with increased cardiometabolic disease risk.

Gynoid storage –

A pear-shaped pattern of fat deposition in the lower half of the body, surrounding the hips, buttocks, and thighs.

Hyperinsulinemia –

Excessive insulin circulating in the blood relative to the level of blood glucose.

increased risk of osteoporosis and other problems. While the standards for essential fat reflect population norms, it is important to recognize that genetic differences exist and that some individuals with low levels of BF may be able to function without any adverse effects or events.

◆ Body Fat Distribution

BF levels and distribution patterns of BF are both sexually and genetically dependent. The specific locations of adipose storage are often referred to as fat depots; significant evidence suggests that fat storage distribution may represent a more important determinant than the degree of adiposity for predicting health risks. Where adipose tissue is stored on the body depends on several variables: genetic predisposition, age, sex, physical activity status, stress hormones, and total fat [23, 47, 49, 50].

Categorically, fat storage is referenced by regional distribution or body tissue sectioning. When analyzed using tissue sections, fat storage is categorized by location as either **subcutaneous**, **intramuscular**, or **visceral**. Subcutaneous fat is the most prevalent form of fat stored on the body, representing approximately 50-70% of total BF. It lies between the dermal layer of the skin and muscle fascia. Centrally located fat is stored below the muscle layer, in and around the organs, and is termed **visceral fat**. Noteworthy differences exist between these storage areas. Visceral adipose tissue is associated with chronic system inflammation, numerous cardiovascular pathologies, and several metabolic disorders [4, 48]. Individuals with large stores of visceral fat significantly increase their risk for obesity-related health problems. Subcutaneous fat further associates with an elevated risk in cases of heavily centralized storage [22]. Normal weight individuals may carry excessive visceral fat and elevated cardiometabolic disease risk similar to their obese counterparts. The term **TOFI** (thin-outside-fat-inside) is used to describe those who disproportionately store visceral fat while maintaining normal weight. This relationship between mortality risk and central adiposity is important to note, particularly for individuals approaching their 5th decade; as humans age, fat begins to mobilize from subcutaneous areas to visceral storage locations, making central evaluation of fat important for exercise professionals for predicting risk and weight loss goals.

Fat depots can also be viewed by body region. When an individual's fat is located around the trunk and above the waist, the storage pattern is referred to as **android storage** or android obesity. Commonly, android storage manifests in an apple-shaped physique. **Gynoid storage**, on the other hand, reflects a greater distribution of fat in the body's gluteal-femoral region below the waist and often manifests in a pear-shaped appearance. As stated above, the body region where fat storage prevails the most directly relates to the degree of health risk. Android BF storage is associated with **hyperinsulinemia**, elevated blood lipids, and

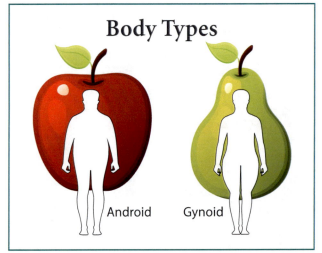

hypertension [4, 12]. On the other hand, gynoid BF storage is associated with reduced health complications; with this said however, once fat levels reach the level of obesity, health risks increase regardless of the storage patterns. The cellular dynamics are explained by each respective area's fat cell characteristics.

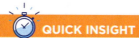

QUICK INSIGHT

CROSS-SEX HORMONE THERAPY

Introduction: Fat distribution is an important secondary sex characteristic which is generally peripheral, or pear-shaped (gynoid), in females and central, or apple-shaped (android), in males. However, during cross-sex hormone therapy (CSHT) total BF increases in male-to-female transitions (MtFs) and decreases in female-to-male transitions (FtMs), approaching BF amounts of the desired sex. However, changes in android or gynoid fat distribution might be a better measure for masculinization and feminization than changes in amount of BF. As yet, the exact effects of CSHT on fat with respect to android and gynoid distribution patterns are unknown [31].

Generally, fat distribution in MtFs changed towards a more female-like fat distribution, with an increase in gynoid fat and a trend towards a decreasing waist to hip ratio. The opposite tended to occur in FtMs, with a decrease in gynoid fat and an increase in android fat and waist-to-hip ratio (WHR).

◆ The Role of Hormones

Several differences exist in fat cells located in various body regions between sexes. It is likely most differences exist due to the body's androgenic hormone concentrations. Each area possesses a differing level of specific hormone sensitivity and responds to endocrine mediation. Estrogen enhances gynoid fat patterning in women while protecting against visceral fat storage, whereas testosterone and other androgens affect android storage characteristics in males. Total fat mass and subcutaneous fat mass each have shown to be inversely associated with a decrease in testosterone [31]. Increased testosterone concentrations during and following puberty are accompanied by decreased abdominal fat storage and increased lean mass in males. Likewise, females experience increases in gynoid storage and total BF mass, with rising estrogen and progesterone levels following the hormonal shifts related to puberty. After a reduction in estrogen production during menopause, females experience an increase in visceral fat deposition.

When the regions are compared by lipolytic behavior (fatty acid release), additional differences become evident [31]. Males have elevated **β-adrenergic receptors** in lower BF cells, which increase the release of free fatty acids from lower body storage in response to catecholamines. Females have higher concentrations of **α2-adrenergic receptors** in lower BF stores, which reduce the lipolytic response to catecholamines [37, 51, 52]. The fat depots above the waist, though more metabolically destructive, are also more metabolic in general. Central fat is easier to lose due to the adrenergic receptor density; thus, during exercise, lipolytic activity is likely to be higher, and central weight loss is favored. This also suggests that lower BF stores in females resist liberating fatty acids into circulation for oxidation and metabolism, making it harder to lose lower BF in females compared to males [51, 52].

DEFINITIONS

β-adrenergic receptors –

Receptors which, upon activation by the catecholamines norepinephrine and epinephrine, promote breakdown and release of triglycerides.

α2-adrenergic receptors –

Receptors involved in the inhibition of fat mobilization from tissue, opposing the effects of activated B-adrenergic receptors.

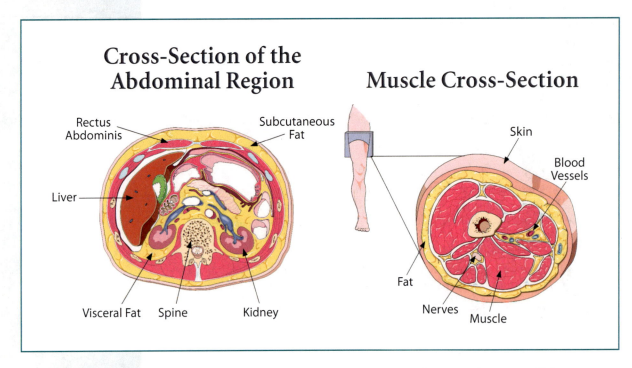

Catecholamine-mediated release in upper BF cells is somewhat comparable between sexes; however, males seem to exhibit a higher free fatty acid release from subcutaneous abdominal fat in response to exercise, although some equivocal data exists. When compared by internal layer distribution, women commonly show higher levels of subcutaneous fat storage, whereas males have shown greater susceptibility to visceral fat storage [51]. This information suggests that both males and females can change their abdominal storage with appropriate exercise and diet, but females will experience greater difficulty in reducing fat storage around the hips, buttocks, and thighs due to a natural resistance to fat mobility compared to males [8, 37, 46]. Therefore, android fat patterning is altered more easily with exercise and dietary strategies than gluteal-femoral fat stores.

Stature-Weight Indices

Fat mass measurement, analysis of fat distribution, and risk for non-communicable diseases can be determined using several indirect methods. Since health risk represents the greatest consequence of obesity and related disorders, identifying total fat mass and regional distribution is important in risk prediction and disease intervention. The methods of assessing BF by mass and distribution range from simple to fairly complex techniques. In some cases, the assessment techniques use only anthropometric measures to provide predictions.

Indirect Methods of Assessing BF → Height-Weight Tables | BMI | Waist Circumference | Waist-to-Hip Ratio

Height Weight Tables

Height-weight tables (HWT) were originally designed to predict mortality rates associated with a person's size in order to determine insurance premiums. If a person was short and heavy, predicted risk was elevated and so were the individual's insurance costs. Data collected in the 1940's and 50's was used to identify the most desirable weight for each height related to the lowest mortality rates. The 1959 tables established weight ranges for different frame sizes to better identify the weight composition with respect to bone thickness. In more recent years, HWT has established a criterion to determine frame size using elbow breadth. The frame size measures were determined from the first two National Health and Nutrition Examination Studies and tabled by sex for reference. The United States Department of Agriculture also publishes height-weight ranges as part of the Dietary Guidelines for Americans, but the table fails to identify frame size and does not separate gender in the weight ranges. HWT have significant deficiencies for health guidance because they incorporate far too many assumptions. Likewise, valuable data that cannot be collected using a scale and a ruler significantly impacts exercise prescription and behavior modification. For these reasons, these tables have been replaced with the BMI in clinical environments.

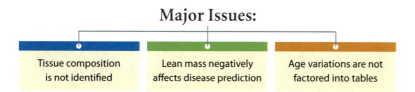

Body Mass Index (BMI)

BMI computes body size into a single measure and represents a more practical utilization of one's anthropometrics to predict risk for disease, health complications, and all risk of mortality. It uses a ratio of body weight compared to body height: $weight(kg)/height(m)^2$. Similar limitations to the HWT exist since body size is the only factor accounted for: although body size is an important predictor of mortality, it does not incorporate body composition measurement. Collision sport athletes and bodybuilders often maintain leaner measures of BF, but are categorized as high risk when using the BMI values due to the total mass. Higher amounts of muscle mass can skew results because excess weight is always considered a negative for stature weight indexing. Among Division I American football players, BMI overestimated the prevalence of overweight and obesity in 50.6% of the cases measured. On the contrary, someone with very little lean mass may present as low risk, when this individual actually has an unhealthy body composition. This is referred to as normal weight obesity or "skinny fat" among layman. Normal weight obesity is expected in 8-10% of the population. Certain height ranges also decrease the accuracy of prediction. Individuals measured at less than five feet in height often have higher BMI scores than their mass represents.

BMI may have some downsides, but it certainly holds merit for health assessment purposes. BMI is more accurate at predicting risk than weight alone and is relatively easy to calculate, even for the nonprofessional. Males and females use the same table, so predictive values are somewhat universal, and it takes very little time to calculate and track changes. Ideal values (lowest mortality) for BMI are 22 kg/m^2 for males and 21 kg/m^2 for females [43]. Values between 18.5 and 24.9 kg/m^2 are considered to be within the healthy weight range. Once BMI becomes less

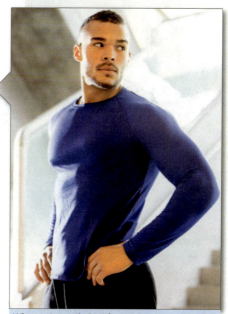

When using only BMI for assessment a large muscular athlete could be confusingly identified as "obese" – making additional direct composition testing preferred to obtain useful data.

than 18 and greater than 25 kg/m^2, health risks increase, with values over 27 kg/m^2 reflecting the greatest number of health-related complications. A BMI of less than 18.5 kg/m^2 is defined as underweight; 25-29.9 kg/m^2 is considered the overweight range, and a measure beyond 30 kg/m^2 indicates obesity. It is important to note that underweight individuals also have increased risk of health problems, and values less than 17 are often used as part of the criteria to evaluate anorexia nervosa.

Classification of Weight by Body Mass Index (BMI), Waist Circumference, and Associated Disease Risks

Category	BMI (kg/m^2)	DISEASE RISK RELATIVE TO NORMAL WEIGHT AND WAIST CIRCUMFERENCE	
		Men <102 cm (40 in.) Women <88 cm (35 in.)	Men >102 cm (40 in.) Women >88 cm (35 in.)
Underweight	< 18.5	---	---
Normal	18.5 - 24.9	---	---
Overweight	25.0 - 29.9	Increased	High
Obese Class I	30.0 - 34.9	High	Very high
Obese Class II	35.0 - 39.9	Very high	Very high
Obese Class III	> 40.0	Extremely high	Extremely high

Relationship Between Body Mass Index and Percentage Body Fat

	Adult Males					Adult Females			
Age	Increased Risk BMI < 18.5	Healthy BMI 18.5 - 24.9	Increased Risk BMI 25 - 29.9	High Risk BMI 30+	Age	Increased Risk BMI < 18.5	Healthy BMI 18.5 - 24.9	Increased Risk BMI 25 - 29.9	High Risk BMI 30+
20 - 39	< 7.9%	8 - 19.9%	20 - 24.9%	> 25%	20 - 39	< 20.9%	21 - 28.9%	29 - 31.9%	> 32%
40 - 59	< 10.9%	11 - 21.9%	22 - 27.9%	> 28%	40 - 59	< 22.9%	23 - 29.9%	30 - 32.9%	> 33%
60 - 79	< 12.9%	13 - 24.9%	25 - 29.9%	> 30%	60 - 79	< 23.9%	24 - 31.9%	32 - 34.9%	> 35%

> **QUICK INSIGHT**
>
> *BMI is the reference value used when population segments are defined by percentages of people who are overweight or obese. In the United States, approximately 40% of the adult population has a BMI greater or equal to 30 kg/m² [19]. Importantly however, even though BMI strongly predicts risk within a population, it may over or underestimate risk for a given individual. Although stature-weight assessments offer a degree of usefulness for predicting disease risk, circumference measures add value to the prediction by measuring regional distribution. Abdominal girth, waist:hip ratio (WHR), waist:height ratio (WHtR), and saggital abdominal diameter provide data regarding central adiposity and also contribute to the prediction of body composition. Combining the height-weight data with circumference values can better identify risk and demonstrate any predictive flaws in the data acquired when either measure is used independently.*

BMI Formulas

$$BMI = \text{Weight in kilograms} \div \text{Height in meters}^2$$
$$BMI = (\text{Weight in pounds} \div \text{Height in inches}^2) \times 703$$

Waist Circumference

Waist circumference has gained strong support for predicting obesity-related risk for disease. The correlation between abdominal adiposity and disease outcomes has made this simple assessment measure quite valuable for identifying need for weight management intervention strategies [3]. For certain populations, including Caucasian males, waist circumferences provide even more utility when employed in conjunction with BMI to predict disease risk because BMI indicates behavior-related fat storage [16]. Visceral fat associates with lower levels of physical activity and behavior traits as opposed to genetic predisposition. Likewise, the measure assists BMI interpretation because large abdominal circumference does not relate to muscle mass hypertrophy; therefore, a distinction can be made between fat mass and muscle mass [35]. Waist-circumference values above 102 cm (40 inches) for males and 88 cm (34.5 inches) for females are associated with a high risk for cardiovascular and metabolic disease. Waist circumference can also be used to estimate body composition, as it directly measures a fat depot that can predict total BF storage.

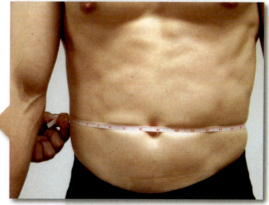

Abdominal circumference measures are taken from the side of the body with the subject standing in an upright posture with feet located under the hips. The reference site for abdominal circumference measurement is the horizontal line of the umbilicus (belly button). The assessment should be performed against bare skin with the tape lying taut and parallel to the floor. The measuring tape should be enough to prevent folds but should not cause cutaneous indentations.

Waist-to-Hip Ratio

Waist-to-Hip ratio (WHR), another circumference measure, also predicts risk for negative health consequences. The predictive value of WHR alone works better than BMI when predicting mortality and cardiovascular disease risk [10,33,41]. However, it may be less effective than waist circumference independently, as the additional variables involved reduce the assessment's ability to specifically evaluate the central adiposity level [10]. This occurs because the measurement is expressed as a ratio comparing hip girth with waist girth. If a person maintains high amounts of subcutaneous fat below the waist, the potential of waist mass to predict true risk is reduced. Pre-pubescent children cannot be accurately assessed using WHR due to the fact that hormonally mediated storage has not yet been established.

WHR is measured in similar fashion as abdominal assessments, and like the waist circumference measurement, no single, universal standard for the measurement sites exists [2]. The WHO recommends measuring the waist circumference midway between the lower rib margin and the iliac crest of the pelvis. For the hip measurement, the suggestion is to use the widest point over the greater trochanter. The Anthropometric Standardization Reference Manual recommends using the torso's narrowest part for the waist measurement and the apex or largest part of the buttocks. Since the norms for WHR were formed from the Anthropometric Standardization Reference Manual, it makes logical sense to use their reference sites. The ratio is calculated by dividing the waist measurement by the hip measurement. The closer the value is to 1.00, the greater the indication of central adiposity and the greater determination for risk. Although ranges exist which are age and sex-specific, values above 0.9 for men and 0.8 for women seem to present the greatest increase in risk for negative health outcomes.

Waist-to-Hip Ratio Norms for Men and Women

Risk for Heart Disease	Low		Moderate		High		Very High	
Age (y)	Men	Women	Men	Women	Men	Women	Men	Women
20 - 29	<0.83	<0.71	0.83 - 0.88	0.71 - 0.77	0.89 - 0.94	0.78 - 0.82	>0.94	>0.82
30 - 39	<0.84	<0.72	0.84 - 0.91	0.72 - 0.78	0.92 - 0.96	0.79 - 0.84	>0.96	>0.84
40 - 49	<0.88	<0.73	0.88 - 0.95	0.73 - 0.79	0.96 - 1.00	0.80 - 0.87	>1.00	>0.87
50 - 59	<0.90	<0.74	0.90 - 0.96	0.74 - 0.81	0.97 - 1.02	0.82 - 0.88	>1.02	>0.88
60 - 69	<0.91	<0.76	0.91 - 0.98	0.76 - 0.83	0.99 - 1.03	0.84 - 0.90	>1.03	>0.90

Body Composition Assessment

Assessment of body composition provides constituent-specific data about fat mass and FFM within the body. The advantage of body composition over stature-weight and circumference references is that it compartmentalizes the tissue. Since FFM contributes positively to health, whereas excess fat does not, it is important to distinguish between the two. Excess fat mass becomes detrimental when stored in abundance and identifying the amount and proportion of fat mass becomes integral for determining strategies for weight management. Identifying the actual amount of fat on the body can help to determine health risk and relative significance based on total and regional storage.

Body composition assessment allows exercise professionals to track the specific changes in the tissue when weight loss or gain occurs. When combined with indicators of fat patterning (i.e. circumference values), disease risk predictability enhances dramatically. Total BF and regional distribution can be evaluated, and the data can be used to provide direction to the formulation of the exercise prescription and need for dietary changes. Body composition assessments use different measures to ascertain the body's density. This is so because body density is used in regression equations to predict BF. Tests to measure or predict body density generally fall into two categories: clinical assessments and field tests. Clinical assessments require precision instruments and controlled settings to estimate body fat. Common clinical tests include dual x-ray absorptiometry (DXA), hydrostatic weighing, air displacement plethysmography, and multi-frequency bioelectrical impedance. Field tests require less sophisticated equipment and are generally easier to implement. Common field tests include girth measurements, skinfold assessment, bioelectrical impedance, and near infrared interactance.

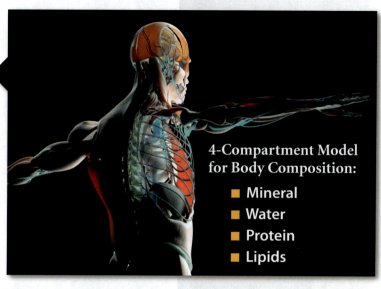

4-Compartment Model for Body Composition:
- Mineral
- Water
- Protein
- Lipids

PRACTICAL INSIGHT

Body composition is often perceived as a psychologically uncomfortable assessment and being self-conscious of one's body when being evaluated by an exercise professional is very common. With roughly 70% of America overweight/obese, body image becomes a relevant consideration in fitness training and during assessments. People are usually not comfortable participating in assessment techniques that require some level of clothing removal. Likewise, very few people want someone to grab and highlight the amount of fat on their bodies. This fact becomes even more evident when the amount of fat carried is significant.

The assessment an exercise professional uses should reflect the client's size, age, and fitness level and consider the psychological stress potentially caused. Using skinfold measurements on an obese client makes very little sense because skinfold measurement accuracy is inversely proportional to the person's body fat level. In most cases, this invasive measure should not be used for obese individuals since data obtained is unlikely to be accurate. If a person is visibly overweight, circumference measures are recommended, especially as this method allows for regional tracking, a more important focus for this population.

Practical Considerations: In some cases, it does not make sense to measure fat at all. For some people, the stress of the experience is not worth the data. A visibly obese person is obviously overfat and both the exercise professional and client are keen to this fact. Why subject them to an assessment that will indicate that an exercise prescription aimed at safe weight loss is recommended? For overweight people, circumference measures, gauging clothing "fit," and tracking weight loss can be the best assessments to identify BF changes.

Clinical Assessments

Clinical assessments are most often completed in laboratories and are not commonly used in traditional exercise settings due to the size and cost of the equipment, the technical expertise required, and time and effort involved. A brief review of each is warranted, however, as these methods are often employed as the criterion reference value by which standard estimation error (SEE) is determined for field tests.

Dual X-ray Absorptiometry

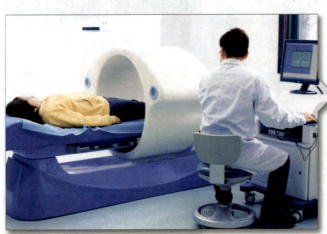

Dual X-ray Absorptiometry (DXA) is commonly used in research settings to assess multiple tissue components, including bone mineral, fat, and lean tissue. X-ray attenuation depends upon tissue characteristics, including thickness, density, and chemical composition. The body tissues weaken the high and low X-ray energies at different magnitudes based on density and chemical composition: these magnitudes are called attenuation ratios. Based on the data provided using these ratios, tissue composition can be identified. DXA is commonly referred to as the 'gold standard' of body composition analysis, with some researchers suggesting it is more accurate than hydrostatic weighing and very close to multi-component estimates. This makes it a popular method for clinical research and comparative measures [26, 38].

Hydrostatic Weighing

Hydrostatic, or underwater, weighing uses Archimedes principle of buoyancy to calculate body density. Fat mass is less dense than water; so, when fat is placed in water, it floats. Based on this concept, the fatter an individual, the greater the propensity to float, and therefore, the less he or she will weigh underwater. The assessment is performed by having the test subject exhale maximally before being submerged and weighed on an underwater scale. This process in and of itself is uncomfortable when done thoroughly and correctly, which is why this assessment is not recommended for children, those with claustrophobia, the elderly, and sick individuals, with some in these groups unable to complete the test [9]. Adjustments for water density are made based on the water temperature and residual volume (remaining volume of air in the respiratory system) in the body. The weight lost under water is proportional to the volume of water displaced by the body volume. Calculations determine body density, which is converted to BF percentage using a population-specific conversion formula. When performed properly, this method of BF assessment is considered quite accurate: second only to DXA when performed among appropriate populations.

Air Displacement Plethysmography

Air displacement plethysmography (ADP), as the name implies, uses air displacement instead of water to estimate volume. This method requires minimal time, client compliance, and technical skill. The BOD POD is the most recognized commercial plethysmography chamber. It works via a pressure-volume inverse relationship in accordance with Boyle's law, which is used to calculate total volume displacement. The predictability level of body density using the BOD POD correlates with hydrostatic weighing but has been shown to underestimate percent BF compared to multi-component methods and DXA [20]. When intra-individual variability was assessed between trials using the BOD POD, researchers suggested to perform at least two trials with measured Thoracic Gas Volume (TGV), with the average of the values reported. As with skinfold assessments, densiometric-based assessments require subjects to be clothed in tight fitting swimsuits to ensure the most accurate measurement; of course, this concern is relevant for those obese and overweight individuals who are reluctant to wear a bathing suit for an assessment [13]. Body temperature, room temperature, and body moisture have also been shown to cause an underestimated measurement when body density is being evaluated in the BOD POD [11, 14].

Field Tests

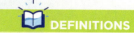

DEFINITIONS

Field tests –

A practical assessment used to predict outcomes of gold standard criterion measures, usually through cheaper, more portable means.

Circumference measurement –

Girth measures at standard anatomical sites around the body, often denoted by distances between bony landmarks.

Exercise professionals are far more likely to utilize **field tests** due to their ease of implementation in practical environments. Field tests vary by assumption and principle, and therefore, have specific procedures associated with their employment. The measurement techniques and equipment needs for each assessment method are subject to the evaluation protocol. The decision to use an assessment should be based on a technician's capabilities, the benefits the data will provide, and the population segment being assessed.

Circumference Measurements

Circumference estimation of body composition employs measurements of select locations to predict BF. The testing methods are easy to perform and require minimal equipment. The assessment device is often no more than a common linen or plastic measuring tape. Commonly referred to as "girth measurements," these techniques simply require the **circumference measurement(s)** of specific anatomical sites. The measured values are then charted, graphed, or equated based on the particular protocol being used. Depending upon the estimation model, girth measurements can predict body composition and help determine regional fat storage. The estimations are based on the positively associated, linear relationship between the circumference values of cited anatomical areas and the amount of BF a person carries.

The ease and non-invasive nature of the procedure for girth measurements make them very practical assessment methods for fitness professionals. When performed correctly with the appropriate prediction equation and comparative data, circumference estimations of BF can have a SEE of ~4% of clinical assessments obtained in a laboratory [53]. Due to the measurements' very essence, they can provide useful information about fat distribution patterns as well as BF changes during weight loss. Clients can see and understand the quantifiable differences found between measurements, which often serve to motivate, even when body weight has not significantly changed. Additionally, the methods have far more useful for measuring and predicting the BF of obese individuals, where calipers and other methods have a less accurate predictive value [44]. One downside is that body fatness in muscular individuals may be over-predicted. When

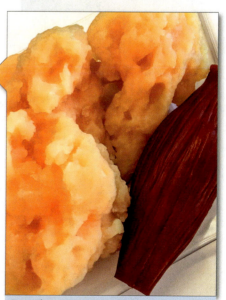

Circumference measurements can accurately reflect changes in body composition because equal quantities (by weight) of body fat and skeletal muscle take up different amounts of space within the body, as muscle is more dense and takes up less space than fat.

performing girth measurements in order to track progress of weight and fat loss, the tester must inform the client to wear the same clothes for each measurement in order to improve test reliability. See the Screening and Evaluation Chapter for a review of the full protocol.

Skinfold Measurements

Subcutaneous fat is the lipid mass that lies between the skin and the muscle tissue. Technicians can "pinch" select sites using the thumb and index finger to create a fold of skin and fat with equal parallel sides, separating the subcutaneous fat from the lean muscle tissue: referred to as a skinfold. Skinfolds taken at specific locations can be measured and summed to predict body density specific to a particular population. Large inter-individual differences exist in the patterning of subcutaneous adipose tissue both within and between sexes [17]. Low intra and inter-rater reliability have been observed in skinfold measurements which may be mitigated by repeated rehearsal and clear, consistent instructions [34]. However, skinfolds remain useful because a linear relationship exists among homogeneous groups. This relationship decreases over a wide range, which suggests that the equations used to convert skinfold into body density must reflect the population being measured [39]. Currently, more than 100 population-specific regression equations are used to predict body density and fatness from skinfold measurements.

Generalized Body Composition Equations

Males

7-Site Formula *(chest, midaxillary, triceps, subscapular, abdomen, suprailiac, thigh)*

Body density
$1.11200000 - 0.00043499 \text{ (sum of seven skinfolds)} + 0.00000055 \text{ (sum of seven skinfolds)}^2 - 0.00028826 \text{ (age)}$

4-Site Formula *(abdomen, suprailiac, tricep, thigh)*

Percent body fat
$0.29288 \text{ (sum of four skinfolds)} - 0.0005 \text{ (sum of four skinfolds)}^2 + 0.15845 \text{ (age)} - 5.76377$

3-Site Formula *(chest, abdomen, thigh)*

Body density
$1.1093800 - 0.0008267 \text{ (sum of three skinfolds)} + 0.0000016 \text{ (sum of three skinfolds)}^2 - 0.0002574 \text{ (age)}$

Body density *(chest, triceps, subscapular)*
$1.1125025 - 0.0013125 \text{ (sum of three skinfolds)} + 0.0000055 \text{ (sum of three skinfolds)}^2 - 0.0002440 \text{ (age)}$

Percentage body fat *(abdomen, suprailiac, triceps)*
$0.39287 \text{ (sum of three skinfolds)} - 0.00105 \text{ (sum of three skinfolds)}^2 + 0.15772 \text{ (age)} - 5.18845$

Females

7-Site Formula *(chest, midaxillary, triceps, subscapular, abdomen, suprailiac, thigh)*

Body density
$1.0970 - 0.00046971 \text{ (sum of seven skinfolds)} + 0.00000056 \text{ (sum of seven skinfolds)}^2 - 0.00012828 \text{ (age)}$

4-Site Formula *(abdomen, suprailiac, tricep, thigh)*

Percent body fat
$0.29669 \text{ (sum of four skinfolds)} - 0.00043 \text{ (sum of four skinfolds)}^2 + 0.02963 \text{ (age)} - 1.4072$

3-Site Formula *(triceps, abdomen, suprailiac)*

Percentage body fat *(triceps, abdomen, suprailiac)*
$0.41563 \text{ (sum of three skinfolds)} - 0.00112 \text{ (sum of three skinfolds)}^2 + 0.03661 \text{ (age)} + 4.03653$

Body density
$1.0994921 - 0.0009929 \text{ (sum of three skinfolds)} + 0.0000023 \text{ (sum of three skinfolds)}^2 + 0.0001392$

The sum of skinfolds offers a fairly reliable prediction of fat mass when the regression model is appropriate. Jackson and Pollock developed a generalized model which categorizes large segments of gender-specific groups varying by age and level of fat mass [39]. Age needs to be factored into the equation, as variations in storage patterns manifest when comparing the young and the old. As a person ages, accumulations of subcutaneous fat are mobilized to more central areas and replaced by visceral fat storage. Therefore, regression equations applied to older populations should be adjusted to match the population. It is important to note that, while skinfold measurements tend to under-predict total BF, the largest errors are associated with the inability to measure visceral adiposity. Clinical data from criterion measures using hydrostatic weighing suggests that skinfold estimation error is approximately 3-4%; however, experienced assessors can consistently produce results within 0.5-2% [21]. Prediction error most commonly results from a technician's testing error. This may be due to inexperience, poor technique, variations in tissue consistency, too much fat mass at the site, or incorrect site identification. To ensure accuracy, an exercise professional should perform numerous individual measurements under the supervision of an expert before using skinfold assessment to measure BF on a client.

When deciding on the sites and protocols for skinfold assessment, it is important to realize that accuracy does not necessarily increase with more test sites. Slight error on each measurement of a seven-site assessment may create significant inaccuracy when the sums are totaled. What may be of more value is how well the assessment identifies and exploits total body storage. Using the Jackson-Pollock generalized equation, three-site assessment allows for measures at each body region [39]. This can identify a high-storage depot that may be missed when using other skinfold models. A good rule of thumb stipulates that the assessment should at least measure one of the primary storage areas related to sex-specific storage. For women, a lower body and triceps site should be included in the assessment, while assessment on males should include either the abdominal or subscapular site due to the propensity for regional storage.

Skinfold assessment should be performed on individuals who are not visibly overweight. Individuals who maintain excessive fat mass or those who have large fat depots at select sites are difficult to measure. This is particularly true when they are also muscular. In some cases, accurate folds cannot be made due to high levels of muscle combined with increased fat mass. This situation causes skin tightness in the area, making it difficult to create a fold. If, for any reason, the assessment cannot be performed with accuracy, the data is of little use. In these cases, an alternate assessment technique should be employed [53]. Skinfold predictability can be complemented using additional girth measurements, in particular, to account for visceral storage [18]. For purposes of reliability, the same tester and test should be used during any follow-up evaluations. There are numerous calipers on the market for skinfold assessment ranging in price from less than $20 to over $300. No matter the price paid for the calipers, the equipment pressure should be calibrated to 10 g/mm^2 to

Skinfold Guidelines

1. Be sure the test subject did not apply skin cream to the sites, or the skin will become slippery and assessment error may occur.

2. Correctly identify the gender specific sites, and mark the fold location for reliable subsequent measures. Generally, the right side of the body is used for assessment.

3. Using the left hand with a thumb down position, straddle the marked site with the index and thumb and push into the fat mass until the underlying muscle can be felt.

4. Firmly grasp the skinfold and pull away from the muscle. The skinfold should have parallel sides. The pinch width is specific to the amount of fat mass.

5. Holding the calipers in the right hand pull the trigger to open the calipers and place the caliper arms on either side of the fold about 1/2 an inch below the fingers in the center of the fold. The caliper arms should be held at a level that forms a 90 degree angle perpendicular to the fold.

6. Maintaining the pressure on the fold with the index finger and thumb release the caliper trigger and assess the measurement within 4 seconds. Do not let go of the fold until the reading has been made and the calipers are withdrawn from the fold.

7. Record the value.

8. Measure each site at least twice for accuracy, allowing at least 15 seconds between subsequent measures of the site. If values differ by more than 1-2 mm, reassess a third time. Average the measures.

9. Add the sum of skinfolds and apply the score to the population specific equation, or chart to identify the predicted percentage of body fat.

ensure a more accurate prediction. The brand used is often based on professional preference and budget. It is not recommended to use calipers that require the tester to manually pinch the fold with the instrument due to tension variations which may over or under compress the fold [39].

Skinfold Sites

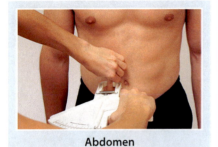
Abdomen

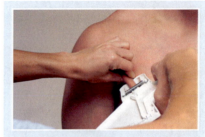
Chest

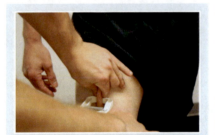
Thigh

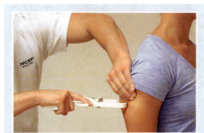
Triceps

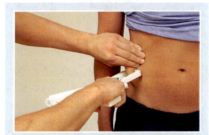
Suprailiac

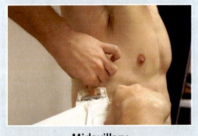
Midaxillary

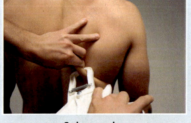
Subscapular

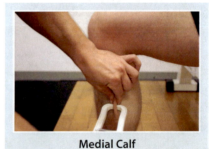
Medial Calf

Site Locations	Fold Orientation	Fold Description
Abdomen	Vertical	Taken 2 cm (approximately 1 in.) to the right of the umbilicus.
Chest (Males only)	Diagonal	The site is one half the distance between the anterior axillary line and the nipple.
Thigh	Vertical	On the front of the thigh, midway between the hip (inguinal crease) and the superior aspect of the patella (kneecap).
Triceps	Vertical	Located halfway between the acromion process (shoulder) and the inferior part of the elbow on the rear mid line of the upper arm.
Suprailiac	Diagonal	Taken with the natural angle of the iliac crest at the anterior axillary line immediately superior to the iliac crest.
Midaxillary	Vertical	Fold is taken on the midaxillary line at the height of the xiphoid (end of sternum).
Subscapular	Diagonal	Just below the lowest angle of scapula, taken on a 45 degree angle toward the right side.
Medial Calf	Vertical	Seated with the right knee flexed and sole of the foot on the floor. The fold is taken on the medial side of the calf at its greatest circumference.

QUICK INSIGHT

Cellulite is not a special fat as many people seem to believe. It is characterized by a dimpled or wrinkled appearance of the skin that occurs when the tissue pressure is increased from compression (sitting) or muscle contractions. Cellulite is simply subcutaneous fat that has herniated into the skin's dermal layer beneath the epidermis. Irregularities in the connective tissue border between the dermis and the fat cells, resulting from tissue weakness, allow fat mass to migrate through the border into the superficial layer [29].

Although cellulite is commonly visible on obese individuals, it can also affect the non-obese. It is estimated to affect 80-90% of females [54]. *The posterolateral thighs and buttocks of females are particularly susceptible due to the quantity of fat stored in that region. Since cellulite is based on connective tissue attachment and compressive pressure, the only way to effectively reduce its appearance is to lower total BF. Many creams and ointments can be purchased to hyperhydrate the area to temporarily mask cellulite, but no over-the-counter or prescription remedies exist to remove it. Acoustic wave therapy has been shown to improve cellulitis through improved local blood-flow, increased collagen and elastin fibers* [29, 54].

DEFINITIONS

Cellulite –

A condition in which fat deposits push through connective tissue under the skin, presenting a dimpled appearance.

Bioelectrical impedance analysis (BIA) –

A measure of the resistance to flow of an electrical current through body tissues used to estimate body composition.

Bioelectrical Impedance

Developed in the 1970's, **bioelectrical impedance analysis (BIA)** employs the conductivity of water to predict body fatness. Since fat contains significantly less water than muscle tissue, the conduction speed of an electrical impulse sent through body tissues provides information as to the magnitude body fat. Numerous instruments, techniques, and population specific equations exist for BIA. New segmental multi frequency (1, 5, 50, 250 500, 1000khz) BIA uses a weak electrical current run through the five segments of the body (trunk, left leg, right leg, left arm and right arm) to identify resistance to the electrical flow, referred to as impedance. Unlike the whole body BIA, this new technology does not utilize gender and age to predict body the body composition and only use the data collected from impedance of body segments. Clinical assessments using BIA have been shown to be the most accurate (SEE 3-5%) in population [7, 42]. Other techniques using BIA have not shown the same level of accuracy, particularly in obese persons [32]. Handheld devices and scales show pronounced differences in accuracy and measurement consistency. Even similar equipment has exhibited variations among manufacturers [42]. Meta-analysis of validation studies found BIA overestimated FFM with scaling errors as BMI increased among the obese: manufacturer equations significantly overestimated FFM and underestimated %BF compared to DXA [30]. Thus, multi-frequency BIA appears to be a more appropriate method for body composition assessment than single frequency BIA methods.

Part of the issue with validity and reliability when using BIA is the numerous factors affecting accuracy and precision [30]. Factors associated with the equipment, environment, client, and equation selection can all influence error. Due to variations in equipment prediction, the same measurement instrument should be used each time to maximize reliability. Even if the measurement is incorrect when compared to more accurate protocols, it should still reliably show change between pre- and post-tests on the same subject, given that his or her body temperature, hydration, and mineral content remain the same [24, 25]. To maintain reliability and enhance assessment accuracy, certain client factors should be considered. Importantly, the client's hydration state needs to be regulated, as an increase or decrease in water volume creates measurement variation. Likewise, the environment needs to be controlled because cold skin temperatures cause under-

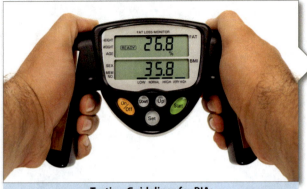

Testing Guidelines for BIA:
- No eating or drinking within four hours of the test
- No exercise or strenuous work within 12 hours of the test
- No alcohol consumption for at least 24 hours before the test
- If possible, void the bowel and bladder before assessment
- Avoid testing during menstruation
- Diuretic medications will invalidate the test

estimation of fat mass. Additionally, the skin thickness at the point of the electrodes influences the assessment. Measurements performed in the original clinical trials were more accurate because the electrodes were placed on the back of the hand and top of the foot, where the skin is not conditioned from friction, and consequently, more permeable to the current. The bottom of the feet and palms of the hands represent the most frictionally conditioned parts of the body, and therefore, are not the best sites for electrode placement. Ironically, almost all devices manufactured for BIA use these undesirable locations for electrode placement.

BIA certainly has its share of shortcomings, but it can be used to track changes effectively outside of clinical environments. The assessments are physically and psychologically benign, and when used in conjunction with girth measures, serve as a viable solution for select populations. Taking the steps to enhance accuracy is important to acquire effective data, and closely observing the testing protocols and using the correct equation reduces error.

Body Composition Continuum

Body composition values fall along the health and physical fitness continuum. As a health-related component of fitness, body composition is associated with a range of positive and negative health outcomes. There does appear to be a threshold where, beyond a certain point, the amount of fat mass on the body begins to negatively affect the biological function of other tissues. Although identifying the exact ideal BF for all men and women has been somewhat elusive for researchers, a reasonable cut off value does seem to exist for each sex. Values above 20% for men and above 30% for women are more greatly associated with negative health outcomes than values below these BF percentages[1]. This of course, considers BF as an independent variable for health risk. When physical activity, diet, and smoking are factored in, the ideal values may fluctuate based on the additional information. A 35-year-old male who smokes and has a BF of 17% presents a much greater risk for disease than a 35-year-old male with 20% BF who does not smoke. Likewise, a female who has 29% BF but routinely eats a healthy diet and performs exercise most days of the week will likely have a lower risk than a sedentary female with a BF of 25%. BF can be viewed in a related but inverse perspective as aerobic fitness. In aerobic fitness, very low numbers increase the risk for disease; with body fat, high numbers associate with negative health consequences. Maintaining values that are moderate, in conjunction with appropriate health and fitness behaviors, will dramatically reduce the risk for possible health problems.

Percent Fat in Men and Women		
Risk Category	Men (% Body Fat)	Women (% Body Fat)
Essential	3 - 5	11 - 14.9
Lean	6 - 10.9	15 - 18.9
Fitness	11 - 15.9	19 - 22.9
Healthy	16 - 19.9	23 - 26.9
Moderate Risk	20 - 24.9	27 - 31.9
High Risk	>25	>32

Percent Fat in Children 6-17 Years Old		
Risk Category	Boys (% Body Fat)	Girls (% Body Fat)
Very Low	<6	12
Low	7 - 10	13 - 15
Optimal Range	11 - 19	16 - 25
Moderately High	20 - 24	26 - 30
High	25 - 30	31 - 35
Very High	>31	>35

BF values can be used for more than predicting health risk. Accurately assessed values can help develop and inform evaluation of an exercise prescription. This is accomplished by converting the weight of fat into a caloric value. The **Target Body Weight Formula** identifies changes in fat weight associated with increased or decreased BF, although it is predominantly used for the latter. If the desired BF is placed in the formula, the end value reflects the new appropriate weight for a client at that particular BF percentage. This calculation can determine the number of calories that need to be expended and can help clients to realize weight loss goals.

>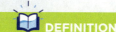
> **DEFINITIONS**
> **Target body weight formula –**
> *A computation of healthy or ideal body weight for goal-setting by inputting current weight and desired body fat percentage.*

Target Body Weight Formula

Fat mass = current body weight × (% body fat ÷ 100)
Fat-free mass (FFM) = current body weight − fat mass

$$\text{Target body weight} = \frac{\text{FFM}}{1 - \frac{\{\text{Desired \% BF}\}}{100}}$$

Example
A 30-year old male weights 185 lbs. and has a body fat percentage of 20%. His goal is to reach 15% body fat. What is his target bodyweight at 15% body fat?

Fat mass = 185 × .20 = 37 lbs
FFM = 185 lbs. − 37 lbs. = 148 lbs

$$\text{Target body weight} = \frac{148}{1 - \frac{\{15\}}{100}} = 174 \text{ lbs}$$

The formula can assist in setting short and long-term weight loss goals for a client, as well as aid in tracking program effectiveness and identifying errors in balance between diet and energy expenditure. Using the predicted value, correct adjustments can be determined for caloric intake and expenditure recommendations.

Using the previous example for a 155 lb. person at the beginning of this section, to change from 20% BF to 15%, he would have to lose approximately 9 lbs. Taking into account that 3,500 calories equals one pound of fat energy, this individual must create a negative caloric balance of 31,500 kcal to lose the 9 lbs. If the goal is one pound of weight loss per week, the client would have to create a negative caloric balance of 500 kcal every day for nine weeks. Five hundred calories equate to about five miles of running, probably an unrealistic goal for a client to accomplish every day. Instead, diet and exercise management can be used together to make sure each day ends with a negative balance of 500 kcal. Realistic goals provide the foundation of exercise adherence. This and other weight loss strategies will be covered in the Weight Management Chapter.

Male	<3%	5%	10%	15%	18%	22%	25%	30%
	Essential		Lean		Early Risk		Obesity	Morbidly Obese
Female	<11%	14%	16%	22%	26%	27%	32%	40%

REFERENCES:

1. Abernathy R and Black D. Healthy body weights: an alternative perspective. *The American journal of clinical nutrition* 63: 448S-451S, 1996.

2. Arnold TJ, Schweitzer A, Hoffman HJ, Onyewu C, Hurtado ME, Hoffman EP, and Klein CJ. Neck and waist circumference biomarkers of cardiovascular risk in a cohort of predominantly African-American college students: a preliminary study. *Journal of the Academy of Nutrition and Dietetics* 114: 107-116, 2014.

3. Balkau B, Deanfield JE, Després J-P, Bassand J-P, Fox KA, Smith SC, Barter P, Tan C-E, Van Gaal L, and Wittchen H-U. International day for the evaluation of abdominal obesity (IDEA): a study of waist circumference, cardiovascular disease, and diabetes mellitus in 168 000 primary care patients in 63 countries. *Circulation* 116: 1942-1951, 2007.

4. Berg AH and Scherer PE. Adipose tissue, inflammation, and cardiovascular disease. *Circulation research* 96: 939-949, 2005.

5. Berz K and McCambridge T. Amenorrhea in the female athlete: What to do and when to worry. *Pediatric annals* 45: e97-e102, 2016.

6. Borrell LN and Samuel L. Body mass index categories and mortality risk in US adults: the effect of overweight and obesity on advancing death. *American journal of public health* 104: 512-519, 2014.

7. Chumlea WC, Guo SS, Kuczmarski RJ, Flegal KM, Johnson CL, Heymsfield SB, Lukaski HC, Friedl K, and Hubbard VS. Body composition estimates from NHANES III bioelectrical impedance data. *International journal of obesity* 26: 1596, 2002.

8. Cinti S. The adipose organ. In: *Obesity:* Springer, 2018, p. 1-24.

9. Claros G, Hull HR, and Fields DA. Comparison of air displacement plethysmography to hydrostatic weighing for estimating total body density in children. *BMC pediatrics* 5: 37, 2005.

10. Dobbelsteyn C, Joffres M, MacLean DR, and Flowerdew G. A comparative evaluation of waist circumference, waist-to-hip ratio and body mass index as indicators of cardiovascular risk factors. The Canadian Heart Health Surveys. *International journal of obesity* 25: 652, 2001.

11. Duren DL, Sherwood RJ, Czerwinski SA, Lee M, Choh AC, Siervogel RM, and Chumlea WC. Body composition methods: comparisons and interpretation. *Journal of diabetes science and technology* 2: 1139-1146, 2008.

12. Fantuzzi G. Adipose tissue, adipokines, and inflammation. *Journal of Allergy and Clinical Immunology* 115: 911-919, 2005.

13. Fields D, Hunter G, and Goran M. Validation of the BOD POD with hydrostatic weighing: Influence of body clothingin. *International journal of obesity* 24: 200, 2000.

14. Fields DA, Higgins PB, and Hunter GR. Assessment of body composition by air-displacement plethysmography: influence of body temperature and moisture. *Dynamic Medicine* 3: 3, 2004.

15. Flegal KM, Kit BK, Orpana H, and Graubard BI. Association of all-cause mortality with overweight and obesity using standard body mass index categories: a systematic review and meta-analysis. *Jama* 309: 71-82, 2013.

16. Ford ES, Maynard LM, and Li C. Trends in mean waist circumference and abdominal obesity among US adults, 1999-2012. *Jama* 312: 1151-1153, 2014.

17. Fosbøl MØ and Zerahn B. Contemporary methods of body composition measurement. *Clinical physiology and functional imaging* 35: 81-97, 2015.

18. Garcia AL, Wagner K, Hothorn T, Koebnick C, Zunft HJF, and Trippo U. Improved prediction of body fat by measuring skinfold thickness, circumferences, and bone breadths. *Obesity Research* 13: 626-634, 2005.

19. Hales CM, Fryar CD, Carroll MD, Freedman DS, and Ogden CL. Trends in obesity and severe obesity prevalence in US youth and adults by sex and age, 2007-2008 to 2015-2016. *Jama* 319: 1723-1725, 2018.

20. Heymsfield SB, Ebbeling CB, Zheng J, Pietrobelli A, Strauss BJ, Silva AM, and Ludwig DS. Multi component molecular level body composition reference methods: evolving concepts and future directions. *Obesity reviews* 16: 282-294, 2015.

21. Heyward V. ASEP methods recommendation: body composition assessment. *Journal of exercise physiology online* 4, 2001.

22. Ibrahim MM. Subcutaneous and visceral adipose tissue: structural and functional differences. *Obesity reviews* 11: 11-18, 2010.

23. Karpe F and Pinnick KE. Biology of upper-body and lower-body adipose tissue—link to whole-body phenotypes. *Nature Reviews Endocrinology* 11: 90, 2015.

24. Kyle UG, Bosaeus I, De Lorenzo AD, Deurenberg P, Elia M, Gómez JM, Heitmann BL, Kent-Smith L, Melchior J-C, and Pirlich M. Bioelectrical impedance analysis—part I: review of principles and methods. *Clinical nutrition* 23: 1226-1243, 2004.

25. Kyle UG, Bosaeus I, De Lorenzo AD, Deurenberg P, Elia M, Gómez JM, Heitmann BL, Kent-Smith L, Melchior J-C, and Pirlich M. Bioelectrical impedance analysis—part II: utilization in clinical practice. *Clinical nutrition* 23: 1430-1453, 2004.

26. Laskey MA. Dual-energy X-ray absorptiometry and body composition. *Nutrition* 12: 45-51, 1996.

27. Lloyd-Jones D, Adams R, Carnethon M, De Simone G, Ferguson TB, Flegal K, Ford E, Furie K, Go A, and Greenlund K. Heart disease and stroke statistics—2009 update. A report from the American Heart Association Statistics Committee and Stroke Statistics Subcommittee. *Circulation*, 2008.

28. Lloyd-Jones D, Adams RJ, Brown TM, Carnethon M, Dai S, De Simone G, Ferguson TB, Ford E, Furie K, and Gillespie C. Heart disease and stroke statistics—2010 update. A report from the American Heart Association. *Circulation*, 2009.

29. Luebberding S, Krueger N, and Sadick NS. Cellulite: an evidence-based review. *American journal of clinical dermatology* 16: 243-256, 2015.

30. Lukaski HC and Siders WA. Validity and accuracy of regional bioelectrical impedance devices to determine whole-body fatness. *Nutrition* 19: 851-857, 2003.

31. Mansour MF, Chan C-WJ, Laforest S, Veilleux A, and Tchernof A. Sex Differences in Body Fat Distribution. In: *Adipose Tissue Biology*: Springer, 2017, p. 257-300.

32. Mialich MS, Sicchieri JF, and Junior AAJ. Analysis of body composition: a critical review of the use of bioelectrical impedance analysis. *Int J Clin Nutr* 2: 1-10, 2014.

33. Myint PK, Kwok CS, Luben RN, Wareham NJ, and Khaw K-T. Body fat percentage, body mass index and waist-to-hip ratio as predictors of mortality and cardiovascular disease. *Heart* 100: 1613-1619, 2014.

34. Nagy E, Vicente-Rodriguez G, Manios Y, Béghin L, Iliescu C, Censi L, Dietrich S, Ortega F, De Vriendt T, and Plada M. Harmonization process and reliability assessment of anthropometric measurements in a multicenter study in adolescents. *International Journal of Obesity* 32: S58, 2008.

35. Nazare J-A, Smith J, Borel A-L, Aschner P, Barter P, Van Gaal L, Tan CE, Wittchen H-U, Matsuzawa Y, and Kadowaki T. Usefulness of measuring both body mass index and waist circumference for the estimation of visceral adiposity and related cardiometabolic risk profile (from the INSPIRE ME IAA study). *The American journal of cardiology* 115: 307-315, 2015.

36. Organization WH. WHO global infobase online. *URL: https://apps who int/infobase/ Obesity aspx[0606 2018]*, 2016.

37. Palmer BF and Clegg DJ. The sexual dimorphism of obesity. *Molecular and cellular endocrinology* 402: 113-119, 2015.

38. Pietrobelli A, Formica C, Wang Z, and Heymsfield SB. Dual-energy X-ray absorptiometry body composition model: review of physical concepts. *American Journal of Physiology-Endocrinology And Metabolism* 271: E941-E951, 1996.

39. Pollock ML and Jackson AS. Research progress in validation of clinical methods of assessing body composition. *Medicine and science in sports and exercise* 16: 606-615, 1984.

40. Roger VL, Go AS, Lloyd-Jones DM, Adams RJ, Berry JD, Brown TM, Carnethon MR, Dai S, De Simone G, and Ford ES. Heart disease and stroke statistics—2011 update: a report from the American Heart Association. *Circulation* 123: e18, 2011.

41. Sahakyan KR, Somers VK, Rodriguez-Escudero JP, Hodge DO, Carter RE, Sochor O, Coutinho T, Jensen MD, Roger VL, and Singh P. Normal-weight central obesity: implications for total and cardiovascular mortality. *Annals of internal medicine* 163: 827-835, 2015.

42. Shafer KJ, Siders WA, Johnson LK, and Lukaski HC. Validity of segmental multiple-frequency bioelectrical impedance analysis to estimate body composition of adults across a range of body mass indexes. *Nutrition* 25: 25-32, 2009.

43. Shah B, Sucher K, and Hollenbeck CB. Comparison of ideal body weight equations and published height weight tables with body mass index tables for healthy adults in the United States. *Nutrition in clinical practice* 21: 312-319, 2006.

44. Shake CL, Schlichting C, Mooney LW, Callahan AB, and Cohen ME. Predicting percent body fat from circumference measurements. *Military medicine* 158: 26-31, 1993.

45. Stein CJ and Colditz GA. The epidemic of obesity. *The Journal of Clinical Endocrinology & Metabolism* 89: 2522-2525, 2004.

46. Tchernof A, Bélanger C, Morisset A-S, Richard C, Mailloux J, Laberge P, and Dupont P. Regional differences in adipose tissue metabolism in women: minor effect of obesity and body fat distribution. *Diabetes* 55: 1353-1360, 2006.

47. Thompson D, Karpe F, Lafontan M, and Frayn K. Physical activity and exercise in the regulation of human adipose tissue physiology. *Physiological reviews* 92: 157-191, 2012.

48. Tilg H and Moschen AR. Adipocytokines: mediators linking adipose tissue, inflammation and immunity. *Nature Reviews Immunology* 6: 772, 2006.

49. Valencak TG, Osterrieder A, and Schulz TJ. Sex matters: The effects of biological sex on adipose tissue biology and energy metabolism. *Redox biology* 12: 806-813, 2017.

50. van Dijk SJ, Molloy P, Varinli H, Morrison J, Muhlhausler B, Buckley M, Clark S, McMillen I, Noakes M, and Samaras K. Epigenetics and human obesity. *International Journal of Obesity* 39: 85, 2015.

51. Votruba SB and Jensen MD. Sex differences in abdominal, gluteal, and thigh LPL activity. *American Journal of Physiology-Endocrinology and Metabolism* 292: E1823-E1828, 2007.

52. Votruba SB and Jensen MD. Sex-specific differences in leg fat uptake are revealed with a high-fat meal. *American Journal of Physiology-Endocrinology and Metabolism* 291: E1115-E1123, 2006.

53. Wang J, Thornton J, Kolesnik S, and Pierson R. Anthropometry in body composition: an overview. *Annals of the New York Academy of Sciences* 904: 317-326, 2000.

54. Zerini I, Sisti A, Cuomo R, Ciappi S, Russo F, Brandi C, D'Aniello C, and Nisi G. Cellulite treatment: a comprehensive literature review. *Journal of cosmetic dermatology* 14: 224-240, 2015.

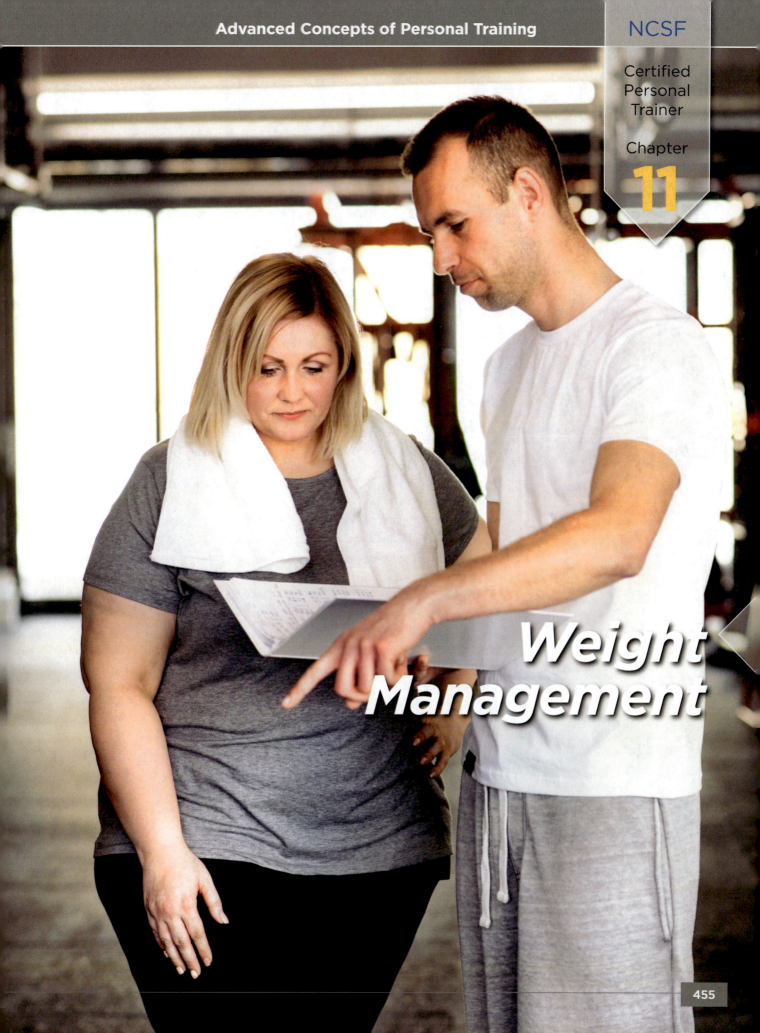

Factors that Impact Weight Management

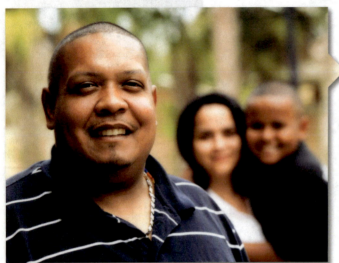

Rising obesity represents an ever worsening health risk, threatening those of all ages in the United States [23]. The current rate of weight gain and the medical costs associated with it have prompted the government to create a formal initiative to combat the alarmingly steady rise in this controllable disease's prevalence [50]. Obesity-related medical costs exceed $150 billion per year while indirect costs related to absenteeism and reduced productivity are estimated to be $8.65 billion annually [1, 27]. Prevalence of obesity is expected to worsen, linear-time trend forecasts suggest over 44% of the population will be obese in 2030 [31]. Of even more concern, a 2014 study of overweight and obesity in children, using data from 1980-2013, found that worldwide, the prevalence of overweight and obesity increased substantially in children and adolescents in both developed and developing countries [41].

The prevalence of overweight and obese Americans has pushed weight management to the forefront of the exercise professional's job responsibilities. Most clients who hire an exercise professional do so in order to accomplish goals related to looking and feeling better. Although the desire to lose weight is often vanity driven, the health outcomes associated with attaining a healthy weight are more far-reaching. In theory, weight loss is a relatively easy task to accomplish since it can be achieved by simply reducing energy consumed and increasing energy expended. However, reality presents a very different picture, with most people finding it very difficult to successfully lose weight and keep it off. Social, economic, physiological, psychological, and emotional factors each play a part in creating barriers to adherence and success in a weight management program [10, 39, 55]. Addressing one factor alone may be ineffective, as the other factors can independently create obstacles, or more likely, be intertwined with and compound the barriers to achievement. Due to the multifactorial nature of the disease, a trainer must understand how each aspect interacts with energy balance and, ultimately, fat reduction.

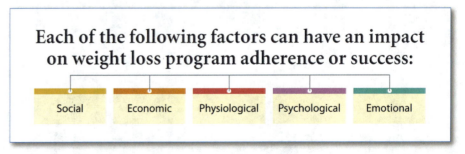

Each of the following factors can have an impact on weight loss program adherence or success:

- Social
- Economic
- Physiological
- Psychological
- Emotional

Social Factors

Social factors that affect weight stem from many different aspects of American tradition, behaviors, and lifestyle activities [32]. From the traditional perspective, food and drink have long been associated with celebrations, family gatherings, special events, and other social engagements. Linked with sensations of pleasure, the tendency for most people is to indulge themselves with more calories than the body needs often occurs during these activities. High calorie beverages, appetizers, large meal sizes, and desserts are all part of normal eating patterns at weddings, holidays, family events, and social gatherings. Likewise, weekend activities often cause variations in eating habits and calorie intake compared to the more structured work week. Visits to restaurants, social clubs, and gatherings with friends routinely dismantle efforts made during the week: calories burned from exercise and conscious dietary restraint are easily replaced in a short period. External influences from these environments often overpower even the most devoted. A casual walk through a sporting event tailgate makes this fact obvious.

To contend with the additional caloric consumption associated with social events, weight management strategies should identify the specific problems affecting the individual and seek appropriate remedies to prevent or decrease the negative actions. A thorough evaluation of individual behaviors can help identify common triggers and problem areas that warrant intervention or education. Some common habits that present obstacles to weight loss are listed in the adjacent image.

Contributing environmental factors can cause people to overeat in social settings. Exercise professionals should acknowledge the risks and obstacles in each situation and provide clients suitable strategies to combat these pitfalls in order to further goal attainment. These strategies should be discussed and documented as an ongoing part of the weight management program.

Economic Factors

Economic factors have increasingly been identified as obstacles to weight management [47]. Recent identification of some of these factors' impact has led to criticism of corporate and government practices [21, 42, 53]. High-calorie, low-cost foods have become a staple of many American diets, particularly for those in the lower socioeconomic income bracket [36]. **Food deserts**, which lack fresh healthy food options such as farmers' markets, reflect areas with impoverished population segments where this risk is intensified [60]. Fast-food restaurants offer convenience, low price, and an abundance of calories. For individuals living within budgetary restraints, fast food is many times an 'essential' dietary option. Higher quality food is more expensive and harder to keep fresh than inexpensive alternatives. Fruits, vegetables, fish, lean meats, and whole grain products require a larger food budget for daily consumption, and they frequently have a shorter shelf life. When shopping on a budget, boxed, processed foods and lower quality foods high in fats and preservatives provide a more cost-effective alternative. Compound this with the fact that sugar and salt are excellent preservatives and individuals with budgetary constraints are seemingly set up for an unhealthy lifestyle. Quite simply, Americans from lower socioeconomic brackets have less opportunity to eat well because access and affordability limit their selections; this situation explains, at least in part,

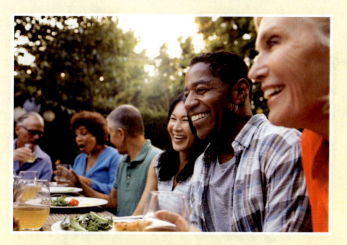

Obstacles to Weight Loss

1. Over-consumption of food in attempts to try all the food dishes presented.
2. Eating large portions by loading the plate at a buffet or self-serve bar.
3. Consuming food and drink in response to boredom or social nervousness.
4. Location eating: close proximity to food increases likelihood of consumption.
5. Pressures to try dishes to acknowledge preparation effort by the party host.
6. Ordering multiple dishes or very large portions based on appetite at restaurants.
7. Not realizing the caloric density of foods prepared by others.
8. Throwing out restrictive habits due to the environment.
9. Allowing alcohol to skew judgment.
10. Eating or drinking in response to peer pressure.

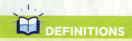

DEFINITIONS

Food deserts –

An area, either in urban or rural environments, in which it is difficult to access affordable nutritious food.

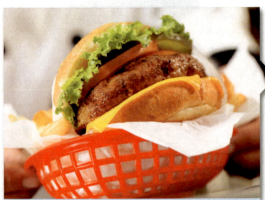

High-calorie, low-cost foods have become a staple of many American diets, particularly for those in the lower socioeconomic income bracket.

DEFINITIONS

Hunger –

The physiological drive to seek food caused by hormonal signaling from peripheral tissues to the hypothalamus.

Hypothalamus –

A region of the forebrain that regulates many vital biological feedback systems by governing the outflow of pituitary-gland hormones and the autonomic nervous system.

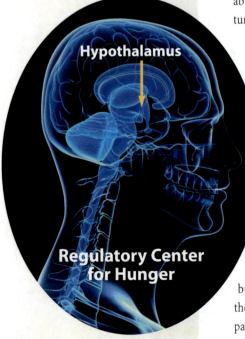

the higher rates of obesity among this population group [61].

The level of nutrition education and overall food knowledge also links with socioeconomic status [13]. Less affluent Americans have limited access to educational resources compared to wealthier classes. Nutritional knowledge is an integral component of health literacy, and low health literacy is associated with poor health outcomes. Consequently, relative familiarity with nutrient value, caloric density, and healthy dietary practices often lags in poorer communities, and information availability is even more limited. For instance, the United States Department of Agriculture (USDA) provides quality education and applications on the internet, but without appropriate resources, this information remains difficult to access. Risk for obesity has been connected to socioeconomic status, and the behaviors learned early in life tend to stay with an individual into adulthood. Those with less opportunity during their early years may be more susceptible to weight gain as adults, regardless of their later economic status [40, 45]. For example, many professional athletes from lower economic backgrounds continue to follow the dietary practices associated with the limited means of their childhood, even as millionaires, illustrating that early behaviors and exposures can have a lifetime impact.

Physiological Factors

Hunger is the primary physiological determinant for eating behaviors. Stimulated by the **hypothalamus**, hunger stems from the physiological drive that signals the need to eat [14]. Although neural signals initiate the process, hunger is a subjective feeling, and therefore does not indicate the exact caloric intake needed. The response to hunger and subsequent satiety, or a feeling of fullness, is multifaceted, and results in the variety of eating responses often observed among humans. Satiation is experienced when the body has consumed adequate food to satisfy its need, thereby shutting off the hunger response. However, due to the large number of variables affecting the body's food-intake regulatory system, it is not a precise mechanism [59]. The sensation of fullness may be attributed to the type of calories consumed, the amount of food in the stomach, or the extent food intake satisfies the demand the brain creates [52]. Due to the variability in the regulatory response, a person may overconsume food before the mechanism to turn off hunger signals activates.

Peripheral mechanisms regulate food consumption via chemoreceptors and hormones [65]. These mechanisms' efficiency is not always consistent, another reason why variations in eating patterns exist [16]. One problem is that calories can be consumed at a rate faster than the food intake information can be processed. Likewise, different types of foods affect the speed and magnitude of satiation [16]. Certain foods trigger peripheral mechanisms more efficiently than others. According to the University of Sydney's satiation index, over a two-hour period, fish, apples, oranges, and potatoes yield more efficient and effective satiety than croissants, cakes, donuts, peanuts, candy bars, and yogurt [25]. Fibrous foods and foods with high levels of resistant starch have also been linked with sensations of fullness due to the bulk they produce in the gut [20]. Biochemical evidence exists that suggests fat and protein content positively effects satiety via hormonal feedback mechanisms from the site of the small intestine. The duration of fullness seems to be tied to gastric emptying time (how long food remains in the stomach), fluid content, and overall bulk. Less energy-dense foods, such as whole fruits and vegetables, carry the most water and the least fat. These foods promote greater satiation than high-energy dense foods with comparably more fat and less water [15].

The Satiety Index

Each of the following foods are rated by how much food people consumed in order to satisfy their hunger.
All are compared to white bread, ranked as "100"

Bakery Products		Snacks and Confectionary		Breakfast Cereals with Milk		Carbohydrate-Rich Foods		Protein-Rich Foods		Fruits	
Croissant	47%	Mars candy bar	70%	Mueslix	100%	White bread	100%	Lentils	133%	Bananas	118%
Cake	65%	Peanuts	84%	Sustain	112%	French fries	116%	Cheese	146%	Grapes	162%
Doughnuts	68%	Yogurt	88%	Special K	116%	White pasta	119%	Eggs	150%	Apples	197%
Cookies	120%	Crisps	91%	Cornflakes	118%	Brown rice	132%	Baked beans	168%	Oranges	202%
Crackers	127%	Ice cream	96%	Honeysmacks	132%	White rice	138%	Beef	176%		
		Jellybeans	118%	All-Bran	151%	Grain bread	154%	Ling fish	225%		
		Popcorn	154%	Oatmeal	209%	Wholemeal bread	157%				
						Brown pasta	188%				
						Potatoes, boiled	323%				

Adapted from S.H.A. Holt, J.C. Brand Miller, P. Petocz, and E. Farmakalidis, "A Satiety Index of Common Foods," *European Journal of Clinical Nutrition*, Sept 1995
Disclaimer: The formula does not account for all known contributing factors for satiety. The formula is derived from a small data set.
The data set is based on subjectively reported, rather than directly measured, criteria.

The signaling effect of hunger can also be manipulated by a variety of factors associated with both physical activities and physical state. Lack of sleep (<6 hours per night) has repeatedly been shown to increase perceived need for food consumption the following day. Obese individuals also experience hunger-driven hormone changes, such as leptin-resistance, which lead to **hyperphagia** due to a poor response by the body's hunger "on-off switch." Interestingly, psychological stress plays two different roles in hunger. Acute psychological stress often causes an anorexigenic response, whereas chronic stress causes a hyperphagic response in conjunction with inflammation.

When hunger is not addressed in a reasonable period, the body's perceived food need will often increase and compound. Regularly consuming low energy-dense foods throughout the day eases the hunger-signaling mechanism, and therefore may reduce total caloric intake. Selecting foods that quickly increase satiation, like apples and oranges, can provide a strategic answer to help regulate eating patterns when used as snacks. The inconsistencies in hunger-satisfaction rates also suggest that foods should be consumed at slower rates and with adequate fluid volumes to allow the body time to recognize the nutrients and use the information to better regulate the chemical shut-off valve in the hypothalamic center of the brain.

Psychological Factors

Appetite differs from hunger in that appetite is the primary psychological mechanism controlling eating, though it does have a relationship with the level of hunger the body experiences [12]. Appetite represents a desire to eat based on the "thought of food" in the presence of hunger, but it can also occur without a physiological mediator. A person's appetite or "craving" may be for a type

DEFINITIONS

Hyperphagia –

An abnormally increased desire for food promoting excessive eating.

Appetite –

A psychological desire to satisfy a need for food, often occurring independently of hunger.

of food, a particular nutrient, or desire stemming from environmental sights, smells, or thoughts. Planning to order a particular meal before getting to a favorite restaurant or craving a hot dog at a ball park represent common examples. Appetite is often blamed for food overconsumption because it links with the psychological perception of satisfaction from food. Many people order a large entrée at a restaurant, but after consuming the appetizer, table breads, and a drink, their actual hunger has subsided. When the additional food is delivered, the pleasurable sights and smells stimulate appetite again, which often, consequently, helps to motivate the person to further indulge in calories they probably do not need; this common pattern holds true for dessert eating as well.

The psychological pleasure of eating contributes greatly to calorically dense diets. Sensations associated with favorite foods cause pleasure-seeking neurotransmitters to be released, driving people to eat [15]. People find pleasure in tastes, textures, and sensations associated with certain foods or the environments where the food is consumed. This association causes people to desire the foods even when they are not hungry or to overconsume the foods after they are full. High-calorie foods rich in fats, sugar, and salt often have the most desirable tastes and, therefore, present major problems in a diet aimed at weight loss [16]. This "hedonic pathway" appears to be less regulated in obese individuals, promoting an increased desire for highly palatable energy-dense food despite already high levels of stored energy [66].

Psychological considerations can also include:

- Behavioral patterns
- Learned eating behaviors
- Environmental cues
- Peception of the monetary value of food

Behavioral eating patterns commonly relate to an association between locations, times, and events. Eating chips or popcorn while watching television or a movie exemplifies this behavior. Events trigger eating responses as well: the Sunday football game, a trip to the fair, and even an ice cream treat while shopping at the mall have food-event associations. Familiar sights, sounds, and scents can trigger appetite without any presence of hunger [24].

Learned eating behaviors also contribute to psychological factors that surround consumption. Eating everything on the plate is a lesson taught early in life that sticks with people into adulthood. In some cases, these behaviors stem from cultural norms that instigate eating patterns and food choices. Families that center their relationships on food and togetherness encourage large portions and longer periods spent eating. There may be expectations to eat as a sign of affection and appreciation among the family members. Providing extra food to a child or spouse is viewed as showing care for that person, as is eating all the food presented to acknowledge the appreciation for the offering.

In some cases, overeating occurs to avoid food waste. The psychological and tangible value assigned to food can drive people to eat portions that they do not want or need. Commonly, people consume all the food presented at a restaurant because they pay for it, even though their hunger is satisfied before completely consuming the meal. People routinely eat the last portions left in the serving containers to avoid having to deal with the leftovers or throw them out. When food in the refrigerator reaches its termination date, it is often prioritized for consumption, so it is not discarded. These psychological variables help shape our relationship with food and contribute to our collective food culture. The American food culture differs greatly from other countries, which often prioritize a food experience built upon a communal meals and meal preparation, longer meal durations, smaller portion sizes, and less guilt [17, 28, 49].

Certain emotions or mental states can also drive people to consume food when they are not hungry. When bored, eating provides people with a diversion. Without an alternate distraction, people often look through the kitchen and eat to pass the time. Likewise, particular emotions can drive people to eat. Depression, low self-worth, or sadness can cause people to find comfort in food or lose control when eating because it provides pleasure [11, 30]. Emotionally driven food consumption may occur with or without hunger. The food choices selected are commonly associated with pleasure and often lead to indiscriminate eating. Exercise professionals should identify these causes to help clients recognize emotionally triggered eating patterns.

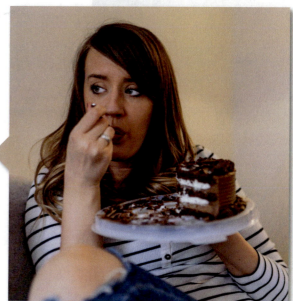

Certain emotions or mental states can drive people to consume food when they are not hungry.

When an individual begins an exercise program, their dietary behaviors may change in one of two ways. Some over-consume unhealthy food as a reward for accomplishing their physical feat. This justification is known as moral licensing and is one reason why exercise without dietary change does not promote weight loss [37]. In other cases, the positive action of participating in an exercise program will lead an individual to consume healthier food. This "positive spillover" response occurs when the motivations for exercising extend to other health behaviors [29]. Whether a person responds to an exercise program with moral licensing or positive spillover plays a critical role in the success of weight management.

Energy Balance and Weight Management Strategies

When individuals routinely consume food in excess of the body's caloric requirements, energy balance can become uneven. Energy balance simply compares the calories consumed versus the calories expended: the old adage is energy in vs. energy out. Since energy can neither be created nor destroyed, as stated in the First Law of Thermodynamics, it must transfer into some form when it enters the body. If the body does not use the consumed energy for enzymatic reactions or convert it into heat and release it into the air, it will likely be stored in the body's cells or become a component of tissue. When the number of calories ingested exceeds the number of calories metabolized, the body experiences a positive caloric balance. Positive caloric balance leads to weight gain because the abundance of energy remains within the body. When the calories consumed match the calories expended, the body is **isocaloric**, or in a neutral caloric balance; consequently, weight should remain unchanged. When the calories expended by the body exceed the number of calories consumed, the body attains a negative balance. Negative caloric balance is necessary for body mass reduction, whether that reduction applies to total body weight, lean mass, and/or body fat.

 DEFINITIONS

Isocaloric –
A balance of calories expended and consumed, promoting weight maintenance.

Energy balance = calories consumed vs. calories expended

Calories consumed > Calories expended	Calories expended > Calories consumed	Calories consumed = Calories expended
potential weight gain from positive caloric balance	potential weight loss from negative caloric balance	weight should remain unchanged: isocaloric balance

◆ Concerns of Significant Caloric Restriction

Undeniably, significant caloric restriction causes weight loss. However, much of this weight loss results from water and lean mass reduction, especially with inadequate protein intake and participation in aerobic exercise [62]. In this scenario, the body employs hormone-driven defense mechanisms: when consumption of calories is inadequate, it turns catabolic. This is likely attributed to survival needs by early humans, who could not eat as regularly as we do today. When food was not available, their bodies, to defend against starvation, reduced metabolic activity by consuming the tissue that required the most calories: muscle. Today, the same phenomenon occurs when the body does not receive adequate nutrients. Significantly cutting calories over time can lead to a reduction in metabolism due to lean mass loss, and when calories drop significantly below **resting metabolic rate (RMR)** (i.e., >300 kcal), the hypothalamus triggers a strong signal to consume food [62].

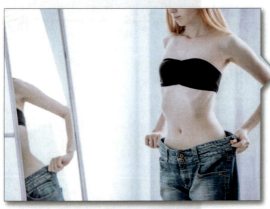

For severely obese individuals, some physicians may prescribe **very low-calorie diets (VLCD)**. These diets are extreme, as they represent values below the recommended minimums. Diets containing only 800-1200 calories should only be prescribed by a medical doctor and require closely monitored nutrient compositions [56]. These diets are inappropriate for active individuals, as they do not support the energy needs of physical activity. They are used in conjunction with metabolic, blood, and vital-sign monitoring in hospital-based settings to prevent any significant negative health consequences. When individuals attempt to duplicate the VLCD plan by utilizing starvation-type diets, they risk damaging the metabolism and placing organs under considerable stress. The minimum recommended caloric intake to maintain adequate nutrient composition is 1200 kcal/day. For many people, this value is still insufficient and can lead to negative outcomes if individual nutrient requirements are not met.

DEFINITIONS

Resting metabolic rate –
The energy required to supply bodily functions during resting conditions.

Very low-calorie diets –
A clinically-supervised dietary plan involving intake below 800 kcal per day, usually achieved through liquid meals.

Yo-yo dieting –
The cyclical loss and gain of weight associated with failing to adhere to strict healthy eating plans.

◆ Yo-Yo Dieting and Intermittent Fasting

Historically, it was presumed that significant physiological detriments occur in individuals who follow low-calorie "fad" diets. Cumulative evidence suggests, however, that there is little detrimental effect of weight cycling on current and future obesity and metabolic risk; therefore, weight loss efforts in individuals with obesity should continue to be encouraged. Since the **Yo-Yo dieting effect** may be linked to a reduced metabolism with age, resistance exercise is a key element in maintaining metabolic health [58]. Due to the restrictive nature of dieting, particularly without exercise, a loss of lean mass may occur that can compound negative effects over time. Lean mass is one of the primary contributors to an individual's metabolic rate and losses can be significant among older adults. The reduction in lean mass associated with dietary practices that solely emphasize caloric restriction potentially increases a person's susceptibility for subsequent fat gain with age.

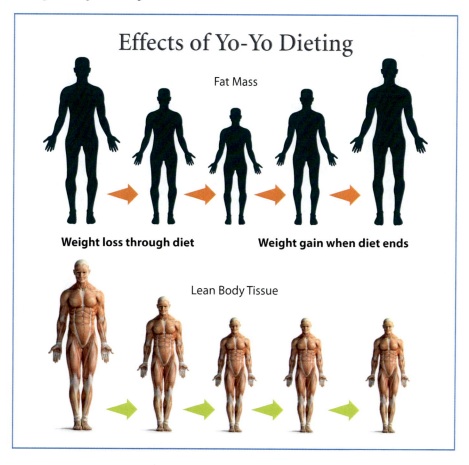

Intermittent fasting strategies represent another form of on-off dietary consumption. Intermittent fasting appears to promote weight loss and may improve metabolic health. The evidence is particularly strong when the eating patterns reduce or eliminate nighttime feeding. Intermittent fasting intervals that affect night time eating may result in sustained improvements in human health via influence on circadian biology and modifiable lifestyle behaviors, such as sleep [43]. Additionally, novel research has demonstrated that changes in gut microbiota play a key role in this phenomenon, and improved nutritional strategies that account for these can reset the weight-rebound clock. Further research indicates both intermittent and periodic fasting results in benefits for preventing certain metabolic disorders, cardiovascular diseases and neurological disorders as Parkinson's and Alzheimer's disease [34].

◆ Food Recalls and Logs

To appropriately manage weight, the correct balance between food timing, caloric expenditure, and caloric intake must be attained routinely. To accomplish successful weight loss or weight gain, the factors which contribute to the balance must be identified and managed correctly. Determining an individual's caloric intake requires some method of dietary-energy

 DEFINITIONS

Intermittent fasting –

An umbrella term for several patterns of fasting and non-fasting over defined periods independent of caloric restriction.

assessment. Several protocols exist to identify or estimate the actual number of calories being consumed in a typical day. They are divided into food logs and food recall assessments. Food recalls are easily implemented and require minimal effort; however, the accuracy of such assessments is limited because they tend to under predict total calories consumed. The assessment requires a client to recall all the food and drink consumed over a selected period. In most cases, a 24-hour recall is used so that the information remains fresh in the client's mind. He or she is asked to record every calorie-containing food or beverage by the serving or portion size consumed. To be valid, the information must be complete, recalled in detail, and measured as precisely as possible. Before employing this method and to help enhance the information's accuracy, exercise professionals should use descriptions, household containers, or models to show clients what serving sizes and normal portions, or food quantities are, in addition to demonstrating the standard household measures. If the client is inaccurate with the quantity of the food or drink consumed, the data collected may be invalid and skew any subsequent recommendations.

Sample Food Log Excerpt

Amount (Serving Size)	Food Description (Cooking Method, Brand Name)	Location (Place, People, Social Environment)	Feeling (Hunger, Anger, Joy)	Time of Day
1 Cup	Kellogg's Corn Flakes	Home Breakfast table	Hungry	8 am
1/2 Cup	Low Fat milk 2%	Home Breakfast table	Hungry	8 am
1 Cup	Decaf Coffee	Home Breakfast table	Hungry	8 am
1	Banana	Home Breakfast table	Hungry	8 am

Food logs use a similar assessment protocol but differ in that the client records the foods as they are consumed. Ideally, a client should take pictures of all food consumed to ensure the accuracy of the data, especially as it relates to portion and serving size. This difference in the data collection methodology significantly increases potential accuracy above the recall method because the recording is done at the time of the intake. Food records can be completed over a 24-hour period, but the preferred method is to use three days of dietary consumption. A multiple-day log's purpose is to identify variations in eating patterns and changes that occur between days in the week versus the weekend. Generally, the days used should represent the beginning, middle, and end of the week. Commonly, Monday, Thursday, and Saturday are designated for review. Including one weekend day helps gauge common differences in eating habits that many individuals display on weekends compared to weekdays. This strategy enhances typical representation as it reflects the dietary and consumption habits consistent with different eating locations and frames of mind.

It is prudent to have the client identify the time and location where the food or drink was consumed, as well as his or her feelings at the time of the behavioral patterns. This combination will help identify intervention strategies. Food records require the same attentiveness and client education as the 24-hour recall. Clients should be clearly instructed on the protocol and advised to be conscious of the common errors found with the assessment. Clients should be convinced that they are not being judged and that their food intake does not reflect negatively upon them.

It is important for goal attainment to have accurate information. Otherwise, it may be a costly waste of time and effort.

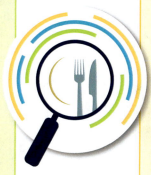

Common Errors in Food Recall or Food Log Assessments
- Incorrect serving size or portion
- Limited familiarity with container sizes or measurements
- Forgotten items
- Falsifying quantities or purposely leaving items out
- Temporarily changing eating habits
- Limited knowledge of mixed food contents or restaurant-prepared foods
- Overlooking use of condiments
- Guessing rather than recalling
- Assessing a non-typical eating pattern

Steps to Improve Recall Accuracy
- Recall the activities in sequence from when they woke up until they went to bed
- Demonstrate the quantity using a tangible measuring model
- Describe the eating experience to improve detail; use drawings to show exact sizes
- Identify what was added to the food, if anything
- Recall the beverages separately
- Recall snacks consumed outside of main meals
- Ask the client if they have recalled everything, or if there is anything they are not sure of

Food recall and log data can be analyzed using several different computer diet-analysis programs, performed manually using food-composition tables, or through easily downloadable mobile applications. Websites, including cronometer.com and myfitnesspal.com, provide a detailed breakdown of foods' energy and nutrient composition. These resources compare nutrient intake with current food recommendations and identifies possible deficiencies that may negatively influence health. Once the data is compiled, it needs interpreting for both quantifiable and non-quantifiable information. Quantifiable information includes the food source and nutrient contents as it indicates total energy. Non-quantifiable information would include location of meal, why it was selected, and the time it was consumed. Both types of data are useful in identifying intake and food-selection patterns or habits.

The data should be evaluated for energy content, energy nutrient distribution, quality food choices, variety, and nutrient balance. Although the total caloric intake will be used in determining energy balance, nutrient quantities should also be closely evaluated for health purposes. These nutrients can paint a broader picture of the diet's value as it pertains to health and may provide details that are useful to subsequent weight-management strategies and recommendations. A diet high in fat, sugar, and processed carbohydrates will likely contribute as much to dietary problems as excess calories.

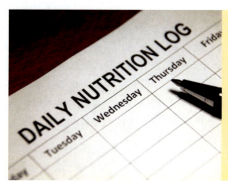

Basic Nutrients to Evaluate
- Percentage of Calories
- Carbohydrates
- Sugar
- Fats
- Proteins
- Saturated fat

Additional Nutrients
- Cholesterol
- Fiber
- Sodium
- Calcium
- Iron
- Water

DEFINITIONS

Total daily energy expenditure –

A measure of the calories expended over a day, often estimated in order to identify daily intake needs.

Thermic effect of food –

The caloric cost above the resting metabolic rate due to digestion and processing of food.

RMR predictions are founded on the principles that:

- *RMR is proportionate to body size*
- *RMR decreases with age*
- *Muscle is more metabolically active than fat*

◆ Metabolism

Identifying caloric intake provides information for half of the energy-balance equation. The next step in completing the evaluation involves determining the total **daily energy expenditure** (**TDEE**). Daily caloric expenditure is calculated by adding an individual's RMR and their voluntary metabolism, created from daily activity participation and the **thermic effect of food** (**TEF**). The sum of the two measures constitutes an individual's daily need. Daily need reflects the number of calories required for an isocaloric, (neutral) balance, representing the quantity of calories needed for weight maintenance.

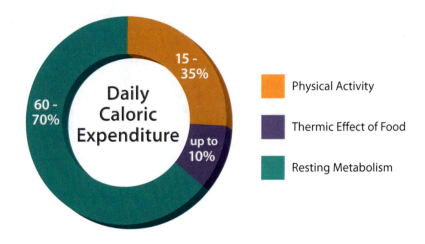

Resting Metabolic Rate

RMR generally represents between 60-70% of the total caloric expenditure in a given day. It is defined as the rate at which the body expends energy to support vital functions, including heart contractions, digestion, and various cellular activities. Together, these processes carry an oxygen cost of 1 MET, or metabolic equivalent [26]. Metabolic rates vary from person to person and are affected by several factors, including genetics, sex, age, height, weight, lean body mass, and hormone activity. In addition, certain conditions can cause increased metabolic activity at rest: fever, stress, starvation, recovery from exertions, and malnutrition. RMR is different than basal metabolic rate (BMR) or overnight metabolic rate. BMR reflects the caloric demands associated with sleep, which requires about 10% less oxygen (0.9 METS) when compared to being awake and resting. BMR's purpose is to lower the metabolism to vegetative state, so the body can focus on cellular recovery.

Several available methods can measure or predict human metabolic rate. In clinical environments, measurements are most commonly performed using indirect calorimetry. Indirect calorimetry uses respiratory measurements of oxygen consumption and carbon dioxide production to calculate caloric expenditure. Although more accurate than predictive equations, the technique is not always practical for exercise professionals because the equipment needed to perform the analysis and a complete understanding of the scientific protocol are not readily available or easy to employ. For logistical purposes, metabolic rate is more commonly predicted from equations. The use of equations to predict RMR allows for close estimations based on known factors.

This relationship is reflected in all equations used to predict RMR. Three commonly used

RMR equations are the Cunningham Lean Mass Equation, Revised Harris-Benedict Equations, and the Mifflin-St Jeor Equation.

The Cunningham Lean Mass Equation can predict RMR when an individual's body composition has been measured and accurately identified. It is not sex specific, as it is calculated by the relative lean mass of an individual, and therefore does not require adjustment for sex-specific differences in fat storage. The value derived from the Cunningham Equation is useful for weight-loss or weight-gain programs because its focus is on the metabolically active lean mass. Identifying and using the quantity of lean mass in the calculation strengthens the prediction of the Cunningham Equation. This is accomplished by reducing the overestimation of RMR found in other equations that use total body weight but do not account for the different contributions of fat mass and fat free mass on metabolism. One limiting factor of the Cunningham Equation is that it does not account for age, which is known to affect metabolism independently of lean mass. Therefore, the predicted value will be more accurate for younger individuals, as this is the population on which it was established.

The Revised Harris-Benedict or Mifflin-St Jeor equations may be more appropriate when lean mass cannot be accurately determined. Unlike the Cunningham Lean Mass Equation, the Harris-Benedict and Mifflin-St Jeor equations are multifactorial, utilizing sex, weight, height, and age to individualize the prediction and account for specific variations. Although it does not differentiate lean mass from fat mass, the equation does use weight and height based on predictive norms for body composition for a given age, and additionally, uses separate sex-specific equations. It is important to note, as with most equations in science, that the calculation in both equations uses the metric system.

RMR represents the largest portion of caloric need but does not completely cover the total daily caloric need. Physical activity generally accounts for 20-30% of a person's daily expenditure but may be even higher among athletes and certain fitness enthusiasts [33, 44]. This value contributes the most variability in total caloric need, and therefore can be the most readily manipulated with the goal of increasing caloric expenditure. Estimating the average energy expenditure related to physical activity can increase error unless it is measured using more direct means. Activity multipliers have been developed to approximate daily need based on daily activity norms. When using the equations to predict daily need, estimates of **calories-per-kilogram** of bodyweight have been established to enhance the prediction's accuracy. Standard deviations of the RMR predictions are usually between 100-200 kcal, which may increase to 300-400 if an inappropriate activity multiplier is selected [19].

Cunningham Lean Mass Equation

RMR = (21.6 × Fat Free Mass in Kilograms) + 370

Example

42 year old female weighing 142 lbs with 24% body fat
142 lbs × .24 = 34 lbs of fat mass
142 lbs − 34 lbs of fat mass = 108 lbs (fat free mass)
108 lbs ÷ 2.2 = 49 kg
RMR = (21.6 × 49 kg) + 370 = 1,428 Calories

Revised Harris Benedict Equations

Males: 66 + (5 × ht) + (13.8 × wt) − (6.8 × age)
Females: 655 + (1.8 × ht) + (9.6 × wt) − (4.7 × age)

- RMR expressed in kilocalories per day
- ht (height) expressed in centimeters
- wt (weight) expressed in kilograms
- age expressed in years

Example Conversions

215 pound male subject
215 ÷ 2.2 lb/kg = 97.7 kg

Sample 6 ft. tall subject
6 ft × 12 inches/ft = 72 inches
72 inches × 2.54 cm/in = 182.9 cm

Sample subject's RMR calculation
RMR = 66 + (5 × ht) + (13.8 × wt) − (6.8 × age)
RMR = 66 + (5 × 182.9) + (13.8 × 97.7) − (6.8 × 50)
RMR = 1,988 kcal per day

Mifflin-St Jeor Equations

Males: (10 × w) + (6.25 × h) − (5 × a) + 5
Females: (10 × w) + (6.25 × h) − (5 × a) − 161

- w = weight in kg (1 pound = 0.45359237 kilograms)
- h = height in cm (1 inch = 2.54 centimeters)
- a = age (in years)

DEFINITIONS

RMR equations – Formulas that incorporate measures of body size and/or body composition used to estimate the caloric expenditure at rest across a 24-hour period.

Calories-per-kilogram – The simplest estimate of caloric needs based solely upon body weight; typical standards are 25 to 30 kcals/kg/day for normal, healthy individuals.

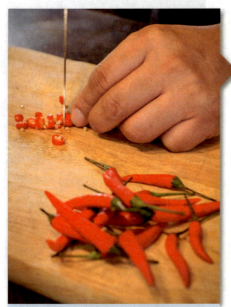

Complex carbohydrates, including whole grains and vegetables, spicy foods high in capsaicin, such as hot peppers, and lean proteins, can all promote increases in daily metabolism.

DEFINITIONS

Thermogenesis –

The process of heat production; quantified by units of kilocalories in human metabolism.

As mentioned earlier, another contributing factor to voluntary metabolism is the TEF or dietary-induced **thermogenesis**. It has been well documented that increasing caloric intake heightens metabolic functions related to digestion, transportation, and nutrient assimilation. More complex foods, foods rich in fiber, digestion-resistant starch, and foods high in capsaicin, like hot peppers, cause increases in metabolic rate above that of the normal American diet [35, 67]. Lean proteins, vegetables, and whole grains are more difficult to break down, and consequently, require more energy to digest. Depending on the diet's contents, the TEF accounts for approximately 5-10% of caloric expenditure [63]. The additional heat produced from the TEF can contribute as much as 12% to total caloric expenditure. Eating a lean diet high in complex carbohydrates, fruits, and vegetables helps contribute to weight loss through these mechanisms.

Subtracting caloric expenditure from caloric intake will provide the energy balance. This important numeric value represents a predictable physiological outcome for the body. For instance, if a person were to consume 2,500 kcal in a day and then expend 2,200 through TDEE, he or she would be said to carry a positive caloric balance, as the net gain for the day reflects a positive difference of 300 kcal. Generally, if this individual continually experiences a positive caloric balance, he or she will gain weight unless some genetically independent variable accounts for the difference. Where this excess energy is stored within the body will depend on the individual's activity and when the food is consumed. If stored as fat, each pound requires 3,500 kcals, whereas lean mass requires 2,500 kcal per pound. Gains in lean mass occur with participation in rigorous, high-volume resistance training, and appropriately timed energy consumption above that of TDEE. An individual who experiences positive caloric balance without the addition of routine resistance exercise will likely gain fat mass at a rate consistent with his or her genetic predisposition.

QUICK INSIGHT

Most people will experience a slight increase in their metabolism when overeating, which is partly due to a response to the food's thermic effect. But this acute adjustment does not completely prevent the potential for weight gain. Individuals who do not dramatically overeat but routinely maintain a positive caloric balance can gain 5 lbs. of weight in a single year; this is often associated with choosing poor food, eating too much in the evening, and getting insufficient physical activity. Creeping obesity refers to the gradual increase in weight from a positive caloric balance as a person ages. It is anecdotally recognized by individuals who have gained a significant amount of weight since their young adult years, without a dramatic (perceived) change in lifestyle.

Creeping Obesity

One Pound Fat Mass = 3,500 kcals

Daily Caloric Need = 2,200 kcals

Daily Caloric Expenditure = 2,100 kcals

Positive 100 kcal/day

•

100 kcal/day × 365 days/year = 36,500 kcals per year

36,500 kcals per year ÷ 3,500 kcals per lb of fat =

10.4 lbs of fat per year

Metabolism depends on how much oxygen the body needs each day. Therefore, the factors that affect the amount of oxygen used can be manipulated to increase a person's net caloric expenditure. RMR is primarily dependent upon a person's size, or more importantly, relative lean mass. Engaging in activities that promote lean mass maintenance or muscle hypertrophy can enhance metabolic expenditure. It is estimated that one pound of active lean mass represents 11-15 calories of expenditure per day among physically active adults. A two-pound addition of lean mass can equate to more than 5,000 additional kcal expended per year among active individuals. Muscle that is not used for work contributes only 6 kcal each day per pound.

Physical activity can represent more than a third of caloric need when intense work is performed. Increasing the physical demands on the body through exercise or adding more activity throughout the day will increase metabolism, simply due to the energy required to support the activity. When vigorous exercise becomes routine, post-exercise recovery demands also increase metabolic function. Excess post-exercise oxygen consumption (EPOC) can contribute positively to mean daily metabolic rate. Intense total body loading using resistance-type exercise and high-intensity, anaerobic-based conditioning impact EPOC the most (6, 48). By comparison, aerobic exercise has a limited effect. The combination of resistance training, routine high-intensity exercise, and a healthy diet rich in complex foods can cause a person's mean metabolism to increase dramatically. Although RMR is approximately 40% uncontrollable, 60% can be manipulated for improved metabolic fitness.

◆ Weight Management Strategies

When effective weight management strategies target weight loss, the energy balance is tipped to the negative side. Most people utilize dietary adjustment as a single means to create a caloric deficit. But, in countless clinical trials, dieting, independent of other lifestyle changes, has proven to be ineffective for long-term weight management. Many dieters also fail to realize that food nutrient content and timing, together, play an important role in the influence hormones have over metabolic outcomes. To assume that a negative balance is exclusively responsible for fat loss is inaccurate and a common misconception. For fat weight to be reduced, diet + nutrient timing + physical activity must all be part of the equation.

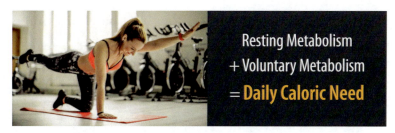

Resting Metabolism + Voluntary Metabolism = **Daily Caloric Need**

The factors that cause weight gain are the same variables that must be controlled for successful weight loss. These variables fall into three primary areas: type and quantity of energy expenditure, type and timing of energy input, and lifestyle behaviors' influence. Each area alone contributes to weight loss or weight gain, but when employed in a unified manner, they present a compound effect that is far more efficacious than when applied independently. Energy output includes all actions that expend calories, including RMR, diet-induced thermogenesis (TEF), daily physical activity, and structured exercise. Energy input includes all energy that enters the body, the form the energy is in, and the specific quantities that are ingested at a given time. In a related vein, influential lifestyle behaviors are all actions that affect the previous two categories.

Variables that must be controlled for successful weight loss include:

Energy output	Energy input	Influential lifestyle behaviors
• RMR • Diet-induced thermogenesis • Daily activity • Structured exercise	• All energy that enters the body • Forms of energy intake • Specific quantities and intake patterns	• Actions that affect input and output

Increasing physical activity in general relates importantly to total caloric output. The most sedentary individuals, outside of the 30-40 minutes of exercise they perform three days a week, may actually have a greater risk for weight gain than those who do not engage in any structured exercise but are physically active throughout most days of the week. This phenomenon occurs because the mean caloric output is higher with ongoing activity than it is with intermittent exercise engagement. This explains why a person who is sedentary at work but follows a structured exercise program may not lose weight, as energy balance is comprised of the sum of the total energy expended throughout the day. In fact, most research agrees that, when using exercise as the key aspect to weight management, a person must complete more than 225 minutes of moderate to vigorous activity a week and that number elevates for notable weight loss among adults.

Expected Initial Weight Loss and Possibility of Producing Clinically-Significant Weight Loss from Different Exercise Modalities[54]

Modality	Weight Loss	Clinically-Significant Weight Loss
Pedometer-based step goal	Range: 0 to 1 kg of weight loss	Unlikely
Aerobic exercise training only	Range: 0 to 2 kg of weight loss	Possible, but only with extremely high exercise volumes
Resistance training only	None	Unlikely
Aerobic and resistance training only	Range: 0 to 2 kg of weight loss	Possible, but only with extremely high volumes of aerobic exercise training
Caloric restriction combined with aerobic exercise training	Range: 9 to 13 kg of weight loss	Possible

Combining structured exercise with regular physical activity improves caloric expenditure dramatically compared to exercise alone. Physical activity can be added into any lifestyle at varying dosages based upon the situation. Biking instead of driving, using the stairs instead of the elevator, and playing tennis instead of going to the movies all exemplify ways to infuse physical activity into an everyday lifestyle.

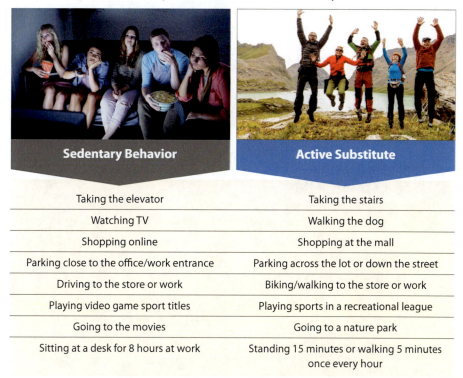

Physical Activity Substitutes for Sedentary Behaviors

Sedentary Behavior	Active Substitute
Taking the elevator	Taking the stairs
Watching TV	Walking the dog
Shopping online	Shopping at the mall
Parking close to the office/work entrance	Parking across the lot or down the street
Driving to the store or work	Biking/walking to the store or work
Playing video game sport titles	Playing sports in a recreational league
Going to the movies	Going to a nature park
Sitting at a desk for 8 hours at work	Standing 15 minutes or walking 5 minutes once every hour

Structured exercise prescribed for weight loss should emphasize continuous activity aimed at maximal caloric expenditure and total body loading. The body burns far fewer calories at rest or stopped than when it is moving. For this reason, aerobic activity is often the first type of activity introduced as a weight loss treatment. Continuous aerobic activity can contribute to significant expenditure when performed at appropriate intensity and duration, especially for someone that has been completely sedentary. However, a common theme among aerobic exercisers is that they do not lose weight. Simply performing an act does not guarantee an outcome. This is also true of resistance exercise, which has been shown to be the most effective training variable when accounting for active lean-mass growth and maintenance. Evaluating levels of training intensity among gym goers shows that the average work intensity fell well below levels necessary for overload-based adaptations. Many individuals expect participation to be adequate for the desired outcomes, which is clearly wrong: the intensity with which the exercise is performed is the most important variable. While continuous exercise is needed for caloric expenditure, resistance training is needed for lean-mass maintenance, suggesting a combination approach is most appropriate for those wishing to decrease their fat stores.

For an exercise plan to yield the greatest contribution to a negative caloric balance, the focus should be on performing the maximum amount of work in the allotted time. Ideally, the actions and modalities used for exercise aimed at weight loss should include both resistance training and aerobic activities. High-intensity interval training, high-intensity (resistance) circuits, and intermittent high intensity total body weight-training stations have all demonstrated positive effects yielding desirable adaptations for fat loss. For newer exercisers, bodyweight activities can be combined initially to form a complete exercise program that flows with minimal transitional rest and low risk for training-based injuries. Aerobic training, resistance training, and flexibility routines can be strategically combined throughout the workout via various techniques to use the full amount of workout time. Maximizing the use of time available for structured activity is a key component of any exercise-related weight-loss strategy, as is progressively increasing training intensity. Individuals who reach elevated levels of fitness burn even more calories during the exercise bout, primarily due to an ability to handle higher exercise intensities for longer durations. The contribution of post-exercise metabolism encouraged by high-intensity training also warrants attention, as it enhances fat utilization throughout the body [7].

Strategies related to energy input for weight loss:

- Prepare food rather than eating out.
- Prepare smaller quantities of food for each meal.
- Eat smaller meals more frequently.
- Place small portions on the serving plate during a meal and wait two minutes before having additional servings; serve food from the kitchen rather than family-style.
- Replace processed foods with whole fruits and vegetables.
- Carry healthy snacks to avoid feeling hungry.
- Use smaller serving containers.
- Avoid close proximity to snack trays and buffet tables.
- Eat slowly during each meal.
- Avoid long periods between meals.
- Be conscious of beverage calories.
- Shop from a premeditated grocery list.
- Select low-calorie or reduced-fat sauces and dressings.
- Serve whole fruits for dessert.
- Offer low-calorie appetizers at social events.
- Do not be overly restrictive of foods; eat in moderation.
- Communicate to others that you are focusing on calorie control.

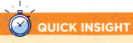

QUICK INSIGHT

SPOT REDUCTION

Weight loss will occur as the body dictates, as determined by the caloric restriction's severity, total energy expenditure, and the individual's genetic predisposition. Exercise cannot dictate lipid metabolism in any particular area. Therefore, what is commonly referred to as "spot reduction" is not possible in humans. Emphasizing leg training will not ensure lower-extremity body-fat loss, just as performing abdominal work will not increase lipid use or fat reduction around the trunk. In general, fat loss patterns are controlled via genetic predisposition rather than by the areas exercised. For example, running may cause one person to initially lose fat around the abdomen, whereas a different person may experience body fat changes in the lower body.

Ineffective gimmicks, novel modalities, pills, and "special exercises" aimed at spot reduction include ab isolation machines, low-frequency electrode units, sweat-suit devices, specialized cardiovascular machines, and cellulite creams. For fat loss to occur, the body must attain a negative caloric balance while maintaining adequate energy to prevent lean mass loss. Essentially, the best advice is to eat less, at the right times, and exercise intensely.

Stress, Social Behaviors, and Weight Management

Adjustments to diet and physical activity compose part of behavioral modification strategies, but they do not represent the full spectrum of behavioral considerations. Stress and social behaviors both affect weight management outcomes, albeit through different means. Unregulated emotional or psychological stress causes adrenal corticoids to be released, increasing available energy: this is a primal response, termed fight or flight. Cortisol functions to provide readily available energy by promoting the breakdown of fat at adipocytes, increasing glucose output from the liver, and breaking down lean tissue to provide substrates for further glucose production. This fuel is meant to support the physical activity required for dire survival situations. However, in modern times, stress often exists without a need for any primal physical action. This chronic stress is associated with overeating, increased substance abuse, and poor sleeping patterns, all of which associate with increases in unwanted body fat. In addition, stress can also increase lipid storage proximal to the liver, increasing visceral fat [4, 5]. Avoiding stress when one can or employing beneficial coping strategies to better manage it reduces its detrimental effects on the body. To properly manage tension, one must know where the potential for stress exists. A complete stress-management approach must be part of any weight management plan and should either create viable strategies to cope with stress or alter the environment to reduce its severity or impact.

Social behaviors do not affect weight management through hormonal means but can present obstacles to diet and physical activity adherence. As stated earlier, social activities often promote increased caloric consumption and are usually not activities that are physical in nature. This increases the likelihood that a positive energy balance will supplant the potential negative contributions of the diet and exercise program to weight loss. Additionally, social environments commonly feature alcohol consumption, which facilitates a feeling of relaxation for many Americans after a long day. At seven (7) kcal per gram, the caloric density of alcohol rivals that of fat but is worse metabolically: it is not a necessary nutrient but actually a weak poison. Alcoholic beverages range between 100 kcals in a light beer to mixed drinks like margaritas and long island teas that can provide a whopping 600 kcals per drink. Four or five alcohol-containing beverages over a weekend can potentially add more calories than are burned in four prior workouts during the week. Likewise, the foods served with alcohol are usually not prepared with health in mind and are also commonly high in calories. Bar foods are high in fat and calories and foods consumed with alcohol have a greater propensity to be stored as lipids compared to when ingested without the presence of alcohol. Few people realize a beer belly is actually metabolically derived: since alcohol buildup in the body will potentially lead to death, the body preferentially metabolizes it first, with absorption starting in the stomach.

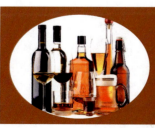

Alcohol use causes three issues:
- Fat oxidation is inhibited in the presence of alcohol.
- Other foods entering circulation are steered toward fat storage.
- Alcohol inhibits protein synthesis (doubly detrimental for trying to maintain or lose weight).

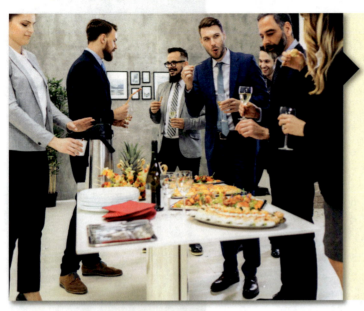

Strategies to Avoid Poor Food Choices and Behaviors When in Social Environments

- Never go out hungry; consume healthy, low-calorie foods before going out.
- Drink water or low-calorie beverages between alcohol-containing beverages.
- Avoid close proximity to high-calorie snack foods.
- Select healthy food choices before committing to bad food choice decisions.
- Try to find social activities that include physical activity or a reduced emphasis on food and drink as the main form of entertainment.
- Add ten minutes of cardiovascular activity for each alcoholic beverage consumed to negate the empty calories.

To reduce the consequences of social behavior for weight loss, alternatives or compensatory actions should be considered. If high caloric consumption is a problem for a client, the personal trainer should devise a plan centered on preventative action. Asking people to stop engaging in socially stimulating environments is likely to end in failure, and in many cases is professionally inappropriate. However, the trainer should educate the client, add accountability, and teach other ways to avoid these pitfalls. Providing strategies to avoid poor food choices and behaviors when in social situations will help reduce the impact of these events. One strategy that has worked is to create a team or provide a medium for social access to individuals with common goals. Setting up group events around activity causes a double benefit among group participants. Avoiding the pitfalls that present as common obstacles to success should be a strategic focus.

QUICK INSIGHT

FAD DIETS

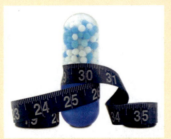

The dramatic elevations in body weight throughout the American population have also dramatically increased the popularity of fad diets. Consumers are bombarded with quick weight loss schemes fueled by media promotion, easy money opportunities for celebrities, and by companies selling the misconception that weight can be reduced quickly with minimal effort. New books and remedies guaranteeing effective weight loss keep the market flooded, routinely driving the message that viable alternatives to caloric restriction and exercise for weight management exist. It should be obvious that singling out a particular energy nutrient or engaging in extreme changes does not work. If any single method did work, only one diet book or strategy would be needed and everyone would gravitate towards it. Some common indications of unsound weight loss promotions include:

- Weight loss due to a "special" supplement or secret ingredients
- Rapid or dramatic results
- A diet advertised as working without exercise
- Emphasis on short-term change
- Dramatic changes to normal patterns
- Celebrity, athlete, or "doctor" endorsed
- Claims of research such as "independent studies prove"
- Claims to replace, or add to, metabolic or hormone function
- Emphasis on one nutrient or limited food choices
- Lack of emphasis on caloric reduction and behavior modification
- Assertion claiming to reduce cellulite or fat in specific locations
- Warnings that if it works "too well" to reduce the dose

◆ Weight Gain

Not every person wants to lose weight. For some people, gaining weight is just as challenging as losing weight is for others. Proper weight gain is accomplished in the same manner as proper weight loss; however, instead of a negative caloric balance, the emphasis falls on intelligently creating a positive energy balance. Seemingly, a positive caloric balance would be easily attained by simply eating high-calorie food; unfortunately, this method often works to increase total body weight but commonly leads to fat gain, rather than added lean mass. Intentional weight gain should come from lean mass, which requires a slower process, as hypertrophy and the synthesis of lean mass is much more complex than storing adipose tissue. This is true because the body resists muscle gain to a certain extent: it is a conservative machine that only uses what is necessary to deal with the stresses placed upon it. Without the use of anabolic drugs, notable increases in lean mass take months to years to accomplish in healthy, trained adults.

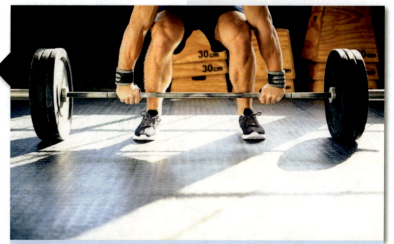

Weight gain goals are often vanity or performance-based; in some cases, however, they are necessary among individuals recovering from a debilitating disease or getting ready for surgery or disease treatment.

Weight gain goals are often vanity or performance based; however, sometimes gaining is necessary, especially in patients that are recovering from a debilitating disease or preparing for surgery or treatment. Healthy weight gain works on an incremental basis, which is inversely consistent with weight loss. If done aggressively, both approaches will yield consequential results. Diets emphasizing excess calorie reduction frequently cause lean mass loss, while diets employing excess caloric consumption cause an increase in fat mass. To avoid both scenarios, controlled changes in the diet and meaningful training activities will provide for the proper tissue adaptation. Weight gain attempts must emphasize hypertrophy training combined with prudent caloric additions to the diet. Adding 150-300 kcal per day with a focus on appropriate protein timing should be sufficient to encourage lean mass increase when joined with hypertrophy training [8]. Recommendations can be more aggressive for individuals who find it extremely difficult to gain weight. For lean individuals who are physiologically resistant to weight gain, it is recommended to employ heavy resistance training with an addition of 500-750 kcals of carbohydrates and protein timed around training [46, 51]. Body composition should be monitored and tracked along with caloric intake to identify variations associated with excess or insufficient intakes.

Protein should represent the majority of the additional calories in the diet, as long as the value stays within the 1.6-2.0 grams-per-kilogram of body weight upper limit. If additional calories are required, they should come from nutrient-dense carbohydrates, such as vegetables and plants, that contain strong phytonutrients and healthy fats. Foods composed of saturated fats are not a good choice as they can lead to an increased risk for negative blood lipid profile adjustments, even without weight gain. Feeding throughout the day, of about 0.3 grams-per-kilogram of body weight after key exercise sessions and every 3-4 hours throughout the day, may also positively contribute to the weight gain goals [9, 38]. For individuals who find it difficult to eat frequently, meal supplements and shakes may aid in fulfilling the calorie requirements. If protein supplements are used, whey protein is ideal for post-exercise consumption and casein protein can be used at night due to its slower absorption rate. Personal preferences will ultimately define the ideal dietary strategy.

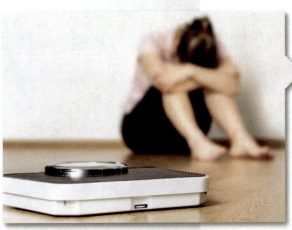

◆ Feeding and Eating Disorders

Whenever clients attempt weight loss, exercise professionals should consciously identify inappropriate behaviors. Disordered eating patterns are commonly associated with weight loss attempts, even in cases involving individuals educated about healthy strategies and wary of inappropriate behaviors. Two of the most common disordered eating patterns include avoidant, or restricted, eating and binge-eating behaviors. Although both behaviors characterize psychiatrically defined and diagnosed eating disorders, individuals who engage in these behaviors are not necessarily suffering from a psychiatric disorder. Hoping to accelerate weight loss, individuals attempting to control calories often engage in episodes of severe restriction. This may be to compensate for overeating, to cause a negative caloric balance, or to prepare for an event characterized by high energy intake. Not uncommonly, people intentionally do not eat all day, knowing they have a party that evening that will provide an abundance of food and drink.

While intermittent fasting has merits, severe restriction promotes an acute internal metabolic milieu, causing a catabolic environment that promotes lean mass loss. Restriction is also likely to lead to rebound bingeing due to a hypothalamic-derived reaction: eating due to the psychological wear on the body from prolonged physiological signals of hunger. Binge eating occurs when people engage in recurring episodes involving consuming large quantities of food very quickly. This commonly occurs due to the stress and fatigue of aggressive dieting or a temporary emotional lapse. For this reason, weight loss should be part of lifestyle changes that are not aggressively applied. Small, consistent changes do not cause significant stress on a person's normal behavior patterns and are thus less likely to trigger an event. When disordered eating patterns become routine, the behaviors may be psychologically motivated beyond the individual's control. Feeding and eating disorders can start from attempts at weight modification that grow into damaging physiological patterns with roots in more significant underlying psychopathology. Feeding and eating disorders are classified as psychological disorders by the American Psychological Association (APA) due to their potential for harm. They are complex, multifaceted conditions that presumably stem from internal conflict and biochemical variations in the brain [18]. Unmet personal needs and issues of control are often linked to compensatory eating behaviors that attempt to cope with the emotional dysfunctions [18].

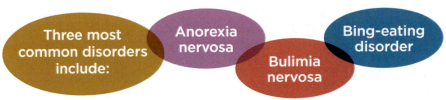

Three most common disorders include: Anorexia nervosa, Bulimia nervosa, Bing-eating disorder

Each has a specific diagnostic criteria listed in the Diagnostic and Statistical Manual of Mental Disorders (DSM) of the APA [3]. A stereotypical physical characteristic does not exist for people with eating disorders except for severe, later-stage anorexia, where a person is visibly emaciated. A person may be of normal weight or even overweight and suffer from the afflictions of any one of the above disorders.

Anorexia Nervosa

Anorexia is probably the most well-known eating disorder. It is characterized by a significant body image disorder, intense fear of becoming fat, and a preoccupation with weight [14].

Although anorexia is most commonly diagnosed in females, nearly 8% of anorexics are male [57]. Anorexia's most obvious symptoms include severe weight loss from caloric restriction, strict dietary practices, and heavy exercise participation. Although anorexics may engage in other compensatory activities, including vomiting and laxative use, caloric restriction is most common [3]. Anorexia is a serious condition that has the highest rate of mortality among psychiatric disorders [64]. It has been reported that 20% of the mortality cases were from suicide [2]. Exercise professionals who suspect an individual may suffer from the disorder should discuss it with the client and recommend counseling. Due to the severity of the disorder, for clients under 18 years of age, the exercise professional should share the suspicions with the individual's designated emergency contact person. The trainer must understand with whom it is appropriate and legal to talk with about the suspected disorder. Individuals suffering from anorexia will not be able to cure themselves and, therefore, require psychological counseling or medical intervention.

Bulimia Nervosa

Bulimia nervosa is more difficult to identify than anorexia because it is shadowed in secrecy; in fact, many bulimics maintain normal weight or may be just slightly overweight [39]. Bulimia is often characterized by binge-eating and purging, seen in about 80% of the cases, or inappropriate compensatory actions, including heavy use of diet pills and laxatives. Illicit drug use is also more common with bulimic conditions. Weight changes may be limited in bulimics, so symptomatic identification is difficult. Estimates suggest that between 1-3% of the population is bulimic, with females showing a greater propensity for the disorder, representing 9 out of every 10 cases [3]. Bulimics may experience episodes of severe compensatory behavior followed by periods of reduced symptomatic activity. Low self-esteem and body dissatisfaction are connected to weight, so body image often dictates the severity of the behavior. Those with anxiety disorders, mood disorders, and who struggle with impulse control are most at risk for bulimia. Fortunately, most bulimics who seek counseling do so on their own to reduce their mental suffering.

Binge-Eating Disorder

Binge-eating disorder is the most common eating disorder and involves the consumption of large amounts of food followed by feelings of guilt, depression, and low self-worth [22]. Binge episodes may occur 1-3 times per week in the mildest cases, 4–7 episodes per week in moderate, 8–13 episodes per week in severe, and extreme 14 or more episodes per week in severe cases [3]. Compensatory actions may be taken but are done so on an irregular basis. Estimates suggest that binge-eating disorder affects 1.2% of the population, including 1.6% of females and 0.8% of males [57]. Binge eaters are more likely to be overweight or obese and experience feeling that they cannot control their eating. Most binge eaters have a long history of dieting or weight loss struggle and are not happy with their bodies [3]. Caucasian women seem to represent the largest group of sufferers, but men and women of all races may suffer from the disorder.

Exercise professionals should be knowledgeable as to the signs and symptoms of feeding and eating disorders, and understand that these three, while the most common, are not the only feeding and eating disorders that exist, according to the APA (American Psychological Association). Individuals who are overly pre-occupied with exercise or feel the need to exercise every time they eat are potential candidates for these dysfunctions. Discussing concerns with clients may shed some light on the situation and help them identify negative behaviors.

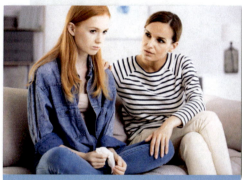

Characteristics of eating disorders:

- Body dissatisfaction
- Emphasis on body weight
- Preoccupation with food and appearance
- Avoidance of eating or noticeable overconsumption
- Depression
- Feelings of guilt, remorse, or self-loathing related to eating behavior
- Body image distortion
- Intense fear of being fat
- Use of laxatives, appetite suppressants, purging, or diuretics
- Use of illegal drugs
- Eating alone
- Exercising excessively
- Smoking cigarettes

REFERENCES:

1. Andreyeva T, Luedicke J, and Wang YC. State-level estimates of obesity-attributable costs of absenteeism. *Journal of occupational and environmental medicine/American College of Occupational and Environmental Medicine* 56: 1120, 2014.

2. Arcelus J, Mitchell AJ, Wales J, and Nielsen S. Mortality rates in patients with anorexia nervosa and other eating disorders: a meta-analysis of 36 studies. *Archives of general psychiatry* 68: 724-731, 2011.

3. Association AP. *Diagnostic and statistical manual of mental disorders (DSM-5®)*: American Psychiatric Pub, 2013.

4. Björntorp P. Do stress reactions cause abdominal obesity and comorbidities? *Obesity reviews* 2: 73-86, 2001.

5. Black PH. The inflammatory consequences of psychologic stress: relationship to insulin resistance, obesity, atherosclerosis and diabetes mellitus, type II. *Medical hypotheses* 67: 879-891, 2006.

6. Børsheim E and Bahr R. Effect of exercise intensity, duration and mode on post-exercise oxygen consumption. *Sports medicine* 33: 1037-1060, 2003.

7. Braun W, Hawthorne W, and Markofski M. Acute EPOC response in women to circuit training and treadmill exercise of matched oxygen consumption. *European journal of applied physiology* 94: 500-504, 2005.

8. Burd NA, Tang JE, Moore DR, and Phillips SM. Exercise training and protein metabolism: influences of contraction, protein intake, and sex-based differences. *Journal of applied physiology* 106: 1692-1701, 2009.

9. Burke L, Burke L, and Deakin V. *Clinical sports nutrition*: McGraw-Hill Education, 2010.

10. Clark MM, Niaura R, King TK, and Pera V. Depression, smoking, activity level, and health status: pretreatment predictors of attrition in obesity treatment. *Addictive behaviors* 21: 509-513, 1996.

11. Colles SL, Dixon JB, and O'brien PE. Loss of control is central to psychological disturbance associated with binge eating disorder. *Obesity* 16: 608-614, 2008.

12. Dagher A. The neurobiology of appetite: hunger as addiction. In: *Obesity Prevention*: Elsevier, 2010, p. 15-22.

13. Dammann KW and Smith C. Factors affecting low-income women's food choices and the perceived impact of dietary intake and socioeconomic status on their health and weight. *Journal of nutrition education and behavior* 41: 242-253, 2009.

14. Dodds W. Central Nervous System Regulation of Appetite in Humans and Pet Animals. *Ann Clin Exp Metabol* 2: 1013, 2017.

15. Drewnowski A. Energy density, palatability, and satiety: implications for weight control. *Nutrition reviews* 56: 347-353, 1998.

16. Erlanson Albertsson C. How palatable food disrupts appetite regulation. *Basic & clinical pharmacology & toxicology* 97: 61-73, 2005.

17. Estima CC, Bruening M, Hannan PJ, Alvarenga MS, Leal GV, Philippi ST, and Neumark-Sztainer D. A Cross-Cultural Comparison of Eating Behaviors and Home Food Environmental Factors in Adolescents From São Paulo (Brazil) and Saint Paul–Minneapolis (US). *Journal of nutrition education and behavior* 46: 370-375, 2014.

18. Fairburn CG and Harrison PJ. Eating disorders. *The Lancet* 361: 407-416, 2003.

19. Frankenfield DC, Rowe WA, Smith JS, and Cooney R. Validation of several established equations for resting metabolic rate in obese and nonobese people. *Journal of the American Dietetic Association* 103: 1152-1159, 2003.

20. Fuller S, Beck E, Salman H, and Tapsell L. New horizons for the study of dietary fiber and health: a review. *Plant foods for human nutrition* 71: 1-12, 2016.

21. Gostin LO. Law as a tool to facilitate healthier lifestyles and prevent obesity. *Jama* 297: 87-90, 2007.

22. Guerdjikova AI, Mori N, Casuto LS, and McElroy SL. Binge eating disorder. *Psychiatric Clinics* 40: 255-266, 2017.

23. Hales CM, Fryar CD, Carroll MD, Freedman DS, and Ogden CL. Trends in Obesity and Severe Obesity Prevalence in US Youth and Adults by Sex and Age, 2007-2008 to 2015-2016. *JAMA* 319: 1723-1725, 2018.

24. Havel PJ. Peripheral signals conveying metabolic information to the brain: short-term and long-term regulation of food intake and energy homeostasis. *Experimental Biology and Medicine* 226: 963-977, 2001.

25. Holt SH, Brand Miller JC, Petocz P, and Farmakalidis E. A satiety index of common foods. *European journal of clinical nutrition* 49: 675-690, 1995.

26. Jette M, Sidney K, and Blümchen G. Metabolic equivalents (METS) in exercise testing, exercise prescription, and evaluation of functional capacity. *Clinical cardiology* 13: 555-565, 1990.

27. Kim DD and Basu A. Estimating the medical care costs of obesity in the United States: systematic review, meta-analysis, and empirical analysis. *Value in Health* 19: 602-613, 2016.

28. Kuijer RG and Boyce JA. Chocolate cake. Guilt or celebration? Associations with healthy eating attitudes, perceived behavioural control, intentions and weight-loss. *Appetite* 74: 48-54, 2014.

29. Lee B, Lawson KM, Chang P-J, Neuendorf C, Dmitrieva NO, and Almeida DM. Leisure-time physical activity moderates the longitudinal associations between work-family spillover and physical health. *Journal of leisure research* 47: 444-466, 2015.

30. Leehr EJ, Krohmer K, Schag K, Dresler T, Zipfel S, and Giel KE. Emotion regulation model in binge eating disorder and obesity-a systematic review. *Neuroscience & Biobehavioral Reviews* 49: 125-134, 2015.

31. Levi J, Segal LM, St Laurent R, Lang A, and Rayburn J. F as in fat: how obesity threatens America's future 2012. 2012.

32. Levine DI. The Curious History of the Calorie in US Policy: A Tradition of Unfulfilled Promises. *American journal of preventive medicine* 52: 125-129, 2017.

33. Manini TM, Everhart JE, Patel KV, Schoeller DA, Colbert LH, Visser M, Tylavsky F, Bauer DC, Goodpaster BH, and Harris TB. Daily activity energy expenditure and mortality among older adults. *Jama* 296: 171-179, 2006.

34. Mattson MP, Longo VD, and Harvie M. Impact of intermittent fasting on health and disease processes. *Ageing research reviews* 39: 46-58, 2017.

35. McCarty MF, DiNicolantonio JJ, and O'keefe JH. Capsaicin may have important potential for promoting vascular and metabolic health. *Open Heart* 2: e000262, 2015.

36. Mello MM, Rimm EB, and Studdert DM. The McLawsuit: the fast-food industry and legal accountability for obesity. *Health Affairs* 22: 207-216, 2003.

37. Merritt AC, Effron DA, and Monin B. Moral self licensing: When being good frees us to be bad. *Social and personality psychology compass* 4: 344-357, 2010.

38. Moore DR, Robinson MJ, Fry JL, Tang JE, Glover EI, Wilkinson SB, Prior T, Tarnopolsky MA, and Phillips SM. Ingested protein dose response of muscle and albumin protein synthesis after resistance exercise in young men–. *The American journal of clinical nutrition* 89: 161-168, 2008.

39. Moroshko I, Brennan L, and O'Brien P. Predictors of dropout in weight loss interventions: a systematic review of the literature. *Obesity reviews* 12: 912-934, 2011.

40. Must A and Strauss RS. Risks and consequences of childhood and adolescent obesity. *International journal of obesity* 23: S2, 1999.

41. Ng M, Fleming T, Robinson M, Thomson B, Graetz N, Margono C, Mullany EC, Biryukov S, Abbafati C, and Abera SF. Global, regional, and national prevalence of overweight and obesity in children and adults during 1980–2013: a systematic analysis for the Global Burden of Disease Study 2013. *The lancet* 384: 766-781, 2014.

42. Olstad D, Teychenne M, Minaker L, Taber D, Raine K, Nykiforuk C, and Ball K. Can policy ameliorate socioeconomic inequities in obesity and obesity related behaviours? A systematic review of the impact of universal policies on adults and children. *Obesity Reviews* 17: 1198-1217, 2016.

43. Patterson RE and Sears DD. Metabolic effects of intermittent fasting. *Annual review of nutrition* 37: 371-393, 2017.

44. Pontzer H, Durazo-Arvizu R, Dugas LR, Plange-Rhule J, Bovet P, Forrester TE, Lambert EV, Cooper RS, Schoeller DA, and Luke A. Constrained total energy expenditure and metabolic adaptation to physical activity in adult humans. *Current Biology* 26: 410-417, 2016.

45. Pulgaron ER. Childhood obesity: a review of increased risk for physical and psychological comorbidities. *Clinical therapeutics* 35: A18-A32, 2013.

46. Res PT, Groen B, Pennings B, Beelen M, Wallis GA, Gijsen AP, Senden JM, and Van Loon LJ. Protein ingestion before sleep improves postexercise overnight recovery. *Medicine & Science in Sports & Exercise* 44: 1560-1569, 2012.

47. Roberto CA, Swinburn B, Hawkes C, Huang TT, Costa SA, Ashe M, Zwicker L, Cawley JH, and Brownell KD. Patchy progress on obesity prevention: emerging examples, entrenched barriers, and new thinking. *The Lancet* 385: 2400-2409, 2015.

48. Schuenke MD, Mikat RP, and McBride JM. Effect of an acute period of resistance exercise on excess post-exercise oxygen consumption: implications for body mass management. *European journal of applied physiology* 86: 411-417, 2002.

49. Shepherd R and Raats M. *The psychology of food choice*: Cabi, 2006.

50. Shortt J. Obesity—a public health dilemma. *AORN journal* 80: 1069-1078, 2004.

51. Snijders T, Smeets JS, van Vliet S, van Kranenburg J, Maase K, Kies AK, Verdijk LB, and van Loon LJ. Protein Ingestion before Sleep Increases Muscle Mass and Strength Gains during Prolonged Resistance-Type Exercise Training in Healthy Young Men–3. *The Journal of nutrition* 145: 1178-1184, 2015.

52. Sørensen LB, Møller P, Flint A, Martens M, and Raben A. Effect of sensory perception of foods on appetite and food intake: a review of studies on humans. *International journal of obesity* 27: 1152, 2003.

53. Story M, Kaphingst KM, and French S. The role of schools in obesity prevention. *The future of children*: 109-142, 2006.

54. Swift DL, Johannsen NM, Lavie CJ, Earnest CP, and Church TS. The role of exercise and physical activity in weight loss and maintenance. *Progress in cardiovascular diseases* 56: 441-447, 2014.

55. Teixeira P, Going S, Houtkooper L, Cussler E, Metcalfe L, Blew R, Sardinha L, and Lohman T. Pretreatment predictors of attrition and successful weight management in women. *International journal of obesity* 28: 1124, 2004.

56. Tsai AG and Wadden TA. The evolution of very low calorie diets: an update and meta analysis. *Obesity* 14: 1283-1293, 2006.

57. Udo T and Grilo CM. Prevalence and Correlates of DSM-5–Defined Eating Disorders in a Nationally Representative Sample of US Adults. *Biological psychiatry*, 2018.

58. van Dale D and Saris WH. Repetitive weight loss and weight regain: effects on weight reduction, resting metabolic rate, and lipolytic activity before and after exercise and/or diet treatment. *The American journal of clinical nutrition* 49: 409-416, 1989.

59. van der Klaauw AA and Farooqi IS. The hunger genes: pathways to obesity. *Cell* 161: 119-132, 2015.

60. Walker RE, Keane CR, and Burke JG. Disparities and access to healthy food in the United States: A review of food deserts literature. *Health & place* 16: 876-884, 2010.

61. Wang Y and Beydoun MA. The obesity epidemic in the United States—gender, age, socioeconomic, racial/ethnic, and geographic characteristics: a systematic review and meta-regression analysis. *Epidemiologic reviews* 29: 6-28, 2007.

62. Weiss EP, Racette SB, Villareal DT, Fontana L, Steger-May K, Schechtman KB, Klein S, Ehsani AA, Holloszy JO, and Group WUSoMC. Lower extremity muscle size and strength and aerobic capacity decrease with caloric restriction but not with exercise-induced weight loss. *Journal of Applied Physiology* 102: 634-640, 2007.

63. Westerterp K, Schoeller DA, and Westerterp-Plantenga MS. Biomarker for energy intake: resting energy expenditure and physical activity. In: *Advances in the Assessment of Dietary Intake*: CRC Press, 2017.

64. Westmoreland P, Krantz MJ, and Mehler PS. Medical complications of anorexia nervosa and bulimia. *The American journal of medicine* 129: 30-37, 2016.

65. Yeo GS and Heisler LK. Unraveling the brain regulation of appetite: lessons from genetics. *Nature neuroscience* 15: 1343, 2012.

66. Yu YH, Vasselli J, Zhang Y, Mechanick J, Korner J, and Peterli R. Metabolic vs. hedonic obesity: a conceptual distinction and its clinical implications. *obesity reviews* 16: 234-247, 2015.

67. Zsiborás C, Mátics R, Hegyi P, Balaskó M, Pétervári E, Szabó I, Sarlós P, Mikó A, Tenk J, and Rostás I. Capsaicin and capsiate could be appropriate agents for treatment of obesity: A meta-analysis of human studies. *Critical reviews in food science and nutrition* 58: 1419-1427, 2018.

Advanced Concepts of Personal Training

NCSF

Certified Personal Trainer

Chapter 12

Exercise Program Components

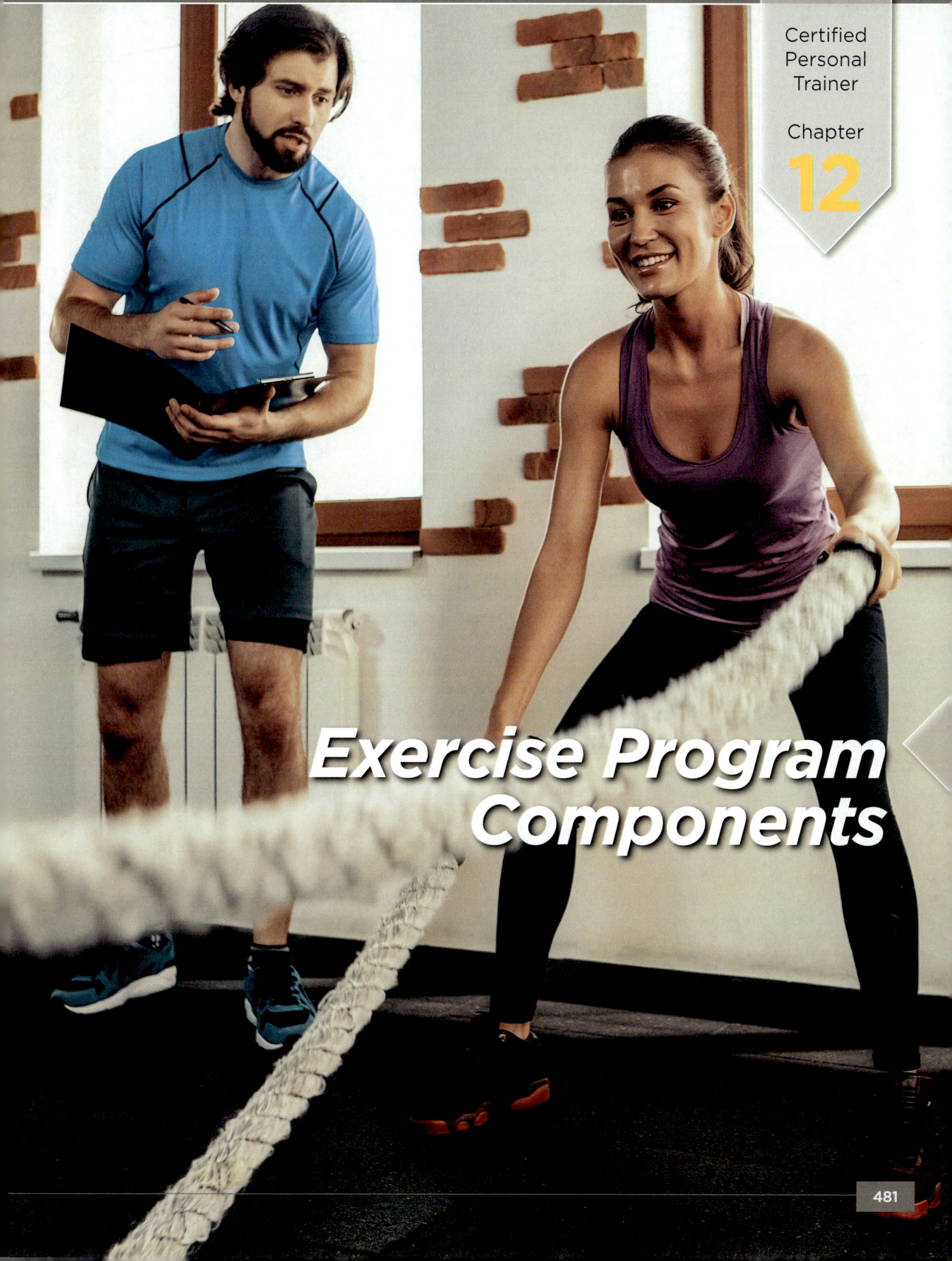

Introduction

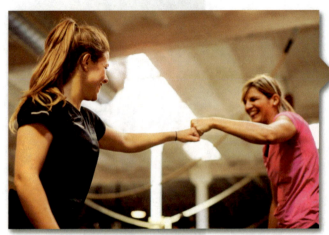

When designing accurate training programs, exercise professionals must consider all the factors and variables that will affect the individual. Designing effective programs presents a challenge because interacting stresses must be accounted for simultaneously to manage desired adaptations. A comprehensive exercise program brings together specifically designed activity components and connects them to achieve an individual's overall program goals. Understanding the body and its adaptive responses more easily yields synthesized results from the stresses the program creates. This allows more rapid goal attainment and generally improves overall outcomes.

The needs analysis stems from the interview, screening, and assessment protocols and heavily informs all program decisions. These initial findings guide the program design to effectively address the client's key needs and goals. To facilitate an efficient process, the guiding principles of exercise program design must be appropriately combined. When correctly balanced, in appropriate proportion and emphasis, they create the desired training effect.

Principles of exercise program design can include the following:

- *Progressive Preparation* – acclimating the body to more challenging work levels
- *Energy Continuum* – the predominant energy system used to fuel the work
- *Exercise Selection* – type of exercise or modality selected
- *Periodization* – phasic adaptational-based system used to maximize desired responses
- *Exercise Order* – sequence of exercises
- *Training Frequency* – number of exercise bouts per week
- *Training Duration* – length of time engaged in physical effort
- *Training Intensity* – level of effort performed relative to capabilities
- *Rest Periods* – duration of time between each physical effort
- *Training Volume* – quantity of total work performed
- *Recovery Periods* – duration of time between exercise sessions

These principles are also viewed as training variables, or components, and can be adjusted to attain the exercise program's desired effect during a particular time duration, or phase. Changes to one or more of these variables can present a completely different physiological outcome, so exercise professionals must clearly recognize the independent characteristics of each. To take it a step further, the interrelationship among variables must also be known to appropriately create a coordinated and supportive program matrix, while simultaneously preventing any conflicts that could be obstacles to adaptation. An easy way to view this program harmony is to consider each component as an ingredient in a recipe. In appropriate quantities, each ingredient complements the others to produce a predictable and desirable outcome. When imbalance or conflict among variables exists, the outcome may be neither completely predictable nor desirable when compared to the intended goal.

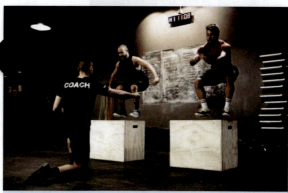

The trainer must motivate and guide the client to follow all components of the program for him or her to be able to reach their goals. One missing ingredient can spoil the entire recipe.

◆ Progressive Preparation

According to the principles of kinetics, mechanical objects function best when resistive forces are reduced or controlled. Objects moving under the duress of resistance do not have the same capacity to accelerate, whether the resistive source is friction, tension, or another constraint. The human body is no different. When body tissue is cold, it resists movement. Cold tissue presents limitations to range of motion (ROM), activation patterns, metabolism, and force production [3, 26, 27]. For the body to function optimally during activity, it must be adequately prepared for the level of stress applied. Most people understand that performing a **warm-up** should precede higher intensity physical activity; however, many individuals fail to understand the scientific rationale for this sequence and the methods necessary for optimal performance. Warm-up is a generic term that describes a preparation period prior to a designated physical activity. It has relevance for virtually any mode of physical activity, whether its intent is health, recreation, or competition. As the name implies, a warm-up increases tissue temperature prior to engaging in elevated levels of physical work.

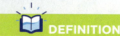 **DEFINITIONS**

Warm-up –

A period of preparation for physical activity characterized by gradual increases in heart rate, respiratory rate, metabolism and body temperature.

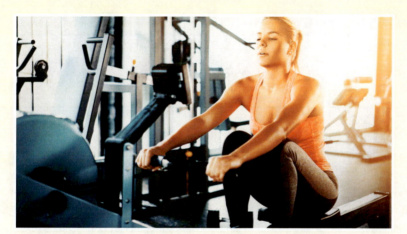

The increase in body temperature from a warm-up assists the function of tissues through several proposed physiological mechanisms, [13, 15, 20, 21, 28] including:

- Increased neural sensitivity, leading to heightened activation and acute potentiating effects.
- Greater economy of movement due to lowered viscous resistance within the active muscle.
- Increased delivery of oxygen to the muscles, since hemoglobin releases oxygen more readily at higher temperatures.
- Heightened capillary activity, causing increased cellular gas exchange.
- Increased nerve transmission, enzymatic activity, and muscle metabolism, due to the effect temperature has on accelerating the rate of bodily processes.
- Increased blood flow, which heightens metabolic processes and muscle temperature.
- Improved ROM capability, seen with increases in muscle and core temperatures.

Scientific observation has shown that increasing muscle temperature speeds the transfer of gases at the cellular level, increases blood flow through vasodilatation and the opening of dormant capillaries, lowers lactate levels, increases oxygen uptake, and increases energy metabolism within muscle [5, 17]. Arguments have been made as to whether these physiological changes reduce injury risk for individuals who employ them as a precursor to activity. That said, it is generally accepted that a warm-up will reduce activity-related injury risks (i.e., sprains, strains) and enhance performance [11, 28]. A key element that supports this notion is that muscle tissue pliability increases as muscle temperature rises and neural response time is accelerated [4, 21, 24]. This allows for increased lengthening of the musculotendinous unit and improved neuromuscular control.

A warm-up provides a further benefit as the blood flow to the cardiac muscle (heart) mirrors the activity's gradual intensity progression [33]. Moving from low to moderate and then moderate to high-intensity activity will help reduce cardiac muscle stress by reducing oxygen deficits in skeletal muscle and lowering lactate build up and reduces risk of thermal strain. This state helps prevent spikes in systolic blood pressure and lessens the risk of abnormal electrical rhythms (**cardiac arrhythmias**). Psychological enhancements accompany warm-up and the associated progressions as well. This preparation period increases mental focus and arousal, which, in turn, can facilitate enhanced motor activity [5, 30]. Directing attention to specific movements, conditions, and environments can lead to improved performance. This combination of mental and physical preparation, when applied, can effectively enhance physical capabilities.

> **DEFINITIONS**
>
> **Cardiac arrhythmias –**
>
> *A group of conditions in which the electrical impulses that coordinate myocardial contraction are disrupted, resulting in irregular, too fast, or too slow heart beats.*
>
> **Gross motor activation –**
>
> *Recruitment patterns that engage large muscle groups, often applied cyclically for locomotion.*

Warm-ups

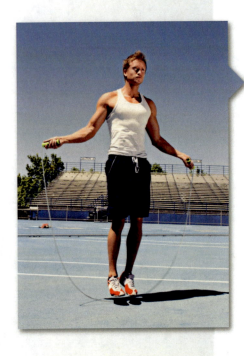

Warm-ups usually fall into one of two categories: general or specific. Each holds merit for inclusion, both before and during daily physical activity. The general warm-up is characterized by **gross motor activation**, designed to increase blood flow and temperature in the working musculature. General warm-ups often utilize basic movement patterns repeated continuously for a set period such as jogging, jumping rope, rhythmic movement patterns, and cycling. The may emphasize specific activation patterns and or mobility work depending on the goals of the exercise bout. Warm-ups usually last anywhere from five to ten minutes, depending on the individual's physical fitness level and the activity that he or she is preparing to perform. Higher-intensity activities require longer warm-up periods prior to their engagement, whereas long-duration, low-tension warm-ups tend to be shorter. The actual warm-up duration is subject to the level of intensity employed in the training. In general, anaerobic warm-ups function at a 2-3:1 (warm-up to work time ratio), whereas aerobic training is a 1:6-10. Higher intensities require significant preparation, so a 10-minute total tension period may require a 20 to 30-minute preparatory session, particularly when training above 85% of maximal intensity. This total time includes all phases of a warm-up. For example, Olympic athletes perform at the highest level and may use gradual, progressive warm-ups lasting approximately thirty minutes for optimal physiological preparation.

Specific Warm-up

Specific warm-ups attempt to utilize actions and musculature that will be used during selected activities and will often resemble, either in whole or in part, the actual activity to be completed. They effectively warm up the muscles and enhance the specific neuromuscular pathways employed by the specific motor patterns of the intense activity [6, 20]. Making use of lighter weights for high repetitions on the bench press before heavier training sets are employed is a common example. Using specific sprint mechanics and submaximal speed sprinting before attempting full-speed sprints is another. Both activities are event specific but still elicit all the aforementioned physiological and psychological responses. In either case, the goal is the same: increase performance while reducing the likelihood of injury.

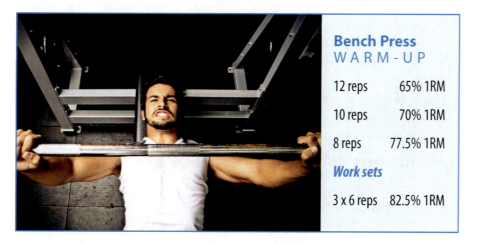

Bench Press WARM-UP

Reps	% 1RM
12 reps	65% 1RM
10 reps	70% 1RM
8 reps	77.5% 1RM
Work sets	
3 x 6 reps	82.5% 1RM

SAMPLE-SPECIFIC WARM-UPS

Bench press:
Set 1: 65% 1RM 10 reps
Set 2: 75% 1RM 8 reps
Sets 3: 5 Work sets

Sprinting:
Set 1: Speed cyle 50% - 75% - 50%
Set 2: Speed cycle 70% - 90% - 70%
Sets 3: Accelerate 80% - 100%

Performance (Sport-Specific) Warm-up

Performance-based warm-ups try to maximize the actions used during the training bout or for a sport. These types of warm-ups are not often employed for general fitness purposes, as they hone in on attainment of specific physical preparation. They include a general movement phase and a movement-specific phase, followed by a neural-specific (preparation) phase [30]. Performance warm-ups are stackable and are sometimes referred to as a staircase. They are commonly used for high-effort performance fitness and for power and strength training sessions. These activities combine continuous movement, employing large muscles with gross sport-specific movements; they are executed by gradually increasing ranges of motion, becoming more specific to the speed and energy system the activity employs. The durations often reach 15-20 minutes before transitioning into the more intense work. An example would be jumping rope for 3 minutes followed by mobility drills, then progressing to muscle activation drills, then engaging in low to moderate-intensity ballistic drills. The intensity used is often 20-25% less than that employed for the actual training. The concept is to focus on skills and motor patterns that will improve the athlete's overall performance.

Functional Warm-up

The fourth warm-up class has been termed the "functional warm-up." The functional training philosophy and its application are rooted in the physical rehabilitation setting. For decades, allied health care professionals have been using this thinking to complement other ther-

> **DEFINITIONS**
>
> **Proprioception –**
> *The ability to sense body movement and position independent of visual input.*
>
> **Movement Economy –**
> *The energy required to move at a given speed or generate a specific amount of power.*

apeutic modalities to improve movement capabilities after an injury occurrence. Functional training utilizes integrated movement patterns that elicit increased joint stability, enhancing **proprioception** while improving energy transfer in the kinetic chain. The goal is to create a more stable and functional joint for improved **movement economy** and mechanical performance. Fitness professionals can, and have, applied this concept to training routines that promote enhanced responses and movement efficiency. Essentially, this mode employs a compilation of mobility, activation, and stability-based exercises selected to meet the needs of the individual.

Applying the functional training concept to the warm-up component presents several advantages. First, the activities accomplish many of the same physiological and psychological benefits as (traditional) general and specific warm-ups but with the added benefit of functional enhancement, including improved posture and movement proficiency. Secondly, the functional warm-up addresses the ever-present injury prevention and spinal-function concerns of sound fitness programming. Although some of the activities employed within a functional warm-up may not fully present in an integrated approach, they can be designated with the term functional because they prevent injury and promote stability. Further clarification and exploration of integrated functional training techniques and the functional training paradigm will be covered under functional resistance training.

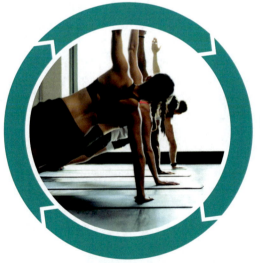

Sample Functional Warm-up in Circuit Format

Phase One
Low-Level Aerobic Activities
Examples: walking, biking, marching
Duration: 3 minutes

Phase Two
Rotator Cuff Activities
Examples: internal, external rotation with resistive bands
Duration: 2 - 4 sets

Phase Three
Abdominal Activities
Examples: crunch, physioball reverse curl-up
Duration: 2 - 4 sets

Phase Four
Low Back Activities
Examples: bridging, back extensions
Duration: 2 - 4 sets

To be classified as a warm-up activity, the actions prescribed should be directed at continuous movement. Walking on a treadmill is continuous, but provides limited value. For instructor-led training sessions or for those with time constraints, this does not constitute a good use of time. A progressive, functional warm-up addresses several areas of need simultaneously, including joint mobility, improved movement proficiency and improved muscle activation patterns. For most people, these areas are a priority and should take precedence over a 10-minute warm-up of walking or biking.

Due to the fact that exercise professionals must show results for their clients' time and money, trainers often neglect activities directed at improving function for actions that will elicit a visual change. Problems arise when underemphasizing certain areas leads to some level of debilitation or deficiency. Back pain, shoulder problems, and similar ailments reduce training participation and effectiveness. Thus, exercise professionals should use warm-up time to address preventative action, while keeping in mind the role of the warm-up in physiological preparation. Utilizing exercises in a **circuit** enables multiple activities to function in a structured format with continuous movement, integrating the specifically designed warm-up effects (e.g., temperature) with the purposes of the functional training model.

> **DEFINITIONS**
>
> Circuit –
>
> *A training method of performing a sequence of exercises across several stations, usually incorporating minimal rest intervals.*

Functional Warm-up Circuits

Circuit 1	2x	Circuit 2	2x
Good morning	12	Good morning w/IYT reach	9
Step back w/OH reach	6/side	Rev lunge w/rotation	6/side
Lateral squat	6/side	Lateral ground sweeps	6/side

ONLINE VIDEO INSTRUCTION

◆ Designing Warm-ups

Any program component should be based on the client's personal profile and needs. This also holds true of warm-up activities. Deciding on the right movement preparation for the client will be based on the intended goal, the training experience, the client's current physical capabilities, and the exercise bout's specific requirements. In some cases, the traditional general warm-up may be most appropriate for a client being introduced to exercise. On the other hand, an experienced exerciser may need a more aggressive preparation due to the higher level of intensity used in his or her training routine. It is not uncommon for some warm-ups to reach intensities that are greater than a new exerciser's entire workout. The movements and level of difficulty should mirror the capabilities of the client while still emphasizing the warm-up concept and purpose.

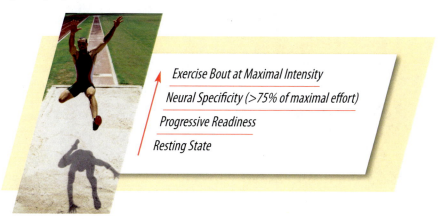

Exercise Bout at Maximal Intensity
Neural Specificity (>75% of maximal effort)
Progressive Readiness
Resting State

Likewise, the specific activities an exercise professional selects to incorporate into the warm-up depend upon several factors often stemming from the activity being used in the current or future exercise session. Warm-up modalities and exercises vary regarding difficulty and intensity, presenting a perfect opportunity for exposure to movements that facilitate progress towards skill mastery. Warm-up segments are ideal for practicing exercises that will be used more aggressively in the future. For instance, body squats are a warm-up level activity but should be mastered before resisted squats are used; the warm-up segment makes for an ideal learning environment due to the intensity and continuous rehearsal process.

The order of operations also becomes a relevant concept in progressive warm-up bouts. Since the purpose of warming-up is to gradually increase temperature, ROM, and intensity relative to the exercise session, it only makes sense that exercise selection reflects this progressive concept. Whether employing warm-ups aimed at performance preparation, functional movements, or general preparation, the sequence of activities should be sensibly ordered. Gross motor movements at a controlled pace will supersede faster, more specific motor actions. The selection of movements should logically support the subsequent activities and serve a desired purpose. Stated simply, preparatory actions should resemble motor recruitment, in whole or in part, consistent with the actions of the exercise bout. Deciding on the program components is the exercise professional's job, and selection should be based on the client's best interest. Professional discretion will ultimately define the choices made for each aspect of the training regimen and will certainly be based on knowledge, personal philosophy, and experience. Gaining comprehension of different modalities and the particular benefits of each can enhance the program offerings and lead to more efficient goal attainment by the client. This concept can be implemented throughout the training session, starting with the warm-up.

◆ Cool downs

Warm-ups are used to progressively prepare the body for activity, whereas a cool down works toward an equal, but opposite goal. The purpose of cooling down at the end of an exercise session is to bring the body back down to a pre-exercise state. The cool down should take place immediately following the exercise bout, using low intensity, rhythmic, large-muscle group activities through full ROM.

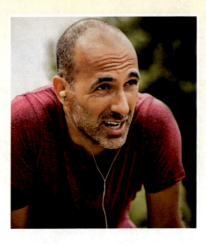

The physiological rationale for the cool down includes the following [31, 32]:

- Prevention of blood pooling
- Promotion of venous blood return, which positively effects cardiac output
- Reduction of blood and muscle lactate
- Reduced concentration of catecholamines in the blood
- Reduced risk of cardiac irregularities post-exercise

Cool downs using dynamic mobility work of continuous full body movement at low-moderate levels should be employed following both moderate to high-intensity anaerobic and aerobic exercise. The actions performed during a cool down promote a continued delivery of oxygen to the tissues that were placed under stress, which may attenuate delayed-onset muscle soreness (DOMS), associated with muscle cell disruption, **cellular ischemia**, and tonic muscular spasm. During exercise, blood is shunted to active skeletal muscle via dilation of local blood vessels. In the absence of a cool down, blood may pool in these tissues which limits venous return and can rapidly reduce cardiac output. A gradual decrease in activity prevents an immediate decline in cardiac output and reduces the risk for symptoms of inadequate circulation such as lightheadedness or dizziness [31, 32]. Although the primary activities should be of a light continuous nature, flexibility exercises, such as static stretching, can also be utilized at the end of the cool down to further promote a more relaxed state and take advantage of the warm tissue. Active recovery seems to demonstrate better outcomes than passive measures; however, massage and soft foam rolling demonstrate added benefits to recovery response and perceived relaxation.

> **DEFINITIONS**
>
> **Cellular ischemia –**
>
> *Restriction of oxygen supply, generally caused by inadequate blood flow, that promotes dysfunction to metabolic activities.*

Cool down Program

Mobility (6x3-5 sec holds per side)	Foam Roll (slow) – massage technique	Static stretch (10-20 sec holds)
Forward lunge with lean	Hip abductors	Proximal hamstring (active isolation) 2x side
Lateral lunge with rotation	Low back	Iron-cross stretch (active-assisted) 2x side
Hip flexors step-back w/rotation reach	Glute/piriformis	Low back stretch

Metabolic System and Programming Considerations

As discussed earlier, the body utilizes different energy systems to form adenosine triphosphate (ATP) for mechanical work. Each system has specialized features that make it ideal for managing specific types of stress. Neural, muscular, or metabolic adaptations will depend on the intensity and duration of the training strategy employed.

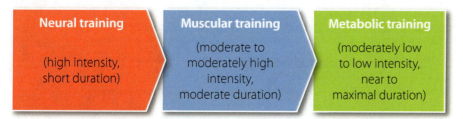

Neural training (high intensity, short duration) → **Muscular training** (moderate to moderately high intensity, moderate duration) → **Metabolic training** (moderately low to low intensity, near to maximal duration)

When training across the metabolic (system) continuum in a single bout of exercise, the energy system and programmatic order should reflect the most intense to the least intense work. Activities aimed at maximal strength and power that emphasize neuromuscular adaptations are

> **DEFINITIONS**
>
> **Compound exercises –**
> *Multi-joint movements involving the concurrent recruitment of several large muscle groups.*

ordered first; this will include the fastest speeds and highest loads (i.e., near to maximal **compound exercises**). Muscle-specific adaptations, including hypertrophy-related strength and strength balance, are secondary. Next, those exercise strategies used to enhance metabolic efficiency or anaerobic capacity are ordered in the final segment of anaerobic training; finally, aerobic exercise is performed last. Changing this order reduces the ability to tax any given system, due to accumulated stress. Granted, many programs do not emphasize all categories of fitness in the same day, but when an individual only trains two or three times a week, it may make sense to be more inclusive of fitness components that span the energy continuum than not.

Metabolic System Continuum

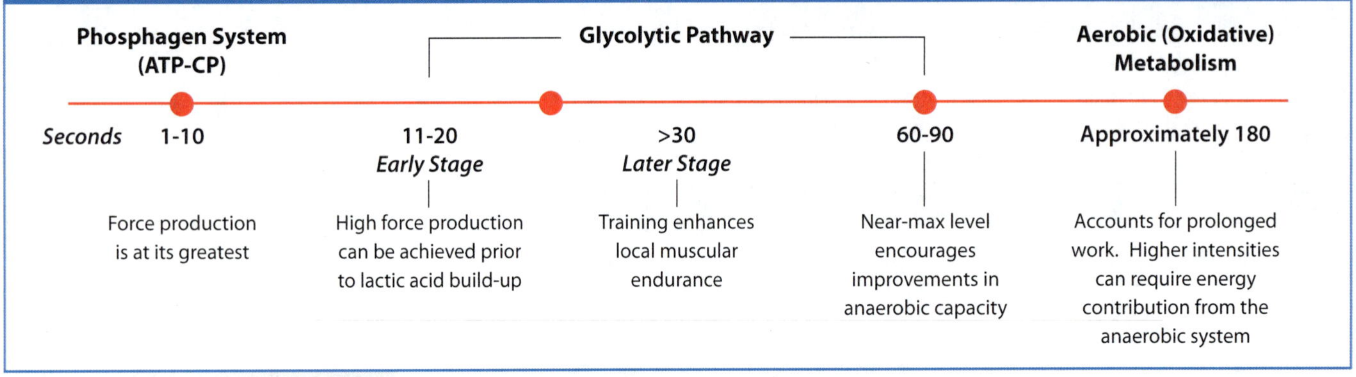

System	Phosphagen System (ATP-CP)	Glycolytic Pathway			Aerobic (Oxidative) Metabolism
Seconds	1-10	11-20 Early Stage	>30 Later Stage	60-90	Approximately 180
	Force production is at its greatest	High force production can be achieved prior to lactic acid build-up	Training enhances local muscular endurance	Near-max level encourages improvements in anaerobic capacity	Accounts for prolonged work. Higher intensities can require energy contribution from the anaerobic system

Rate of ATP Synthesis is Dependent Upon Substrate

Substrate	Relative Rate	
Phosphocreatine	100	Direct ~P transfer, no substrate oxidation required.
Glycogen *(anaerobic glycolysis)*	55	Phosphorolysis, G-1-P formed without use of ATP yielding 3 ATP/glucosyl group, "tree structure" gives many simultaneous reaction sites.
Glucose *(aerobic glycolysis)*	23	Limited by rates of membrane glucose transport, glycolysis, and mitochondrial oxidation.
Fatty Acids	10	Lipolysis only at interface between oil droplet and cytosol, limited by transport and mitochondrial oxidation.

Goal	Adaptation	Energy System	Emphasis
Power	Neural	Phosphagen system	Velocity-force
Maximal strength	Neuromuscular	Phosphagen system	Maximal force
Hypertrophy/strength balance	Muscular	Glycolytic system	Time-tension
Anaerobic capacity/metabolic fitness	Metabolic	Glycolytic system	Force-velocity capacity
Aerobic fitness	Metabolic	Oxidative system	CRF/metabolic specificity

Clearly, the metabolic system defines the capacity for work when expressed by time and intensity. Matching the energy system with the goal is fundamental to proper, scientifically based exercise programming. Straying from the correct energy system or duration within that system can compromise results. For instance, lifting a weight for 15 repetitions to failure compared to five repetitions to failure will have completely different results when applied over a training cycle, as reflected by adaptations associated with nerves, hormones, enzymes, and, subsequently, muscle tissue. Knowing these systems is not only advantageous for exercise programming, but necessary for goal attainment.

Exercise Program Components

◆ Exercise Selection

Exercise selection is equally important for proper program design. Once the goal of the training has been identified, a trainer can then select the modalities and specific movements needed to maximize the energy system and best address the needs analysis. Much like the options available for the exercise program, the specific exercises the program employs have numerous variables to consider. Aerobic training most frequently utilizes a single modality performed for an extended period of time, such as jogging, biking, swimming, or stair climbing. However, this is not the only available option, as any continuous activity can become a cardiovascular workout if the principle aspects apply. Creative exercise programming may utilize any group of movements executed in a continuous fashion that result in the maintenance of elevated heart rates for the entire training period. The exercise modality may change ten or fifteen times during the specified exercise period, but if it matches the intensity and demands of the energy system, it is acceptable and appropriate for the goals of training aerobically. The main guidelines to consider are client-specific characteristics and the targeted heart rate for the entire period. Cardiovascular circuit training exemplifies how many movements can be synergistically applied to form an aerobic workout, as long as the heart rate remains elevated for the workout duration.

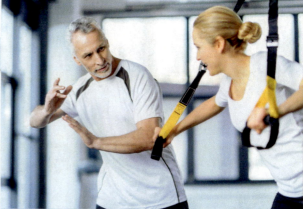

A well-developed needs analysis will provide the best guide for optimizing exercise selection.

Anaerobic training is far more complicated because it includes so many options and subcategories of those options, as it spans across energy systems. The needs analysis will once again provide the best guide for the exercise selection. Deficiency or a desire to improve in any particular area justify selecting from the group of exercises that specifically focus on that adaptation, whether it be for strength, power, speed, flexibility, or balance. Once the category of exercises has been identified, the client-specific criteria should be applied to the decision-making process. For instance, if a client has weak glutes, it would make sense to employ the back squat exercise, but if he or she also has tight hip flexors, a reverse lunge would make more sense, as it addresses both issues. Each factor identified in the needs analysis may classify a particular exercise as advantageous or inappropriate, depending on the training goals and the client's capabilities.

Although many more options for training are available to today's fitness professionals than in the past, each selection will still require the support of research and practice-based evidence. Where novel modalities may lack research support, the characteristics of the movement actions and intensities they require will categorize exercises and modalities, delineating their usefulness and limitations. Reviewing the exercise usages, benefits, and disadvantages will help an exercise professional when deciding on the best solution to meet the individual client's need. Many of these findings will be reviewed in the following chapters and provide insight as to logical choices for specific situations.

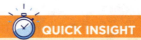

QUICK INSIGHT

SKILL ACQUISITION AND MOVEMENT ECONOMY

The first step in implementing any exercise program or fitness activity is to teach the client to become proficient in the actions appropriate to the training regimen. Although not a designated principle of programming, this work is a fundamental component in exercise instruction. Often referred to as the preparation phase of training, clients are taught how to properly execute each movement with correct biomechanical technique. Using physical and verbal cues, exercise professionals can help clients become proficient at each exercise movement. Progressing a client toward more complex or resisted exercises before the techniques have been mastered often leads to a breakdown in form. Common consequences of poor form are repetitive **microtrauma**, *which manifests into acute inflammatory syndrome at, or around, an articulation or joint, limiting results from the training* [3, 18, 24, 29]. *Personal trainers should accept nothing less than perfect movement execution during each training bout. Exercise professionals who allow clients to perform exercises incorrectly are being negligent in their job performance.*

In sports, athletes routinely practice actions and movement sequences that they will perform on the field or court. They do this so they can become more efficient at managing the forces for precise execution during a competitive situation. By rehearsing the activity over and over again, the body learns to coordinate motor patterns via enhancements in neural efficiency. Once the pattern is learned, the nerves maintain a type of motor history, so every time the situation calls for the motor pattern, the body knows exactly what to do. This phenomenon explains why people do not forget how to ride a bike or throw a ball when they become adults, even though they may not have performed the actions routinely since they were age 10.

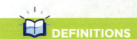

DEFINITIONS

Microtrauma –

Extremely localized injury to muscle fibers, tendons, ligaments, or bones, which may cause low levels of inflammation with, or without, the presence of symptoms.

◆ Exercise Order

As mentioned earlier, when exercise selection causes different energy systems to be used in the same training bout, the sequence should be based on logical consideration. The primary concern relates to specific need. If a person has deficiencies or health risks that can be improved upon with training, exercises or activities related to these deficiencies should be prioritized. Traditionally, aerobic exercise is performed after resistance training when the two are combined in a single training period at high intensity.

The reason for this order is threefold:

1) Aerobic training decreases levels of muscle glycogen, and consequently, will reduce the client's ability to maximally stimulate the muscle during the resistance-training portion of the exercise session.

2) Lactate in the system allows for training at higher heart rates with lower measures of RPE.

3) Aerobic training prior to resistance training seems to downregulate the mTOR pathway related to skeletal muscle hypertrophy [23].

However, if aerobic training tops the priority list based on the needs analysis, then it should precede anaerobic training in the exercise session to enable maximal effort during this modality. Hypertensive clients, those with low CRF, or those with risk factors for heart disease will benefit most from aerobic-based activities; however, these clients still need resistance exercise as well as it benefits insulin sensitivity and muscle function. This determination, drawn from the needs analysis, would warrant changing traditional exercise order [19, 29, 34].

When aerobic and anaerobic activities combine in a single bout for a healthy person with no underlying conditions, the order of exercises selected for the program will generally follow a consistent, preset format. In most cases, the order will be as follows:

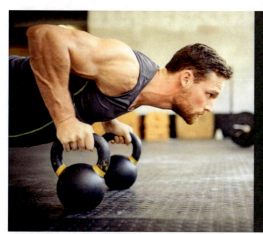

1. General Warm-up
2. Mobility Training
3. Neural Readiness
4. Ballistic Activities *(Phosphagen)*
5. Intermittent Resistance Training *(Phosphagen, Glycolytic)*
6. Anaerobic Metabolic Training *(Glycolytic, Aerobic)*
7. Aerobic Training *(Aerobic)*
8. Dynamic Stretching
9. Static Stretching

The type of anaerobic activities will vary by the client and may or may not include all of the different training options in a single session, but the energy systems and intensity used will ultimately determine the order. Furthermore, due to varied loads and movement speed and complexity, anaerobic exercise has additional characteristics that define the actual order used in the exercise session. Velocity-based movements, compound multi-joint, heavy, and complex activities are ordered first, transitioning to actions of moderate weight or those compound movements which require less total mass; these are followed by lighter, single-joint, isolated exercises, which tend to be last in a training session. The size and number of muscle groups used should always be considered along with the force employed to correctly order operations, with the larger muscle groups taking precedence over smaller groups in the

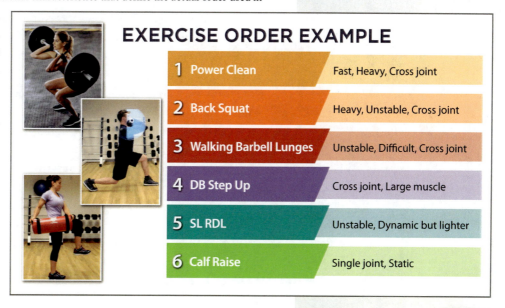

EXERCISE ORDER EXAMPLE

#	Exercise	Characteristics
1	Power Clean	Fast, Heavy, Cross joint
2	Back Squat	Heavy, Unstable, Cross joint
3	Walking Barbell Lunges	Unstable, Difficult, Cross joint
4	DB Step Up	Cross joint, Large muscle
5	SL RDL	Unstable, Dynamic but lighter
6	Calf Raise	Single joint, Static

exercise sequence. For instance, leg exercises precede arm exercises, and cross-joint hip movements will precede cross-joint shoulder movements. This method ensures that the most physiologically challenging activities are completed first in the exercise bout, before fatigue can contribute to a limitation in force production or the ability to maintain proper technique. These concepts will be further explored in the chapter devoted to anaerobic exercise prescription.

◆ Training Frequency

The number of times a person engages in a particular activity per week represents participation frequency. Frequency contributes importantly to the exercise program, as it plays a role in the rate and degree of the adaptation response and, when properly applied, can help to prevent **overtraining syndrome** [9, 14]. The stress stimulus forms the basis for the physiological adaptation response, and frequency factors into the volume of stress to which the body is exposed. When the stress is excessive, the outcome is negative. On the other hand, when the stress is inadequate or too infrequent, the outcome remains insignificant because the body manages it through acute adjustments rather than chronic adaptations. Guidelines exist that will help define appropriate frequency, based on the client's available time, relative capabilities, and **training tenure**, as well as his or her goals. A common frequency choice in exercise programming for general health attainment is ≥3 sessions per week; however, while structured exercise performed three times per week will provide many health benefits, it would be ignorant to use this value to define the appropriate frequency for all exercise programs. Since frequency factors into training-volume stress across multiple days, it becomes very important for managing not only neuromuscular adaptations that require high intensity but also cardiovascular adaptations that require fairly significant time exposure per week.

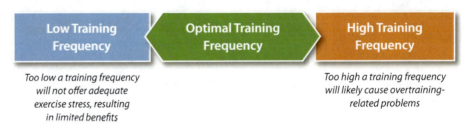

Too low a training frequency will not offer adequate exercise stress, resulting in limited benefits

Too high a training frequency will likely cause overtraining-related problems

Generally speaking, when all factors are properly balanced to avoid overtraining, the more frequent the exercise participation, the greater the rate and magnitude of the adaptations. But before adopting the "more is better" philosophy, a few key elements must be clarified. First, a tolerable upper limit to stress exists before the body reaches the exhaustion phase of Selye's General Adaptation Syndrome [8, 12]. This tolerable upper limit is affected by individual factors, as well as the type, intensity, and duration of the exercise. Jogging at a moderate level most days of the week for 30 minutes will provide more health benefits than jogging at the same intensity three times per week [10]. But this is not true of higher intensity. Training at elevated intensities across maximal attainable distances most days of the week would cause overtraining effects [25]. Even elite runners train at their maximal distances only a couple times per week and complement this exhaustive training with shorter running distances of varying intensities throughout the week. This illustrates the need for balance between intensity, duration, and frequency [22]. This scenario is also true of resistance training. Bodybuilders train up to six days in a week, but they vary the targeted muscle groups so that each muscle has an appropriate opportunity to recover before exposing it to high stress again. If a new exerciser were to attempt a competitive

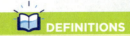

Overtraining syndrome –

A condition caused by an intolerable accumulation of training stress resulting in systemic inflammation, psychologic and neuroendocrinologic symptoms, and performance decrements observed for >2 months.

Training tenure –

The period of time an individual has performed exercises relevant to the exercise prescription.

body builder's workout, he or she would risk getting rhabdomyolysis. This identifies that frequency is also a factor of training experience and physical condition.

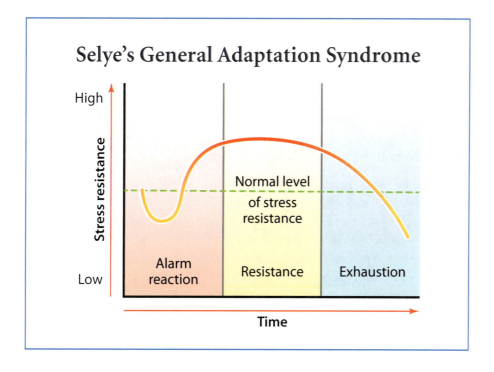

◆ Training Duration

The amount of time a person is exposed to training stress in a single period of exercise is referred to as the duration of training and is often measured by actual time-under-tension. The reason time-under-tension represents a more relevant marker of measurement is that rest interval adds to time. Decisions regarding training duration, like frequency, are both intensity and goal specific, but again, the client's capabilities and time availability contribute to the decision-making process. Unlike frequency, however, duration is subject to energy storage, tolerable stress, and relative rate of fatigue. The higher the intensity, the faster an exerciser depletes his or her glycogen reserves, and the earlier the exercise bout will lose effectiveness. Fatigue becomes the most significant factor defining the limit of the exercise session's length, but adaptations are also duration-specific due to differences in the energy systems. To elicit anaerobic adaptations, the duration of time a muscle is placed under stress is relatively short; in fact, a normal weightlifting bout equates to 9-12 minutes of total time-under-tension. On the contrary, the duration of stress required for chronic aerobic adaptations exceeds this value by 3-7 times. Duration differences also exist within the specific energy systems, depending on the intended goal. Strength training requires very heavy loads (85-100% 1RM), applied for short periods of time.

When the total work is tallied, it may add up to only 5 minutes of actual resistance training, even though the training session lasted an hour. As mentioned earlier, rest intervals play a role in total duration, and, therefore, since 2-5 minutes of rest is required to repeat heavy resistance training sets, this dramatically extends the exercise bout. Be that as it may, adaptation is related

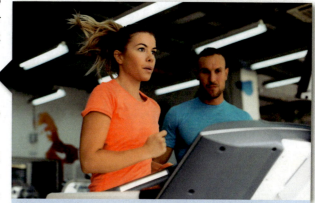

The amount of time a client is exposed to training stresses in a single bout is referred to as the duration of training. This is often measured by actual time-under-tension.

to the contact time with the resistance, not the total time spent in a gym. Strength training requires time for rephosphorylation of the high-energy phosphate bonds for repeat training effort. After 5 minutes, phosphocreatine recovery may be 80% of starting stores. With that in mind however, all anaerobic training need not focus on maximal strength: when hypertrophy is the desired outcome, the duration of time-under-tension increases significantly relative to the time spent in the exercise bout. The actual amount of weight lifted per repetition drops to moderate levels (70-85% 1RM), but the repetition ranges must increase to compensate for the difference. This places high levels of mechanical stress on the tissue for longer periods of time, a necessary element to increasing anabolic hormone response. Hypertrophy training duration may be two or three times that of strength training, even though both modalities utilize the anaerobic energy system and feature similar exercise selections.

Regardless of whether one performs the majority of work in the anaerobic or aerobic system, a consistent relationship exists between training duration and training intensity. The more intense the work, the shorter the duration of time in which it can be performed. To the contrary, the lighter the work load, the longer the activity can be performed. Aerobic training performed at low intensity can last hours, but when the intensity rises, the ratio of time to exhaustion is inverted. A trainer must account for the balance between intensity and duration for effective exercise program design because adaptations relate specifically to intensity and time-under-tension. In the context of the time-tension relationship, trainers should consider that adequate fuel storage and hydration directly affect exercise performance duration. An appropriate and effective exercise prescription will not be fully attainable if the exerciser presents low initial energy storage at the training bout's onset.

> **DEFINITIONS**
>
> **Maximal capacity –**
>
> *The highest workload an individual can sustain; defined by maximal oxygen consumption (VO₂max), 1-repetition max (1RM) or volitional failure.*

◆ Training Intensity

Training intensity predicts exercise-induced adaptations more than any other factor. Although it cannot truly exist independently in an exercise prescription, the training intensity sets the foundations for the physiological stress and hormonal response. It also indicates how long the activity can be performed, how much rest and recovery are needed to support it, and how often it can be performed. Since each bout has an intensity-duration relationship, balancing these two factors is fundamental to successful goal attainment. The specific intensity-duration ranges necessary for adaptations are covered within the Programming for Anaerobic and Aerobic Training Chapter, but some general guidelines do exist when viewed from a broad perspective of program design. For most active individuals, "exercise level" training begins at 60% of **maximal capacity**. Anything under that value is considered physical activity with limitations in adaptation potential. Deconditioned and diseased populations may see benefits below that level, as their physical capability remains low, but for a healthy adult, intensities below 60% do not provide enough stress to elicit an adaption from the body and are managed by acute metabolic and hormone adjustments.

Intensity has two relevant issues that need to be discussed, as they determine the degree to which it is employed in an exercise regimen. The first issue is the physical aptitude and abilities of the client. These considerations imply that safety and the relative capabilities and tolerance of the client must be carefully considered in any exercise program. Inappropriately intense exercise will often cause movement compensation, compromise biomechanical technique, and may yield injury. This situation can also become a psychological barrier to exercise participation due to the perceived levels of discomfort. The desired adaptation composes the other key consideration for programming intensity. As mentioned earlier, the "time duration of intensity" should match the load, energy system, and rest interval requirements for specific adaptations. If these factors are not properly coordinated, they will throw off the body's (intended) adaptation response.

Two factors determine appropriate intensity for application in a program:

- **Client's physical aptitude and safety** — Excessive exercise may cause injury or psychological barriers
- **Energy system utilized** — Each system has different fatigue rates, as well as intensities and durations that can be employed; any mismatch will impede goal attainment

◆ Rest Intervals

Rest intervals, or rest periods, impact the adaptation response more than most would believe. The performance of repeat actions at set intensities will be delineated by energy-system-specific factors. So, while the definition of rest interval for exercise is the "duration of time between each act of physical effort," the metabolic system is the criterion that defines the actual time. High-intensity burst activities quickly use up the tissues' more powerful energy stores. Once these energy provisions are used, or the associated metabolic byproduct accumulation becomes inhibitive, the action can no longer be repeated at the set intensity. To repeat the action at the same high level, the body must allow the cell to recover during the rest cycle: in this case, allowing rephosphorylation to occur and the acidic energy byproducts to be removed[1]. This suggests that rest intervals are not arbitrary but rather, relative to the energy system's proficiency. Interestingly, training that exposes individuals to energy-system taxation provides the adaptations that promote more efficient recovery. So, the more an energy system is used, the better it functions in response to repeat (consistent) stress, and in many cases, will lead to the reduction of the rest interval needed for repeat action.

> **DEFINITIONS**
>
> **Rest intervals –**
>
> *The time duration between physical effort that influences energy system contribution, recruitment capacity, subsequent performance, and training adaptation.*

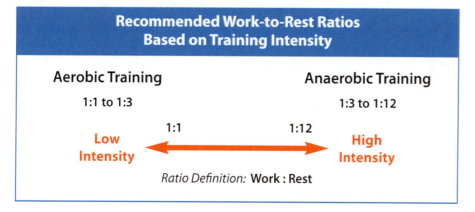

Recommended Work-to-Rest Ratios Based on Training Intensity

Aerobic Training: 1:1 to 1:3 (Low Intensity, 1:1)
Anaerobic Training: 1:3 to 1:12 (High Intensity, 1:12)

Ratio Definition: Work : Rest

In aerobic training, the rest interval may be between a 1:1 or 1:3 work-to-rest ratio, depending on the training system and desired outcome. In anaerobic bouts, that value jumps to 1:3 to

1:20 depending on the resistance used and the intended outcome. For example, when running one-mile repeats that last seven minutes, the rest interval will be equivalent to the measured running times, in this case, seven minutes, which would represent a 1:1 work-to-rest ratio. In bouts of heavy resistance training, such as a 5RM squat, the recovery may be over 2 minutes, even though the movement only takes 15-20 seconds to perform; this reflects a work-to-rest ratio between 1:6-1:8. The anaerobic system dictates an inverse relationship due to the excessive demands of byproduct management, as both rest and intensity increase linearly. For example, at max levels of the anaerobic system, the shorter the duration of time under tension (1-3 reps), the longer the recovery to repeat the action (3-5 minutes). In the squat example, the recovery from a 1RM squat may double the recovery time of a 10 RM squat effort, which makes sense when considering the relative intensities of each effort: 1RM load represents 100%, 10RM load equates to about 75% of that 1RM. When determining the rest interval to use in an exercise program, all of the relevant factors should be taken into consideration to ensure that the program delivers the intended results.

◆ Training Volume

Clearly, the selected intensity and the other programming variables share an interdependent relationship. It has been established that the exercise intensity level defines rest intervals, training duration, frequency, and **training volume**. This remains true both of a single bout of exercise as well as over the course of the training cycle. Training volume measures total work performed. It combines sets, repetitions, and loads lifted. Training volume is calculated by multiplying the number of sets by the number of repetitions by the weight lifted per repetition. For instance, an individual who weighs 155 lbs. and completes four sets of body weight lunges for ten repetitions would have his or her training volume expressed as (4 sets x 10 reps x 155 lbs. body weight) = 6,200 lbs. The goal is to approximate desired volumes per day or week consistent with appropriate intensity levels to facilitate adequate recovery.

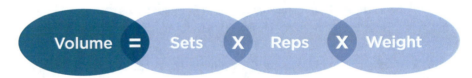

This calculation will help determine **progressive overload** for ongoing adaptations and will support programmatic considerations, including determining appropriate training duration and frequency. High volumes and intensities require increased recovery to reflect this demand; likewise, with lower volume and intensity, recovery durations should be reduced accordingly. One important caveat, however, is to always consider intensity and volume separately and collectively; do not simply combine them into a single factor. The reason for this is that tissue has physical taxation limits. Consider the following scenario: an individual can back squat 350 lbs.; if this person squats 5 sets of 15 repetitions using 100 lbs., it equates to a training volume of 7,500 lbs. (using less than 30% 1RM); now, compare that volume-intensity relationship to 5 sets of 5 repetitions using 300 lbs.: the volume is 7,500 lbs. (using more than 85% 1RM). The latter regimen will certainly require more rest and recovery based on the intensity, even with the consistent volume. This explains why cardiovascular circuit activities can be performed almost every day, whereas heavy weight lifting requires rest days, even if the two totals result in the same volume over a week.

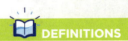

DEFINITIONS

Training volume –

A measure of work performed during an exercise bout, taking into consideration the intensity and either the frequency or duration of movement – in resistance training it is calculated by Sets x Reps x Load.

Progressive overload –

The gradual increase in training stress to elicit a targeted physiological adaptation.

◆ Recovery Period

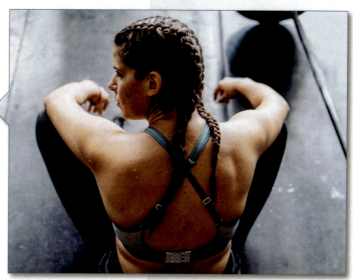

The recovery period is the duration of time between exercise bouts. It may reflect a four-hour period between aerobic and anaerobic training in the same day or a multiple-day period between subsequent bouts of resistance training for a muscle group. During the period of recovery, energy sources depleted from the exercise bout can be replenished (i.e., glycogen), while cellular adaptations occur in the tissue based on the signaling effect of the stress experienced during the previous workout. Adaptations to the duress take place when the stress is eliminated, during sleep, for example, making recovery as important as the exercise. Simply stated, recovery periods are necessary for improvements. If the body experiences constant stress, it will become exhausted and begin to break down, as seen with overtraining syndrome. Injury, illness, and other negative side effects of overtraining can quickly occur with inadequate recovery. However, too much recovery is not positive either; when the exercise volume drops below certain thresholds, adaptations are reduced.

◆ Exercise Principles

The thoughtful interaction of exercise programming principles can create an effective arrangement of adaptation-specific stress. The difficulty most exercise professionals have is balancing these applications in a complementary fashion, so the design is logical, timely, client-appropriate, and outcome-based. To help ensure the program (matrix) makes sense, each component should be evaluated for consistency with the **principles of exercise** across a phase of training. This task is usually done over 1-3 months to ensure that safe and effective improvements are ongoing and consistent with the goals. The principles of exercise are **specificity**, **overload**, and **progression**. Collectively, these determinants ensure that exercise stress reflects the program goals: by definition, that the exercise provides adequate stress or overload for the desired adaptation response. In addition, the exercise must be applied consistently in a progressive manner so that the body continues to improve. The exercise principles steer the program components to properly account for the necessary inclusion and quantity of exercise stress.

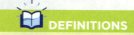

Principles of exercise –

Concepts that function to guide exercise programming in order to achieve desired outcomes.

Fundamental Principles of Exercise:		
Specificity	**Overload**	**Progression**
For a desired adaptation to occur in the body, stress must be appropriately and specifically applied	A training stress that challenges a physiological system above the level to which it is accustomed	Stress applied must continually be perceived as new for any physiological system to adjust

Principle of Specificity

The principle of specificity is very logical in its application. This tenet states that, for a physiological system to adapt, the stress demand must be appropriately and explicitly applied to that physiological system. Essentially, the adaptations relate specifically to the amount and type of applied physiological stress. If the proper amount of stress is placed on a system in an appropriate manner, the system will respond by changing to try to meet the stress. The principle of specificity guides the exercise selection and other components of programming to ensure the proper elements exist to match the desired goal.

Principle of Overload

The overload principle is defined as training stress which challenges a physiological system of the body above the level to which it is accustomed. Overload is applied by manipulating one or more of the training components, with the most commonly modulated components being intensity, duration, and rest intervals; however, possible adjustments that can be used to overload a system are not limited to these three factors alone. The exercise selection, training volume, velocity of movement, and frequency can also be modified to create a more physiologically taxing training experience. When the body no longer perceives overload, it achieves a fixed state, and the adaptation response discontinues. This phenomenon is often referred to as staleness or a **training plateau**. Planned variations within the exercise program allow for the constant application of overload though changes in the type or level of the stress: these ensure continued improvement by the body's physiological systems.

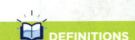

DEFINITIONS

Training plateau –

A decrease in noticeable progress occurring when the body no longer responds to a training stimulus.

Stress –

A disruptive stimulus eliciting a physiological response.

The principle of overload can be applied by manipulating various training components, such as:

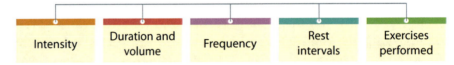

Intensity | Duration and volume | Frequency | Rest intervals | Exercises performed

Principle of Progression

The planned, incremental increase in exercise **stress** is referred to as "progressive overload," which is structured to promote continued adaptations. The principle of progression suggests that the stress applied must continually be perceived as "new" to the physiological system to elicit a stress-induced adaption response. Progressions within an exercise program are intended to continually tax the system; however, the adjustments to stress should not be excessive. Large increases in physical stress above what those to which the system has already adjusted create a disparity between the rate of the adaptation process and the stress level the system can maintain, called strain. Rapid progression rates are not sustainable and can very quickly lead to failure along the stress-adaptation-response pathway. When overload becomes unmanageable, the system inhibits and may even reverse the intended stress response, potentially leading to injury.

Progressions are individual-specific and rates of change vary depending on previous exposure to the stress and the current physical state of the individual. New exercisers with limited training experience often present a faster rate of improvement; these early increases in performance and efficiency develop through nervous system adaptations. On the contrary, individuals who have reached high levels of adjustment to a particular stress progress at a much slower rate relative to the percentage of change experienced; this an illustration of the law of diminishing returns: the closer you are to peak performance, the more energy is required to make even small improvements. Another key factor in applying the principle of progression is

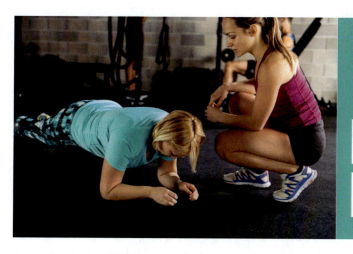

The magnitude of progressions employed in a training program will be influenced by several factors, including:
- Training tenure (experience)
- Current physical condition
- Genetic potential
- Nutrition and recovery

the person's level of fitness. Individuals who are in better physical condition can manage more stress, compared to less physically fit individuals. As a rule of thumb, increases in exercise stress should be approximately 2-5% per week. Some more aggressive practitioners have suggested progressions as high as 10% per week, but the likelihood of sustaining a consistent adaptation rate of this magnitude, without any deleterious effects, is unlikely.

Initial Improvement in Physical Fitness Level but Lack of New Overload Causes Little Change

Continued Improvement in Physical Fitness Level Due to Progressive Overload

Periodization

Periodization represents the concept that the body adapts more efficiently when the adaptations are strategically built upon each other. It reflects a logical method of organizing training into sequential phases and cyclical time periods to allow for residual adaptation responses to staircase progressively. When designed appropriately, a periodized training program increases the potential for achieving specific performance goals and minimizes overtraining potential. Periodized training plans are proposed as superior to non-periodized training plans for health, fitness, and performance outcomes. It would seem intuitive that one needs to establish system function (e.g., cardiovascular, musculoskeletal) and movement competency in order to be healthy and that a healthy person can then make further improvements upon these to become fit. Once the individual achieves a base level of fitness, he or she can begin to focus on performance. Skipping over any phase of the developmental progression (function, health, fitness, and

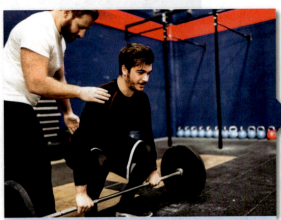

Periodization represents the concept that the body develops more efficiently when adaptations are strategically built upon each other.

performance) would not be realistic or necessarily positive, especially in the long term.

As previously stated, each preceding phase of training entails specific goals which function to support the subsequent phase. General preparatory acts, such as movement competence, specific activation patterns, and ROM precede more enduring attainments, such as stability and sustained activation, which themselves are precedents that support maximal force and velocity attainment. Using periodized phases within a defined training cycle allows progressive overload to be applied specifically to a defined purpose and then augmented to achieve the next goal or level of training. The desired adaptive response associated with training is referred to as **supercompensation**. Supercompensation represents the acute response elicited from the training stress as the body attempts to maintain internal order or "training homeostasis." Orderly manipulation of stress-specific applications allows for predictable outcomes with each outcome, or adaptation, having a shelf life. Physical attributes respond at different rates and are sustained for different time periods, depending on the variables of stress applied. For instance, VO_2max and maximal speed exhibit much more sensitivity than strength, hypertrophy, and flexibility to detraining effects.

DEFINITIONS

Supercompensation –

The process of adapting to a training stimulus, resulting in an improved performance capacity.

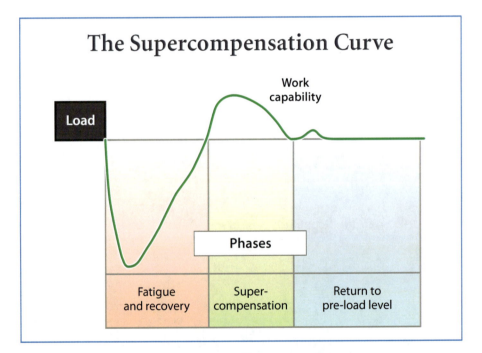

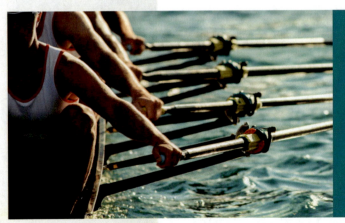

Longevity of common residual training effects:

Aerobic endurance effects:	30 +/- 5 days
Maximal strength effects:	30 +/- 5 days
Anaerobic endurance effects:	18 +/- 4 days
Strength endurance effects:	15 +/- 5 days
Maximal speed effects:	5 +/- 3 days

In periodization, the outcomes are arranged in a series of cycles and phases that takes the calculated residuals developed in a previous phase, or cycle, and employs them for the next phase, or cycle. Knowledge of interdependent characteristics that affect health and performance-related fitness provides for efficient and effective programming plans that are timely and help prevent overtraining. With proper application of supercompensation theory, an individual will be better suited for ongoing training, assuming adequate recovery and that the new stress is properly timed. When the variable components of programming are suitably manipulated, the work level is appropriate, and the corresponding recovery is adequately achieved, intentional and progressive improvements will occur.

Exercise Program Safety Factors

Program development represents one side of the equation; program implementation and instruction characterizes the other side. The act of implementation brings additional factors for consideration. These do not necessarily play a direct role in the program components or the exercise principles themselves but are necessary considerations for proper program execution. Ensuring that these factors are appropriately managed will increase client safety and reduce the risk of liability associated with the training program. One of the exercise professional's most important jobs is to make sure all participants remain safe when engaged in supervised physical activity. It is well known that physical exertion comes with inherent risks for injury; however, exercise professionals can dramatically minimize this danger by accounting for potential problems. The concept of a safe environment spans across all conditions and areas of training that affect the client. These include the client's acute condition, the ambient temperature and relative humidity, internal and external area safety hazards, the training space and surrounding areas, properly functioning equipment, and adequate instruction and supervision. Each factor has independent relevance that can compound when other factors are also unaccounted for during the exercise session.

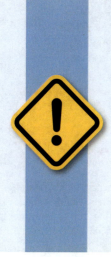

Factors to consider for creating a safe training environment

- Client's acute condition : hydration, mental distraction, illness, hypoglycemia, excess fatigue, postural adjustments, etc.
- Environmental temperature and humidity
- Establishing a clear work space *(e.g., no dumbbells or equipment to trip over)*
- Equipment operating condition
- Proper supervision (e.g., spotting, verbal or tactile cues, correct equipment use)

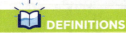

DEFINITIONS

Contraindications –

A factor that makes a particular training method inadvisable due to the harm it may cause the individual.

Humidity –

The amount of water vapor in the air; can lead to excessive, counter-productive sweating by reducing the capacity for evaporation.

The client's acute condition depends on several daily variables, which may or may not contribute to concerns during training. Some acute considerations include mental distraction or lack of focus, acute illness, dehydration, glycogen depletion, medication, drug or alcohol use, hypoglycemia, hyponatremia, and excessive fatigue. Any one of these daily variables can lead to injury during physical activity performance, and they are therefore considered relative **contraindications** to exercise participation. If an exercise professional recognizes that a client is not functioning properly or is experiencing an issue that may increase risk for injury, the activity should be discontinued and rescheduled for another day, provided the problem has subsided. Failure to follow this protocol constitutes poor professional judgment and, in some cases, may be deemed professional negligence.

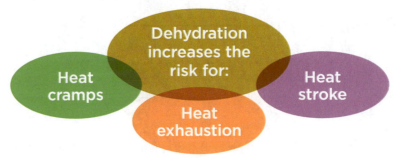

When analyzing the environmental conditions for safety, the first external factors often assessed are the temperature and relative **humidity** of the training environment. In some cases, pollution and altitude may also be factors, but these challenges to exercise are less common in most environments. High temperatures and humidity create physiological stress that increases dehydration and heat-related illness risk. Mechanisms that regulate internal temperature can become relatively dysfunctional as heat loss from evaporation and convection become diminished due to the environmental conditions [2, 18]. Training in controlled conditions indoors often alleviates any concerns related to temperature. However, with outside training, temperature

---

HEAT EXHAUSTION | HEAT STROKE

Symptoms
- Faint or Dizzy
- Headache
- Profuse Sweating
- Irritability
- Weak, Rapid Pulse
- Shallow Breathing
- Pale, Cool, Clammy Skin
- Nausea or Vomiting
- Muscle Cramps

Treatment
1. Have victim lie down in a cool shaded or air-conditioned area.
2. Drink water if victim is conscious.
3. Use caution when victim stands up, apply cold compresses.

Symptoms
- Absence of Sweating
- Pulsating Headache
- Hot, Red, Dry Skin
- High Body Temp: Above 103°
- Nausea or Vomiting
- Strong, Rapid Pulse
- Confusion
- Convulsions
- May Lose Consciousness

Treatment
1. **DIAL 911**
2. Take action to cool victim by any means. Place victim in a cool area, wrap in wet towel, sponge victim with cool water.

and humidity must be considered. During summer months, selecting the most appropriate time of the day is often the easiest and most controllable component involved in managing these conditions. Preplanning and having a contingency plan are necessary aspects to consider in dealing with environmental conditions.

The training space and the equipment used for exercise performance must also be accounted for and evaluated for safety prior to participation. Before the exercise is performed, the training area should be assessed to ensure it does not present any possible risks to the client and is large enough to accommodate the activities. This includes establishing a clear work space, accounting for other people working in close proximity, and keeping an eye on concurrent activities within the environment.

The equipment being used constitutes another possible safety issue within the training area. All equipment should be evaluated for proper function, making sure moving parts and cables are not damaged or excessively worn and ensuring all nuts and bolts are secure. Friction over time loosens connections and can actually disengage pieces of machinery and other training equipment. If the equipment uses additional safety apparatuses, such as clips, stoppers, range-limiting devices, or components that need to be secured or weighted down, these should be properly employed during each performance to help reduce the risk in case the client fails during the exercise. If a piece of equipment's ability to function properly is in question, avoid using it until it has received proper maintenance. Additionally, the client's capabilities should be evaluated before deciding on the equipment used within the program. For instance, hypertensive clients should avoid compression equipment like the leg press, and stability equipment may not be appropriate for clients with balance limitations or acute vestibular disruption from a cold.

Exercise professionals can further enhance the safety and effectiveness of the training environment by providing proper supervision and instruction. Spotting clients, evaluating their movements for poor mechanics and signs of fatigue, and providing instructional cues to enhance movement proficiency will all contribute to better training practices. Setting controls and providing motivation and assistance will improve the client's performance, while concurrently reducing safety-related issues. Exercise professionals should be very active during the training session, observing the client and managing the environment for maximum safety.

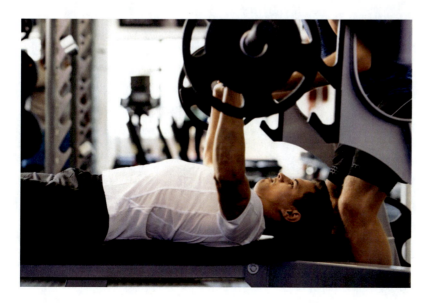

REFERENCES:

1. Allen DG, Lamb GD, and Westerblad H. Skeletal muscle fatigue: cellular mechanisms. *Physiological reviews* 88: 287-332, 2008.

2. Armstrong LE, Casa DJ, Millard-Stafford M, Moran DS, Pyne SW, and Roberts WO. Exertional heat illness during training and competition. *Medicine & Science in Sports & Exercise* 39: 556-572, 2007.

3. Bergh U and Ekblom B. Influence of muscle temperature on maximal muscle strength and power output in human skeletal muscles. *Acta physiologica scandinavica* 107: 33-37, 1979.

4. Bigland-Ritchie B, Thomas C, Rice C, Howarth J, and Woods J. Muscle temperature, contractile speed, and motoneuron firing rates during human voluntary contractions. *Journal of Applied Physiology* 73: 2457-2461, 1992.

5. Bishop D. Warm up I. *Sports medicine* 33: 439-454, 2003.

6. Bishop D. Warm up II. *Sports medicine* 33: 483-498, 2003.

7. Blumenstein B. *Psychology of sport training:* Meyer & Meyer Verlag, 2007.

8. Carfagno DG and Hendrix JC. Overtraining syndrome in the athlete: current clinical practice. *Current sports medicine reports* 13: 45-51, 2014.

9. Dankel SJ, Mattocks KT, Jessee MB, Buckner SL, Mouser JG, Counts BR, Laurentino GC, and Loenneke JP. Frequency: the overlooked resistance training variable for inducing muscle hypertrophy? *Sports Medicine* 47: 799-805, 2017.

10. Eckel RH, Jakicic JM, Ard JD, De Jesus JM, Miller NH, Hubbard VS, Lee I-M, Lichtenstein AH, Loria CM, and Millen BE. 2013 AHA/ACC guideline on lifestyle management to reduce cardiovascular risk: a report of the American College of Cardiology/American Heart Association Task Force on Practice Guidelines. *Journal of the American College of Cardiology* 63: 2960-2984, 2014.

11. Fradkin AJ, Zazryn TR, and Smoliga JM. Effects of warming-up on physical performance: a systematic review with meta-analysis. *The Journal of Strength & Conditioning Research* 24: 140-148, 2010.

12. Fry RW, Morton AR, and Keast D. Overtraining in athletes. *Sports Medicine* 12: 32-65, 1991.

13. Gerbino A, Ward SA, and Whipp BJ. Effects of prior exercise on pulmonary gas-exchange kinetics during high-intensity exercise in humans. *Journal of Applied Physiology* 80: 99-107, 1996.

14. Grgic J, Schoenfeld BJ, Davies TB, Lazinica B, Krieger JW, and Pedisic Z. Effect of resistance training frequency on gains in muscular strength: a systematic review and meta-analysis. *Sports Medicine:* 1-14, 2018.

15. Güllich A and Schmidtbleicher D. MVC-induced short-term potentiation of explosive force. *New Studies in Athletics* 11: 67-84, 1996.

16. Issurin VB. New horizons for the methodology and physiology of training periodization. *Sports medicine* 40: 189-206, 2010.

17. Koga S, Shiojiri T, Kondo N, and Barstow TJ. Effect of increased muscle temperature on oxygen uptake kinetics during exercise. *Journal of Applied Physiology* 83: 1333-1338, 1997.

18. Lopez RM and Jardine JF. Exertional Heat Illnesses. In: *Sport and Physical Activity in the Heat:* Springer, 2018, p. 313-329.

19. MacDonald HV and Pescatello LS. Exercise Prescription for Hypertension: New Advances for Optimizing Blood Pressure Benefits. In: *Lifestyle in Heart Health and Disease:* Elsevier, 2018, p. 115-136.

20. McGowan CJ, Pyne DB, Thompson KG, and Rattray B. Warm-up strategies for sport and exercise: mechanisms and applications. *Sports medicine* 45: 1523-1546, 2015.

21. Nakano J, Yamabayashi C, Scott A, and Reid WD. The effect of heat applied with stretch to increase range of motion: a systematic review. *Physical Therapy in Sport* 13: 180-188, 2012.

22. O'keefe JH, Patil HR, Lavie CJ, Magalski A, Vogel RA, and McCullough PA. Potential adverse cardiovascular effects from excessive endurance exercise. *Mayo Clinic Proceedings.* Elsevier, 2012, p. 587-595.

23. Ogasawara R, Sato K, Matsutani K, Nakazato K, and Fujita S. The order of concurrent endurance and resistance exercise modifies mTOR signaling and protein synthesis in rat skeletal muscle. *American Journal of Physiology-Endocrinology and Metabolism* 306: E1155-E1162, 2014.

24. Pearce AJ, Rowe GS, and Whyte DG. Neural conduction and excitability following a simple warm up. *Journal of science and medicine in sport* 15: 164-168, 2012.

25. Porter HJ, Davis JJ, and Gottschall JS. Exercise Time and Intensity: The Ideal Ratio to Prevent Overtraining and Maximize Fitness. *Medicine & Science in Sports & Exercise* 50: 651, 2018.

26. Ranatunga K, Sharpe B, and Turnbull B. Contractions of a human skeletal muscle at different temperatures. *The Journal of physiology* 390: 383-395, 1987.

27. Sapega AA, Quedenfeld TC, Moyer RA, and Butler RA. Biophysical factors in range-of-motion exercise. *The Physician and Sportsmedicine* 9: 57-65, 1981.

28. Shellock FG and Prentice WE. Warming-up and stretching for improved physical performance and prevention of sports-related injuries. *Sports Medicine* 2: 267-278, 1985.

29. Shiotsu Y and Yanagita M. Intervention Study on the Exercise Order of Combined Aerobic & Resistance Training in the Elderly. *Journal of Sports Science* 5: 322-331, 2017.

30. Silva LM, Neiva HP, Marques MC, Izquierdo M, and Marinho DA. Effects of Warm-Up, Post-Warm-Up, and Re-Warm-Up Strategies on Explosive Efforts in Team Sports: A Systematic Review. *Sports Medicine:* 1-15, 2018.

31. Takahashi T, Okada A, Hayano J, and Tamura T. Influence of cool-down exercise on autonomic control of heart rate during recovery from dynamic exercise. *Frontiers of Medical and Biological Engineering* 11: 249-259, 2001.

32. Van Mechelen W, Hlobil H, Kemper HC, Voorn WJ, and de Jongh HR. Prevention of running injuries by warm-up, cool-down, and stretching exercises. *The American Journal of Sports Medicine* 21: 711-719, 1993.

33. Vega RB, Konhilas JP, Kelly DP, and Leinwand LA. Molecular mechanisms underlying cardiac adaptation to exercise. *Cell metabolism* 25: 1012-1026, 2017.

34. Zanettini R, Bettega D, Agostoni O, Ballestra B, Del Rosso G, Di Michele R, and Mannucci PM. Exercise training in mild hypertension: effects on blood pressure, left ventricular mass and coagulation factor VII and fibrinogen. *Cardiology* 88: 468-473, 1997.

Advanced Concepts of Personal Training

NCSF Certified Personal Trainer

Chapter 13

Anaerobic Resistance Training

Anaerobic Resistance Training

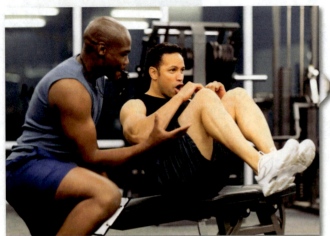

The time-tension relationship and total resistance used for training heavily determine chronic adaptations in both the anaerobic or aerobic energy systems. Often times anaerobic training in considered synonymous with resistance training, but the reality is "exercise" uses some sort of resistance regardless of the energy system employed. Resistance can be bodyweight against gravity, wind, water or inclination or it can be an external load as seen in free weight lifting and machine training. The magnitude of the resistance is the main influence that affects all the other related factors, and therefore, it must be quantified and controlled to create the desired adaptive response. Resistance employed for aerobic exercises is not quantified by a weight or load but rather expressed as the percentage of maximal oxygen used by the body to perform the work; thus, it is response specific. On the other hand, anaerobic resistance often uses external weights and loads and is quantified as a percentage of maximal force produced or velocity attained by the body. In some cases, it is the combination of the two. For an activity to be considered anaerobic resistance training, the force the body overcomes to perform a task must exceed the energy production capabilities of the aerobic systems.

◆ Role of Anaerobic Resistance Training

Anaerobic resistance training provides a significant number of benefits associated with health and life quality. Whereas aerobic exercise strongly correlates with cardiorespiratory health and lifespan, anaerobic training (sprinting and lifting) has a much greater impact on the functional aspects of the body. Adaptations in the nervous system, musculoskeletal system, endocrine system, and even the cardio-metabolic systems can all be managed through anaerobic-based training programs.

Positive adaptations and benefits of resistance training:		
	Nerve	Improved recruitment, synchronicity, responsiveness and firing rate
	Muscle	Fat-free mass maintenance, hypertrophy, improved tissue quality
	Connective tissue, including bone	Increased strength and mass, enhanced bone mineral density (BMD), improved tissue quality
	Cardiovascular system	Improved metabolic efficiency, increased capillary density, stroke volume, and vascular health (shear stress/eNOS) production)
	Metabolic system	Improved cell efficiency, enhanced byproduct management, mitochondria proliferation
	Endocrine system	Improved insulin sensitivity, heightened anabolic affinity (hormones and receptors), attenuated catabolic activity

Resistance Training and Musculoskeletal Health

Without adequate loading over time, the neural, muscular, and skeletal systems decline with age, increasing risk for musculoskeletal disease. The loss of lean mass is associated with a reduction in bone quality, muscular strength, and anaerobic power, all of which directly correlate to quality of life (QOL). Earlier chapters suggested these physical attributes are necessary for proper human function and even more important for the aging population's functional independence. Disconcertingly, physical activity among younger populations has declined: today's 20 to 30-year old individuals now have similar levels of physical activity to their 40 to 50-year old counterparts, promoting a heightened risk of skeletal-muscle loss with age. In fact, lean mass decline can begin before age 30 in sedentary populations [81]. Among older Americans, this common occurrence is significantly and independently associated with functional impairment and disability. Part of the reason the decline impacts human health so greatly involves the interrelationship of body systems'. Bone health depends upon muscle strength; muscle strength is contingent on the lean mass quantity and (neuro) motor-unit recruitment and activation efficiency. All are affected by loading and movement velocity.

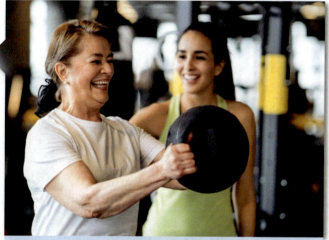

Resistance training can prevent the onset of sarcopenia; studies have also shown that strength, balance, agility, and jump training all help prevent functional decline among older populations.

Resistance training can help prevent the onset of age-associated muscle loss (sarcopenia) [83, 94]. Studies have shown that strength, power, balance, agility, and jump training (especially in combination) prevent functional decline in the elderly [14, 19, 94]. In addition, studies have demonstrated the positive effect of external loading in the structure of the weight-bearing bone, indicating that exercise helps prevent bone fragility [88]. These studies emphasize that adequate maintenance of muscle strength, particularly in the lower limbs, is crucial for proper balance and suggest that dynamic balance is an independent predictor of a standardized QOL estimate [50].

In addition to decline in functional capabilities, the fear of falling is pervasive among older people and is an independent risk factor for decreased mobility and loss of QOL [20, 28]. Lack of body confidence can have severe implications for physical and health-related deficits, as very functional older adults reduce total movement due to fear of falling. The marked deficits in the strength and health status found among independent and healthy seniors who report being fearful of falling underscores the seriousness of this psychological barrier as a potential risk factor and making balance confidence an important predictor of falls in older adults [21, 55, 90]. The Centers for Disease Control reported in 2014 that one older adult falls every second of every day; the report found these falls to be the number one cause of deaths and injuries among older Americans [5]. Individuals who engage in multicomponent training programs including resistance training result in greater improvements in self-reported balance confidence and physical capabilities, which may negate the psychological impact age can have on activity participation by reducing fears of falling or injury [13].

Resistance Training & Bone Density

Earlier text stressed the importance of weight-bearing and resistance exercises in preventing reductions in bone mass with age. Resistance training and physical activity yield anabolic effects on bone tissue, as underscored by strong evidence correlating bone mass and the relative strength of the attached musculature [51, 95]. Bone loss can occur at any age, but the onset of bone mass decline is fairly consistent among adults after the age of 30, with the most significant loss occurring in older age [97]. Resistance training aimed at improving total body strength can considerably reduce the risk of premature bone loss and the development of osteopenia and osteoporosis. This effect occurs due to the mechanical load placed upon the musculoskeletal system, and age does not limit these improvements. Pre-pubescent children, adolescents, and adults have all demonstrated gains in bone quality with weight-bearing exercise and high impact movements, as these activities stress the bone and elicit the desired adaptations; this is especially important for those with increased risk of bone disease [44, 95].

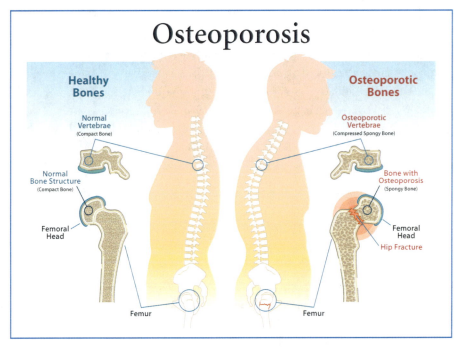

Bone stress continues to stimulate bone health throughout the lifespan when (adequate) stress is routinely applied. Exercise-stimulated increases in bone diameter diminish the risk of fractures by mechanically counteracting the thinning of bones and may halt bone porosity [28, 37]. Recommendations for resistance exercise aimed at improving bone mass or preventing increased bone porosity include selecting dynamic, ground-based activities that exceed threshold intensity and occur with a regular frequency [28]. Additionally, using an unusual loading pattern on the bones can contribute to improved adaptation by stimulating varied muscle group recruitment. The activities should be supported by adequate energy intake, calcium, and vitamin D [34]. Loading the musculoskeletal system to help fight against degenerative bone diseases is recommended for every movement once an individual has attained an appropriate level of fitness, except in movements of loaded spinal flexion. It should also be noted that individuals who have a vertebral or hip fracture, or history of fractures, represent a special case, and should be referred to a professional with specialized training in osteoporotic injury [30].

Improved Body Composition and Insulin Sensitivity

Resistance training's impact on structural tissue progresses under proper loading conditions, and these adaptations support body-compartment health. Humans are made up of minerals, protein, fat, and water, and all of these compartments are affected by resistance exercise: muscles, tendons, and ligaments strengthen, bones thicken, water storage increases in muscle tissue, and body fat is altered. Resistance training has demonstrated importance in several ways related to body composition particularly for disease prevention. Both weight control and routine movement are essential factors in decreasing the risk for inflammation and metabolic syndrome. Studies analyzing the effects of resistance training on body composition have found it to increase energy expenditure and preserve lean mass, thus promoting changes in body composition as well as body weight when energy intake is controlled and maintained at a constant level [63, 93]. Other studies have identified that resistance training yields positive effects on body composition but does not cause significant changes in fat mass. Not surprisingly, the greatest effects have been demonstrated when aerobic exercise, resistance training, and caloric control are combined [45, 71]. With this said, resistance training is likely more important for managing endocrine responses than for its beneficial health effects related to body fat. Obesity promotes inflammatory chemicals which wreak havoc on the cardiovascular system. Resistance training attenuates inflammation and improves insulin sensitivity in muscle mass and adipose tissues [16, 60]. This is particularly relevant for obese individuals, who live in a chronic low-grade inflammatory state, which can actually be compared, in some ways, to metabolic cancer [62, 85]. Currently, this (inflammatory) metabolic state threatens the life-expectancy of more than 33% of all Americans. Resistance training not only prevents this condition but can reverse it, and, unlike aerobic exercise, yields more pronounced metabolic benefits [85]. Additionally, and importantly, resistance training aids in managing dietary-induced circulating growth factor in the body. Several research trials have indicated that obese subjects who engage in routine, dynamic strength training experience improvement in whole-body insulin sensitivity [85]. This has also been shown to be true for children [26].

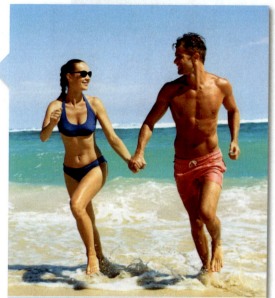

The greatest effects on body composition have been demonstrated when aerobic exercise, resistance training, and caloric control are all strategically combined.

QUICK FACT

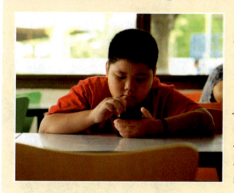

Insulin resistance is considered the primary defect in the pathophysiology of obesity-related disorders in children, such as type II diabetes [26]. Performing resistance training only twice a week for a 16-week period significantly increased insulin sensitivity and strength in overweight, adolescent Latino males, independent of changes in body composition [80].

Insulin sensitivity augmentation has value for non-obese elderly as well. As mentioned earlier, aging is associated with sarcopenia, or a loss of muscle mass, and consequently, the metabolic quality of skeletal muscle tissue, which leads to reduced daily function. In addition, age-related muscle changes also lead to an increased risk for developing insulin resistance and type II diabetes. Insulin resistance results in the muscle's inability to respond to insulin's anabolic effects and can exacerbate sarcopenia and accelerate the loss of independence. Loss of muscle mass and strength could be the main mechanism connecting chronic disease to physical disability [48]. Physiological decline associated with age-related decrease in physical activity is a primary threat to older individuals. In addition to improving muscular strength, resistance training also advanced insulin-stimulated glucose uptake in healthy individuals, healthy elderly individuals, and individuals with metabolic syndrome, diabetes, and other chronic diseases [17, 18, 33, 86].

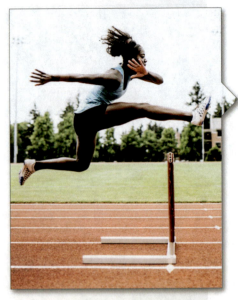

Improved Range of Motion and Movement Economy

Free-weight resistance training has significant implications for movement proficiency when compared to aerobic training. Aerobic training reduces flexibility in the trunk, hips, and knees because the movements lack full range during this type of exercise; resistance exercise yields the opposite effect when performed through proper range of motion (ROM). In fact, in trained distance runners, the addition of resistance training added improvements of up to 8% in **running economy** and significant improvements in marathon performance [46]. Among the elderly, resistance exercise improved flexibility and mobility and led to enhancements in gait speed and balance [12]. While research trials often select homogenous groups for evaluation, all people advance in their movement economy with resistance training, whether the goals are related to athletic or functional performance. Several clinical trials indicate that resistance training programs using 60-80% of 1RM effectively improve ROM when performed for only 6 to 10 week periods, resistance programs which employ combined movements promote significant gains in mobility regardless of age [24]. These enhancements likely relate to both muscular (fascia) and neuromuscular characteristics.

> **DEFINITIONS**
>
> **Running economy** –
> *Energy demand for a given velocity of submaximal running, represented by the steady-state consumption of oxygen (VO_2) and the respiratory exchange ratio.*

Improved Quality of Life & Function

Adequate strength and power strongly correlate to functional independence in older adults. Research findings demonstrate that resistance exercise can augment multiple domains of functional fitness, even among previously sedentary, elderly individuals [31,35,38]. When disabled older women with coronary heart disease participated in an intense resistance training program, they experienced improved physical capacity over a wide range of activities of daily living (ADLs). These benefits extended beyond muscular strength, as improvements in other components of fitness were also observed, including endurance, balance, coordination, and flexibility gains [10,40]. The resistance training program's intensity seems to facilitate a strong dose-response: strength gains and functional improvements increase with intensity of the exercise. This is consistent with other research findings, which support supervised moderate and high-intensity training for healthy older adults. Lower intensity levels using traditional resistance training models, regardless of volume, have not been shown sufficient to achieve optimal improvements in functional performance. Supervised, high-intensity, free-weight-based resistance training for healthy older adults appears to be as safe as lower-intensity training but is much more effective for physiological and functional improvements [84]. This also applies to children and young adults. Velocity and loading conditions are optimized when the intensities exceed low-to-moderate levels. When velocity increases with higher intensities, the effects increase even more.

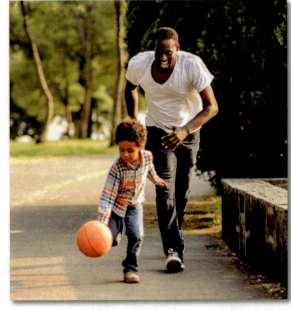

PRACTICAL INSIGHT

RESISTANCE TRAINING AND CALORIC EXPENDITURE

Resistance training has been shown to improve strength and increase muscle mass but has taken a back seat to aerobic training for weight loss. However, research has shown time and time again that resistance training is an equal or even more important aspect of weight management. Adding lean mass causes a proportionate increase in resting and active metabolism. Each kg of muscle mass provides an additional 13 kcal increase in resting metabolism per day [39]. This value becomes more significant when the tissue is actively stressed, contributing to enhancement in total-body oxygen utilization. The added mass forces the body to perform more work every time it moves, further increasing daily energy expenditure. Resistance training offers an added advantage, as it also associates with excess post-exercise oxygen consumption (EPOC) [36]. When exercise VO_2 and exercise duration were matched, circuit resistance training (high-intensity) was associated with a greater metabolic expenditure associated with EPOC [9]. Another significant finding was that the **respiratory exchange ratio (RER)**, an estimation of the cellular level measurement of CO_2/O_2, also referred to as **respiratory quotient (RQ)**, decreased from 0.85 to 0.75, demonstrating greater reliance on fat utilization following intense circuit exercise when compared to the measured RQ at a normal resting rate taken before the circuit training program. The effect that varied types of resistance training have on the body has been demonstrated in numerous studies. Although exercise duration is a factor, high-intensity anaerobic training demonstrates the most significant impact on EPOC [36, 91]. From this information, it can be surmised that routine participation in high-intensity resistance exercise can have a notable, positive effect on mean resting metabolic rate (RMR) values.

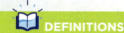

DEFINITIONS

Respiratory exchange ratio (RER) –

The ratio of the amount of carbon dioxide (CO_2) produced and oxygen (O_2) consumed, determined by comparing exhaled gases to that of ambient air; used to estimate the respiratory quotient at submaximal intensities.

Respiratory quotient (RQ) –

The ratio of carbon dioxide consumed and oxygen produced at the site of the tissue, used to identify the relative oxidation contribution of fat, carbohydrate, and protein.

Training for a Desired Outcome

Unlike aerobic exercise, where only a few parameters affect the adaptations, anaerobic training programs must use detail-oriented care to ensure they attain specific, desired outcomes. Therefore, in addition to selecting a modality, exercise professionals should select multiple exercises based on client need, and these should be performed in an appropriate order, with each exercise accompanied by a designated (adaptation-specific) load, speed, and consequent rest interval. In addition, the exercise programmer must be mindful that the systems affected by resistance training have different sensitivities to the applied stress. For instance, neuromuscular adaptations related to anaerobic training are specific to the magnitude and velocity of the force (load and speed); however, this factor has fewer implications for muscle architecture and metabolic adaptations. Dissecting the specific goals and matching the stress specificity to the adaptations significantly aids in the process of programming.

In general, the goals of resistance training fall under one of the following adaptation categories:

| Function or Physical Readiness (General Preparation) | Anaerobic Endurance | Hypertrophy | Strength | Power |

In many cases, training regimens reflect adaptation phases. A program may, or may not, include all phases across a training period, as some programs place a significant emphasis on only one or two of these categorical areas. Interestingly, the less experienced the exerciser, the more a holistic, or general, approach is employed, whereas more elite exercisers require specific emphasis to continue desired adaptations. This is partly explained by the fact that new exercisers experience many simultaneous adaptations because all exercise stress is fairly novel, so change comes more easily. Experienced exercisers, on the other hand, confront the Law of Diminishing Returns, and therefore, must work harder for the same percentage of change because adaptation potential lessens as more progress is made toward their genetic endpoint.

Anaerobic Programming – Categorical Emphasis

Function or General Physical Readiness
This is the first objective that should be accomplished, as movement competence must be established before setting any fitness goals. Function places emphasis on establishing correct movement patterns, proper strength balance across joints, proper activation of force couples and prime movers, baseline stability, flexibility, and mobility in preparation for more challenging stress. In many cases, body weight is the preferred first load employed to enhance neuromuscular control.

Anaerobic Endurance
Once an individual has established proper musculoskeletal health, the actions can be further challenged by volume. Adjustments to the time under tension (TUT) and recovery periods allow for ongoing improvement in select movements while increasing musculo-metabolic proficiency. This category pushes movement competence to repeatability, requiring longer periods of activation under load and greater ROM across movements.

Hypertrophy
Optimal health requires a certain amount of lean mass. While the body inherently resists adding excess muscle mass, modest increases can occur following specific training. Planned programs featuring high volume and moderate load are ideal for increasing protein synthesis beyond the basic recovery from physical activity. Unlike training for strength and power, when training for hypertrophy, the nervous system serves a reduced role, exchanging maximal speed or force for stress on the metabolic system.

Strength
Strength constitutes the maximum amount of force a muscle can produce in a single effort, and this category increases focus on maximal, balanced force. Muscle strength comes from two factors: increased total mass and neuromuscular efficiency. Therefore, the categorical emphasis centers upon motor unit recruitment, with factors such as force-couple efficiency, reduced restriction, and maximal joint stability when using large muscle groups. Loads are elevated and TUT is specific to muscle architecture changes or nervous system enhancements.

Power
Power is the speed of work. Therefore, this category emphasizes ballistic or plyometric exercise with a goal of fast-twitch fiber recruitment and nervous system proficiency. The individual's relative characteristics will drive programmatic decision making, but velocity of movement is the focus. Force requirements increase exponentially with loaded, velocity-based movements; intensities may be a little as 5% for speed work and as high as 90% for Olympic exercise when programming for improvements in power. Since power is a performance metric, an individual must first demonstrate adequate measures of function and health-related fitness before engaging in these movements that promote high levels of tension and stress.

◆ Goals of Resistance Training

Each desirable adaptation response to resistance exercise has defining characteristics required of the stress used for its attainment. Resistance training outcomes are similar to the outcomes that occur when cooking. If all the ingredients a recipe calls for are included in correct proportion, mixed correctly, and timed appropriately, the food will come out as desired. However, if any ingredients are changed, reduced, increased, or forgotten, or the mixing technique or cooking time is adjusted, the outcome is not always predictable or desirable. Resistance training program design and the subsequent adaptations work the same way. To cause the desired adaptation using resistance training, the correct recipe of exercise and its related factors is required. If any part of the recipe changes, the adaptation response is affected. The following section provides the evidence-based training stress necessary for the intended adaptation.

Repetition-Specific Maximums

• 1 RM	100%	• 7	82.5%
• 2	95%	• 8	80%
• 3	92.5%	• 9	77.5%
• 4	90%	• 10	75%
• 5	87.5%	• 11	72.5%
• 6	85%	• 12	70%

This table identifies estimated percent intensities for multi-repetition maximums. Percent intensity (% 1RM) is used to achieve the appropriate resistance training adaptation response, or goals. Goals include general fitness, anaerobic endurance, hypertrophy, strength and power.

◆ General Fitness Training – Physical Readiness

Resistance training for function borrows attributes from all anaerobic training categories to lay the foundations for improved performance. Since the emphasis focuses on establishing a base of physical qualities and skills, the adaptive focus is placed on all of the components of fitness. This suggests that all aspects that positively affect muscular fitness are employed to some degree within the training program. Fitness components have a spectrum of characteristics and applications beyond those needed for normal function, and these are individually specific to health and life quality. The primary goal of function-based training is to encourage appropriate levels of fitness within each of the respective components while also developing movement competence across a repertoire of exercise activities. The information captured during the screening and evaluation period can help determine starting points and exercise selection.

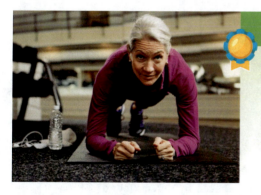

General Fitness Training Goals

- Movement competence for biomechanical foundations
- Proper activation
- Improved central stability, peripheral stability, and ROM

Using parameters associated with foundational health-related fitness categories, a trainer can blend activities within the program in a logical, sequential order. To maximize use of time and adaptation, chosen exercises should benefit more than one fitness area at a time. Resistance training machines are easy to use but do not often provide this benefit as the environment is too controlled. Since adaptations sought relate specifically to the stress and the environment in which the stress is applied, competent trainers often prefer closed-chain exercises that use unilateral stances, which better promote mobility and stability. The client's capabilities and needs will guide the selection and number of exercises programmed for any categorical emphasis, as well as the intensity and total volume. As a minimum, to ensure a proper stimulus, function-based training should be performed at least three days per week, employing a total body workout concept. When possible, one day of recovery between exercise sessions should be arranged. Workouts can be performed on consecutive days, but the movements employed should be complementary to the whole-body approach. Due to the reduced emphasis on load when programming for physical readiness, recovery concerns tend to be less of a factor compared to strength or hypertrophy training. A program aimed at function presents a prolific range of options, so any number of variables can be adjusted to match the client's need and schedule.

GENERAL FITNESS TRAINING GUIDELINES

General Fitness		
Intensity	50-70% 1RM (glycolytic)	
Frequency	3-5x/week	
Volume	30-36 sets/day	
Mode	Multiple modality	
Reps	8-20	
Rest Interval	30-60 seconds	
Endocrine	Limited GH, testosterone, adrenal hormones	

EMPHASIS: Improved Health & Fitness

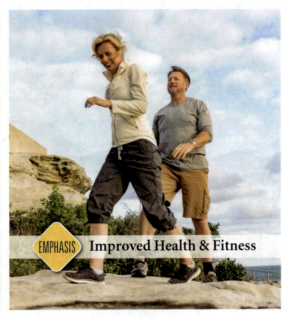

A client-specific general exercise program allows for creative application of stress. When general fitness is the goal, trainers can utilize any anaerobic training systems, so long as they are safe for the individual and logically fit the exercise program. Since body composition constitutes part of the health-related components of fitness, the total caloric output should be considered and managed. Many individuals use resistance training specifically for weight loss purposes, but that component represents just one part of this category's goal. Varying intensity and sets and utilizing activities that combine two exercises into one can effectively improve the rate of progress toward goals. Although numerous options are available for ever-changing workouts, the applied stress should still allow for frequent enough exposures to the exercise so that adaptations can occur, and movement proficiency can be secured. Making too many changes within a workout program may limit success because the individual may never develop movement proficiency. The neuromuscular system adapts based on a **dose response**, so a particular exercise or movement should be performed for at least 3 consecutive weeks before altering it or changing it to a different exercise. Clients want to see improvements and rehearsing these motor patterns frequently will ensure they are engrained within the nervous system. When compared to muscular or metabolic system programs, this approach yields the most rapid adaptive response.

DEFINITIONS

Dose response –

The degree of physiological response is related to the amount or dose of a given stimulus.

General Fitness Sample Program

Exercise	Sets x Reps	Intensity	Rest Interval	System
Dynamic warm-up Kneeling opposite raise Wide-leg goodmorning Split-stance reaches Lateral squat with reach	2x12 or 7 per side	Light (20-30%)	Transitional	Circuit
Modified deadlift	4x6	Lift to form	60 sec	
Front squat to MB overhead press	3x8	8-12 lb ball	60 sec	Combination
Supine pull-ups	4xamap	Bodyweight	45 sec	
Bench push-ups	3x8	Bodyweight	45 sec	
Lateral squat walks w/front raise	2x4 each way	10 lb plate	30 sec	Combination
Split-stance RDL	3x8	Light mod	40 sec	
Low box step-ups Rev flyes	12 2x10	Bodyweight Light	40 sec	Superset
Leg curl on ball Wide-leg mountain climbers Band face-pulls	2x10 8 per side 12	Bodyweight	Transitional	Circuit
5 min dynamic stretch				

Key: MB- Medicine Ball; Amap- As many as Possible; RDL- Romanian Deadlift

◆ Anaerobic Endurance Training

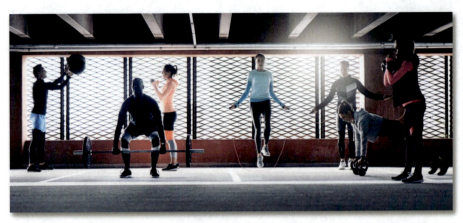

The definition of anaerobic endurance implies that the rate of force decline ultimately determines a muscle's ability to perform prolonged work at a sustained intensity. This category follows a foundational fitness period because anaerobic endurance is affected by several baseline factors such as:

- **Exposure to longer durations of resistive stress** *(local and systematic, enduring characteristics)*
- **Central and peripheral stability** *(stabilizing characteristics)*
- **The muscle's absolute strength** *(force capacity)*
- **Neural efficiency** *(motor patterning and rehearsal)*
- **Aerobic capacity** *(oxygen capacity and utilization)*
- **Anaerobic energy-system efficiency** *(metabolic tolerance and conditioning)*

While this category is often considered specific to endurance athletes, skipping over this phase and all of the aforementioned adaptational responses would be naïve. **Training tenure** is a key predictor in anaerobic performance outcomes. The neuromuscular system must experience an increase in stress to stimulate adaptation, and this period provides an opportunity for further movement rehearsal to proceed in a progressive manner. Secondarily, the lower intensities used in this category promote a foundational bridge to be able to use higher loads later, based on the gain in movement proficiency and other enduring characteristics of the neuromuscular system.

> **DEFINITIONS**
>
> **Training tenure –**
>
> *Denotes the level of training and experience an individual possess related to a stress.*

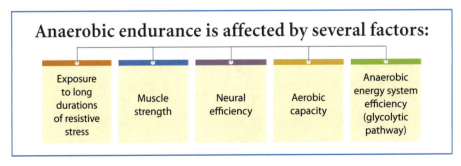

Anaerobic endurance is affected by several factors: Exposure to long durations of resistive stress; Muscle strength; Neural efficiency; Aerobic capacity; Anaerobic energy system efficiency (glycolytic pathway)

Many people express surprise at finding out that muscular strength plays a large role in anaerobic endurance characteristics; however, when analyzed closely, the reason becomes quite clear. The stronger a muscle becomes, the less intense the absolute submaximal work; as an individual's strength increases, the body perceives the same load to be "easier or lighter" because it represents a lower relative percentage. Consider the following example: two men are asked to bench press 100 lbs. as many times as possible to test their respective muscular endurance. One man has a maximal bench press of 150 lbs., while the other has a maximal bench press of 300 lbs. Which of these men could bench press 100 lbs. more times? The answer lies in their respective strength. The 100 lbs. resistance would be 66% of the first man's 150 lbs. bench-press maximum, or 1RM, whereas it would only represent 33% of the second man's 300 lbs. bench-press 1RM. It is obviously easier to lift 33% of a maximum for a high number of repetitions than to lift 66% of the maximum. Notably, strength and its complementary stabilizing characteristics do not compose the only factors in local muscles' anaerobic endurance. The glycolytic pathway's efficiency and the individual's respective buffering and aerobic capacities would also come into play. The ability to remove hydrogen and clear lactate from the blood and tissue remains necessary to continue force production and depends on oxygen utilization. If lactate production exceeds lactate removal, the cell's acidity will increase, inducing fatigue-causing force output to decline quickly.

Utilizing components of anaerobic endurance training proves very useful for many clients. It provides numerous adaptive benefits for several types of clients, including those who are fit but new to resistance training. The phase's key value lies in developing movement proficiency with resisted exercises while building a base for future progressions. Anaerobic endurance training also provides a good start to a weight loss program, with an aim of increasing total work and caloric expenditure per time segment and represents a useful place to resume training for those returning to exercise after extended time off. Endurance sport enthusiasts often gravitate to this reduced-rest, interval type of training as well; however, while it can serve as an appropriate supplement, research has demonstrated strength and power training yields far better performance results for both race times [3].

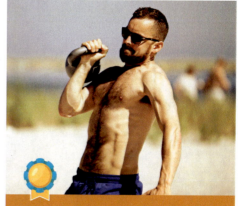

Anaerobic Endurance Training Goals

- Improve neural/movement competency (motor rehearsal)
- Align strength balance across joints
- Improve mobility
- Increase TUT across activation segments
- Improve metabolic conditioning
- Increase total work per time segment

ANAEROBIC ENDURANCE TRAINING GUIDELINES

Anaerobic Endurance

Intensity	50-70% 1RM (glycolytic)
Frequency	3-5x/week
Volume	30-45 sets/day
Mode	Multiple modality
Reps	12-25
Rest Interval	Short as tolerated
Endocrine	Minimal GH, epinephrine

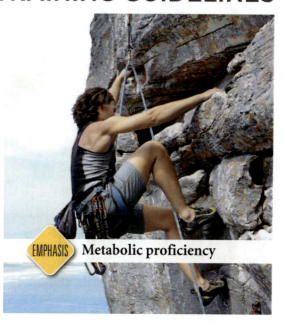

EMPHASIS Metabolic proficiency

Anaerobic endurance training's potential exercise palette provides for a level of diversity. Although individual muscle groups may be emphasized within this category, they are often used to supplement training movements, as the outcomes of isolated training do not align ideally with the aforementioned goals. In general, the aim should be to optimize movement while addressing areas that are weaker or where deficits exist to help remove imbalances. Muscle strength balance across joints is of particular importance and should be specifically emphasized in this category of training. Total repetition, or movement segment time, often ranges from 30-45 seconds per set, but may extend to a minute in length among experienced exercisers.

Anaerobic Endurance Sample Program

Exercise	Sets x Reps	Intensity	Rest Interval	System
Dynamic warm-up Goodmorning w/T-reach Reverse step-back w/OH reach Lunge w/lateral lean Ground sweeps	2x12 or 7 per side	Light (20-30%)	Transitional	Circuit
Neutral grip deadlift	3x6	Lift to form	60 sec	
Bulgarian squats	4x6 side	Lift to form	60 sec	
DB back flys	4x12	Bodyweight	45 sec	
DB chest press	3x15	Bodyweight	45 sec	
Glute-ham raise	3x8	Bodyweight	40 sec	
Lateral lunge w/ rotational reach	2x6 each way	8 lb MB	30 sec	Combination
45 degree cable pull-down Bench sit-ups	2x15 15	Light-moderate Bodyweight	40 sec between sets	Superset
MB floor to ceiling reach Band pull-a-parts Lateral box step-overs DB Curl to Press	3x12 3x15 3x7 each side 3x10	Bodyweight Light	Transitional	Circuit
5 min dynamic stretch				

Key: MB- Medicine Ball; Amap- As many as Possible; RDL- Romanian Deadlift; DB- Dumbbell

◆ Hypertrophy Training

Hypertrophy training is used to increase the mass of a muscle for any number of reasons. Individuals often pursue mass gains for aesthetic purposes, but hypertrophy may also be aimed at disease or musculoskeletal management, attenuating impact forces in sports, or counteracting natural aging processes. Although numerous systems and techniques exist that can be used to cause a muscle to grow, they all must follow a consistent theme of promoting muscle protein synthesis. For a muscle to increase in size, it must be stimulated by a cascade of stresses that signals a response from anabolic hormones. Recalling from earlier chapters, specific types of stress release anabolic hormones by triggering certain signaling pathways. The more muscle tissues the hormones target and the higher the tissues' affinity for the hormones, the greater the hypertrophic response will be, assuming adequate energy and nutrition are available to support tissue growth. This identifies the need to stimulate the recruitment of many motor units when training for muscle growth. This increased recruitment facilitates the process of muscle remodeling in large quantities of tissue, as described in earlier chapters. Single bouts of exercise performed a couple of times per week are inadequate for notable improvements in muscle growth. Rather, a minimum of 10 sets per week, per muscle group is necessary for modest changes in lean mass, with each muscle group being trained at least twice per week[77,78]. Most programs use 30-40 sets per exercise bout, with 4-6 days a week of training. Training bouts are often split into areas of emphasis with off-setting days of recovery. Commonly, body parts are selected based on the overlap of muscle actions, such as chest and triceps, back and biceps etc. This volume makes such a regimen difficult to function as the primary emphasis for most personal training clients, since many do not book sessions for 4-6 days; however, some positive changes in body mass are commonplace in the first 4 months of training due to initial physiological adjustments to exercise.

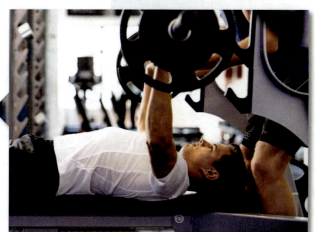

Hypertrophy training aims to enhance total muscle mass and potentially optimize body composition.

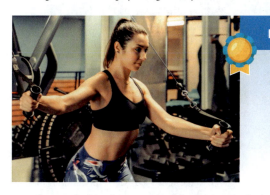

Hypertrophy Training Goals

- Promote protein synthesis
- Increase loading capabilities to moderate-heavy (70-85% 1RM)
- Optimize total muscle balance
- Improve endocrine adaptations
- Enhance the glycolytic pathway

A second obstacle to emphasizing hypertrophy in personal training programs is that the gains are based on volume, intensity, frequency, TUT, and tenure. Specific requirements for hypertrophy training mandate that exercises trigger a high, mechanically-induced, metabolic stress response. This may occur from the quantity of muscle mass employed to move a heavy resistance, as seen in deadlifts (mechanical tension). Alternately, it may stem from the metabolic environment created by the time-tension relationship involved. Moderate-resistance exercise performed to volitional failure paired with minimal rest achieves an ideal metabolic condition to stimulate anabolic hormone release. Pushing higher intensities through the glycolytic pathway is a key element in this process. This training category commonly employs isolation-based training, focusing solely on a single muscle group to trigger the metabolic response and a cascade of hormonal events. Of importance, the exercises should be performed to failure, with rest periods set as short as tolerable for the weight used. This combination of stress augments human growth hormone and leads to subsequent gains in lean mass in a fashion superior to any other training arrangement. Many exercisers fail to see the results they desire from hypertrophy training because 1) the rest intervals are too long or 2) the resistance is either too light, or too heavy. Essentially, the blend of moderately heavy (70-85% 1RM) loads pushed to volitional failure, for periods >20 seconds with short rest intervals encourages the low blood pH known to stimulate the desired hormone response [20, 32]. To ensure that the appropriate rest interval is followed, a stop watch should be used between sets. More intense sets of exercise should use the 60-90 second recovery, assuming maximal effort is performed to failure; moderate intensity sets should use 30-60 second recovery periods [96]. The short rest periods make body building physiologically very uncomfortable, explaining why most exercisers take too much time between sets, and, consequently, don't experience the anabolic effects they were hoping for in response to the training.

HYPERTROPHY TRAINING GUIDELINES

Hypertrophy		
	Intensity	70-85% 1RM (glycolytic)
	Frequency	4-6x/week
	Volume	High (30-40 sets/day)
	Mode	Compound and Isolated Lifts
	Reps	8-12 (8-10 high anabolic)
	Rest Interval	30-60 sec (up to 90 sec)
	Endocrine	Testosterone, GH, cortisol, epinephrine, IGF-1

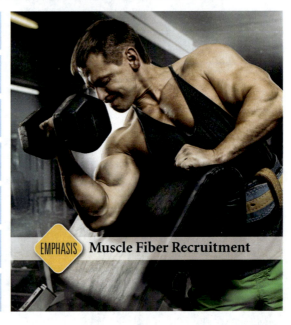

EMPHASIS: Muscle Fiber Recruitment

Since gains in muscle mass are also consistent with higher-intensity total body exercise movements, it makes sense to blend major compound exercises with isolation-based exercise. Exercises involving larger muscle groups (i.e., legs and back) elicit a greater hormonal response under loads greater than 80% 1RM. Since muscle hypertrophy depends on hormone response and the hormone response is systemic, exercises involving larger muscle groups will also benefit the small muscle groups. This suggests that back squats, deadlifts, bench press, military press, bent-over rows, and other **compound movements** should be employed as often as possible within considerations for adequate recovery. The heaviest lifts often attain maximal benefit by increasing volume using a pyramid-style, staircasing effect for preparation; this means 4-6 sets of increasing intensity across an exercise. This style of training presents another limiting factor for most personal training situations, because it requires much more time. Higher intensities demand longer rest intervals and recovery time. Additionally, training experience has real implications for growth rate. Experienced body builders show greater mass gains following 18

> **DEFINITIONS**
>
> **Compound movements** –
>
> *Actions involving two or more joints and the recruitment of large amounts of muscle mass across several muscle groups.*

months of training compared to their initial 18 months. This suggests promoting adaptations towards gaining muscle mass proceeds relatively slowly as it requires high-volume, fairly heavy resistance, and elevated discomfort tolerance.

Hypertrophy Training Sample Program

Exercise	Sets x Reps	Intensity	Rest Interval	System
Dynamic warm-up Goodmorning w/IYT reach Reverse lunge w/OH reach Forward lunge w/rotation Lateral ground sweeps	2x12 or 7 per side	Light (20-30%)	Transitional	Circuit
Bench press	4x8-10	Lift to form	75 sec	
Incline DB press	3x8	Lift to form	60 sec	
Speed push-ups Cable flyes	3x 10 sec 12	Bodyweight Load to form	60 sec	Superset
Tricep pull-overs Tricep rope pull-downs	3x 10 3x15	Lift to form Load to failure	45 sec	Superset
Cable kickbacks	3x15	Light-moderate	20 sec	
Cable rotation V-situps	2x8 side 12	Lift to form Bodyweight	30 sec	Superset
5 min dynamic stretch				
Key: MB- Medicine Ball; Amap- As many as Possible; RDL- Romanian Deadlift; DB- Dumbbell; OH- Overhead				

PRACTICAL INSIGHT

Hypertrophy for the personal training client is definitely attainable, but accomplishing this goal does come with limitations. Utilizing the aforementioned guidelines for a hypertrophic response will increase mass on a previously untrained client with only two or three training days per week. This hypertrophic response appears within approximately 4-6 weeks (20, 79). In significantly detrained individuals, this change may occur more rapidly. The difficulty regarding hypertrophic improvements lies in continuing to make progress in mass gains following the initial adaptation, due to the previously mentioned time restrictions. Deconditioned clients will reap relatively greater improvements in mass in a shorter time period, compared those who have been trained for several months or years. Additionally, although personal training should focus on reaching client goals, many other important needs warrant priority in the exercise session. Solely emphasizing hypertrophy training may limit the attainment of more important health pursuits within the program. One common concern related to hypertrophy or resistance training is the fear of getting too massive. This trepidation is more common in women, which often leads to selecting light resistance when training or avoiding resistance training altogether; however, due to their low levels of testosterone, females face a greater challenge than men with respect to adding muscle mass. In fact, an addition of 1-2 lbs. of muscle with an equal weight loss from fat will actually make a person smaller, even though bodyweight remains unchanged, due to the density of lean tissue.

Strength Training

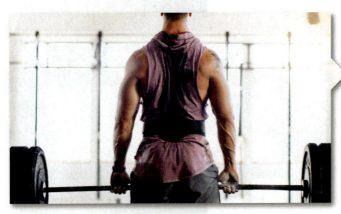

Muscular strength is defined by the ability to produce a maximal contractile force. But, in the context of free-moving conditions, (functional) strength is really the ability to accomplish tasks against different types of resistance which may employ a specific joint or combination of joints across a predetermined ROM. It is really only during specific strength training and physical therapies that movements are isolated to a set joint angle against resistance. The ability to produce a maximal contractile force therefore applies to a specific purpose. Numerous factors can affect the force production capabilities of the body: some independent, others co-dependent (or relational). A single muscle's contractile force is independent, as it is a factor of the cross-sectional muscle size as well as total recruitment, speed of recruitment, and proficiency of the motor units involved. When muscles work together for movements, the cooperation, or relational factors, become much more relevant. **Force couples**, stabilizers, and **kinetic chain** efficiency all affect the resultant force output, with the most common limiting factor to producing a movement being the sustained force of local and global joint stabilizers.

Resistance movements that challenge the maximal capabilities of all involved tissues will yield the greatest adaptive response. Adaptations for increased strength include heightened neural efficiency, and to a lesser degree, increased mass. Strength adaptations include some level of architectural adjustments in the muscle cell, but these are secondary to the neural changes. Based on the adaptations that lead to increased force output, training for maximal strength requires high levels of resistance across multiple joint segments to optimally promotes greater motor unit recruitment and **central-peripheral stability**. These maximal forces rapidly drain the phosphagen energy system, limiting the performance duration to 15-20 seconds. This suggests that repetition ranges aimed at "strength" are relatively low, often less than six. When 6-10 repetitions are used, the purpose of the exercise and the load shift from targeting the neural system to anabolic benefits and the enduring characteristics of stabilizers. Because the phosphagen system takes priority when performing heavy resistance training to increase strength, longer rest periods are necessary to fully re-phosphorylate adenosine triphosphate (ATP) and creatine phosphate. This requires 2-5 minutes of rest between maximal bouts. A common tactic in strength training is to reduce the exercise variety and increase the sets: for example, performing 4-6 sets of compound exercises. When appraised by the total number of exercises employed (4-6 total exercises), strength training sessions initially seem to use shorter durations; however, after accounting for the required rest intervals needed between sets, these will become fairly long training bouts.

 DEFINITIONS

Force couples –

The synergistic action of opposing or adjacent muscles to produce a rotational action; i.e., upper trapezius and serratus anterior contracting to promote scapular rotation.

Kinetic chain –

An engineering term used to describe the relationship between adjacent body segments whereby movement at one joint produces or affects movement at another joint through the transfer of energy.

Central-peripheral stability –

Refers to the ability to recruit a pattern of necessary musculature in order to maintain structural integrity of the trunk (central) and limbs (peripheral) while managing internal and external forces.

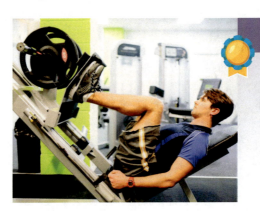

Strength Training Goals

- Maximize multi-joint loading capabilities
- Increase total force output
- Enhance central-peripheral stability
- Improve kinetic-chain proficiency
- Improve nervous system proficiency (motor unit recruitment, firing rate, and synchronicity)

Very heavy resistance training limits muscle growth stimulation due to the reduced volume, so programming hypertrophy sets to follow the maximal strength sets is warranted if that is part of the goal. Since strength increases proportionately with muscle cross-sectional area, increases in muscle mass will equate to improvements in force production.

With this understood, the size related gains in strength have limitations; for instance, bodybuilders do not exhibit the high strength levels of competitive powerlifters for two primary reasons:

- **They do not properly train the neural characteristics for maximal force production**
- **They isolate muscle groups using machines and other tactics which reduce stabilizer strength**

Individuals who emphasize absolute strength training movements create more efficient force production capabilities that can be more easily transferred, compared to individuals who perform only hypertrophy training. This difference occurs because the stress stimulus and environment are adaptation specific. The nervous system's enhancement of force production becomes even more evident when previously sedentary individuals begin strength training. In these cases, initial gains are significant and occur fairly rapidly due to the previously inefficient state of the neuromuscular system. Motor patterning occurs through the rehearsal of resisted movements, which causes the nervous system to improve at producing forces across the movement range. In the first 3-5 weeks of training, the nervous system is primarily responsible for resultant improvements in strength [64, 79]. This is valuable for personal training because it demonstrates noticeable improvements that the clients can observe, adding to motivation and compliance, as they can move more resistance at the same or lower relative rate of perceived exertion (RPE).

STRENGTH TRAINING GUIDELINES

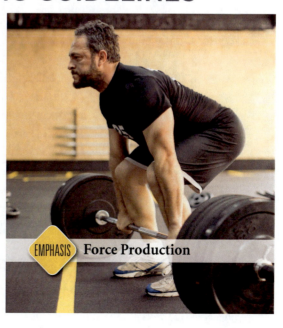

Maximal Strength		
	Intensity	75-95% 1RM (phosphagen/glycolytic)
	Frequency	3-5x/week
	Volume	Low (18-30 sets/day)
	Mode	Cross joint lifts
	Reps	3-5 (nervous) 6-10 (muscle)
	Rest Interval	Glycogen 60-90 sec Phosphagen 2-5 min
	Endocrine	GH, testosterone

EMPHASIS Force Production

Strength training movements are often compound, thereby coordinating large quantities of mass to move resistance. The use of large muscles for high-intensity training stimulates the release of testosterone in larger quantities, compared to small muscle group use. This factor aids in developing greater strength over time. Additionally, closed-chain, cross-joint exercises strengthen the muscles used for central and peripheral stabilization to a much greater degree compared to exercise performed on resistance machines. Both ground-based and non-ground based exercises require additional body control for proper performance, thereby increasing stability and leading to improved strength performance. Some examples include the squat, deadlift, military press, pull-up, and dips. These movements require the exerciser to prevent body sway, so forces can be more efficiently directed to the vertical component of the lift. Trunk muscles stabilize these movements and correlate to all closed-chain force capabilities.

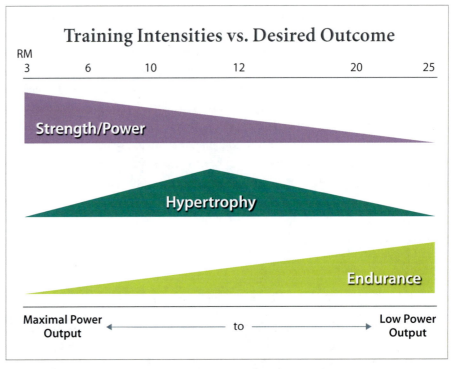

Strength training for new clients should be modified, reducing emphasis on the specificity of absolute strength prescription that would be employed for an experienced weightlifter. As with any new stress, clients should be appropriately acclimated and properly instructed. Inexperienced exercisers should focus on mastery of skill and movement proficiency. The most common training error is attempting to progress strength training when a proper base has not yet been established. Increasing repetition ranges and total number of sets usefully increases the proficiency that derives from motor rehearsal. All exercises should be performed with perfect technique before a new stress is considered and incorporated.

Strength Training Sample Program

Exercise	Sets x Reps	Intensity	Rest Interval	System
Dynamic warm-up Goodmorning w/IYT reach Rev lunge w/MB rotation Forward lunge to MB press MB squat swings	2x12 or 7 per side	Light (20-30%)	Transitional	Circuit
Box jumps	3x5	Bodyweight	90 sec	
Back squat	4x6-10	75-85% 1RM	120 sec	
Leg press	3x6-8	Load to form	120 sec	
RDL	3x6	Load to form	90 sec	
BB reverse lunges	4x5 side	Load to form	60 sec	
Nordic hamstrings Hanging leg raises	4x6 4x8	Bodyweight	60 sec	Superset
MB slams	3x15 sec	8-10 lb. MB	45 sec	
Adductor slides Lunge slides	2x10 sec side	Bodyweight	Transitional	Superset
5 min dynamic stretch				

Key: MB- Medicine Ball; RDL- Romanian Deadlift; BB- Barbell

◆ Power Training

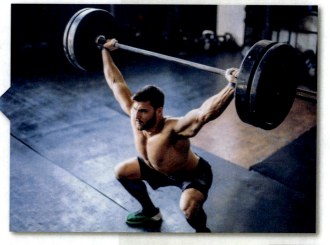

Training for power differs from training for hypertrophy or strength, with the greatest distinction being the rate of movements. Power training typically uses ballistic actions (momentum forces) to generate large amounts of force, beyond those which an individual could produce using controlled dynamic contractions. The movements are performed rapidly, thereby increasing the stress placed upon the tissue. Even light resistance can cause considerable force demands upon the muscle and connective tissues due to the high velocities attained during power training. Recalling earlier discussions, if a light object is accelerated, the force required to decelerate or stop it is much greater than the object's weight, because this weight is magnified by the rate of movement or velocity. A 5 lb. medicine ball is easy to press off the body, but to project it across the room requires much more acceleration force. Likewise, the person catching the mass must provide a deceleration force much greater than the 5 lbs. that the ball weighs due to the velocity of the moving weight. The same principle holds true when the body accelerates through space. Performing body weight squats requires much less acceleration and deceleration force compared to the same ballistic movement, jump squats, which require much more to propel the body rapidly across a maximal distance.

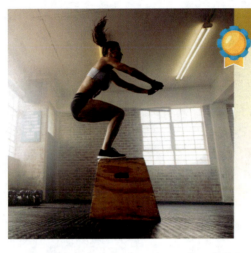

Power Training Goals

- Increase fast-twitch fiber firing rate and recruitment
- Improve force coupling/energy transfer rate
- Enhance movement economy through neural efficiency and the stretch-shortening cycle
- Develop optimal acceleration-deceleration balance
- Improve reactive stability across central and peripheral systems

DEFINITIONS

Plyometrics –

A method of training involving repeated rapid lengthening and contracting of muscles for the purpose of increasing power; denotes an amortization phase of <0.3 seconds.

Ballistics –

Actions that exhibit maximal concentric acceleration over a brief contraction time.

Amortization phase –

Also known as the transition or contact phase; constitutes the period of time between the concentric and eccentric phases of a plyometric exercise wherein the stretch-shortening cycle is exploited to maximize power production.

Training for improved power uses two distinct categories: **plyometrics** and **ballistics**. The distinctions between the two centers on contraction speed. An **amortization phase** that maintains propulsion contact for <0.3 seconds are plyometric; contractions that require longer resisted contact are ballistic. This is easily illustrated when viewed in application. Sprinting at maximal velocity is plyometric, as the speed is maintained at a high level and each foot-to-ground contact occurs at a rate <0.3 seconds. Harnessing oneself to a drag sled loaded with 45 lbs. and then trying to 'sprint' the same distance would significantly slow the body's horizontal velocity down, causing the maximal pull speed to become ballistic, as each propulsion contact time is consequently slower.

| Common plyometric exercise categories: | Depth jumps | Box jumps | In-place jumps | Upper/lower body rebounds |

In ballistic-power training, resistance slows down the movement so that each amortization phase becomes longer than 0.3 seconds. The rate of action and resultant force though, still exceed what is needed to simply move the resistance from point A to point B. Another example is seen with weighted jump shrugs. When using 5 lb. dumbbells, the ground contact speed may be plyometric, but when the weight increases to 30 lb. dumbbells, the same movement becomes ballistic, because of the amount of time it takes to get back off the ground between each jump. While the rate of force may be maximal in both cases, the forces that the muscles must overcome are different, and therefore, the movement velocity is different. Ballistic movements tend to require more total motor recruitment and often cause a more rapid fatigue rate when compared to the same number of dynamic voluntary movements. In many cases, maximal power using ballistic movements can only be performed for a low number of repetitions before compromising movement velocity. Similar to maximal strength training, rest intervals employed for power training need to be long enough to allow for full recovery. Without adequate recovery, subsequent sets and repetitions will be performed at slower velocities, reducing the power output and consequent adaptation. One strategy used to train for maximum power is to use lighter resistance across less repetitions but to perform every movement maximally. This allows for higher velocities and shorter tension times to attenuate the fatigue rate, thereby reducing the time needed to fully recover but still achieving close to peak power. Since power development relies on neural adaptations, the volumes do not need to be high. Olympic lifts and maximal height jumps for instance, rarely exceed 5-6 repetitions per set; low-repeat jumps are done for time (10 sec), and most drag training and sled pushes are done for distances of only 30 yards. Based on these time factors, it should be clear that power training relies predominantly on the phosphagen system for energy, and just like strength training, increases in volume come from the addition of more sets, not repetitions.

POWER TRAINING GUIDELINES

Power		
	Intensity	30-50% 1RM (glycolytic) or 60-95% 1RM (CP)
	Frequency	2-4x/week
	Volume	Varied by activity (moderate)
	Mode	Olympic lifts, ballistics, plyometrics
	Reps	2-5 (CP) 8-20 (glycolytic)
	Rest Interval	30-240 seconds
	Endocrine	GH, testosterone, epinephrine

EMPHASIS: Acceleration

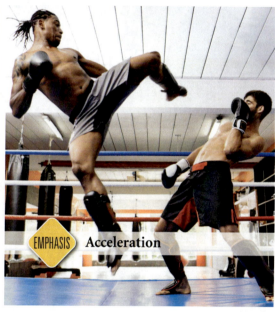

The modes of training for power include the Olympic lifts, jump training, weighted throws, sled pulling and pushing, bands, and resistance-swing exercises. A common movement pattern chosen for power training entails hip/knee extension and hip/knee flexion because the muscles involved in these movements can produce impressive acceleration forces. Power exercise modalities have recently gained popularity in many personal training settings, but are much more widespread in programs directed at athletic performance. When using traditional power training, the sets and repetitions match the resistance and the speed of the movement. As mentioned above, high-intensity plyometrics use low-repetition schemes combined with more sets; likewise, high-speed movements, such as medicine ball rebounds, often use time as the metric for volume, often employing fewer sets and more rest to ensure power output remains greater than 90%. The specific TUT of the training also varies by the same factors. In many cases, power-based exercises are used in conjunction with strength exercises to cover different training stresses in the same workout.

Power can be incorporated into personal training programs directed at multiple populations by simply changing the movement velocity and/or load. For example, single-leg box step-ups for a novice exerciser may progress to an accelerated rate to make them ballistic, whereas after practicing controlled sit-to-stand bench squats, an older adult client may progress to rapidly rising from the seated position, which would then qualify as a power progression. Both cases require high levels of relative power output due to the increased movement rate. Another strategy used to train power characteristics employs an applied hybrid model to increase safety by adding controlled eccentric movements followed by rapid concentric contractions. In the example of the older adult performing the rapid chair stands, the hybrid model would require the client to rise from the chair as quickly as possible and then return to the seated position using a traditional, controlled rate of descent during the eccentric phase. A medicine-ball chest pass also exemplifies the hybrid model. The client can accelerate the ball from the chest to pass it to his or her trainer, who then hands it back to repeat the action. In these hybrid models, the power training comes through concentric acceleration without the demands or safety issues associated with the eccentric deceleration component (recall that muscle damage increases with prolonged or high-velocity eccentric contractions). With proper instruction, more advanced clients can certainly perform fitness/skill-level-appropriate drops and jumps and medicine ball throws. Of course, client-specific considerations will apply.

Power Training Sample Program

Exercise	Sets x Reps	Intensity	Rest Interval	System
Dynamic warm-up Goodmorning w/MB reach Three reach squat Lateral lunge w/rotation MB swings to OH squat	2x12 or 7 per side	Light (30-40%)	Transitional	Circuit
Clean pulls	3x4	Progressive loads	90 sec	
Hang cleans	4x3-4	Lift to form	120 sec	
Back squat Squat jumps	3x4 12	> 85%	120 sec	Contrast set
Lateral ballistic box step-ups for height	3x6 per side	Bodyweight	75-90 sec	
Jump pull-ups	4x 10 sec	Bodyweight	75 sec	
Rebound push-ups	3x7	Light-moderate	60 sec	
KB swings Lateral bounds	2x4 per side 2x4 per side	Lift to form Bodyweight	60 sec	Superset
Nordic hamstrings MB pullover to stand	4x 6 8	 10 lb. MB	60 sec	Superset
5 min dynamic stretch				

Key: MB- Medicine Ball; OH - Overhead; KB- Kettlebell

Training Systems

Clearly, different demands placed on the muscular system present different adaptation responses within the tissues. The human body can achieve seemingly limitless movement options and can produce forces across a broad range of velocities while also engaging multiple systems when performing work. Thus, a vast number of methods exist that can elicit a desirable training response. Trainers must identify the specific demand-result relationship needed to affect the adaptations' magnitude and the rate at which those adaptations occur. Within resistance exercise, several **training systems** have demonstrated improved effectiveness in producing desired results in one or more of the anaerobic-based fitness components. Each training system offers unique characteristics that produce specific responses from the targeted physiological systems. The rationale for including a particular system depends on the demand's emphasis and the known adaptations it makes possible. In some cases, training systems may be concomitantly employed in an exercise bout, whereas in others, training systems may not be used at all. The decision to implement any of the systems will hinge upon the same considerations as the other program components.

> **DEFINITIONS**
>
> **Training systems –**
> *Training methods used to strategically exploit different categories of stress to emphasize specific improvements in strength, power, hypertrophy, or metabolic efficiency.*

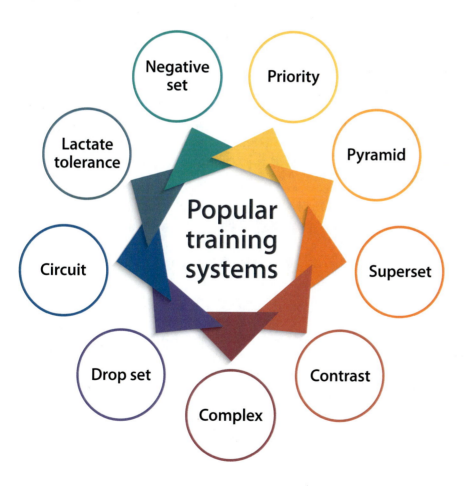

Priority System

The priority system, a logic-based approach to exercise training and programming, suggests performing exercises for deficient muscle groups at the beginning of an exercise session to ensure they receive adequate attention at times of maximal energy availability. This system is commonly used during the general preparation or foundational phases of an exercise program. Muscles that present restrictions, or are subject to imbalance or force-activation deficits, attain "priority" in the exercise order, even if they normally would be trained later in an exercise bout (e.g., leg curls). The priority system makes particular sense for new clients or those who have experienced negative consequences due to their musculoskeletal deficiencies. Normally, the priority system has special relevance for those possessing significant function or health issues, which is similar to the manner in which athletic training and physical therapy emphasize only exercises aimed at select pathologies.

This approach may also supersede the typical energy system order of operations. For instance, anaerobic-based phosphagen and glycolytic exercises would come before aerobic exercise when training; however, if an individual suffers from a controlled disease or requires greatly improved cardiorespiratory endurance, aerobic exercise may precede anaerobic exercise. Modalities aimed at ROM or improved mobility may also require a shift in exercise order based on the priority of the situation.

Pyramid System

The original pyramid system was employed by bodybuilders for muscle hypertrophy in order to cover a broad range of recruitment stimulus. It utilized a very high-volume group of sets, requiring exercisers to increase weight while decreasing repetitions in each subsequent set. At the lowest end of the repetition range, the sets ascended in an opposite manner, decreasing the weight while increasing the repetitions. This allowed bodybuilders to use high and moderate loads to cover the most anabolic repetition ranges [6-15]. This system is not very practical for most other training goals and is likely inappropriate for personal training due to time and frequency limitations.

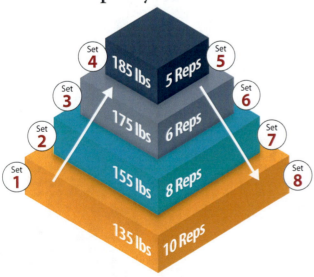

Example Pyramid Model

The modern pyramid system utilizes the principle of neuromuscular preparation, or Treppe effect, to increase the amount of force a muscle can produce by employing neuromuscular conditioning sets. This system is actually only a half pyramid and works by increasing the resistance for each subsequent set as the repetitions are reduced. It functions similarly to a specific warm-up but staircases the loading as the neuromuscular system gets primed for increasing resistance. The repetitions and weight amounts used depend upon the defined strength goal. In some cases, the early sets are not performed to volitional failure in preparation for the heavier workloads. Other techniques utilize resistance selected for maximal performance of each set within the defined repetition scheme. Pyramid training is very effective, primarily for improvements in maximal strength, but it may also be used to complement hypertrophy training, with rep schemes descending from 12 to 6 repetitions. The actual number of repetitions selected for the pyramid system will vary based on the client's capabilities and intended goals. One advantage to this method is that it allows for a wider range of repetitions and resistive stress compared to traditional work sets, which commonly use the same number of repetitions for each set, the classic 3 sets of 10 repetitions for instance.

Superset System

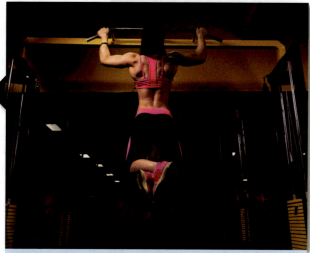

Supersets possess utility for endurance, hypertrophy, strength, and power improvements, suggesting they function as a diverse programmatic tool.

The superset system entails a simple design that can be very effective for accomplishing multiple training goals. It has utility for endurance, hypertrophy, strength, and power improvements, suggesting it functions as a diverse programmatic tool. The general concept is to perform one set of exercise immediately followed by a different exercise, with only transitional rest: the time it takes to transition from one exercise to the other between the sets. Because any two exercises can be placed together, trainers can create a plethora of combinations. The intended training adaptations will determine the exercise selection for the superset. If endurance is the goal, the emphasis should be placed on creating an ischemic condition. Anaerobic endurance will often use multi-set durations totaling 60-90 seconds: for example, 30 seconds of slide board lunges paired with 30 seconds of slide board adduction. When hypertrophy is the goal, the superset will combine two exercises that target the same muscle group or overlap the primary and secondary movers. This enables prolonged tissue stress by increasing the total TUT to stimulate greater muscle fiber recruitment. Chest press with chest flies, or shoulder press with side raises exemplify common supersets. Note that the exercise order mandates that the heavier, more challenging exercise be performed prior to the lighter, more isolated activity. In some cases, a pre-fatigued state dictates the order based on safety; in this case, consider combining supine triceps extension (skull crushers) and close-grip bench press. The sets and reps employed are consistent with the anabolic recipe for hypertrophy, and volitional failure is commonly used among bodybuilders to promote the longest TUT possible with the load.

Sample Supersets for Different Goals

Hypertrophy	Strength	Fitness/caloric expenditure
Combines two exercises targeting the same muscle group to stimulate greater fiber recruitment	Combined opposing muscle groups or lower and upper body exercises so that prime movers/stabilizers do not become fatigued from the initial set	Any combination can be used as long as it is consistent with goal
Bench press and push-ups	**Back squat and seated row**	**Triceps dips and bicep curls**

To facilitate strength improvement, the superset captures the enduring characteristics of the employed joint's stabilizers. In heavy-load supersets, the same local stabilizers should not be used, as they will become a pronounced limiting factor for the load used in the second set. Early phases of training often use opposing muscle groups (agonists:antagonists) or take advantage of using lower and upper-body exercises so that the prime mover and stabilizers do not suffer fatigue from the previous set. If general fitness or caloric expenditure is the desired outcome, then any combination consistent with the program goals is appropriate and can be combined as long as it makes sense.

Supersets may become more complex by adding a third exercise, referred to as the tri-set system. When a third exercise adds additional stress, considerations should be made for fatigue throughout the set and any respective stability limitation. Utilizing three exercises that stress the same postural muscle groups or articular stabilizers may lead to fatigue-related compensation and consequent performance breakdown. For this reason, the three exercises' requirements and how they work as a tri-set should be reviewed before they are joined and implemented in a program. This is particularly true when using heavier resistance or higher movement complexity. In general, tri-sets challenge the metabolic system and are common in high-intensity training (HIT) programs. Exercise combinations for less trained or novice clients should split the body into its respective thirds using an exercise for each of the upper, lower, and trunk musculatures. If a client is well-conditioned, other combinations can be utilized based on the individual's performance capabilities.

Sample Tri-sets

Beginner	Seated floor reach	Body squats	Side raise
Intermediate	Step-ups	Push-ups	Abdominal crunch
Advanced	Pull-ups	Lunge	Body dips

The repetition ranges of supersets and tri-sets can vary between exercises to cater to increasing demands or remain constant: the guiding determinations are both safety and effectiveness. The supersets may also be performed by time segments, such as 2 sets of 20 seconds, rather than repetition ranges. Using a time-based approach to sets allows exercisers to self-pace their efforts. Individuals who train at higher intensities will likely pass ventilatory threshold, making the perceived effort rather high on the **Borg scale**. Individual variables will ultimately serve as the defining factor for the program's activity selection.

> **DEFINITIONS**
>
> **Borg scale –**
>
> A scale of perceived exertion ranging from 6 "no feeling of exertion" to 20 "very, very hard" developed by Dr. Gunnar Borg as a simple way to measure heart rate; multiplying the score by 10 gives an approximate heart rate for young adults.

RPE	Description
6	Rest
7	Very, Very Light
8	
9	Very Light
10	
11	Fairly Light
12	
13	Somewhat Hard
14	
15	Hard
16	
17	Very Hard
18	
19	Very, Very Hard
20	"Exhaustion"

The Borg's RPE scale is often used to determine work intensities among those on medications that may alter heart rate (HR) responses, clients without access to a HR monitor, or those who do not assess their HR during training. The original scale runs from 6-20 as seen in the graphic; adding a zero loosely reflects HR (beats/min). A modified scale includes values from 0-10, with 0 being no exertion at all [7].

Contrast System

The contrast system is founded on the superset concept, but as the name suggests, the exercises chosen are specifically selected to utilize contrasting stresses. The system works by creating a (neurological) conditioning set, using near maximal loads in a controlled manner, immediately followed with a replicating movement of low loads at very high speeds. This contrasting superset maximizes fast-twitch recruitment and challenges stability elements at both ends of the force-velocity curve. Based on this information, it should make sense that the system is commonly used for performance enhancement, emphasizing the combination of neuromuscular crossover between strength and power. The first set of an exercise is performed using a near maximal set of less than 6 repetitions, followed by a duplicate movement using low resistance, at maximal speed – 5 reps of squat at 85% of 1RM superset (contrasted) with 5 max speed jump squats.

Sample Contrast System

Weighted Back Squat superset	Bench Press superset	Dumbbell Pull-overs superset
with	with	with
Jump Squats	Medicine Ball Chest Pass	Medicine Ball Chop Rebounds

The slow, heavy component recruits fast-twitch fibers based on the application of dynamic voluntary contractions for strength, while the fast, light component utilizes more power-based recruitment factors to recruit the remaining pool of fast twitch fibers. These techniques are physiologically demanding and often require complete rest periods. It should be noted that some texts refer to contrast training as crossing energy systems rather than working in a consistent system.

Complex System

Complex training has also been defined differently, depending on the source. In some cases, it refers to a grouping or "complex" of movement patterns such as a lunge or bar complex. In other cases, and more commonly in the literature, complex training combines a heavy-loaded conditioning set, followed by a plyometric or ballistic activity that employs the predisposed "conditioned" muscle groups. Often the grouping includes a very heavy compound leg movement (>85% 1RM), such as a squat, followed by a jump, bound, or sprint. The idea is based on the physiological phenomenon known as post-activation potentiation (PAP). PAP is a neural gain in the excitability threshold as a residual effect of a previously high excitation level, as seen with heavy movements. The complex system is a special type of superset in that the rest period between exercises may be either as short as 30 seconds or as long as 12-minutes to employ maximal gain; however, per logistical concerns, 4 minutes of recovery is most often used. It should also be noted that in order to elicit the PAP response, the heavy load's conditioning contractions should not be maximally fatiguing; thus, set and repetition schematics in this system always use integers of less than five at up to 98% capacity: 3 reps of 90% front squat (98% capacity), rest 4 minutes, then 40-yard maximal speed sprint.

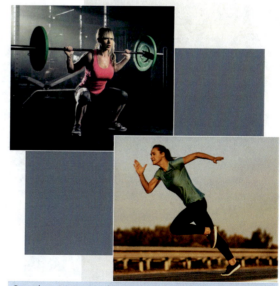

Complex training combines a heavily-loaded conditioning set, followed by a plyometric or ballistic activity that employs the predisposed "conditioned" muscle groups.

> **DEFINITIONS**
>
> **Volitional failure –**
>
> *Achieved during a set of repetitions when the muscle can no longer perform the action using correct form.*

Drop Set/ Strip Set System

Drop sets, or strip sets, represent another hypertrophy-emphasizing technique that increases the demands on a select muscle or group. The system uses 2-3 performances of the same exercise with only the time it takes to drop or "strip" the weight down, which serves as the "transitional" rest. Essentially, each set is performed for a designated number of repetitions or **volitional failure** before the weight is lowered for the subsequent set. In many cases, it is combined with a pyramid set, where three progressive sets are employed with normal rest, and the 4th "set" is stripped down from the heaviest to the lightest load employed.

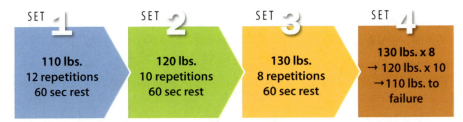

SET 1	SET 2	SET 3	SET 4
110 lbs. 12 repetitions 60 sec rest	120 lbs. 10 repetitions 60 sec rest	130 lbs. 8 repetitions 60 sec rest	130 lbs. x 8 → 120 lbs. x 10 → 110 lbs. to failure

Performing thirty to forty consecutive repetitions may seem like endurance training, but the response is actually hypertrophic when performed to a max, even though the load decreases throughout the set. This occurs because the relative intensity remains at near maximal level at all times during the performance. The associated metabolic stress and subsequent ischemic conditions trigger an anabolic endocrine response based on the high concentration of lactate and hydrogen in the tissue. Performing a drop set by decreasing the weight 3x for a total of thirty repetitions to volitional failure each time, induces a completely different adaptive response than performing thirty repetitions using the same resistance for an entire set. The drop set/strip set system works due to maximal tolerable intensity, rather than a submaximal load repeated for a predetermined repetition number.

Circuit System

The circuit training system has gained popularity in many fitness facilities due to the potential for high caloric expenditure, tolerable resistance levels across the whole body, and relatively short workout duration. In most resistance training circuits, 12-15 exercises are performed for a predefined time period, or repetition range, before moving to the next exercise. When used for fitness training, the exercise selection commonly employs one exercise for each major muscle group. Rest periods are normally 15-30 seconds or the transitional time between exercises. The circuits may be performed continuously for a designated time period or may be done for a certain number of cycles. The client's exercise tolerance often stands as the best gauge to use when programming circuit sets and repetition schemes. Some circuits mix cardiovascular activities in between the resistance training exercises to encourage elevated HRs, caloric expenditure, and inter-set muscle recovery. When using the circuit system, any exercise can be introduced into the exercise sequence, as long as it is appropriate for the client. If higher intensity is planned in the circuit, the order should be consistent with that of strength training, ordering harder, more complex movements first and descending to isolated, limited-range activities later.

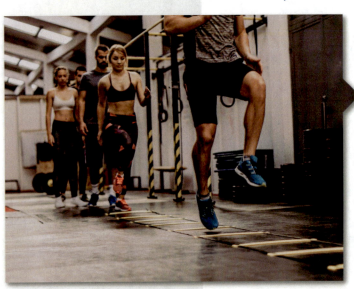

Circuit System Benefits

- High caloric expenditure
- Use of tolerable resistance
- Allows for effective use of time

Lactate Tolerance System

The lactate tolerance system represents an interesting twist to the circuit training concept. With this unique system, an individual's lactate tolerance is built or tested using a group of selected exercises, each of which is assigned a number of repetitions. The training goal is to complete all repetitions of all the exercises in the shortest period of time. The difficulty lies in tolerating the lactic acid and hydrogen produced during the performance of high-quantity repetitions. In some cases, a client will be able to complete an individual exercise's repetition requirements in two or three sets; in other cases, it may take four or five sets due to fatigue onset. In either case, the training system allows for a complete exercise bout in a very short period of time. The duration of any rest period between sets depends upon the exerciser's ability to recover and/or tolerate discomfort. This allows the same training bout to be individualized, based on relative condition.

The number of exercises and repetitions selected will be determined by the client's strength, endurance, and aerobic capabilities. One of the hardest components of lactate tolerance training is achieving a balance: pacing the body to perform at a level where the repetitions are completed as quickly as possible, versus simply attempting to go as fast as possible, where fatigue hinders exercise technique and forces the participant to stop. The client determines how many repetitions to perform based on rate of perceived exertion, then moves to a different exercise. A good introduction of the system is to designate a maximum number of repetitions per set so the client does not "over-fatigue" while attempting to perform all the repetitions in a single exertion and then require prolonged rest before continuing. This training system works effectively for well-conditioned clients and athletes. The same exercise bout can be used repeatedly throughout a multi-week training cycle with the goal of reducing the time to completion each week. This benchmark serves as a useful tracking tool to gauge the client's adaptation response to the training program.

Sample Lactate Tolerance System:
- 50 modified pull-ups
- 80 bench push-ups
- 80 stability ball leg curls
- 40 medicine ball slams
- 60 air squats

Negative Set System

The negative set system was popularized by early strength athletes attempting to maximize force production and TUT at supramaximal intensities for specific lifts. The concept behind the training technique is the body's ability to produce more force during the eccentric contraction than it can during the concentric phase of the movement. The technique requires exercisers to "negatively" lift a resistance that is greater than their 1RM – usually 110%-130%

of maximum – by performing a controlled eccentric movement, followed by a spot-assisted, concentric movement [22].

The negative system is generally not appropriate for personal training clients when using intensities such as those described above, but the concepts of controlled eccentrics can be used safely and effectively in some more appropriate situations. For instance, a spot-assisted concentric phase of the pull-up followed by an unsupported, slow eccentric contraction, or stepping off a box to land in a decelerated squat are common uses.

Exercise Considerations

When designing anaerobic training sessions, trainers should carefully ensure that exercise stress aligns with the individual performing the program, and that it is safe and effective. Most people can engage in light to moderate physical activity without any significant risk, but when exercise intensity rises or volume increases, potential problems can result. In some cases, programmatic adjustments can attenuate the stress quantity resulting from multiple training sessions; at other times, the adjustments are made based on individual-specific factors, such as age or current physical condition. Regardless, exercise professionals should weigh each factor and make decisions to ensure the program components are effective but always safe.

Concurrent Training

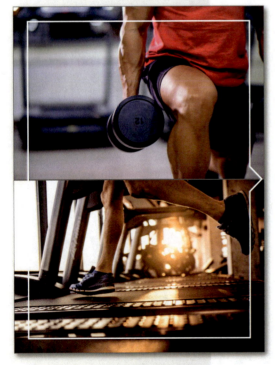

Although many different types of modalities and techniques can be used together in a comprehensive fitness regimen, some adaptive conflicts exist that warrant extra program deliberations. Recalling the principles of training specificity, anaerobic and aerobic training induce distinct neuromuscular adaptations. The adaptation response is specific to the intensity and the time-tension relationship, which is where the problem lies when combining aerobic exercise with (anaerobic) strength, hypertrophy, or power training. Aerobic training, for example, increases mitochondrial and capillary density and decreases the quantity of glycolytic enzymes for more oxidative enzymes. In contrast, anaerobic training reduces mitochondrial density and marginally impacts oxidative enzyme concentration but dramatically increases activity and concentration of the glycolytic and phosphagen related enzymes. Initially, both training modalities will induce the transformation of fast-twitch, type IIx muscle fibers into type IIa fibers, but endurance training reduces mass over time [74]. This effect results from different hormonal responses to the two training modalities: where anaerobic training elicits a greater anabolic hormone release, aerobic training stimulates the more catabolic adrenal hormones, as more energy is needed.

Interestingly, aerobic sports performance is always complemented by resistance training for strength and power, which results in improvements in economy. This has been demonstrated by gains in both short and long-term endurance capacity in both sedentary and trained individuals [4, 27, 67, 73] as well as improvements in lactate threshold. On the contrary, aerobic training inhibits maximal power and strength and can negatively affect muscle mass. Continuous aerobic training negatively impacts force output and mass via changes to neuromuscular adaptations (asynchronous firing patterns), neural recruitment pathways, and a heightened catabolic hormone profile. Individuals looking to increase mass, strength, or power should avoid long bouts of aerobic training for these reasons. Essentially, the training magnitude should be consistent with the desired outcome. If improving a 10k running time is the goal, then anaerobic power and strength training should be used to complement the endurance training. If hypertrophy and strength form the training base, anaerobic conditioning drills and short intervals should be employed instead of low-intensity, steady-state training. This is not to suggest that a person should avoid aerobic training altogether, as it is fundamental to health. Rather, one should tailor the volumes to acceptable levels to allow for the desired adaptations to become dominant.

Age

Earlier text discussed the issue of lean mass loss with age (sarcopenia) and the consequential effect it is has on power and strength production. The effects of age on anaerobic measures has been analyzed in healthy subjects using both open and closed-chain exercises. Age differences in specific strength between young and old persons were observed even when adjustments were made for total lean mass. Older adults demonstrated as much as a 41% lower power output across varying loads [70]. Additionally, older adults experienced a faster rate of fatigue, with a 24% decline in peak velocity over a 10RM [70,72]. Other studies have reported similar results, suggesting older adults possess less capacity to sustain maximum concentric velocity during repetitive contractions than their younger counterparts [2,15]. Locomotion speed correlates well with function, so the slower a person moves, the greater the risk of disability; this programming consideration attains particular importance for the older individual. Velocity impairments negatively impact several functional measures, including mobility, movement competence and power (rate of sit to stand), and dynamic stability (center-of-mass management, balance recovery), which are all associated with QOL, independence, and fall risk among older adults.

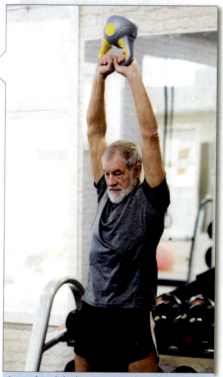

Age-related decline in strength and power can be attributed to changes in muscle architecture, including the loss of type II fiber mass/efficiency.

Age-related reductions in concentric and eccentric maximal contractile force occur in men and women alike, with no differences between the gender groups at any particular velocities [72]. Gender-specific, age-related declines in strength for men and women have been suggested to be 30% and 28% for concentric contractions and 19% and 11% for eccentric contractions, respectively [57,69]. Interestingly, when compared to similarly age-matched men, women tend to demonstrate a reduced rate of decline in eccentric peak torque with age, while experiencing an enhanced capacity to store and utilize elastic energy [23]. Age-related decline in muscle strength and power results from muscle atrophy, sarcopenia, and changes in the muscle architecture, leading to lower muscle quality [25]. The loss of type IIa fibers, a reduction in myosin ATPase, and loss of myosin-heavy chain proteins within the contractile unit denote the primary architectural causes of age-related decline in muscle strength, power, and size [25,68]. Resistance training performed by older adults produces similar improvements in muscle strength, compared to young adults, underscoring the importance of this type of training for the aged individual. Due to anabolic hormonal decline with age, cross-sectional muscle-fiber improvements are generally limited to 10-30%, but the nervous system maintains responsiveness to training stimuli. This explains why strength improves to a greater magnitude than hypertrophy, with previously untrained individuals experiencing >100% increase in 1RM [59]. Likewise, men and women demonstrate a similar ability to increase strength with age. These findings suggest that starting resistance training earlier in life yields better muscle quality in later years.

How early is early, when considering the timepoint that an individual should begin resist-

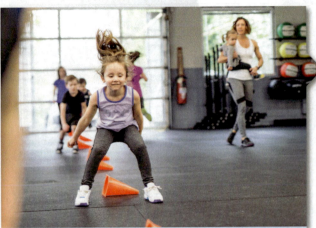
Body weight exercises using pushing, pulling, climbing, and ballistic activities in play-based programs are encouraged and well-received among children and adolescents.

ance training? Changes in human fiber-type characteristics are said to be dynamic and activity-specific until approximately age six; but that statement alone that does not support maximal weightlifting efforts for children [58]. It is commonly suggested that when children can consistently follow instructions, they can engage in exercise-related training activities. This usually coincides with organized sports play. A common fallacy suggests that children should not engage in resistance exercise, as it may stunt their growth. This is a myth that has existed for decades, bred by the misconception that weight-bearing exercise can damage growth plates. Documentation of this risk is non-existent, as studies have found that the forces placed upon children's bones while they were at play exceeded the forces exerted on the bones during resistance training by a factor of ten and it is regarded as an opportune time to build bone mass and increasing bone density [58].

Measures of eccentric impact force observed at play exceed the concentric force capabilities of children, so the myth is clearly false. Since children are, invariably children, the emphasis on anaerobic-based training should be developmentally oriented, as the clear majority of childhood adaptations occur in the nervous system. And, while this is the most obvious scientifically based rationale, many reasons exist suggesting that children should not be placed on body-building-based hypertrophy programs. For one, resistance training bores children once the initial novelty wears off, so body weight exercises using pushing, pulling, climbing, and ballistic activities in play-based programs are encouraged and well received when organized into recreation. Children do well using short-burst activities and can manage several minutes of work. Exercise professionals should be particularly cognizant of body temperature as well as the external environment when programming for younger individuals, making sure to provide adequate break time with hydration stations. Children do not have well-developed thermoregulatory systems and can overheat much more easily than adults. Trainers must remember that they are not little adults: they do not have the attention span or hormonal profile of adults, so effective adult programs including HIT, high-intensity interval training (HIIT), bodybuilding, and maximal strength training are inappropriate.

Gender

Gender differences exist in both the ability to produce force and the magnitude of the adaptive response experienced with anaerobic training. An average adult female's maximal total body strength is approximately 40% less than the average male's [92]. Interestingly, gender-based regional strength differences between the upper and lower body have been identified. Upper-body force capacities of an average female are just over half (55%) of the force capacity that an average male can produce. However, when lower body measures were observed and compared, females, regardless of weight, were able to produce 75% of the force of their male counterparts. Even more interesting, when lower body force capacity was normalized by lean mass, the disparity between genders disappears, suggesting that female lower body strength is at least comparable if not equal to males, according to these lean mass values [29, 43]. Women maintain higher fat mass values compared to men, which contributes to the discrepancy found in relative measures at similar body weights. The additional lean mass contributes to greater force output capabilities in men. The observed distinc-

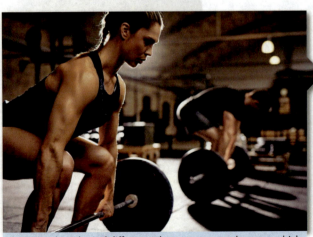
There are physiological differences between men and women which alter the rate and magnitude of certain adaptations.

tion between men and women is likely based on the mass distribution associated with hormone differences. Men show larger upper body muscle mass than women, but when lower body lean mass is compared, the differences are again reduced [72]. Additionally, the rate at which women and men add strength is similar, relative to lean mass. This is why exercise programs for males and females do not differ in the prescriptions used for a desired anaerobic adaptation.

When gains in lean mass are compared over the initial eight weeks of resistance training, no gender difference exists. This observation is consistent with the duration of time before hypertrophic adaptations take place, as well as the role the nervous system plays in early strength improvements. When longer studies were used, women showed a decreased ability to add lean mass when compared to men, particularly in the upper body. Following prolonged resistance training, females showed only small changes in mass, measured by site-specific circumference values (0.16 -0.2 inches) [54, 61]. Researchers conclude that the increase in muscle mass is met by a proportionate reduction of fat mass at the selected, measured regions. These findings suggest that most women can perform routine resistance training with little worry of increasing specific body-segmental circumference measures.

Anabolic hormones increase notably via training in both genders, but the concentration difference between men and women is significant. Men show a 10-15x greater testosterone concentration compared to women in response to the same resistance workout but remain fairly similar with regard to growth hormone release [52, 82]. The difference in testosterone levels and hormone receptor concentrations at target tissues likely accounts for the major differences in muscle hypertrophy between men and women. The role testosterone plays in muscle hypertrophy may be illustrated by the mass attained by female body builders who use anabolic hormones, thereby negating the typical gender-based hormonal differences.

Women who show larger than average increases in mass may possess:

- Higher than normal anabolic hormone levels
- A high testosterone-to-estrogen ratio
- Genetic predisposition towards muscularity
- Greater tolerance to resistance exercise [103]

Overtraining

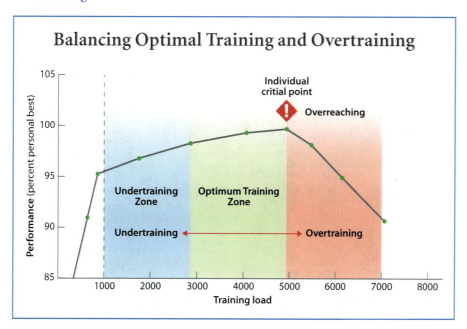

While most people do not exercise enough, some exercise too much and too often. Both aerobic and anaerobic exercise, when practiced excessively, can become too stressful for the body to recover from over time. Certainly, a single exhaustive bout of exercise performed at intensities

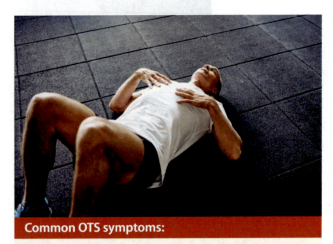

Common OTS symptoms:

- Persistent heavy, stiff, and sore muscles (consistent over multiple days): not the same as DOMS
- Persistent fatigue, washed-out/burned out feeling
- Decreased performance capacity and intensity/ability to maintain the training regimen
- Increased susceptibility to infections, colds, headaches
- Nagging and somewhat chronic injuries
- Sleep disturbances
- Decreased mental concentration and restlessness
- Increased irritability and depression
- HR variations, elevated resting HR, suppressed exercise HR (sympathetic - tachycardia, parasympathetic - bradycardia)
- Loss of appetite and weight loss
- Bowel movement changes
- Absence of menstruation

 DEFINITIONS

Overreaching (NFO) –

A short-term detriment in performance as a result of increased training stress which may take several days or a few weeks to restore.

that significantly exceed the limits of the system can be physiologically detrimental, but this situation occurs more often due to negligence or inexperience. Excessive bouts of ongoing exercise can push the body to experience a cumulative overstress effect. This causes a phenomenon called non-functional **overreaching** (NFO), defined as acute maladapted physiology, which presents as a category of symptoms associated with the overstressed condition. If overreaching is not managed appropriately with proper dietary and recovery strategies, it becomes non-functional and can lead to potentially chronic stress, termed overtraining syndrome (OTS). Overtraining is a detrimental state characterized by a condition of prolonged maladapted physiology, where symptoms signal underlying hormonal, immunologic, neurologic, and psychologic disturbances. OTS can last months and have significant physiological and psychological implications for sufferers. Often, a musculoskeletal injury, such as a stress reaction or stress fracture(s) results as a culmination of the distress.

Managing training volumes and assuring adequate recovery helps avoid overtraining. A key element is the state of the body during stress applications. Hypo-hydration combined with inadequate nutrient storage can leave the body vulnerable, as can inadequate sleep. Additionally, a rapid return or shift to high volume/intense training following periods of not training or working at low volume/intensity can quickly result in NFO and related musculoskeletal injuries. Due to the lower training volumes used in personal training, OTS is a less frequent issue, but among fitness competitors and endurance athletes, NFO and OTS are common. Literature reviews suggests there are more than 100 signs and symptoms of NFO and OTS, but fatigue, performance decline, and mood disturbances are the most prominent and are always included. The following figure provides the most commonly reported signs and symptoms of these conditions.

Sympathetic vs Parasympathetic Overtraining Symptoms

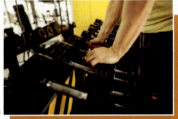
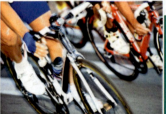

Sympathetic
- Performance decrements
- Easily fatigued
- Restlessness/excitability
- Disturbed sleep
- Weight loss
- Accelerated resting HR
- Delayed recovery
- Associated with anaerobic activity

Parasympathetic
- Performance decrements
- Easily fatigued
- Depression, inhibition
- Sleep undisturbed
- Constant weight
- Bradicardic (decreased) HR
- Good recovery capability
- Associated with aerobic activity

Detraining

Detraining represents a de-conditioning process that reverses the adaptations gained from previous exercise participation. Once the application of stress is absent or reduced, the muscle begins to return to its pre-trained state. Anaerobic training adaptations have better residuals than aerobic adaptations, exhibiting a slower reversal rate. Detraining due to the cessation of resistance stress causes:

- A reduction in muscle mass and fiber size
- Increased capillary and mitochondrial density
- Increased body fat percentage
- Increased aerobic enzyme with concurrent reductions in anaerobic-enzyme concentration
- Loss of muscle strength, power, and endurance
- A reduction in neuromuscular efficiency [65, 66]

The degree to which any of these myo-physiological characteristics change depends upon the individual's training age, the quantity and intensity of other activities performed, and how long the resistance activity has been abandoned. Individuals trained at high intensities return to pre-training values at a slower rate [28]. In fact, whereas aerobic detraining effects can occur in one week, a week off from intense anaerobic training has demonstrated improvements in measured force and power output when following a long training cycle. These improvements are likely due to the adaptations associated with resistance training that occur during recovery. Overtraining occurs very commonly with resistance training due to the heavy stress placed on the tissue. Therefore, extended rest intervals can be incorporated at the end of 8 to 12-week training cycles to yield positive effects.

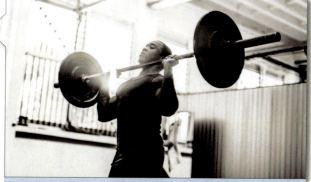

Detraining represents a de-conditioning process that reverses the adaptations gained from previous training. Once the application of stress is taken away, or reduced, the body begins to return to its pre-trained state.

When training stops, the initial effects are not dramatic, except for measures of top speed and velocity among elite athletes; however, following 3 weeks of detraining, peak power output and mean power output decrease by approximately 9% and 10%, respectively [53, 56]. Total force production is also notably affected. Strength experiences an initial decline after 3 weeks, but usually remains above control values for very long periods due to neural plasticity [8, 65]. Training-induced changes in fiber cross-sectional area are reversed, but strength performance decline related to the muscle atrophy is limited, suggesting that, at least initially, little change in neural pathway efficiency occurs. Fiber distribution remains unchanged during the initial weeks of inactivity, but oxidative fibers may increase within 8 weeks of detraining in resistance-trained individuals, while a shift toward glycolytic dependence is seen in those who are aerobically trained [66]. Hormonal changes include a reduction in insulin sensitivity, possible changes in testosterone and growth-hormone levels, and a reversal of short-term, training-induced adaptations in fluid-electrolyte-regulating hormones.

Following 12 weeks of detraining, significant decline in muscle mass and fiber cross-sectional area occurs, with a noted shift from the type IIa fibers back to either type I oxidative, or type IIx fast glycolytic fibers: essentially reversing the process initiated with training [1, 6, 8]. This shift likely contributes to observable muscle atrophy. Peak torque remains above initial values, but upper body measures have demonstrated significant reductions in strength, by as much as 6-10% in young adults and 11-15% in older adults. Interestingly, long-duration studies of detraining (>30 weeks) suggest a considerable decline in strength occurs following 4 months of detraining [8]. This suggests that a detraining threshold may exist before the magnitude of the decline becomes accelerated. Older women show particular sensitivity to detraining from resistance exercise programs.

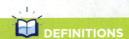

DEFINITIONS

Reversibility principle –

Any adaptation that takes place as a result of training will gradually be reversed with the stoppage of training.

 QUICK FACT

The **reversibility principle** *dictates that athletes lose the beneficial effects of training when they stop working out. Conversely, it also means that detraining effects can be reversed when athletes resume training. Detraining occurs within a relatively short time period after an athlete ceases to train.*

The detraining effect is most pronounced for aerobic metabolism, with compromise occurring within one week of cessation. Among distance runners, a 14-day training interruption led to a reduction in VO_2max of approximately 1 MET, a faster rate of time-to-exhaustion, and an increase in both maximal HR and sub-maximal steady-state HR at 75 and 95% VO_2max [66]. Other evidence of detraining included a decrease in both resting plasma volume and insulin-stimulated glucose disposal. Elite cyclists measured over a 5-week training cessation period experienced increases in body mass and large drops in physiological and hematological values. In less-trained individuals, significant reductions in VO_2max have been reported to occur within 2-4 weeks of detraining [65]. This initial, rapid decline associates with a reduced maximal cardiac output, as mediated by a reduction in stroke volume with little or no change in maximal HR. A decrease in blood volume appears to contribute to stroke volume and VO_2max decline during the initial weeks of detraining. Additionally, changes in left ventricular function, hemoglobin content, and skeletal muscle capillarization also contribute as mediating factors. When detraining extends beyond 2-4 weeks, further declines in VO_2max appear to result from reduced oxygen extraction and lessened thermoregulatory efficiency. Additionally, skeletal muscle oxidative enzyme activity, while not directly linked to changes in VO_2max, appears to be a metabolic agitator to carbohydrate metabolism and increased RPE.

The negative effects associated with detraining can be avoided, or at least limited, by employing a reduced-training strategy. The training volume can be reduced as long as training intensity is maintained at the highest attainable level [29]. Marked reduction in volume requires the use of heavy total-body, cross-joint exercises to maintain mass, power, and strength. To reduce detraining's effect on aerobic exercise, high-intensity intervals can be employed effectively. HIT and HIIT have both demonstrated a marked effect at fitness maintenance with reduced training volume. Muscle isolation should also be avoided during periods of low frequency, and exchanged for compound, higher-intensity lifts.

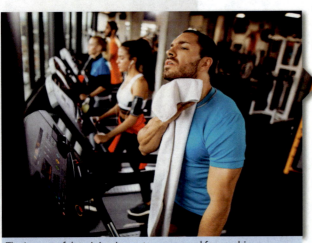

The impact of detraining is most pronounced for aerobic adaptations, with compromise to VO_2max, stroke volume, capillary density, mitochondrial density, and aerobic enzyme activity all occurring within a single week.

Common Injuries Associated with Training

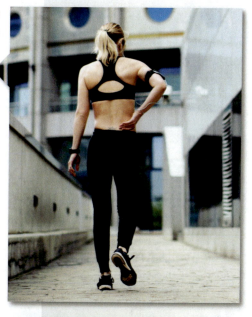

High-intensity activities, including sports, produce a significant number of injuries among participants. NCAA reports suggests that incidence of acute and chronic injury occurs in more than 70% of student-athletes. Many of the injuries occur with high-velocity movement and contact between players, but overuse injuries are the most common. Overuse injuries are, in a sense, chronic conditions, brought on by cumulative trauma or repetitive use and distress. On the other hand, acute injuries typically occur in response to a single traumatic event, while overuse injuries result from repetitive minor traumas that occur with over exposure to stress without adequate healing time. While preventative actions can reduce the risk of all injuries during physical activity, much more can be done to account for and prevent overuse injuries than is possible with respect to acute injuries.

Interestingly, overuse injuries resulting from aerobic endurance training show much greater prevalence than injuries associated with resistance training and related anaerobic-based activities. It has been reported that resistance-trained individuals experience one injury per 1,000 training hours, with most reports implicating the greatest risk for the shoulders, low back, and knees. Muscle strains and chronic inflammation of tendons (tendonitis) represented the most common reported issues. Resistance-based activities performed with proper warm-up and instruction and appropriate loading demonstrate a low risk associated with participation. In many cases, the injuries stem from lack of mobility, musculoskeletal imbalances, or poor biomechanics employed during exercise. According to the literature, resistance-based exercise can do more to prevent injuries than to cause them.

Muscle Strains

Muscle strains account for many of the common injuries associated with physical activity participation. Strains occur when the muscle tissue is stretched into significant deformation or the fibers tear due to excessive tension. Muscle strains, colloquially referred to as "pulled" or "torn" muscles, may occur in response to anything that places sudden or unaccustomed forces upon the muscle tissue.

Additional factors that increase susceptibility to muscle strain include being overweight, inflexible, immobile, physically inactive, or in poor overall physical condition. Although evidence is equivocal, the absence of a warm-up before exertion may increase injury risk as well. Strains are often recognized by an immediate sharp pain at the site of an injury. In the hours that follow, the tissue becomes swollen, stiff, and tender to contact due to inflammation. If the muscle is severely torn, bruising and discoloration occur in and around the injury site. Strains are usually evaluated by degree of severity:

- A **first-degree** strain causes localized pain and discomfort that usually subside in about a week or two. General healing time for a first-degree strain is approximately six weeks.
- **Second degree** strains occur when the tissue is significantly damaged; these are associated with increased pain and tenderness. These injuries often sideline or limit activity for several weeks to several months depending on the severity and the site of injury.

Common causes of muscle strains:

- Lifting heavy objects
- Unstable joint segments during exertion
- Poor lifting mechanics
- Muscle imbalances
- Exertion in an unfamiliar position
- Placement of deconditioned muscle groups under high stress
- Lack of an adequate warm-up
- Overstretched tissue

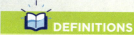

DEFINITIONS

Muscle strains –

The stretching or tearing of a muscle or a tendon; the fibrous cord of tissue that connects muscles to bones; occur when muscles are stretched beyond their limits or are forced to contract too strongly.

In many cases, the tissue heals in about 2-3 months, depending on severity.

■ **Third degree** strains are also called complete tears. They present significant trauma to the tissue, with pain persisting for several weeks to months following the injury. The susceptibility of re-strain is very high during the recovery process. Once the pain subsides, many people feel they have healed, which is not true, as the architectural structures have not been completely remodeled. The lack of pain in the presence of tissue that is still being repaired can often lead to exertion beyond the tissue's capacity, resulting in re-injury. The best predictor of tissue injury is having a prior injury.

PRACTICAL INSIGHT - HAMSTRING STRAINS

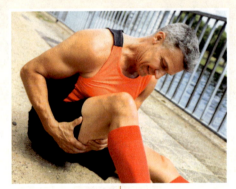

Hamstrings are the most common site for strains, or "pulled muscles." The issue lies in the dual role the hamstrings play as they cross both the hip and the knee. Hamstrings function with the glutes to extend the hip and the gastrocnemius to flex the knee. When the knee extensors dominate the knee flexors (> 3:2 ratio) in force potential, the knee and hamstring experiences added risk of injury, which is further amplified across the hamstrings when knee flexor strength and hip extensor strength also become imbalanced. Most strains to the hamstring occur when significant force is exerted across the hip and knee simultaneously, as in sprinting, causing a strain of the biceps femoris. Injury prevention research has shown that emphasis should be placed on eccentric knee flexion to reduce the risk of hamstring strains. More significant strains occur when the hip is flexed and the knee is forcefully extended. This causes a high strain, as the hamstrings are fully stretched and placed under force, resulting in the most traumatic hamstring injuries. Over-aggressive ballistic and facilitated stretching of the hamstring have been implicated for increased risk among predisposed individuals.

Early management of a muscle strain includes the use of cryotherapy to alleviate pain and reduce inflammation [49]. It is important that the affected limb is elevated and compressed to help manage inflammation, and that the strained muscle not be placed in a shortened or flexed position. Ice applications should be done for 15-20 minutes several times per day following the injury but should not be applied directly to the skin in order to avoid skin irritation. Heat should not be an acute therapy but can be used later in the treatment when moving back to activity. Over-the-counter, anti-inflammatory medications, including aspirin, can be used to manage pain and will improve mobility by reducing inflammation; however, these meds should not be used to manage pain with the intent of a premature return to activity. Other strategies to manage the injury include PRICE therapy: protection, rest, ice, compression, and elevation can help the affected muscle in several ways. Protecting the strained muscle from further injury and resting the tissue allow the healing process to occur. Ice can be directly applied early, followed by ice massage later in the treatment. Ace bandages or compression wraps can help support the tissue and reduce swelling. Avoid tightly wrapping the bandage to allow for adequate blood flow. Elevation helps reduce the swelling simply due to the effect of gravity. When returning to activity, use longer warm-ups and acclimate the tissue before jumping back into intense training. Low-level cardiovascular exercise is often used for leg injuries to encourage blood flow.

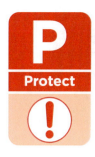

Protection	**Rest**	**Ice**	**Compression**	**Elevation**
immediately following an injury, it is important to protect the injured body part from further damage	avoid painful activities involving the injury site	the application of ice or cold to the injured body part reduces inflammation	means of reducing swelling and excessive bleeding in the injured area	elevation above the level of the heart immediately following an injury helps to minimize the amount of swelling and pain

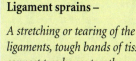

Ligament sprains –

A stretching or tearing of the ligaments, tough bands of tissue that connect two bones together at a joint, often reducing the stability of a joint.

Return to play –

Injury-specific protocols dictate the point in the recovery from an injury when a person is able to return to playing sports or participate in an activity at a pre-injury level

Mechanoreceptor –

A sensory receptor that detects mechanical pressure from touch, vibration and tension; acts to communicate changes in pressure to the central nervous system.

Low back pain –

One of the most common forms of musculoskeletal discomfort occurring as a result of one or more conditions effecting the bones, nerves, muscles, discs, or tendons of the lumbar spine.

Ligament Sprain

Ligament sprains compose another common soft tissue injury and often occur during participation in physical activity. Whereas strains affect the muscle tissue, connective-tissue sprains affect joints. Damage to ligaments usually occurs when the joint becomes unstable during activity or after a fall or sudden movement that violently pulls or twists a body segment. The ankle joint is one of the most common sites for sprains, particularly when decelerating force is applied to uneven surfaces during running or jumping.

When the connective tissue becomes significantly deformed under excessive tension or tears due to violent force, immediate localized pain and rapid joint swelling occur. Significant ligament trauma causes small blood vessel tears, which leads to bruising. The natural defense mechanism of the body to protect the injured area promotes excessive joint stiffness, tenderness, and difficulty moving the injured joint. When a joint injury occurs, it should be immediately treated with the PRICE therapies. The sooner ice can be applied, the better swelling, pain, and stiffness can be managed. Similar to strains, sprains are also categorized by severity. Due to the semi-avascular nature of ligaments compared to muscle tissue, healing takes more time. First-degree and mild second-degree sprains often heal themselves given adequate time and rest. Ligament tears require medical attention. Severe tearing or complete rupture of the ligaments often requires surgical repair, as damage caused by high-level sprains can lead to significant instability, improper alignment, and tissue damage, making the joint particularly vulnerable to future injury. Therefore, if significant pain and instability are experienced, particularly with bruising, clients should be immediately referred to a medical professional for diagnosis and treatment. Follow up or **return to play** procedures for ankle sprains, in particular, include **mechanoreceptor** education to prevent chronic ankle rolls in the future.

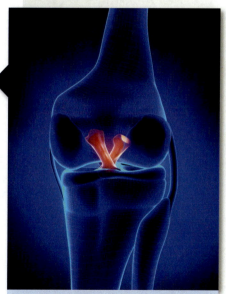

Due to the semi-avascular nature of ligaments compared to muscle, full healing takes a longer period of time.

Low Back Pain

It is estimated that 90% of adults experience acute or chronic **low back pain** at some point. Low back pain is characterized as localized pain, muscle tension, and/or stiffness below the rib

In most cases, the tissue is predisposed to injury due to a combination of:

- Too much stress
- Overuse, particularly from biomechanically compromised movements
- Muscle imbalances
- Lack of flexibility
- General deconditioning
- Overstretched tissue

DEFINITIONS

Sciatica –

Refers to pain, numbness, or tingling radiating along the path of the sciatic nerve due to pressure or impingement; a large nerve, it extends from the lower back down to the back of each leg.

Central stability –

The ability to maintain active control of spinal and pelvic posture during dynamic movement in order to facilitate force transfer across the trunk.

Pelvic floor –

The layer of muscles spanning the bottom of the pelvis that support the pelvic organs and stability of the pelvic region.

Lumbar stenosis –

A narrowing of the space surrounding the spinal nerves of the lower back with subsequent compression often leading to leg pain.

Scoliosis –

A congenital sideways curvature of the spine that occurs most often around puberty.

Spondylitis –

Describes several inflammatory conditions affecting the vertebral joints that may, over time, lead to the fusion of vertebrae.

Spondylosis –

A stress fracture of a specific portion of the vertebra, the pars interarticularis, usually due to repeated hyperextension of the lumbar spine.

Spondylolisthesis –

The anterior slipping of one vertebra relative to an adjacent vertebra; seen with bilateral spondylosis in a specific region.

cage and above the gluteal fold and may present with or without **sciatica**. The high number of unanchored joints along the spine coupled with a vertical and oblique muscle system creates the perfect environment for a host of potential interdependent problems. Low back pain is implicated as the most common complaint among weightlifters, as the injury can be triggered by a variety of situations experienced in resistance training.

The resultant repetitive microtrauma leads to spinal muscle strain or injury to the ligaments that support the spine. Over time, muscle strain and stretched ligaments may lead to structural alterations and disc degeneration, leading to spinal positions that increase potential for further injury and chronic pain.

Spinal flexor-to-extensor imbalance is considered a predisposition to injury, as are tight/overactive hip flexors. In lieu of using the inner unit to stabilize the spine, overactive hip flexors and spinal erectors anchor and stabilize the spine using an anterior tilt of the pelvis during lifting tasks. The use of the back extensors and hip flexors inhibits the local postural stabilizers of the spine, or core system, needed for **central stability**. Lack of **pelvic floor** involvement impedes central stability and increases low back stress during resistance exercise and locomotion. To minimize risk of low back pain, abdominal flexion capability should equal the force produced through trunk extension, or a 1:1 ratio. However, many people present with a strength balance ratio of 1:3 (flexion:extension) when the strength of abdominal flexion is compared to that of lumbar extension. Acute and chronic back pain can lead to greater susceptibility for future damage. Back pain causes people to change normal movement patterns to relieve the distress. Variations in lifting posture can promote undesirable lifting mechanics. In many cases, compensatory actions force non-injured back tissues to absorb additional stress, adding to an even greater risk for injury. Spinal column deviations, such as **lumbar stenosis** and **scoliosis**, may contribute to pain with certain activities, while vertebral defects, such as **spondylosis**, **spondylitis**, **spondylolysis**, and **spondylolisthesis** can cause disk irritation, vertebral slippage, and impingement discomfort when aggravated.

PRACTICAL INSIGHT

The therapy for low back pain will depend on the cause, and in many cases, acute low back problems will go away with rest in 7-10 days. Pain persisting beyond a week warrants medical evaluation, as a serious injury may be present. Additionally, lower back injuries that cause numbness or weakness in a limb should be evaluated immediately by a physician. Low back pain represents the most debilitating injury in persons under the age of 45. Therefore, appropriate attention and management upon early onset is important to prevent a chronic syndrome. Interestingly however, many of the self-reported therapies employed contribute to the problem. Individuals with low back pain will often attempt to strengthen the low back muscles to discourage the pain. In reality though, the front musculature contains the key to the back musculature. Exercise professionals using corrective exercises to help alleviate non-pathological low back pain should stretch the thoracolumbar fascia hip flexors and hamstrings and strengthen the rectus abdominis. Additionally, cross activation patterns, including opposite raises and quadruped stability work should be employed, as core muscle activation helps reduce back stress. Weight loss, particularly for those with android obesity, also helps alleviate symptoms.

Shoulder Impingement Syndrome

Shoulder impingement syndrome is a common condition affecting the glenohumeral joint, often seen in sports and activities which employ repetitive overhead movements. The condition's prevalence increases with age. Repeated arm movement overhead can cause the rotator cuff tendons to contact the outer end of the shoulder blade where the clavicle attaches, called the acromion. When this happens, the rotator cuff tendons become inflamed and swollen (tendonitis). The swollen rotator cuff can get trapped and pinched under the acromion. All these conditions can inflame the bursa in the shoulder area. As mentioned previously, a bursa is a fluid-filled sac that provides a cushion between the bone and tissues, such as skin, ligaments, tendons, and muscles, with inflammation of the bursa known as bursitis. Subacromial impingement can occur as a result of:

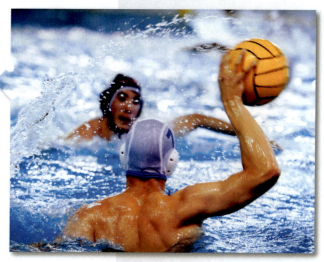

- An unstable shoulder joint
- Rotator cuff and scapular stabilizer weaknesses
- Posterior capsule tightness
- Postural distortions
- Improper lifting technique
- Increased joint pressure, causing tissue compression and friction

Impingement often leads to pain expressed as a "pinching" sensation with overhead movement. Chronic impingement syndrome can cause significant muscle damage, bone deformation, and mechanical dysfunction. In some cases, bone spurs, calcification of tendons, or changes in the normal contour of the bone, a hooked acromion, may be present.

Impingement syndrome has increased in prevalence among younger Americans due to **technology postures**. Forward shoulders and exaggerated kyphotic positions change the resting scapular angle, which, in turn, changes the shoulder joint-complex system. Remember the glenoid fossa, or cup of the shoulder, is part of the scapulae. Underactive rhomboids and the lower fibers of the trapezius muscles further contribute to a progressive anterior migration of the humeral head. Shoulder flexion with internal rotation (overhead kettle bell swings and close grip upright row) should be avoided, as these coupled joint actions increase the risk of subacromial impingement syndrome; to promote proper shoulder balance, an even greater emphasis should be placed on internal rotator cuff mobility and scapular stabilizer muscle function.

> **DEFINITIONS**
>
> **Technology postures –**
>
> *The common positions individuals attain when using technology such as smart phones and computers that contribute to musculoskeletal complications from a forward flexed spinal position.*

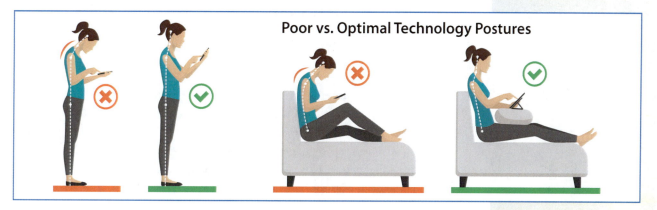

Poor vs. Optimal Technology Postures

If pain occurs during shoulder movements, the activity should be discontinued immediately and replaced with actions that do not present discomfort. If shoulder discomfort continues, ice and anti-inflammatory medicines can be used to reduce swelling and rest given to provide recovery. If the pain continues past 10 days, a medical professional should evaluate the injury. Therapeutic exercises for shoulder complex strengthening and ROM may improve the condition and can be prescribed by a therapist. Persistent symptoms may warrant a cortisone injection to reduce associated pain. Most people who experience impingement syndrome find relief with medication, corrective exercises, and temporary avoidance of repetitive overhead activity. Those suffering from chronic impingement syndrome should be evaluated for musculoskeletal damage and perhaps, more specifically, rotator cuff injury.

Rotator-Cuff Injury

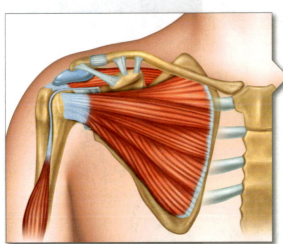

The four muscles that make up the rotator cuff (supraspinatus, infraspinatus, subscapularis, and teres minor) are vulnerable in both active and sedentary populations. Active individuals usually experience inflammation, calcium build-up in the tendon, and tears due to multiple contributing factors, such as muscular imbalances. This is particularly true in sport movements when high-force acceleration is associated with inadequate decelerative neuromuscular control. In most cases, rotator cuff injuries are not caused by an independent factor, but rather a combination of contributing factors. Repetitive stress from overuse often leads to impingement, causing tissue abrasion and inflammation. The damaged tissue causes compression syndrome and further erosion, which weakens the tissue and can lead to tears. Repetitive activities, including volleyball, baseball, tennis, and swimming are all associated with rotator cuff problems. Improper weight lifting technique, long-term postural distortions, and inadequate or imbalanced rotator strength and mobility can also lead to problems with resistance-trained individuals.

Usually caused by a combination of contributing factors:

Repetitive stress from overuse and/or consistent overhead activities	Damaged and inflamed tissues result in compression syndromes and erosion of connective tissue	Improper weight lifting technique and inadequate rotator cuff strength

Rotator-cuff injuries can be managed using ice, rest, therapeutic exercise, and stretching. Avoiding the activities that cause the problem is indicated to prevent further damage. With torn tissue, surgery may be necessary to correct the damage. Ongoing pain and movement limitation warrant medical referral for proper diagnosis and treatment. The majority of rotator cuff injuries can be prevented with adequate strengthening exercises and regular activities that encourage improved mobility.

Tendonitis

As mentioned earlier, tendonitis is an acute inflammation of the tendon, which frequently occurs due to repetitive overuse or excessive strain or may stem from sudden trauma caused by unmanageable force vectors. Tendonitis most often results from overuse during repetitive actions or sport movements, including those performed while weight training or playing tennis, golf, and throwing sports. The hinge joints of the elbow and knee are commonly associated with this ailment, resulting from resistance-based exercise.

Bicep Tendonitis at the Shoulder

With resistance training, tendonitis may occur due to muscle imbalance, acute high volume, repetitive biomechanical error, or other soft tissue disorders. Likewise, joint disorders, including arthritis and gout, can increase one's propensity for developing tendonitis. Tendonitis is more common in adults over 40 years of age but can affect anyone. The reduction in aging tendons' functional quality that results from reduced force tolerance and elasticity make these individuals more susceptible to tears. Treatment of tendonitis is consistent with other soft tissue injuries. Initial treatment includes avoiding activities that aggravate the problem, anti-inflammatory medications, ice therapy, and resting the injured area. Neoprene sleeves are common for elbow and knee issues. Avoiding any activity that led to the problem or causes discomfort is very important to prevent a chronic syndrome. If conditions do not improve, a physician may recommend cortisone injections or physical therapy; surgery is rarely needed.

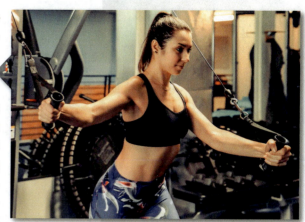

 QUICK INSIGHT

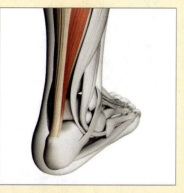

For many years, most tendon pain has been referred to as tendonitis (i.e., lateral epicondylitis, bicipital tendonitis, plantar fasciitis), but in reality, tendinopathy is a better umbrella term because the suffix "pathy" indicates a disease or disorder. Tendinopathy literally means a disease or disorder of a tendon, so it is now typically used to describe any problem involving a tendon. The suffix 'itis' in medical terminology means inflammation; therefore, in literal terms, tendonitis means inflammation of a tendon. Tendonitis is an accurate diagnosis for an acute injury when the tendon is overloaded, causing pain and swelling from tears in the injured tissue. Tendinosis is much more common and a more appropriate name for many of injuries associated with chronic non-inflammatory degeneration of a tendon. This degeneration can include changes to the structure or composition of the tendon, which often results from repetitive micro-traumas or failure of the tissue to heal following a tendon rupture.

 DEFINITIONS

Exertional-rhabdomyolysis –

The breakdown and necrosis of skeletal muscle caused by extreme physical exertion.

Rhabdomyolysis

Formerly an extremely uncommon occurrence rarely seen outside of extreme military training in high-temperature environments, **exertional-rhabdomyolysis** has established a name in the fitness industry. Boot camps, HIIT programs, and even spin classes have created resistance-based metabolic rigors that prove to be too much for the muscular system to handle. The result of these intense, acute bouts cause destruction of the muscle cell, which leaks its contents into circulation. Activities that have caused documented cases of exercise-induced rhabdomyolysis range from low-resistance (10-15 lbs. weights), high-volume circuit training, to low and high-intensity spin classes, to American football practice, to a fairly newly researched phenomenon involving blood flow restriction training [11, 41, 75, 87]. Regard-

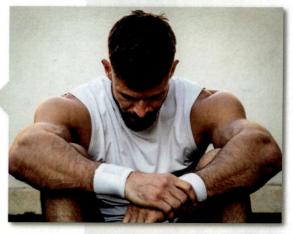

less of the type of activity, the theme that is consistent in most documented cases of exertional-rhabdo is "too much too fast:" whether this be intensity, volume, or advanced exercises that one is unaccustomed to, or has not done over an extended period of time [76]. Common symptoms include extreme muscle cramps and/or prolonged muscle pain, coupled with dark or tea-colored urine and sustained weakness [42, 89]. Exertional-rhabdo can have very serious consequences: organ damage, severe ischemia, cardiac arrhythmia, and even death. It is characterized by the breakdown and necrosis of skeletal muscle after engaging in extreme physical activity; high temperature and dehydration are often implicated as well. Although several different mechanisms can lead to skeletal muscle cell damage and death, the common final pathway is an increase in intracellular, free-ionized calcium in the cytoplasm and mitochondria at a level much higher than normal. This creates a cascade of events that releases intracellular contents into circulation, causing pain, swelling, and potential organ damage.

Mild cases of exertional-rhabdo often go undiagnosed and are usually attenuated with proper hydration and rest. Individuals suffering from severe symptoms (dark, tea-colored urine), need to seek immediate medical attention for intravenous hydration to protect the kidneys from damage. Physicians will also track circulatory creatine kinase (CK) levels, myoglobin levels, kidney function, hydration status, and electrolyte values until the values return to normal, which usually takes 48-72 hours; however, in extreme cases, symptoms can subside despite highly elevated levels of CK that last up to 18 days after the acute incident [47]. Causes of exertional-rhabdo are preventable and should not occur in professionally developed training programs. Any exercise professional that creates programs that injure participants assumes an elevated liability risk. Causing a participant to incur rhabdomyolysis would be strong grounds for a professional negligence lawsuit.

REFERENCES:

1. Andersen LL, Andersen JL, Magnusson SP, Suetta C, Madsen JL, Christensen LR, and Aagaard P. Changes in the human muscle force-velocity relationship in response to resistance training and subsequent detraining. *Journal of Applied Physiology* 99: 87-94, 2005.

2. Baudry S, Klass M, Pasquet B, and Duchateau J. Age-related fatigability of the ankle dorsiflexor muscles during concentric and eccentric contractions. *European journal of applied physiology* 100: 515, 2007.

3. Beattie K, Carson BP, Lyons M, Rossiter A, and Kenny IC. The effect of strength training on performance indicators in distance runners. *The Journal of Strength & Conditioning Research* 31: 9-23, 2017.

4. Bell G, Syrotuik D, Martin T, Burnham R, and Quinney H. Effect of concurrent strength and endurance training on skeletal muscle properties and hormone concentrations in humans. *European journal of applied physiology* 81: 418-427, 2000.

5. Bergen G. Falls and fall injuries among adults aged≥ 65 years—United States, 2014. *MMWR Morbidity and mortality weekly report* 65, 2016.

6. Bogdanis GC. Effects of physical activity and inactivity on muscle fatigue. *Frontiers in physiology* 3: 142, 2012.

7. Borg G. Psychophysical scaling with applications in physical work and the perception of exertion. *Scandinavian journal of work, environment & health*: 55-58, 1990.

8. Bosquet L, Berryman N, Dupuy O, Mekary S, Arvisais D, Bherer L, and Mujika I. Effect of training cessation on muscular performance: A meta-analysis. *Scandinavian journal of medicine & science in sports* 23: e140-e149, 2013.

9. Braun W, Hawthorne W, and Markofski M. Acute EPOC response in women to circuit training and treadmill exercise of matched oxygen consumption. *European journal of applied physiology* 94: 500-504, 2005.

10. Brochu M, Savage P, Lee M, Dee J, Cress ME, Poehlman ET, Tischler M, and Ades PA. Effects of resistance training on physical function in older disabled women with coronary heart disease. *Journal of Applied Physiology* 92: 672-678, 2002.

11. Brogan M, Ledesma R, Coffino A, and Chander P. Freebie rhabdomyolysis: a public health concern. spin class-induced rhabdomyolysis. *The American journal of medicine* 130: 484-487, 2017.

12. Buchner DM, Cress ME, De Lateur BJ, Esselman PC, Margherita AJ, Price R, and Wagner EH. The effect of strength and endurance training on gait, balance, fall risk, and health services use in community-living older adults. *The Journals of Gerontology Series A: Biological Sciences and Medical Sciences* 52: M218-M224, 1997.

13. Büla CJ, Monod S, Hoskovec C, and Rochat S. Interventions aiming at balance confidence improvement in older adults: an updated review. *Gerontology* 57: 276-286, 2011.

14. Byrne C, Faure C, Keene DJ, and Lamb SE. Ageing, muscle power and physical function: a systematic review and implications for pragmatic training interventions. *Sports Medicine* 46: 1311-1332, 2016.

15. Caserotti P, Aagaard P, and Puggaard L. Changes in power and force generation during coupled eccentric–concentric versus concentric muscle contraction with training and aging. *European journal of applied physiology* 103: 151-161, 2008.

16. Conn VS, Koopman RJ, Ruppar TM, Phillips LJ, Mehr DR, and Hafdahl AR. Insulin sensitivity following exercise interventions: systematic review and meta-analysis of outcomes among healthy adults. *Journal of primary care & community health* 5: 211-222, 2014.

17. Cornelissen VA, Fagard RH, Coeckelberghs E, and Vanhees L. Impact of resistance training on blood pressure and other cardiovascular risk factors: a meta-analysis of randomized, controlled trials. *Hypertension* 58: 950-958, 2011.

18. Cornelissen VA and Smart NA. Exercise training for blood pressure: a systematic review and meta-analysis. *Journal of the American Heart Association: Cardiovascular and Cerebrovascular Disease* 2, 2013.

19. Cruz-Jentoft AJ, Landi F, Schneider SM, Zúñiga C, Arai H, Boirie Y, Chen L-K, Fielding RA, Martin FC, and Michel J-P. Prevalence of and interventions for sarcopenia in ageing adults: a systematic review. Report of the International Sarcopenia Initiative (EWGSOP and IWGS). *Age and ageing* 43: 748-759, 2014.

20. Damas F, Phillips S, Vechin FC, and Ugrinowitsch C. A review of resistance training-induced changes in skeletal muscle protein synthesis and their contribution to hypertrophy. *Sports medicine* 45: 801-807, 2015.

21. Denkinger MD, Lukas A, Nikolaus T, and Hauer K. Factors associated with fear of falling and associated activity restriction in community-dwelling older adults: a systematic review. *The American Journal of Geriatric Psychiatry* 23: 72-86, 2015.

22. Doan BK, Newton RU, Marsit JL, Triplett-mcbride NT, Koziris LP, Fry AC, and Kraemer WJ. Effects of increased eccentric loading on bench press 1RM. *The Journal of Strength & Conditioning Research* 16: 9-13, 2002.

23. Edwen C, Thorlund JB, Magnusson SP, Slinde F, Svantesson U, Hulthen L, and Aagaard P. Stretch–shortening cycle muscle power in women and men aged 18–81 years: Influence of age and gender. *Scandinavian journal of medicine & science in sports* 24: 717-726, 2014.

24. Fatouros IG, Kambas A, Katrabasas I, Leontsini D, Chatzinikolaou A, Jamurtas AZ, Douroudos I, Aggelousis N, and Taxildaris K. Resistance training and detraining effects on flexibility performance in the elderly are intensity-dependent. *The Journal of Strength & Conditioning Research* 20: 634-642, 2006.

25. Faulkner JA, Larkin LM, Claflin DR, and Brooks SV. Age-related changes in the structure and function of skeletal muscles. *Clinical and Experimental Pharmacology and Physiology* 34: 1091-1096, 2007.

26. Fedewa MV, Gist NH, Evans EM, and Dishman RK. Exercise and insulin resistance in youth: a meta-analysis. *Pediatrics*: peds. 2013-2718, 2013.

27. Ferrauti A, Bergermann M, and Fernandez-Fernandez J. Effects of a concurrent strength and endurance training on running performance and running economy in recreational marathon runners. *The Journal of Strength & Conditioning Research* 24: 2770-2778, 2010.

28. Foster C and Armstrong M. What types of physical activities are effective in developing muscle and bone strength and balance? *Journal of Frailty, Sarcopenia and Falls* 3: 58-65, 2018.

29. Frontera WR, Hughes VA, Lutz KJ, and Evans WJ. A cross-sectional study of muscle strength and mass in 45-to 78-yr-old men and women. *Journal of applied physiology* 71: 644-650, 1991.

30. Giangregorio L, Papaioannou A, Heinonen A, Cheung A, Laprade J, Ashe M, MacIntyre N, Shipp K, McGill S, and Ravi J. Intensity is a subjective construct. *Osteoporosis international: a journal established as result of cooperation between the European Foundation for Osteoporosis and the National Osteoporosis Foundation of the USA* 27: 2391, 2016.

31. Gianoudis J, Bailey C, and Daly R. Associations between sedentary behaviour and body composition, muscle function and sarcopenia in community-dwelling older adults. *Osteoporosis International* 26: 571-579, 2015.

32. Gonzalez AM, Hoffman JR, Stout JR, Fukuda DH, and Willoughby DS. Intramuscular anabolic signaling and endocrine response following resistance exercise: implications for muscle hypertrophy. *Sports medicine* 46: 671-685, 2016.

33. Gordon B, Benson A, Bird S, and Fraser S. Resistance training improves metabolic health in type 2 diabetes: a systematic review. *Diabetes research and clinical practice* 83: 157-175, 2009.

34. Gordon CM, Zemel BS, Wren TA, Leonard MB, Bachrach LK, Rauch F, Gilsanz V, Rosen CJ, and Winer KK. The determinants of peak bone mass. *The Journal of pediatrics* 180: 261-269, 2017.

35. Gray M, Powers M, Boyd L, and Garver K. Longitudinal comparison of low-and high-velocity resistance training in relation to body composition and functional fitness of older adults. *Aging clinical and experimental research*: 1-9, 2018.

36. Greer BK, Sirithienthad P, Moffatt RJ, Marcello RT, and Panton LB. EPOC comparison between isocaloric bouts of steady-state aerobic, intermittent aerobic, and resistance training. *Research quarterly for exercise and sport* 86: 190-195, 2015.

37. Hart NH, Nimphius S, Rantalainen T, Ireland A, Siafarikas A, and Newton R. Mechanical basis of bone strength: influence of bone material, bone structure and muscle action. *Journal of musculoskeletal & neuronal interactions* 17: 114, 2017.

38. Hartman MJ, Fields DA, Byrne NM, and Hunter GR. Resistance training improves metabolic economy during functional tasks in older adults. *Journal of strength and conditioning research* 21: 91, 2007.

39. Heymsfield S, Peterson C, Bourgeois B, Thomas D, Gallagher D, Strauss B, Müller M, and Bosy–Westphal A. Human energy expenditure: advances in organ–tissue prediction models. *Obesity Reviews*, 2018.

40. Hollings M, Mavros Y, Freeston J, and Fiatarone Singh M. The effect of progressive resistance training on aerobic fitness and strength in adults with coronary heart disease: a systematic review and meta-analysis of randomised controlled trials. *European journal of preventive cardiology* 24: 1242-1259, 2017.

41. Honda S, Kawasaki T, Kamitani T, and Kiyota K. Rhabdomyolysis after High Intensity Resistance Training. *Internal Medicine* 56: 1175-1178, 2017.

42. Huerta-Alardín AL, Varon J, and Marik PE. Bench-to-bedside review: Rhabdomyolysis–an overview for clinicians. *Critical Care* 9: 158, 2004.

43. Hughes VA, Frontera WR, Wood M, Evans WJ, Dallal GE, Roubenoff R, and Singh MAF. Longitudinal muscle strength changes in older adults: influence of muscle mass, physical activity, and health. *The Journals of Gerontology Series A: Biological Sciences and Medical Sciences* 56: B209-B217, 2001.

44. Joana J and Silva J. The effect of high-and low-impact physical activity on bone mineral density: A literature review. *Annals of Physical and Rehabilitation Medicine* 61: e401, 2018.

45. Johannsen NM, Swift DL, Lavie CJ, Earnest CP, Blair SN, and Church TS. Combined aerobic and resistance training effects on glucose homeostasis, fitness, and other major health indices: a review of current guidelines. *Sports Medicine* 46: 1809-1818, 2016.

46. Joyner MJ. Modeling: optimal marathon performance on the basis of physiological factors. *Journal of Applied Physiology* 70: 683-687, 1991.

47. Kahanov L, Eberman LE, Wasik M, and Alvey T. Exertional rhabdomyolysis in a collegiate American football player after preventive cold-water immersion: a case report. *Journal of athletic training* 47: 228-232, 2012.

48. Kalyani RR, Corriere M, and Ferrucci L. Age-related and disease-related muscle loss: the effect of diabetes, obesity, and other diseases. *The lancet Diabetes & endocrinology* 2: 819-829, 2014.

49. Kaminski TW, Hertel J, Amendola N, Docherty CL, Dolan MG, Hopkins JT, Nussbaum E, Poppy W, and Richie D. National Athletic Trainers' Association position statement: conservative management and prevention of ankle sprains in athletes. *Journal of athletic training* 48: 528-545, 2013.

50. Karinkanta S, Heinonen A, Sievänen H, Uusi-Rasi K, and Kannus P. Factors predicting dynamic balance and quality of life in home-dwelling elderly women. *Gerontology* 51: 116-121, 2005.

51. Kelley GA, Kelley KS, and Tran ZV. Resistance training and bone mineral density in women: a meta-analysis of controlled trials: LWW, 2001.

52. Kraemer WJ, Gordon S, Fleck S, Marchitelli L, Mello R, Dziados J, Friedl K, Harman E, Maresh C, and Fry A. Endogenous anabolic hormonal and growth factor responses to heavy resistance exercise in males and females. *International journal of sports medicine* 12: 228-235, 1991.

53. Kraemer WJ, Koziris LP, Ratamess NA, Hakkinen K, Triplett-mcbride NT, Fry AC, Gordon SE, Volek JS, French DN, and Rubin MR. Detraining produces minimal changes in physical performance and hormonal variables in recreationally strength-trained men. *Journal of Strength and Conditioning Research* 16: 373-382, 2002.

54. Kraemer WJ, Nindl BC, Ratamess NA, Gotshalk LA, Volek JS, Fleck SJ, Newton RU, and Häkkinen K. Changes in muscle hypertrophy in women with periodized resistance training. *Medicine and science in sports and exercise* 36: 697-708, 2004.

55. Landers MR, Oscar S, Sasaoka J, and Vaughn K. Balance confidence and fear of falling avoidance behavior are most predictive of falling in older adults: prospective analysis. *Physical therapy* 96: 433-442, 2016.

56. Lemmer JT, Hurlbut DE, Martel GF, Tracy BL, EY IV FM, Metter EJ, Fozard JL, Fleg JL, and Hurley BF. Age and gender responses to strength training and detraining. *Medicine & Science in Sports & Exercise* 32: 1505-1512, 2000.

57. Lindle R, Metter E, Lynch N, Fleg J, Fozard J, Tobin J, Roy T, and Hurley B. Age and gender comparisons of muscle strength in 654 women and men aged 20–93 yr. *Journal of applied physiology* 83: 1581-1587, 1997.

58. Lloyd RS, Faigenbaum AD, Stone MH, Oliver JL, Jeffreys I, Moody JA, Brewer C, Pierce KC, McCambridge TM, and Howard R. Position statement on youth resistance training: the 2014 International Consensus. *Br J Sports Med* 48: 498-505, 2014.

59. Macaluso A and De Vito G. Muscle strength, power and adaptations to resistance training in older people. *European journal of applied physiology* 91: 450-472, 2004.

60. Mann S, Beedie C, Balducci S, Zanuso S, Allgrove J, Bertiato F, and Jimenez A. Changes in insulin sensitivity in response to different modalities of exercise: a review of the evidence. *Diabetes/Metabolism Research and Reviews* 30: 257-268, 2014.

61. Martel GF, Roth SM, Ivey FM, Lemmer JT, Tracy BL, Hurlbut DE, Metter EJ, Hurley BF, and Rogers MA. Age and sex affect human muscle fibre adaptations to heavy–resistance strength training. *Experimental physiology* 91: 457-464, 2006.

62. Mendelson M, Michallet AS, Monneret D, Perrin C, Estève F, Lombard P, Faure P, Lévy P, Favre–Juvin A, and Pépin JL. Impact of exercise training without caloric restriction on inflammation, insulin resistance and visceral fat mass in obese adolescents. *Pediatric obesity* 10: 311-319, 2015.

63. Miller T, Mull S, Aragon AA, Krieger J, and Schoenfeld BJ. Resistance Training Combined With Diet Decreases Body Fat While Preserving Lean Mass Independent of Resting Metabolic Rate: A Randomized Trial. *International journal of sport nutrition and exercise metabolism* 28: 46-54, 2018.

64. Moritani T. Neuromuscular adaptations during the acquisition of muscle strength, power and motor tasks. *Journal of Biomechanics* 26: 95-107, 1993.

65. Mujika I and Padilla S. Detraining: loss of training-induced physiological and performance adaptations. Part I. *Sports Medicine* 30: 79-87, 2000.

66. Mujika I and Padilla S. Detraining: loss of training-induced physiological and performance adaptations. Part II. *Sports Medicine* 30: 145-154, 2000.

67. Nader GA. Concurrent strength and endurance training: from molecules to man. *Medicine and science in sports and exercise* 38: 1965, 2006.

68. Nair KS. Age-related changes in muscle. *Mayo Clinic Proceedings*, 2000, p. S14-18.

69. Neder JA, Nery LE, Silva AC, Andreoni S, and Whipp BJ. Maximal aerobic power and leg muscle mass and strength related to age in non-athletic males and females. *European journal of applied physiology and occupational physiology* 79: 522-530, 1999.

70. Newton RU, Häkkinen K, Häkkinen A, McCormick M, Volek J, and Kraemer WJ. Mixed-methods resistance training increases power and strength of young and older men. *Medicine & Science in Sports & Exercise* 34: 1367-1375, 2002.

71. Nindl BC, Harman EA, Marx JO, Gotshalk LA, Frykman PN, Lammi E, Palmer C, and Kraemer WJ. Regional body composition changes in women after 6 months of periodized physical training. *Journal of Applied Physiology* 88: 2251-2259, 2000.

72. Petrella JK, Kim J-s, Tuggle SC, Hall SR, and Bamman MM. Age differences in knee extension power, contractile velocity, and fatigability. *Journal of Applied Physiology* 98: 211-220, 2005.

73. Piacentini MF, De Ioannon G, Comotto S, Spedicato A, Vernillo G, and La Torre A. Concurrent strength and endurance training effects on running economy in master endurance runners. *The Journal of Strength & Conditioning Research* 27: 2295-2303, 2013.

74. Putman CT, Xu X, Gillies E, MacLean IM, and Bell GJ. Effects of strength, endurance and combined training on myosin heavy chain content and fibre-type distribution in humans. *European journal of applied physiology* 92: 376-384, 2004.

75. Ramme AJ, Vira S, Alaia MJ, VAN JDL, and Rothberg RC. Exertional rhabdomyolysis after spinning: case series and review of the literature. *The Journal of sports medicine and physical fitness* 56: 789-793, 2016.

76. Scalco RS, Snoeck M, Quinlivan R, Treves S, Laforét P, Jungbluth H, and Voermans NC. Exertional rhabdomyolysis: physiological response or manifestation of an underlying myopathy? *BMJ open sport & exercise medicine* 2: e000151, 2016.

77. Schoenfeld BJ, Ogborn D, and Krieger JW. Dose-response relationship between weekly resistance training volume and increases in muscle mass: A systematic review and meta-analysis. *Journal of sports sciences* 35: 1073-1082, 2017.

78. Schoenfeld BJ, Ogborn D, and Krieger JW. Effects of resistance training frequency on measures of muscle hypertrophy: a systematic review and meta-analysis. *Sports Medicine* 46: 1689-1697, 2016.

79. Seynnes OR, de Boer M, and Narici MV. Early skeletal muscle hypertrophy and architectural changes in response to high-intensity resistance training. *Journal of applied physiology* 102: 368-373, 2007.

80. Shaibi GQ, Cruz ML, Ball GD, Weigensberg MJ, Salem GJ, Crespo NC, and Goran MI. Effects of resistance training on insulin sensitivity in overweight Latino adolescent males. *Medicine and science in sports and exercise* 38: 1208, 2006.

81. Short KR, Vittone JL, Bigelow ML, Proctor DN, Coenen-Schimke JM, Rys P, and Nair KS. Changes in myosin heavy chain mRNA and protein expression in human skeletal muscle with age and endurance exercise training. *Journal of applied physiology* 99: 95-102, 2005.

82. Staron R, Karapondo D, Kraemer W, Fry A, Gordon S, Falkel JE, Hagerman F, and Hikida R. Skeletal muscle adaptations during early phase of heavy-resistance training in men and women. *Journal of applied physiology* 76: 1247-1255, 1994.

83. Stewart V, Saunders D, and Greig C. Responsiveness of muscle size and strength to physical training in very elderly people: a systematic review. *Scandinavian journal of medicine & science in sports* 24: e1-e10, 2014.

84. Straight CR, Lindheimer JB, Brady AO, Dishman RK, and Evans EM. Effects of resistance training on lower-extremity muscle power in middle-aged and older adults: a systematic review and meta-analysis of randomized controlled trials. *Sports Medicine* 46: 353-364, 2016.

85. Strasser B, Arvandi M, and Siebert U. Resistance training, visceral obesity and inflammatory response: a review of the evidence. *Obesity reviews* 13: 578-591, 2012.

86. Strasser B, Siebert U, and Schobersberger W. Resistance training in the treatment of the metabolic syndrome. *Sports medicine* 40: 397-415, 2010.

87. Tabata S, Suzuki Y, Azuma K, and Matsumoto H. Rhabdomyolysis after performing blood flow restriction training: a case report. *Journal of strength and conditioning research* 30: 2064-2068, 2016.

88. Theou O, Stathokostas L, Roland KP, Jakobi JM, Patterson C, Vandervoort AA, and Jones GR. The effectiveness of exercise interventions for the management of frailty: a systematic review. *Journal of aging research* 2011, 2011.

89. Tran M, Hayden N, Garcia B, and Tucci V. Low-intensity repetitive exercise induced rhabdomyolysis. *Case reports in emergency medicine* 2015, 2015.

90. Trombetti A, Reid K, Hars M, Herrmann F, Pasha E, Phillips E, and Fielding R. Age-associated declines in muscle mass, strength, power, and physical performance: impact on fear of falling and quality of life. *Osteoporosis international* 27: 463-471, 2016.

91. Tucker WJ, Angadi SS, and Gaesser GA. Excess postexercise oxygen consumption after high-intensity and sprint interval exercise, and continuous steady-state exercise. *Journal of strength and conditioning research* 30: 3090-3097, 2016.

92. Vanderburgh P, Kusano M, Sharp M, and Nindl B. Gender differences in muscular strength: an allometric model approach. *Biomedical sciences instrumentation* 33: 100-105, 1997.

93. Verheggen R, Maessen M, Green D, Hermus A, Hopman M, and Thijssen D. A systematic review and meta-analysis on the effects of exercise training versus hypocaloric diet: distinct effects on body weight and visceral adipose tissue. *Obesity Reviews* 17: 664-690, 2016.

94. Vlietstra L, Hendrickx W, and Waters DL. Exercise interventions in healthy older adults with sarcopenia: A systematic review and meta-analysis. *Australasian journal on ageing*, 2018.

95. Watson SL, Weeks BK, Weis LJ, Harding AT, Horan SA, and Beck BR. High-Intensity Resistance and Impact Training Improves Bone Mineral Density and Physical Function in Postmenopausal Women With Osteopenia and Osteoporosis: The LIFTMOR Randomized Controlled Trial. *Journal of Bone and Mineral Research* 33: 211-220, 2018.

96. Willardson JM. A brief review: factors affecting the length of the rest interval between resistance exercise sets. *The Journal of Strength & Conditioning Research* 20: 978-984, 2006.

97. Wright NC, Looker AC, Saag KG, Curtis JR, Delzell ES, Randall S, and Dawson-Hughes B. The recent prevalence of osteoporosis and low bone mass in the United States based on bone mineral density at the femoral neck or lumbar spine. *Journal of Bone and Mineral Research* 29: 2520-2526, 2014.

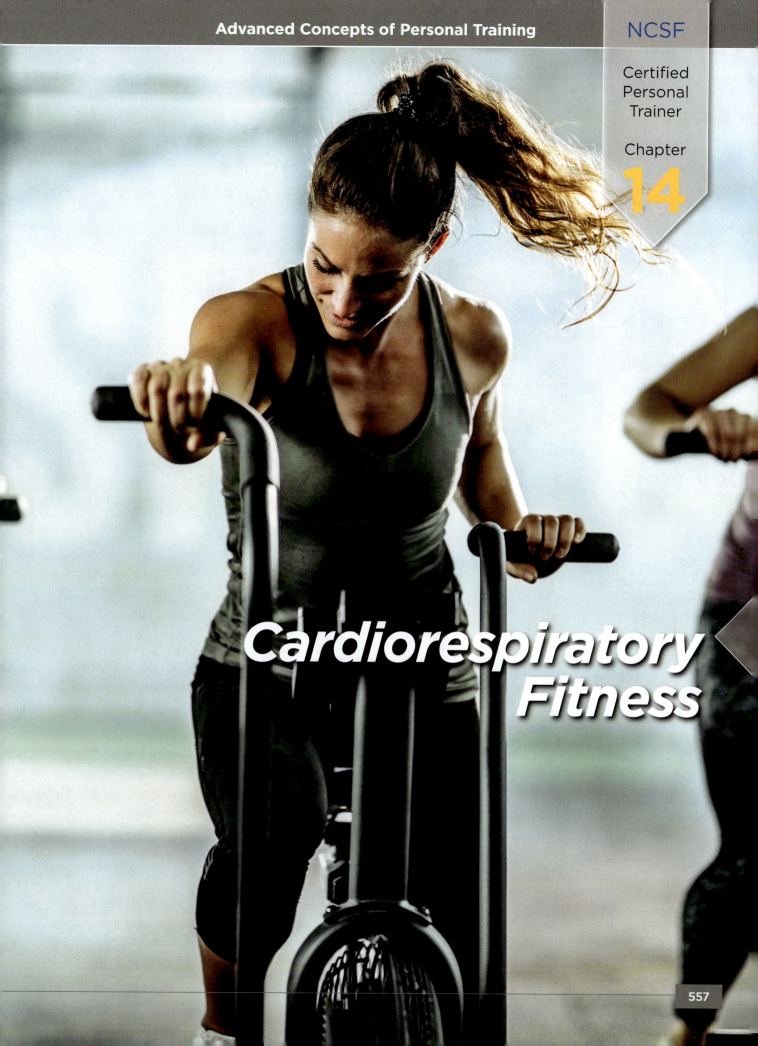

Advanced Concepts of Personal Training

NCSF Certified Personal Trainer

Chapter 14

Cardiorespiratory Fitness

Cardiorespiratory Fitness

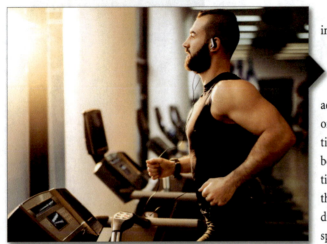

It has been well-documented that cardiorespiratory fitness (CRF) positively influences lifespan and quality of life, independent of other factors [38]. This relationship alone supports routine participation in aerobic activities to encourage adequate cardiovascular health throughout a person's life. Recalling key aspects of cardiovascular physiology from the earlier text, aerobic exercise yields the greatest positive adaptations on the structures and organs responsible for maintaining adequate blood and oxygen supply to the tissues. These include the heart, lungs, vascular system, and muscles. The body's ability to efficiently deliver oxygen-rich blood to all its tissues and the tissues capacity to use the oxygen to make adenosine triphosphate (ATP) are the foundation of cellular function and longevity. Since most Americans will die of cardiovascular or related diseases, aerobic system efficiency warrants specific attention in all exercise programs for health and fitness.

However, as with any health component, considerable variation exists between people, even those of the same age and background. Numerous factors determine a person's CRF level, so an evaluation of a client's aerobic capacity is needed to ascertain his or her relative ability to use oxygen. This evaluation also helps to establish exercise tolerance, interests, and exercise program starting points

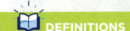

◆ Assessing Cardiorespiratory Fitness

Following the screening process for exercise participation, it is prudent to assess clients in some capacity to identify their relative CRF. Test selection decisions will be based on:

- The client's specific characteristics
- The exercise professional's knowledge and experience in testing
- Other logistical considerations that affect the outcome

> **DEFINITIONS**
>
> **Submaximal tests –**
>
> *A category of assessment methods in which test protocols do not reach the maximal capacities of the systems; maximal measures are predicted by incorporating physiological responses to these submaximal workloads.*

As mentioned previously, **submaximal tests** are far more common in personal training settings, as opposed to maximal tests, and when administered properly, these submaximal tests can provide useful data for the exercise prescription. Individuals new to exercise or those who have limited experience with aerobic training present additional issues for testing. For instance, it would be inappropriate to ask a new exerciser to execute a 1-mile maximal run test. The person would most likely perform poorly regardless of effort, experience significant distress, and the results would be useless. Being overly aggressive with the selected assessment activities can easily turn a person away from exercise participation, especially if exercise and fitness training are novel experiences. In addition, given the relative psychological states of new exercisers, they are likely to associate anxiety with the assessments and may possess some level of intimidation related to the new experience, particularly if they have not performed well in similar activities in the past.

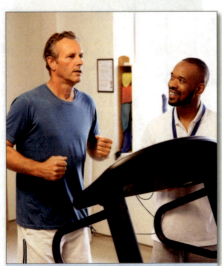

CRF test selection should be based on the client's proficiency, goals, and specific needs.

Selecting the appropriate test for a client does not need to be complicated. Each test has criteria distinctions that designate whether it is a viable option for the client. Submaximal test modalities offer different advantages and disadvantages, depending on the client's characteristics. Matching the test with the client's capabilities will provide quality, valid data. If the trainer selects an appropriate assessment and adheres strictly to the protocol, the tests should provide useful data. In some cases, the data will offer a prediction of oxygen consumption capabilities (VO_2max). In others, the performance is charted, and a category of fitness is determined. In either case, the exercise prescription will likely be based on heart rates for intensity determination rather than VO_2 or MET intensities; this is so because the latter two require specific knowledge of oxygen usage employing premeditated calculations or the use of equipment that determines intensity via those means. Although it serves as an accurate method to gauge aerobic training intensities, using percentage of VO_2max for the purposes of prescribing exercise is usually limited to cardiac rehabilitation programs.

Step tests
- Easy to implement using limited equipment
- Valid for general population, often over-predict fit individuals
- Metronome-paced test are considered superior to non-paced protocols
- Unsuitable for moderate to high-level obese, or very deconditioned clients
- Leg strength is a relevant factor, as is rhythm during cadence tests

Walk/jog tests
- Easy to implement with limited equipment
- Viable for deconditioned or new exercisers with no experience
- Validity is affected by motivation, exercise tolerance, and distance accuracy
- Over-predicts fit individuals

Run tests
- Easy to implement using limited equipment
- Viable for fit or conditioned individuals only
- Validity affected by test experience due to pace, client motivation, running economy, and distance accuracy

Bike tests
- Relatively difficult to implement because equipment and technical expertise are required
- Viable for multiple populations, but a moderate level of fitness is required
- Validity is high with strict protocol adherence
- Leg strength is a highly relevant factor

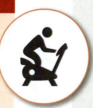

Measuring Intensity Through Heart Rate

Heart rate is the ideal measure for determining intensity because it has a linear relationship with aerobic work. During aerobic training, the harder a person exerts him or herself, the more oxygen is required to satisfy the demand. As a result, the heart must beat more frequently to

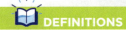

DEFINITIONS

Heart rate training zone (HRTZ) –

A heart rate range relative to an individual's heart rate max that should be maintained during cardiovascular training to obtain targeted adaptations.

Graded exercise test (GXT) –

An evaluation of cardiorespiratory capacity in which periodic increases in intensity are employed to achieve maximal or sub maximal workloads, often using a treadmill or cycle ergometer.

correspond with the increased need for oxygenated blood. This relationship allows oxygen use, or VO_2, to be measured indirectly by tracking the heart rate response to exercise. This can be visualized as the body overcoming applied resistance when no obvious, quantifiable resistance exists. As seen with jogging, biking, and swimming, the heart lets one quantify the work. Oxygen used when running at 150 beats · min-1 is similar to playing basketball at the same heart rate. Therefore, the modality does not really matter; it is the resistance the body must overcome that the heart responds to, and this is measured by the number of responsive beats. The term **heart rate training zone (HRTZ)** defines the heart rate range that a person should maintain while performing work in order to maximize the adaptive response to aerobic exercise.

To determine the HRTZ, trainers should first measure or predict the individual's maximum heart rate (MHR). A direct measurement always provides superior validity, but is not practical for most training situations. Direct measurement requires a person to perform a maximal aerobic test, which is most commonly a **graded exercise test (GXT)**, performed on a treadmill. The problem with maximal GXTs is that the required equipment, expertise, and client effort often create logistical issues for the average personal training situation. For this reason, trainers more commonly employ predictive formulas to determine MHR. The classic formula to predict maximum heart rate subtracts a person's age from 220, expressed as the formula (220 - age) = MHR. The value is considered the highest attainable heart rate for an individual at a given age. This formula's major problem is that it suggests that everyone of a certain age has the exact same maximum heart rate [38]. However, the standard deviation for the MHR equation is 10-12 beats · min-1. If using bell curve theory, this would suggest the formula's accuracy for 68% of the population at any given age. Using the same theory, the remaining 32% of the population's MHR would either be under or over the predicted value by somewhere between 10-24 beats · min-1, depending on the specific location along the curve. This prediction clearly lacks precision, and therefore, may throw off the training zone's accuracy, consequently leading to the reduced effectiveness of the training [19].

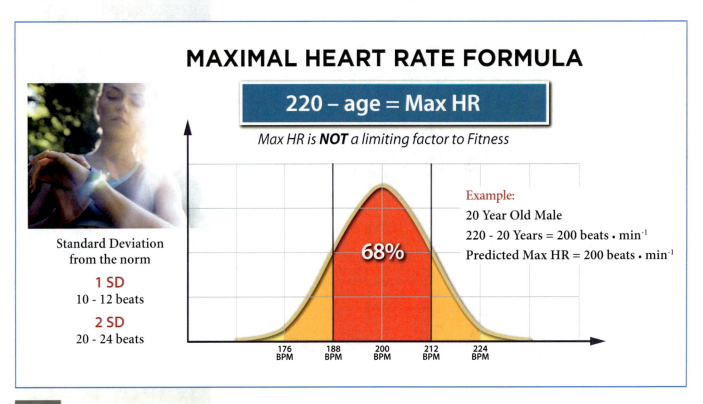

> **QUICK FACT**
>
> *An important note with MHR: a higher number is not always better. In fact, elite athletes experience a mild decline in maximal heart rate as an adaptation. Their bodies extract oxygen so proficiently from the blood that more beats are not beneficial, and therefore, the reduction in maximal heart rate spares energy.*

Rate of Perceived Exertion

To improve the MHR formula, trainers can compare heart rate measures with the values of the Rate of Perceived Exertion (RPE) Scale. RPE is based on Borg's research into monitoring exercise by perception of effort, rather than cardiovascular measures. Borg found that when combining local factors, such as perceived strain and discomfort, and central factors, including respiration rate and relative heart rate, work level can be identified. In his original scale, the numbers 6-20 reflected heart rates of 60-200 beats · min^{-1}. A correlation exists between the scale defined for perceived effort and exercise intensity [14, 34]. A value of 12-14 on the RPE scale correlates with 60-80% of the heart rate reserve (HRR), with 13-14 being closely related to lactate threshold [34]. Using the combined method of age-predicted max heart-rate based training zones and RPE, a person expected to be within a specific target zone should match the zone defined by perceived exertion when training above an intensity of 50% MHR [12]. When the zones align, the measured heart rates can be documented for improved accuracy to generate the exercise prescription. A caveat to RPE is that it uses relative perception: a person can perceive himself or herself to be working "hard" when, by all physiological measures, he or she is not. This phenomenon is called exercise tolerance, which is an individual's interest in a work rate based on psychophysiological factors. In short, some people do not like the level of discomfort needed for exercise-related adaptations.

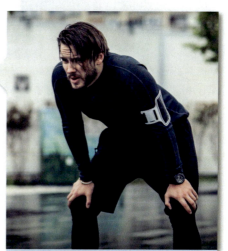

One way to improve the MHR formula is to compare the HR measures with the values of the RPE scale.

Rate of Perceived Exertion (RPE)

BORG RPE	MODIFIED RPE	BREATHING	% OF MHR*	EXERCISE TYPE
6	0	No Exertion	50%-60%	Warm up
7	0			
8	1	Very Light		
9	1			
10	2	Deeper but comfortable breathing. Able to hold a conversation	60%-70%	Recovery
11	2			
12	3			
13	3	Aware that breathing is harder; able to talk but difficult to hold conversation	70%-80%	Aerobic
14	4			
15	5	Starting to breathe hard and getting uncomfortable	80%-90%	Anaerobic
16	6			
17	7	Deep and forceful breathing. Uncomfortable and not wanting to talk	90%-100%	VO$_2$ Max
18	8			
19	9	Extremely hard		
20	10	Maximum exertion		

*% of maximum heart rate

Researchers have come up with other formulas that may increase the accuracy of heart rate prediction for specific populations. Research findings indicate that age, obesity, fitness, and smoking status all contribute to prediction error when using the traditional MHR formula [49]. Therefore, modified formulas to predict max heart rates have surfaced, each of which holds statistical merit for the respective population for which it is designed. The following formulas (below) can take the place of the traditional MHR formula for the select populations. Even with the improved accuracy associated with these formulas, standard deviations still exist that can affect the accuracy of the predicted training zone. Exercise professionals should utilize the RPE scale and other indicators to contend with the inherent variability associated with MHR prediction. Additionally, exercise professionals should be aware of medications that affect heart rate and should always document a client's medications. Certain drugs, such as beta blockers, and calcium channel blockers, may suppress heart rate, while other drugs, such as stimulants that are used to treat attention-deficit hyperactivity disorder (ADHD), act to increase heart rate, rendering these measures inaccurate indicators of work. In these cases, RPE should be used in lieu of heart rate to prescribe exercise training zones.

Multifactor General Population Formula for Max Heart Rate

Men
Max HR = 203.9 − (0.812 x age) + (0.276 x RHR) − (0.084 x kg) − (4.5 x smoking code)

Women
Max HR = 204.8 − (0.718 x age) + (0.162 x RHR) − (0.105 x kg) − (6.2 x smoking code)

Age = years
RHR = resting heart rate
Kg = body weight in kilograms
Smoking code = (1) for smoker, (0) nonsmoker

Obese Individuals
Max HR = 200 − (0.5 x age)

Older Adults
Max HR = 208 − (0.7 x age)

Example
68 Year Old Male • 161 lbs • RHR 75bpm • Current Smoker

Max HR = 203.9 − (.812 x 68) + (.276 x 75) − (.084 x 73) − (4.5 x 1)
Max HR = 203.9 − 55.2 + 20.7 − 6.1 − 4.5
Max HR = 159 bpm

One method used to help gauge intensity is to monitor ventilation rates. The talk test is an informal, subjective method of qualifying predicted MHR values based on one's ability to communicate. The method requires subjects to exercise at an intensity at which conversation is comfortable. The intensity is gradually increased until the exerciser has difficulty maintaining regular conversation. At this point, the individual is at, or near, ventilatory threshold. Ventilatory threshold describes a non-linear increase in respiration that corresponds with higher levels

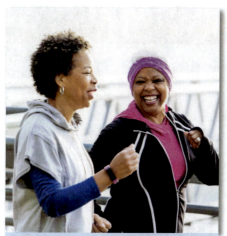

The talk test is an informal, subjective method of qualifying predicted MHR values based on one's ability to communicate while exercising.

of exercise intensity due to increased blood temperature and blood pH reduction. Respiration rises linearly with intensity until the ventilatory threshold is reached, at which time respiration experiences an exponential climb. Research has demonstrated a close correlation between the Talk Test and VO_2 and heart rate intensities at ventilatory threshold [25, 52]. The talk test can be used with the RPE scale to increase the accuracy of HRTZs. An RPE value of 14 generally equates to the value found in the Talk Test performance when conversation becomes difficult [52].

Heart Rate Training Zones

The predicted maximum heart rate can help prescribe exercise intensity by creating HRTZs, and different formulas can calculate the training zones. The two most widely used formulas are the MHR formula and the HHR method. The MHR formula is very easy to implement and is the method used to create most exercise intensity charts found on popular brands of cardiovascular equipment. This formula though, has one major drawback: it suggests that all people of the same age have the same fitness level. Not only can error exist in predicting one's max heart rate, but additional error can arise from the fact that training zones based solely on maximum heart rate do not account for an individual's current fitness level. It is important to remember that all people of the same age do not have similar heart rates at the same respective training intensities.

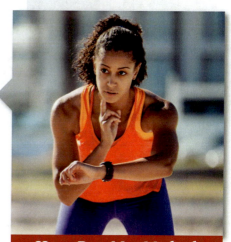

Heart Rate Max Method
- (220 – age) x Training Intensity
- Assumes all people the same age should train in the same range

Heart Rate Reserve Method

The HHR method is another predictive formula that can be used when prescribing training zones. It is considered superior to the MHR method for determining individual HRTZs, as it factors in an additional cardiovascular-based variable, resting heart rate (RHR). Previously in the text, the relationship between RHR and cardiorespiratory efficiency was established, and it was further identified that lower RHR generally indicates higher stroke volume and, consequently, a more efficient heart. The HHR formula employs this relationship to make individual adjustments in the training heart-rate estimates. HRR is calculated by subtracting an individual's RHR from predicted MHR.

The HRR method then requires that the HRR be multiplied by the desired training intensity. The product of that equation is added to the RHR to estimate the HRTZ. HRR works on the premise that training heart rates must lie somewhere between the lowest value (RHR) and the highest value (maximal heart rate) at which the heart can beat. Due to individual variations, that range will differ for most people: a more fit individual will have a broader range between the resting and maximal heart-rate value, while a person with a low level of CRF will have a narrower HRR range, helping to account for fitness differences.

Heart Rate Reserve Method

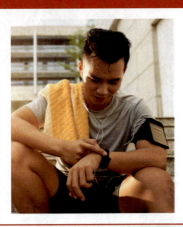

Heart Rate Reserve = Max HR − Resting HR

Training HR = (HRR × Training Intensity expressed as a percentage) + RHR

Example
20 Year Old Male • Max HR 200 beats·min⁻¹ • RHR 60 beats·min⁻¹

200 beats · min⁻¹ − 60 beats · min⁻¹ = 140 beats · min⁻¹
(140 beats · min⁻¹ × 0.60) + 60 beats · min⁻¹ = 144 beats · min⁻¹
(140 beats · min⁻¹ × 0.80) + 60 beats · min⁻¹ = 172 beats · min⁻¹

Training Zone = 144 − 172 beats · min⁻¹

Adequate aerobic stimulus for cardiovascular improvements varies by individual. General guidelines suggest that the intensity must be at least 40% of VO_2max for any cardiovascular adaptations to occur [58]. This value though, is insufficient for performance improvements for the majority of the population. The following ranges will be appropriate for improvements in health and fitness for most.

Recommended Training Intensities

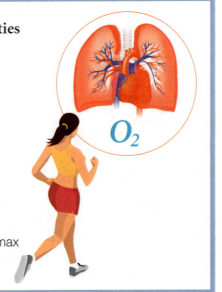

Training Intensity Ranges for Deconditioned Individuals

40-60% VO_2max
50-60% Heart Rate Reserve
60-70% Heart Rate Max

Training Intensity Ranges for Healthy Individuals

60-80% Heart Rate Reserve or VO_2max
75-90% Heart Rate Max

The specific intensity used will be based on a variety of factors, including current fitness level, exercise tolerance, training experience, risk factors for disease, and the client and exercise program goals. VO_2 and HRR do not correlate perfectly, especially at lower intensities, so mild adjustments for deconditioned individuals are made in the intensity selection for this population [13, 17, 59]. Deciding on the exact intensity to employ for a client resembles the procedure for other health-related components. A period of acclimation is recommended to familiarize clients with exercise and to help foster routine engagement in the activity. When creating the exercise prescription, the exercise principles should be properly applied so that the progressive overload is appropriate for the client. Starting or progressing too aggressively can lead to attrition and overuse injury.

Types of Aerobic Training

A variety of aerobic training modes can be used to elicit the desired adaptation response. In general, aerobic training uses either steady-state work within targeted heart rate zones or varying interval heart rates with zones that reflect the intended adaptation. Steady-state has historically been the most common method of aerobic training employed across the population, as it is well-tolerated and can be performed at low intensities. It requires exercisers to perform at a set pace without varying the resistance or movement factors to maintain a steady heart rate. The term steady-state refers to the heart rate's consistency during the performance of work. Heart rate adjustments within five beats per minute suggest that aerobic pathways are maintained at a constant level because the oxygenated blood supply is meeting the demands of the cells.

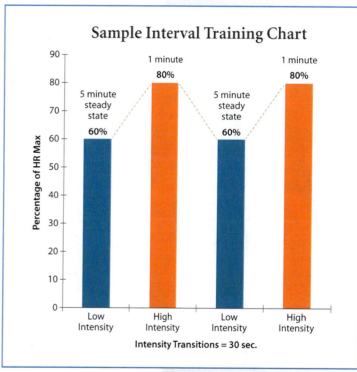

On the other hand, interval training takes advantage of variations in heart rate and resistance or speed. The heart rates fluctuate based on the intensity of the work at a given time. Interval training represents a more effective method for attaining higher exercise intensities and, therefore, greater exercise-induced adaptations. It is also well tolerated when the interval intensities and duration match participant capabilities. The foundation of programming interval-based exercise lies in the premise that the body will always adapt to the highest perceived stress when chronically applied, even though the time spent in the highest intensity ranges may be limited when compared to the total activity duration. It is much easier to push the body at high intensities for short periods of time, compared to attempting to maintain higher steady-state levels for the exercise session's duration. Using intervals, a client can reach exercise intensities he or she otherwise would not be able to experience or maintain. It is suggested that, when applied properly, interval training yields a greater adaptation response compared to steady-state training performed for the same time period [45, 66].

High-Intensity vs. Low-Intensity Training

Intensity selection also depends upon desired outcome. Higher-intensity training optimizes the cardiorespiratory system for performance and contributes significantly to caloric expenditure [39].

When compared to high-intensity work, moderate intensities are useful for [40]: Health attainment | Caloric expenditure | Disease prevention | Reduced risk for injury

However, many exercisers prefer moderate-intensity activity because it is more tolerable for sustained periods compared to training at higher intensities [24]. For those with health issues that prevent the use of more elevated intensity levels, low-intensity, high-volume aerobic training is recommended as it helps acclimate them to exercise.

In some circles, low-intensity exercise has been recommended for weight loss due to its emphasis on lipid metabolism. Although it is true that sleep, rest, and low-intensity activity utilize fat as a primary fuel source for aerobic metabolism, the total calories expended during activities of low metabolic demand remain considerably fewer than the caloric expenditures associated with higher-intensity activities [1, 37]. Therefore, even though low-intensity exercise burns a higher percentage of calories from fat, the total number of both fat calories and total calories burned is actually lower [69]. Individuals who attempt to lose weight by training in the "fat-burning zone" actually limit their ability to burn calories, which is the primary factor that affects weight loss [31]. Compared to moderate and high intensities, low-intensity exercise reduces caloric expenditure, cardiovascular adaptations, and in some cases, with duration being the key variable, reduces the total amount of fat utilized during the exercise bout [1, 69].

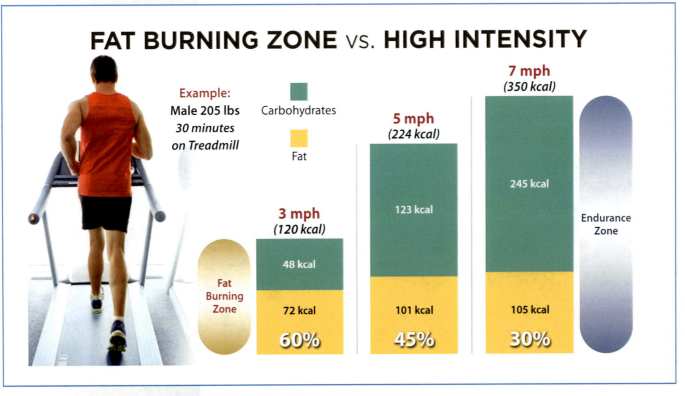

The term "fatmax" describes the specific exercise intensity at which the maximal rate of lipid oxidation occurs. During exercise, this occurs at around 51-53% VO_2max in endurance-trained athletes [44, 54]. Endurance athletes will train their long distances at this intensity to optimize the specific adaptations that occur in response to long, slow distance (LSD) and to spare glycogen. However, due to their less efficient metabolic systems, sedentary individuals demonstrate lower maximal fat oxidation rates and reach fatmax at lower intensities: measured at 43-51% VO_2max [44]. Improved enzyme efficiency, hypertrophy of slow-twitch fibers, and improved lipid oxidation all associate with LSD training and are considered base adaptations of CRF. Intervals on the track and tempo-based runs maximize the heart's efficiency, increase lactate tolerance, improve buffering, and promote increased capillary density, but should only be performed by those whose capabilities warrant higher intensities. In effect, higher-volume, lower-intensity distance training improves the oxygen extraction component, whereas high intensities promote improvements in the oxygen delivery component.

Consistent with defining the appropriate training intensity, the goals of the exercise program outcomes will dictate the training frequency and duration. Unlike other exercise types, aerobic training requires a bit more frequent and consistent participation to optimize results and prevent detraining effects [33, 51]. For health improvements, aerobic activities should be performed most days of the week, equaling at least 14-20 calories per kilogram of body weight across that duration [9, 26]. The same can be said when training for performance, but intensities vary more dramatically. At a minimum, aerobic activity should be performed three or four days per week [33, 50]. For improvements in CRF, deconditioned individuals should accumulate a minimum of 30 minutes of aerobic activity most days of the week, while healthy individuals should engage in aerobic exercise for 30-90 minutes, 3-5 days per week [50]. In addition, vigorously intense activities should be performed for 10-15 minutes at least twice per week by healthy individuals. Interestingly, deconditioned participants show almost equal benefit when the 30-minute time period is divided up into multiple sessions throughout the day (3 x 10 minutes), as long as the heart rates remain above the minimum threshold for CRF improvements [9]. Additionally, deconditioned individuals have shown improvements with a participation of 2-3 sessions per week [65]. However, experienced exercisers require higher volumes and intensities for tangible improvements.

> **QUICK INSIGHT**
>
> **$VO_2max = CO \times (A-V)\ O_2$ difference**
>
> VO_2max is the highest level for which cells can function using oxygen for fuel. VO_2max is a function of oxygen delivery efficiency as determined by cardiac output and the oxygen-extraction efficiency, referred to as $(A-V)\ O_2$ difference: the difference in oxygen content between the arteries and the veins. Training for improved CRF should emphasize adaptations in the oxygen delivery (higher intensity) or adaptations to improve the extraction of the oxygen (lower intensity). Variations in training intensity and duration can account for all of the necessary adaptations.

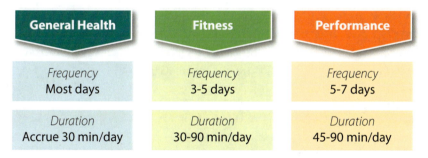

From an overall health standpoint, training at higher intensities most days of the week may initiate a cost-benefit imbalance due to the elevation in risk for musculoskeletal injury that occurs with more frequent, longer bouts of aerobic exercise. Likewise, regular training beyond 80% VO_2max has been correlated with greater injury risk [35, 63]. Longer-duration bouts and high intensities are, in fact, necessary for higher-end performance and competition-level training. But, if the goal is health and fitness, then training at roughly 80% of VO_2max, 4-5 days per week, for approximately thirty minutes is appropriate. Interestingly, the regimen generally recommended for health (60-80% VO_2max) is called the 'junk zone' for performance. Again, the adaptations associated with long, slow distance require roughly 45-65% VO_2max, whereas intervals and repeat track distances require >85% VO_2max. This makes sense when you look at an endurance event like the marathon. Competitors want to spare glycogen by maximizing the advantage of a moderate fatmax level during the first 20 miles and then rely heavily on the anaerobic system to run as fast as possible for the last six miles. Competitive distance runners benefit most from improvements in the aerobic-anaerobic relationship.

Energy Expenditure

An energy expenditure of 200-400 kcal per day marks CRF improvement consistent with the other aerobic prescription guidelines for health [39, 61]. When aerobic exercise is performed for a duration and intensity that meets or exceeds 14 kcal per kilogram of body weight per week, the body experiences improved health. Calories per training bout, or those expended when performing aerobic activity, seem to be part of the multifactorial threshold for health [26]. The relationship between calories and aerobic training stems from the oxidation value of energy. Approximately five (5) kcal of energy are released per liter of oxygen used. Therefore, measuring calories expended in an exercise bout or oxygen used by the body during the exercise period will identify the work performed. In fact, energy expenditure can be represented in numerous ways that all reflect the amount of oxygen or calories used while performing activity.

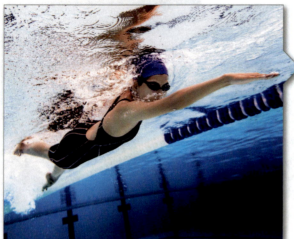

Energy expenditure equaling 200-400 kcals each day is recommended for CRF improvements and overall health.

Many people get confused concerning the various energy systems' contributions when calories are discussed because calories burned are determined by the energy and the quantity of oxygen used during the activity. Since aerobic-based exercise utilizes constant movement and a fairly-simple quantification of oxygen used, caloric expenditure is easily displayed on exercise equipment or can be calculated based on the size of the individual and resistance (speed) at which he or she moves during the event. Anaerobic exercise requires force demands that cannot be satisfied by oxygen for fuel: hence the term "anaerobic" (an=without + aerobic=air or oxygen). So how is caloric expenditure determined? The body experiences an oxygen debt when working anaerobically, which is paid back during the rest interval. During a set of squats or maximum sprints, ADP and lactate build up in the cells as they use anaerobic-based energy. During the rest interval, oxygen is used in the process of clearing glycolytic waste products like lactate and for rephosphorylation of high-energy phosphagens. Therefore, oxygen is used during resistance training during recovery, but not necessarily relied upon heavily to support force production work.

Understanding METs

The different ways to express energy expenditure allow for multiple variables that can fully predict how much work is being done, how much oxygen is needed, and how many calories are burned during the activity. One of the more common ways to convey the demands of an activity is through a unit referred to as a MET, or metabolic equivalent. An activity's MET intensity reflects the magnitude of work performed by the body relative to rest. Therefore, one MET represents the value of oxygen used when the body rests and equals the derived unit: 3.5 ml of oxygen per kg of body weight per minute (3.5 ml · kg^{-1} · min^{-1}).

| Expressed as 3.5 ml · kg^{-1} · min^{-1} | Minutes reflect time of activity | Kilograms represent body weight | Milliliters identify the O_2 used |

This value is the same for every person. It becomes relative to an individual by factoring in weight and the time spent at that relative oxygen demand. If an activity is performed above a resting level, which is 1 MET, then the MET value changes to reflect each oxygen level (3.5) until the cell can no longer use oxygen for fuel. For instance, casual walking is generally performed at 2.8 METs; working at a desk is 1.5 METs, while washing and waxing a car is 4.5 METs. When multiplied by the 3.5 ml · kg^{-1} · min^{-1} unit, each of these values is converted to the activity's specific oxygen demand when time and weight are considered. Once the total oxygen utilized has been determined, the total calories expended can be calculated, given that each liter (L) of oxygen used equates to ~5 kcal burned.

MET Example One

Example: 220 lb. (100 kg) man sitting in a chair for 60 minutes (1 MET)

$$3.5 \text{ ml} \cdot \text{kg}^{-1} \cdot \text{min}^{-1} \times 100 \text{ kg} = 350 \text{ ml} \cdot \text{min}^{-1}$$

$$350 \text{ ml} \cdot \text{min}^{-1} \times 60 \text{ min} = 21{,}000 \text{ ml}$$

$$21000 \text{ ml} \times \frac{.001 \text{ L}}{\text{ml}} = 21 \text{ L}$$

$$21 \text{ L} \times 5 \text{ kcal} \cdot \text{L}^{-1} = 105 \text{ kcal}$$

The example above shows that when the relative individual variables are factored in, the MET value can be expressed as a measure of oxygen use and calories expended. In the case above, the 220 lb. man sitting in the chair for an hour would require 21 liters of oxygen, or 105 calories, for his tissues to function. This ability to express the values based on known variables allows identification of how much oxygen or energy is needed to perform a particular task. The above equation can also be used to identify oxygen demand and calories for any level of work when the necessary variables are known. In fact, this is the same formula that aerobic exercise equipment uses to provide exercisers with the calories they expend during a workout.

One of the first values requested of an exerciser when starting on an electronic aerobic machine is his or her weight. The machine quickly converts the pounds entered to kilograms and adds this value into the equation. The next value the machine often requests is the amount of time the exercise will be performed. This number is also entered into the equation. The last bit of information used is the speed setting or intensity level selected. The machine has MET intensities built into its default program data, based on the level or speed selected. The following example demonstrates the machine's conversion of information to provide the user with a caloric value.

MET Example Two

Example: 220 lbs. (100 kg) male exercising at level 8 on a Stairclimber for 30 minutes

Weight: $220 \text{ lbs.} \div \frac{1 \text{ kg}}{2.2 \text{ lbs.}} = 100 \text{ kg}$

Intensity: Level 8 = 10 METs *(Default value based on resistance and speed)*

Time: 30 minutes

1 MET = 3.5 ml · kg^{-1} · min^{-1}

$$\frac{10 \text{ MET} \times 3.5 \text{ ml} \cdot \text{kg}^{-1} \cdot \text{min}^{-1}}{1 \text{ MET}} = 35 \text{ ml} \cdot \text{kg}^{-1} \cdot \text{min}^{-1}$$

$$35 \text{ ml} \cdot \text{kg}^{-1} \cdot \text{min}^{-1} \times 100 \text{ kg} = 3500 \text{ ml} \cdot \text{min}^{-1}$$

$$3500 \text{ ml} \cdot \text{min}^{-1} \times 30 \text{ min} = 105{,}000 \text{ ml}$$

$$105{,}000 \text{ ml} \times \frac{.001 \text{ L}}{\text{ml}} = 105 \text{ L}$$

$$105 \text{ L} \times 5 \text{ kcal} \cdot \text{L}^{-1} = 525 \text{ kcal}$$

This equation works for any activity that has been scientifically measured for work. Clinicians have analyzed hundreds of activities to provide MET intensities for use in determining oxygen demand and energy expenditure. In some cases, the activities are weight-bearing, like the stair climbing example, where the exerciser must lift his or her body weight as part of the resistance. In others, such as biking, the weight of an individual is not a relevant factor in determining the oxygen demand. Activities where bodyweight is a factor when determining work express the value as ml · kg^{-1} · min^{-1}, whereas in non-weight-bearing activities, the oxygen is expressed as L · min^{-1}.

The exercise bike uses revolutions per minute (RPMs) and the selected resistance to determine the MET intensity. The subsequent energy expenditure is based on how long that MET intensity is performed. This explains why a person who weighs 150 lbs. and exercising at level 5 on the stationary bike will burn the same number of calories as a person weighing 200 lbs., presuming each person pedals at the same intensity for the same time period. Based on size, the smaller exerciser performs more relative work when the liters of oxygen are normalized to milliliters per kilogram of body weight per minute.

Common Expressions of Energy Expenditure	
Liters of oxygen per minute	L · min^{-1}
Calories per minute	Kcal · min^{-1}
Milliliters of oxygen per kilogram of bodyweight per minute	ml · kg^{-1} · min^{-1}
Metabolic equivalent of oxygen	METs
Calories per kilogram of bodyweight per minute	Kcal · kg^{-1} · hr^{-1}

During weight-bearing exercise, the amount of bodyweight determines the work being performed. The person's weight most often represents the vertical and horizontal resistive force that must be overcome to perform the movement. This variable becomes a factor when exercisers working out on this type of equipment lean on the guide rails or support bars to make the exercise easier. Any weight alleviated from the resistance to the movement and applied to the machine guide rails no longer contributes to the vertical or horizontal component of work, essentially reducing the number of actual calories burned. If 30% of the body weight is removed from the leg's resistance force, the resultant calories used the machine displays are 30% higher than the actual number burned. Commonly, exercisers set the machine on high training levels and compensate by resting on the machine to manage the work rate. This causes people to perceive a caloric expenditure during the exercise that may be as much as 50% above the true value burned.

Similar pitfalls exist for non-weight-bearing machines. The MET value determined by the selected training level is based on a default RPM speed (rotations per minute), normally about 70 RPMs (numbers may vary). When exercisers select training levels that are too difficult, they compensate by peddling slower, which negates the workload. Most machines are not technologically advanced enough to identify the change and recalculate the value, even though a light often flashes to signify a lower than desired RPM rate. However, most exercisers will acknowledge their work rate as consistent with the machine's data display, which is often an over-prediction of actual calories burned.

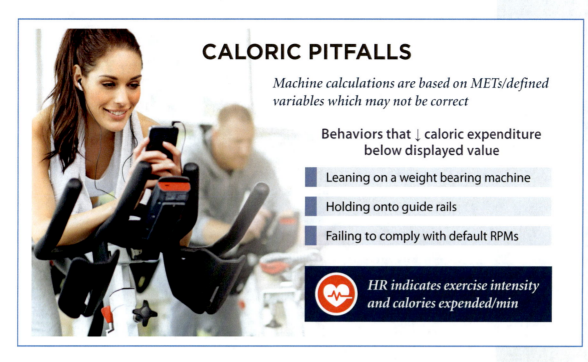

When METs are applied to a person's predicted or measured VO_2max to determine work rate or training zones, the amount of work the individual can tolerate becomes increasingly evident. The math required to convert VO_2max into METs is simple. One MET equals 3.5 ml · kg^{-1} · min^{-1}, and relative VO_2max is expressed using the same units. Therefore, to identify a person's maximum MET-intensity capabilities, simply divide the VO_2max by 3.5 ml · kg^{-1} · min^{-1}. Once this maximal MET value is identified, it can be used to determine the individual's realistic energy expenditure capacity.

For example, if a 37-year-old male weighing 200 lbs. was identified through aerobic testing to have a VO_2max of 46.5 ml · kg^{-1} · min^{-1} his maximal MET intensity would be 13 METs. Using the VO_2reserve (VO_2r) method, one would then subtract one (resting) MET from the METmax to identify the trainable range: 46.5 ml · kg^{-1} · min^{-1} – 3.5 ml · kg^{-1} · min^{-1} = 43 ml · kg^{-1} · min^{-1}.

$$43 \text{ ml} \cdot \text{kg}^{-1} \cdot \text{min}^{-1} \div \frac{3.5 \text{ ml} \cdot \text{kg}^{-1} \cdot \text{min}^{-1}}{1 \text{ MET}} = 12.25 \text{ METs}$$

If the individual wanted to lose weight, the length of time needed can easily be figured out based on their respective capacity. A healthy person is expected to train at an intensity between 60% and 80% HRR, or VO_2r. The individual's VO_2r was 43 ml · kg^{-1} · min^{-1}, or 12.25 METs.

$$60\% \times 12.25 \text{ METs} = 7.35 \text{ METs}$$
$$80\% \times 12.25 \text{ METs} = 9.8 \text{ METs}$$

The training intensity value suggests this individual should perform aerobic exercise at a work rate between 7.35 and 9.8 METs. Assuming this person could sustain the lower level for 30 minutes, the predicted aerobic training contribution to weight loss can be calculated.

$$7.35 \text{ MET} \times \frac{3.5 \text{ ml} \cdot \text{kg}^{-1} \cdot \text{min}^{-1}}{1 \text{ MET}} = 25.7 \text{ ml} \cdot \text{kg}^{-1} \cdot \text{min}^{-1}$$

$$25.7 \text{ ml} \cdot \text{kg}^{-1} \cdot \text{min}^{-1} \times 91 \text{ kg} = 2{,}338 \text{ ml} \cdot \text{min}^{-1}$$

$$2{,}338 \text{ ml} \cdot \text{min}^{-1} \times 30 \text{ min} = 70{,}140 \text{ ml}$$

$$70{,}140 \text{ ml} \times \frac{.001 \text{ L}}{\text{ml}} = 70.1 \text{ L}$$

$$70.1 \text{ L} \times 5 \text{ kcal} \cdot \text{L}^{-1} = 350 \text{ kcal}$$

Based on these findings, a healthy male individual can realistically be expected to burn 350 kcal in an aerobic exercise bout in the training program's early stages. This prediction is very helpful because the expected caloric expenditure identifies the rate at which weight loss can occur via exercise capacity and the amount of dietary adjustments that must be made to compensate for the value. When a client has a 12 MET capacity or higher, eliciting the desired training response and reaching weight loss goals becomes easier because the person has a high capacity to expend energy. When clients are deconditioned and present MET capacities lower than 10 METs, it becomes increasingly difficult to reach the same weight loss goals [10].

METs & Daily Caloric Expenditure

METs can also be used in the energy balance equation to identify daily caloric expenditure. As stated above, the average daily caloric expenditure is more relevant than any single aspect involved in high-energy expenditure when it comes to weight management. Therefore, identifying the mean energy expenditure value helps to identify the need for additional physical activity if weight loss and health are to be attained. In the same way one can use food logs to identify the caloric intake for a day, activity logs help calculate the caloric expenditure. Recording the activity and the participation duration provides the data necessary to calculate the daily energy expenditure. The chart shows a 24-hour activity recall for a 39-year-old female weighing 152 lbs.

The example represents a total daily oxygen use of 475 liters of oxygen or $1.65 \text{ kcal} \cdot \text{min}^{-1}$. Adding additional activity to this individual's lifestyle would increase the calories expended per day. Simply increasing daily oxygen use by an average of only one liter per hour would increase the caloric expenditure by 120 kcal. Encouraging more movement throughout the day can dramatically enhance the likelihood for a successful weight loss program [2, 57]. Additionally, those individuals who attain a minimum expenditure of 1,000-2,000 kcal per week from physical activity notably increase their health and reduce their risk for disease [2].

Using METs to Determine Daily Caloric Expenditure

Time	Activity	MET	Kcal
8:00 - 8:30 am	Showered and dressed	2.5	91
8:30 - 8:50 am	Ate breakfast	1.5	36
8:50 - 9:30 am	Drove to work w/traffic	2.0	97
9:30 - 9:40 am	Walk to office	3.0	36
9:30 - 10:45 am	Sat at desk	1.5	136
10:45 - 12:00 am	Meeting	1.5	136
12:00 - 1:00 pm	At lunch	1.5	109
1:00 - 2:30 pm	Sat at desk	1.5	163
2:30 - 2:50 pm	Walk to other office	3.0	72
2:50 - 5:00 pm	Presentation (standing)	2.3	361
5:00 - 5:15 pm	Walk to car	3.0	54
5:15 - 5:35 pm	Drove home	2.0	48
5:35 - 6:00 pm	Washed-up and changed	2.5	76
6:00 - 6:45 pm	Ate dinner	1.5	82
6:45 - 11:00 pm	Watch TV	1.0	308
11:00 - 11:10 pm	Self-care	1.0	12
11:10 pm - 8:00 am	Sleep	0.9	576
Total Energy Expenditure			**2,393**

Modes of Aerobic Training

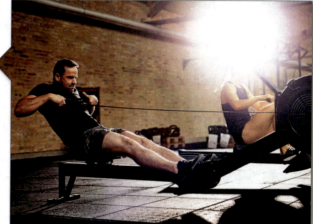

Physical activity can come from a variety of exercise modalities. Aerobic exercise activities aimed at improving CRF include numerous equally effective forms. The key factors are duration, intensity, frequency, and energy expended per session. This suggests that any continuous, rhythmic activity that utilizes large muscle groups can be included in the CRF program. The exercise or mode selected should be based on the client's capabilities, interests, and experience. Each mode has advantages and disadvantages which should be evaluated and matched to the client. Identifying the activities that the client finds to be fun or most tolerable will help ensure compliance and adherence to the training prescription. If several modes are of interest to the client, the exercise prescription should include a mixture of activities. Commonly referred to as cross-training, programming a variety of aerobic activities reduces boredom, lessens risk of overuse injury, and emphasizes different muscle groups, helping to reduce the risk of muscular imbalances. These modes can even be combined in a single training session. Running, rowing, and biking for instance, can each be utilized in 10-minute segments for a 30-minute workout. The variation in mode and musculature used allows for higher training intensity due to improved mental focus. Boredom becomes a factor in any long-duration activity performed on a frequent basis. Therefore, varying the modes reduces the consequences of mental staleness commonly experienced with single-mode, steady-state training.

◆ Systems of Training

Similar to anaerobic training, any of the selected modes of aerobic training present varied systems that can elicit improved adaptive responses. Each system varies by specific factors that modify the intensity, such as speed, terrain, or resistance. These systems can be used independently or in a coordinated fashion, depending on the program goals and the client's interests.

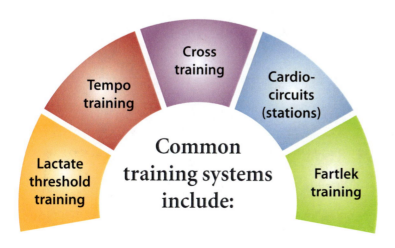

Common training systems include:
- Lactate threshold training
- Tempo training
- Cross training
- Cardio-circuits (stations)
- Fartlek training

Lactate Threshold and Tempo Training

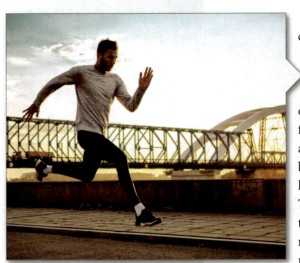

Lactate threshold training employs tactics that vary the amount of anaerobic contribution during the aerobic exercise bout. Conditioned individuals use this technique to push training levels for improvements in stamina and lactate tolerance. Lactate threshold is the point where lactate production equals the rate of lactate clearance. This state uses contributions from both energy systems (aerobic and anaerobic), but the anaerobic system's limiting effects are accommodated for via buffering mechanisms, which allow steady-state heart rate to be maintained and the work to be performed without consequence. When the pace is increased beyond the lactate threshold, the contribution from anaerobic metabolism can no longer be compensated for via the buffering mechanisms used for lactate turnover. This causes lactate and excess hydrogen ions produced from anaerobic metabolism to accumulate in the local musculature, which increases discomfort, ventilation rate, and perceived exertion, eventually forcing the exerciser to slow down to a recovery pace or to stop. It is suggested that exercisers should attempt to train using a pace at, or just below, lactate threshold for optimal cardiorespiratory adaptations [20, 21]. This type of training is called "tempo training." Many endurance athletes will use steady-state tempo pace on certain training days. Then, on other days, they cross the lactate threshold, using intervals to push the energy system to tolerate greater demands and to improve VO_2max. Lactate intervals generally last between 2-5 minutes, depending on the intensity reached and the condition of the exerciser. This method of training should only be used by individuals acclimated to the training intensity [21].

Cross Training

Cross training, as mentioned earlier, utilizes different exercise modes for aerobic improvements. In some cases, the exercise mode varies by exercise session. In other cases, different modes are used within the same workout. The benefits include reduced risk of overuse of a particular muscle or group, reduced risk of boredom, utilization of different muscle groups for improved condition, and better mental focus during the exercise session from the different exercise stimuli. Cross training can also be employed in cycles to help maximize the efficiency of a particular exercise mode. For example, over a 12-week training cycle, three different approaches may be used for each four-week period. Biking can be used for the first segment, attempting to improve aerobic conditioning in the legs without impact, before switching to stair climbing in the second four-week period, and then jogging for the last segment of the cycle. This method allows adaptations specific to the mode to take place and encourages improvement in neural efficiency while the client still benefits from the residuals of the other activities.

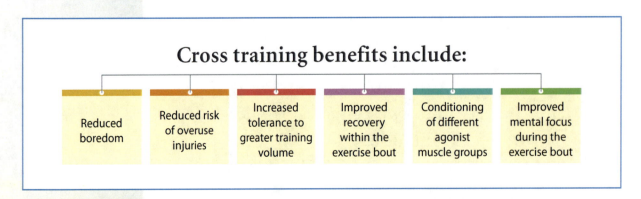

Cross training benefits include: Reduced boredom | Reduced risk of overuse injuries | Increased tolerance to greater training volume | Improved recovery within the exercise bout | Conditioning of different agonist muscle groups | Improved mental focus during the exercise bout

Cardio Circuit Training

Cardio circuit training is aerobic conditioning that utilizes different exercise types, and often total-body contributions during the exercise session. Cardio circuits require exercisers to perform steady-state aerobic activity with intermittent resistance training activities. A common example would be a parcourse, which employs jogging at a set pace along a designed fitness trail, stopping at designated locations along the route to perform calisthenics, pull-ups, push-ups, or other anaerobic activities, before continuing on the jog at the steady-state pace to the next activity stop. Parcourses often exist at local community parks. These courses can be mimicked in fitness facilities by switching from aerobic activity to resistance training movements with only transitional rest. In most cases, an exercise will be selected for each body part and performed every three minutes during the exercise routine. Cardio-circuits work very well in the personal training environment because they can be used to address several facets of the exercise program in an ongoing, aerobic-based exercise session.

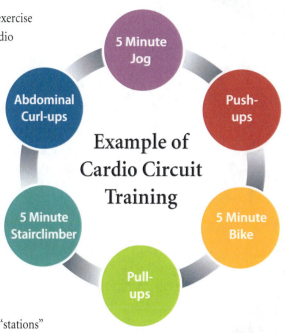

The next level up in intensity is referred to as "training stations." These "stations" are performed to anaerobic capacity before jogging to the next station. Often, 4-rounds (sets) of four to six exercises are used in a continuous basis lasting up to 20 minutes (4 sets x 4 exercises x 60 seconds each + 4 minutes of jogging). These are perceived as very difficult, as lactate levels remain high throughout the training bout and are better suited for intermediate to advanced exercisers.

Fartlek Training

Fartlek is a Swedish term meaning "speed play." **Fartlek training** is essentially a type of interval training that uses steady-state pace with periodic variations in speed and/or positive and negative incline grades. The biggest difference compared to standard interval training is the variation in speeds and distances used within the interval segment, along with the changes in the surface angle. A common example is a jog along a street with sprints interspersed between light poles, then a run up a flight of stairs. However, Fartlek training is not limited to jogs and sprints; true Fartlek training takes advantage of a variety of surfaces, uphill running, sprints, and downhill over-speed segments at different intervals in between (recovery) steady-state pace. The distances used and segment speeds will be determined by the training goals and the client's capabilities. These are often used in spring and fall periods when outside training is most conducive.

> **DEFINITIONS**
>
> **Fartlek training –**
> *Swedish for "speed play", a training method that blends interval and aerobic training by using unstructured fluctuations of higher and lower intensity efforts.*

Aerobic Training Considerations

Genetics

Participants in routine aerobic exercise can generally increase their VO_2max by 10-30%, with an average improvement of approximately 15% [62]. The improvement amount depends upon pre-training status, exercise tolerance, level of participation, and genetics. Of these factors, the largest variation is attributed to genetics, which accounts for as much as 50% of the differences [7, 8, 68].

Genetics largely drive adaptive responses in maximal cardiac output and oxygen extraction capabilities; individuals with the following show the greatest improvements [36, 43, 68]:

- Larger stroke volumes
- Greater concentrations of type I fibers
- Greater mitochondria and capillary density
- Higher myoglobin concentrations
- More efficient neural and metabolic pathways

Certain individuals are physiologically more efficient in aerobic pathways, and therefore present the most dramatic improvements in training [70].

Age

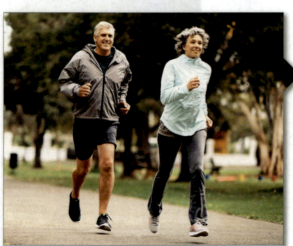

Healthy, sedentary adults experience a decline of their VO_2max by about 1% per year after age 25.

Healthy, sedentary adults experience a decline of approximately 1% per year in maximal aerobic capacity after age 25. The combination of inactivity, weight gain, and age-related decline in muscle mass and maximal heart rate all contribute to the loss of aerobic efficiency [22, 32]. In trained males, the rate of loss is attenuated to approximately 0.5% per year; interestingly however, among trained females, aerobic decline remains consistent with their sedentary counterparts [6, 22]. With that understood, individuals who attain higher levels of aerobic fitness early in life and consistently work to maintain those levels will obviously experience higher values throughout their lifespans, thereby preventing the early onset of functional decline. When previously sedentary, older adults engage in aerobic activity, they experience similar improvements compared to younger individuals (10-20%) [70]. However, due to their lower starting values, older adults have difficulty reaching high levels of aerobic fitness. The adaptations in older men and women are different, as older men show improvement in both maximal cardiac output and oxygen extraction from increased capillary and mitochondria density; on the other hand, improvements in aerobic efficiency in older women are solely limited to improvements in oxygen extraction [29].

Environmental Factors

External factors stress the body, and these include environmental conditions: heat, humidity, and altitude all exert potentially adverse effects during physical activity. Heat provides considerable stress to the body's internal environment, as the core temperature must remain constant. When muscle tissues contract, they produce heat, which must also be released from the body to prevent dangerous elevations in the core environment.

The human body cools itself via four methods:

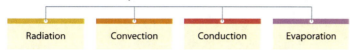

Radiation | Convection | Conduction | Evaporation

Radiation causes heat from the body to pass via air into colder solids that lie in close proximity. It works in the same fashion that sunlight warms the earth. Convection works in a similar way, but the heat is transferred into the air. When it is windy, heat is mobilized from the skin into the air that passes over the body. Conduction represents heat loss to a colder object that contacts the body or heat transferred from deep tissues to the skin. Jumping into cold water illustrates this concept very well. In fact, heat loss to water is 25 times that of heat loss to air at the same temperature [11]. The last method of heat loss is the body's primary defense against overheating. The evaporation process passes water through the skin and evaporates it into the air, causing a cooling effect. Heat is also lost through respiratory water vapor. All four mechanisms cooperate to regulate body temperature.

In hot environmental conditions, heat loss via radiation, convection, and conduction becomes less effective and can be completely inhibited. This leaves evaporation as the only functioning mechanism to remove body heat. As a result, the body mobilizes extracellular fluid to the skin in the form of sweat for evaporation and subsequent cooling; however, this leads to acute dehydration, causing the water content of the blood (plasma) to decrease. Exercise in the heat becomes incrementally more difficult as blood volume drops, which causes it to become denser. This blood plasma reduction forces the heart to work harder to move the blood, thereby making exercise more difficult, even though the pace remains the same. This problem is exacerbated when heat combines with high humidity. In these conditions, the evaporation process decreases significantly because the ambient air/water vapor pressure is consistent with that of the skin. Sweat is produced, but it cannot effectively evaporate into the air to help cool the

Acclimation to Environments

Acclimation to heat and altitude is important for outdoor training. Changes take place when the body is exposed to different environments over an extended period. With ongoing exposure, the body makes physiological adjustments that provide greater heat and altitude tolerance. In the case of heat acclimation, sweat threshold decreases, while sweat rate and production increase and expand the sweat distribution across a broader surface, allowing for greater evaporation [53]. Correspondingly, plasma volumes increase to account for the improvements in sweat efficiency, and the sodium concentration in sweat is reduced. The cardiovascular system also improves circulation and cutaneous blood flow to distribute more heat to the skin. These adaptations allow the body to more efficiently remove heat and enhance performance in hot environments. Generally, it takes 7-12 exposures for this acclimation process to take effect. The altitude acclimation process can take longer, requiring days to weeks depending on the height of exposure (>5000m). Changes occur in response to signaling from the carotid body, the major chemoreceptor responsible for detecting decreases in O_2 tension in arterial blood. The immediate response to acute hypoxia is mediated through the peripheral chemoreceptors, which increase ventilation. Chronic exposure to hypoxia causes greater release of the hormone erythropoietin (EPO) from the kidney, stimulating the production of red blood cells by the bone marrow. This increases the blood's oxygen carrying capacity to improve delivery. Oxygen extraction adaptations occur via increasing the number and size of the mitochondria, as well as facilitating changes in enzyme expression.

> **DEFINITIONS**
>
> **Positive feedback loop –**
>
> *A cyclic process in which the body's response to a stimulus results in a further amplification of the stimulus.*
>
> **Hypoxia –**
>
> *Deficiency in the amount of oxygen reaching the tissues.*

body. This presents a **positive-feedback loop** which forces the body to increase sweat rate to cool down the ever-increasing core temperature, ultimately contributing to even more water loss. As a result, exercise in high heat and humidity can be dangerous, as it increases risk of heat illness and thermoregulatory shut-down.

Physiological adjustments to training in the heat include:
- An earlier onset of sweating
- Increase in sweat production
- Distribution of sweat expands across a broader surface
- Increase in plasma volumes
- Reduction of sodium concentration in sweat
- Improvements in cutaneous blood flow, distributing more heat to the skin
- Improved overall thermoregulatory function

Altitude

Altitude level also affects exercise and training performance. At higher altitudes, the oxygen concentration of air is lower, leading to a reduction in available oxygen that can be extracted during respiration. When physical activity is performed at higher altitude, stress becomes apparent, as an individual's respiratory and heart rates must increase to deliver the same amount of oxygen to peripheral tissues. Due to the progressive decline in the partial pressure of oxygen as elevations rise, the higher a person climbs, the more difficult it becomes to perform all activities, including breathing. At extreme heights, such as Mt. Everest in Nepal, climbers have died from **hypoxia** as their blood oxygen concentrations drop into lethal ranges.

The disadvantage of altitude becomes an advantage when the body has acclimated to the environment [4, 23]. Slow progressions in activity at higher altitudes over several weeks cause physiological adjustments in hemoglobin and red blood cell concentrations via increase in EPO, and these become advantageous upon return to sea level. Many athletes live and train in Colorado to acclimate to the high altitudes. When they return to lower terrestrial levels to compete, these athletes can better remove carbon dioxide, possess larger hemoglobin mass, higher red blood cell concentrations which allow for higher arterial oxygen levels (increase oxygen carrying capacity), and finally, also increase muscle capillary and mitochondrial density (increased extraction and utilization) [27, 46]. All of these factors improve aerobic performance.

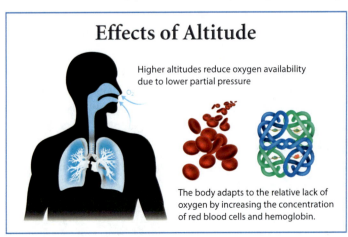

Effects of Altitude

Higher altitudes reduce oxygen availability due to lower partial pressure

The body adapts to the relative lack of oxygen by increasing the concentration of red blood cells and hemoglobin.

Biological Sex Factors

Physiological sex differences account for about a 15% disparity between VO_2max measures in adult men and women. The physiological differences found between genders account for the discrepancy between maximal attainable values [30, 55]. Females have:

- Smaller hearts
- Lower stroke volumes
- Lower hemoglobin concentrations
- Less muscle mass relative to size
- Higher body fat values (on average) compared to men [40]

During submaximal work at the same absolute VO_2, females experience higher heart rates and higher cardiac output to compensate for the gender-related differences [67]. Notably however, females do experience the same relative improvements to aerobic training as do men [18].

Recovery

Recovery needs to be a consideration any time the body performs work at elevated intensities because of the damaged tissue and changes in the cellular environment associated with increased metabolic activity. For healthy, active individuals, exercise performed at low steady-state intensities (50-60% HRR) does not significantly disrupt the muscle-metabolic state. Hydrogen-ion accumulation is attenuated via a slower rate of ATP hydrolysis, and a greater reliance is placed on lipid metabolism. Therefore, the re-synthesis of high-energy phosphate (ATP), oxygen replenishment, and other recovery mechanisms occur rather quickly with rest. When greater concentrations of lactate accumulate due to high glycogen volumes and high-energy phosphate utilization during high-intensity work, the recovery process benefits from a longer active cool down. Active recovery increases blood flow to the working myocytes, increasing the rate of lactate transfer to neighboring oxidative muscle cells and raising mobilization of blood lactate to the liver, thereby increasing the rate of glycogen re-synthesis.

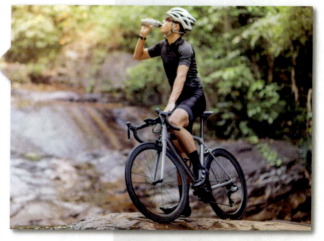

Muscle fatigue entails another factor in recovery. Repeated bouts of exercise utilizing the same muscle groups can cause repetitive microtrauma in tissue not acclimated to the frequency or intensity of training, which increases requirements of rest for recovery. New exercisers can benefit from the one-day-on, one-day-off method, as progressions are steadily applied over an early training cycle. Individuals who train for aerobic performance often use six or seven consecutive days of training, which creates significant stress on soft and bony tissue. To compensate for the stress, variations in distance and speed aid in recovery from one bout to the next. A full day of rest every 7-9 days is a generally accepted practice for trained individuals focusing on endurance performance. Using cross-training techniques can also aid in recovery if multiple days occur without rest. Non-weight-bearing activities, such as swimming and biking, can replace running, as the eccentric component of these activities, which is a major contributor to recovery requirements, is less intense than that experienced with running.

Detraining

The absolute cessation of aerobic activity has deleterious effects on aerobic endurance adaptations in a relatively short period of time.

Trained individuals experience a decline in aerobic performance within the first few weeks of detraining; this is primarily due to:

- A reduction in blood plasma
- An increased reliance on carbohydrates for fuel due to the consequent drop in lipid metabolism enzymes
- A decrease in insulin sensitivity and GLUT4 content
- The reduction of stroke volume and left ventricle mass back to pre-trained levels [16, 42, 47, 48, 60, 64]

If training ceases for three or more weeks, oxygen extraction drops due to mitochondria loss in the muscle cells [5]. When training volumes decrease, similar reductions occur but at a slower rate. To prevent periods of reduced volume from affecting VO_2max, intensities must be elevated to provide an overload stimulus to the system. Reductions in training volume from 6 days to 3 days can be relatively negated by increasing the intensity to maximal tolerable levels. For example, if a training volume of 4 days per week at 70% HRR for 30 minutes is reduced to two days per week, the intensity should increase to 80-85% HRR. This can be accomplished using interval training and lactate threshold steady-states. Even if the intensities cannot be maintained for long periods of time, the body must experience this level of stress to mitigate any negative changes to its current condition.

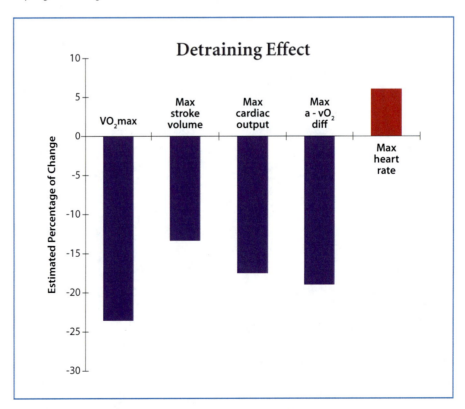

Preventing Common Overuse Injuries

As mentioned earlier, risk of injury is inherent to any increase in physical activity. Due to the repetitive nature of aerobic training, overuse injuries are not uncommon. These injuries often stem from a variety of factors: starting off too aggressively, abruptly increasing progressions, muscle imbalances and lack of range of motion, incorrect or new footwear, and uneven running surfaces. Common injuries associated with aerobic training include chondromalacia, plantar fasciitis, IT Band syndrome, acute low back pain, and shin splints.

Chondromalacia

Chondromalacia is a common injury associated with repeated impact. The condition occurs from damage to the articular hyaline cartilage of the patella on the surface of bone. It can be caused by trauma, overuse, poor joint alignment, or muscle imbalances. It often occurs at the knee cap and is referred to as chondromalacia patella (CMP), from patellar misalignment causing rubbing against the lower end of the thigh, damaging the cartilage underneath the knee cap. The level of damage varies from slight surface abnormalities in the cartilage surface to complete wear of the tissue, exposing the bone. Chondromalacia can also occur from blunt trauma, which tears off either a small piece of articular cartilage or a large fragment containing a piece of bone. The latter often requires invasive surgery to fix.

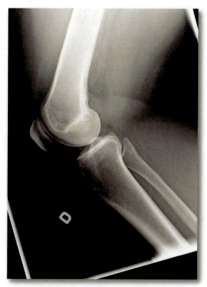

No specific, universally accepted treatment for chondromalacia exists. However, clients or patients presenting with chondromalacia can see improvement by focusing on knee stability, strengthening of the vastus medialis via closed-chain exercises, and other exercises aimed at improving stabilizing and connecting structures at and around the ankle and knee joints [28]. Non-impact aerobic exercises can be used for aerobic conditioning if the knee is not bent more than 90°. Therapeutic modalities include rest, non-steroidal anti-inflammatory medication, and ice therapy. If these treatments fail to improve the condition, arthroscopic surgery may be used to smooth the surface of the articular cartilage and remove cartilage fragments that cause irritation.

Plantar Fasciitis

Plantar fasciitis is the most common cause of heel/foot pain from aerobic activity. A flat, ligamentous band, the plantar fascia, connects the calcaneous (heel bone) to the distal phalanges (toes). This fascia supports the foot arch. When the tissue becomes strained, it becomes swollen and irritated, causing pain in the heel or bottom of the foot when weight is placed upon it. The exact cause of the tissue damage is not known, but it is likely attributed to repeated small tears in the plantar fascia during normal stride when the plantar fascia stretches upon foot strike.

Common variables that contribute to overuse injuries include:

- Initiating a training program too aggressively
- Previous injury
- Poor technique
- Lack of flexibility
- Poor joint alignment
- Muscle imbalances
- An abrupt increase in foot impact repetitions during exercise
- Improper footwear (arch support)
- Uneven gait caused by running on an uneven surface
- Inadequate warm-up protocol

Plantar fasciitis can be caused by various factors such as:

- Tight calves
- Achilles tendinosis
- An abrupt increase in training volume
- Improper arch support
- Prolonged walking or running
- Obesity

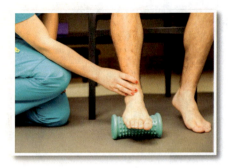

Remedies for plantar fasciitis include stretching the fascia, stretching the calves, myofascial release using a golf ball or similar object, anti-inflammatory medication, massage, foot splints, orthotics or arch supports, and rest [41].

Iliotibial Band Syndrome

Iliotibial band syndrome (ITBS) is common among runners and is responsible for more than 10% of all running-related overuse injuries. The injury occurs in the ligament that runs along the lateral aspect of the thigh, connecting the top of the hip to the lateral femoral epicondyle, presenting as lateral knee pain.

The tissue can become inflamed by:

- IT band, quadratus lumborum, or gluteus medius tightness
- Uneven gait caused by running on uneven surfaces
- High total weekly mileage among runners
- Muscular weaknesses of the quad, hamstrings, or gluteal muscles
- Inadequate warm-up protocols
- Increasing training distances too quickly [3, 15]

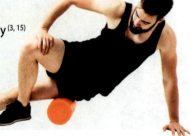

The condition can usually be improved in a matter of weeks by rest, stretching the IT band, myofascial release therapy, and ice and heat therapies. Additionally, it is important to avoid the situations that caused the problem in the first place. It is recommended that therapies be employed for up to six weeks, even if the pain subsides.

Low Back Pain

Aerobic exercise may cause low back pain (LBP) in some participants. Causes range from muscular imbalance, lack of flexibility, lack of mobility, poor movement biomechanics, and poor movement postures, to general deconditioning and android obesity or any combination of the aforementioned factors. Individuals new or returning to exercise are often predisposed to acute pain responses when attempting prolonged activities that have not previously been experienced or have not been experienced for a period of time. The muscles in the back are often ill-prepared for the stress from the postural positions maintained during continuous exercise. Gait discrepancies during walking and running may also contribute to the problem.

In most cases, acute low back pain is treated using traditional therapies for LBP from other causes. Stretching the back and tight hip muscles, strengthening the abdominals and related structures, and heat therapies can all improve the condition. If exercise using erect posture is the probable cause, switching to biking or swimming may alleviate the symptoms.

Shin Splints

Shin splints, or medial tibial stress syndrome, is a common condition that includes pain and tenderness over the middle or lower part of the shin bone. The condition is usually caused by overuse, leading to inflammation of the anterior tibialis muscle and the lateral-anterior muscle compartment. Shin splints can be caused by a variety of different factors, including:

- Sudden increases in training volume
- Running on uneven surfaces
- Lower extremity biomechanical abnormalities
- Improper foot wear
- General overtraining

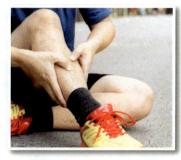

> **DEFINITIONS**
>
> **Shin splints –**
>
> *A common term for medial tibial stress syndrome, a condition characterized by pain along the inner edge of the tibia; caused by an inflammatory response to improper running mechanics or sudden increases in training volume.*

The exact location of the pain may also vary between the medial or lateral aspect of the shin. Medial shin splints are usually caused by excessive pronation or flat feet and are common with activities that cause repetitive pounding. Shin splints are often treated using rest, massage, ice therapy, and stretching and strengthening techniques. Stretching and strengthening the muscles of the lower leg help reduce incidence from muscle imbalance and tightness. Ice therapy and longer warm-ups have shown to be effective as well. Footwear and running surfaces should also be evaluated as possible causes. If the injury persists, it is cause for medical referral to assess if a stress fracture has occurred.

REFERENCES:

1. Astorino TA and Schubert MM. Changes in fat oxidation in response to various regimes of high intensity interval training (HIIT). *European journal of applied physiology* 118: 51-63, 2018.

2. Bailey DP. Sedentary Behavior in Human Health and Disease. *Frontiers in physiology* 8: 901, 2017.

3. Beals C and Flanigan D. A review of treatments for iliotibial band syndrome in the athletic population. *Journal of Sports Medicine* 2013, 2013.

4. Bergeron MF, Bahr R, Bärtsch P, Bourdon L, Calbet JAL, Carlsen KH, Castagna O, González-Alonso J, Lundby C, and Maughan R. International Olympic Committee consensus statement on thermoregulatory and altitude challenges for high-level athletes. *Br J Sports Med* 46: 770-779, 2012.

5. Bishop DJ, Granata C, and Eynon N. Can we optimise the exercise training prescription to maximise improvements in mitochondria function and content? *Biochimica et Biophysica Acta (BBA)- General Subjects* 1840: 1266-1275, 2014.

6. Bortz IV WM and Bortz WM. How fast do we age? Exercise performance over time as a biomarker. *The Journals of Gerontology Series A: Biological Sciences and Medical Sciences* 51: M223-M225, 1996.

7. Bouchard C, Malina RM, and P'Russe L. *Genetics of fitness and physical performance:* Human Kinetics, 1997.

8. Bouchard C, Sarzynski MA, Rice TK, Kraus WE, Church TS, Sung YJ, Rao D, and Rankinen T. Genomic predictors of the maximal O_2 uptake response to standardized exercise training programs. *Journal of applied physiology* 110: 1160-1170, 2010.

9. Braun L. Exercise physiology and cardiovascular fitness. *The Nursing clinics of North America* 26: 135-147, 1991.

10. Brooks AG, Withers RT, Gore CJ, Vogler AJ, Plummer J, and Cormack J. Measurement and prediction of METs during household activities in 35-to 45-year-old females. *European journal of applied physiology* 91: 638-648, 2004.

11. Brychta R and Chen K. Cold-induced thermogenesis in humans. *European journal of clinical nutrition* 71: 345, 2017.

12. Buckley J, Sim J, Eston R, Hession R, and Fox R. Reliability and validity of measures taken during the Chester step test to predict aerobic power and to prescribe aerobic exercise. *British Journal of Sports Medicine* 38: 197-205, 2004.

13. Byrne NM and Hills AP. Relationships between HR and VO_2 in the obese. *Medicine & Science in Sports & Exercise* 34: 1419-1427, 2002.

14. Chen MJ, Fan X, and Moe ST. Criterion-related validity of the Borg ratings of perceived exertion scale in healthy individuals: a meta-analysis. *Journal of sports sciences* 20: 873-899, 2002.

15. Chicorelli AM. Iliotibial Band Syndrome. In: *Orthopedic Surgery Clerkship:* Springer, 2017, p. 347-348.

16. Coyle EF, Hemmert M, and Coggan AR. Effects of detraining on cardiovascular responses to exercise: role of blood volume. *Journal of Applied Physiology* 60: 95-99, 1986.

17. da Cunha FA, Farinatti PdTV, and Midgley AW. Methodological and practical application issues in exercise prescription using the heart rate reserve and oxygen uptake reserve methods. *Journal of Science and Medicine in Sport* 14: 46-57, 2011.

18. Deschenes MR, Hillard MN, Wilson JA, Dubina MI, and Eason MK. Effects of gender on physiological responses during submaximal exercise and recovery. *Med Sci Sports Exerc* 38: 1304-1310, 2006.

19. Duncan GE, Sydeman SJ, Perri MG, Limacher MC, and Martin AD. Can sedentary adults accurately recall the intensity of their physical activity? *Preventive Medicine* 33: 18-26, 2001.

20. Faria EW, Parker DL, and Faria IE. The science of cycling. *Sports medicine* 35: 285-312, 2005.

21. Faude O, Kindermann W, and Meyer T. Lactate threshold concepts. *Sports medicine* 39: 469-490, 2009.

22. Fitzgerald MD, Tanaka H, Tran ZV, and Seals DR. Age-related declines in maximal aerobic capacity in regularly exercising vs. sedentary women: a meta-analysis. *Journal of applied physiology* 83: 160-165, 1997.

23. Girard O, Amann M, Aughey R, Billaut F, Bishop DJ, Bourdon P, Buchheit M, Chapman R, D'hooghe M, and Garvican-Lewis LA. Position statement – altitude training for improving team-sport players' performance: current knowledge and unresolved issues. *Br J Sports Med* 47: i8-i16, 2013.

24. Glass SC and Stanton DR. Self-selected resistance training intensity in novice weightlifters. *Journal of Strength and Conditioning Research* 18: 324-327, 2004.

25. Goldberg L, Elliot DL, and Kuehl KS. Assessment of exercise intensity formulas by use of ventilatory threshold. *Chest* 94: 95-98, 1988.

26. Gordon NF, Scott CB, Wilkinson WJ, Duncan JJ, and Blair SN. Exercise and mild essential hypertension. *Sports medicine* 10: 390-404, 1990.

27. Gore CJ, Sharpe K, Garvican-Lewis LA, Saunders PU, Humberstone CE, Robertson EY, Wachsmuth NB, Clark SA, McLean BD, and Friedmann-Bette B. Altitude training and haemoglobin mass from the optimised carbon monoxide rebreathing method determined by a meta-analysis. *Br J Sports Med* 47: i31-i39, 2013.

28. Habusta SF and Bhimji SS. Chondromalacia Patella. 2017.

29. Hagberg JM, Goldberg AP, Lakatta L, O'connor FC, Becker LC, Lakatta EG, and Fleg JL. Expanded blood volumes contribute to the increased cardiovascular performance of endurance-trained older men. *Journal of Applied Physiology* 85: 484-489, 1998.

30. Harms CA. Does gender affect pulmonary function and exercise capacity? *Respiratory physiology & neurobiology* 151: 124-131, 2006.

31. Hetlelid KJ, Plews DJ, Herold E, Laursen PB, and Seiler S. Rethinking the role of fat oxidation: substrate utilisation during high-intensity interval training in well-trained and recreationally trained runners. *BMJ open sport & exercise medicine* 1: e000047, 2015.

32. Hollenberg M, Yang J, Haight TJ, and Tager IB. Longitudinal changes in aerobic capacity: implications for concepts of aging. *The Journals of Gerontology Series A: Biological Sciences and Medical Sciences* 61: 851-858, 2006.

33. Huang G, Wang R, Chen P, Huang SC, Donnelly JE, and Mehlferber JP. Dose–response relationship of cardiorespiratory fitness adaptation to controlled endurance training in sedentary older adults. *European journal of preventive cardiology* 23: 518-529, 2016.

34. Irving BA, Rutkowski J, Brock DW, Davis CK, Barrett EJ, Gaesser GA, and Weltman A. Comparison of Borg-and OMNI-RPE as markers of the blood lactate response to exercise. *Medicine and science in sports and exercise* 38: 1348-1352, 2006.

35. Jones BH and Knapik JJ. Physical training and exercise-related injuries. *Sports medicine* 27: 111-125, 1999.

36. Joyner MJ and Coyle EF. Endurance exercise performance: the physiology of champions. *The Journal of physiology* 586: 35-44, 2008.

37. Knechtle B, Müller G, and Knecht H. Optimal exercise intensities for fat metabolism in handbike cycling and cycling. *Spinal cord* 42: 564, 2004.

38. Kodama S, Saito K, Tanaka S, Maki M, Yachi Y, Asumi M, Sugawara A, Totsuka K, Shimano H, and Ohashi Y. Cardiorespiratory fitness as a quantitative predictor of all-cause mortality and cardiovascular events in healthy men and women: a meta-analysis. *Jama* 301: 2024-2035, 2009.

39. Leaf DA and Reuben DB. "Lifestyle" interventions for promoting physical activity: a kilocalorie expenditure-based home feasibility study. *The American journal of the medical sciences* 312: 68-75, 1996.

40. Lewis DA, Kamon E, and Hodgson JL. Physiological differences between genders implications for sports conditioning. *Sports medicine* 3: 357-369, 1986.

41. Lim AT, How CH, and Tan B. Management of plantar fasciitis in the outpatient setting. *Singapore medical journal* 57: 168, 2016.

42. Madsen K, Pedersen PK, Djurhuus MS, and Klitgaard NA. Effects of detraining on endurance capacity and metabolic changes during prolonged exhaustive exercise. *Journal of Applied Physiology* 75: 1444-1451, 1993.

43. Maughan R. The limits of human athletic performance. *Annals of transplantation* 10: 52-54, 2005.

44. Maunder E, Plews DJ, and Kilding AE. Contextualising maximal fat oxidation during exercise: Determinants and normative values. *Frontiers in physiology* 9, 2018.

45. Milanović Z, Sporiš G, and Weston M. Effectiveness of high-intensity interval training (HIT) and continuous endurance training for VO_2max improvements: a systematic review and meta-analysis of controlled trials. *Sports medicine* 45: 1469-1481, 2015.

46. Millet GP, Roels B, Schmitt L, Woorons X, and Richalet J. Combining hypoxic methods for peak performance. *Sports medicine* 40: 1-25, 2010.

47. Mujika I and Padilla S. Detraining: loss of training-induced physiological and performance adaptations. Part I. *Sports Medicine* 30: 79-87, 2000.

48. Mujika I and Padilla S. Detraining: loss of training-induced physiological and performance adaptations. Part II. *Sports Medicine* 30: 145-154, 2000.

49. Narita K, Sakamoto S, Mizushige K, Senda S, and Matsuo H. Development and evaluation of a new target heart rate formula for the adequate exercise training level in healthy subjects. *Journal of cardiology* 33: 265-272, 1999.

50. Organization WH. *Global recommendations on physical activity for health*: World Health Organization, 2010.

51. Pedlar CR, Brown MG, Shave RE, Otto JM, Drane A, Michaud-Finch J, Contursi M, Wasfy MM, Hutter A, and Picard MH. Cardiovascular response to prescribed detraining among recreational athletes. *Journal of Applied Physiology* 124: 813-820, 2017.

52. Persinger R, Foster C, Gibson M, Fater DC, and Porcari JP. Consistency of the talk test for exercise prescription. *Medicine & Science in Sports & Exercise* 36: 1632-1636, 2004.

53. Racinais S, Alonso J-M, Coutts AJ, Flouris AD, Girard O, González-Alonso J, Hausswirth C, Jay O, Lee JK, and Mitchell N. Consensus recommendations on training and competing in the heat. *Scandinavian journal of medicine & science in sports* 25: 6-19, 2015.

54. Randell RK, Rollo I, Roberts TJ, Dalrymple KJ, Jeukendrup AE, and Carter JM. Maximal fat oxidation rates in an athletic population. *Med Sci Sports Exerc* 49: 133-140, 2017.

55. Rivera-Brown AM and Frontera WR. Principles of exercise physiology: responses to acute exercise and long-term adaptations to training. *Pm&r* 4: 797-804, 2012.

56. Santos R, Mota J, Okely AD, Pratt M, Moreira C, Coelho-e-Silva MJ, Vale S, and Sardinha LB. The independent associations of sedentary behaviour and physical activity on cardiorespiratory fitness. *Br J Sports Med*: bjsports-2012-091610, 2013.

57. Smith L, Ekelund U, and Hamer M. The potential yield of non-exercise physical activity energy expenditure in public health. *Sports medicine* 45: 449-452, 2015.

58. Swain DP and Franklin BA. VO_2 reserve and the minimal intensity for improving cardiorespiratory fitness. *Medicine & Science in Sports & Exercise* 34: 152-157, 2002.

59. Swain DP and Leutholtz BC. Heart rate reserve is equivalent to% VO_2 reserve, not to% VO_2max. *Medicine and science in sports and exercise* 29: 410-414, 1997.

60. Swoboda PP, Garg P, Foley JR, Fent GJ, Chew PG, Brown LA, Saunderson CE, Dall'Armellina E, Greenwood JP, and Plein S. 12 Cardiac effects of complete enforced detraining assessed by cardiovascular magnetic resonance: BMJ Publishing Group Ltd and British Cardiovascular Society, 2018.

61. Sykes K, Choo LL, and Cotterrell M. Accumulating aerobic exercise for effective weight control. *The journal of the Royal Society for the Promotion of Health* 124: 24-28, 2004.

62. Vieira MdCS, Boing L, Leitão AE, Vieira G, and de Azevedo Guimarães AC. EFFECT OF PHYSICAL EXERCISE on the CARDIORESPIRATORY FITNESS OF MEN-A SYSTEMATIC REVIEW AND META-ANALYSIS. *Maturitas*, 2018.

63. Walther M, Reuter I, Leonhard T, and Engelhardt M. Injuries and response to overload stress in running as a sport. *Der Orthopade* 34: 399-404, 2005.

64. Waring CD, Henning BJ, Smith AJ, Nadal-Ginard B, Torella D, and Ellison GM. Cardiac adaptations from 4 weeks of intensity-controlled vigorous exercise are lost after a similar period of detraining. *Physiological reports* 3: e12302, 2015.

65. Wenger HA and Bell GJ. The interactions of intensity, frequency and duration of exercise training in altering cardiorespiratory fitness. *Sports medicine* 3: 346-356, 1986.

66. Weston KS, Wisløff U, and Coombes JS. High-intensity interval training in patients with lifestyle-induced cardiometabolic disease: a systematic review and meta-analysis. *Br J Sports Med:* bjsports-2013-092576, 2013.

67. Wiebe CG, Gledhill N, Warburton D, Jamnik VK, and Ferguson S. Exercise cardiac function in endurance-trained males versus females. *Clinical journal of sport medicine: official journal of the Canadian Academy of Sport Medicine* 8: 272-279, 1998.

68. Williams AG, Wackerhage H, and Day SH. Genetic testing for sports performance, responses to training and injury risk: practical and ethical considerations. In: *Genetics and Sports:* Karger Publishers, 2016, p. 105-119.

69. Yoshioka M, Doucet E, St-Pierre S, Almeras N, Richard D, Labrie A, Despres J, Bouchard C, and Tremblay A. Impact of high-intensity exercise on energy expenditure, lipid oxidation and body fatness. *International Journal of obesity* 25: 332, 2001.

70. Zhang T, Zhang C-F, Jin F, and Wang L. Association between genetic factor and physical performance. *Yi chuan= Hereditas* 26: 219-226, 2004.

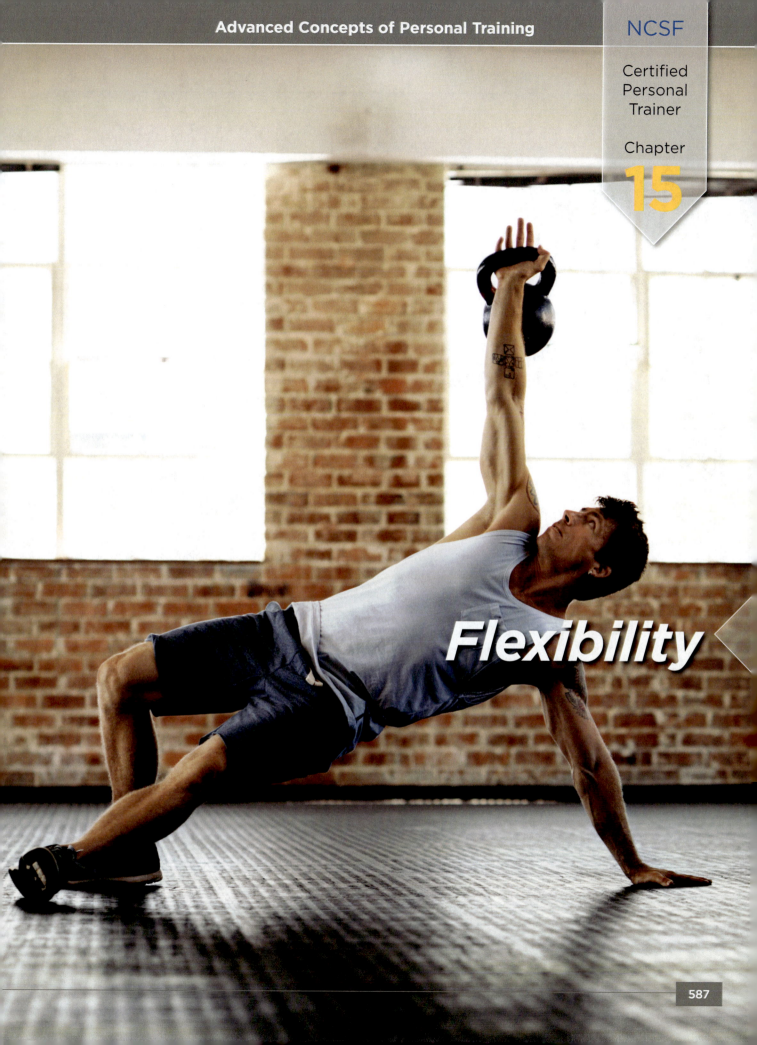

Introduction to Flexibility

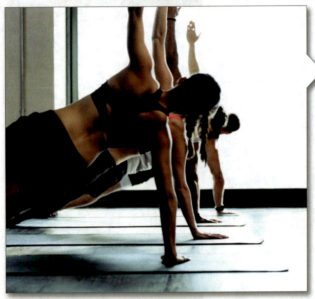

Flexibility incorporates numerous definitions that depend upon different points of reference. Webster's Dictionary defines the term as, "to bend, or having the ability to be bent." In fitness, flexibility is most often defined as the ability of a joint to move through a full **range of motion** (**ROM**). However, even this discipline-specific description is short sighted, as joint ROM requires a reference to a plane of motion and limb angle (flexed vs extended). For the purposes of this book, **flexibility** constitutes the ROM attained at a single joint in one direction. The reference point is important because a joint may have high levels of flexibility in one direction but low levels in another. **Mobility** is another term often (erroneously) interchanged with flexibility. Mobility is the attainable ROM accomplished across fascial lines, as multiple joints are involved and movements may also be multi-planar. The ability to raise a single arm overhead in the frontal plane assesses flexibility of the latissimus dorsi, whereas an overhead squat assesses mobility of several muscles across several joints, including the latissimus dorsi. The measurement may be quantified by angular units or degrees of movement. If the measurement is linear, it is often expressed as a distance covered in centimeters or inches. Regardless of how movement range is quantified, it still reflects the ability of a joint or group of joints to move in relation to the respective axes.

When determining the body's movement capabilities, flexibility is assessed before mobility, as individual joint information identifies potentials for multiple-joint limitations and interactions. Likewise, joint movement may differ when comparing bilateral joints (i.e., the right and left shoulder). Bilateral discrepancies are common, as attainable movements on one side may not be equaled in range at the opposite joint. This suggests that measurement of one or more joint movements does not validly predict total body flexibility or possibly even bilateral flexibility.

> **DEFINITIONS**
>
> **Range of motion –**
>
> The full movement potential of a joint measured by linear or angular distance between two limits.
>
> **Flexibility –**
>
> The range of motion in a joint achieved in a single direction.
>
> **Mobility –**
>
> The range of motion achieved during multi-joint actions in which several groups of connective tissue structures interplay to effect movement.

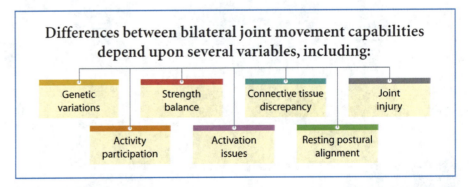

Differences between bilateral joint movement capabilities depend upon several variables, including: Genetic variations, Strength balance, Connective tissue discrepancy, Joint injury, Activity participation, Activation issues, Resting postural alignment.

When mobility is assessed, bilateral disparities often contribute to compensation. Asymmetrical body positions increase risk for injury, as they often compromise joint biomechanics during loading by placing undue stress on connective tissues, enabling and perpetuating abnormal recruitment patterns, and creating faulty stability. Measuring and correcting flexibility issues improves mobility, as the skeleton becomes better aligned. Mobility exercises can enhance bilateral symmetry, but when a significant bilateral ROM deficit exists on one side, it should be addressed independently before emphasis is placed on cooperative movement.

Flexibility and mobility are inherent components to movement capabilities, and therefore play major roles in human function and the ability to attain health and fitness through physical activity, exercise, and sport. Interestingly, though flexibility is a primary determinant in the body's ability to move, it receives very little attention in many exercise programs. Flexibility's importance is highlighted by the fact that it is one of the five categories of health-related components of fitness, yet receives limited appreciation for what it offers. Most personal training clients expect visual changes in their physiques as a quantifiable measure of training effectiveness. Common goals of many programs involve losing body fat and improving muscle "tone." Anecdotally speaking, a strong psychosocial association seems to exist between exercise and vanity. Most individuals who exercise cite a desire to look better for their efforts and take pleasure in the attention they receive when others notice the positive changes that have taken place. Vanity-derived outcomes rank 3rd among top reasons for exercise participation in the United States. Flexibility levels and training adaptations are difficult to quantify upon visual observation and do little to improve a person's appearance: an improvement in flexibility does not equal six-pack abs. Due to this fact, most exercise professionals, potential clients, and fitness enthusiasts pay much more attention to muscular enhancements and body fat reduction. When markers of improvement are vanity-related, flexibility and mobility will likely take a back seat in the exercise prescription. Exercise professionals must avoid this common mistake when programming to appropriately serve their clients' best interests. Understanding flexibility's benefits can help clarify the importance of including routine flexibility and mobility training in the exercise prescription.

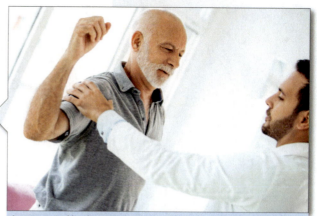

Asymmetrical body positions created by bilateral ROM disparities (shoulder, hip) increase the risk for injury by placing undue stress on connective tissues and promoting faulty movement patterns.

◆ The Importance of ROM

The attainable ROM affects a joint's performance and functionality. Therefore, maintaining an optimal level of flexibility and strength across a joint allows for efficient movement, especially at higher movement velocities, and improves joint health. Likewise, proper **functional range** alleviates the consequences associated with poor ROM, including discomfort, pain, movement limitations, abnormal activation patterns, and injury. The maintenance of flexibility over the span of a lifetime associates with a decrease in functional decline and greater independence [20, 60]. One of the most detrimental outcomes of ROM decline is limitation in movement capabilities, which correlates with decreased activity, quality of life, and premature death. As stated earlier, the series of events that leads to reduced flexibility becomes problematic, as rigidity reduces physical activity participation. This creates a positive feedback loop, as reduced physical activity further limits ROM, reducing physical activity even more. Recall, a positive feedback loop can be a vicious cycle in which the response (limited ROM) caused by the initial stimulus (reduced physical activity) perpetuates the progressive cycle as physical activity decreases even more, further limiting ROM until independence is no longer feasible. As a result, the progressive downward spiral leads to chronic pain, dysfunction, and reduced quality of life [15, 60].

DEFINITIONS

Functional range –

Minimum range of motion necessary to comfortably and effectively perform activities of daily living.

Benefits of Flexibility

- Increased movement range
- Reduction in the rate of functional decline
- Postural symmetry
- Stress reduction
- Reduced tension
- Muscle relaxation
- Reduced incidence of muscle cramps
- Reduced risk of injury
- Relief of muscle pain
- Improved quality of life

A lack of flexibility is implicated in a variety of musculoskeletal injuries. One key factor is postural symmetry. Tight muscles pull on bony structures, distorting their normal alignments. When the kinetic chain is compromised, soft tissues become stressed due to force variations that do not exist when the joint aligns properly. This presents two problems that promote joint injury. The first is that the alignment change causes compensational movement deviation, leading to undue stress on connecting structures [62]. This is why a runner with a hip joint injury can develop a knee injury if he or she continues to train without allowing the hip to properly heal. The second problem is that the body is subjected to ongoing forces that can lead to exhaustive strain. Some common examples of alignment alterations are an anterior shoulder shift, called upper-cross syndrome, and pelvic instability due to compromised pelvic tilting. These musculoskeletal misalignments can cause acute joint discomfort and may lead to chronic pain. Low-back pain, in particular, is often associated with lack of flexibility in the muscles that act on the hip and lumbar spine [2, 21, 36, 40]. Additionally, tight and shortened musculature is subject to injury when the joint forcibly moves through a functionally unattainable movement range at high velocities or under high levels of force. Lack of flexibility related to musculoskeletal imbalances often lies at the root of muscle strains and connective tissue sprains in sports [18, 35].

Improved ROM and participation in flexibility routines have been shown to positively affect stress. Reduced muscular and fascial tension through improved tissue relaxation associate with self-reported stress reduction [6, 12, 38]. Likewise, the activities employed to address ROM and mobility, such as yoga, have shown to affect acute stress responses [52, 65]. The proposed mechanisms include the alleviation of tension, psychomotor distraction, and an overall state of relaxation. This information further supports the use of flexibility for improved health and well-being.

| Activites that emphasize flexibility reduce musculoskeletal stress via: | Alleviation of tension | Reduction of psychomotor distraction | Improved state of overall relaxation |

Hypermobility

When a person can attain an abnormal range of motion at a joint they are often said to be "double jointed" or to have extreme flexibility. In fact, neither concept is accurate. Flexibility refers to tissue extensibility or physiologically controlled range of motion at a joint. Hypermobile joints do not indicate tissue flexibility as much as a lack of stability, referred to as laxity. Therefore, the ability of an articulation to separate upon voluntary control is actually caused by excessive joint laxity. **Hypermobility** is undesirable as it indicates the joint system's integrity is compromised. Individuals with hypermobility at a joint should attempt to strengthen the attached musculature to increase joint stability, thus reducing the risk of possible injury.

DEFINITIONS

Hypermobility –

Movement capacity of a joint beyond the normal range of motion; often compromises joint stability.

Properties of Soft Tissue

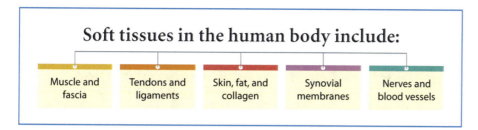

Elasticity

The soft tissues listed in the figure all possess some stretch quality or deformation potential. The property that allows stretched tissue to return to its original, or pre-stretched, form is referred to as the tissue's elasticity. A rubber band that is stretched can be significantly deformed from its starting position, but when the forces that pull the band into a stretched position are removed, the rubber band returns to its initial static position and shape. The ability to return to its original form is based on the rubber band's elastic properties. The pliable properties of soft tissue work similarly and allow the tissue to be deformed beyond its resting state for short periods of time. The length attained is a factor of the relationship between the internal force generated by the tissue, called resistive force, and the external force causing it to lengthen. When low resistive force exists within the tissue and the external lengthening force rises above the tissue's internal force threshold, the tissue will lengthen according to the external lengthening force's magnitude.

Plasticity

Plasticity is the property of a tissue to become permanently deformed, or to attain a new length after being stretched. Appropriate levels of tissue-stretching force applied routinely can cause the connective tissue to assume a chronic plastic state or new permanent length. This explains how tendons adapt to flexibility programs. Due to the limited elastic properties of tendons, they improve in range by permanently lengthening. If the external forces far exceed the resistive forces, the tissue may be lengthened beyond its elastic limit. When this occurs, the tissue may be damaged and permanently deformed. An example of a negative consequence of plasticity is the permanent lengthening of spinal ligaments from the long-term application of stress due to poor seating posture [10, 11]. When this occurs, the system's integrity is compromised, and injury becomes likely.

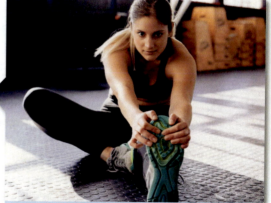

Plasticity refers to the ability of tissue to become permanently deformed or to attain a new length after being stretched. Based on this property, routine flexibility training can cause connective tissues to assume a new permanent length.

Viscosity

Another property affecting soft tissue is variable fluid resistance, referred to as viscosity. This property is not as constant as elasticity or plasticity but varies depending on acute tissue factors. When something is viscous, it adds to the tissue's resistance to change. When viscosity decreases, so does the resistive force present in the tissue. This concept justifies warming up before stretching. Warming a tissue up before stretching will reduce the tissue's viscosity, consequently increasing its elastic response. Changes in viscosity are temporary and do not directly contribute to chronic or plastic tissue adaptations to flexibility training [37, 59, 66]. Decreased viscosity though, can indirectly reduce resistance, allowing for greater ROM during the flexibility program's performance, potentially lessening injury risk. Viscoelasticity describes the tissue's behavior related to external load and internal conditions and properties.

Factors Affecting Joint Range of Motion

Muscle Factors

Although the nervous system mediates tension within the muscle, myogenic mechanisms (mechanisms arising from within the muscle itself) also contribute to both an increase and decrease in ROM. The variations in ROM are, in part, related to the myofibrils within the muscle fibers. The number of sarcomeres and their ability to lengthen contributes to a muscle's ROM. The sarcomeres' lengthening ability seems to depend on the elastic properties of the titin filaments [32, 33, 57]. Titin filaments are the non-contractile protein filaments which make up the sarcomere ends [33]. On the other hand, the contractile filaments, actin and myosin, do not change in length because they require extreme rigidity to produce force. These characteristics allow the contractile proteins to maintain their force generating qualities while still allowing the myofibril to reach greater lengths. If actin and myosin were to possess elastic properties, they would stretch under the application of stress, losing their length-tension relationship, and consequently, their force generating capabilities.

The sarcomeres also play a role in a tissue's passive length. When muscle tissue is immobilized in a lengthened position using a cast, sarcomeres are added along the myofibril at the end of the muscle toward the tendon [12, 53]. The opposite effect occurs when a muscle is arrested in a shortened position. The sarcomere numbers and length reduce to comply with the truncated position. Based on these findings, it can be surmised that muscle fiber elasticity is a factor of the number of sarcomeres along a myofibril and their respective ability to lengthen. For the muscle to reach maximal length, the tissue must be in a relaxed state. Muscle relaxation is a passive act that occurs when the muscle no longer receives neural signals for tension. Most researchers agree that muscle relaxation is contingent upon the removal of calcium from troponin, causing disassociation of the contractile proteins [13]. Muscles elongate passively as a result of external forces because the fibers cannot lengthen themselves when ATP is not hydrolyzed on the myosin head. These forces may be due to a contraction of an antagonist muscle group, gravity, momentum force, or the force provided by a partner when stretching. A muscle's contractile component can be elongated by up to 65% above the resting sarcomere length, which allows for a wide ROM [50]. The muscle's ability to relax when being stretched is a factor of its **extensibility** characteristics.

The amount of force necessary to lengthen a relaxed muscle is called passive tension. The greatest contributor to the lengthening resistance of a relaxed muscle is related to titin, a major component of cytoskeleton and the connective fascia within the tissue, including the epimysium,

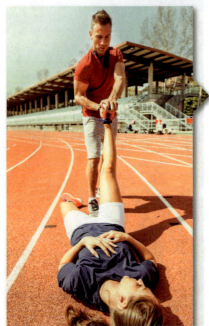

At the physical level, data collected from motion analysis provides a better understanding of a player's response to competition, training, and recovery.

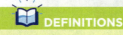

DEFINITIONS

Extensibility –

The capability of a muscle to be stretched based on the limitations of the tissue's structure.

perimysium, and endomysium [12, 34]. High-density foam rolling and acupressure techniques are often used to reduce myofascial restriction before stretching. The term myofascial deformation describes limits to stretch potential associated with a deformed pennate state which adds tension. These deformed areas are often sensitive and trigger pain upon pressure, called "trigger points." Performing self-myofascial release activities before training can help re-pennate the tissue and remove the added restriction.

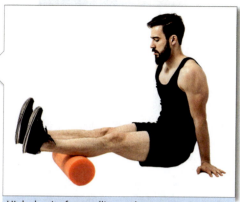

High-density foam rolling and acupressure techniques are often used to reduce myofascial restriction before stretching.

Static stretching techniques are used as part of a cool down because the tissue is warm, and the activities promote a parasympathetic response. Cool downs return the tissue to a relaxed state. When muscle tissue is stretched in a relaxed state, its resistive properties are reduced. The acute response to a flexibility routine is a reduction in passive tension. This explains why participating in a flexibility program enables a person to attain a greater ROM than he or she was capable of previously. This is referred to as an elastic response. When the flexibility training occurs on a routine basis, the muscles' elastic properties increase, and in turn, the passive tension decreases, leading to improved ROM by way of a plastic response.

Connective Tissue Factors

Collagen represents approximately 33% of the protein structural component in the body. It presents limitations due to its inherent properties: high tensile strength and inextensibility. Collagen is the primary constituent of joint capsules, tendons, and ligaments, as their functional roles require very limited extension. The more collagen in an area, the more resistant the tissue is to being elongated or deformed [23]. These properties contribute to the greatest limitation in joint ROM. In fact, the connective tissue that comprises a joint's capsule provides almost 50% of the resistance to the joint's movement [23, 44].

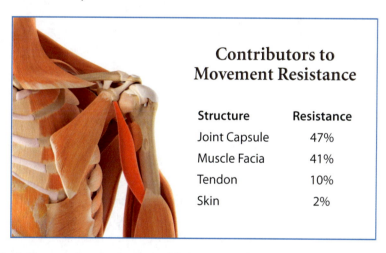

Contributors to Movement Resistance

Structure	Resistance
Joint Capsule	47%
Muscle Facia	41%
Tendon	10%
Skin	2%

Elastic fibers, on the other hand, provide for a greater degree of elongation. They are commonly associated with collagen fibers. When elastic fibers are found in greater quantity than collagen fibers, the specific tissue will have enhanced lengthening characteristics. The elastic properties allow extended tissues to return to their prior state following a stretch. Elastic tissue is present in different concentrations within the muscle fascia and plays a major role in determining the muscle's relative extensibility. Compared to tendons and ligaments, which are primarily composed of collagen, muscle connective tissue has higher quantities of elastic fibers. This elastic component allows the muscle to stretch. In addition, the elastic fibers in the tissue perform several important functions, including conserving tone during muscle relaxation, enhancing coordination during rhythmic motion of the body, accommodating excessive force, and returning tissues to their original form following deformation from force application.

Connective fascia makes up nearly one-third of the body's muscle mass. It serves several functions, including providing shape and a connective framework; it also provides fiber, blood vessel, and nerve alignment and even force transfer to the whole muscle. Under a passive stretch, the muscle fascia contributes the second greatest level of resistance to the movement.

QUICK INSIGHT

MYOFASCIAL RELEASE TECHNIQUE

When muscle tissue undergoes significant stress, the myofascial alignment can be altered due to multidirectional restriction[22]. These restrictions can cause the tissue to adopt a level of dysfunction and may manifest in pain. In some cases, the discomfort is localized. However, since fascia is continuous, tissue restrictions can affect other areas. In some cases, the pain is related to myofascial trigger points, which appear to be associated with the formation of pain circuits in the spinal cord in response to the disturbance of the nerve endings and abnormal contractile mechanisms at multiple dysfunctional sites[29].

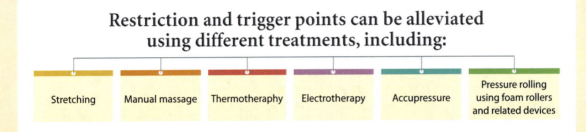

Restriction and trigger points can be alleviated using different treatments, including:

- Stretching
- Manual massage
- Thermotheraphy
- Electrotherapy
- Accupressure
- Pressure rolling using foam rollers and related devices

When myofascial restriction is significant, acupressure and myofascial release techniques, such as high pressure rolling of the affected area, can return the compromised neurophysiological state of the tissue to its functional pathways[8]. Foam rollers, rolling sticks, and related devices have gained popularity in addressing myofascial restriction, associated with physical activity and sport. The devices can provide self-massage, which has proved to be an effective means of soft tissue care. When the tissue alignment is not compromised by restriction and neural physiological mechanisms function properly, tissue performance will improve.

Neural Factors

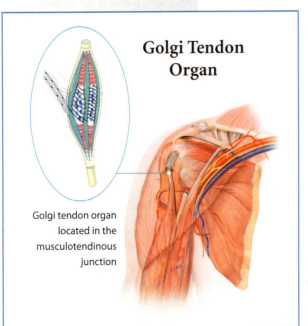

Golgi Tendon Organ

Golgi tendon organ located in the musculotendinous junction

Three primary proprioceptors are used for neural management of the soft tissue that relates to ROM: the muscle spindles, Golgi tendon organs (GTO), and the joint mechanoreceptors[42]. The muscle spindles lie parallel to the muscle fibers in the belly of the muscle. They serve as the primary stretch receptor, identifying the stretch length and velocity. When a stretch is applied in a slow, controlled manner, the muscle spindles remain dormant, allowing the tissue to extend. When the velocity of the stretch increases, the muscle spindles activate to prevent the tissue from being overstretched by adding resistive tension. For this reason, high-speed movements and **ballistic stretching** techniques do not allow the muscle tissue to relax due to counter-tension development, which attempts to reduce the potential attainable length to prevent injury[27, 43, 49]. Muscle spindles activate before the tissue is stretched beyond the point where damage may occur.

DEFINITIONS

Ballistic stretching –
Achievement of maximal range of motion using the momentum of a moving body or limb.

GTO's are located in the musculotendinous junction. Although recent clinical attention has identified several roles of these receptors, an important function for tissue protection is the **autogenic inhibition** response to excessive force [54]. The receptors identify rapid changes in muscle force and operate by inhibiting the muscle contraction to promote tissue relaxation. This occurs to prevent forces that would damage the tissue during active stretching [54]. Essentially, if the force magnitude gets too high, the receptors inhibit signaling to the contracted muscle in order to protect the joint and soft tissue from hyper-elongation.

Mechanoreceptors are found in synovial articulations in four varieties, which serve a number of functions to sense joint changes. Some of these functions include:

- Signaling direction, amplitude, and joint movement velocity
- Regulating changes in joint pressure
- Contributing to postural and kinesthetic sensation
- Facilitating the central nervous system (CNS) in regulating muscle tone
- Producing an inhibitory effect on pain
- Measuring quick changes in the joint movement
- Producing reflex inhibition of muscles acting on the joint
- Signaling pain reception within a joint

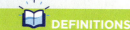

DEFINITIONS

Autogenic inhibition –

The reduction in excitability of a muscle upon the development of high tension; self-induced by the muscle due to negative feedback signaled by activation of its Golgi tendon organs.

Reciprocal inhibition –

Relaxation of musculature on one side of a joint to accommodate a contraction of opposing musculature.

These mechanisms contribute to the neural controls that protect a joint and help it to work efficiently. The combination of roles performed by the joint mechanoreceptors help facilitate improved ROM attainment when proper stretching methods are employed.

Another neural factor that influences tissue elongation is the relationship between agonist-antagonist pairs called reciprocal innervation. When a muscle or muscle group contracts, the antagonist muscle or muscle group's alpha motor neuron is automatically reciprocally inhibited, causing antagonistic relaxation. This **reciprocal inhibition** causes the hamstring muscles to relax during quadriceps contraction, and this reflex prevents the agonist muscle group from having to overcome antagonistic tension in addition to the resistance it accelerates against when attempting to go through a full ROM. Reciprocal innervation at the level of the nervous system (CNS and Alpha mN) allows for coordinated muscle action. It has implications for flexibility because the excitatory impulses lead to greater relaxation in the stretched muscle if the reciprocating muscle contracts. Reciprocal inhibition is often used to describe the accompanying contract-relax techniques of active isolation stretching, where paired opposites are flexed and stretched simultaneously (e.g., contract the quadriceps to increase the relaxation of the hamstrings during a straight-leg hip-flexion stretch).

Age

Like other body tissue, muscle experiences a functional decline with age due to changes in quality and quantity. The actual age at which this functional attenuation occurs varies by contributing factors, including genetics, health status, relative fitness level, and the quantity, frequency, and type of physical

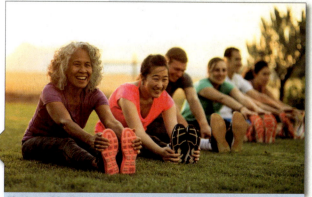

The loss of flexibility with age is attributed to a reduction in sarcomeres along the muscle's length, as these are replaced with lipids and collagen fibers in a process referred to as fibrosis.

activity performed [16, 67]. The latter may have the greatest impact, as physically inactive individuals seem to experience a more rapid decline, further worsened by disease and injury. Sarcopenia accelerates this process, as the size and number of muscle fibers are reduced. Reduced muscle mass negatively affects power, strength, endurance, speed, and flexibility.

The loss of flexibility with age is attributed to a reduction in sarcomeres along the muscle's length, as these are replaced with lipids and collagen fibers [17]. Through a process called fibrosis, the tissue loses its resiliency due to biochemical alterations in which connective-tissue stiffness increases via an addition in the number of cross linkages (collagen). The tissue also experiences a series of mineralization processes, including calcification, which further reduces elasticity. A healthy level of flexibility attained during youth is much easier to maintain over a lifespan, as compared to initiating a flexibility program as an adult, particularly in the later years. Early research suggested an optimal time to begin flexibility training. Termed the "critical period," significant improvements occur between the ages of 7 and 11 years of age with maximal values attained by 15 years of age [45]. This does not suggest that individuals above the age of 15 cannot benefit from flexibility training, but rather that adopting physical fitness-related behaviors early in life increases the likelihood that health-related fitness will extend into the later years, and functional decline will be delayed. Flexibility and mobility training should be a valued part of all physical fitness programming, regardless of the client's age.

Sex

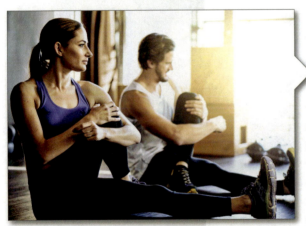

Historically, it was believed that females were more flexible than males. Although supported by some clinical evidence, this statement certainly lacks conclusiveness and does not verify potentials [28, 55]. Simply selecting two random individuals on the street could quickly disprove this theory, as numerous factors can invalidate this claim. In the defense of the researchers, factors exist that support the conclusion, as females are more likely to display greater ROM in some movements compared to males. Although variations exist, the female pelvis is noticeably broader at the top and narrower at the bottom, allowing scientists to determine the gender of skeletons that were buried long ago. This marked sex difference allows for greater pelvic ROM. Additionally, females show greater range in elbow extension due to differences in the curvature of the olecranon process (the proximal end of the ulnar bone), and some show greater trunk flexibility, attributed to shorter leg length and a lower center of gravity [48, 58]. This being said, a person's birth gender will neither ensure nor prevent healthy flexibility.

Females display greater ROM in specific movements compared to males due to anatomical variances:	Pelvis is broader at the top and narrower at the bottom, allowing for greater ROM
	Greater ROM through elbow extension is due to differences in the olecranon process
	Greater trunk ROM is attributed to relatively shorter leg lengths and lower centers of gravity

Females may also experience ROM adjustments due to hormonal effects and physical changes related to pregnancy. It is well documented that peripheral joint laxity increases during pregnancy, and it has been postulated that the hormone relaxin promotes tissue pliability;

however, evidence does not support this claim. In fact, research suggests the changes in peripheral joint laxity do not seem to correlate well with maternal estradiol, progesterone, or relaxin levels [7, 25]. Nonetheless, exercise professionals should be aware of the orthopedic risks of joint laxity during and immediately following pregnancy and structure exercise programs accordingly.

Body Mass

It has been suggested that an increase in muscle mass reduces the tissues' ROM. Taken at face value, this is not at all accurate. These flexibility limitations have been discussed and several mechanisms have been suggested by which flexibility may be reduced. Notably, none of these included the hypertrophy of a muscle fiber, which always possesses the same elastic properties, regardless of the cross-sectional area. This misconception is most likely associated with some of the factors associated with hypertrophy training. When heavy resistance is moved through a limited ROM, the muscle adapts to the environment. Routinely performing limited range movements may lead to reduced flexibility. Heavy bench pressing and bilateral rows have both been implicated in reduced ROM in the upper back and shoulder. Individuals who perform load-appropriate resistance training through full ROM will not lose the lengthening qualities of muscle tissue. In fact, resistance training can improve flexibility when performed correctly [16, 51]. Unilateral activity seems to improve ROM more than bilateral movements due to the separation of the limbs, attainable ROM of the external load, and stabilization of attached structures.

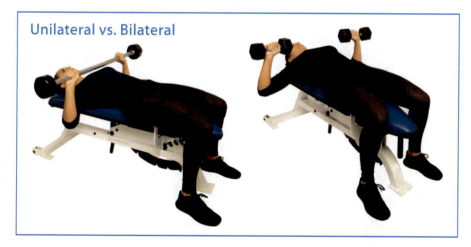

The popularity of steroid use may also lead people to believe resistance training and muscle mass make you less flexible. In addition to the aforementioned possibilities, individuals who use steroids often dramatically increase muscle mass beyond a normal attainable level, influencing the ROM by soft-tissue approximation. The excessive sizes reached by today's bodybuilders may limit movement range due to a muscle-bound phenomenon. Although these individuals would benefit from a flexibility routine, their excessive hypertrophy may become a physical obstacle to movement.

Muscle is not the only tissue that can present obstacles to movement range. Excessive fat mass stored in both visceral and subcutaneous areas can limit a person's ability to move. This is particularly true for central storage, as the midsection collides with other body segments when bending in a seated position. Obesity can have indirect effects as well. Obese individuals tend to participate in less physical activity, move through more limited ranges, and experience musculoskeletal problems, such as lower back pain and orthopedic limitations. Remember, physical activity is one of the leading factors that affect flexibility. These factors further contribute to a reduction in ROM and can manifest into significant limitations in movement capabilities if untreated.

Immobility

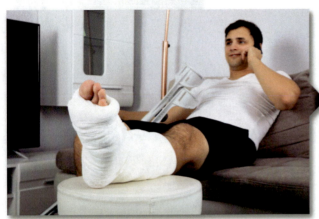

Immobility substantially and negatively affects muscle tissue. Significant strength and flexibility losses can occur in a relatively short period of time [26]. Of particular concern is the loss of elasticity in the connective tissue elements, as the effects are not limited to the tissue structures. Chemical structure changes are also relevant, as they can result in reduced spacing between collagen fibers. When fiber proximity reaches the point that contact occurs between the collagen fibers, cross linkages develop between them [4, 64]. This reduces extensibility, and consequently ROM.

Pain

When stretching protocols are employed, discomfort and pain tolerance influence the ranges attainable. The positions achieved when stretching to full ROM can cause different levels of discomfort, depending on pain inhibition, which is modulated by **nociceptors** in the tissue. Individuals present variations in discomfort tolerance, and thus, the tissue length attained and time held in the stretched position may be limited by a person's relative pain threshold. Warming up tissue prior to stretching is fundamental to flexibility training and promotes a reduction to elongation resistance via decreased viscosity and a lower level of discomfort at submaximal ranges.

 DEFINITIONS

Nociceptors –
Sensory receptors that respond to potentially damaging stimuli and relay a message to higher brain centers, promoting the feeling of pain.

Injury

Musculoskeletal injuries that result in loss of ROM usually are either the result of acute trauma or chronic overuse of a joint [56].

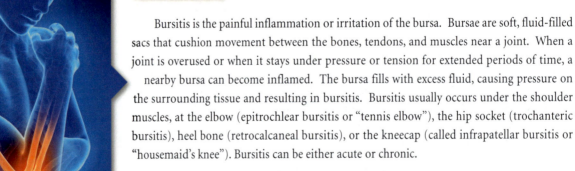

Common injury-related ROM problems include [43, 51, 74]: Bursitis · Tendonitis · Impingement syndromes · Fasciitis

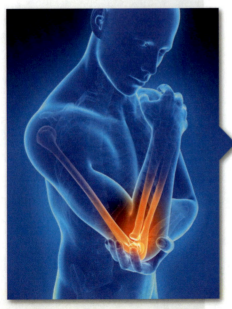

Bursitis is the painful inflammation or irritation of the bursa. Bursae are soft, fluid-filled sacs that cushion movement between the bones, tendons, and muscles near a joint. When a joint is overused or when it stays under pressure or tension for extended periods of time, a nearby bursa can become inflamed. The bursa fills with excess fluid, causing pressure on the surrounding tissue and resulting in bursitis. Bursitis usually occurs under the shoulder muscles, at the elbow (epitrochlear bursitis or "tennis elbow"), the hip socket (trochanteric bursitis), heel bone (retrocalcaneal bursitis), or the kneecap (called infrapatellar bursitis or "housemaid's knee"). Bursitis can be either acute or chronic.

Movement pain associated with bursitis often leads to compensatory actions and limitations in range to avoid the pain. Most commonly, bursitis is caused by trauma. Some specific factors possibly resulting in bursitis include [39, 41]:

- Overuse or injury to joint areas
- Incorrect posture at work or rest
- Poor conditioning before exercise or sports participation
- An abnormal or poorly positioned joint or bone (such as leg length differences) that stresses soft tissue structures

Tendonitis describes inflammation, swelling, and irritation of a tendon, a painful condition felt most at the tendon insertion site. Tendons are bands of fibrous material that attach muscle to bone. When these structures are irritated, they can swell and become acutely inflamed, causing tendonitis. Tendonitis most commonly occurs in tendons associated with increased use. More common types of tendonitis include: biceps tendonitis, Achilles tendonitis, patellar tendonitis, rotator cuff tendonitis, and elbow tendonitis [63].

Tendonitis can result from several different etiologies. However, overuse of the tendon during work or physical activity is the most common cause. Tennis and golf commonly cause tendonitis of the elbow when the activities are performed with incorrect biomechanics. Direct injury to the tendon can also result in tendonitis, as can various inflammatory conditions, such as rheumatoid arthritis [3]. Lastly, aging can make one more prone to developing tendonitis: as one ages, the tendons lose their elasticity, making them more susceptible to irritation and inflammation. Chronic tendonitis reduces activity and movement range, leading to pain and discomfort.

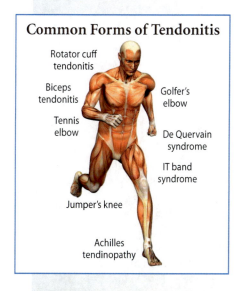

Common Forms of Tendonitis
- Rotator cuff tendonitis
- Biceps tendonitis
- Tennis elbow
- Golfer's elbow
- De Quervain syndrome
- IT band syndrome
- Jumper's knee
- Achilles tendinopathy

Impingement syndromes involve painful entrapments of a tendon between the bony aspects of a joint. The most common example is shoulder impingement syndrome. With this condition, the supraspinatus tendon, subacromial-subdeltoid bursa, and/or the biceps tendon becomes entrapped between the humeral head and the coracoacromial arch. Similar to the other injuries, pain limits attainment of full ROM.

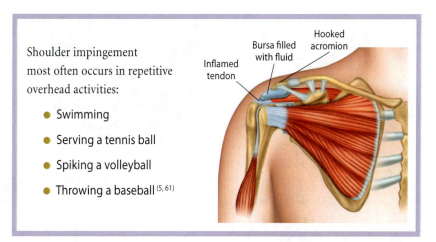

Shoulder impingement most often occurs in repetitive overhead activities:
- Swimming
- Serving a tennis ball
- Spiking a volleyball
- Throwing a baseball [5, 61]

Fasciitis occurs when the fascia that covers a surface of underlying tissue becomes inflamed. Though fasciitis can potentially occur with any fascia, the most prevalent is plantar fasciitis. Plantar fasciitis results when the long, fibrous, plantar fascia ligament along the bottom of the foot develops tears in the tissue, causing pain and inflammation. The discomfort of plantar fasciitis is usually located close to where the fascia attaches to the calcaneus, or heel bone. The

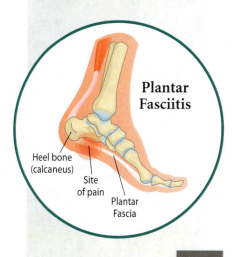

Plantar Fasciitis

most common cause is an overload of physical activity or exercise. Excessive running, jumping, or other activities can easily place repetitive or excessive stress on the tissue and lead to tears and inflammation, resulting in moderate to severe pain that limits activity and movement range [30].

Disease

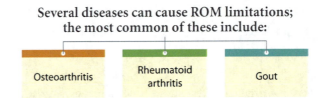

Several diseases can cause ROM limitations; the most common of these include:
- Osteoarthritis
- Rheumatoid arthritis
- Gout

Osteoarthritis (OA) is a degenerative disorder of aging that can affect any joint; it is most commonly diagnosed in the hips, knees, toes, and spine and is often associated with previous injury [14]. OA increases water content and decreases protein makeup of cartilage, thereby decreasing the elastic modulus. The cartilage begins to degenerate, becoming soft and flaking into the joints, losing its ability to cushion. This results in rubbing and friction between the joints, causing joint surface erosion, leading to reactive bone formation. **Osteophytes** (outgrowths of new bone), commonly called "spurs," form at the joint surface edges, and the joint capsules and synovial membranes thicken. The joint spaces begin to narrow and lose stability, leading to pain, inflammation, and limited mobility. In addition to aging, obesity represents a significant factor that may contribute to the development of OA. Other factors are repetitive joint stress, infection, and previous joint injury [9, 19, 31].

Rheumatoid arthritis is an inflammatory disorder of unknown etiology. Its symptoms are generally caused by a person's immune system attacking his or her joints, resulting in inflammation. RA is characterized by symmetric, erosive synovitis (joint inflammation), and in some cases extra-articular involvement (involvement outside of the joint).

Most people with RA experience a chronic, fluctuating course of disease, that despite therapeutic measures, may result in [1, 47]:

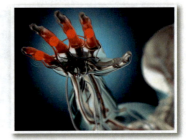

- Progressive joint destruction
- Deformity
- Disability
- Premature death

RA-associated inflammation damages the synovial joints of the wrists, shoulders, knees, ankles, and feet. Rheumatoid nodules that form close to the joints and other skin problems may be present in approximately 25% of RA patients and usually signal the most rapid, progressive form of the disease. Rheumatoid nodules usually develop where pressure is applied, including the sacrum and elbows. RA is debilitating and can significantly compromise movement capabilities associated with joint dysfunction.

Gout is a form of arthritis that primarily affects older males. It appears very quickly, often overnight, causing intense swelling and pain. The ball of the big toe is the most common site for gout. Gout is a condition in which uric acid, a by-product of metabolism normally flushed from the body in the urine, rises above normal levels. When a person has gout, the uric acid

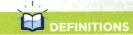

DEFINITIONS

Osteophytes –

Bony outgrowths, or spurs, associated with the degeneration of cartilage at a joint.

forms crystals which are deposited in the joints. These uric acid crystal deposits give rise to inflammation, in turn causing pain, swelling, and redness, which may limit attainable ROM in the affected joint. Gout occurs more frequently in countries that have a high standard of living and is most likely related to diet and alcohol use. The disease can usually be treated easily with medicine and can be prevented by changes in an individual's diet.

While these conditions are associated with movement discomfort and exercise avoidance, it is important for effected patients to continue to exercise to improve day-to-day functioning. Exercise is believed to be the most effective non-pharmaceutical treatment for osteoarthritis, lowers symptoms of rheumatoid arthritis, and may prevent future gout flare-ups.

Factors Affecting Flexibility

- Knowledge of stretching techniques
- Time availability
- Identified deficiencies
- Client's pain tolerance and interest
- Imbalances
- Injury
- Orthopedic limitations
- Disease

Testing Flexibility

The variability between joint ROM indicates that a battery of flexibility assessments should be used to determine if any deficiencies exist. Ideally, each joint should be assessed through each primary movement. Goniometer, inclinometer, and flexometer devices can be used to directly evaluate the joint ROM with quantifiable data. If direct measurement is unattainable, indirect assessments can be performed to assess the functional ROM in different joint movements. In some cases, indirect measures use assistive flexibility devices that provide data feedback such as the sit-and-reach box. In other cases, the movements are quantified using visual/recorded observation and/or tape measurement to determine attainable range.

Direct measurement using a goniometer can effectively assess flexibility but requires significant anatomical knowledge. The goniometer is a protractor-like device that uses a stationary arm fixed at zero degrees with a movable arm that is aligned with the bone of the movement limb or body segment. The goniometer's axis of rotation is aligned over the joint axis and the arms of the instrument are placed over bony landmarks along the longitudinal axis of body segments. The technique requires the body segment to move through its full ROM and then to be held in a static position, at which time the goniometer is placed upon the respective bony landmarks and the

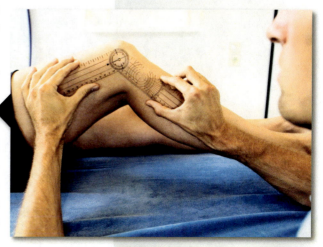

degree of movement is measured and recorded. Norms exist for normal ROM for each specific joint action at each of the articulations. This assessment method provides quality data that can be used for evaluation of range and represents a baseline measurement that can be used comparatively during later evaluations.

Similar to other administrator-reliant protocols, validity and reliability depend upon strict adherence to protocol as well as technical expertise. Primary errors include improper alignment of the rotational axis and incorrect identification of bony landmarks. Some joints, particularly in the lower body, present more difficulty in attaining true validity compared to upper body measures. When weighed against radiography and other techniques used to produce internal bodily images (X-rays, CT scans, MRI), properly employed goniometer techniques show high levels of validity. Indirect measurement methods are more popular in non-clinical settings due to their relative ease of use, as well as the limited technical skill and equipment required. In most cases, a linear measuring instrument, such as a tape measure, is used to quantify the ROM attained in a select battery of field tests. The sit-and-reach and its successors, including the V sit-and reach, modified sit-and-reach, back saver sit-and-reach, and modified back saver sit-and-reach have been used as principal measures of flexibility in physical fitness assessments. These tests help assess low back and hamstring ROM, often as predictors of low back pain risk. The validity of these tests has been scrutinized with respect to measurement and predictability of low-back pain incidence. For this reason, many professionals have gravitated away from these tests and migrated to other testing protocols.

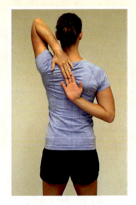

Assessment protocols that employ cross-joint movement have gained in popularity; the following are commonly used among athletic and general populations *(See Assessment Chapter)*:

- Apley back scratch test
- Single straight-leg hip flexion test
- Thomas test
- Trunk flexion/extension tests
- Overhead squat assessment

Additionally, spine and hip assessments have been used to draw conclusions as to movement proficiency related to the lumbo-pelvic hip complex (LPHC) in several planes and across fascial lines. A tracking system using objective measurement devices allows for the identification of changes over a term.

◆ Types of Flexibility Training

Implementing flexibility in a program, like other fitness components, requires the organization of aggregate factors into a structured, premeditated format. The goal of flexibility training is to attain chronic adjustments in the tissue's ability to lengthen using progressively applied stretching techniques. These applications should emphasize reducing the resistance within a muscle during elongation, while encouraging the greatest yield from the tissue's elastic properties. The following text will review different effective techniques to promote flexibility enhancements. The first step to performing full-ROM activities is to ensure that the tissue is in optimal condition to be stretched. This suggests participation in appropriate warmup activities to encourage a reduced tissue viscosity and promote extensibility. As mentioned earlier, employing myofascial release techniques can also reduce fascial restriction that may limit the tissue's optimal elastic properties. Applying acupressure, self-myofascial release techniques, or hard-foam rolling to a tender area before a general warmup of the tissue can add to the flexibility performance. Warm-up modalities should be performed before all stretching activities.

Several techniques can enhance ROM. They are classified into one of two groups: active stretching or passive stretching. In active stretching, the client supplies the force to lengthen the tissue. In passive stretching, an external force supplies the means for moving the body segments. This force may be generated from a partner, gravity, or stretching device.

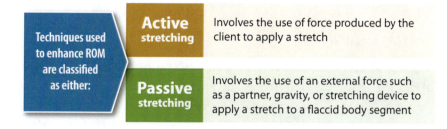

Two categories of flexibility techniques exist within these group classifications. These categories are static flexibility techniques, meaning the tissue is lengthened and held for a designated period of time, and dynamic flexibility techniques, which include activities that require movement across the ROM.

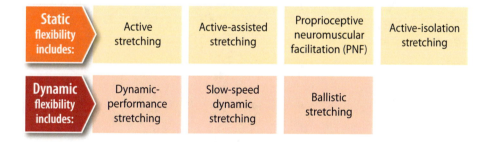

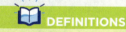

DEFINITIONS

Stretch reflex –

A reflexive contraction of a muscle induced by rapid stretch; triggered by excitation of the muscle spindles and a subsequent feedback loop to the spinal cord resulting in rapid excitation of the stretched muscle and inhibitory signaling of the opposing muscle.

All hold some degree of merit for improving flexibility. The method selected will depend on one's level of knowledge and expertise with a given technique, client appropriateness, time for implementation, and where the activity falls within the exercise program.

Static Stretching

Static stretching is likely the most popular technique employed for flexibility. The basic protocol requires a person to lengthen the tissue in a slow, controlled manner to its terminal ROM and then hold the static position attained. It is important to perform the movement slowly to avoid eliciting the **stretch reflex** that will inhibit the attainment of full ROM via proprioceptive modulation. Once the desired position has been reached, the client should concentrate on relaxing the tissue. Slow, controlled breathing techniques may help manage the discomfort experienced by some clients and aid in improving the tissue's relax-

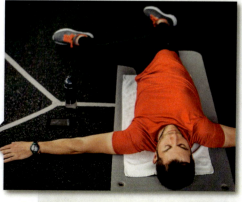

ation state. Several studies have analyzed the different durations of static stretches, and it has been consistently found that the greatest ROM is attained in the first 15-30 seconds. Due to static stretches being a "relative max," pain tolerance is seemingly the determining factor for how long an effective stretch can be held. If one employs a static stretch technique in order to maximize tissue elongation, the duration of the greatest ROM attainable should be maintained for 30 seconds for optimal effect. However, if pain tolerance is low, 2-4 repetitions may achieve the same results. Static stretching beyond four repetitions has not been shown to induce further elongation [24].

Static stretching is ideally performed at the end of a workout routine rather than at the beginning. This choice makes sense, as static stretching reduces power and force output when performed before resistance training or power-based activities. Even relatively short bouts of static stretching before strength and power movements can be detrimental to performance [46]. At the end of the workout, following the cool down, static stretching yields positive results and may aid in recovery.

Active-Assisted Stretching

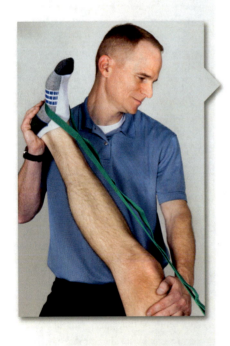

Active-assisted stretching utilizes the same basic premise as the static stretch, but it employs added force to increase the attainable range. The force may come from using the arms to pull the limb or body segment in a direction that increases tissue elongation, a partner adding pressure to the body to increase the stretch, or utilizing an external device, such as a stretch cord or towel, to provide greater range attainment. The duration of the static hold is the same, 30 seconds. Caution must be taken to avoid overstretching the tissue. This is of particular importance when a partner contributes additional force. Communication must be clear and concise so that the partner stretches muscle through only a healthy range. If a personal trainer is going to employ active-assisted stretching techniques with his or her clients, he or she should first explain the process and convey the importance of ongoing communication to avoid potential injury. Static stretching without assistance should be practiced before utilizing the active-assisted technique, so the client becomes comfortable with the protocol and identifies his or her respective limitations.

Active isolation is another hybrid model that uses a combination of active stretching and neural factors. This technique requires the client to actively reach a full ROM by contracting the antagonist muscle (opposite of the muscle being stretched) to elicit a reciprocal inhibitory effect. Once full ROM is reached, the partner holds the body segment, and the client relaxes. Now in the stabilized, lengthened position, the client again contracts the agonist muscle in an attempt to increase the stretch, which the partner lightly assists. The position is held for 6 seconds. The contraction is then released and a passive stretch is applied to the tolerable range and held for 15 seconds. Sustained contractions can be used, but a progressive model seems to work more effectively, plausibly due to the duration of tolerable discomfort.

Proprioceptive Neuromuscular Facilitation

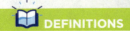

Proprioceptive neuromuscular facilitation (PNF) –

A group of stretching techniques that utilize autogenic and/or reciprocal inhibition to maximize range of motion.

Proprioceptive neuromuscular facilitation (PNF) is basically a hybrid between static and dynamic flexibility because it utilizes different aspects from each protocol. The technique is widely used in clinical settings for rehabilitation of injuries but has gained popularity among fitness professionals due to its marked effects. PNF stretching is generally employed using a partner. Due to the risks associated with the technique, an appropriate level of expertise is required. PNF stretching should only be performed by individuals well-versed in the technique.

PNF protocols vary slightly in the techniques used to attain a maximal ROM. The basic technique utilizes a passive stretch to full tolerable range, which is then held for 10 seconds. Following the 10 second hold, a contract-relax technique is used in which the trainer applies active–assisted pressure, which the client must resist as he or she contracts the stretched muscle. This static tension segment is held for 6 seconds. The excessive tension stimulates the GTOs, causing autogenic inhibition, effectively educating the proprioceptors that the new end ROM is safe to attain. At the end of the 6 second contraction, the limb is again passively stretched by the partner to the furthest attainable range and then held for the tolerable limit or 30 seconds.

Another commonly-employed PNF stretching technique takes advantage of a slightly different contract–relax sequence, in which the client actively or passively reaches a full ROM. Once the full tolerable ROM is attained, the partner stabilizes the body segment in the stretched position. This position is then held for 10 seconds. At the end of the 10 seconds, the client contracts the stretched muscle against the partner. The trainer should instruct and educate the client to the fact that the client should not change any body positions to gain leverage, as any extraneous bodily movement will decrease the stretch's effectiveness. Equally important, the partner assisting the stretch should have a sturdy position to prevent the body segment from moving or knocking him or her off balance. In many cases, the joints which present mechanical advantage for the client will cause slight bodily movements from the original position. The contract phase should last 6 seconds. Again, the partner should passively stretch the limb to the fullest attainable range and the position should be held for the tolerable limit or 30 seconds. In some techniques, the final passive stretch is assisted by the client's active contraction of the opposing muscle group to further move the body segment in the direction of the stretch. This method takes advantage of reflex inhibition and seems to present the greatest flexibility gains related to PNF techniques.

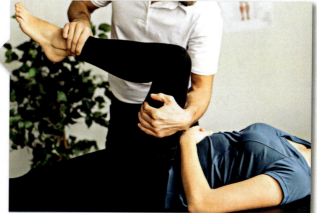

Although PNF stretches provide notable results, the technique has its limitations. It requires a competent partner, and the procedures must be strictly adhered to in order to reduce the injury risk.

Although PNF provides notable results, the technique has its limitations. The procedure requires a competent partner and the procedures must be strictly adhered to in order to reduce injury risk. Even when the protocol is followed precisely, injury is more likely to occur with PNF than with a traditional static stretch. Clients must be thoroughly instructed to listen to their bodies and comply with an appropriate pain threshold. Some clients strive to perform so well that they ignore warning signs and may injure themselves in the process. Additionally, some clients do not like the technique due to the severity of discomfort. If this is the case, the procedure should be exchanged for a more acceptable one.

Dynamic Flexibility

Dynamic flexibility works in the same way in which all physical activity encourages better movement ability. When tissues are routinely moved through a full ROM, they maintain their

DEFINITIONS

Dynamic flexibility –

The act of briefly achieving full range of motion through controlled muscle contraction; often used for movement preparation.

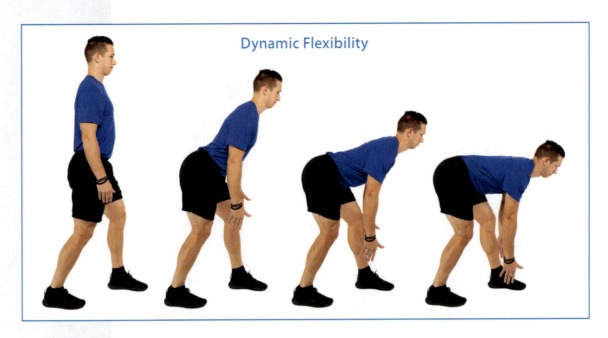

Dynamic Flexibility

elastic properties. Dynamic flexibility is advantageous because it allows the body to gain flexibility from movements that can be employed before or during an exercise program. Dynamic flexibility gained popularity in track and field events and was adopted by many other sports as an effective model for preparation before an event or practice. It has also migrated into exercise programs as a way to improve flexibility during a limited-duration exercise session. Dynamic flexibility is often used for corrective strategies following a general warm-up, or in some cases, is used as a movement-specific warmup modality, mimicking the activities to follow.

Dynamic stretching activities use a variety of movements that are similar to a particular sport or utilize the muscles emphasized in a specific activity. The movements employed for dynamic stretching often exaggerate the joint actions that will be used in the subsequent training bout to facilitate motion at the greatest attainable range. Some common examples are high knee or straight leg marches, step-overs using a hurdle, and long-step lunges. These movements often have upper body actions added to the activity to promote fascial line continuity (e.g., lunge with contralateral cross reach or lateral lean). Dynamic stretches are performed in a controlled fashion so as not to elicit a response from the muscle spindles, which will limit the stretch.

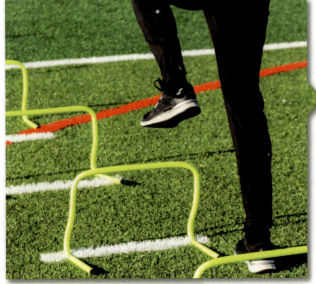

Slow-speed dynamic stretching is very similar to the dynamic performance stretching technique but uses slower, more isolated movements that are held for short periods. Some common examples are slow deep squats, broad step-backs, and floor-to-ceiling reaches. The techniques possess similarities to active yoga, often using a designated time or count to complete each repetition to ensure a controlled eccentric and concentric contraction occurs without any reflex response. Slow-speed dynamic stretching can utilize any movement through a full ROM, so the options are limitless. If the movements are not being used as a specific warm-up modality, it makes sense to select movements that are not normally performed. Utilizing actions that are performed infrequently will help maintain flexibility in all the movement planes. Cooldowns often utilize this technique prior to static stretching.

Dynamic stretches	Dynamic performance stretches	Slow-speed dynamic stretches
• Allow ROM gains related to specific movements employed during training • Popular in sports as an effective preparation model • Provide for both a warm-up and improved ROM outcomes	• Use a variety of sport- or exercise-specific movements that functionally stretch musculature to be utilized • Movements are often exaggerated to attain the greatest ROM • Examples: high knee marches, hurdle step-overs	• Slower, more isolated movements are utilized • Designated time for each repetition can ensure controlled contractions and no activation of the stretch reflex response • Examples: deep squats, single-leg squats

Ballistic Stretching

Ballistic stretching is often considered a contraindicated method of stretching due to its potential risk for injury. The technique requires the body segment to move through a full ROM while under momentum force. Bouncing toe touches, leg and arm swings, and high-knee swings all represent common examples. Karate and ballet have centered on ballistic stretching as a key component to flexibility enhancement. The technique does improve ROM but with potential risk for injury. Proponents suggest the technique mimics the actions used in the events for which the individual trains, whereas opponents cite the movements' destructive potential for tissue and joints. The main argument against ballistic stretching, beside the stress it causes to the muscle, connective tissue, and joints, is that the velocities used never allow the tissue to relax. The fast, jerky movements employed cause the stretch reflex to create tension in the muscle, which is the direct opposite of the desired effect. With all the viable techniques available for safe flexibility training, including ballistic stretching in a personal training program is not necessarily the most prudent decision for those wishing to increase ROM beyond their current limits.

Programming Flexibility

Numerous factors determine how flexibility activities are programmed for a client. Each must be considered to optimize the routine's effectiveness and ensure progress towards the programmatic goals. As with all programming, addressing the deficiencies is prioritized. Muscle imbalances across the joint, involving both specific strength and flexibility, may lead to injury; therefore, prioritizing the major issues will help to prevent further decline and consequences associated with the condition. Time is also an issue that may set program limitations, as most exercise sessions are arbitrarily assigned to 60 minutes. As mentioned, optimal duration for most stretches is 30 seconds, which is consistent with the set duration for many exercises. Selecting a stretching sequence that addresses all the major movements is prudent and consistent with the circuit system. If the time available for flexibility is relatively short, the routine may focus on a particular area of inflexibility. One key point to remember is not to disregard any body

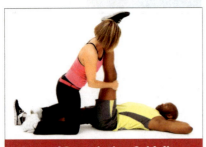

General Prescription Guidelines

Mode:
Static or Dynamic

Volume:
10-12 movements, 2-4 sets, 15-30 sec static holds, 5-10 sec contraction durations for PNF and 6-12 sec holds

Dynamic:
Accumulate 1-2 minutes of stretch time per muscle group

Intensity:
Tolerable discomfort, no pain

Duration:
15-30 minutes

Frequency:
Minimum 2-3 days/week, most days if possible

movement for any broad length of time, or the tissues involved will lose flexibility.

Flexibility routines may be performed independently of other activities, but in most cases involving a personal trainer, they will be planned with aerobic and anaerobic exercises in a more comprehensive program matrix. Basic frequency recommendations are similar to minimums for resistance training: stretch each muscle group twice per week and alternate the stretches to vary the planes of movement. If time is limited, build dynamic activities into the workout to focus on the areas that would otherwise be static-stretched independently. For instance, a weighted squat can be exchanged for weighted Bulgarian squats to increase hip flexor movement range. Additionally, if maximal force output is not a concern, clients can stretch antagonist muscle groups during the rest intervals of strength training exercises (e.g., leg extensions followed by hamstring stretches during the rest interval). Stretching the antagonist muscle group following a lift can take advantage of transitory reciprocal innervation and maximize training session time.

If the client presents orthopedic problems, such as injuries or disease-related joint issues, evaluation and recommendations by a qualified medical professional may be warranted. Selecting activities that do not pose an injury threat and will not exacerbate a problem is important, so third-party guidance may be a relevant consideration to avoid liability related to flexibility programming. Additionally, if a client does not like a particular stretching style due to relative discomfort, it may be substituted with another technique to promote compliance. Regardless, pain, whether perceived or actual, should be avoided during any stretching activity.

Consider the following model for an integrated programming approach to increase and maintain ROM in a daily exercise routine:

Dynamic warm-up – Promote progressive movement range across planes and facial lines. Accumulate 3-5 minutes of time-under-tension.

Examples: split-stance good morning, lateral lunge with cross-rotational reach, reverse lunge with contralateral reach

ROM promoting resistance exercises – Include 3-5 exercises that promote maximal range under loaded conditions. Perform 2-4 sets of 6-12 repetitions.

Examples: forward lunge with overhead press, reverse lunge with contralateral row, Bulgarian squat with plate rotation

Cool down – These movements should resemble, in whole or in part, the exercise performed during the training bout. They should be unloaded and performed through a full ROM. Hold terminal positions for 5-10 seconds. Total time-under-tension should accumulate to 30 seconds (per side if unilaterally performed).

Examples: lateral lunge with ground reach, split-stance ground reach, good morning with T-reach, broad lunge with hip extension (overhead reach and lateral lean)

Static stretches – Select exercises based on the greatest needs. Those exercises that demonstrate limitations to movement should be preferentially selected. Perform lower body stretches prior to upper body stretches. Perform 3-5 exercises while accumulating 30-second holds.

Examples: active hamstring, active iliopsoas, active glute, and active lower-back stretches on a bench

Summary Flexibility Training Protocols

- Explain the techniques and protocols to the client and establish open communication
- Perform an appropriate warm-up
- Select at least one activity per major muscle group or joint action
- Order deficient areas first and perform others in order of need
- Perform 2-4 sets of 30 second holds or accumulate the duration with multiple sets; start slow and progress to greater ranges
- Use multiple planes of movement with each muscle group
- Require strict protocol adherence
- Use dynamic flexibility before static flexibility
- Establish static stretching proficiency before including PNF
- Stretch to tolerable discomfort, not pain
- Use controlled breathing in a rhythmic pattern
- Record any pains experienced during the movements and look for compensatory actions

◆ Common Flexibility Techniques

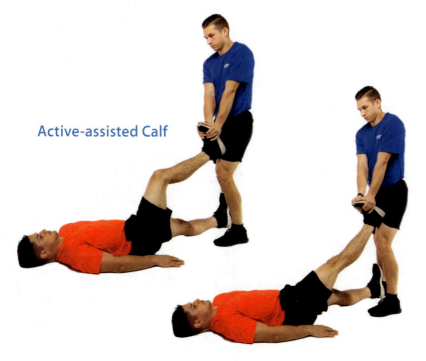

Active-assisted Calf

Chapter 15 — NCSF Advanced Concepts of Personal Training

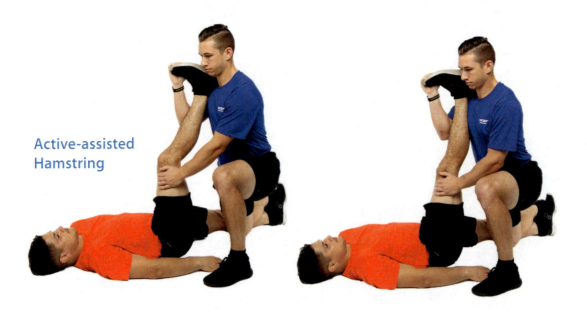

Active-assisted Hamstring

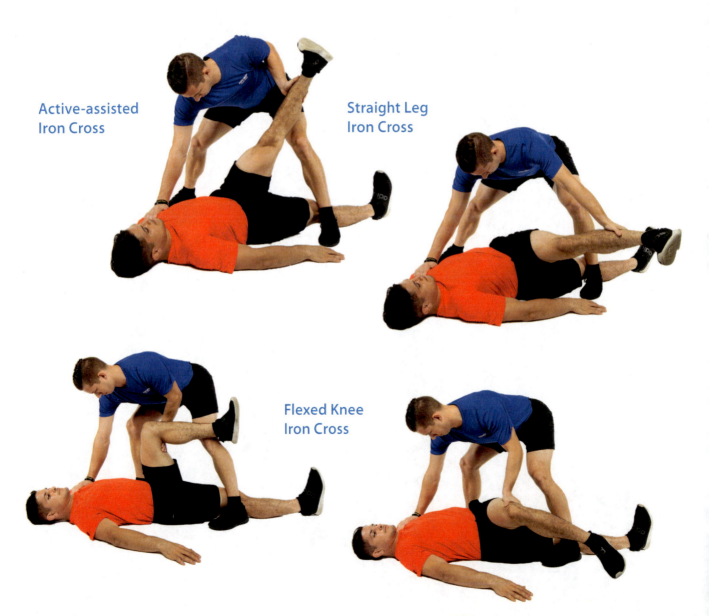

Active-assisted Iron Cross

Straight Leg Iron Cross

Flexed Knee Iron Cross

Flexibility

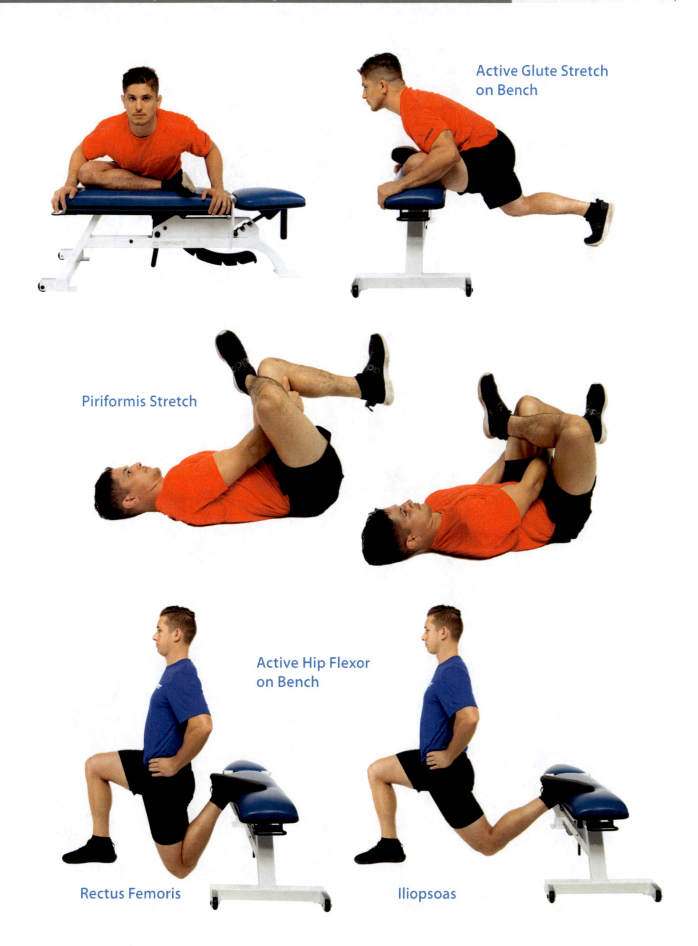

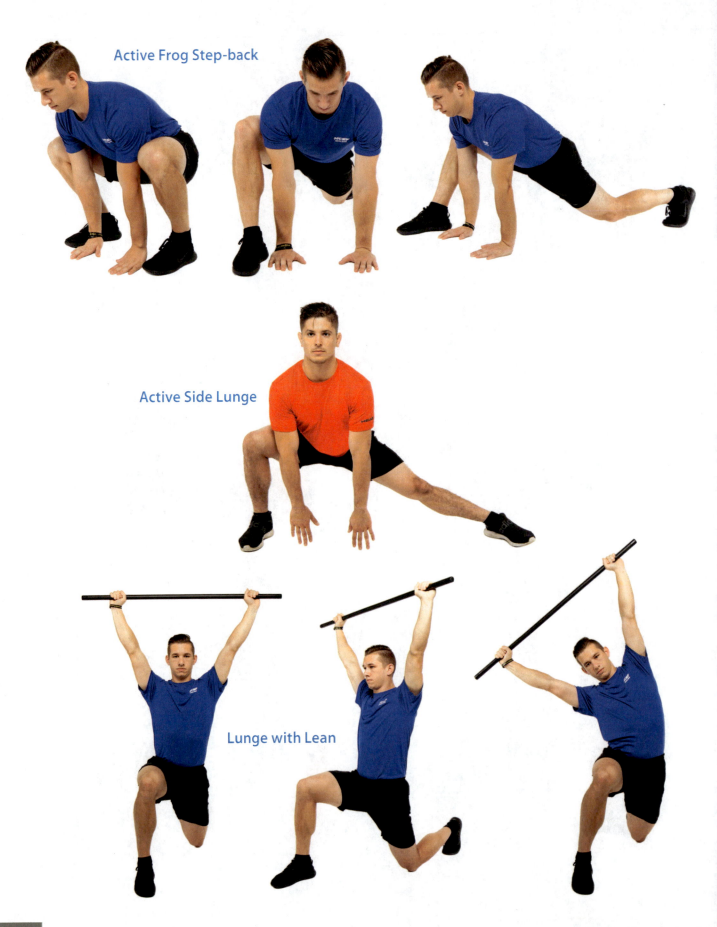

Active Frog Step-back

Active Side Lunge

Lunge with Lean

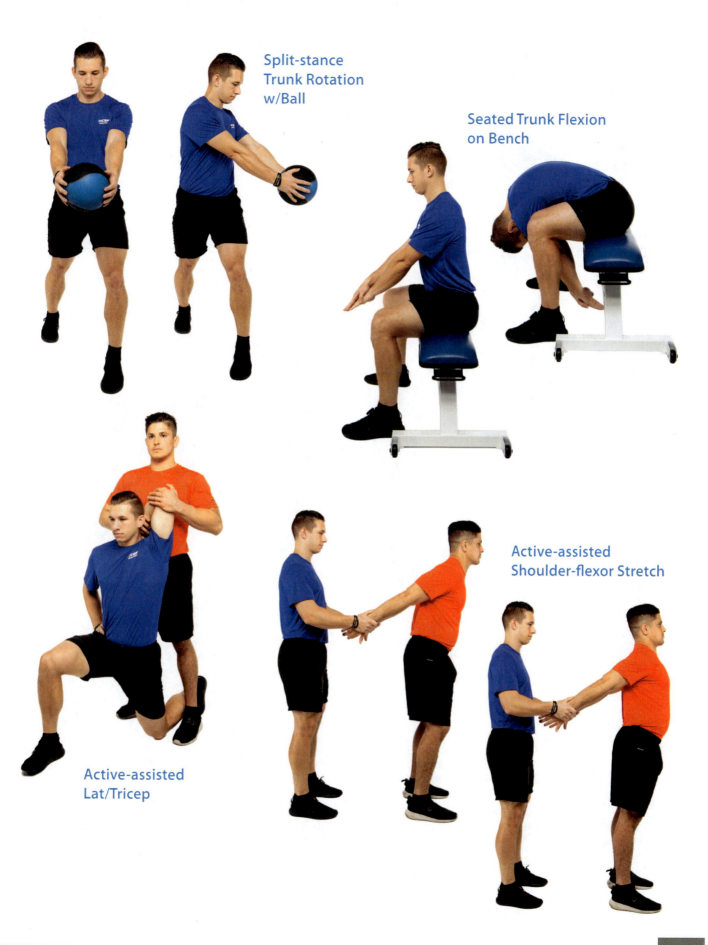

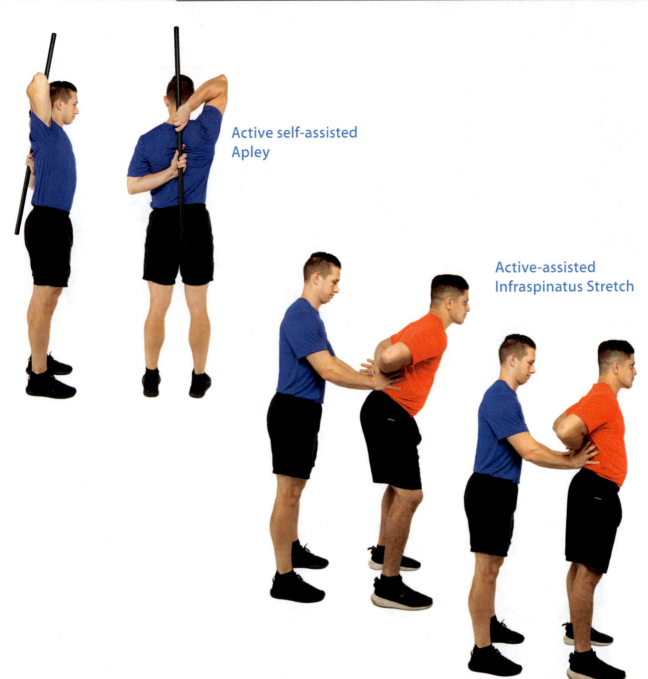

Active self-assisted Apley

Active-assisted Infraspinatus Stretch

REFERENCES:

1. Aletaha D, Neogi T, Silman AJ, Funovits J, Felson DT, Bingham III CO, Birnbaum NS, Burmester GR, Bykerk VP, and Cohen MD. 2010 rheumatoid arthritis classification criteria: an American College of Rheumatology/European League Against Rheumatism collaborative initiative. *Arthritis & Rheumatism* 62: 2569-2581, 2010.

2. Allegri M, Montella S, Salici F, Valente A, Marchesini M, Compagnone C, Baciarello M, Manferdini ME, and Fanelli G. Mechanisms of low back pain: a guide for diagnosis and therapy. *F1000Research* 5, 2016.

3. Almekinders LC and Temple JD. Etiology, diagnosis, and treatment of tendonitis: an analysis of the literature. *Medicine and science in sports and exercise* 30: 1183-1190, 1998.

4. Baker JH and Matsumoto DE. Adaptation of skeletal muscle to immobilization in a shortened position. *Muscle & Nerve: Official Journal of the American Association of Electrodiagnostic Medicine* 11: 231-244, 1988.

5. Braman JP, Zhao KD, Lawrence RL, Harrison AK, and Ludewig PM. Shoulder impingement revisited: evolution of diagnostic understanding in orthopedic surgery and physical therapy. *Medical & biological engineering & computing* 52: 211-219, 2014.

6. Carlson CR and Hoyle RH. Efficacy of abbreviated progressive muscle relaxation training: A quantitative review of behavioral medicine research. *Journal of consulting and clinical psychology* 61: 1059, 1993.

7. Charlton WP, Coslett-Charlton LM, and Ciccotti MG. Correlation of estradiol in pregnancy and anterior cruciate ligament laxity. *Clinical Orthopaedics and Related Research®* 387: 165-170, 2001.

8. Dommerholt J, Chou L-W, Finnegan M, and Hooks T. A critical overview of the current myofascial pain literature–April 2018. *Journal of bodywork and movement therapies*, 2018.

9. Duclos M. Osteoarthritis, obesity and type 2 diabetes: The weight of waist circumference. *Annals of Physical and rehabilitation Medicine* 59: 157-160, 2016.

10. Franz S and Finnerup NB. Diagnostics and Treatment of Pain in Spinal Cord Injury. In: *Neurological Aspects of Spinal Cord Injury:* Springer, 2017, p. 283-302.

11. Frost H. Skeletal structural adaptations to mechanical usage (SATMU): 4. Mechanical influences on intact fibrous tissues. *The Anatomical Record* 226: 433-439, 1990.

12. Gajdosik RL. Passive extensibility of skeletal muscle: review of the literature with clinical implications. *Clinical biomechanics* 16: 87-101, 2001.

13. Gehlert S, Bloch W, and Suhr F. Ca2+-dependent regulations and signaling in skeletal muscle: from electro-mechanical coupling to adaptation. *International journal of molecular sciences* 16: 1066-1095, 2015.

14. Geyer M and Schönfeld C. Novel insights into the pathogenesis of osteoarthritis. *Current rheumatology reviews* 14: 98-107, 2018.

15. Giné-Garriga M, Roqué-Fíguls M, Coll-Planas L, Sitjà-Rabert M, and Salvà A. Physical exercise interventions for improving performance-based measures of physical function in community-dwelling, frail older adults: a systematic review and meta-analysis. *Archives of physical medicine and rehabilitation* 95: 753-769. e753, 2014.

16. Girouard CK and Hurley BF. Does strength training inhibit gains in range of motion from flexibility training in older adults? *Medicine and science in sports and exercise* 27: 1444-1449, 1995.

17. Goffaux J, Friesinger GC, Lambert W, Shroyer LW, Moritz TE, McCarthy JM, Henderson WG, and Hammermeister KE. Biological age--a concept whose time has come: a preliminary study. *Southern medical journal* 98: 985-993, 2005.

18. Granata KP and England SA. Stability of dynamic trunk movement. *Spine* 31: E271, 2006.

19. Greene MA and Loeser RF. Aging-related inflammation in osteoarthritis. *Osteoarthritis and cartilage* 23: 1966-1971, 2015.

20. Hessert MJ, Gugliucci MR, and Pierce HR. Functional fitness: maintaining or improving function for elders with chronic diseases. *FAMILY MEDICINE-KANSAS CITY-* 37: 472, 2005.

21. Hildebrandt M, Fankhauser G, Meichtry A, and Luomajoki H. Correlation between lumbar dysfunction and fat infiltration in lumbar multifidus muscles in patients with low back pain. *BMC musculoskeletal disorders* 18: 12, 2017.

22. Hong C-Z and Simons DG. Pathophysiologic and electrophysiologic mechanisms of myofascial trigger points. *Archives of physical medicine and rehabilitation* 79: 863-872, 1998.

23. Hurschler C, Loitz-Ramage B, and Vanderby R. A structurally based stress-stretch relationship for tendon and ligament. *Journal of biomechanical engineering* 119: 392-399, 1997.

24. Ingraham SJ. The role of flexibility in injury prevention and athletic performance: have we stretched the truth? *Minnesota medicine* 86: 58-61, 2003.

25. Khowailed IA, Petrofsky J, Lohman E, Daher N, and Mohamed O. 17β-estradiol induced effects on anterior cruciate ligament laxness and neuromuscular activation patterns in female runners. *Journal of Women's Health* 24: 670-680, 2015.

26. Kisner C, Colby LA, and Borstad J. *Therapeutic exercise: foundations and techniques:* Fa Davis, 2017.

27. Konrad A, Stafilidis S, and Tilp M. Effects of acute static, ballistic, and PNF stretching exercise on the muscle and tendon tissue properties. *Scandinavian journal of medicine & science in sports* 27: 1070-1080, 2017.

28. Krombholz H. Physical performance in relation to age, sex, birth order, social class, and sports activities of preschool children. *Perceptual and motor skills* 102: 477-484, 2006.

29. Kuan TS, Hong CZ, Chen JT, Chen SM, and Chien CH. The spinal cord connections of the myofascial trigger spots★,★★. *European Journal of Pain* 11: 624-634, 2007.

30. Landorf KB. Plantar heel pain and plantar fasciitis. *BMJ clinical evidence* 2015, 2015.

31. Lieberthal J, Sambamurthy N, and Scanzello CR. Inflammation in joint injury and post-traumatic osteoarthritis. *Osteoarthritis and cartilage* 23: 1825-1834, 2015.

32. Lindstedt S, LaStayo P, and Reich T. When active muscles lengthen: properties and consequences of eccentric contractions. *Physiology* 16: 256-261, 2001.

33. Lindstedt S and Nishikawa K. Huxleys' missing filament: form and function of titin in vertebrate striated muscle. *Annual review of physiology* 79: 145-166, 2017.

34. Linke WA. Titin gene and protein functions in passive and active muscle. *Annual review of physiology* 80: 389-411, 2018.

35. McQuade KJ, Turner JA, and Buchner DM. Physical fitness and chronic low back pain. An analysis of the relationships among fitness, functional limitations, and depression. *Clinical orthopaedics and related research*: 198-204, 1988.

36. Mikkelsson LO, Nupponen H, Kaprio J, Kautiainen H, Mikkelsson M, and Kujala UM. Adolescent flexibility, endurance strength, and physical activity as predictors of adult tension neck, low back pain, and knee injury: a 25 year follow up study. *British journal of sports medicine* 40: 107-113, 2006.

37. Murphy JR, Di Santo MC, Alkanani T, and Behm DG. Aerobic activity before and following short-duration static stretching improves range of motion and performance vs. a traditional warm-up. *Applied Physiology, Nutrition, and Metabolism* 35: 679-690, 2010.

38. Nakamura M, Ikezoe T, Nishishita S, Umehara J, Kimura M, and Ichihashi N. Acute effects of static stretching on the shear elastic moduli of the medial and lateral gastrocnemius muscles in young and elderly women. *Musculoskeletal Science and Practice* 32: 98-103, 2017.

39. Raas C, Attal R, Kaiser P, Popovscaia M, and Zegg M. Treatment and outcome with traumatic lesions of the olecranon and pre-patellar bursa: a literature review apropos a retrospective analysis including 552 cases. *Archives of orthopaedic and trauma surgery* 137: 823-827, 2017.

40. Renkawitz T, Boluki D, and Grifka J. The association of low back pain, neuromuscular imbalance, and trunk extension strength in athletes. *The Spine Journal* 6: 673-683, 2006.

41. Renström P and Johnson RJ. Overuse injuries in sports. *Sports Medicine* 2: 316-333, 1985.

42. Riemann BL and Lephart SM. The sensorimotor system, part II: the role of proprioception in motor control and functional joint stability. *Journal of athletic training* 37: 80, 2002.

43. Sady SP, Wortman M, and Blanke D. Flexibility training: ballistic, static or proprioceptive neuromuscular facilitation? *Archives of physical medicine and rehabilitation* 63: 261-263, 1982.

44. Schwartz M, Leo P, and Lewis J. A microstructural model for the elastic response of articular cartilage. *Journal of biomechanics* 27: 865-873, 1994.

45. Sermeev B. Development of mobility in the hip joint in sportsmen. *Yessis Review* 2: 16-17, 1966.

46. Simic L, Sarabon N, and Markovic G. Does pre-exercise static stretching inhibit maximal muscular performance? A meta-analytical review. *Scandinavian journal of medicine & science in sports* 23: 131-148, 2013.

47. Singh JA, Saag KG, Bridges Jr SL, Akl EA, Bannuru RR, Sullivan MC, Vaysbrot E, McNaughton C, Osani M, and Shmerling RH. 2015 American College of Rheumatology guideline for the treatment of rheumatoid arthritis. *Arthritis & rheumatology* 68: 1-26, 2016.

48. Smith LK, Lelas JL, and Kerrigan DC. Gender differences in pelvic motions and center of mass displacement during walking: stereotypes quantified. *Journal of women's health & gender-based medicine* 11: 453-458, 2002.

49. Smith LL, Brunetz MH, Chenier TC, McCammon MR, Houmard JA, Franklin ME, and Israel RG. The effects of static and ballistic stretching on delayed onset muscle soreness and creatine kinase. *Research quarterly for exercise and sport* 64: 103-107, 1993.

50. Son J, Indresano A, Sheppard K, Ward SR, and Lieber RL. Intraoperative and biomechanical studies of human vastus lateralis and vastus medialis sarcomere length operating range. *Journal of biomechanics* 67: 91-97, 2018.

51. Stone MH, Fleck SJ, Triplett NT, and Kraemer WJ. Health-and performance-related potential of resistance training. *Sports Medicine* 11: 210-231, 1991.

52. Tekur P, Singphow C, Nagendra HR, and Raghuram N. Effect of short-term intensive yoga program on pain, functional disability and spinal flexibility in chronic low back pain: a randomized control study. *The journal of alternative and complementary medicine* 14: 637-644, 2008.

53. Tinklenberg J, Beatka M, Bain JL, Siebers EM, Meng H, Pearsall RS, Lawlor MW, and Riley DA. Use of ankle immobilization in evaluating treatments to promote longitudinal muscle growth in mice. *Muscle & nerve*, 2018.

54. Trajano GS, Nosaka K, and Blazevich AJ. Neurophysiological mechanisms underpinning stretch-induced force loss. *Sports Medicine* 47: 1531-1541, 2017.

55. Trost SG, Pate RR, Dowda M, Saunders R, Ward DS, and Felton G. Gender differences in physical activity and determinants of physical activity in rural fifth grade children. *Journal of school health* 66: 145-150, 1996.

56. Valovich McLeod TC, Decoster LC, Loud KJ, Micheli LJ, Parker JT, Sandrey MA, and White C. National Athletic Trainers' Association position statement: prevention of pediatric overuse injuries. *Journal of athletic training* 46: 206-220, 2011.

57. Wang K, McCarter R, Wright J, Beverly J, and Ramirez-Mitchell R. Viscoelasticity of the sarcomere matrix of skeletal muscles. The titin-myosin composite filament is a dual-stage molecular spring. *Biophysical Journal* 64: 1161-1177, 1993.

58. Wang SC, Brede C, Lange D, Poster CS, Lange AW, Kohoyda-Inglis C, Sochor MR, Ipaktchi K, Rowe SA, and Patel S. Gender differences in hip anatomy: possible implications for injury tolerance in frontal collisions. Annual Proceedings/Association for the Advancement of Automotive Medicine. *Association for the Advancement of Automotive Medicine*, 2004, p. 287.

59. Weppler CH and Magnusson SP. Increasing muscle extensibility: a matter of increasing length or modifying sensation? *Physical therapy* 90: 438-449, 2010.

60. Whitehurst MA, Johnson BL, Parker CM, Brown LE, and Ford AM. The benefits of a functional exercise circuit for older adults. *Journal of strength and conditioning research* 19: 647, 2005.

61. Wilk KE, Obma P, Simpson CD, Cain EL, Dugas J, and Andrews JR. Shoulder injuries in the overhead athlete. *journal of orthopaedic & sports physical therapy* 39: 38-54, 2009.

62. Wilson G, Wood G, and Elliott B. The relationship between stiffness of the musculature and static flexibility: an alternative explanation for the occurrence of muscular injury. *International journal of sports medicine* 12: 403-407, 1991.

63. Wilson JJ and Best TM. Common overuse tendon problems: a review and recommendations for treatment. *Am Fam Physician* 72: 811-818, 2005.

64. Wisdom KM, Delp SL, and Kuhl E. Use it or lose it: multiscale skeletal muscle adaptation to mechanical stimuli. *Biomechanics and modeling in mechanobiology* 14: 195-215, 2015.

65. Youkhana S, Dean CM, Wolff M, Sherrington C, and Tiedemann A. Yoga-based exercise improves balance and mobility in people aged 60 and over: a systematic review and meta-analysis. *Age and ageing* 45: 21-29, 2015.

66. Zakas A, Doganis G, Zakas N, and Vergou A. Acute effects of active warm-up and stretching on the flexibility of elderly women. *Journal of sports medicine and physical fitness* 46: 617, 2006.

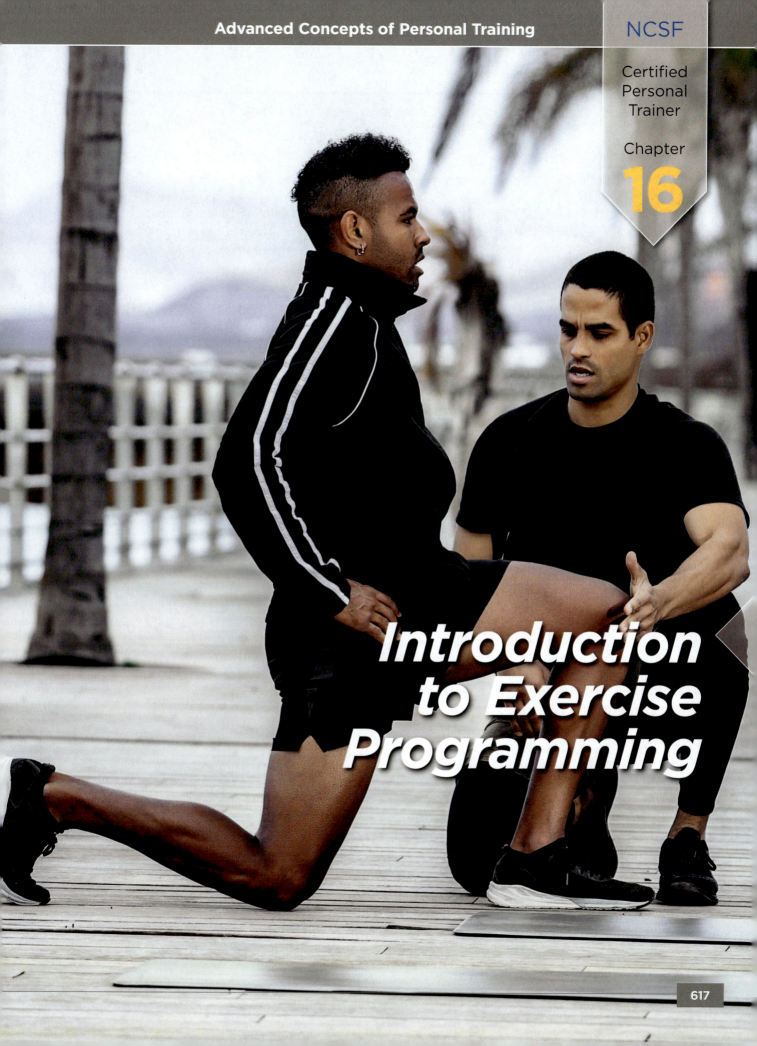

Advanced Concepts of Personal Training

NCSF Certified Personal Trainer

Chapter 16

Introduction to Exercise Programming

Program Design

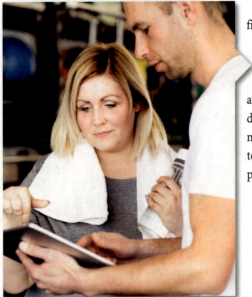

Exercise prescription is defined as a premeditated, structured format employing quantified stress, which is applied in appropriate dosages in a manner that stimulates the body's physiological systems to adapt. This suggests that each action the exercise program defines has a specific purpose related to the intended outcome. To successfully create an exercise prescription, an exercise professional must identify the physiological needs of the client and determine the specific exercise components that will target them. This requires a multi-dimensional review of all factors involved [10, 11]. Writing an effective exercise program is the most difficult task required of exercise professionals because one must understand all the factors that create the need and identify what exercises will encourage the adaptations that provide the greatest benefits. These must then be organized in a complementary manner.

Exercise programming for even the average person can become somewhat complicated due to:

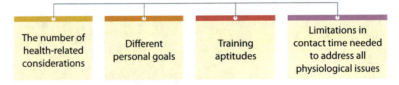

- The number of health-related considerations
- Different personal goals
- Training aptitudes
- Limitations in contact time needed to address all physiological issues

Programming for individual clients may present a variety of challenges for the exercise professional; however, this obstacle can be managed effectively by using the proper approach. A thorough needs analysis, as addressed in previous chapters, is the essential first step for identifying and ranking each client's requirements. Recording each finding provides the basis for the program's decision-making process and will be used as a starting point to evaluate the program components' outcomes along the way.

QUICK INSIGHT

The traditional approach to exercise programs applies the FITT principle. FITT represents F-frequency, I-intensity, T-time, and T-type. This principle suggests that all programming is based on frequency (number of training days), duration (total time of exercise), intensity (difficulty of the exercise), and type (mode of exercise). In personal training, client finances and available time can limit frequency, and the duration traditionally reflects only one hour of work. This leaves the areas of intensity and mode to the trainer's discretion. Due to the limited frequency and duration common to personal training, most programming must combine all the aspects of a comprehensive program into 120-180 minutes (or 2-3 sessions) per week. This only represents 1.2-1.8% of the week.

Maximizing a client's exercise (contact) time vitally impacts goal attainment. In an exercise program's early stages, the rest interval may necessitate complete recovery. After the client attains improved fitness status, different activities can be used during the rest interval to work on progressive skills. For instance, if a chest press is completed and a sixty-second rest period is used between sets, it may be an opportune time to work on active rest techniques, such as stability, dynamic flexibility, or low-level, therapeutic back activities. If future progressions will require activities which involve balance, a client could be acclimated to standing on a single foot, or practice stabilizing on a stability disc. Exercise professionals should always look for ways to promote improvements and maximize available contact time.

◆ Prioritizing Needs

The easiest way to become proficient in exercise program design is to:

1. Be able to identify the most important findings during a comprehensive screening and evaluation.
2. Prioritize the defined needs.
3. Understand which activities and exercises address the problems, based on physiological adaptation response.
4. Implement the exercise principles and program components in a manner that will foster goal achievement.

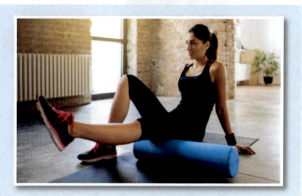

Broad categories requiring improvement that the needs analysis highlights can be refined to create a more specific list of objectives. Then, the trainer identifies solutions that can provide the necessary adaptation-based stress in the most efficient manner that also works within the reasonable capabilities of the client. In most cases, a developmental plan will follow the health, function, fitness continuum to address all issues en route to total goal attainment. This becomes relevant, as most exercise professionals find that the needs analysis identifies health and function issues not related to the client's initial goals. The prevention of disease and age-limiting factors should be prioritized, as these issues relate directly to mortality rates. Deficiencies in health-related fitness and musculoskeletal imbalances should also be ranked among the most important issues. In many cases, one element of an exercise program can provide many benefits and address more than one area of concern simultaneously [8]. For instance, aerobic exercise will aid in cardiorespiratory fitness, while also contributing to reductions in weight and blood pressure [2,4]. Given this fact, time management becomes critical to ensure that the necessary issues and defined goals are managed within the limited contact time an exercise professional has with a given client.

◆ Needs Analysis

A needs analysis helps categorize the relevant findings of a client evaluation. This includes the initial interview, screening protocols, behavior questionnaire, resting assessment battery, physical fitness assessments, and client interview. Any of these utilities may provide data that is identified as important for the client's function, health, or fitness. Areas that affect health and function must become a priority because they represent causes of physical decline, including the presence of disease. These factors attain crucial importance, as the program aim must include efforts that prevent disease foremost. Once these have been addressed, areas of fitness become a priority. Negative fitness-related issues promote premature aging and impact movement proficiency. Therefore, the exercise prescription's ultimate goal should be progression from health attainment toward higher fitness-related measures, as they are more positively associated with health and performance and better physical capabilities.

Making a list of the findings will aid in identifying solutions during the program process. Due to the overlap in reducing negative consequences while promoting positive adaptations,

Making a list of needs-analysis findings can aid in identifying client-specific solutions to use during an exercise program.

systems can be split into categories. Under the health and function category, the three areas of concern are musculoskeletal, cardiovascular, and metabolic health. Skeletal malalignments, such as upper or lower cross syndrome, must be identified and addressed before any advances in fitness can be made because they limit movement and promote injury. Heart rate and blood pressure must be evaluated for cardiovascular function to ensure they are stable and do not present a risk for cardiovascular event. Note that these areas are positively affected by exercise and warrant the implementation of both aerobic and anaerobic activities. Programs may be specialized and modified based on the individually identified issues, and clients with any diagnosed disease will need specific attention to the disease factors. This will be addressed under guidelines for special populations.

Health and fitness-related assessments often present with both high and low marks because people vary in their fitness levels by category, and fitness needs may be more associated with one or more areas. This suggests an individual may score high in one health and fitness related category and low in others. The following demonstrates a sample needs evaluation and an initial action plan.

Health and Function	Assessment
Musculoskeletal	Posture, functional tests (straight-leg hip flexion, Apley test)
Cardiovascular	Resting heart rate and resting blood pressure
Metabolic	Body mass index, central girth, body composition, blood glucose levels

Health and Fitness	Assessment
Cardiorespiratory fitness	Cardiovascular assessments
Muscular fitness	Anaerobic strength, endurance (capacity), power tests
Movement fitness	Stability, flexibility, mobility

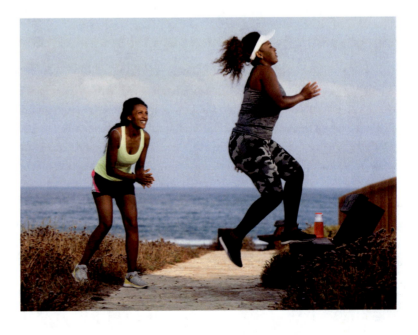

Needs evaluation

Assessment	Issue	Solution	Exercises	Notes
Posture: Plumb line	Forward chin Slight forward shoulder	Strengthen mid/lower trapezius and rhomboids	Y-reaches and T-reaches Seated low and high row Reverse flyes Single-arm row	Tight hamstrings prevent bent-over row: mix Y and T-reaches with good morning (GM)
Flexibility: Failed Apley test Failed Thomas test Failed single-leg hip flexion test	Tight internal rotators Tight hip flexors Tight hamstrings	Stretch pectoralis and subscapularis Stretch rectus femoris and iliopsoas Stretch proximal and distal hamstring	Supinated T-reaches Bulgarian squats Straight-leg and mobility lunges Split-stance good morning Active isolation stretch for each	Focus on lower body unilateral exercises Address flexibility of each in warm-up and cool down
Mobility: Overhead (OH) squat	Tight latissimus dorsi Under-active glutes and rectus abdominis Poor central stability	Stretch latissimus dorsi Strengthen gluteus maximus and rectus abdominis Improve core stability	I-reaches Step-ups, reverse lunges, glute bridges and hip kickbacks Closed-chain abdominal work	No bilateral work until pelvic stability is established Increase OH lifts
Strength balance:	Weak hamstrings Weak trunk flexion Weak glutes	Increase knee flexion strength Increase abdominal strength Increase glute strength	Leg curls (stable and unstable) Modified RDLs Glute-ham raise Eccentric Nordic hamstrings	Cautious of excess back extension
Cardiovascular fitness:	VO_2max 37 ml kg min	Increase CRF	Establish 20 minutes accumulative work in HRTZ	HRTZ minimum 132 beats · min^{-1}
Body Composition:	23%	Reduce body fat	>1000 kcal expenditure week	57 METS of activity
Anthropometrics:	Central girth 41 inches	Reduce total weight	Establish 60 mins accumulative physical activity each day	Provide specific activity list weekly

*HRTZ = Heart Rate Training Zone, CRF = Cardiorespiratory Fitness

◆ Preparation Phase

Early chapters in the text discussed phasic application of stress. Since the body cannot manage a bombardment of all types of stress at the same time, it makes sense to identify the major issues first and establish a plan to restore the issues to functional levels (prioritization model). This means a general preparation or physical readiness phase may be drawn out over several weeks to months before adding any significant challenges, in terms of intensity, towards fitness. Most new exercisers will progress from a period of corrective exercise and strength balance aimed at achieving optimal body function, to more enduring muscular characteristics and kinetic chain enhancements in preparation for increased application towards higher fitness in later phases.

The preparation phase generally aims to accomplish four things:

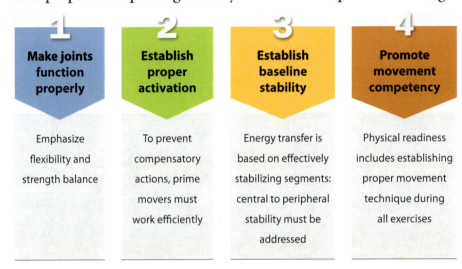

1. Make joints function properly	2. Establish proper activation	3. Establish baseline stability	4. Promote movement competency
Emphasize flexibility and strength balance	To prevent compensatory actions, prime movers must work efficiently	Energy transfer is based on effectively stabilizing segments: central to peripheral stability must be addressed	Physical readiness includes establishing proper movement technique during all exercises

Due to the wide array of issues challenging many new exercisers, as well as the relatively low volume of training associated with personal training settings, traditional exercise approaches do not fit well in the preparation phase. Applying different training systems – circuits, tri-sets and supersets, blended with combination exercises – best serve this phase for enhancing tolerable volume to achieve goal-oriented outcomes. The nature of the activities employed should emphasize motor rehearsal while progressively accounting for the phase's other goals. Generally, resistance loads are light to moderately light (50-70% capacity) because the emphasis falls on the details of proper technique or moving proficiently through full ranges of motion. Additionally, the lower loads provide for different positional applications (e.g., asymmetrical, unilateral, unfamiliar loads) and higher repetition attainment when multiple movements combine. The phase's clear goals and efforts are focused on resolving physical problems.

The following table identifies some common methods that can be used when programming for this phase. Musculoskeletal issues are listed in the table's first column; the second column shows a remedy in the form of a movement. Once the exerciser can perform this motion competently and repeatedly, the trainer can apply a new stress. Challenges to the movement will likely come in the form of resistance, stability, or an increase in ROM. Mastery of the new challenge will signal the trainer to add another stress, based on client-specific factors.

Issue	Remedy	Progression 1	Combination
Underactive glute	Reverse lunge	Add: ipsilateral load	Progressive reverse lunge with MB rotation
Limited spinal rotation	Split stance rotation	Add: medicine ball (MB)	
Tight iliopsoas	Straight-leg lunge with contralateral glute activation	Add: bilateral overhead reach	

MB = Medicine ball

The preparation phase relies heavily on the progressive warm-up segment to aid in reducing movement restriction. Contrary to later phases (strength/power), in the periodization model, when warm-up activities will be determined by the primary exercise selection and written secondary to the program's core aspects. Programming the preparation and anaerobic endurance phases starts out with writing the warm-up based on client-specific considerations and then writing the main program exercises. Certainly, general corrective "cookie cutter" plans exist; however, they lack an individualized approach, and many times do not address a new exerciser's needs. The following table provides an example of the programmatic process to writing a corrective warm-up.

Issue	Solution	Exercise	Combination
Kyphotic exaggeration	Strengthen rhomboids/mid traps; Stretch internal rotators	Wide grip rows; Supinated T-reach	Split-stance GM march with supinated T-reach
Tight hamstrings	Increase knee extension ROM	Wide-leg GM	
Tight latissimus dorsi	Increase shoulder flexion ROM	Split-stance OH reach	
Tight hip flexors	Unilaterally activate glutes while lengthening hip flexor	Forward lunge	Forward lunge with alternate reach
Overactive low back	Increase ROM in spinal flexion	Deep squat spinal flexion; increase lumbar spinal flexor strength	Wide leg ceiling-to-heel reach with posterior pelvic tilt
Weak trunk flexors	Activate rectus abdominis	Standing straight-arm crunch; activate rectus abdominis for 3 second holds	

OH = Overhead, ROM = Range of Motion, GM = Good morning

Introduction to Exercise Programming

Warm-ups in the early phases should be progressive and attempt to emphasize 5-7 issues. Programs should avoid too much variety in order to establish quality movement patterns. Additionally, the selected exercises should showcase activities that will progress into the core aspects of the program in later phases. For instance, a forward lunge with rotation of a PVC bar practiced in early phase warm-ups may eventually become walking lunges with rotation of a 20 lb. straight bar in the primary workout.

Trainers should also consider introducing multi-planar movement during the preparation phase. Actions that take place in all three planes ensure adequate muscle activation, cooperation, and better mobility. In the lower body, lateral squats and side lunges should be instructed, using double or single anchors to ensure proper biomechanics, and in later phases, the client may progress to walking movements with swings that can include the diagonal vectors. Upper body movements in the early phases tend to use longer resistance arms with less weight and focus on bodyweight exercise, whereas these resistance arms shorten as the training focus progresses towards strength and power and more weight is employed.

The following table illustrates some progressive exercise models. Individual movement competence will determine the actual level of adjustment and the duration of time employed to master these before the program advances. Some individuals can skip steps within a progression, while others will require more time before any additional sequences are considered. Programmed progressions should be fluid, seamless, and never forced. Likewise, if a motion induces compensation, it should be regressed to the prior level or adjusted to ensure only quality movements are performed.

Preparation Phase	Anaerobic Endurance Phase	Hypertrophy/ Strength Phase	Strength/ Power Phase
Dumbbell (DB) fly	DB fly on ball	Standing cable fly	Ballistic band fly
Bench push-up	DB chest press	Barbell (BB) bench press	Bench press contrast with MB chest pass
Single-step lateral squat	Alternating step lateral squat with MB	Alternating step with BB lateral squat	Lateral squat walks with KB swing
DB lunges	DB walking lunges	Walking lunges with plate rotations	Ballistic lunges

DB = Dumbbell, MB = Medicine ball, KB = Kettlebell

Exercise selection stems from the needs analysis. In most cases, several different exercises can serve the same adaptive purpose, though some tend to fit better than others in certain phases, depending on the specific adaptation goals. Aligning the activities with the client's aptitude and skill aids in refining the selection. Recall from earlier text that the preparation phase tends to use more closed-chain, unilateral exercises performed using body weight or open-circuit loading. These exercises' characteristics promote localized activation, range of motion (ROM), peripheral and central stability, and movement competence, all established goals of this phase.

Another concern in the early phases relates to oxygen efficiency. Most new exercisers do not have high levels of CRF and often present with VO_2max values and rate pressure products that do not allow for anything more than light to moderate exercise intensity. Of additional consequence is that aerobic metabolism requires more **time-under-tension (TUT)** than resistance training, so those clients that see an exercise professional twice a week will have much more difficulty establishing an acceptable metabolic-fitness foundation. One way to contend with this is to orient the entire exercise training regimen toward cardiovascular-based exercises. Since the resistance used in these movements is less intense, cardio-resistance-based circuits can be combined with aerobic interval circuits to cover 50% of the exercise bout. This provides significant benefits for both foundational health and fitness, as it potentially affects all the health-related components of fitness simultaneously while still addressing the phase-specific goals. The following table shows an example of this concept.

> **DEFINITIONS**
>
> **Time-under-tension (TUT) –**
>
> *The time a muscle spends under load during a set.*

Circuit 1	Box step-up (left leg), MB chest pass, Box step-up (right leg), MB floor to ceiling chop	3 x 15 sec (30 sec between rounds)
Circuit 2	MB squat to press, modified pull-up, leg curl on ball, modified push-up	2 x 20 sec (30 sec between rounds)
Aerobic superset	Stationary bike, rower	5-min bike, 500m row, 5-min bike; must attain steady state heart rate in each
Total time-under-tension		21 minutes

MB = Medicine Ball

Following the aerobic segment, the body should be brought back to baseline metabolism. Cool downs are necessary for clearing metabolic leftovers, attenuating myofascial tension, and returning blood to the heart. During the preparation phase, many of the initial cooldown activities resemble, in whole or in part, the training movements that have been used previously. A dynamic application of mobility should be emphasized first. Then, foam massage-type rolling of the fascia is followed by static stretching of the most restricted areas. Generally, hip flexors, hip extensors (glutes and hamstrings), calves, trunk extensors and rotators, and internal and external shoulder rotators top the charts as areas of inflexibility. The flexibility assessments will reflect the areas requiring the most attention and specific emphasis. It cannot be overstated that lack of flexibility and mobility are significant impediments to adaptation and must be addressed early and often in the training phases.

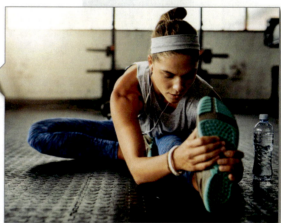

Cool downs are necessary for clearing metabolic leftovers, attenuating myofascial tension, and returning blood to the heart.

When constructing a personal training program, trainers can reverse the periodization model in a unique way in comparison to the typical design of sports models. In periodization for sport conditioning, the season of play dramatically affects the program phases. Athletes work around the season rather than the season and training regimen working around the athlete's development. For personal training clients, the phases of training do not have to change until the phase's specific goals have been met. Since the trainer bases all decisions on the client's progress, the phases can be manipulated to best meet the individual's current needs. Therefore, a phase may be lengthened or shortened depending on the accomplishments achieved and goals fulfilled in each phase.

It was stated earlier that the preparation phase may last months for deconditioned or older adults. A 60-day preparation phase, for instance, is completely appropriate if progress is steadily being made, and the individual is improving in the areas of need.

Sample Program – Preparation Phase

Warm-up – 2 sets of 30 sec for each exercise
- GM
- Step back with I-reach
- Ground reach with trunk flexion
- GM with T-reach
- Reverse lunge with OH reach
- Lateral lunge with rotation reach

Time: 6 minutes

Activation-specific drills – 2 x 10 for each exercise
- Glute bridge
- Band pull-downs (scapular plane)
- Prone T-pulls on bench

Time: 3 minutes

Core Workout: Primary Exercises

Exercise	Load	Sets	Reps	Rest	System
DB modified deadlift	Load to form	3	up to 12	45 sec	Superset
Bench push-ups	Body weight				
MB OH reverse lunge	6lb. MB	3	up to 12	45 sec	Superset
Standing cable row	Load to form				
Lateral step-up	20 lbs.	3	up to 10	45 sec	Superset
Standing DB press					
Leg curl	30 lbs.	4	up to 15	60 sec	Tri-set
Bench hip bridge	BW				
Bench (prone) reverse flies	8 lbs.				
Bike + row	4 METs	2	7.5 min (each)		Transitional

Time: 35 minutes

Cool down – 2 x 6 reps (3 per side) with 5 sec holds

Lunge with lateral lean	2x	Circuit
Hip flexor step back		
Lateral lunge ground reach		

Time: 3 minutes

Active isolation stretch: distal and proximal hamstring	2x15 sec
Partner-assisted hip-flexor stretch	2x15 sec
Partner-assisted pectoralis stretch	2x15 sec

Time: 1.5 minutes

Foam roll low back, IT band, glute
Time: 3 minutes

Total activity time: 51.5 minutes

GM = Good morning, OH = Overhead, DB = Dumbbell, MB = Medicine ball, BW = Bodyweight

◆ Anaerobic Endurance Phase

Anaerobic endurance is a logical continuation of the preparation phase's activities. As with all transitional phases, certain aspects will progress, while others remain consistent. Too much variety in the preparation phase can be detrimental to a client's progress towards proficiency in high quality movement patterns. Where many of the exercises will remain the same between phases, changes will most often occur in how much weight is used, how the exercises are loaded (i.e.; asymmetrical, overhead, unfamiliar), and the rest interval between sets. The program goals also remain consistent, with some added components, like stabilizer endurance, strength, and improved kinetic chain proficiency, used to prepare for the transition to the next phase.

The primary goals of the anaerobic endurance phase:

Continue to promote proper activation, strength balance, and ROM

Increase central and peripheral stability segments

Enhance ground reaction force transfer and kinetic chain proficiency

Increase mobility and movement competency: train movements (emphasis), not muscles

Although trainers can stress each of these goals independently, addressing multiple goals via coordinated efforts saves time and aligns more appropriately with how the body learns. As mentioned previously, the warm-up phase presents the perfect opportunity to introduce movements which can be used as 'practice activities' to secure movement proficiency. Once mastered, these same activities can be made more challenging and will eventually migrate from the warm-up to become aspects of the training's core. A GM with forward I-reach, for instance, can be developed to include using two light DBs or plates. Light load adjustments and unfamiliar loading through the use of light weights, resistance bands, PVC pipe, sand bags, and medicine balls all make excellent additions to progress movements during this phase. The goal is movement mastery, so the duration of time the activities are used in the warm-up will depend on the client's development via motor rehearsal. The following table demonstrates some progressive options for increasing the demand of an activity while still focusing on the details of quality movement execution.

Preparation phase warm-up circuit	Anaerobic endurance warm-up circuit	Demand of the activity
GM with I-reach	GM with I-reach using 2.5 lb. plate raise	Increases demands in posterior chain
Reverse lunge	MB OH reverse lunge	Increases demands in central stabilizers
Lateral lunge with rotation	Lateral lunge with MB rotation	Challenges lateral stability and ROM

GM = Good Morning, OH = Overhead, MB = Medicine ball

> **DEFINITIONS**
>
> **Residual adaptations –**
> *Physiological training effects that are retained for a period of time after ceasing a particular form of training.*

The previous table clearly denotes that the exercises' base movements change little, if at all, but the progressions from one phase to the next will elicit an increase in the activity's demand via the stressors added. Premature and overaggressive progressions represent the most common problems endemic to program adjustments. An effective method for progression through phases is to build on the **residual adaptations** through movement adjustments. If for instance, a supine hip bridge was used in the preparation phase, consider adding some challenge to the glute activation by performing the activity unilaterally from the ground or bilaterally on a bench. In both cases, the demand increases, but the exercise selection's purpose remains the same: glute activation. As mentioned before, changing the loading location is also a common theme of this phase. The following table shows some typical examples.

Preparation phase	Anaerobic endurance	Demand of the activity
Step-up	Step-up with ipsilateral (shouldered) sand bag	Increases demands in prime movers and challenges central stability
Walking lunge	Walking lunge with a front-loaded position	Increases demands in anterior chain
DB reverse lunge	Reverse lunge to DB press	Challenges central and peripheral stability

DB = Dumbbell

Since the anaerobic endurance phase consists predominantly of open circuit, unilateral movements, it provides for numerous exercise combinations. Lunges can join with presses, side raises, cable pulls, and rotational activities; Bulgarian squats and step-ups can be employed similarly or partnered with a variety of arm and trunk movements or unfamiliar loading schematics. These are complementary exercises when programmed as supersets. Combination and multi-movement exercises can also be used in circuits but tend to be overly fatiguing, thereby making supersets a preferred training system in this phase. This is particularly true with efforts at or above 70% of maximal capacity. Repetition ranges continue to be towards the higher end of the spectrum, as movement rehearsal is still emphasized. While the common training intensity ranges from 60-80% of 1RM, superset loads in this phase are generally programmed at less than 75% 1RM. Similar to the preparation phase, tri-sets and circuits can be used to enhance cardiovascular benefit. All the while, the aerobic base should continue to be emphasized. Performing 20-30 minutes of fairly continuous movement provides the most benefit.

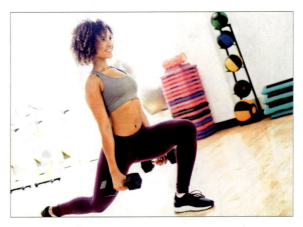

Sample Program – Anaerobic Endurance Phase

Warm-up – 2 sets of 30 sec for each exercise
GM T-reach
Broad step-back with alternate reach
Lateral ground sweeps with trunk flexion
Split-stance GM with Y-reach
Reverse lunge with rotation
Lateral squat with MB swing
Time: 6 minutes

Activation-specific drills – 2 x 10 for each exercise
Supine bench bridge
Band pull-aparts
Prone M-reach with 2.5 lb. plates on incline bench
Time: 3 minutes

Core Workout: Primary Exercises

Exercise	Load	Sets	Reps	Rest	System
3/4 squat to neutral grip press Modified pull-up	15 lbs. BW	4	up to 10	45 sec	Superset
Walking lunge (front hold) Standing cable chest press	8 lb. MB Load to form	3	up to 12	45 sec	Superset
DB Romanian deadlift T-bar row Bench push-ups	20 lbs. 25 lb. plate BW	3	up to 10	60 sec	Tri-set
Leg curl on ball Seated trunk rotation Ab curl-up to press	BW 6 lb. MB 10 lbs.	3	up to 15	60 sec	Tri-set
Climb, row, bike	5 METs	1	5 min (each)		Transitional

Time: 35 minutes

Cool down – 2 x 6 reps (3 per side) with 5 sec holds
Lunge with alternate reach — 2x — Circuit
Bulgarian squat
Broad lateral squats with reach
Time: 3 minutes

Active isolation stretch: distal and proximal hamstring — 2x15 sec
Partner-assisted hip-flexor stretch — 2x15 sec
Partner-assisted pectoralis stretch — 2x15 sec
Time: 1.5 minutes

Foam roll low back, IT band, glute
Time: 3 minutes

Total activity time: 51.5 minutes

GM = Good morning, MB = Medicine ball, BW = Bodyweight

◆ Hypertrophy-Strength

The hypertrophy-strength phase gets its name from the fact that increases in lean mass improve muscle's relative force output. In this phase, residual adaptations associated with increases in ROM, mobility, and stability from the prior phases support the decision to employ more resistance for select exercises. Hypertrophy phases often emphasize muscles over movement, and use moderate time-tension relationships, generally lasting 20-45 seconds (6-15 repetitions). In personal training scenarios, a logistical conflict exists when the emphasis is gaining lean mass, as the training volume tends to be far too low to yield significant change. The set-rep parameters can be consistent, but to attain the minimum threshold for (significant) hypertrophic adaptations from training, at least 10 sets per muscle group should be accumulated per week. To accomplish this with a 3 day per week resistance training regimen, increasing emphasis on specific training systems helps reach the goal.

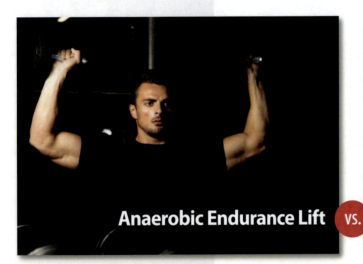
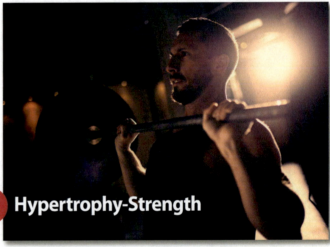

Anaerobic Endurance Lift vs. **Hypertrophy-Strength**

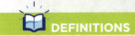

Accumulative fatigue –

Occurs when the effects of one workout builds up and transfers to the next training session.

During the hypertrophy-strength phase, pyramids, compound sets, and strip sets will be used to complement traditional hypertrophy supersets. Tri-sets and circuits can still be used, but because loading intensities increase to 70-85% 1RM, they are less commonly employed. As more exercises are introduced to a set (i.e., superset, tri-set, circuits), the resistance must be lighter to maintain form due to **accumulative fatigue**. Another characteristic of this phase involves the increase in closed-circuit, bilateral exercises. While unilateral exercises encourage peripheral stability and increased activation across a broader ROM, bilateral actions promote greater strength gains, as heavier loads can be utilized.

Goals of the hypertrophy-strength phase include:

 Improve force transfer across the kinetic chain

 Increase lean mass

 Increase force output

 Challenge stability with mobility

Warm-ups in this phase represent a combination of corrective strategies along with more movement-specific resistance preparation. This provides and represents an ideal time to practice lifts, movements, and exercises that will be used in the subsequent exercise bouts or in later phases. The following table reflects some examples of these changes. Hypertrophy-strength phases tend to last 3-5 weeks when performed on the heavy side (80-90% of 1RM) of the resistance spectrum, but may last 6-10 weeks when used in a progressive development process, with less emphasis on near maximal loading to volitional failure. The reason the duration (in weeks) is less than other phases is the body cannot tolerate maximal lifting combined with maximal TUT for a very long period before overtraining occurs. The body recovers more efficiently to lower exercise load, compared to higher loads, when the volumes match.

Warm-up Exercise	Purpose	Prepare For:	Progress To:
MB squat swings	Improve central stability and pelvic control	Back squats	OH-bar squats
Reverse lunge with MB OH press	Improve mobility in lats, glutes, and hip flexors	Axial-loaded lunges	Lunge to DB press
MB OH forward lunge with lateral lean	Prevent medial-lateral femoral sway; stretch lateral sling and IT band	BB front squats and BB front-loaded lunges	BB OH lunge

GM = Good Morning, OH = Overhead, MB = Medicine ball, BB = Barbell, DB = Dumbbell

Implementation of more traditional exercises occurs in the hypertrophy-strength phase. This phase also begins the crossover from glycolysis (moderate loads across moderate repetitions) to the phosphagen system (heavier loads across fewer repetitions). When performed with the intent of maximizing lean mass, the emphasis intends to trigger anabolic hormone response. Recall from earlier chapters that this requires heavy compound exercises, including squats, deadlifts, leg press, bench press, and military press with limited rest to promote greater anabolic concentrations in the blood, and isolated muscle activity to stimulate ischemic responses from the tissue to trigger growth factor release.

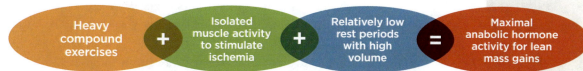

When programs include six days of training per week, trainers commonly pair muscle groups to attain adequate volume in order to achieve maximal total recruitment of each area of the body. As previously mentioned, pairing chest and triceps or back and biceps often characterizes traditional bodybuilding approaches. In a three day program, this becomes impractical; in personal training scenarios, it makes better sense to perform a total body "with emphasis" plan. While a total body day helps meet weekly volume requirements, the "emphasis" of each day reflects a theme (push, pull, lower body, etc.). The program may have "total body with push" emphasis on Monday, "total body with leg" emphasis on Wednesday, and "total body with pull" emphasis on Friday. This allows for greater total volume across the whole body when the goal is adding lean mass and provides the opportunity to accumulate 10 sets per muscle group in 3 1-hour personal training programs. The following table demonstrates the nuances of this program modification.

Traditional Body Building – Chest and Triceps	Total Body with Push Emphasis
Bench press *12, 10, 8, 6, 10*	BB front squat to OH press *3x6*
Incline DB press *4x8*	Bench press *4x10*
Dips *3x failure*	Lunge to OH DB press *4x5 per side*
DB push-ups s/s cable flys *4x12/10*	Bench push-up to slide pike *3x failure*
Supine triceps extension s/s close-grip bench *4x failure*	Chest flys s/s rear deltoid pulls *3x10/10*
Triceps push-down *5x10*	Triceps pull-over s/s high-to-low cable cross pulls to arm extension *3x8/10-12*
Cable triceps kickback *3x12 side*	Incline sit-up to DB press *4x10*
Total TUT: 16 minutes Total workout time: 42 minutes	Total TUT: 13.5 minutes Total workout time: 37 minutes

DB = Dumbbell, BB = Barbell, OH = Overhead, S/S = Superset, TUT = time-under-tension

The rest interval is a key element in the development of strength and mass. For strength, longer rest intervals are appropriate. Hypertrophic adaptations require shorter rest intervals to promote cellular ischemia in efforts to trigger a growth-factor response. The lowest amount of recovery time needed to repeat the exercise set with proper form represents a guide to rest intervals, which is normally between 30-90 seconds, depending on the individual and load. Rep schemes of 6-8, at 80-85% 1RM, may require 90 seconds of recovery, particularly for stronger individuals, whereas a set of 10-12 repetitions loaded appropriately at 70-75% 1RM will likely require only 30-45 seconds recovery for well-trained individuals.

Aerobic training during these later phases generally shifts from modality adjustments to intensity adjustments. Since the increase in resistance requires more recovery between sets, less time is available for tri-sets and circuits that are part of the aerobic plan. Thus, higher intensity interval-based aerobic exercise becomes the dominant training system employed in this phase, as clients should now be able to tolerate higher intensities above steady state values. Even 15 minutes of interval training can have profound adaptive effects when high intensities are reached. Another training system of choice that may be used during this phase is the introduction of anaerobic conditioning drills with 1:1-1:3 work-rest ratios. Repeat sprints (running or biking), cone drills, and lactate stations can be employed to add to caloric deficit while raising heart rates for those at the intermediate training level.

Due to the significant blood flow dynamics associated with localized muscle emphasis, a proper cool down is crucial. Dynamic mobility activities and foam rolling are relevant inclusions from this phase forward. Likewise, to take advantage of the metabolic environment, a planned recovery drink or food should be arranged within 30-45 minutes of exercise

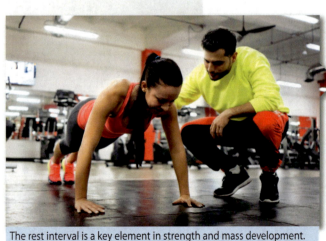

The rest interval is a key element in strength and mass development. For strength, longer rest intervals allow maximal force production due to the maximal energy made available through more recovery time. Hypertrophic adaptations require shorter rest intervals to promote cellular ischemia in efforts to trigger a growth-factor response.

cessation. The more emphasis that is placed on specific muscles, the more recovery becomes a priority. Recovery should start with a sufficient cooldown, followed by adequate, balanced fluid and energy provisions.

Sample Program – Hypertrophy-Strength Phase (Pull Emphasis)

Warm-up – 2 sets of 30 sec for each exercise
- Wide leg floor to ceiling reach
- MB OH forward lunge
- OH squat
- 3-reach deadlift
- Lunge with rotation to OH reach
- OH squat with MB swing

Time: 6 minutes

Activation-specific drills – 2 x 10 for each exercise
- Ballistic reverse T-flys
- Band M-pulls

Time: 2 minutes

Core Workout: Primary Exercises

Exercise	Load	Sets	Reps	Rest	System
BB front squat to press	45 lb. bar	4	up to 8	60 sec	Combination
Bent-over row	Load to form	3	up to 8	60 sec	
Reverse lunge with cable row	20 lbs.	2	6 per side	45 sec	Combination
Lateral KB swings	15 lbs.	2	4 per side	30 sec	
Lat pull down	60 lbs.	3	up to 10	45 sec	Superset
High-bar row	45 lbs.				
Seated row	BW	3	up to 15	45 sec	Superset
Straight bar curls	30 lbs.				
Abdominal pull-over	6 lb. MB	4	up to 6 each	30 sec	Transitional
Eccentric Nordic hamstrings	BW				
Row	5-8 METs	1	17 min		Intervals

Time: 25 minutes

Cool down – 2 x 6 reps (3 per side) with 5 sec holds
- Lunge with lateral lean   2x   Circuit
- Lateral lunge with rotation
- Supine straight-leg march

Time: 3 minutes

Active isolation stretch: distal and proximal hamstring	2x15 sec
Iron cross stretch	2x15 sec
Active-assisted lat/triceps stretch	2x15 sec

Time: 1.5 minutes

Foam roll low back, IT band, glute

Time: 3 minutes

Total activity time: 40.5 minutes

MB = Medicine ball, OH = Overhead, BB = Barbell, KB = Kettlebell, BW = Bodyweight

◆ Strength-Power

Strength-power training phases may emphasize strength or power preferentially but inherently suggest a shift toward increased movement velocity. Since strength is the application of force, and power is the speed at which force is applied, a common theme in this phase is increasing the speed of work. Dynamic voluntary contractions tend to become ballistic in nature. The exercises may remain consistent, but the load is reduced while movement speed increases. This is appropriate for a large variety of clients when matched appropriately, as power is an important functional component of fitness and indicator of independent living. Exercise selection and implementation are defined by client capabilities. For instance, a 70-year-old male may perform sit-to-stand repetitions for time, whereas a 17-year-old high school athlete may perform squat jumps.

Notably, an integrated approach to strength and power can best serve individuals when the training goal is health and fitness rather than athletic development. Understanding that power is a rate of work, programming in these phases should help transfer competent, controlled movements from previous phases into faster paced actions. Consider some of the following transitions or phasic exercise progressions.

Strength	Power
Back squat	Squat jumps
BB walking lunges	Lunge jumps
Incline bench press	Incline MB pass
Push-ups	Speed or clap push-ups
Cable trunk rotation	MB alternating side pass

BB = Barbell, MB = Medicine ball

In general, only proficient actions are used for ballistic movements because load is exchanged for speed, and ballistic activities may cause harm if not performed correctly. Step-ups for instance, should be performed with perfect technique under load before introducing ballistic step-ups or jumps. Likewise, intensity should not increase dramatically as the exercises migrate towards power. If jumps are used, a person must be able to land efficiently before attempting ballistic jumps and plyometrics. Building up movement capabilities and skill efficiency prevents injury. Box jumps should start at 12 inches with competent stretch shortening movement and soft landings before moving up to 15 or 18 inches. A common error, as with all power movements, is being overly aggressive with the exercises or intensity programmed. As a general rule, body weight is used before external loading. Loading is never heavy: normally <10% of body weight is used for loads when weighting ballistic exercise, as body weight is key to the resistance. Many personal trainers err by arbitrarily adding weight to fast paced exercises instead of calculating appropriate training loads, forgetting the goal of movement quality.

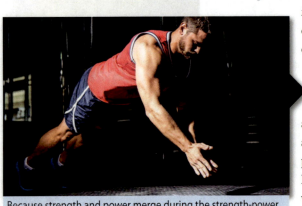

Because strength and power merge during the strength-power phase, the repetitions attained during each set tend to be more time-specific rather than a defined numerical range of repetitions.

When strength and power merge, the repetitions attained during the set tend to be more time specific rather than a defined numerical range of repetitions. In most cases, power-based exercises rely on the phosphagen system, so the activities tend to last <20 seconds and require longer rest intervals; this is particularly true with higher intensities. Some common examples include:

- Ballistic push-ups performed at max speed for 15 seconds with 90-second rest periods
- Power cleans using 4 repetitions at 80% 1RM with a 2-minute recovery
- High-knee lateral cone step using intervals of 10 seconds on, 30 seconds off.

The activity complexity, velocity of movement, and load determine the number of sets, time-under-tension (reps) and load assignments for the exercise. Trainers should prefer increasing the number of sets of an exercise over increasing repetitions per set to add volume in this phase. If the load is only body weight, then the time-tension relationship may increase with no change to the rest intervals. Contrarily, when resistance is added, both parameters must be adjusted: time tension will be reduced while recovery is increased. Again, the demands on the energy system, training experience, and overall fitness will be qualifying determinants.

In most personal training scenarios, power is used in an integrated fashion and will not solely be emphasized across all exercises performed in a single training bout. Reducing loads and adding speed is a common theme across populations and can be accomplished with a number of training modalities. Bands replace cables for fast movement, MBs replace DBs and BBs, as they can be thrown and slammed, slide boards are used for traditional leg exercises and novel equipment, such as kettlebells and ropes, can be implemented as well. Certainly, Olympic lifts and plyometrics can be used if an exercise professional has received proper training in teaching the exercises proficiently, and the client maintains adequate mobility and joint health to perform the activities. Olympic exercises though, are often reserved for those training for higher performance levels.

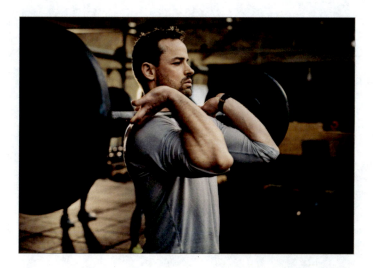

Sample Program – Strength-Power (Lower Body Emphasis)

Warm-up – 2 sets of 30 sec for each exercise

MB floor to ceiling reach	Hip-flexor march
MB reverse lunge with rotation	Lunge with MB press
OH squat swings	Lateral MB squat swings

Time: 6 minutes

Activation-specific drills – 2 x 10 for each exercise

Ballistic MB squat pass
Band OH squat pulls

Time: 2 minutes

Core Workout: Primary Exercises

Exercise	Load	Sets	Reps	Rest	System
Back squat	75, 80, 85% 1RM	4	10, 7, 5, 5	90 sec	Contrast
Squat jump	6 lb. MB	Last 2 sets	6		
Jump pull-ups	BW	3	AMAP	60 sec	
Lateral ballistic box step-over	BW	2	15 sec side	30 sec between legs	
Speed push-ups	BW	3	up to 10	45 sec	Superset
Inverted row	BW				
Leg curl on slide	BW	3	15 sec	45 sec	Superset
Slide adduction	BW				
Hanging leg raises	BW	4	up to 6 each	30 sec	Superset
Alternating reverse lunge with band rotation	Light band		20 sec		
Jog/run	5-8 METs	1	15 min		Intervals

Time: 38 minutes

Cool down – 2 x 6 reps (3 per side) with 5 sec holds

Lunge with rotation	2x	Circuit
RDL march		
T-march with hip extension		

Time: 3 minutes

Active isolation stretch: distal and proximal hamstring	2x15 sec
Low back stretch	2x15 sec
Active-assisted glute stretch	2x15 sec

Time: 1.5 minutes

Foam roll low back, IT band, glute

Time: 3 minutes

Total activity time: 53.5 minutes

MB = Medicine ball, OH = Overhead, BW = Bodyweight, AMAP = As many as possible

◆ Progressions and Re-assessments

The characteristics of training each phase demonstrate the variety of exercise possibilities that exists in programming for diverse populations. Personal training clients may require different methods and systems to best address their individual issues. Numerous program options must necessarily cater to the various client characteristics, which often result in programs as diverse as the clients themselves. Traditional approaches to personal training follow a modified body builder/strength program that ineffectively meets most client's needs. Although the stress of 8-10 exercises performed using 3 sets of 10 repetitions will cause adaptations, this schema does not provide for the many individual needs of the average client.

Writing exercise prescriptions requires ongoing, appropriate management of both the needs assessment and the client's defined goals. An individualized approach is necessary for client specific, long-term success. Testing results and re-evaluation criteria should be incorporated into the program and used to inform the creation of the prescribed stress [5, 9]. Personal trainers should recall the use of effective goal strategies, focusing on daily and weekly objectives to stay on track for both short and long-term goal attainment. Goal attainment quantification should remain consistent with the tests and evaluation criteria used to assess and re-assess the training program's effectiveness. A recommended approach will use movements and systems in the program that are similar to, or the same as, those used in the testing protocols. This strategy will provide for quantified improvements that the clients can see, fostering a positive psychological impression about their capabilities and progress. When setting the goals, exercise professionals must be conscious of time constraints and the dose-response gradient of physiological adaptations. The nervous system responds quickly to stress, whereas the muscular, metabolic, and cardiovascular systems experience a slower adaptation process.

Neural efficiency often contributes to a rapid adaptation rate in the first 4-6 weeks, provided adequate volume is used. As explained previously, during the initial training phases, clients may experience improvements beyond the norm, and progressions can be matched to support these adjustments. However, the emphasis should still be on skill acquisition and motor learning rather than resistance-based overload. Once the body reaches its initial improvement response (usually the initial 3-4 weeks), shifting to a progression rate of 2.5% per week is usually an appropriate goal for progressive overload. This value adequately provides a functional target that the body can adapt to on an ongoing basis [1]. Aggressive progressions of more than 2.5-5% usually lead to faulty movement patterns, incorrect performance via aberrant neuromuscular compensation, and an increase in the potential for injury. Perpetual monitoring of individual performances will help define the best progression rate for each client. The body adapts to stress based on the duration of exposure, intensity, mode of exercise, and frequency of application. Therefore, the number of times a client engages the program components per week will influence the rate of adaptation and subsequent progression, provided intensity is appropriate. A client who participates at a higher training volume will progress at a proportionately faster rate than if he or she uses lower volume; of course, this is an inherent problem when clients train only twice a week [3, 6, 12, 13].

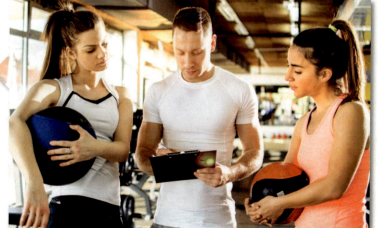

Writing exercise prescriptions requires appropriate and ongoing management of the needs analysis and defined goals; an individualized approach is necessary for client specific, long-term success. Progressive changes and re-testing are also integral to optimizing and continuing adaptations.

◆ Duration of Program Phases and Cycles

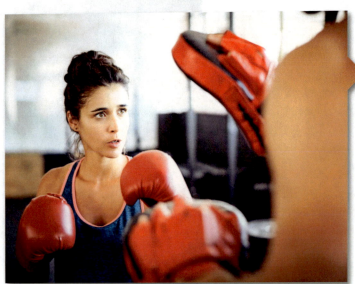

Exercise programs may be aimed at eliciting any number of adaptive responses. The specific adaptation and magnitude of improvement desired will determine what efforts (time and type) are necessary to achieve the sought-after effect. As adaptations are attained, the program must continue to progress to create a new perceived stress in order for the next level of physiological improvement to occur. Regarding the priority of the adaptations, programs evolve from different emphases and foci toward new directions. The priority focus should continually address defined physiological need and specific goal attainment. Recalling the characteristics of effective goal setting, a designated time-period exists in which efforts should concentrate on achieving short and long-term goals. Programming activities and components, including the application of progressive overload and physiologically specific stress, should reflect a calculated time period, or training cycle.

Training cycles are categorized by time or outcomes:

- Macrocycles may last 6-12 months
- Mesocycles tend to last less than 3 months
- Microcycles may include any number of weeks for an acute goal

Normally personal training employs mesocycles, where two or more training phases are applied over 3-6 weeks [7]. Utilizing a designated length of time allows for a premeditated and structured plan for the appropriate application of stress. The quantified periods of planned stress also allow for retesting the emphasized components at the end of the training cycle to identify the programming's effectiveness and to set the next training cycle's values.

When the needs list is extensive, the training cycles may employ specific emphases in a building-block approach (periodization) and change at the beginning of each new cycle. For instance, the initial training cycle may consist of a 6-week preparation and anaerobic endurance phase to emphasize motor learning, movement patterning, baseline endurance, and general conditioning in preparation for more challenging training protocols. The next training cycle may modify the phases to emphasize specific movement strength and more coordinated activities requiring 8 weeks of training to attain the necessary adaptation response. The actual training cycle length will be based on the client contact time, fitness status, training experience, and training aptitude. If a client does not comply with the initially programmed frequency, the training cycle may have to be lengthened to allow for adequate exposure to the exercise stress. Concentrating on specific goals, rather than taking a broad approach to address everything at one time, increases the likelihood of timely goal attainment. This is not to suggest selecting only one or two issues and ignoring the rest of the needs list but rather implies planned emphasis, based on a system of priority.

◆ Program Tracking

Program components should be tracked on a daily basis to gauge the program's effectiveness and to monitor for any problems that may present themselves during the training. Exercise professionals should record each performance so that progressive overload can be properly applied in each training bout, and movement proficiency can be evaluated. Once exercise adaptation has occurred, the body will require a new perceived stress to support continued improvements. This is where many exercisers fail, as they continue to use the same stress routinely. This explains why a person may spend more time in the gym without experiencing any change to his or her physique or measured performance. Tracking also holds value in identifying how effective each program component is at addressing its intended purpose. If certain areas of improvement are noticed, the programmed activities are serving their intended role in those areas. If other areas do not show progress, then the applied stress is incorrect on some level. Trainers should review the intensity, volume, rest interval used, and specificity of the stress to identify the problem. If tracking is not used, these errors may not be recognized until the end of the training cycle. This error wastes both time and effort. Identifying these obstacles early on allows for productive program adjustments. Likewise, if results are relatively slow, the stress should be analyzed to determine its adequacy. In many cases, adaptations occur to the initial exercise stress and adjustments to new progressions are either overly aggressive or insufficient to stimulate the next level of physiological attainment.

Program tracking is also necessary from a liability standpoint. If a personal trainer finds him or herself involved in litigation, the program components are often reviewed for appropriateness. If the documented programming information is limited or non-existent, it becomes difficult to defend correct procedure, as no tangible proof exists. Trainers must document and maintain program records, a standard of all professional training services. Additionally, using programs to identify client improvements instills confidence in one's professional capabilities and can be used for motivation in the program. For example, clients who do not show improvements in body composition may want to give up or assume the personal trainer is not fully competent. Providing reinforcement through other adaptation improvements may be the justification needed to keep clients motivated and on track.

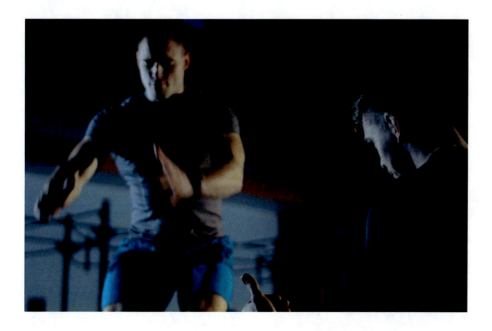

REFERENCES:

1. Bird SP, Tarpenning KM, and Marino FE. Designing Resistance Training Programmes to Enhance Muscular Fitness. *Sports Medicine* 35: 841-851, 2005.

2. Bouaziz W, Vogel T, Schmitt E, Kaltenbach G, Geny B, and Lang PO. Health benefits of aerobic training programs in adults aged 70 and over: a systematic review. *Archives of gerontology and geriatrics* 69: 110-127, 2017.

3. Braith R, Graves J, Pollock M, Leggett S, Carpenter D, and Colvin A. Comparison of 2 vs 3 days/week of variable resistance training during 10-and 18-week programs. *International Journal of Sports Medicine* 10: 450-454, 1989.

4. Ciolac EG. High-intensity interval training and hypertension: maximizing the benefits of exercise? *American journal of cardiovascular disease* 2: 102, 2012.

5. Fletcher GF, Balady GJ, Amsterdam EA, Chaitman B, Eckel R, Fleg J, Froelicher VF, Leon AS, Piña IL, and Rodney R. Exercise standards for testing and training: a statement for healthcare professionals from the American Heart Association. *Circulation* 104: 1694-1740, 2001.

6. Grgic J, Schoenfeld BJ, Davies TB, Lazinica B, Krieger JW, and Pedisic Z. Effect of Resistance Training Frequency on Gains in Muscular Strength: A Systematic Review and Meta-Analysis. *Sports Medicine:* 1-14, 2018.

7. Hartmann H, Wirth K, Keiner M, Mickel C, Sander A, and Szilvas E. Short-term Periodization Models: Effects on Strength and Speed-strength Performance. *Sports Medicine* 45: 1373-1386, 2015.

8. Johannsen NM, Swift DL, Lavie CJ, Earnest CP, Blair SN, and Church TS. Combined aerobic and resistance training effects on glucose homeostasis, fitness, and other major health indices: a review of current guidelines. *Sports Medicine* 46: 1809-1818, 2016.

9. Kraemer WJ and Ratamess NA. Fundamentals of resistance training: progression and exercise prescription. *Medicine and science in sports and exercise* 36: 674-688, 2004.

10. Peterson MD, Rhea MR, and Alvar BA. Applications of the dose-response for muscular strength development: a review of meta-analytic efficacy and reliability for designing training prescription. *Journal of Strength and Conditioning Research* 19: 950, 2005.

11. Pollock ML, Franklin BA, Balady GJ, Chaitman BL, Fleg JL, Fletcher B, Limacher M, Piña IL, Stein RA, and Williams M. Resistance exercise in individuals with and without cardiovascular disease: benefits, rationale, safety, and prescription an advisory from the committee on exercise, rehabilitation, and prevention, council on clinical cardiology, American Heart Association. *Circulation* 101: 828-833, 2000.

12. Rhea MR, Alvar BA, Burkett LN, and Ball SD. A meta-analysis to determine the dose response for strength development, 2003.

13. Schoenfeld BJ, Ogborn D, and Krieger JW. Effects of Resistance Training Frequency on Measures of Muscle Hypertrophy: A Systematic Review and Meta-Analysis. *Sports Medicine* 46: 1689-1697, 2016.

Advanced Concepts of Personal Training

NCSF Certified Personal Trainer

Chapter 17

Working with Special Populations

Working with Special Populations

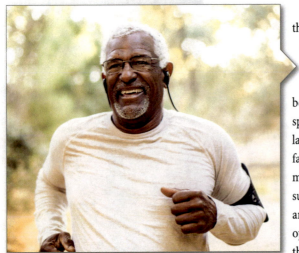

Special populations represent defined subgroups of the general population that present with certain acute or chronic conditions that may or may not be pathophysiological. Take for instance, two separate time periods in life, childhood, and pregnancy, that present specific physiological conditions that are not abnormal; however, constituents of these groups fall under a special subgroup because the physiology associated with the developmental time period dictates special considerations for physical activity (PA) that differ from the general population. Similarly, individuals in pre-disease states and those with diagnosed disease fall under a special subgroup because of physiological variances that may warrant modification from regular exercise prescriptions. In all cases, the term 'special' suggests evaluating and monitoring the individual for specific physiological indices and modifying programmatic components to promote positive adaptations that optimally improve the respective condition, or at the very minimum, do not worsen the condition. For the hypertensive client, this means lowering blood pressure (BP) and heart disease (HD) risk; for the child, this means age-appropriate assessments and PA regimens; for the pregnant female, this means maintaining health and fitness while reducing (exposure) risks for the unborn child.

Exercise professionals have a fiduciary responsibility to maintain adequate competency relative to the individuals they service. In some cases, the risks associated with certain conditions warrant higher levels of competency than is measured by a personal trainer certification exam. In such cases, exercise professionals should seek additional education and training before working with higher-risk, special populations. For the purposes of this text, the following diseases and conditions are presented as controlled with or without medication, and, as such, reflect individuals with stable conditions who can and should exercise. For those with pre-existing disorders, medical referral is often recommended before initiating PA, and in some cases, physicians will define parameters based on relative factors or medications. These requirements have been outlined under the "Screening and Evaluation" section of this text.

◆ Exercise & Asthma

Asthma is a chronic, inflammatory pulmonary disorder that causes recurrent spasmodic episodes and is characterized by hyperirritability or a reversible obstruction of the airways, known colloquially as asthma attacks. The disease is classified as a chronic obstructive pulmonary disorder (COPD) caused by smooth muscle contraction and airway reactivity, leading to bronchospasms. The narrowing of the airway passages due to constriction is further worsened by the swelling of the windpipe lining and an increase in mucus produced along the tract, which makes it difficult to breathe. Major episodes of asthma can restrict breathing to a point that becomes life threatening. Over 3,500 Americans die each year from asthma, with the highest incidence among African-Americans [20]. Of the nearly 25 million asthmatics in the United States, more than one fourth of them are under 18 years of age [18]. Indirect costs of asthma

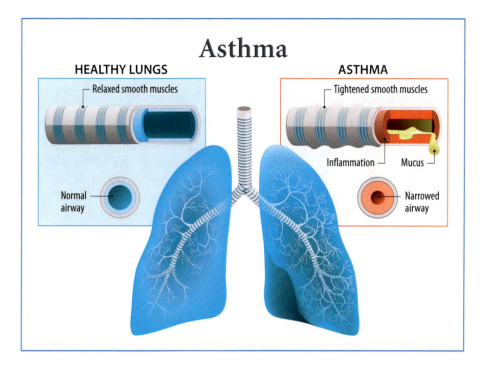

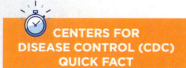

CENTERS FOR DISEASE CONTROL (CDC) QUICK FACT

Current asthma prevalence is higher among adults with obesity than among those with normal weight for all races and Hispanic origin groups.

include missed work or skill days from sickness or death, and lost work output exceeds $56 billion annually in the United States, with a direct cost of $3,300 per person in America [19].

Asthma symptoms include shortness of breath, coughing, wheezing, and labored respiration. Asthma is induced by several mechanisms, including allergens, chemical irritants, smoke, pollutants, cold air, and exercise. **Exercise-induced asthma (EIA)** occurs when the PA triggers the onset of symptoms, particularly when training exceeds ventilatory thresholds. EIA affects most asthmatics and is considered a significant barrier to activity participation and overall health among the young and old alike.

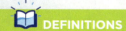

DEFINITIONS

Exercise-induced asthma (EIA) –

A narrowing of the airways in the lungs in response to strenuous physical exertion, also known as exercise-induced bronchoconstriction.

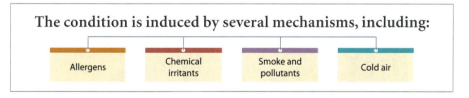

The condition is induced by several mechanisms, including: Allergens, Chemical irritants, Smoke and pollutants, Cold air

Asthma can be managed effectively via preventative strategies, medication, and regular exercise. Preventing the onset of asthma requires several environmental considerations. Steering clear of poorly ventilated rooms, minimizing allergen exposure from dust, mold, animal dander, and avoiding cold air or smoke all reduce the incidence of asthma. Exercise has demonstrated significant improvements in asthmatics' physical-fitness measures. Many asthmatics avoid PA for fear of initiating an asthmatic episode, but routine exercise participation has been shown to reduce the occurrence of asthmatic conditions and should be part of the overall management strategy [60].

Asthma and Exercise – Special Considerations for Children

Exercise should be introduced to asthmatics early on to reduce the psychosocial impact the disorder can have on children. Children with moderate or severe asthma present lower measures of aerobic capacity, lower left-ventricular mass, and impaired

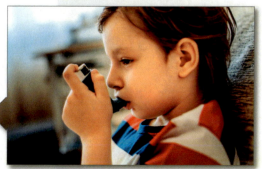

systolic function compared to healthy children of the same age [84]. This may partially explain why they report participating in fewer physical activities. In addition, children with asthma have a higher risk for being overweight and experience higher levels of emotional difficulties compared to healthy children [47, 80]. Interview reports demonstrate that both children and their parents identify asthma as a barrier to the child's health [94].

Exercise can effectively prevent many asthma-related problems. Therefore, strategies to promote exercise within this population should be explored to protect children from mental and physical health limitations. Asthmatic children who exercise have shown the ability to achieve a level of performance similar to that of healthy children when they participate in comparable levels of exercise [83]. Studies comparing the two groups found improvements in maximal aerobic oxygen consumption and anaerobic threshold. Asthmatic children experience the additional benefits of improved ventilatory capacity and decreased **hypercapnia**: elevated levels of CO_2 in the blood. When anaerobic activities were performed using one-minute sprints, both mild and moderately asthmatic children demonstrated parity in exercise tolerance compared to healthy children [23]. Perhaps the most significant finding is that asthmatics experience reduced incidence of EIA with regular exercise participation, and in many cases, EIA is not triggered during the participation [68]. It is recommended that asthmatic children be encouraged to participate in both aerobic and anaerobic exercise activities to promote improvements in health and fitness. It is not uncommon for symptomatic children to become asymptomatic adults.

Asthma and Obese Adults

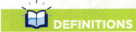

DEFINITIONS

Hypercapnia –
Excessive carbon dioxide (CO_2) levels in the blood, usually a result of inadequate respiration.

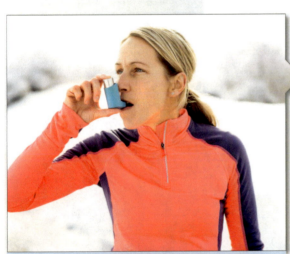

Routine exercise participation reduces the occurrence and severity of exercise-induced asthma.

Several studies have shown that, among adults, obesity is associated with an increased risk of asthma diagnosis, more frequent asthma-related health care use, and greater symptom or severity burden [100]. With routine exercise participation, adults demonstrate similar improvements as children. Adults new to exercise present deficiencies consistent with asthmatic children. Researchers attribute reduced physical condition as a more prominent factor in limiting exercise performance than the obstruction of airflow [36]. Adults are likely to experience the same mental barriers to exercise expressed by children. Fear of an asthmatic episode may be the greatest reason for avoiding exercise participation.

Similar to asthmatic children, routine exercise participation in adults reduces occurrence and severity of EIA. Interestingly, when acute exercise measures are compared to healthy controls, asthmatics show consistent endocrine and metabolic responses and similar tidal volume (the volume of air inhaled and exhaled with each breath) but demonstrate reduced breathing frequency [41]. Tidal volume maintenance may compensate for airflow obstruction, and therefore, allow for the successful participation in aerobic activities by asthmatics. Individuals with mild and moderate asthma can attain high measures of oxygen consumption and with appropriate training and medications, can successfully participate in endurance sports at a competitive level [41].

Even when intensity is high (80-90% maxHR), trained asthmatics have a reduced occurrence of EIA. Following supervised, high-intensity training, adult asthmatics reported a reduced fear of experiencing breathlessness during exercise and less anxiety related to higher-intensity exercising. Asthma symptoms during various forms of exercise abate significantly with routine aerobic exercise participation. Other studies have reported that regular sub-maximal exercise has improved quality of life (QOL), exercise capacity and reduced need for medication and overall symptoms in both adults and children [68]. When comparing land and water-based exercise, similar findings were noted [29]. Aerobic exercise on land and in water resulted in reduced incidence of EIA during and after the training sessions, similar improvements in aerobic capacity, as well as reduced total symptoms [29]. Water-based environments may present more favorable conditions to the asthmatic, as the air tends to be warmer and humidified compared to land-based training. Nonetheless, the research findings around asthmatics and exercise suggest that multiple forms of training will promote similar effects so long as the exercise intensity is consistent.

Physical fitness training programs can be designed to improve both anaerobic and aerobic fitness in asthmatic clients. Regular participation increases physical fitness measures and lowers ventilation rate during mild and moderate exercise, thereby lowering the incidence and likelihood of triggering an EIA event. Additionally, exercise exhibits a profound psychological effect on exercise confidence, perception of breathlessness, and reduced anxiety toward an EIA event. Although no change in lung function seems to occur in response to exercise, the corresponding benefits of routine PA provide significant improvements in overall health. Personal trainers need to be familiar with the signs and symptoms of asthma, conditions and environments that induce or trigger the onset of symptoms, and medications prescribed to manage the condition when working with asthmatic clients. Forms or documents used for pre-exercise screening should include items that identify clients with asthma and whether they use medication in the treatment of the disorder. Individuals who use medication to control asthma must be required to comply with recommendations for use before exercise or possess their prescribed inhaler when exercising in the event that EIA or any other asthmatic episode occurs. When implementing exercise strategies, personal trainers should use longer warmups, be sure that the environment is appropriate (avoid cold environments), and avoid activities in areas of poor ventilation. Additionally, personal trainers should attempt to manage environmental conditions to reduce the risk of an event, and always ensure that before the commencement of the training session, medication is on-hand and accessible.

General recommendations for asthmatics:

- Evaluate the training environment for common asthma triggers
- Employ longer warm-up and cool down periods to acclimate the body to changing physiological conditions
- Swimming, cycling, and walking are less likely than running to trigger an event
- Participating in sports that use stop-and-go activities (e.g., tennis, volleyball, and basketball) are less likely to trigger EIA when compared to long, continuous activity
- High-intensity exercise triggers EIA more often than moderate-intensity exercise; intensities of 60-80% HRR are recommended when prescribing aerobic training
- Steady-state endurance training is less likely than intervals to trigger a response
- Encourage controlled nasal breathing whenever possible
- Maintain appropriate medications on site and have an emergency plan

◆ Diabetes & Exercise

Diabetes is a primary health problem in America with a bleak outlook: the rate of diabetes has almost doubled in the past 20 years, with up to 14% of all Americans having the disease [21]. According to the latest reports from the CDC, 30.3 million Americans have diabetes, with nearly another 85 million US citizens functioning in a prediabetic state [21]. People with diabetes suffer an increased risk of serious health complications, including vision loss, HD, stroke, kidney failure, amputation of toes, feet, or legs, and premature death. The National Diabetes Statistics Report suggests diabetes and its related complications accounted for $245 billion in total medical costs, lost work, and wages in 2012. This figure is up from $174 billion in 2007.

Diabetes is characterized by high blood-glucose levels due to sugar regulation impairment within the body. Type I diabetes, previously termed

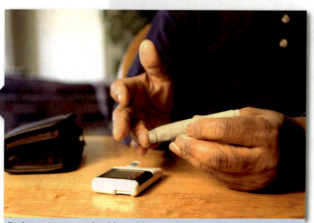

Diabetes is a major health problem in US; its prevalence has almost doubled in the past 20 years, with up to 14% of all Americans suffering from the disease.

Juvenile Diabetes, is an autoimmune disorder where the body produces antibodies against the Islet cells of the pancreas, causing a reduction in, or more commonly, the cessation of insulin production. Type I diabetes is often referred to as Insulin-Dependent Diabetes Mellitus due to the need to supply insulin via an external source, as the body cannot produce it. Type II diabetes occurs more commonly and is characterized by insulin insensitivity and beta cell dysfunction in the later stages of the disease. Several mechanisms cause Type II diabetes, including genetic predispositions, obesity, sedentary lifestyle, and poor diet. Obesity alone puts adults over 25 years of age at 4X the risk of developing diabetes compared to those with normal weights[8]. In some cases, pregnant females develop the disease due to genetic predisposition, advanced maternal age, pre-diabetic condition before pregnancy exacerbated by pregnancy, and obesity. Gestational diabetes mellitus (GDM) is a temporary diabetic condition that occurs during pregnancy. It will often subside following delivery but increases the risk for later development of Type II diabetes.

Type I diabetes	• Autoimmune disorder characterized by the production of antibodies that attack the Islet cells of the pancreas; reduces or stops insulin production • Often referred to as Insulin Dependent Diabetes Mellitus due to the need to supply insulin via an external source
Type II diabetes	• Characterized by insulin insensitivity and beta cell dysfunction in later stages • Caused by several mechanisms including genetic predisposition, obesity, sedentary lifestyle, and poor diet • Pregnant females can develop gestational diabetes mellitus (GDM)

QUICK INSIGHT

According to the Gallup-Healthways Well-Being Index, obese adults between the ages of 25 and 64 are at least four times more likely to have been diagnosed with diabetes than those who are normal weight. By their mid-to-late 30s, 9.3% of obese adults have been diagnosed with diabetes, compared with 1.8% among those who are normal weight.

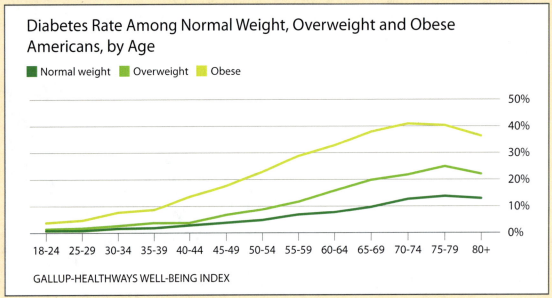

These results are based on nearly 500,000 interviews conducted in the U.S. from 2014 through 2016 as part of the Gallup-Healthways Well-Being Index.

PA plays a significant role in improving symptoms of diabetes. During exercise, cellular glucose uptake increases significantly, resulting in reduced circulating levels of glucose without the presence of high insulin concentrations. This insulin-like effect of active muscle tissue reduces the requirements for insulin to regulate glucose, thereby improving blood glucose levels in diabetics.

Low cardiorespiratory fitness is a powerful and independent predictor of mortality in diabetics [99]. Individuals with Type II diabetes often incur the greatest risk due to the presence of compounding factors including dyslipidemia, inflammatory obesity, and hypertension, the latter of which commonly leads to early mortality from cardiovascular disease (CVD). Aerobic training performed at an intensity of 50%-75% VO_2max for at least 30 minutes has been shown to improve cardiorespiratory function in diabetics [101]. In addition, aerobic exercise participation positively impacts visceral and subcutaneous adiposity, insulin response, and plasma triglyceride levels [101]. Improvements in blood-glucose-marker dynamics and CRF measurements have been found in as little as 14 to 20 minutes when high intensities are used during exercises. Consideration of exercise duration is especially important because most people do not exercise long enough at self-selected intensities to see marked improvements in these measures [51].

Resistance training (RT) yields similar, and in some cases, more profound effects than aerobic training on diabetes and blood-glucose kinetics [46]. With regard to acute responses, RT exercise effectively improved integrated glucose concentration. Compared to aerobic training, Type II diabetics who participated in 4 months of strength training significantly improved blood glucose levels and insulin resistance, reduced low-density lipoproteins (LDL) and triglycerides, and increased high-density lipoproteins (HDL) over diabetic subjects who performed only aerobic training for the same time period [14].

When aerobic and resistance activities were combined in an exercise circuit, positive adaptations on glucose control, insulin action, muscular strength, and exercise tolerance were observed. In a related review, circuit training significantly impacted indices of glycemic control, cardiorespiratory fitness, muscular strength, and body composition [69]. Following 8 weeks of circuit training, submaximal heart rate (HR) and BP were reduced, skinfold and waist to hip measures significantly decreased, **glycosylated hemoglobin** (a measure of disease control) and fasting blood-plasma glucose were lowered, while functional capacity, muscular strength, lean body mass, and glycemic control all increased significantly [52,69]. Based on these and other findings, it seems that both RT and aerobic training are necessary components to an effective exercise program for those with diabetes. These modes can be performed independently or combined in a circuit training program. Although exercise remains a staple for proper management of the disease, certain conditions may be exacerbated by exercise participation. Diabetics should undergo a thorough medical examination prior to initiating an exercise program so that a physician can rule out any possible factors that may lead to macro or microvascular complications or injury. Within this screen, it is particularly important to analyze the disease effects upon the heart, kidneys, eyes, and nervous system.

High-risk diabetics require appropriate supervision and program modification to address the heightened risk of cardiovascular incident and tissue damage associated with compromised vascular dynamics. The American Diabetic Association (ADA) provides guidelines and recom-

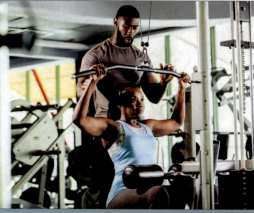

Benefits of exercise on diabetes:

- Improved insulin sensitivity
- Improved glucose regulation
- Improved blood lipid profile
- Reduced visceral fat storage
- Improved cardiovascular fitness
- Improved muscular fitness
- Reduced loss of muscle mass
- Reduced risk for cardiovascular disease
- Reduced risk for peripheral vascular disease
- Reduced risk for heart attack and stroke
- Improved quality of life (QOL)

DEFINITIONS

Glycosylated Hemoglobin (HbA1c) –

A measurement of the amount of hemoglobin to which glucose is bound; used as an indicator of long-term glucose control.

Additional screening criteria used to determine risk for injury or complications among diabetics include:

Age >35 years

Obesity > 25 years

Presence of Type I Diabetes > 15 years

Presence of Type II Diabetes > 10 years

Presence of additional risk factors for HD

Presence of microvascular disease, including retinopathy and nephropathy

Peripheral vascular disease

Autonomic neuropathy

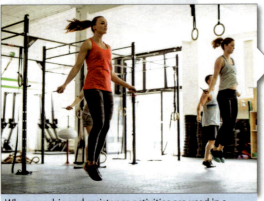

When aerobic and resistance activities are used in a circuit fashion for diabetics, positive adaptations on glucose control, insulin action, muscular strength, and exercise tolerance are usually observed.

mendations to aid in managing exercise programs for Type I and II diabetics. The differences between the classifications of the disease are also included in the recommendations for safe participation. Due to the fact that Type I diabetics do not produce insulin, it must be injected, usually subcutaneously, to regulate blood glucose. Exercise profoundly affects cellular uptake of glucose, and when insulin is injected prior to exercise, the combination of heightened cellular absorption can lead to dangerously low levels of blood glucose, a condition known as hypoglycemia. This can cause light-headedness, fainting, or, on rare occasions, diabetic coma. For this reason, Type I diabetics are required to monitor metabolic indices and plan insulin use around PA participation. Type I diabetics should not exercise within one hour of taking insulin, and insulin injection sites should not be at, or near, the location of the prime mover for the exercise.

Type I diabetics can compete at elite performance levels with appropriate management of the disease. Team Novo Nordisk is a group of Type I diabetics that compete worldwide in cycling, running, and triathlon events. NFL quarterback Jay Cutler and Olympic swimmer Gary Hall, Jr. have competed their entire careers with Type I diabetes. With prolonged and more intense exercise, carbohydrate regulation becomes more important, so planned pre-exercise meals and adequate carbohydrate availability need to be accounted for during prolonged exercise to avoid hypoglycemia. Diabetics do not all respond the same way to exercise, and therefore, individual attention is necessary. Tracking the techniques that promote the best performance and glucose regulation response can aid in formulating the ideal management strategy. Record insulin injection time and dosage, food by ingestion time and quantity of carbohydrates, and intensity/duration measures to identify specific outcomes.

Type II diabetics do not have the same concerns related to hypoglycemia from injected insulin, but rather, must regulate carbohydrate intake and monitor blood glucose to avoid exercise-related complications. Type II diabetics may present more difficulty with exercise management due to the fact that the disease often entails low levels of physical fitness, obesity, and additional cardiovascular risk factors. Higher-risk Type II diabetics should be acclimated to exercise with similar precautions for those with cardiovascular risk, as well as specific considerations for the presence of microvascular complications. In addition, different medications for Type II diabetes exist and each has a unique action. Type II diabetic medications work by increasing insulin production (Sulfonylurea, Meglitinide), sensitizing the body to circulating insulin present in the blood (Metformin), helping insulin to work better in the muscle and fat cells (Thiazolidinedione), or acting to regulate carbohydrate digestion (Alpha-glucose Inhibitor). Due to the different mechanisms of action, physician recommended adjustments may need to be made before exercise participation, and clients need to comply strictly with medication instructions.

General recommendations for Type I diabetics

- Maintain proper identification of the condition
- Avoid exercise if fasting glucose levels are > 200 mg/dl and ketosis is present
- Use caution if fasting glucose levels are > 300 mg/dl without ketones
- Monitor blood glucose before and after exercise and identify when changes to food or insulin are needed
- Track glycemic response to exercise conditions for future reference
- Use carbohydrates (CHO) to avoid hypoglycemia
- Keep fast-acting CHO available during and after exercise
- Pay close attention to signs of fatigue and metabolic shifts during exercise
- Avoid high intensities when using new exercises

General recommendations for Type II diabetics

- Maintain proper pre-exercise metabolic control
- Consume adequate fluids
- Perform regular PA most days of the week
- Include client-appropriate aerobic and anaerobic activities
- Focus on caloric expenditure (minimum goal of 1,000 kcal/week) and weight loss
- Initiate exercise with appropriate acclimation periods
- Work up to aerobic intensities of 60-80% HRR
- Modify exercise activities for microvascular complications
- Comply with medication recommendations and monitor blood indices appropriately

Retinopathy (small vessel disease of the eyes)
- Avoid exercises that produce high blood pressure (BP), particularly high-intensity, compressive RT (e.g., leg press)
- Do not use activities that lower the head below the waist, such as yoga
- Do not use activities that may jar the head, such as plyometrics

Nephropathy (small vessel disease of the kidneys)
- Avoid moderate to heavy weightlifting
- Avoid high-intensity aerobic activity
- Avoid holding one's breath during exercise (notably raises BP)
- Maintain adequate hydration

Peripheral Neuropathy (small vessel disease of nerve tissue)
- Avoid exercise that causes pounding/repetitive stress to the feet
- Select non-weight-bearing exercises
- Ensure proper footwear is always worn during PA

◆ Exercise & Cardiovascular Disease

Exercise has become a universally accepted component for cardiac rehabilitation and therapy for CVD. For more than 30 years, aerobic exercise has been an integral part of post-cardiac event rehabilitation and has been used as a key strategy in improving aerobic capacity, while reducing the risks associated with **comorbidities**. RT performed in circuit formats has gained popularity as a component of cardiopulmonary rehabilitation programs, particularly among diabetics. Each type of CVD has specific characteristics which determine the type and extent of safe activity. Participation levels and recommended guidelines will depend on the specific disease-related factors, such as the progressive stage of disease, degree of damage or symptoms, the current state of the individual, and the presence of other health-limiting factors. In most cases, individuals with disease can participate in PA, although the actual mode, intensity, and volume of participation will vary according to the relative level of health risk.

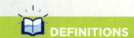

Comorbidities –

The presence of additional diseases or disorders occurring with a primary disease or disorder; associated with worse health outcomes and more complex clinical management.

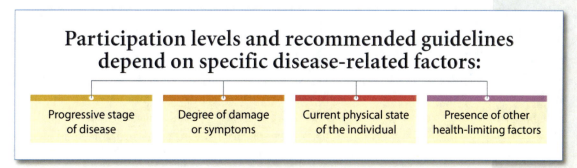

Participation levels and recommended guidelines depend on specific disease-related factors:
- Progressive stage of disease
- Degree of damage or symptoms
- Current physical state of the individual
- Presence of other health-limiting factors

Exercise and Hypertension

Hypertension is characterized by high BP in the circulatory arteries. The guidelines from the American Heart Association (AHA) and the American College of Cardiology (ACC) now define high BP as 130 mm Hg or higher for the systolic blood pressure (SBP) measurement, or 80 mm Hg or higher for the diastolic blood pressure (DBP) measurement. Therefore, BP measures at or above 130/80 mmHg, are now considered hypertensive. High circulatory BP:

- Causes turbulent blood flow and excessive stress along the inner lining of blood vessels, resulting in endothelial lesions
- Leads to the formation of atherosclerotic plaque and the onset of coronary artery disease (CAD)
- Can also lead to kidney damage, stroke, and chronic heart failure

Hypertension is an epidemic and incurs a markedly increased risk of developing cardiovascular disorders. For individuals with mild or moderate hypertension, all current treatment guidelines emphasize the role of nonpharmacological interventions, such as modifications to diet and participation in routine PA. A large number of studies have demonstrated that regular aerobic exercise reduces the incidence of hypertension and plays a significant role in managing the early stages of the disease [75]. In addition to preventing hypertension, regular aerobic exercise has been found to lower BP up to an average of 9 mmHg in both systolic and diastolic measures, while improving blood lipid profiles and insulin sensitivity [51]. It also improves endothelial function and platelet activation and attenuates inflammatory response. For individuals with stage 1 hypertension (130-139/80-89 mmHg) with no other coronary risk factors and no evidence of cardiovascular disease, exercise and dietary management are the initial treatment, generally lasting twelve months [4]. Individuals with diabetes, cardiovascular disease, or more marked elevations in BP (>180/105 mm Hg) should add endurance exercise training to their treatment regimen only after initiating pharmacologic therapy. Endurance exercise training appears to elicit even greater reductions in BP in medicated patients with hypertension [1].

To train hypertensive persons, dynamic exercise of moderate intensity is preferable, with a rate of perceived exertion (RPE) of 12-14, at 40-70% VO_2max, (e.g. brisk walking, cycling) for 30-60 minutes, 3-5 times per week based on the common recommendations of various professional committees and organizations in their scientific statements [75]. This approach is well-tolerated and appears to be more effective in lowering BP in general at the magnitude of 1-9 mmHg [75]. Training at somewhat moderate intensities (40-70% VO_2max) appears to lower BP as much as exercise at higher intensities. This may be important in specific hypertensive populations with lower levels of cardiorespiratory fitness, especially considering adherence to exercise [1]. With that said, recent research findings suggest that overweight, middle-aged men (45 years old) with hypertension saw a decreased SBP of 1.5 mmHg and DBP of 0.6 mmHg for every 10% increase in exercise intensity over 40% VO_2max. Further research into high-intensity interval training (HIIT) has shown that those with the highest BP values benefit the most from HIIT's lowering effects, indicating that levels of exertion appear to lower BP in a

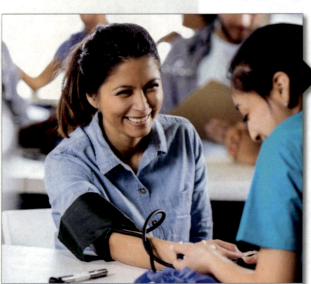

Regular aerobic exercise has been found to lower BP by an average of 9 mmHg in both systolic and diastolic measures.

dose-response relationship [66]. Since physically active and fit individuals with hypertension have markedly lower rates of mortality than sedentary, unfit, hypertensive individuals, aerobic exercise should be used to manage the disease while serving to improve cardiorespiratory fitness. When addressing program priorities in the exercise prescription among clients with hypertension, cardiorespiratory training should be emphasized to reduce risk for morbidity and mortality.

>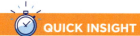
> ### QUICK INSIGHT
> #### POST-EXERCISE HYPOTENSION
>
> *Aerobic activity aimed to treat hypertension does not have to be performed in long bouts of continuous training as previously recommended. Research has indicated that several ten-minute sessions of brisk walking throughout the day provided the same benefits as 30 minutes of continuous walking at the same intensity[157]. The relative intensity and cumulative total duration of work seem to be more important than the activity duration per session. This suggests that individuals with hypertension can manage the disease with short, planned bouts of exercise throughout the day, rather than being required to use a single, long-duration workout session. Personal trainers can use this information to acclimate clients to routine exercise, as well as prescribe "homework" without the full commitment of long-duration exercise sessions.*

The amount of research regarding RT exercise and hypertension is scarce when compared to aerobic training, which may be why the benefits associated with RT and hypertensives are less certain. Both high-intensity aerobic training and RT exercise can cause dramatic, acute increases in BP, followed by significant drops in BP, termed **post-exercise hypotension (PEH)**. Exercise prescription guidelines released by Current Hypertension Reports include a combination of 30+ minutes of moderate aerobic exercise on most, but preferably all days of the week, as well as RT of at least 2-5 times per week totaling at least 150 minutes of total exercise per week for the treatment of hypertension [4, 76].

DEFINITIONS

Post-exercise hypotension (PEH) –

A phenomenon of prolonged reduction in resting blood pressure in the minutes and hours following an acute exercise bout.

Previous recommendations and guidelines have centered on aerobic training for treating hypertensive individuals due to the substantiated evidence surrounding its benefits. New guidelines do not dismiss the important benefits of aerobic training, but new research has emerged also implicating RT as another means, outside of prescribed medication, of reducing BP [76]. This case in point illustrates why certified personal trainers and exercise professionals have a fiduciary obligation to their clientele to stay up-to-date in the field of exercise science so that they can better use their tools and skills and acquire new strategies to help their clients become healthy and disease free.

General guidelines for hypertension

- Aerobic exercise – accumulate 40-60 min at 50-75% VO_2 max 3-5 days per week
- Can lower systolic and diastolic measures of BP by 9 mmHg over time
- Improves endothelial function and platelet activation, and lowers negative inflammatory responses
- Does not have to be a single, long-duration bout; several 10-min sessions provide the same benefits as 30 minutes of continual walking
- RT – use 12-15 repetitions, preferably in circuit format; avoid heavy RT (>70% 1RM) and holding one's breath
- Reduce salt intake
- Attain adequate potassium intake (90 mmol/day)
- Reduce body weight if necessary
- Limit or avoid alcohol

Exercise and Coronary Artery Disease (CAD)

CAD is the most common form of HD and accounts for the most disease-related deaths in the United States. It is characterized by the narrowing, hardening, and blockage of coronary vessels from atherosclerotic plaque build-up. It is commonly attributed to several factors, including obesity, physical inactivity, high BP, poor lipid profile, and smoking. Based on these risk factors, a multi-factorial approach is necessary to reduce the risk of progressive atherosclerosis, which leads to coronary-artery occlusion and heart attack.

Coronary Artery Disease is commonly attributed to several factors including:

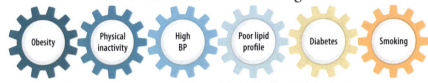

Obesity • Physical inactivity • High BP • Poor lipid profile • Diabetes • Smoking

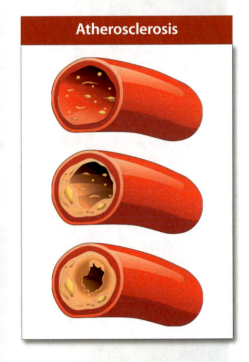

Atherosclerosis

Aerobic training and general increases in PA have been recommended as an integral part of prevention and treatment therapies. Exercise improves cardiovascular risk factors by reducing dyslipidemia, sympathetic tone, insulin resistance, and inflammation, while enhancing fibrinolysis, normalizing endothelial function, and retarding atherosclerosis in the vessels [22, 53]. Individuals with established CAD demonstrate improvements in symptoms of angina and congestive heart failure (CHF) and experience attenuation of exercise-induced ischemia. Due to the strong evidence for exercise's benefit for cardiovascular disease prevention and rehabilitation, it is recommended that it be included in multidimensional therapy for cardiovascular disease [39].

Regular aerobic exercise results in increased exercise capacity, improved circulatory function, and lower myocardial oxygen demand, leading to cardiovascular benefits. It is recommended that individuals with CVD who have been cleared for exercise gradually build up to 30 accumulated minutes of aerobic exercise at least 5 days per week, for a total of at least 150 minutes of exercise. If exercise intensity is vigorous, the recommended volume of exercise decreases to 25 minutes, performed at least 3 days per week [2, 39]. The initial exercise goal is to attain a work rate that results in the expenditure of 100 to 200 kcal per exercise session. Exercise at this level has been shown to reduce SBP and HR at rest. While performing submaximal work, exercise can increase the level of physical work capacity, reduce the myocardial oxygen cost at rest and during performance of submaximal exercise, aid in the reduction of body fat with a concomitant increase in muscle mass, and reduce plasma triglyceride levels. When combined with pharmacologic intervention and diet therapies, the benefits are more significant. Studies show that aerobic exercise, combined with cholesterol reducing agents such as statins, can lead to atherosclerotic plaque regression [35].

As an adjunct to endurance training, individuals with CAD can benefit from RT via:

- Improved muscle strength and endurance
- Increased metabolism and cardiovascular function
- Enhanced psychosocial well-being and QOL
- Concurrent reductions of cardiovascular risk factors [13, 39, 45]

Individuals with disease that present good cardiac performance capacity may include RT without any restraints as part of cardiac rehabilitation programs for CAD. However, based on the current data, RT is not recommended for all persons with HD. Individuals with CAD should be clinically screened and perform a symptom-limited, maximal, graded exercise test prior to engaging in RT. Individuals who have characteristics associated with an increased risk of cardiac event during exercise should avoid heavy RT.

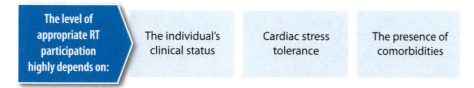

Persons with myocardial ischemia and/or poor left ventricular function should not engage in RT, as these exercises may lead to cardiac-wall motion disturbances and severe ventricular arrhythmias. Intra-arterial BP measurements in cardiac patients have demonstrated that, during low-intensity RT (40-60% maximum voluntary contraction) with 15-20 repetitions, only modest elevations in BP occur [96]. The BP response to low-intensity weight training is similar to the values seen during moderate endurance training and can be safely utilized in medically cleared clients with CAD [96].

RT activities may include any number of modalities consistent with standard strength training. Activities aimed at improving functional strength support activities of daily living and may enhance daily PA participation. Body weight exercises, free weights, elastic bands, and other resistive modalities may be used to exercise major muscle groups in cardiopulmonary rehabilitation. Resistive training workloads should be determined by gradual acclimation to movement proficiency. Higher repetition schemes with light resistance encourage improved neuromuscular movement patterns and present minimal effect on the BP response.

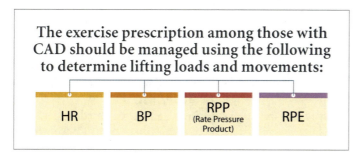

Circuit weight training is an ideal method for implementing strength training activities in cardiac-compromised clients, as it has been reported to:

- Improve strength
- Increase lean body mass
- Enhance self-efficacy
- Potentially decrease risk factors for CAD
- Allow for performance of daily strength tasks more safely, efficiently, and with greater self-confidence [12, 25]

Circuit training has become an accepted component of exercise programs for populations with cardiac risk. Although reports are somewhat limited, studies have shown that high-risk clients can increase fitness in a fashion similar to healthy populations. Furthermore, the hemodynamic responses to circuit weight training suggest that it is a clinically safe and acceptable form of exercise for most individuals with CAD [12]. Circuit training activities should be client-specific and adapted to acceptable MET levels of work output. Cardiovascular measures should be monitored during the training, and adjustments should be made based on HR response and RPE. Longer warm-ups prior to engagement and increased periods of transitional rest should be utilized based on RPE. Closed-chain, body-weight exercises effectively enhance fitness components that may transfer to daily life activities. Proper breathing techniques should be monitored to avoid breath holding, and isometric abdominal contractions should be avoided. In general, one exercise for each major muscle group can be used with approximately 15-20 repetitions. Programs should start out with single sets and may be moved to two sets per muscle group as a client improves in function and work capacity [87]. PA and exercise play a vital role in preventing the top killer in America, HD.

General Recommendations for CAD

- Aerobic exercise
- Accumulate up to 40-60 minutes of low intensity aerobic activity most days of the week. Increase to a frequency of 3-4 sessions per week, at an intensity of 40-75% HRR for 20-40 minutes
- Use 10 minute warm-up and cool down periods
- Resistance training
- Introduce resistance training using closed-chain, body weight activities: 1 set, 15-20 repetitions
- Circuits may include one exercise per muscle group to start and gradually progress at a client-appropriate pace
- Cardiovascular measures should be monitored, and RPE should be used to gauge intensity
- Medications should be accounted for and used in accordance with physician recommendations
- Flexibility should be encouraged, utilizing proper breathing techniques
- Avoid heavy resistance, isometric training, and breath holding during activities

Congestive Heart Failure (CHF)

CHF is caused by an enlargement of the left ventricle and central portion of the heart in response to CAD and the strain against vascular peripheral resistance. This myocardial hypertrophic adaptation decreases the filling capacity of the ventricles, altering the heart's efficiency in mobilizing blood through the chambers and leading to significant reduction in stroke volume (SV), as well as reduced valve function. The compromised cardiac output (CO) limits oxygen availability, consequently decreasing work capacity. Individuals with CHF demonstrate poor cardiovascular status and impaired exercise capacity due to both cardiac limitations and peripheral maladaptations of the skeletal musculature. The reduced work capacity often leads to significant peripheral muscle atrophy and functional decline.

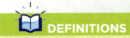

DEFINITIONS

Congestive Heart Failure (CHF) –

A chronic progressive condition resulting in the inability to pump adequate blood to the body.

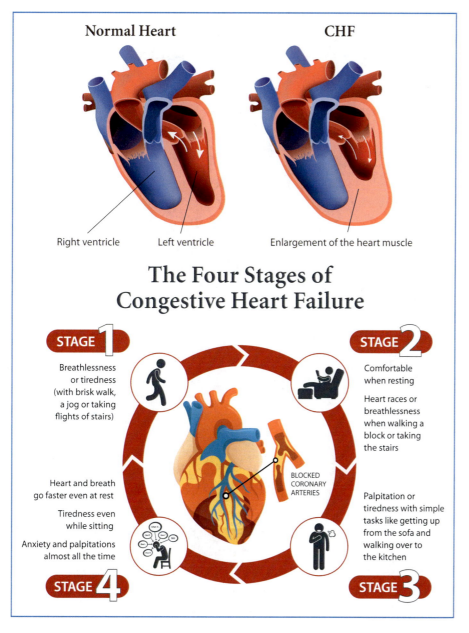

According to researchers, individuals with CHF who participate in an exercise training program:

- Improve circulation and skeletal muscle oxygen delivery and utilization
- Increase the heart's pumping capacity
- May positively affect heart enlargement
- Reduced hospitalization and mortality
- Improved quality of life [33, 44, 62, 82]

Due to the related pathology and low levels of exercise tolerance endemic to CHF, individuals with this condition have limited activity selection. Walking and stationary cycling have both been shown to be tolerable and lead to improvements in aerobic capacity [33]. Initially, lower-intensity, steady-state training should be used but can be exchanged for interval training with documented improvements in function. Interval training has demonstrated a positive effect upon peripheral musculature, above that seen with steady-state training, without inducing greater cardiovascular stress. At present, an optimal parameter for measuring intensity has not been established, but the intensity range of 40-80% peak oxygen consumption has been applied successfully [33]. A heart rate reserve (HRR) of 60-80% may be used in conjunction with RPE to guide exercise intensity. RPE is generally a better measure of intensity than HR, given that most clients with CHF take medicines (B-Blockers and Ca^{++} channel blockers) that suppress the HR response. Due to the inability to sustain work for long time periods, initial exercise should utilize 40-50% peak VO_2 with exercise duration lasting at least 3-5 min per session, performed several times daily [64]. Progression order should emphasize duration before frequency, with intensity being the last stage of progression.

Peripheral muscular weakness is of significant concern with CHF clients. Recent scientific evidence suggests that the application of specific resistance exercise activities is safe and induces significant and important metabolic and functional adaptations in the peripheral skeletal muscles [78]. These adaptations are valuable in addressing the issues of muscle weakness and atrophy facing the majority of CHF patients.

Appropriate RT has been shown to do the following for clients with CHF:

- Improve exercise tolerance and peak oxygen consumption
- Stimulate changes in muscle composition and muscle hypertrophy
- Lead to alterations in skeletal muscle metabolism
- Contribute to improvements in muscular strength and endurance, particularly when applied in combination with aerobic exercise [78, 97]

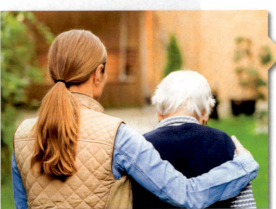

Peripheral muscular weakness is of significant concern with CHF clients, so RT must be modified to effectively train the skeletal muscles without producing significant cardiovascular stress.

RT activities must be modified to cater to the specific limitations of individuals with CHF. The exercise program's main focus is to effectively train the skeletal muscles without producing significant cardiovascular stress. Therefore, RT activities differ for clients with CHF compared to prescriptions for other cardiac impairments. RT should emphasize small muscle groups, using short bouts of work and appropriate repetitions to avoid excessive cardiac muscle stress [65].

When performing dynamic-strength exercises, the movements should be slow and controlled, at intensity values of 50-60% of one repetition maximum. The number of repetitions can range between 15 and 20, or as tolerated, but work durations should not exceed 60 seconds [97]. Following the performance of the exercise, adequate recovery periods should be utilized. In general, a recovery period greater than twice the set duration is necessary. Individuals who present very low cardiac reserve may be required to lift very limited loads, such as small free weights (2-6 lbs.) or utilize elastic bands with 8-10 repetitions. Exercise machines may also be used effectively by clients with CHF. It is important to understand that CHF represents a wide spectrum of disability. Some CHF clients will tolerate close to normal training stress, whereas others may be severely limited. With such variability in this population, these clients must get medical clearance and the personal trainer must adhere closely to physician recommendations.

> **General recommendations for CHF**
> - Short bouts of aerobic activity at 40-50% peak O_2 capacity, performed several times/day for durations of at least 3-5 min/session
> - An appropriate aerobic exercise program can improve circulation, increase the pumping capacity of the heart, and positively affect heart enlargement
> - Incorporate RT using smaller muscles at intensities of 50-60% 1RM; perform as tolerated with longer rest intervals than a healthy client
> - RPE scale should be employed for clients since most will be on medicines that block the HR response
> - Excessive stress should be avoided due to a limited work capacity
> - Progressions should mirror individual tolerance and work capacity

Exercise during Pregnancy

PA, including structured exercise, can provide numerous benefits for the health and fitness of the expectant mother [153]. Pregnant females who engage in moderate exercise demonstrate:

- Improvements in cardiorespiratory fitness
- Reduced maternal weight gain
- Reduced musculoskeletal discomfort (including reduced incidence of low back pain during and following pregnancy)
- Reduced postural compromise
- Decreased incidence and severity of varicose veins (dilated veins due to valvular incompetence) and thrombosis
- Reduced risk for preterm birth
- Fewer complications during delivery and shorter delivery lengths [204]
- Reduced risk for pregnancy-related disorders
- Improved glucose tolerance
- Improved psychological well-being and subjective body image
- Quicker recovery from the stresses and strains of delivery [74]

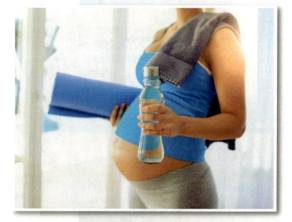

Recommendations concerning exercise during pregnancy have gone through significant changes during the past four decades. Today, considerable support touts the beneficial effects of moderate exercise during pregnancy, even in formerly inactive women. It is now suggested that healthy pregnant women can engage in numerous types of PA, using gestational, age-adapted exercise for safe and effective support of maternal and fetal health. In most cases, pregnant women should practice exercise in a moderate, submaximal range based on individual criteria and physician approval, but women have trained using high intensities into the third trimester without complication. Exercise has demonstrated a variety of effects on the pregnant woman, the developing fetus, and the placenta. The naturally occurring physiological adjustments related to pregnancy on the maternal cardiorespiratory system include increases in oxygen consumption, CO, HR, SV, and plasma volume. These hormonally driven alterations improve aerobic capacity without the addition of any PA-related adaptations.

> *Major physiological changes that occur during pregnancy:*
>
> - In general, maternal resting oxygen consumption (VO_2) and CO increase in the early stages of pregnancy.
>
> - HR becomes progressively elevated through gestation, with a concurrent increase in SV until the third trimester, at which time it begins to decline until term; the decline is likely attributed to diminished venous return.
>
> - Plasma volume increases earlier and to a greater magnitude than red blood cell volume, resulting in mild blood dilution and a decline in its oxygen-carrying capacity; this occurs despite increased red blood cell production, which warrants a compensatory increase in dietary iron intake.
>
> - Pulmonary shifts cause tidal volume to increase with an unchanged rate of breathing, causing increased ventilation during pregnancy; however, residual volume (lung volume after maximum expiration) decreases, especially in the third trimester, due to elevation of the diaphragm by the fetus.
>
> - There is a gestation-proportionate increase in metabolism associated with increased mass.

Recommendations concerning exercise during pregnancy have gone through significant changes in recent years. Today, there is considerable support for the beneficial effects of moderate exercise during pregnancy, even among formerly inactive women.

When exercise is performed during pregnancy, exercise-induced cardiopulmonary changes remain essentially the same or are slightly exaggerated compared to non-pregnant females. Females maintain aerobic work capacity during pregnancy and may experience exercise performance improvements related to the hormonal effects on the cardiovascular system. Typical training adaptations associated with exercise also occur during pregnancy. The increase in oxygen reserve seen in early pregnancy drops as term approaches; this reduction in oxygen reserve is related to the reductions in SV as mentioned above, suggesting that maternal exercise may present a greater physiological stress in the third trimester [70]. Relatively minor changes occur in the blood concentrations of O_2 and energy substrates during prolonged exhaustive exercise, demonstrating no loss in exercise performance due to metabolic alterations. In addition, despite a temperature increase of 1-2° C, little evidence exists for significant fetal metabolism alteration, cardiovascular hemodynamics, or blood catecholamine concentrations [70, 74]. Early research on animals suggested that a risk of neural-tube defects may be present due to exercise-induced hyperthermia; however, several studies have deemed this unlikely in humans due to a more efficient heat management system [43]. These observations suggest that acute exercise normally does not represent a major distress for either the fetus or mother in uncomplicated pregnancies.

Reduced Risk for Complications

Evidence-based guidelines indicate that participation in regular PA is an important component of a healthy pregnancy [43]. In addition to promoting physical fitness, exercise may assist in preventing or treating maternal-fetal diseases as well as maintaining healthy gestational weight gain. Women who are the most physically active demonstrate the lowest prevalence of GDM. This has important implications, as preventing the occurrence of GDM using PA and proper diet may decrease the incidence of obesity and type II diabetes in both mother and offspring following birth. GDM is the most common medical complication of pregnancy [54]. Women with GDM incur elevated risk for numerous maternal health complications, and their infants suffer increased hazard of death and morbidity [54].

Physically active women are also less likely to develop **pre-eclampsia** during pregnancy, compared to sedentary females [27]. Pre-eclampsia occurs in 2-7% of all pregnancies and is a leading cause of maternal and fetal morbidity and mortality. Although not fully understood, it is proposed that pre-eclampsia may be caused by the following: abnormal placental development, predisposing maternal constitutional factors, oxidative stress, immune maladaptation, and genetic susceptibility. Exercise may reduce risk for developing pre-eclampsia via several mechanisms, including the stimulation of placental growth and vascularity, a reduction of oxidative stress, and exercise-induced reversal of maternal endothelial dysfunction. Whatever the actual preventative mechanism, PA constitutes an important part of reducing pre-eclampsia risk.

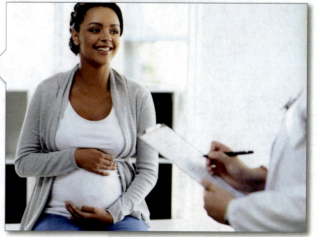

DEFINITIONS

Pre-eclampsia –

The development of elevated blood pressure and protein in the urine after the 20th week of pregnancy.

Weight gain is expected during pregnancy but is generally less than 30 lbs. Today, many women get pregnant when they themselves are already overweight or obese. Unfortunately, maternal obesity associates with reproductive complications, including an increased risk of infertility and miscarriage. When combined with proper diet, exercise reduces the probability of obesity-related complications during pregnancy. Regular exercise following conception has been shown to prevent gestational weight gain and reduce post-partum weight retention [71].

Institute of Medicine Weight Gain Recommendations for Pregnancy			
Pre-pregnancy Weight Category	Body Mass Index	Recommended Range of Total Weight Gain (lbs.)	Recommended Rates of Weight Gain in the Second and Third Trimesters (lbs.) (Mean Range [lbs./week])
Underweight	Less than 18.5	28–40	1 (1–1.3)
Normal Weight	18.5–24.9	25–35	1 (0.8–1)
Overweight	25–29.9	15–25	0.6 (0.5–0.7)
Obese (includes all classes)	30 and greater	11–20	0.5 (0.4–0.6)

Fetal Considerations

Aerobic PA during pregnancy may be important in maintaining infant birth weight within the normal range. Studies suggest that aerobic exercise strongly and inversely associates with fetal growth ratio. In cross comparisons, infants born to women with the highest levels of PA weighed an average 21 ounces less than infants born to sedentary women. It is suggested that women who engage in regular and appropriate PA throughout pregnancy have leaner babies than sedentary mothers [17]. Although exercise results in an elevation of fetal HR and breathing rate, training has not proved to incur increased risk of negative pathological consequences [61]. Other measures of fetal condition have also demonstrated very little risk to the fetus with exercise participation at appropriate levels. Women who train during pregnancy experience improved delivery outcomes, which manifest in fewer signs of stress during delivery and better general condition of newborns (e.g., higher Apgar scores) [56].

Training Considerations

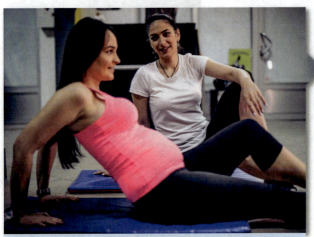

The level of training that is defined as appropriate for a pregnant female is specific to the individual and based on numerous physiological and genetic factors.

The level of training defined as appropriate for a pregnant female is specific to the individual and based on numerous physiological and genetic factors. To date, no upper level of intensity and training volume has been determined for pregnant women, with any guidelines only offering recommendations that previously sedentary females start with moderate intensity, and that if women were regularly participating in vigorous PA prenatal, it is safe to continue this practice, provided they remain healthy and discuss appropriate reductions in intensity with their healthcare providers [30]. Moderate-intensity aerobic exercise has been shown to be safe during pregnancy. Although impairment of sufficient oxygen and substrate supply to the fetus has not been demonstrated with aerobic activity, it is usually recommended to perform exercise in a submaximal range, with different countries providing recommended ranges of anywhere between 60% to 90% of maxHR [30].

One study analyzed the effects of high versus moderate-volume training on 42 healthy, athletic females who had performed exercise regularly prior to conception [55]. The women were split into one of two exercise groups and followed while they performed standardized exercise programs from gestational week 17 until 12 weeks postpartum. No complications were found in either the high or moderate-volume groups. Researchers concluded that well-trained women can benefit substantially from training at high volumes during an uncomplicated pregnancy [55]. The physiological adaptations to exercise during pregnancy appear to protect the fetus from potential harm, and the benefits of continued activity during pregnancy appear to outweigh any potential risks. All decisions about participation in PA during pregnancy should however be made by women in consultation with their medical advisers [19]. Restriction of PA should be dictated by obstetric and medical indications. Health care providers should inform pregnant women of potential risks and individualize exercise prescription and recommendations to reflect the safest level of participation.

In addition to aerobic exercise, maternal participation during pregnancy in other types of exercise has demonstrated positive outcomes. Studies of RT that incorporates moderate resistance and avoids maximal isometric contractions have shown no adverse outcomes for maternal exercisers, while showing improvements in strength and flexibility [3]. Moderate resistance exercise may provide additional benefits, preventing back pain and muscle strain during pregnancy. It seems that expecting women can participate in many fitness-related activities without consequence, provided that consideration is given to contraindications and warning signs.

Conditions that make exercise contraindicated during pregnancy:

- Certain types of heart and lung diseases
- Cervical insufficiency or cerclage
- Being pregnant with twins or triplets (or more) with risk factors or history for preterm labor
- Placenta previa after 26 weeks of pregnancy
- Premature contractions or labor
- Preterm labor or ruptured membranes (water has broken) during this pregnancy
- Pre-eclampsia or pregnancy-induced hypertension
- Severe anemia
- Persistent bleeding
- Thyroid disease
- Pre-existing cardiopulmonary pathologies

General Recommendations

Although a wide range of physical activities seem to be safe for pregnant females, some considerations must be applied. The overall health of a woman, including obstetric and medical risks, should be evaluated before prescribing an exercise program. Each activity should be reviewed individually for its potential risk, and women should discuss their intentions for PA with their primary health care provider. The physiologic and morphologic changes of pregnancy may interfere with the ability to engage safely in some forms of PA. Increases in body weight, the forward shift of the center of gravity, and the ligamentous laxity experienced during pregnancy can increase the risk of injury (3). Contact sports, activities requiring significant balance or that increase the risk of falling, and activities with a high potential for injury are not suitable during pregnancy.

> The physiological and morphological changes of pregnancy may interfere with the ability to safely engage in some forms of PA due to risk for injury:
>
> Increases in BW
>
> Forward shift of the center of gravity
>
> Ligamentous laxity

ACTIVITIES TO AVOID DURING PREGNANCY

- Any activity or sport involving a high risk of falling, trauma, or collisions/blunt force trauma to the abdomen (especially during the 2nd and 3rd trimester)
    - Contact sports, including, but not limited to, ice hockey, boxing, soccer, and basketball
    - Falling risk activities including, but not limited to, downhill snow skiing, water skiing, surfing, off-road or high-speed road cycling, gymnastics, horseback riding, and skydiving
- Exercise in hot or humid environments, such as "hot yoga" or "hot Pilates," or while having a fever, which may cause overheating and cause irreversible fetal damage
- Activities at altitude or depth, due to the risk of altitude sickness or decompression sickness from which the fetus is not protected
    - Scuba diving
    - Activities performed above 6,000 feet (if not accustomed to high altitude)
- Sedentary behavior and motionless standing, which are associated with adverse maternal outcomes
- Exercising in the supine position in late pregnancy has raised concerns, as supine CO decreases compared to the lateral position at rest; the reported 25% decrease in uterine blood flow during supine exercise is caused by uterine obstruction of the inferior vena cava [74]

> **General summary recommendations for pregnant individuals**
>
> - Consult your primary health care provider before beginning an exercise program.
> - Maintain adequate hydration at all times and ensure adequate caloric intake during pregnancy and lactation.
> - Stop exercise upon experiencing fatigue; never train to exhaustion.
> - Weight-bearing exercises can produce a greater decrease in O_2 reserve than non-weight bearing activities, so adjust intensities accordingly.
> - Beware of joint laxity during activity selection.
> - Immediately report vaginal spotting, bleeding, or any other adverse symptom to your primary physician.
> - Avoid all dangerous activities and high-risk training in general during high-risk pregnancies (e.g., having twins).

Children & Exercise

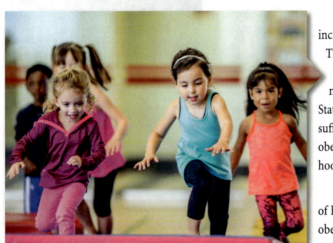

Over the past few decades, the prevalence of overweight and obesity has increased dramatically among children and adolescents in the United States. The number of overweight children between ages 2 and 5 has more than doubled since the 1970s. In school-aged children (6-19 years of age), that number has almost tripled. Today, 1 out of every 3 children in the United States is overweight or obese [37]. Children and adolescents who are overweight suffer a high susceptibility to becoming obese adults. In addition, the level of obesity found in adults relates to childhood weight: this identifies why childhood obesity is the number one health concern among American parents [42].

Overweight children and adolescents are at risk for an increased number of health problems during their youth and into adulthood. Overweight and obese children experience an elevated danger of developing risk factors associated with cardiovascular disease, including hypertension, hypercholesterolemia, dyslipidemia (high TG, low HDL), and Type II diabetes. In a population-based sample of 5 to 17-year-olds, almost 60% of overweight children had at least one CVD risk factor, while 25% of overweight children had two or more CVD risk factors [48]. Less common health conditions associated with increased weight in children include asthma, hepatic steatosis (fatty degeneration of the liver), and sleep apnea (intermittent breathing cessation). Additional consequences of childhood and adolescent obesity or overweight status stem from psychosocial-related factors. Overweight children and adolescents are targets of early and systematic social

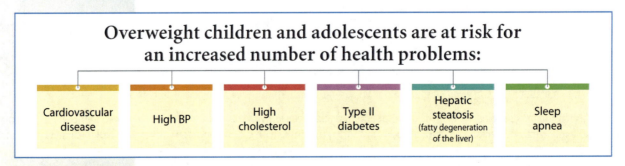

Overweight children and adolescents are at risk for an increased number of health problems:

- Cardiovascular disease
- High BP
- High cholesterol
- Type II diabetes
- Hepatic steatosis (fatty degeneration of the liver)
- Sleep apnea

discrimination [98]. They report lower self-esteem than non-overweight children and may develop impaired social function, a condition which often persists into adulthood [98].

Exercise and routine PA can have a pronounced effect on the health and fitness of children and adolescents. Children can benefit from all types of activity, including strength training, flexibility, and aerobic conditioning.

Routine participation in exercise and sports-related activities can:

- Improve cardiovascular fitness
- Enhance bone health
- Reduce susceptibility to weight gain
- Improve glucose tolerance
- Reduce the risk of the early development of health problems [77]

Differences Between Children & Adults

Although children and adults experience similar benefits from aerobic and RT, physiological differences exist between these populations. The muscle characteristics of children are quantitatively and qualitatively different from those of adults. Performance differences between adults and children seem to be metabolically and hormonally mediated. Children are similar to adults in the ability to use the immediate anaerobic energy system. They tolerate short, intense exercise similarly to adults but demonstrate a greater ability to recover [63]. This is likely due to lower peak power outputs, attributed to less muscle mass and lower stimulation of type II fibers. Additionally, faster phosphocreatine re-synthesis, greater oxidative capacity, better acid-base regulation, faster readjustment of initial cardiorespiratory parameters, and higher removal of metabolic by-products in children could also explain their faster recovery following high-intensity exercise.

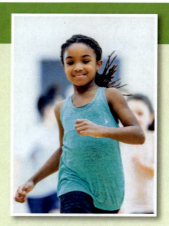

Children have a greater ability to recover from short, high-intensity exercise, likely due to:
- Lower peak power output
- Less muscle mass
- Lower stimulation of type II muscle fibers
- Faster phosphocreatine resynthesis
- Greater oxidative capacity
- Better acid-base regulation
- Faster readjustment of initial cardiorespiratory parameters
- Higher removal of metabolic by-products

When the glycolytic pathway is employed during exercise, children demonstrate a reduced performance capacity compared to adults [9]. Until they reach puberty, children seem to maintain an immature glycolytic system in terms of both fuel storage and enzyme concentration [91]. The reduced activity of phosphofructokinase-1 (PFK-1) and lactate dehydrogenase (LDH) enzymes (two key enzymatic reactions in glycolysis) likely limit the rate of glycolytic ATP generation in children. This assumption is supported by a lower production of muscle lactate relative to adults, suggesting less reliance on this energy system during the performance of work.

Comparing aerobic metabolism, children are better in terms of achieving steady-state HR during endurance activities [91]. Children are well adapted to prolonged exercise of moderate intensity due to efficient utilization of lipids, as demonstrated by lower respiratory exchange ratio values during moderate endurance exercise. Data indicate that children rely more on fat oxidation than adults, which is likely attributed to increased free fatty acid mobilization, greater glycerol release, and increases in growth hormone release in prepubescent children during exercise [89]. This also explains why children, who require a positive caloric balance for growth, best regulate weight through PA, whereas adults must use diet and exercise to manage body composition.

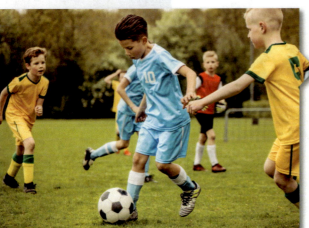

Children are well adapted to prolonged exercise of moderate intensity due to efficient utilization of lipids. Programming and activities should be fun, engaging, and of appropriate intensity.

Differences between adults and children are also observed within the cardiovascular system. Children demonstrate higher HRs with lower SV and total CO at a given submaximal work rate [91]. Likewise, at maximal exercise intensities, HRs are higher, while SV and CO remain lower in children compared to adults [91]. Physiological differences, including heart size and blood volume, likely account for the differences in SV. Heart rate recovery occurs at a faster rate in children compared to adults, which may be due to higher blood pH from the greater reliance on lipid metabolism during steady-state exercise.

Thermoregulation in response to exposure to hot and cold environments also differs between children and adults [96]. Many physical and physiological changes occur during growth and maturation that can affect thermoregulation during resting and active states. In most cases, the physical and physiological differences between children and adults explain the different responses to thermal stress. The primary physiological difference affecting the thermoregulation of heat between children and adults is related to the sweating mechanism. Children produce less sweat and have a lower sweat rate per gland, even though the heat-activated sweat glands are present in higher densities than in adults [50]. The lower sweating rate per gland may be explained by the smaller sweat gland size, a lower sensitivity of the sweating mechanism to thermal stimuli, and possibly a lower sweat gland metabolic capacity. Additional differences in thermoregulation between children and adults include metabolic, circulatory, and hormonal disparities [50]. Adults have a much higher surface-area-to-mass ratio than children, allowing for greater heat loss to the environment, thereby placing less reliance on evaporative cooling. Likewise, children have a lower blood volume than adults, which may limit the internal transfer of heat to the body's surface for dry release. Children are also at a thermodynamic disadvantage when walking or running in heated environments due to higher metabolic costs of locomotion and greater cardiovascular strain from a lower CO and less hemoglobin. The increased physiological demand leads to more rapid increases in internal temperatures when exercising in the heat [50].

Thermoregulatory functions are also different among children:

- The major difference is related to the sweating mechanism: children produce less sweat, possibly due to smaller sweat gland size, a lower sensitivity of the sweating mechanism to thermal stimuli, and lower sweat gland metabolic capacity

- Adults have a higher surface-area-to-mass ratio, allowing for greater heat loss into the environment

- Children have lower blood volume, limiting the internal transfer of heat to the body's surface

- Children are at a disadvantage when walking or running in the heat due to a higher metabolic cost of locomotion and greater cardiovascular strain from lower CO and hemoglobin blood concentrations

Program Considerations

Children can perform aerobic exercise using prescriptions that are similar to adults. With running, children experience a reduced HR, but training zones can be used to reflect appropriate intensity and pace. Cycling response is similar between children and adults, so no adjustment is required [92]. The key to getting children active in aerobic-based training is to select activities that they enjoy. If the activity is not perceived as fun, it is not likely they will engage in it on a routine basis. Pushing children into structured exercise rather than activities that are perceived as play may turn them off to participation in the future. Children should pick their own activities and be encouraged to perform either intermittent, high-intensity work or moderate, steady-state, paced training to take advantage of their physiological differences.

Children can also benefit from routine RT activities. Previous research has shown that children can increase their muscular strength and muscular endurance as a result of regular participation in a progressive RT program. Interestingly, when performed two times per week with only single sets per exercise, higher-repetition schemes (>12 repetitions) using lighter resistance provide better results than lower-repetition prescriptions (6-8 repetitions) using heavier loads [31]. When high-repetition training (13-15 repetitions) was compared to moderately heavy RT (6-8 repetitions), and contrast training (totaling 12-16 repetitions) similar results occurred [31]. Dramatic and almost identical improvements were found in the high-repetition resistance and contrast training above the heavier resistance loads. Motor rehearsal is a key element in the developmental process, so it makes sense to use higher repetitions and routine rehearsal of activities.

Children do not experience the same dramatic endocrine response as adults with heavy RT due to immature hormonal glands. Adaptations to strength training in children are neurally driven. Therefore, higher-repetition activities provide for greater motor enhancements when compared to low-repetition training. Children should be encouraged to focus on motor efficiency rather than heavy RT for optimal improvements. Following puberty, adolescents can engage in repetition schemes that are similar to adults, but again, the emphasis should be on proper technique rather than maximal attainable loads. Children demonstrate significant adaptation response to routine strength training, even at limited volumes [59]. One day of strength training on child-sized weight machines per week using one set of 10-15 repetitions for 12 exercises demonstrated limited gain in upper body strength, but a 14% improvement in lower body strength [31]. When a second day of strength training was added per week, significant improvements were found in all measures. These findings support the concept that muscular strength can be improved during the childhood years with limited volume, and that a frequency of 2-3 per week is required for improvements in children participating in an introductory strength training program [59].

Anytime RT in youth is discussed, risk of stunted growth due to damage of the epiphyseal plates is mentioned. However, several extensive research studies have discredited this dated belief by demonstrating that not only were these concerns unwarranted, there were no deleterious effects of RT when exercise was programmed and performed properly. Interestingly, young athletes who engaged in RT have shown decreased risks and frequencies of fracture and soft tissue injuries, which is usually attributed to their increased

Aerobic training

- Children can train at steady-state levels similar to adults
- Avoid extended periods of activity
- Children can perform short bouts (10 min) of intense aerobic exercise on an intermittent basis
- Emphasize enjoyable activities that stimulate play
- Be cautious of overheating and make sure children remain fully hydrated

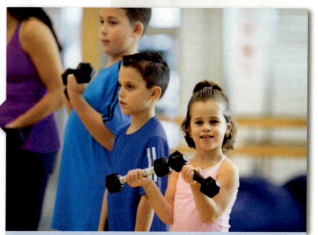

Anytime RT among youth is discussed, the risk of stunted growth due to damage of the epiphyseal plates is mentioned. However, extensive research has discredited this belief and actually shown young athletes who perform RT to have lower risks for fractures and soft tissue injuries.

Working with Special Populations

bone strength, BMD, and tendon strength [7, 57, 73]. When it comes to RT in children and preventing training-based injuries, the crucial aspects that play the biggest roles are teaching the youth engaged in activity proper technique and making sure they have supervision by trained professionals, who, when it is appropriate, can program appropriate progressive overload [72].

Anaerobic training

- Age-appropriate exercise can start when children begin organized sports (Olympic weightlifting often begins at 10-11 years)
- Higher-repetition schemes are more effective for pre-pubescent children
- Encourage motor learning and proper technique
- In general, two sets are sufficient for improvements in strength and endurance
- Multi-joint activities that develop motor skills are preferred over isolated training
- It is not recommended that children lift loads greater than their 8 RM to emphasize motor function and control
- Progressive overload should emphasize increased repetitions rather than load
- Pubescent adolescents can follow similar prescriptions as adults, but the emphasis should be on motor learning and efficient movement patterns

Exercise & the Elderly

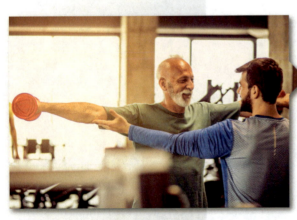

Age-related losses in physiological capacities contribute to the elderly population's decline in physical function. Attenuation of aerobic capacity, balance, muscular fitness and power have significant implications for aging adults. A general lack of PA contributes to a 10%-30% loss of biological function between the ages of 40 and 65, with the most pronounced decline affecting the physically inactive [90]. Further decline may be related to disease, genetic and environmental factors, poor mental health, or pre-existing injuries, including chronic low back pain.

The elderly who are sedentary possess an elevated susceptibility to:

- Hypertension and CAD
- Diabetes and obesity
- Osteoporosis and risk for falling and breaking a bone
- Depression
- Limitations related to structural changes in the connective tissues [5]

Fifty percent of individuals between 65 and 74 years of age report at least one physical limitation, with 30% reporting significant limitations [25]. It is suggested that >65% of individuals over 65 have hypertension, and at least 30% have been diagnosed with HD or obesity [34]. In many cases, the limitations older adults experience stem from a decrease in muscle mass and range of motion (ROM) due to limited PA.

Recall that sarcopenia means the age-related loss of muscle mass and function [34]. The loss of power, reduction in walking or gait speed, and reduced strength in older age appear to be caused by both muscular and neural factors [130]. Following age 60, the decline accelerates, leading to a pronounced loss of function. Although all older adults experience some level of decline, sedentary older adults experience the greatest reduction in muscle quantity and quality, physical performance and QOL [93]. This situation is worsened by the steady decline in aerobic capacity. Strength training increases muscle strength and muscular power in the elderly, thus counteracting part of the age-related loss [93]. Improvements, however, depend on the initial strength of the elderly person. The benefit of strength training is greatest in frail elderly and the very old, although all older adults can benefit from strength training. Considering the growing segment of the elderly population, the focus on sarcopenia and measures to counteract it are becoming increasingly more important. Combining resistance and aerobic training together have the greatest impact on health on sarcopenia in adults, compared to either type of training alone [5, 95].

Benefits of Exercise

Independent older adults gain significant functional benefits from both aerobic and strength training activities. Aerobic exercise results in improvements in functional capacity and may reduce BP and risk of developing type II diabetes in the elderly. Adaptations to routine aerobic exercise occur similarly between younger and older men and include increased CO and oxygen extraction capabilities [38]. The adaptations in older women, however, are almost exclusively related to improvements in oxygen extraction capabilities [88]. Although comparisons between the young and the old identify differences in maximal oxygen extraction and CO, older adults may improve their aerobic capacity by 10%-30% with routine aerobic exercise. The yearly decline in maxHR accounts for the greatest reduction in CO with age, while decline in oxygen extraction capabilities are likely attributed to the progressive loss of lean mass in the elderly.

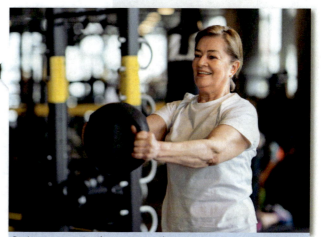

Resistance exercise demonstrates the greatest capacity to thwart functional decline among the elderly. It is also of great use for reducing the risk for osteoporotic fractures.

Resistance exercise demonstrates the greatest capacity to arrest decline and substantially improve physical function in the elderly [16, 40, 58]. It has been clearly demonstrated that skeletal muscle in older, untrained men and women will respond with significant strength gains, accompanied by considerable increases in muscle fiber size and capillary density [6, 67, 86]. Maximal working capacity, VO_2max, and serum lipid profiles also benefit from high-intensity RT. RT has been shown to significantly increase energy requirements, insulin sensitivity, and also positively impacts multiple risk factors for osteoporotic fractures in previously sedentary, post-menopausal women [49]. Interestingly, overall PA seems to increase in those participating in exercise programs compared to sedentary controls. This may be related to increased physical confidence and a reduced concern for falling [11]. Fun and enjoyment of social interactions are emphasized as the main motivation to join physical activities [28]. In the frail elderly, if only one type of training is being selected, strength training is recommended above aerobic training as it presents remarkable effects. When aerobic training is performed in lieu of, or without RT, the loss of lean mass is significantly greater, which seemingly perpetuates one of the main effects of sarcopenia. So, though aerobic training benefits any sedentary person, for the elderly, the best overall results come from participating in both RT and aerobic training.

RT demonstrates the greatest capacity to slow age-related functional decline:

- Significant strength gains
- Considerable increases in fiber size and capillary density
- Increased maximal work capacity and VO_2max
- Improved serum lipid profile
- Improved insulin sensitivity
- Reduced risk for osteoporotic fractures in post-menopausal women
- Increased physical confidence and reduced concern over falling
- In the frail elderly, strength training is considered superior to aerobic training for maintaining adequate function in performing daily tasks

Considerations for Training

Aerobic activity can be prescribed in the same manner as it would be for healthy young adults but most often requires an acclimation phase in the lower end of the normal training zones. Deconditioned older adults can start by accumulating 35-45 minutes of exercise performed throughout the day before progressing to continuous, low end (50%-60% HRR) steady-state training, or a multi-component training with a goal of accumulating 2 to 3 hours of moderate intensity training per week [26]. Healthy older adults should also begin at appropriate lower-end starting points before being progressed to higher exercise intensity.

Flexibility training should be encouraged for older adults, following adequate warm-up periods. Static stretching is beneficial when performed 2-3 days per week, using all the major muscle groups [26]. Functional-based activities, particularly those performed with a closed-chain through full ROMs, can also contribute to improved mobility [32]. Encouraging tasks of daily activity by employing multi-planar movements in training can improve balance, movement competence, and dynamic ROM. Limitations should be identified, and dynamic movements and static stretching should be used to encourage improved ROM in deficient areas.

Older adults are particularly susceptible to limited ROM in the following movements due to postural adjustments common with age:

A combo of the following has been shown to greatly enhance functional independence and QOL in older adults:

- Aerobic activity
- Strength training
- Balance, power, and flexibility exercises
- Increased general daily activity

- Trunk extension
- Trunk rotation
- Shoulder flexion
- External humeral rotation

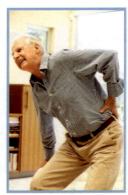

Working with Special Populations

RT is an integral part of the exercise prescription for older adults. Heavy, moderate, and low intensity RT protocols have shown to be effective in improving muscular strength and lean mass maintenance in this population [10, 24, 79]. This suggests that RT at any intensity can benefit older adults. Additionally, improvements in muscular strength and endurance can be attained with limited exercise volume, something that exercise professionals should consider when initiating an exercise program for the elderly. Similar to children, training the major muscle groups twice per week at moderate intensity is sufficient for improvement among new exercisers [10]. Likewise, for new exercisers, RT consisting of only single sets provides adequate stress to significantly enhance muscle function and physical performance during early training phases [74].

The aging neuromuscular system is highly responsive to RT. Therefore, following the initial adaptations to strength programs, older adults should be encouraged to participate in higher-volume work. In most cases, the elderly are most challenged by daily tasks that require the ability to generate short bursts of energy anaerobically. The performance of daily tasks, such as rising from a chair, climbing stairs, or lifting or reaching for an object, requires muscle strength, dynamic balance, and power. High levels of physical function are associated with elevated levels of anaerobic power in older adults. Since muscle power recedes at a faster rate than strength with age, it is necessary to emphasize power training in programs for the elderly where appropriate [63]. Peak muscle power may be improved using light, moderate, or heavy resistances, which allows for different options based on the client's capabilities. Research suggests that using high velocity resistance training may be the most effective strategy to achieve simultaneous improvements in muscle strength, power, and endurance in older adults [63]. It is important to realize that the high intensity is relative to the client's maximal values, which are often relatively low. Individual capacity will determine the most appropriate exercise prescription.

Functional limitations are obstacles that prevent one from engaging in daily activities which directly relate to QOL, such as independence and the ability to play with children. Middle-aged to older-aged adults who are sedentary present with more physical limitations than those who are active. The primary goal of a training program for an elderly person should focus on preventing premature death, followed by increasing QOL. Including training to help mitigate fall risk is a direct preventative method to help with achieving this goal. Twenty-seven percent of elderly individuals who experienced a severe fracture from falling died within one year of being hospitalized, with most of these deaths occurring within the first 3 months [15]. Including static and dynamic balance training, brisk walking, and muscular strengthening exercises have all been shown to decrease the risks of falling in the elderly population [85]. Prudent personal trainers and exercise professionals would do well to encourage and include these types of activities with their clients.

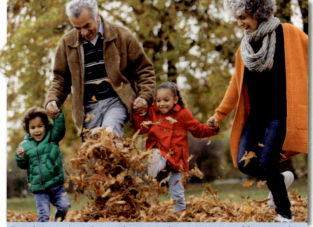

Regular exercise is key to thwarting the progression of functional limitations that prevent older adults from engaging in basic daily activities, maintaining independence and being able to play with children.

Exercise plays an important role in enhancing the QOL of the older adult. Improved physiological and psychological function helps to maintain personal independence and reduces the effects of aging. One of the largest obstacles to helping older adults is getting them to start participating in physical activities. The importance of PA cannot be overstated, as those who accumulate at least 7 hours of PA per week have a 40% lower chance of dying early than those who accumulate less than 30 minutes of activity. Initially, many older persons have low physical confidence and fear they will become injured by engaging in physical activities. However, vigorous activity is not required to make a substantial impact on mortality risk: all that is needed is 2.5 hours (150 minutes) of moderate-intensity activity to reduce the risk of dying early [36, 81]. Exercise professionals should understand that older adults must be educated to the importance of PA, individually encouraged to participate, and appropriately supported during and after participation to ensure sustained involvement.

Resistance Training
- 2-3 sessions/week, 8-10 exercises, 10-15 repetitions; progressions similar to young adults
- Encourage functional activities using full range of motion (especially loaded, closed-chain movements) and appropriate power activities
- Healthy older adults can perform heavy RT, but should avoid holding their breath and using isometric contractions

Aerobic Training
- Deconditioned older adults should accumulate 30-40 minutes in 10-min sessions most days of the week using 50-60% HRR
- For healthy older adults, 60-80% HRR for 30-60 minutes is appropriate

Flexibility
- Static stretching through a pain-free range should be performed 2-3 times per week, using 2-3 sets of 15-30 sec holds
- Encourage appropriate breathing techniques
- Dynamic ROM activities should be employed for 2-3 sets, 10-15 repetitions
- Employ spinal extension and outward rotation activities

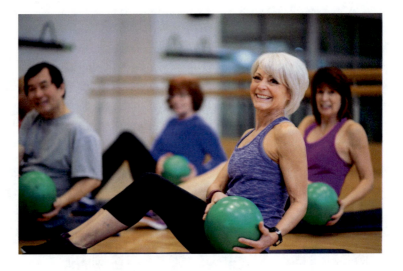

REFERENCES:

1. Abdullah MR, Eswaramoorthi V, Musa RM, Maliki M, Husin AB, Kosni NA, and Haque M. The Effectiveness of Aerobic Exercises at difference Intensities of Managing Blood Pressure in Essential Hypertensive Information Technology Officers. *Journal of Young Pharmacists* 8, 2016.

2. Anderson L, Oldridge N, Thompson DR, Zwisler A-D, Rees K, Martin N, and Taylor RS. Exercise-based cardiac rehabilitation for coronary heart disease: Cochrane systematic review and meta-analysis. *Journal of the American College of Cardiology* 67: 1-12, 2016.

3. Artal R and O'toole M. Guidelines of the American College of Obstetricians and Gynecologists for exercise during pregnancy and the postpartum period. *British journal of sports medicine* 37: 6-12, 2003.

4. Ashor AW, Lara J, Siervo M, Celis-Morales C, Oggioni C, Jakovljevic DG, and Mathers JC. Exercise modalities and endothelial function: a systematic review and dose–response meta-analysis of randomized controlled trials. *Sports medicine* 45: 279-296, 2015.

5. Bauman A, Merom D, Bull FC, Buchner DM, and Fiatarone Singh MA. Updating the evidence for physical activity: summative reviews of the epidemiological evidence, prevalence, and interventions to promote "active aging". *The Gerontologist* 56: S268-S280, 2016.

6. Bechshøft RL, Malmgaard-Clausen NM, Gliese B, Beyer N, Mackey AL, Andersen JL, Kjær M, and Holm L. Improved skeletal muscle mass and strength after heavy strength training in very old individuals. *Experimental gerontology* 92: 96-105, 2017.

7. Bedoya AA, Miltenberger MR, and Lopez RM. Plyometric training effects on athletic performance in youth soccer athletes: a systematic review. *The Journal of Strength & Conditioning Research* 29: 2351-2360, 2015.

8. Bell JA, Kivimaki M, and Hamer M. Metabolically healthy obesity and risk of incident type 2 diabetes: a meta-analysis of prospective cohort studies. *Obesity reviews* 15: 504-515, 2014.

9. Beneke R, Hutler M, Jung M, and Leithauser RM. Modeling the blood lactate kinetics at maximal short-term exercise conditions in children, adolescents, and adults. *Journal of applied physiology* 99: 499-504, 2005.

10. Borde R, Hortobágyi T, and Granacher U. Dose–response relationships of resistance training in healthy old adults: a systematic review and meta-analysis. *Sports medicine* 45: 1693-1720, 2015.

11. Brawley LR, Rejeski WJ, and King AC. Promoting physical activity for older adults: the challenges for changing behavior. *American journal of preventive medicine* 25: 172-183, 2003.

12. Butler R, Palmer G, and Rogers F. Circuit weight training in early cardiac rehabilitation. *The Journal of the American Osteopathic Association* 92: 77-77, 1992.

13. Caruso F, Arena R, Phillips S, Bonjorno Jr J, Mendes R, Arakelian V, Bassi D, Nogi C, and Borghi-Silva A. Resistance exercise training improves heart rate variability and muscle performance: a randomized controlled trial in coronary artery disease patients. *Eur J Phys Rehabil Med* 51: 281-289, 2015.

14. Cauza E, Hanusch-Enserer U, Strasser B, Ludvik B, Metz-Schimmerl S, Pacini G, Wagner O, Georg P, Prager R, and Kostner K. The relative benefits of endurance and strength training on the metabolic factors and muscle function of people with type 2 diabetes mellitus. *Archives of physical medicine and rehabilitation* 86: 1527-1533, 2005.

15. Cenzer IS, Tang V, Boscardin WJ, Smith AK, Ritchie C, Wallhagen MI, Espaldon R, and Covinsky KE. One-Year Mortality After Hip Fracture: Development and Validation of a Prognostic Index. *Journal of the American Geriatrics Society* 64: 1863-1868, 2016.

16. Chou C-H, Hwang C-L, and Wu Y-T. Effect of exercise on physical function, daily living activities, and quality of life in the frail older adults: a meta-analysis. *Archives of physical medicine and rehabilitation* 93: 237-244, 2012.

17. Clapp 3rd J. Exercise and fetal health. *Journal of developmental physiology* 15: 9, 1991.

18. Control CfD and Prevention. Asthma FastStats. *Atlanta, GA: National Center for Health Statistics Available at< http://www cdc gov/nchs/fastats/asthma htm> Accessed on May 1, 2016.*

19. Control CfD and Prevention. Asthma-related missed school days among children aged 5–17 years. *Available from:)(Accessed January 10, 2017) https://www cdc gov/asthma/asthma_stats/missing_days htm View in Article| Google Scholar*, 2015.

20. Control CfD and Prevention. Most recent asthma data. *cdc gov [Internet] Feb*, 2017.

21. Control CfD and Prevention. National diabetes statistics report, 2017. *Atlanta, GA: Centers for Disease Control and Prevention*, 2017.

22. Cornelissen VA and Fagard RH. Effects of endurance training on blood pressure, blood pressure–regulating mechanisms, and cardiovascular risk factors. *Hypertension* 46: 667-675, 2005.

23. Counil F-P, Varray A, Matecki S, Beurey A, Marchal P, Voisin M, and Préfaut C. Training of aerobic and anaerobic fitness in children with asthma. *The Journal of pediatrics* 142: 179-184, 2003.

24. Csapo R and Alegre L. Effects of resistance training with moderate vs heavy loads on muscle mass and strength in the elderly: A meta-analysis. *Scandinavian journal of medicine & science in sports* 26: 995-1006, 2016.

25. Currie KD, Bailey KJ, Jung ME, McKelvie RS, and MacDonald MJ. Effects of resistance training combined with moderate-intensity endurance or low-volume high-intensity interval exercise on cardiovascular risk factors in patients with coronary artery disease. *Journal of science and medicine in sport* 18: 637-642, 2015.

26. de Souto Barreto P, Morley JE, Chodzko-Zajko W, Pitkala KH, Weening-Djiksterhuis E, Rodriguez-Mañas L, Barbagallo M, Rosendahl E, Sinclair A, and Landi F. Recommendations on physical activity and exercise for older adults living in long-term care facilities: A taskforce report. *Journal of the American Medical Directors Association* 17: 381-392, 2016.

27. Dempsey FC, Butler FL, and Williams FA. No need for a pregnant pause: physical activity may reduce the occurrence of gestational diabetes mellitus and preeclampsia. *Exercise and sport sciences reviews* 33: 141-149, 2005.

28. Devereux-Fitzgerald A, Powell R, Dewhurst A, and French DP. The acceptability of physical activity interventions to older adults: A systematic review and meta-synthesis. *Social Science & Medicine* 158: 14-23, 2016.

29. Emtner M, Finne M, and Stålenheim G. High-intensity physical training in adults with asthma. A comparison between training on land and in water. *Scandinavian journal of rehabilitation medicine* 30: 201-209, 1998.

30. Evenson KR, Barakat R, Brown WJ, Dargent-Molina P, Haruna M, Mikkelsen EM, Mottola MF, Owe KM, Rousham EK, and Yeo S. Guidelines for physical activity during pregnancy: comparisons from around the world. *American journal of lifestyle medicine* 8: 102-121, 2014.

31. Faigenbaum AD, Loud RL, O Connell J, Glover S, O Connell J, and Westcott WL. Effects of different resistance training protocols on upper-body strength and endurance development in children. *Journal of Strength and Conditioning Research* 15: 459-465, 2001.

32. Fatouros IG, Kambas A, Katrabasas I, Leontsini D, Chatzinikolaou A, Jamurtas AZ, Douroudos I, Aggelousis N, and Taxildaris K. Resistance training and detraining effects on flexibility performance in the elderly are intensity-dependent. *The Journal of Strength & Conditioning Research* 20: 634-642, 2006.

33. Fleg JL, Cooper LS, Borlaug BA, Haykowsky MJ, Kraus WE, Levine BD, Pfeffer MA, Piña IL, Poole DC, and Reeves GR. Exercise training as therapy for heart failure: current status and future directions. *Circulation: Heart Failure* 8: 209-220, 2015.

34. Flegal KM, Kruszon-Moran D, Carroll MD, Fryar CD, and Ogden CL. Trends in obesity among adults in the United States, 2005 to 2014. *Jama* 315: 2284-2291, 2016.

35. Franklin BA and Lavie CJ. Impact of statins on physical activity and fitness: ally or adversary? *Mayo Clinic Proceedings*. Elsevier, 2015, p. 1314-1319.

36. Freiberger E, Sieber C, and Pfeifer K. Physical activity, exercise, and sarcopenia–future challenges. *Wiener Medizinische Wochenschrift* 161: 416-425, 2011.

37. Fryar CD, Carroll MD, and Ogden CL. Prevalence of obesity among children and adolescents: United States, trends 1963–1965 through 2009–2010. *National Center for Health Statistics* 1960, 2012.

38. Giada F, Bertaglia E, De Piccoli B, Franceschi M, Sartori F, Raviele A, and Pascotto P. Cardiovascular adaptations to endurance training and detraining in young and older athletes. *International journal of cardiology* 65: 149-155, 1998.

39. Gielen S, Laughlin MH, O'Conner C, and Duncker DJ. Exercise training in patients with heart disease: review of beneficial effects and clinical recommendations. *Progress in cardiovascular diseases* 57: 347-355, 2015.

40. Giné-Garriga M, Roqué-Fíguls M, Coll-Planas L, Sitjà-Rabert M, and Salvà A. Physical exercise interventions for improving performance-based measures of physical function in community-dwelling, frail older adults: a systematic review and meta-analysis. *Archives of physical medicine and rehabilitation* 95: 753-769. e753, 2014.

41. Hallstrand TS, Bates PW, and Schoene RB. Aerobic conditioning in mild asthma decreases the hyperpnea of exercise and improves exercise and ventilatory capacity. *Chest* 118: 1460-1469, 2000.

42. Han JC, Lawlor DA, and Kimm SY. Childhood obesity. *The Lancet* 375: 1737-1748, 2010.

43. Hayman M, Brown W, Ferrar K, Marchese R, and Tan J. SMA Position Statement for Exercise in Pregnancy and the Postpartum Period. 2016.

44. Hirai DM, Musch TI, and Poole DC. Exercise training in chronic heart failure: improving skeletal muscle O2 transport and utilization. *American Journal of Physiology-Heart and Circulatory Physiology* 309: H1419-H1439, 2015.

45. Hollings M, Mavros Y, Freeston J, and Fiatarone Singh M. The effect of progressive resistance training on aerobic fitness and strength in adults with coronary heart disease: a systematic review and meta-analysis of randomised controlled trials. *European journal of preventive cardiology* 24: 1242-1259, 2017.

46. Holten MK, Zacho M, Gaster M, Juel C, Wojtaszewski JF, and Dela F. Strength training increases insulin-mediated glucose uptake, GLUT4 content, and insulin signaling in skeletal muscle in patients with type 2 diabetes. *Diabetes* 53: 294-305, 2004.

47. Hong SJ, Lee MS, Lee SY, Ahn KM, Oh JW, Kim KE, Lee JS, and Lee HB. High body mass index and dietary pattern are associated with childhood asthma. *Pediatric pulmonology* 41: 1118-1124, 2006.

48. Horgan G. Healthier lifestyles series: 1. Exercise for children. *The journal of family health care* 15: 15-17, 2005.

49. Hurley BF and Roth SM. Strength training in the elderly. *Sports Medicine* 30: 249-268, 2000.

50. Inbar O, Morris N, Epstein Y, and Gass G. Comparison of thermoregulatory responses to exercise in dry heat among prepubertal boys, young adults and older males. *Experimental physiology* 89: 691-700, 2004.

51. Jelleyman C, Yates T, O'Donovan G, Gray LJ, King JA, Khunti K, and Davies MJ. The effects of high–intensity interval training on glucose regulation and insulin resistance: a meta–analysis. *Obesity reviews* 16: 942-961, 2015.

52. Johannsen NM, Swift DL, Lavie CJ, Earnest CP, Blair SN, and Church TS. Combined aerobic and resistance training effects on glucose homeostasis, fitness, and other major health indices: a review of current guidelines. *Sports Medicine* 46: 1809-1818, 2016.

53. Joyner MJ and Green DJ. Exercise protects the cardiovascular system: effects beyond traditional risk factors. *The Journal of physiology* 587: 5551-5558, 2009.

54. Kampmann U, Madsen LR, Skajaa GO, Iversen DS, Moeller N, and Ovesen P. Gestational diabetes: A clinical update. *World journal of diabetes* 6: 1065, 2015.

55. Kardel KR and Kase T. Training in pregnant women: effects on fetal development and birth. *American Journal of Obstetrics & Gynecology* 178: 280-286, 1998.

56. Kramer MS and McDonald SW. Aerobic exercise for women during pregnancy. *Cochrane database of systematic reviews*, 2006.

57. Lesinski M, Prieske O, and Granacher U. Effects and dose–response relationships of resistance training on physical performance in youth athletes: a systematic review and meta-analysis. *Br J Sports Med*: bjsports-2015-095497, 2016.

58. Liu C-j and Latham NK. Progressive resistance strength training for improving physical function in older adults. *The Cochrane database of systematic reviews*: CD002759, 2009.

59. Lloyd RS, Faigenbaum AD, Stone MH, Oliver JL, Jeffreys I, Moody JA, Brewer C, Pierce KC, McCambridge TM, and Howard R. Position statement on youth resistance training: the 2014 International Consensus. *Br J Sports Med*: bjsports-2013-092952, 2013.

60. Lucas SR and Platts-Mills TA. Physical activity and exercise in asthma: relevance to etiology and treatment. *Journal of Allergy and Clinical Immunology* 115: 928-934, 2005.

61. May LE, Glaros A, Yeh H-W, Clapp III JF, and Gustafson KM. Aerobic exercise during pregnancy influences fetal cardiac autonomic control of heart rate and heart rate variability. *Early human development* 86: 213-217, 2010.

62. McKelvie RS, Teo KK, McCartney N, Humen D, Montague T, and Yusuf S. Effects of exercise training in patients with congestive heart failure: a critical review. *Journal of the American College of Cardiology* 25: 789-796, 1995.

63. McKinnon NB, Connelly DM, Rice CL, Hunter SW, and Doherty TJ. Neuromuscular contributions to the age-related reduction in muscle power: mechanisms and potential role of high velocity power training. *Ageing research reviews* 35: 147-154, 2017.

64. Meyer K. Exercise training in heart failure: recommendations based on current research. *Medicine and science in sports and exercise* 33: 525-531, 2001.

65. Meyer K. Resistance exercise in chronic heart failure-landmark studies and implications for practice. *Clinical and investigative medicine* 29: 166, 2006.

66. Molmen-Hansen HE, Stolen T, Tjonna AE, Aamot IL, Ekeberg IS, Tyldum GA, Wisloff U, Ingul CB, and Stoylen A. Aerobic interval training reduces blood pressure and improves myocardial function in hypertensive patients. *European journal of preventive cardiology* 19: 151-160, 2012.

67. Moore DR, Kelly RP, Devries MC, Churchward-Venne TA, Phillips SM, Parise G, and Johnston AP. Low-load resistance exercise during inactivity is associated with greater fibre area and satellite cell expression in older skeletal muscle. *Journal of cachexia, sarcopenia and muscle*, 2018.

68. Morton AR and Fitch KD. Australian association for exercise and sports science position statement on exercise and asthma. *Journal of Science and Medicine in Sport* 14: 312-316, 2011.

69. Mosher PE, Nash MS, Perry AC, LaPerriere AR, and Goldberg RB. Aerobic circuit exercise training: effect on adolescents with well-controlled insulin-dependent diabetes mellitus. *Archives of physical medicine and rehabilitation* 79: 652-657, 1998.

70. Mottola MF and Artal R. Fetal and maternal metabolic responses to exercise during pregnancy. *Early human development* 94: 33-41, 2016.

71. Muktabhant B, Lawrie TA, Lumbiganon P, and Laopaiboon M. Diet or exercise, or both, for preventing excessive weight gain in pregnancy. *Cochrane database of systematic reviews*, 2015.

72. Myers AM, Beam NW, and Fakhoury JD. Resistance training for children and adolescents. *Translational pediatrics* 6: 137, 2017.

73. Negra Y, Chaabene H, Hammami M, Hachana Y, and Granacher U. Effects of high-velocity resistance training on athletic performance in prepuberal male soccer athletes. *The Journal of Strength & Conditioning Research* 30: 3290-3297, 2016.

74. Olson D, Sikka RS, Hayman J, Novak M, and Stavig C. Exercise in pregnancy. *Current sports medicine reports* 8: 147-153, 2009.

75. Pescatello LS, MacDonald HV, Ash GI, Lamberti LM, Farquhar WB, Arena R, and Johnson BT. Assessing the existing professional exercise recommendations for hypertension: a review and recommendations for future research priorities. *Mayo Clinic Proceedings*. Elsevier, 2015, p. 801-812.

76. Pescatello LS, MacDonald HV, Lamberti L, and Johnson BT. Exercise for hypertension: a prescription update integrating existing recommendations with emerging research. *Current hypertension reports* 17: 87, 2015.

77. Poitras VJ, Gray CE, Borghese MM, Carson V, Chaput J-P, Janssen I, Katzmarzyk PT, Pate RR, Connor Gorber S, and Kho ME. Systematic review of the relationships between objectively measured physical activity and health indicators in school-aged children and youth. *Applied Physiology, Nutrition, and Metabolism* 41: S197-S239, 2016.

78. Ponikowski P, Voors AA, Anker SD, Bueno H, Cleland JG, Coats AJ, Falk V, González–Juanatey JR, Harjola VP, and Jankowska EA. 2016 ESC Guidelines for the diagnosis and treatment of acute and chronic heart failure: The Task Force for the diagnosis and treatment of acute and chronic heart failure of the European Society of Cardiology (ESC). Developed with the special contribution of the Heart Failure Association (HFA) of the ESC. *European journal of heart failure* 18: 891-975, 2016.

79. Raymond MJ, Bramley-Tzerefos RE, Jeffs KJ, Winter A, and Holland AE. Systematic review of high-intensity progressive resistance strength training of the lower limb compared with other intensities of strength training in older adults. *Archives of physical medicine and rehabilitation* 94: 1458-1472, 2013.

80. Reichenberg K and Broberg A. Eotional and behavioural problems in Swedish 7-to 9-year olds with asthma. *Chronic respiratory disease* 1: 183-189, 2004.

81. Rom O, Kaisari S, Aizenbud D, and Reznick AZ. Lifestyle and sarcopenia—etiology, prevention, and treatment. *Rambam Maimonides medical journal* 3, 2012.

82. Sagar VA, Davies EJ, Briscoe S, Coats AJ, Dalal HM, Lough F, Rees K, Singh S, and Taylor RS. Exercise-based rehabilitation for heart failure: systematic review and meta-analysis. *Open heart* 2: e000163, 2015.

83. Santuz P, Baraldi E, Filippone M, and Zacchello F. Exercise performance in children with asthma: is it different from that of healthy controls? *European Respiratory Journal* 10: 1254-1260, 1997.

84. Shekerdemian L and Bohn D. Cardiovascular effects of mechanical ventilation. *Archives of disease in childhood* 80: 475-480, 1999.

85. Sherrington C, Whitney JC, Lord SR, Herbert RD, Cumming RG, and Close JC. Effective exercise for the prevention of falls: a systematic review and meta-analysis. *Journal of the American Geriatrics Society* 56: 2234-2243, 2008.

86. Snijders T, Nederveen JP, Joanisse S, Leenders M, Verdijk LB, Van Loon LJ, and Parise G. Muscle fibre capillarization is a critical factor in muscle fibre hypertrophy during resistance exercise training in older men. *Journal of cachexia, sarcopenia and muscle* 8: 267-276, 2017.

87. Sparling P, Cantwell J, Dolan C, and Niederman R. Strength training in a cardiac rehabilitation program: a six-month follow-up. *Archives of physical medicine and rehabilitation* 71: 148-152, 1990.

88. Spina RJ, Ogawa T, Kohrt WM, Martin 3rd W, Holloszy J, and Ehsani A. Differences in cardiovascular adaptations to endurance exercise training between older men and women. *Journal of Applied Physiology* 75: 849-855, 1993.

89. Stoedefalke K. Effects of exercise training on blood lipids and lipoproteins in children and adolescents. *Journal of sports science & medicine* 6: 313, 2007.

90. Trombetti A, Reid K, Hars M, Herrmann F, Pasha E, Phillips E, and Fielding R. Age-associated declines in muscle mass, strength, power, and physical performance: impact on fear of falling and quality of life. *Osteoporosis international* 27: 463-471, 2016.

91. Turley KR. Cardiovascular responses to exercise in children. *Sports Medicine* 24: 241-257, 1997.

92. Turley KR and Wilmore JH. Cardiovascular responses to treadmill and cycle ergometer exercise in children and adults. *Journal of Applied Physiology* 83: 948-957, 1997.

93. Verlaan S, Aspray TJ, Bauer JM, Cederholm T, Hemsworth J, Hill TR, McPhee JS, Piasecki M, Seal C, and Sieber CC. Nutritional status, body composition, and quality of life in community-dwelling sarcopenic and non-sarcopenic older adults: A case-control study. *Clinical Nutrition* 36: 267-274, 2017.

94. Vila G, Hayder R, Bertrand C, Falissard B, De Blic J, Mouren-Simeoni M-C, and Scheinmann P. Psychopathology and quality of life for adolescents with asthma and their parents. *Psychosomatics* 44: 319-328, 2003.

95. Villareal DT, Aguirre L, Gurney AB, Waters DL, Sinacore DR, Colombo E, Armamento-Villareal R, and Qualls C. Aerobic or resistance exercise, or both, in dieting obese older adults. *New England Journal of Medicine* 376: 1943-1955, 2017.

96. Vincent KR, Vincent HK, Braith RW, Bhatnagar V, and Lowenthal DT. Strength training and hemodynamic responses to exercise. *The American journal of geriatric cardiology* 12: 97-106, 2003.

97. Volaklis KA and Tokmakidis SP. Resistance exercise training in patients with heart failure. *Sports Medicine* 35: 1085-1103, 2005.

98. Wadden TA and Stunkard AJ. Social and psychological consequences of obesity. *Annals of Internal Medicine* 103: 1062-1067, 1985.

99. Wei M, Gibbons LW, Kampert JB, Nichaman MZ, and Blair SN. Low cardiorespiratory fitness and physical inactivity as predictors of mortality in men with type 2 diabetes. *Annals of internal medicine* 132: 605-611, 2000.

100. Weiss ST. Obesity: insight into the origins of asthma. *Nature immunology* 6: 537, 2005.

101. Wilmore JH, Green JS, Stanforth PR, Gagnon J, Rankinen T, Leon AS, Rao D, Skinner JS, and Bouchard C. Relationship of changes in maximal and submaximal aerobic fitness to changes in cardiovascular disease and non [ndash] insulin-dependent diabetes mellitus risk factors with endurance training: The HERITAGE Family Study. *Metabolism-Clinical and Experimental* 50: 1255-1263, 2001.

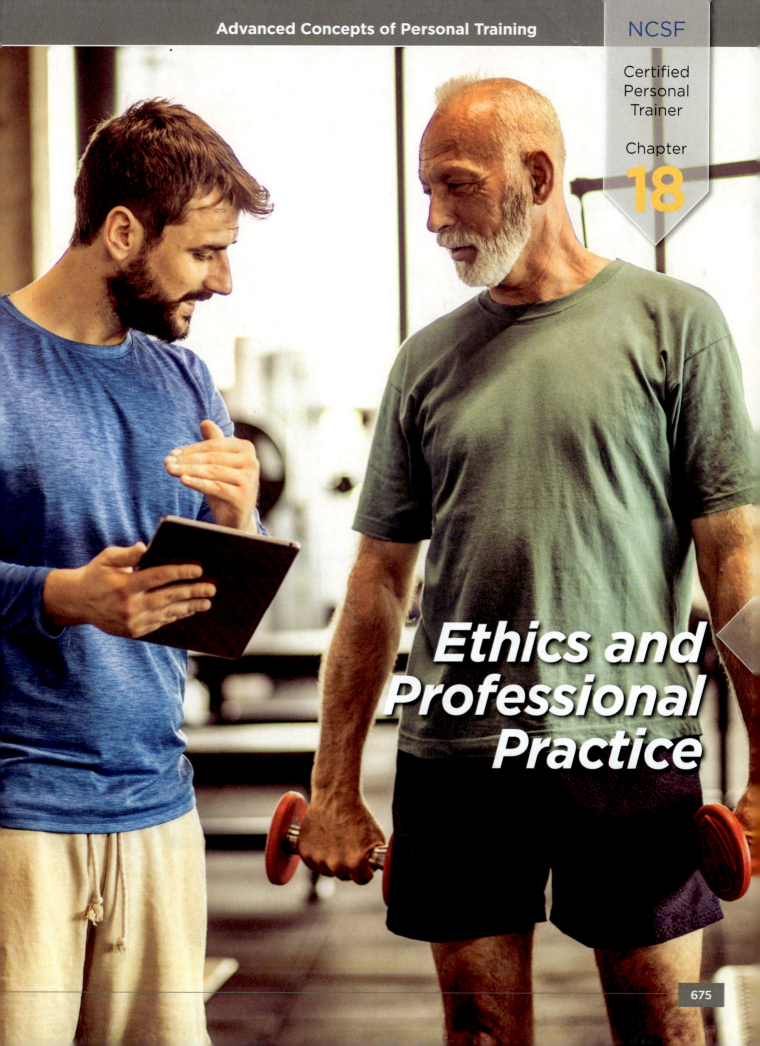

What Makes a Professional

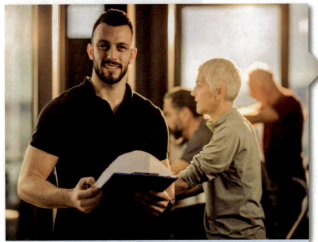

Establishing the highest level of professionalism within the fitness industry ensures growth and future opportunity within the field.

The personal trainer profession is evolving into a recognized and respected supporting cog in the allied health care system. The industry's ongoing development depends on increasing trainer competence and elevating standards of practice [5, 8]. Establishing the highest level of professionalism within the field will ensure growth and future opportunity within the industry as a whole. Professionalism starts with the desire to advance within one's chosen field [8]. Striving to reach the profession's highest level leads to success and demonstrates strong personal character [3, 4]. To perform optimally within a profession, one must identify the qualities exemplified by the most successful and respected practitioners.

Professionalism is defined as the conduct, aims, or qualities that characterize a profession or a professional person. It is not just attained by the desire to achieve in one's chosen field, but also originates from performing routine actions, complying with industry standards, and managing external perceptions [2, 19]. Importantly, consumers often judge professionalism and competence via their external perceptions. Perception is commonly defined by outward appearance, ability to communicate, remaining updated within the field, and conveying confidence in one's capabilities. For many people, appearance is the first measure of professionalism [19]. To some, attention to detail and appearance indicates how seriously and attentive an exercise professional will be to other components of the job. Proper grooming and appropriate attire conveys respect for both one's self and the profession as a whole. Therefore, exercise professionals should routinely make a conscious effort to look professional by dressing appropriately.

The second attribute linked to perception of professional competence is effective communication. Language usage is often considered a facet of both social and cognitive intelligence, and communication skills are valuable when working with people, as these skills are not only

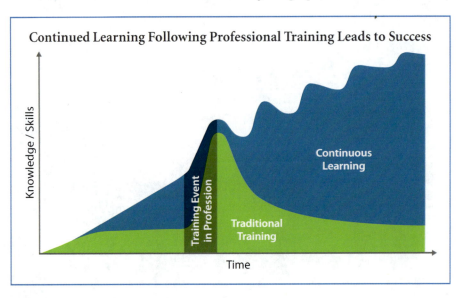

used to pass information, but also to convey emotions. Physical and verbal messages can express care, support, empathy, interest, and enthusiasm [18]. All of these features are central to effective personal trainer services. Professional exchanges should be clear, accurate, concise, and relevant. In some cases, trainers may be tempted to say only what the listener wants to hear when the factual results of assessments may be perceived as unpleasant. Nonetheless, these facts must be conveyed, but should be delivered so that they do not deflate the client. Thus, employing proper judgment and tact are crucial to being a good communicator.

Inquiry is a third characteristic often attributed to successful practice and entails the continued pursuit of knowledge and professional development. Abundant new information, research, methods, and protocols regularly emerge within the fitness industry, so not even the most expert trainers can know everything at any point in time. New information refuting or endorsing "established knowledge" arises every day and practices regularly evolve to include updated techniques. However, trainers must be interested in improving their knowledge and competency to remain current in such a dynamic profession. They must also maintain and hold current professional credentials. Ongoing professional development and competency maintenance requires continued education, which explains the requirements set by certification and licensing boards that mandate credentialed professionals to report continuing education units (CEUs) or continuing education credits (CECs) at the end of a certification cycle.

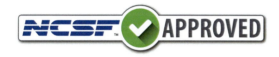

Confidence is another quality that people look for in a professional when gauging competence. Although less tangible, confidence is still observable. This self-assurance stems from a belief in one's abilities and knowledge, **self-efficacy**, and experience. When someone does not exude confidence, others perceive a deficiency in ability. This is not to suggest that a lack of skill actually exists, but rather that others trust those individuals who possess conviction and believe in their capacity to perform effectively. Many cases exist that involve individuals who may have a limited knowledge base on a topic or field but are seen as experts solely because they project confidence in their message. Dedicated and well-informed professionals should learn how to confidently communicate their competency so that others will accurately perceive the ability and knowledge they possess.

The measure of professionalism encompasses more than personal characteristics and presentation, as it is also based on actions, principles, and an individual's decision-making process. Professional actions demonstrate effectiveness, convey aptitude, and identify a practitioner as skilled, diligent, and resourceful [9]. When a person acts in a professional manner, he or she exemplifies the traits expected of the model practitioner. Regardless of the career, effective people present similarities within their daily routines and professional behaviors.

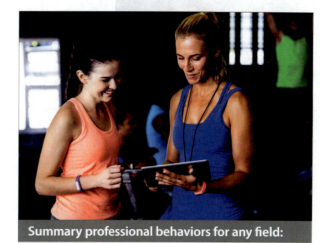

Summary professional behaviors for any field:

- Punctuality and awareness of one's schedule
- Responding to emails, phone messages, and outstanding commitments in a timely fashion
- Accurate and clear communication
- Upholding commitments
- Premeditating actions
- Performing routine follow-up actions
- Providing prompt feedback
- Documenting operations
- Implementing an organized system
- Accessing resources as needed
- Thinking critically in an unbiased fashion
- Accepting responsibility
- Being task driven
- Identifying and improving deficiencies
- Proactively addressing issues and conflicts

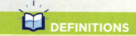

DEFINITIONS

Self-efficacy –

A belief in one's ability to be successful in certain situations or accomplish a task.

Professional Principles

Professional principles support the actions and decisions that enable a practitioner to develop the behaviors appropriate to the chosen career. Each profession entails a slightly different application of professional principles, determined by governing bodies, employer requirements, and consumer expectations and demands. Professional principles provide the framework for conformity to an industry standard. They are used to adapt the proper behavior and attitude toward the relevant job tasks and enable the developing professional to identify the competencies required to become an effective contributor to the profession.

Professional principles are determined by: Governing bodies | Employer requirements | Consumer expectations and demands

Interpersonal Relations & Communication

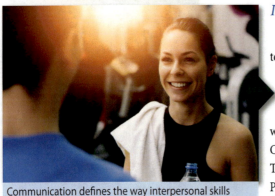

Communication defines the way interpersonal skills are applied to maintain good relations within the work environment; in addition, it often defines how a person is viewed as both a professional and a person.

The basic principles of communication define the way interpersonal skills are applied to maintain good relations within the work environment. They include using professional language when speaking with clients and colleagues and properly disseminating information. Commonly termed "soft skills," these personal attributes and actions often define how one is viewed as both a professional and a person. In many cases, the way one is perceived will affect success and growth potential within a work environment. Clients will often divulge personal and private information to exercise professionals. Thus, it is important to consider the client's privacy rights under the Health Insurance Portability and Accountability Act of 1996 (HIPAA), as well as professional standards [1]. Anything a client shares with a personal trainer, including but not limited to personal life matters and medical information, should be kept secure and only revealed to the appropriate professionals when necessary and appropriate.

Professional Compliance

The principle of compliance means making decisions based on established professional norms. Providing evidence-based information and practicing and acting in a manner concurring with defined standards and guidelines falls under this principle's purview. All allied health fields establish best practice standards and scope of profession norms and boundaries. Adhering to professional standards promotes effective outcomes and leads to reduced liability risk. Non-compliance with recognized standards is commonly associated with negative outcomes and may limit professional advancement in the wake of employer or board sanctions.

Professional Judgment & Autonomy

Professional judgement represents the ability to make considered decisions or come to sensible conclusions. In many cases, civil and criminal legal implications are based on judgement considered prudent and thoughtful. This judgement is based on preconceived values, which guide the decision-making process to protect the profession's stakeholders, including those who receive professional services. Autonomy suggests self-governance in accordance with the governing body's highest expectations, and this principle supports professional accountability. Therefore, all professionals must make independent decisions based on the best interest of the stakeholders affected by those decisions.

Professional Ethics

Ethics represent moral principles that govern a person's behavior. The principle of professional ethics obligates those acting in a defined role to make an ethical covenant with society to exercise judgment in the best interest of all others they are serving in a professional capacity. It encompasses all the principles and standards that underlie one's responsibilities and conduct in a field of expertise and is extended to all stakeholders of the profession. It requires practitioners to act in a fiduciary role to fulfill the highest ideals and core values of both the profession and discipline. Professional ethics are defined by the body of the profession, generally in the form of a regulatory body that oversees practitioners. A code of ethics represents a set of expectations or rules used to objectively evaluate a professional's actions.

Self-Discipline

This principle reflects a structured approach to the management of professional activity, as it places expectations on premeditated and conscience-driven professional ethics. Self-discipline entails both restraint, diligence, and personal control and is a key attribute among those in leadership positions. It also indicates one's aptitude for ongoing compliance with the rigors of the profession.

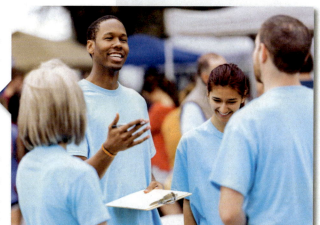

Self-discipline entails both restraint and diligence; it identifies personal control, is a key attribute among those in leadership positions, and demonstrates one's aptitude for ongoing compliance with the rigors of the profession.

The principles of a profession embody the professional standards by which practitioners perform their trade [10]. The personal trainer must abide by a standardized code of conduct that, at a minimum, ensures safe and professional practice. Professional standards allow for critical evaluation and the accountability of the practitioner to all stakeholders of the profession. Most of these standards incorporate clearly articulated requirements and specific guidelines defining correct practice. These requirements and guidelines are developed in accordance with evidence-based criteria, social responsibility, and uniformly accepted norms [12]. All NCSF-certified professionals are expected to comply with the certification board's code of ethics and professional practices.

Professional Standards

Professional standards distill expectations of what constitutes sound and proper practice by identifying fundamental ethical considerations, while addressing more specific acts of professional conduct. Secondarily, they may serve as a basis for judging the merit of a formal complaint pertaining to violations of professional and/or ethical standards. Defined principles provide guidance for professional behaviors, activities, and decision-making processes and serve as a framework for self-evaluation. They outline the benchmarks as defined by peers within the profession and should be used as the foundation on which to build a professional practice. Equally important to note is that professional standards evolve with the profession they serve, and therefore provide ongoing contributions to the profession's integrity, and ultimately respect.

Common professional standards of the personal training profession:

- Valid assessment and documented attainment of the minimal competency standards
- Proper representation of one's academic achievements, skills, and abilities
- Practicing within the defined scope of the profession
- Commitment to continued learning and maintenance of professional competency
- Protection of client privacy by not disclosing information to third parties, unless required by law
- Maintaining appropriate files and documenting all professional activity
- Providing proper screening and evaluation and acquiring medical clearance when needed
- Referring clients to appropriate health care practitioners as needed
- Establishing and delivering the highest quality services
- Implementing strategies and management services in accordance with evidence-based criteria
- Avoiding conflicts of interest, improper dissemination of information, and false representation
- Calling attention to unethical, illegal, and unsafe behaviors by other professionals

Every day, fitness professionals must make decisions regarding different aspects of their job responsibilities. In some cases, the decisions are simple and imply minimal consequences, while other decisions may have serious repercussions. The ability to make the right decision in a situation is based on several factors that stem from the aforementioned composite of what makes a quality professional. Professional decision-making is actually a formatted, cognitive process which uses analytical and critical thinking to determine the ideal conclusion for a situation, conflict, or problem [7].

Professional decision-making requires one to evaluate a problem, gather information, develop alternative solutions, weigh each alternative objectively, and select the best choice based on the facts presented. Essentially, decision-making leads to the selection of a course of action and is a reasoned process based on known and potential factors and assumptions. Structured, rational decision making composes an important part of all science-based professions. Knowledge in a given area forms the foundation for making informed decisions. Where low levels of knowledge exist, external input must be sought to make the correct decision. As one's level of expertise increases, intuitive decision making may replace a more structured approach because the professional can better recognize a set of indicators from experience in similar situations [13, 20]. Expertise suggests the ability to define a course of action without weighing all the alternatives or seeking outside support, secondary to accrued knowledge and experience.

The Professional Decision-Making Process

 Identify the problem: Is it a goal, challenge, or opportunity?

 Gather information: Collect facts and data, differentiate opinion and assumptions, consider professional boundaries, and identify the stakeholders

 Develop alternatives: Establish criteria, consider all the aspects, and look at precedents

 Weigh the alternatives: Identify the advantages and disadvantages, benefits, and consequences of each option

 Record your findings and use for future decision making

 Analyze the outcome and learn from past actions

 Monitor the effect: Analyze the process or the result: could anything be improved upon?

 Implement the solution: Premeditate a plan, properly communicate, and adapt to the situation or individual

 Select the best course of action: Prioritize by appropriateness, suitability, and benefits vs. consequences

Following this process will create the best solution for the problems endemic to professional situations. With experience, application of previous learning to common problems creates an increased level of professional proficiency and expertise. Experts have dealt with many situations, deliberated on all the alternatives, and learned from the outcomes. The decision-making process combines both on-the-job learning and more traditional knowledge attainment. This explains why inquiry is a fundamental component of effective professionalism.

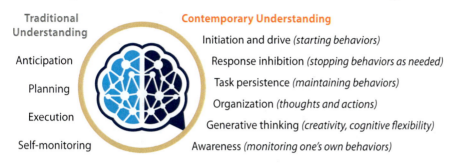

The decision-making process recruits many aspects of cognitive function, and ethics is an inherent component in professional decision-making. Personal ethics and professional ethics may differ, but they share a single foundation. Ethics is defined as a system of moral principles within each person that is applied to behavior [14]. Professional ethics are the moral principles pertinent to a profession which determine acceptable practices. These include actions, communications, and behaviors. In most cases, governing organizations will define ethical conduct based on peer-determined criteria which protect the profession's primary stakeholders. Ethics help to formulate the standards of practice, and therefore are often categorized with specific components of the profession.

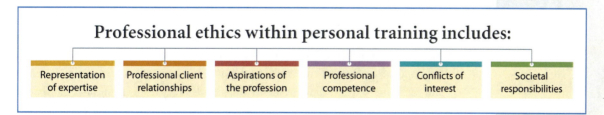

Representation of Expertise

Personal trainers are expected to be honest and trustworthy. This includes factually representing one's academic background, degrees, and experience. It has been suggested that nearly one-third of the resumes presented for American jobs do not accurately represent the individual, or contain falsifications of some kind [15]. Obviously, professional ethics require being truthful in all forms of communication. In the fitness industry, a common questionable practice involves the assignment of a credential or distinction without valid assessment of competency. For instance, taking a weekend course that provides a certificate or certification does not represent the attainment of expertise. Often, the distinction of "specialist" or "certified" is used to make the education course more marketable. However, a credential must be backed by a validly constructed, psychometrically analyzed, and proctored examination. Though a course may provide some valuable information on a subject and help one improve his or her craft, representing oneself as an expert after a weeklong or weekend course is inappropriate. With that said, it would be acceptable to market oneself as having completed educational course work in that particular area within the discipline. Additionally, credentials expire. If a role certification or task-specific credential has lapsed, the professional must either immediately update it or remove the credential as part of the biographical representation, resumé, and/or advertisement. A person representing themselves as certified when her or she is not is subject to claims of false advertising and related professional liability-based lawsuits.

Professional Client Relationships

In a professional role, the personal trainer makes an ethical covenant with all stakeholders of the profession to act in their best interest. This suggests placing the others' welfare in the center of the professional domain. The client/professional relationship, in particular, has an ethical basis and is built on confidentiality, trust, and honesty [11, 16, 17]. This requires the establishment of boundaries: limits that allow for safe connection between individuals. With defined boundaries, appropriate levels of human intimacy and the maintenance of trust are possible. Unclear boundaries can lead to inappropriate relationships. The professional is in a position of power because the expectation of trust rests on the assumption that the professional will operate in the client's best interest. Boundary violations occur when the power of trust is misused and/or abused. If, at any time, ethics may be compromised by the dynamics of the client/professional relationship, the personal trainer has the responsibility to withdraw from providing professional services.

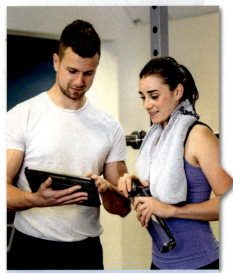

The trainer-client relationship requires the establishment of appropriate boundaries to allow for safe connection during service provision and the maintenance of trust.

Duty of the Profession

In addition to the responsibility a personal trainer has to the client, he or she also has obligations to the profession. The ethics of aspiration represent one's effort to attain a level of aptitude consistent with the defined professional standards and to represent the profession based on its ideals and core values. Compliance with the industry's standards and code of conduct is an ethical responsibility of all personal trainers. When the members of a profession strive to reach a higher standard, the entire profession reaches new benchmarks, leading to advancement for all. Performing at a sub-par level by not complying with accepted standards is unethical when considering personal responsibility to the profession.

Professional Competence

It is the personal trainer's ethical responsibility to remain current in the knowledge and skills of the occupation. Personal trainers owe it to the stakeholders of the profession to attain appropriate competency and to elevate, or at least maintain, abilities and skills throughout one's career. Individuals who possess professional credentials are mandated by the governing body to earn continued education credits to maintain their certified or licensed status. With regard to considerations for professional ethics, personal trainers should identify their deficiencies and focus efforts on improving competency within these areas of weakness. Taking coursework that provides new challenges and leads to improved skill and comprehension is the ethical path, whereas collecting continued education credits in other manners, such as through professional contacts or falsification of professional activities in any way, constitutes unethical practice.

Conflicts of Interest

The personal trainer must also avoid conflicts of interest. A conflict of interest (often based on self-interest) is defined as an influence that compromises one's objectivity in professional decision making [18]. Conflicts of interest interfere with unbiased judgment and may lead to concessions that are not in the best interest of others [6]. Potential conflicts of interest may arise from commercial promotions of fitness or health-related products and services which may create, or appear to create, an inappropriate, undue influence, generating bias unrelated to product merit. The trainer should be aware of this potential tension and offer fitness advice that is accurate, balanced, complete, and devoid of bias. When the trainer receives anything of substantial value, including royalties, from companies in the healthcare industry, such as a manufacturer of supplements and fitness devices, this fact should be disclosed to clients and colleagues.

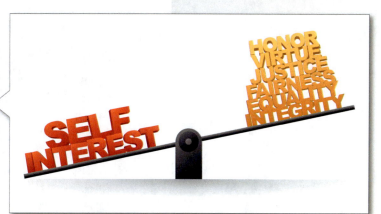

Societal Responsibilities

Responsibility to society is also of ethical concern to the professional personal trainer. Personal trainers should support and participate in those health programs, practices, and activities that contribute positively and in a meaningful and effective way to the welfare of individual clients, the health and fitness community, or the public good. Personal trainers who provide expert testimony in courts of law recognize their duty to testify truthfully and should not bear witness to matters about which they are not knowledgeable. Exercise professionals should be prepared to have any testimony given in a judicial proceeding subjected to peer review by an institution or professional organization to which they belong. Moreover, it is unethical for a trainer to accept compensation contingent upon the outcome of litigation.

Profession advocacy is another societal responsibility incumbent on exercise professionals. In addition to complying with best practices for the profession, all exercise professionals should promote it. Questions of character can sway perception of a profession, so practicing exercise professionals must support their profession in a manner that sheds a positive light on the industry.

Risk Management

Ethics, standards, and guidelines provide the framework for professional practices. In addition to accounting for the consistent delivery of service, the peer-defined, minimal-acceptable standards guide risk management, particularly as they pertain to litigation. In this vein, the protection of the stakeholders is the primary objective of health and fitness professionals [8]. This is accomplished through the anticipation, recognition, and control of risk in occupational environments. Like decision making, consideration for risk and how to manage it requires a structured process. The comprehensive framework for risk assessment and management includes several stages of analysis. Put simply, it is a process of reviewing historical precedence related to the outcome of different strategies, looking at the probability of incidence, analyzing the factors that contribute to risk, and identifying control mechanisms that affect the probability of occurrence [15].

Three general categories of risk which a personal trainer must manage:

- Participant risk
- Environmental risk
- Professional risk

Being proactive is the first step to managing risk. This means being aware of possible hazards and areas where they commonly exist. There are generally three categories of risk with which a personal trainer must contend. They include participant risk, environmental risk, and professional risk [2]. Moreover, within these categories exist internal and external risk factors. External risks are sources that a trainer has no direct control over but may be able to predict. This may have to do with changes in business dynamics, such as the reduction in training hours over the holiday season, or be related to the danger of a client getting hit by an object dropped by a third party in the weight room. Although no direct control over the risk exists, proactively analyzing the situation and predicting the possibility of an adverse circumstance arising allows one to better reduce the likelihood of the negative event. Internal risks are those over which a personal trainer has a level of control. The effect or level of control over the danger is based on all the activities incurred in a risk management program.

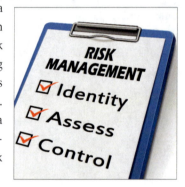

Participant Risk

Of the three categories of risk, participant risk is of significant concern because it is most commonly linked with direct liability and legal action. Injury is inherent in physical activity and this hazard exists daily. Personal trainers must contend with this issue by implementing appropriate risk-management behaviors: properly screening participants, using client-appropriate protocols, maintaining safe work environments, and instructing proper technique.

Environmental Risks

Environmental risks affect one's business, and changes in the industry environment can lead to financial shifts. For instance, a poor economy may reduce consumer spending, and those who once had expendable income for personal training may no longer be able to afford the service. A hurricane, flood, car accident, or injury may all be forms of environmental risk that can adversely affect a personal trainer's ability to participate successfully in his or her trade. The degree of risk and the ratio of external to internal risk factors can be analyzed to determine what actions can be used to mitigate the effect of any issues arising from environmental risk.

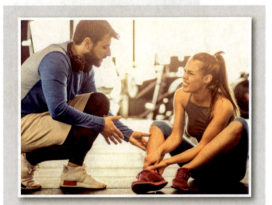

Risk for injury is inherent to all physical activity, but it can be minimized with:

- Proper screening of participants
- The use of client-appropriate protocols
- Maintaining a safe work environment
- Instructing proper technique

Professional Risks

Professional risks directly relate to one's professional activity. Every employee has a risk of being fired for one reason or another, but by consistently performing at a high standard, the risk is well-managed and may never become an issue. Professional risks may come from employers, competition in a business environment, or changes within the profession. Forgetting to renew one's personal trainer or CPR certification may increase professional liability by removing the mechanisms which protect against a particular risk. Likewise, not maintaining professional liability coverage may increase susceptibility to a negative financial outcome.

Each area of risk presents different and unique situations that must be managed. In some cases, the risk is related to an independent and relatively rare circumstance, and therefore may not require ongoing effort to manage. In other cases, the risk may be experienced every day, requiring a structured and consistent action or behavior as a staple in one's daily professional activities. The goal of risk management is to identify, prevent, and minimize problems. Assessing each situation will help identify and stratify dangers and the circumstances that may increase a particular hazard's prevalence. With this information, a management plan to adequately address each possible problem is created. This process serves as an internal audit of one's business activities and commonly leads to dramatic improvements in the overall delivery of service, more efficient use of resources, better business management, and an improved grasp of one's professional career or business.

The Six Steps of Risk Management

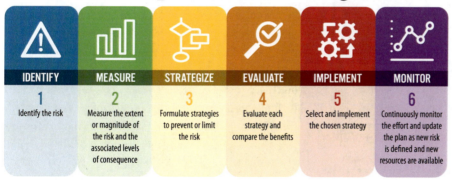

1. **IDENTIFY** — Identify the risk
2. **MEASURE** — Measure the extent or magnitude of the risk and the associated levels of consequence
3. **STRATEGIZE** — Formulate strategies to prevent or limit the risk
4. **EVALUATE** — Evaluate each strategy and compare the benefits
5. **IMPLEMENT** — Select and implement the chosen strategy
6. **MONITOR** — Continuously monitor the effort and update the plan as new risk is defined and new resources are available

The six steps of risk management should be applied to each facet of one's professional career in order to quantify the potential risk that exists. Many personal trainers do not realize the potential pitfalls they experience every day because they lack awareness of risk and do not fully understand its potential magnitude. The more educated a professional becomes about his or her field and work environment, the more evident the inherent dangers become. Professional governing bodies are most often comprised of individuals with high levels of expertise in the field of practice. Part of that capability lies in understanding the dynamics of the profession and pitfalls associated with practicing within the trade. To address this issue, standards and protocols are formed by peer committees to help the profession contend with risk. Personal trainers should become proficient in the standards of conduct and practice, as well as the skill-set protocols defined by the profession as necessary for delivery of safe and effective professional services. Mitigating risk is an ongoing, multifaceted process. In the context of the personal training profession, numerous strategies can reduce potential dangers and aid in effective delivery of a quality product. For most situations, clearly defined best approaches have been developed from a historic perspective but have strong relevance in today's personal training environments. Other situations beyond these may require a level of resourcefulness and research to find an effective management strategy that may have been used by other vocations for similar situations.

> **The Best Risk Management Plans:**
>
>
>
> 1. Are structured by comprehensive and sound principles, which provide the integral framework of the plan.
> 2. Consider the problem and the risk within the full context of the situation, using a broad perspective. This is done by acknowledging, incorporating, and balancing the multi-dimensions of risk.
> 3. Ensure the highest degree of reliability for all components of the risk management process so accuracy is validated, as assumption itself is a risk.
> 4. Commit to routine implementation of strategies and the ongoing process of tracking outcomes.
> 5. Change with the identification of new facts and resources.

Emergency Plan

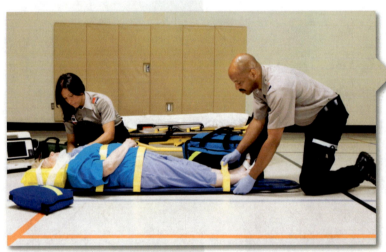

Identifying threats to safety is the first step in ensuring that proper planning and procedures can be determined for the best outcome. An emergency response plan is a sound practice and entails a system of actions used to provide a safe environment for stakeholders. Different training environments may indicate different preparatory and emergency response systems to provide the highest reasonable level of safety for participants. A group of policies with supportive procedures should be created for each of the environments used for professional practice, as threats often differ. For instance, a fire drill is more likely relevant for inside activities, whereas an emergency response protocol for a heat stress condition is more likely related to outside environments.

Areas of emergency risk: Medical | Fire | Severe weather | Physical threat

Being proactive enables exercise professionals to be aware of conditions that could pose an increased risk to participants. Proactive behaviors include evaluation, planning, and practice. Evaluation suggests auditing environments, equipment, and participants regularly to determine safety compliance. A safety compliance list should be used routinely to ensure that all the proper safety practices are being followed. Planning requires premeditated actions that function systematically to ensure a safe outcome. Establishing a written game plan for different scenarios improves the likelihood that adherence to the specific safety practices will be employed during emergencies. Practicing the plan involves the actual engagement of discussing and reviewing all the procedures to ensure they function in the intended manner. This procedure also allows for trouble shooting the plan and ensuring its efficiency and effectiveness. It is recommended that emergency plans consult and involve all parties to ensure all understand their responsibilities.

Types of emergency exercises:

- **Discussion-based exercises:** *Familiarize participants with current plans, policies, agreements, and procedures; may be used to develop new plans, policies, agreements, and procedures.*
- **Operations-based exercises:** *Validate plans, policies, agreements, and procedures, clarify roles and responsibilities, and identify resource gaps in an operational environment.*

Scope of Practice

Although no licensure exists in personal training, the **scope of practice** has been defined to acknowledge acceptable and unacceptable activities based on credentialed qualifications and education. A personal trainer's emphasis is on improving health and physical fitness while acting to prevent disease, premature aging, and the onset of health problems. Personal trainers are not able to diagnose medical problems or serve the role of any other defined health care provider, including but not limited to the following: physical therapists, athletic trainers, registered dietitians, and rehabilitation therapists. Acting outside the scope of practice is unethical, and in many cases illegal; it can lead to negligence and/or professional liability lawsuits.

Standard Protocols

Personal trainers must achieve proficiency in the profession's standardized protocols and guidelines. These standards and guidelines have been established for safe and effective practice in the client's best interest. A professional may forego a standardized approach when this is justified by adequate evidence. However, when activities fall outside the norm, the danger of negative consequences increases. The actual hazard and extent of the consequences should be evaluated before making a professional decision.

Emergency/Safety Procedures

In addition to the protocols mentioned above, personal trainers owe their clients a **duty of care**, which is often what is called into question during litigation. To satisfy their legal requirements, personal trainers must comply with established safety protocols and implement the necessary safety and emergency procedures, as warranted by a given situation. Taking the time to ensure a client's safety and defining emergency procedures in the event of a serious situation contributes greatly to reducing liability risk.

Documentation

In any health-related profession, documentation is required and necessary for effective delivery of services. Documenting test outcomes, tracking program activities, and maintaining client files are all required of the personal trainer. This allows for optimal data use as a criterion for program decision making. If an incident occurs that requires evidence concerning the nature of the professional activities, personal trainers must present their documentation during a legal proceeding. Improperly documenting activities, not documenting at all, and improperly storing sensitive information which compromises client privacy, all dramatically increase related risk. Some common documents used by personal trainers to manage risk and effectively deliver services include informed consent, screening

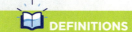
DEFINITIONS

Scope of practice –

The services that a qualified health care professional is deemed competent to perform and is permitted to undertake in keeping with the terms of his or her professional credential and/or license.

Duty of care –

The legal responsibility to avoid behaviors that could reasonably be foreseen to cause harm to others.

Common documents used to manage risk and deliver optimal service:

- Informed consent
- Screening forms, notes, and findings
- Program documents and tracking records
- Accident report forms
- Emergency plans
- Equipment safety check forms

forms, screening notes and findings, program documents and tracking records, accident/incident reporting forms, emergency plans, and equipment safety check forms. Documents should be maintained for one year past the statute of limitations of the state where the services were rendered.

Program Implementation

It is expected that personal trainers comply with standard operational procedures to initiate client participation in an exercise program. This includes following the guidelines for screening, program decision making, physical evaluation, and program activity management. The everyday activities supervised by personal trainers should be performed with the highest regard for client safety. This includes instruction, supervision, and spotting, as well as implementing components such as warm-up and cool down routines. Taking short cuts or not focusing on the job at hand may lead to increased risk.

Liability Coverage

Personal trainers should maintain an appropriate amount of personal liability insurance in the event that a lawsuit is filed, and the verdict is not favorable. A general rule of thumb is to maintain enough coverage that one's professional practice will not be at risk of functioning uninsured, or going out of business due to a lawsuit. Validly credentialed professionals can purchase $2 million of coverage for about $200 per year.

Although the ideal situation in any profession is never to experience any negative consequences associated with one's job, inevitably, some risk factors will create a situation that must be managed. When risk management evolves into situation management, the goal should be to minimize the effects of the problem. Taking the right steps during and immediately following an occurrence will aid in alleviating the problem or limiting the extent of the damage. Personal trainers should establish a plan to deal with each situation that has a high probability of occurring or which will have the greatest impact on a professional career.

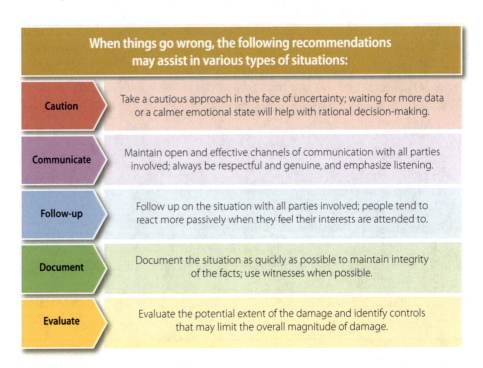

When things go wrong, the following recommendations may assist in various types of situations:

Caution	Take a cautious approach in the face of uncertainty; waiting for more data or a calmer emotional state will help with rational decision-making.
Communicate	Maintain open and effective channels of communication with all parties involved; always be respectful and genuine, and emphasize listening.
Follow-up	Follow up on the situation with all parties involved; people tend to react more passively when they feel their interests are attended to.
Document	Document the situation as quickly as possible to maintain integrity of the facts; use witnesses when possible.
Evaluate	Evaluate the potential extent of the damage and identify controls that may limit the overall magnitude of damage.

REFERENCES:

1. Act A. Health insurance portability and accountability act of 1996. *Public law* 104: 191, 1996.

2. Chiu W-Y, Lee Y-D, and Lin T-Y. Innovative services in fitness clubs: personal trainer competency needs analysis. *International Journal of Organizational Innovation (Online)* 3: 317, 2011.

3. Cruess RL and Cruess SR. Teaching professionalism: general principles. *Medical teacher* 28: 205-208, 2006.

4. Cruess RL, Cruess SR, and Steinert Y. *Teaching medical professionalism: supporting the development of a professional identity:* Cambridge University Press, 2016.

5. De Lyon AT, Neville RD, and Armour KM. The role of fitness professionals in public health: a review of the literature. *Quest* 69: 313-330, 2017.

6. DeAngelis CD. Medical professionalism. *Jama* 313: 1837-1838, 2015.

7. Dhami MK. Psychological models of professional decision making. *Psychological Science* 14: 175-180, 2003.

8. George M. Interactions in expert service work: Demonstrating professionalism in personal training. *Journal of Contemporary Ethnography* 37: 108-131, 2008.

9. Healy LM. *International social work: Professional action in an interdependent world:* Oxford University Press, USA, 2008.

10. Keffer JH. Guidelines and algorithms: perceptions of why and when they are successful and how to improve them. *Clinical chemistry* 47: 1563-1572, 2001.

11. Kelly TM. *Professional Ethics: A Trust-Based Approach:* Lexington Books, 2018.

12. Lester S. Professional standards, competence and capability. *Higher Education, Skills and Work-based Learning* 4: 31-43, 2014.

13. Nimkulrat N, Niedderer K, and Evans M. On understanding expertise, connoisseurship, and experiential knowledge in professional practice. *Journal of Research Practice* 11: 1, 2016.

14. Phalen RF. *Core Ethics for Health Professionals: Principles, Issues, and Compliance:* Springer, 2017.

15. Prater T and Kiser SB. Lies, lies, and more lies. *SAM Advanced Management Journal* 67: 9, 2002.

16. Rasoal D, Skovdahl K, Gifford M, and Kihlgren A. Clinical ethics support for healthcare personnel: An integrative literature review. *Hec Forum*. Springer, 2017, p. 313-346.

17. Schick IC and Guo L. Ethics committees identify success factors: A national survey. *Hec Forum*. Springer, 2001, p. 344-360.

18. Siedentop D and Van der Mars H. Introduction to physical education, fitness, and sport. 2004.

19. Smith Maguire J. The personal is professional: Personal trainers as a case study of cultural intermediaries. *International Journal of Cultural Studies* 11: 211-229, 2008.

20. Wieten S. Expertise in evidence-based medicine: a tale of three models. *Philosophy, Ethics, and Humanities in Medicine* 13: 2, 2018.

GLOSSARY OF TERMS

A2-adrenergic receptors – Receptors involved in the inhibition of fat mobilization from tissue, opposing the effects of activated B-adrenergic receptors.

Acclimation – A physiological adjustment by an organism in response to an environmental change such as altitude, temperature, humidity or systemic pH.

Accumulative fatigue – Occurs when the effects of one workout build up and transfer to the next training session.

Acetyl CoA – Compound that functions as a coenzyme in various biological reactions and is formed as an intermediate for the metabolism of carbohydrates, fats, or proteins in the mitochondria; it is critical in the first step of the Krebs Cycle.

Acne vulgaris – A common, chronic skin disease involving blockage and/or inflammation of hair follicles and their accompanying sebaceous gland.

Actin – The thin myofilament within sarcomeres used to create tension inside muscle cells.

Action potential – A wave-like change in the electrical properties of a cell membrane that functions as a signal to promote a cascade of events including muscular contraction.

Activities of daily living (ADLs) – The fundamental skills typically needed to manage basic physical needs comprised of the following areas: grooming/personal hygiene, dressing, toileting/continence, transferring/ambulating and eating.

Acute angina – A short-term chest pain caused by reduced blood flow to the heart. It is often precipitated by exertion and associated with cardiovascular disease.

Acute peripheral fatigue – Occurs when cells experience dysfunction due to a metabolic reduction in pH; acid limits enzyme activity, requiring buffering compounds before work can be re-initiated.

Adenosine triphosphate (ATP) – The primary energy source created within the mitochondria of muscle cells via various metabolic processes. ATP facilitates performance of mechanical work.

Adequate Intakes (AI) – Formerly the Estimated Safe and Adequate Daily Dietary Intake, it is the recommended average daily-intake level, based on observed or experimentally determined approximations or estimates of nutrient intake by a group or groups of apparently healthy people.

Adipocytes – Cells that primarily compose adipose tissue, specialized in storing energy as fat.

Adipokines – A special type of cytokine released by adipose (fat) tissue to communicate energy needs and other information to various organs, including the brain, liver, immune system, and skeletal muscle; dysregulation of these signalers has been implicated in obesity, type 2 diabetes mellitus, and cardiovascular disease.

Adipose tissue – The storage form of fat tissue in the human body, which can be broken down for the liberation of necessary energy.

Adrenal cortex – The outer portion of the adrenal glands that secretes steroidal hormones such as cortisol and aldosterone.

Adrenal medulla – The inner portion of the adrenal glands that converts the amino acid tyrosine into the catecholamines for release into the bloodstream.

Adrenergic – Relates to nerve cells in which epinephrine or norepinephrine act as neurotransmitters.

Aerobic system – Metabolic pathway wherein the mitochondrion utilizes fats, pyruvate from carbohydrates, and amino acids from protein to produce ATP in the presence of oxygen.

Aerobic – The metabolic processes of energy production that require the presence of oxygen, also known as oxidative metabolism.

Afferent stimuli – Sensory information carried inward toward the brain and spinal cord from sensory and motor nerves throughout the body, as opposed to efferent stimuli, which carry information from the brain to the peripheral nerves.

Agility – A rapid whole-body movement with change of velocity or direction in response to a stimulus.

Agonist – The muscle that contracts and shortens during a given movement/exercise to resist/accelerate the load (e.g., biceps during a biceps curl).

Air displacement plethysmography – A scientifically-validated method to measure human body composition that predicts body density based on volume and weight.

Alanine – A non-essential amino acid known for increasing immunity and providing energy for the brain, central nervous system, and muscles.

Albumin – A blood protein produced in the liver that functions as a transporter for various molecules including FFA, hormones, and calcium.

Alveoli – The tiny, thin-walled, capillary-rich sacs found in the lungs where the exchange of oxygen and carbon dioxide takes place.

Alzheimer's disease – A neurodegenerative disorder, or type of dementia, often occurring during older age, that causes progressive irreversible mental deterioration, memory loss, diminished cognition, and eventual loss of independence due to generalized degeneration of the brain.

Amenorrhea – The absence of menstruation in a woman of childbearing age.

Amino acids – Organic molecules consisting of hydrogen, carbon, oxygen, and nitrogen that combine to form the basic elements of proteins.

Amortization phase – Also known as the transition or contact phase; constitutes the period of time between the concentric and eccentric phases of a plyometric exercise wherein the stretch-shortening cycle is exploited to maximize power production.

Anabolic hormones – Compounds involved in stimulating protein synthesis and tissue growth (muscle, organs, connective tissue); anabolism is associated with building tissues in general.

Anaerobic capacity – The total amount of energy for work obtainable from the anaerobic sources, measured in all-out efforts; the capacity to run the body systems without using oxygen.

Anaerobic system – One of two major metabolic pathways, the ATP-PC Phosphagen system or anaerobic glycolysis, that produces energy without the presence of oxygen. Anaerobic systems provide the energy for high power, high intensity activities.

Anaerobic – Those metabolic processes of energy production that do not require the presence of oxygen.

Androgenic hormone – A generic term used to describe any natural or synthetic steroid-based hormone that controls the development and maintenance of masculine characteristics (e.g., facial hair, deepening of the voice).

Androgenic-anabolic steroids (AAS) – Synthetically produced variants of the naturally occurring male sex hormones.

Android storage – Central (or apple shaped) fat pattern associated with increased cardiometabolic disease risk.

Aneurism – An excessive localized enlargement of an artery (or abnormal dilation) caused by the weakening of an arterial wall due to issues such as hypertension and atherosclerosis or genetics; this bulge can rupture and cause life-threatening situations or sudden death when occurring within the brain or other integral organs.

Angiogenesis – The development of new blood vessels as an adaptation-specific response to aerobic training, resulting in greater capillary density and improved oxygen-extraction capacity.

Antagonist – The muscle that relaxes and lengthens during a given movement/exercise to allow full contraction of the working muscle(s) (e.g., triceps during a biceps curl).

Anterior pelvic tilt – A forward rotational movement of the iliac crests of the pelvis, originating from the lumbosacral joint, which impacts the curvature of the spine.

Antioxidants – Can be man-made or natural substances that may prevent or delay some types of cell damage; it is found in foods and available as dietary supplements.

Aorta – The main artery of the body, supplying oxygenated blood from the left ventricle to the circulatory system.

Apolipoprotein A-I (ApoA-I) – The primary protein component of high-density lipoproteins (HDL); it plays specific roles in the metabolism of cholesterol and lipids and functions; ApoA-I can impact cellular inflammation and oxidation actions within circulation, having an effect on vascular structures.

Appetite – A motivational drive to obtain food, often influenced by one's experiences and environment.

Aromatization – Chemical reaction process by which excess testosterone is converted to estrogen in order to maintain a homeostatic environment.

Arrhythmia – A potentially-dangerous abnormal heart rhythm which can be caused by physical exertion or without activity in cases where there is an issue with the cardiovascular system, or in the presence of disease.

Arteries – The large, muscular-walled blood vessel structures that transport oxygenated blood away from the heart to the tissues.

Arterioles – The smaller, thinner-walled arteries that serve as the connecting structures to capillaries.

Arteriosclerosis – A thickening and hardening of the arterial walls from chronic conditions such as high blood pressure, old age, or negative behaviors, such as smoking.

Asymmetrical loading – Loading is not symmetrical in the sagittal and frontal plane.

Asynchronous motor unit firing – A neuromuscular adaptation presenting itself within type I muscle fibers in response to repeated bouts of prolonged activity which helps preserve energy and prevent premature fatigue.

Atheroemboli – Also known as a cholesterol embolism or blue toe, this condition occurs when cholesterol is released from an atherosclerotic plaque, travels as an embolus in the bloodstream, and ends up lodging (as a clot) in a specific area causing dangerous obstruction.

Atherogenic – A term used to describe dynamics which promote the formation of fatty plaques in vascular structures (arteries).

Atherosclerosis – Refers to the deposit and buildup of fats, cholesterol, and other substances (known as plaque) in and on arterial walls, which can restrict blood flow and lead to heart attack or stroke.

Atherothrombotic disease – Describes disease characterized by atherosclerotic lesion disruption which results in a dangerous blood clot(s) and occlusion of vascular structures; this condition is the major cause of acute coronary distress (i.e., heart attack) and the leading cause of mortality among industrialized nations.

Atria – The two upper chambers in the heart that receive blood from the veins and push it into the ventricles; the left atrium receives oxygenated blood from the lungs while the right atrium receives deoxygenated blood from venous circulation.

Atrophy – The wasting away of an organ, muscle, or other bodily tissue; it is often associated with the loss of muscle mass due to inactivity.

Attention-deficit/hyperactivity disorder – A chronic condition marked by persistent inattention, hyperactivity, and potential impulsivity; often begins in childhood and progresses into adulthood.

Autogenic inhibition – The reduction in excitability of a muscle upon the development of high tension; self-induced by the muscle due to negative feedback signaled by activation of its Golgi tendon organs.

Autoimmune disorders – A type of disease in which the body produces antibodies to attack its own tissues, leading to the deterioration and potential death of cells, glands, or organs; examples include lupus, multiple sclerosis, rheumatoid arthritis, etc.

Autonomic nervous system (ANS) – A component of the nervous system responsible for bodily functions that are not consciously controlled, such as breathing, heart function, and digestive processes.

A-V O_2 difference – The difference in oxygen saturation when comparing the arteries and veins (blood leaving and returning to the heart); it indicates the level of oxygen uptake efficiency of working muscles and other tissues.

B-adrenergic receptors – Receptors which, upon activation by catecholamines norepinephrine and epinephrine, promote breakdown and release of triglycerides.

Balance – The ability to manage forces which act to disrupt stability.

Ballistic stretching – Achievement of maximal range of motion using the momentum of a moving body or limb.

Ballistics – Actions that exhibit maximal concentric acceleration over a brief contraction time.

Baroreceptors – The specialized receptors that detect changes in blood pressure and blood flow in order to inform the CNS to either decrease or increase blood pressure or heart rate. Baroreceptors are located in the aorta and carotid arteries.

Beta oxidation – The process by which fats are oxidized, or broken down, in the mitochondria to produce acetyl CoA.

Beta-hydroxy beta-methylbutyrate (HMB) – A metabolite of the essential amino acid leucine. As a dietary supplement, it is reported to enhance gains in strength and lean body mass associated with resistance training.

Bioelectrical impedance analysis (BIA) – A measure of the resistance to flow of an electrical current through body tissues used to estimate body composition.

Bioenergetics – Describes the various processes of energy/macronutrient use within the body and relates to the function of various energy systems for fuel provision during exercise.

Blood pressure – A measure of the force or lateral pressure exerted by the circulating blood against the arterial walls; it is modulated in response to activity, nutrition, and health status; defined as CO x TPR.

Blood viscosity – A measure of the thickness and stickiness of blood caused by variable quantities of various blood constituents; elevated viscosity measures can serve as a strong predictor for cardiovascular events.

Body composition – A health-related component of fitness, indicated by the ratio of fat mass to fat-free mass within the body, often expressed as a percentage of body fat.

Body mass index (BMI) – Stature weight index determined by a person's weight in kilograms divided by their height in meters squared; used to predict risk for disease and mortality.

Bone mass – This represents the surface area of bone and total tissue volume.

Bone mineral density (BMD) – The mineral content in a given volume of bone, used as a measure of bone health as well as to diagnose diseases, such as osteoporosis.

Borg scale – A scale of perceived exertion ranging from 6 "no feeling of exertion" to 20 "very, very hard" developed by Dr. Gunnar Borg as a simple way to measure heart rate; multiplying the score by 10 gives an approximate heart rate for young adults.

Brain-derived neurotrophic factor (BDNF) – A protein-based compound released by nerves or brain support cells, such as astrocytes, that binds to a receptor on a nearby nerve cell to promote brain neuron survival by facilitating growth, maturation, and maintenance of these cells.

Branched-chain amino acids (BCAAs) – Essential nutrients (leucine, isoleucine, and valine) that the body obtains from proteins found in food, especially meat, dairy products, and legumes.

Bronchodilator – A substance that dilates, or opens, the bronchi and bronchioles and decreases resistance in the respiratory airway, thereby increasing airflow to the lungs.

Bursa – A small fluid-filled sac that reduces friction between connective and bony tissues during movement.

Caffeine – A central nervous-system stimulant.

Calcium – The most abundant mineral in the body; it is required for vascular contraction and vasodilation, muscle function, and other body functions including bone rigidity.

Calorie – The basic unit of heat measurement, defined as the heat required to raise the temperature of 1 gram of water 1 degree Celsius.

Calories-per-kilogram – The simplest estimate of caloric needs based solely upon body weight; typical standards are 25 to 30 kcals/kg/day for normal, healthy individuals.

Cancer – An abnormal growth of cells which tend to multiply in an uncontrolled way and sometimes spread (metastasize) to other tissues; the term cancer does not refer to a single pathology but rather includes more than 100 distinctive diseases that can involve any tissue of the body and may present many different forms in each specific body area.

Capillaries – The smallest vascular structures with the thinnest walls, which allow for oxygen and nutrient transport as well as waste product removal from muscles, organs, and other tissues.

Carcinogenic – A substance having the potential to promote cancer formation in the body.

Cardiac arrhythmias – A group of conditions in which the electrical impulses that coordinate myocardial contraction are disrupted, resulting in irregular, too fast, or too slow heart beats.

Cardiac fibrosis – Refers to an abnormal thickening and stiffening of the heart valves (primarily tricuspid) and/or heart muscle walls, which can indicate a progression towards heart failure.

Cardiac muscle – A type of involuntary, mononucleated, striated muscle found exclusively within the heart.

Cardiac output (CO) – The total volume of blood available for use by all bodily tissues, dictated by heart rate and stroke volume.

Cardiomyopathies – A disease of the heart muscle that makes it harder for the heart to pump blood to the rest of the body, which can lead to heart failure.

Cardiorespiratory fitness – A health-related component of physical fitness, defined as the ability of the circulatory, respiratory, and muscular systems to supply oxygen during sustained physical activity.

Catabolic – A state in which the body is breaking down molecules in metabolism.

Catecholamines – Potent neurotransmitters that help the body respond to stress or elicit "fight-or-flight" reactions: e.g., dopamine, epinephrine, norepinephrine.

Cellular ischemia – Restriction of oxygen supply, generally caused by inadequate blood flow, that promotes dysfunction to metabolic activities.

Cellular permeability – The ability of nutrients and other substances to pass through the cellular wall: the greater the permeability, the greater the transfer of nutrients and other compounds.

Cellulite – A condition in which fat deposits push through connective tissue under the skin, presenting a dimpled appearance.

Center of gravity – A point within a given object such as the human body where the line of gravitational pull is equal in all directions; for example, the center of gravity for the body should be directly down the midline of the body in the frontal plane if the body is symmetrical on both sides.

Central fatigue – Occurs with insufficient or systemic depletion of CHOs, resulting in reduced motor unit recruitment and firing rate: reflects a conscious and subconscious brain decision to reduce the intensity of exercise until energy replenishment and/or recovery have provided energy for the re-initiation of work.

Central nervous system (CNS) – The central processing unit for the nervous system, consisting of the brain and spinal cord; the CNS is responsible for integrating all sensory information and sending nerve impulses that regulate appropriate responses.

Central stability – The ability to maintain active control of spinal and pelvic posture during dynamic movement in order to facilitate force transfer across the trunk.

Central-peripheral stability – Refers to the ability to recruit a pattern of necessary musculature in order to maintain structural integrity of the trunk (central) and limbs (peripheral) while managing internal and external forces.

Cerebrovascular disease – A collective term referring to diseases that impact the brain and its blood vessels: includes stroke, aneurysms, and vascular malformations.

Chondrocytes – The only cells found within healthy cartilage which produce and maintain the cartilage's matrix integrity; they assist in amplifying the cushioning effect of cartilage during impact forces placed upon joints.

Circuit – A training method of performing a sequence of exercises across several stations, usually incorporating minimal rest intervals.

Circumference measurement – Girth measures at standard anatomical sites around the body, often denoted by distances between bony landmarks.

Closed kinetic chain exercises – Exercise in which force is applied to a distally-fixed position or object.

Closed skills – Motor skills performed in a stable or predictable environment (e.g., bowling).

Closed-circuit system – This involves the use of a single, connected load such as a barbell when performing an exercise; these systems generally reduce peripheral stability requirements and the potential range of motion, thereby increasing the potential for loading.

Coefficient of digestibility – The proportion of food that is digested compared to what is absorbed, expressed as a percentage.

Comorbidities – The presence of additional diseases or disorders occurring with a primary disease or disorder; associated with worse health outcomes and a more complex clinical management.

Complete protein – A source of protein that contains adequate proportions of all nine of the essential amino acids.

Complete tetanus – This indicates the achievement of a sustained muscular contraction due to a rate of repeated stimulation (twitches), which prevents relaxation.

Compound exercises – Exercises that involve more than one joint and multiple muscle groups.

Compound lipids – Lipids conjoined with other substances: phospholipids, glycolipids, sulpholipids, lipoproteins.

Compound movements – Actions involving two or more joints and the recruitment of large amounts of muscle mass across several muscle groups.

Concentric – A muscle contraction where the working tissues apply enough force to overcome applied resistance so that the tissues shorten as they contract; this process often occurs among the muscles involved during the acceleration phase of a lift.

Congestive heart failure (CHF) – Characterized by an enlargement of the left ventricle and central portion of the heart in response to coronary heart disease and strain against vascular peripheral resistance (high blood pressure); the hypertrophic adaptations cause reduced blood flow through the heart, reduced valve function and a significant reduction in stroke volume that significantly limits oxygen availability and work capacity.

Contraindications – A factor that makes a particular training method inadvisable due to the harm it may cause the individual.

Coordination – The ability to control and use multiple body parts and/or senses at the same time efficiently.

Core temperature – The operating temperature of an organism which is normally maintained within a narrow range; typically obtained most accurately through rectal measurement.

Cori cycle – Name given to the process of lactate and pyruvate recycling in the liver to produce new glucose.

Coronary artery disease (CAD) – A disease of the coronary arteries often due to atherosclerosis; it leads to an obstruction of coronary circulation, potentially resulting in a dangerous cardiovascular event; it is also known as atherosclerotic heart disease or ischemic heart disease.

Corrective exercise – Activities aimed at restoring or improving joint function via neuromuscular and musculoskeletal system improvements.

Cortisol – Regulates numerous metabolic and cardiovascular functions as well as helping to manage blood pressure; it is released in response to exercise stress and low blood glucose concentrations; a chronic elevated cortisol level is associated with overtraining.

Creatine kinase – An enzyme which can catalyze creatine phosphate into creatine and a free phosphate ion to liberate immediate energy within the phosphagen energy system.

Creatine monohydrate – Used as a dietary supplement to improve muscle strength and athletic performance. Creatine is a naturally occurring chemical in the body and is commonly found in the diet via the consumption of red meat and seafood.

Creatine phosphate (CP) – An inorganic compound found in skeletal muscle tissue capable of storing and providing high-energy phosphate elements to fuel muscular contractions; along with ATP and CP, it comprises the immediate substrate of the phosphagen system.

Creeping obesity – Obesity resulting from an incremental weight gain over a period of time, usually attributed to sustained caloric intake coupled with a decrease in physical activity.

Cross bridges – These consist of a myosin head that projects from the surface of the thick myofilament and binds to the surface of the thin myofilament (actin) in the presence of calcium ions.

Cross-sectional study – A type of observational study that analyzes data collected from a specific population or populations at a specific point in time to obtain "cross-sectional" data for comparisons; often examine the relationship between disease and other variables of interest that exist in a defined population.

Cytokines – Various substances secreted by components of the immune system to modulate tissue functions or have an impact on other cells; these can serve as signalers, growth factors, or facilitators of inflammatory actions.

Cytosol – The cytoplasmic fluid which surrounds all organelles within a cell.

Daily values (DV) – A nutrition-label guide to the nutrients in one serving of food, based on a 2,000-calorie diet for healthy adults.

Deaminate – The process by which the liver breaks down a protein by removing an amino group for use as potential fuel; glutamate is also deaminated in the kidneys.

Deep vein thrombosis (DVT) – Deep vein blood clots that can cause serious circulation blockage and potential death from pulmonary embolism (blockage of pulmonary arteries).

Dehydration – Occurs when the body loses more fluid than is taken-in; signs and symptoms include increased thirst, headache, dry skin, dizziness, increased heart rate and BP, decreased urine output and dry mouth.

Dehydroepiandrosterone (DHEA) – A hormone produced by the adrenal glands that, in turn, helps produce other hormones, including testosterone and estrogen. Synthetic versions are available for supplementation and are reported to ward off chronic illness and improve physical performance.

Delayed onset muscle soreness (DOMS) – Muscle soreness expedited by an inflammatory response to cellular damage, ischemia, and tonic spasms which presents 24-72 hours following an intense bout of exercise; common causes include performing new (unaccustomed) exercises, heavy eccentric work, and high work volume.

Dementia – A chronic disorder of various mental processes caused by brain disease or injury that is characterized by memory disorders, personality changes, and impaired reasoning; the term is often used for a decline in mental ability severe enough to limit performance of daily living activities.

Depression – A mood disorder that causes a persistent feeling of sadness and loss of interest; it can impact how a person feels, thinks, and behaves and can lead to a variety of emotional and physical problems.

Derived lipids – Substances derived from simple and compound lipids by hydrolysis.

Diabetes – A group of metabolic diseases (type 1 and 2) that involve insulin and glucose mismanagement; this results in a chronic state of excess sugar in the bloodstream, which causes numerous physical issues affecting the nervous system, vascular structures, and various organs.

Diastole – The heart's relaxation phase in which the atrial chambers fill with blood (diastolic phase).

Diastolic blood pressure – The pressure within arteries in between heart beats when the ventricles are relaxed and filling with blood; it presents as the second value within blood pressure measurements (120/80 mmHg).

Dietary reference intakes (DRI) – An umbrella term encompassing specific standards for dietary intake; the quantity of each nutrient needed for proper function and health is defined in one of the DRIs.

Disaccharides – The carbohydrate formed when two monosaccharides bond to each other: sucrose, lactose, and maltose.

Distress – A negative form of stress that influences physiological or psychological health; it can be caused by excessive stress of any type or forms of stress which are not associated with improving one's well-being, such as anxiety or lack of sleep.

Dose response – The degree of physiological response is related to the amount or dose of a given stimulus.

Duty of care – The legal responsibility to avoid behaviors that could reasonably be foreseen to cause harm to others.

Glossary of Terms

Dynamic flexibility – The act of briefly achieving full range of motion through controlled muscle contraction; often used for movement preparation.

Dynamic posture – Biomechanical proficiency, or lack thereof, during movements of the body such as locomotion, stepping, jumping etc.; assessment allows for the detection of faulty movement patterns, strength imbalances and risk for injury during given activities.

Dyslipidemia – A term used to indicate poor blood lipid profile measurements: elevated low-density cholesterol, low levels of high-density cholesterol, elevated total cholesterol levels or sub-optimal cholesterol ratio; it is a risk factor for cardiovascular disease and stroke.

Dyspnea – Difficult or labored breathing; shortness of breath due to some inefficiency or disease.

Eccentric – A muscle contraction where the resistive force is greater than the force applied by the muscle so that it lengthens as it contracts; this contraction often occurs among the muscles decelerating resistance during a lift.

Electrolytes – Minerals (sodium, calcium, potassium, chlorine, phosphate, magnesium) found in blood, urine, tissues and other bodily fluids that help balance the amount of water and pH level in the body based on osmolar relationships.

Electron transport chain – A group of compounds which expedite a series of oxidation-reduction reactions for eventual aerobic production of ATP within the mitochondria.

Embolic disease – Describes diseases where an embolus (blockage-causing material such as blood clots, lipids, or even air bubbles) inside vascular structures causes occlusion at some point in the body resulting in ischemia and potential cellular death (e.g., deep vein thrombosis, pulmonary embolism).

Emergency plan – A comprehensive plan for dealing with emergency situations that may arise during exercise testing and eprformance. This plan should include a list of possible emergencies, consequences, required actions, written procedures and the resources available in a particular facility.

Emotion – A component of the integrated model of function which relates to the impact of psychological condition on movement efficiency.

Endomysium – A thin sheath of connective tissue that covers each separate muscle fiber within a fascicle.

Endorphins – A group of hormones secreted from the brain and central nervous system. They have a number of physiological functions and effects on the body and are released in relatively high quantities following exercise, activating opiate receptors that cause analgesic and pleasurable sensations.

Endothelium – A thin layer of flat epithelial cells that line blood vessels. These cells allow for the diffusion of oxygen and waste products; the lining of blood vessels, when damaged, is associated with plaque build-up.

Endurance – The ability of a muscle group to execute repeated muscle actions over a period of time sufficient to cause muscular fatigue or to maintain a specific percentage of the 1 Repetition Maximum (1-RM) for a prolonged period of time.

Energy yielding nutrients – Macronutrients (carbohydrates, protein, fats) that provide the body with energy, measured in calories.

Enzymes – Protein-based components produced by cells that function to catalyze (speed up) a biochemical reaction.

Epidemiological studies – A form of research that focuses on the patterns, causes, and effects of health and disease conditions within specific populations (e.g., age groups, racial/ethnic groups, sexes).

Epimysium – A dense collection of collagen fibers that covers the entire surface of muscle.

Epinephrine – A catecholamine hormone, also known as adrenaline, that is secreted by the adrenal glands during conditions of stress to increase blood circulation, ventilation, and carbohydrate metabolism to prepare skeletal muscles for exertion.

Epiphyseal plates – The transverse cartilage plates, located near the end of long bones and responsible for increases in vertical growth during childhood and adolescence.

Ergogenic aid – Any product that offers a mental or physical edge while exercising or competing, also called performance enhancers.

Essential amino acids – Nine (9) amino acids that cannot be produced by the body and must be consumed in the diet.

Essential body fat – Necessary fat present in nerve tissues, bone marrow, and organs. Loss of this fat compromises physiological function.

Estimated average requirement (EAR) – The average daily nutrient-intake level estimated to meet the requirement of half the healthy individuals in a particular group; this value is needed in order to set the RDA values.

Estrogen – A steroid hormone that promotes the development and maintenance of female secondary characteristics (e.g., breast tissue).

Eustress – A positive, desirable form of stress that influences physiological or psychological health; it's source can be events such as exercise or working towards obtainable goals within one's occupation.

Excess post-exercise oxygen consumption (EPOC) – A measurable increase in the rate of oxygen consumption following strenuous activity due to a deficit created by the work; it increases metabolism for hours after the bout as dictated by the duration, type, and intensity of the exercise.

Excitation-contraction coupling – This describes the process in which an action potential propagates across the sarcolemma triggering release of calcium by the sarcoplasmic reticulum to initiate a muscular contraction.

Exercise – Planned, structured, and repetitive bodily movements performed to improve or maintain one or more components of physical fitness.

Exercise-induced asthma (EIA) – A narrowing of the airways in the lungs in response to strenuous physical exertion, also known as exercise-induced bronchoconstriction.

Exertional-rhabdomyolysis – The breakdown and necrosis of skeletal muscle caused by extreme physical exertion.

Extensibility – The capability of a muscle to be stretched based on the limitations of the tissue structures.

Fartlek training – Swedish for "speed play", a training method that blends interval and aerobic training by using unstructured fluctuations of higher and lower intensity efforts.

Fascia – The most superficial layer of muscle composed of a fibrous connective tissue that encapsulates the underlying layers to form individual muscles; fascia provides shape consistent with the arrangement of the muscle tissue to enhance intramuscular tension and regulate transfer of force across joints.

Fascicle – A bundle of wrapped muscle fibers.

Fat-burning zone – Lower-intensity training (<65% of VO_2max) where the predominant fuel source is fat, as aerobic pathways can maintain the workload; not necessarily an optimal weight loss method as the relative quantity of total calories burned remains low compared to higher intensities.

Fat-free mass – All tissues within the human body that contain no fat.

FatMax – Is the highest intensity of work that can be performed where fat is the primary fuel for energy; it is also known as the aerobic limit.

Fat-soluble vitamins – Vitamins that are soluble in fat and predominantly stored in the body, primarily in the liver. Excess supplemental amounts can cause adverse health effects.

Female athlete triad – The interrelationship of menstrual dysfunction, low energy availability (with or without an eating disorder) and decreased bone mineral density; relatively common among young women participating in sports.

Fibrinolysis – A process that occurs naturally inside the body to break down (fibrin) blood clots that can be induced by medications or occur as a result of stress or disease.

Fibrocartilage – Tough connective tissue composed of a dense matrix of fibers serving as a shock absorber for structures exposed to high forces.

Field tests – A practical assessment used to predict outcomes of gold standard criterion measures, usually through cheaper, more portable means.

Fight-or-flight response – An acute increase in adrenal hormone activity which expedites enhancements in cardiac output, blood flow, and energy metabolism to rapidly deal with a perceived stress.

Fixed compensation – Chronic biomechanical compensation which cannot be alleviated with proper instruction or cueing.

Flexibility – A health-related component of fitness, indicated by the ability of a muscle to move through a range of motion at a single joint in a single plane.

Food deserts – An area, either in urban or rural environments, in which it is difficult to access affordable nutritious food.

Force closure – The support of soft tissues which help maintain positional integrity of a joint.

Force couples – The synergistic action of opposing or adjacent muscles to produce a rotational action; i.e., upper trapezius and serratus anterior contracting to promote scapular rotation.

Form closure – The efficiency of the structural aspects of articulating segments; primarily consists of skeletal and connective tissues.

Free fatty acids – Liberated lipid molecules found in the blood plasma that represent ~10% of fat in the body; due to the insolubility of fat, FFA must be bound and transported through the blood by the protein albumin.

Free radicals – Highly unstable molecules, naturally formed during exercise or when the body converts food to energy; it can cause oxidative stress, triggering cellular damage.

Frontal plane – The plane of movement split by the midaxillary line which breaks the body into front and back halves; applicable actions often involve abduction and adduction and require side-to-side movement of the body or joints (e.g., lateral lunge).

Functional range – Minimum range of motion necessary to comfortably and effectively perform activities of daily living.

Functional-based activities – Activities aimed at improving the body's ability to efficiently manage various aspects of daily living, including physical activity, without undue resistance.

Gait – The set of characteristics observed when a person walks or locomotes in other fashions; gait can include factors such as stride length, stride frequency, and various compensatory movements.

Gastric emptying – The process of emptying food from the stomach; strongly influence by the volume and composition of gastric contents.

General peripheral fatigue – Occurs with a lack of energy in working tissues due to low pre-exercise stores or localized depletion of anaerobic energy stores; acute rest intervals will not help, as muscular energy provisions are too low.

Genetic predisposition – Increased propensity towards a conditioning or outcome based on one's inherited genes.

Geriatric – Used as a reference term for older populations or people, especially with regard to their health care or special needs.

Gestational diabetes mellitus – Defined as any degree of glucose intolerance with the onset of or during a pregnancy; the condition is caused by metabolic disruption due to weight gain and hormonal actions facilitated by the placenta that cause release of compounds that counteract insulin.

Global muscle systems – Larger muscles responsible for motion and regional stability that tends to function in a phasic manner.

Glucagon – Hormone released from the pancreas to promote the breakdown of glycogen to glucose in the liver to aid in blood sugar homeostasis.

Gluconeogenesis – The creation of new glucose in the liver from other organic molecules, such as pyruvate, lactate, glycerol, and amino acids.

Glucose – A simple sugar molecule that provides the primary source of metabolized fuel for the glycolytic energy system.

Glutamine – The most abundant amino acid found naturally in the body; it is produced in the muscles and distributed by the blood to the organs that need it. Athletes supplement with glutamine for enhanced exercise performance.

Glycemic index – A measure of the blood-glucose-raising potential of the carbohydrate content of a food. A value of 100 represents the standard or the equivalent of pure glucose.

Glycemic load – An index that simultaneously describes the blood-glucose-raising potential of the carbohydrate in a food and the quantity of carbohydrate in a food; it is calculated by multiplying the glycemic index by the amount of carbohydrate in grams provided by a food and dividing the total by 100.

Glycemic response – The effect a food or meal has on blood glucose following consumption.

Glycogen – Storage form of carbohydrates in the body which is broken down to fuel mechanical work: primary storage sites include skeletal muscles and the liver.

Glycolysis – Metabolic process involving the breakdown of sugars (glucose) through a series of reactions to provide energy (ATP) during anaerobic work.

Glycosylated hemoglobin (HbA1c) – A measurement of the amount of hemoglobin to which glucose is bound; used as an indicator of long-term glucose control.

Gold standard – A method of describing the proportion of components that comprise the body, including fat, muscle, bone, and water; often represented by body fat percentage, the proportion of fat mass to fat free mass.

Golgi tendon organs (GTOs) – Special kinesthetic receptors located near muscle-tendon junctions which send reflexive signals to the spinal cord to regulate muscle tension; they function to protect tissue from overstraining and injury using autogenic inhibition.

Goniometer – An instrument used to measure joint angles or range of motion of a specific joint.

Gout – A type of inflammatory arthritis that promotes joint redness, swelling, and pain; there are various nutritional triggers such as dehydration, sugary beverages, alcohol, red meat or seafood and it may also be instigated by surgery; if left untreated it can cause irreversible joint and/or kidney damage.

Graded exercise test (GXT) – An exercise test which uses progressive stages to measure/estimate maximal oxygen consumption capacity; this type of test is often used to assess cardiovascular fitness.

Gross motor activation – Recruitment patterns that engage large muscle groups, often applied cyclically for locomotion.

Growth hormone (GH) – Promotes cell division and proliferation by facilitating protein synthesis; it protects glycogen reserves and limits carbohydrate metabolism by mobilizing lipids for fuel during exercise and plays a role in recovery.

Glossary of Terms

Guarana – A substance derived from the seeds of a South American tree, which has among the highest caffeine concentration of any plant.

Gynecomastia – A swelling of the breast tissue in boys or men caused by an imbalance of the hormones estrogen and testosterone.

Gynoid storage – A pear-shaped pattern of fat deposition in the lower half of the body, surrounding the hips, buttocks, and thighs.

Health – The condition of being sound in body, mind, or spirit and free from physical pain, illness, or disease.

Heart rate training zone (HRTZ) – A heart rate range relative to an individual's heart rate max that should be maintained during cardiovascular training to obtain targeted adaptations.

Hematocrit – The percentage of blood that consists of red blood cells: the most commonly used erythrocyte test.

Hemoglobin – A protein found in red blood cells that helps to transport oxygen to tissues.

Hemorrhagic stroke – Occurs as a result of a weakened blood vessel rupture (aneurysm) in or on the surface of the brain; it is most commonly caused by prolonged and uncontrolled high blood pressure.

High density lipoprotein (HDL) – Sometimes called "good" cholesterol due to particle activity, it absorbs cholesterol and carries it back to the liver, which then flushes it from the body. High levels can lower risk for heart disease and stroke.

Homeostasis – The body's tendency to seek a constant, desirable range of conditions that maintain equilibrium within all physiological systems.

Homocysteine – An amino acid that is produced by the body by chemically altering adenosine; it can be a marker of increased CVD risk.

Humidity – The amount of water vapor in the air; can lead to excessive, counterproductive sweating by reducing the capacity for evaporation.

Hunger – The physiological drive to seek food caused by hormonal signaling from peripheral tissues to the hypothalamus.

Hyaline cartilage – Tough yet elastic connective tissue found in various parts/joints of the body which allows for minimal movement, depending on the surrounding anatomy.

Hydrogenation – Chemical reaction in which hydrogen reacts to an organic compound. In the context of food processing, it refers to the saturation of unsaturated liquid oils with hydrogen atoms.

Hypercapnia – Excessive carbon dioxide (CO_2) levels in the blood, usually a result of inadequate respiration.

Hyperglycemia – An abnormally high blood glucose level; it is a hallmark sign of diabetes, which can potentially damage bodily tissues, including vascular structures.

Hyperinsulinemia – A condition in which excess levels of insulin are found in circulation relative to blood glucose; it often indicates progressive insulin resistance as a precursor to diabetes.

Hypermobility – Movement capacity of a joint beyond the normal range of motion; often compromises joint stability.

Hyperphagia – An abnormally increased desire for food promoting excessive eating.

Hypertension – High blood pressure: a condition that has a negative impact on the cardiovascular system due to excessive pressure exerted upon arterial walls that causes damage over time.

Hyperthermia – Abnormally high body temperature caused by failure of the heat-regulating mechanisms of the body to deal with the heat from the environment. Signs and symptoms include fatigue, syncope, cramps, exhaustion and heat stroke.

Hypertrophy – An increase in muscle fiber size.

Hypoglycemia – A low blood sugar level that occurs when glucose concentrations drop below a critical concentration in the blood; where the metabolic demands of the brain and central nervous system cannot be met.

Hyponatremia – Refers to a below-normal plasma sodium concentration (<135 mmol/L); it can be caused by excessive water consumption and is most commonly seen during endurance training in the heat.

Hypoperfusion – Essentially a shock response in a given tissue due to inadequate oxygen and nutrient supply which can quickly result in cellular death.

Hypothalamus – A region of the forebrain that coordinates the autonomic nervous system and governs the endocrine system via the pituitary gland; it directs homeostatic maintenance activities such as eating, drinking, body temperature regulation, sleep, and emotional responses.

Hypothermia – A potentially dangerous decrease in body temperature below normal levels which can lead to diminished neuromuscular control, frostbite, or death: body temperature below 95.0 °F (35.0 °C).

Hypothyroidism – An abnormally low activity of the thyroid gland which results in "slow metabolism" and, usually, weight gain; it can result in retardation of growth and mental development.

Hypovolemia – State of decreased blood volume that can result in multiple organ failure die to inadequate circulating volume and subsequent inadequate perfusion.

Hypoxia – A state of oxygen deficiency in a given tissue, muscle or organ; this condition can be caused by intense work or a myriad of pathophysiological issues, such as cardiovascular disease.

Iliotibial (IT) band syndrome – Common overuse injuries involves inflammation of the IT band due to chronic friction against the femur and lateral aspect of the knee joint.

Incomplete protein – A source of protein lacking in one or more of the essential amino acids.

Incretin – A group of metabolic hormones that stimulate a decrease in blood glucose levels; they are released after eating and augment the secretion of insulin emitted from pancreatic beta cells of the islets of Langerhans.

Inner unit – Collective group of local spinal and pelvic stabilizers: includes the transverse abdominis, diaphragm, posterior internal oblique, pelvic floor, and multifidus.

Insoluble fiber – A fiber found in wheat bran, vegetables, and whole grains; it adds bulk to stool and helps food pass more quickly through the stomach and intestines.

Insulin – A hormone produced by the pancreas that serves various functions, including blood glucose control and tissue growth; insulin dysfunction is related to diabetes.

Insulin-like growth factor 1 (IGF-1) – Considered to be a central signaling hormone released from the liver that initiates muscle growth following resistance training.

Intermittent fasting – An umbrella term for serval patterns of fasting and non-fasting over defined periods independent of caloric restriction.

Interstitial spaces – Fluid-filled spaces between tissues that allow for the transfer of oxygen, nutrients, waste products, hormones, neurotransmitters, and other compounds.

Intervertebral disc – A fibrocartilaginous disc that serves as a cushion between the vertebra of the spinal column.

Intramuscular fat – Lipid deposits stored within skeletal muscle fibers.

Ischemic (ischemia) – A low oxygen state usually due to obstruction of the arterial blood supply or inadequate blood flow leading to hypoxia in the tissue.

Ischemic stroke – Occurs as a result of an obstruction within a blood vessel that supplies oxygenated blood to the brain; this blockage type accounts for the vast majority of stroke cases.

Isocaloric – A balance of calories expended and consumed, promoting weight maintenance.

Isokinetic contraction – This signifies a constant speed of movement regardless of the muscular force applied; training requires specialized laboratory equipment, which is primarily used for rehab and research purposes.

Isometric contraction – Tension is created but no changes in joint angles occur; it often occurs in stabilizers during movement to regulate body segment/joint positioning.

Isotonic contraction – Tension remains while joint angles change; this contraction is seen during most exercises/activities that include a concentric (acceleration) and eccentric (deceleration) component.

Joint capsule – A connective tissue enclosure that surrounds specific joints and consists of an outer fibrous membrane and an inner synovial membrane, assisting in joint protection and stability.

Joint – A point of articulation between two or more bones that allows for a functional connection and various amounts of motion, depending on local anatomical features.

Ketosis – A normal but potentially dangerous metabolic process when it progresses to severe ketoacidosis; ketosis occurs when the body does not have enough glucose for energy and burns stored fats instead. This results in circulating acid build-up caused by ketones. This condition can be caused by dietary measures, such as a low-carb diet, or diseases like diabetes.

Kinetic chain – The chain of force transfer across motion segments of the body.

Krebs cycle – A series of enzymatic reactions that occur in the mitochondria involving aerobic metabolism of acetyl compounds which produce ATP for cellular energy; it is also known as citric acid cycle or the tricarboxylic acid (TCA) cycle.

Kyphosis – Excessive convex curvature of the thoracic spine presenting as a bowed or rounded back.

Kyphotic – A convex curvature of the spine, as seen in the thoracic segment.

Lactate threshold – Reflects the maximal intensity at which steady state can be maintained: the intensity at which lactate accumulation begins to exceed lactate removal; muscle and blood lactate concentrations begin to increase exponentially; it is proposed as the best and most consistent predictor of endurance performance.

Lactic acid (lactate) – Energy substrate produced as an end-product of glycolysis that can be used by various tissues of the body as fuel to continue ongoing work (e.g., aerobic cells, heart); it serves as a buffer for hydrogen ions created by sugar metabolism.

L-arginine – Essential amino acids obtained from the diet (found in red meat, poultry, fish, dairy); l-arginine changes into Nitric Oxide.

Leptin – A type of cytokine released from adipose tissue that serves a role in fat storage regulation in the body; leptin dysfunction is associated with obesity and metabolic issues, giving it the common nickname of "obesity hormone."

Liability – The state of being responsible for something, especially by law; a personal trainer maintains a fiduciary responsibility to function in the best interest of the client.

Ligament sprains – A stretching or tearing of the ligaments, tough bands of tissue that connect two bones together at a joint, often reducing the stability of a joint.

Ligaments – Tough fibrous bands of connective tissue that support internal organs and attach adjacent bones at articulation sites; due to limited blood supply, self-repair is difficult following an injury.

Linoleic acids – Essential polyunsaturated fatty acid (PUFA) belonging to the omega-6 fatty acids group.

Linolenic acids – Essential polyunsaturated fatty acid (PUFA) belonging to the omega-3 fatty acids group. Highly concentrated in certain plant oils and has been reported to reduce inflammation and help prevent certain chronic diseases.

Lipase – A specific enzyme capable of breaking down lipid molecules (fat stores) in the body.

Lipids – Various classes of organic compounds composed of fatty acids or their derivatives; dietary sources include oils, fats, waxes, and cholesterol, while endogenous (internal) sources include free fatty acids, triglycerides, lipoproteins, and phospholipids.

Lipogenesis – The process of fatty acid and triglyceride synthesis from glucose or other substances, stimulated by a diet high in carbohydrates.

Lipolysis – The breakdown of triglycerides from fat storage in the body for potential liberation into circulation to serve energy needs.

Lipolytic effects – Causing lipolysis, the breakdown of lipids into glycerol and free fatty acids.

Lipoproteins – Protein-based compounds that transport various forms of lipids, such as cholesterol, in the bloodstream; there are high and low-density lipoproteins which serve various functions and have different implications related to the risk for heart disease.

Local muscle systems – Musculature essential for localized joint stability and neutral joint positioning.

Longitudinal studies – A form of observational research in which data is gathered for a given sample of a population over a period of time to examine long-term effects or relationships; these studies can last years or even decades.

Lordosis – Excessive concavity or inward curvature of the lumbar spine.

Lordotic – A concave curvature of the spine, as seen in the lumbar segment.

Low back pain – One of the most common forms of musculoskeletal discomfort occurring as a result of one or more conditions effecting the bones, nerves, muscles, discs, or tendons of the lumbar spine.

Low density lipoprotein (LDL) – Sometimes called "bad" cholesterol, it makes up most of the body's cholesterol. High levels raise risk for heart disease and stroke due to the small size of the lipoprotein.

Lower cross syndrome – Lower body distortion characterized by an undesirable anterior tilt of the pelvis.

Lumbar stenosis – A narrowing of the space surrounding the spinal nerves of the lower back with subsequent compression often leading to leg pain.

Lumen – When referring to an artery or vascular structure, this term describes the inside open space of the tubular structure.

Maximal capacity – The highest workload an individual can sustain; defined by maximal oxygen consumption (VO_2max), 1-repetition max (1RM) or volitional failure.

Mean arterial pressure (MAP) – The average arterial pressure during one cardiac cycle.

Mechanoreceptor – A sensory receptor that detects mechanical pressure from touch, vibration and tension; acts to communicate changes in pressure to the central nervous system.

Metabolic equivalent (MET) – A measurement of energy use expressed as multiples of the resting metabolic rate; one MET equals an oxygen uptake rate of 3.5 ml of O_2 per kg of body weight per min of work (3.5 ml·kg-1·min-1).

Metabolic syndrome – Recognized as a cluster of interrelated conditions–high blood pressure, poor glucose management, excess body fat (especially around the waist), systemic inflammation, and abnormal cholesterol levels–that significantly increases one's risk for heart disease, stroke, and diabetes.

Microtrauma – Extremely localized injury to muscle fibers, tendons, ligaments, or bones, which may cause low levels of inflammation with, or without, the presence of symptoms.

Minerals – Micronutrients that the body needs in small amounts that must be obtained through diet.

Mitochondria – An organelle responsible for significant energy production and metabolic processes within each cell.

Mobility – The ability to move cooperative body segments through full, unrestricted range of motion.

Monocytes – Large phagocytic (cells which can ingest other cells) white blood cells released from the immune system to deal with invading pathogens such as bacteria, viruses, and fungi; these cells are transported to sites throughout the body in response to inflammation.

Monosaccharides – The simplest form of carbohydrate: glucose, fructose, and galactose.

Monounsaturated fatty acids – "Good" fat: molecules with one unsaturated carbon bond in the molecule.

Mortality – Tefers to death that occurs in a population or other group. It is often utilized as a term in research studies that examine rate of death due to a specific disease or ailment.

Motor neuron – A nerve cell within the peripheral nervous system that propagates electrical impulses to working musculature to regulate contractions and bodily movement.

Motor rehearsal – Repeated exposure to a movement pattern which enhances efficiency over time due to increased neuromuscular proficiency.

Motor unit – A motor neuron and all of the muscle fibers it innervates.

Movement economy – The energy required to move at a given speed or generate a specific amount of power.

Muscle hypertrophy – An increase in size of skeletal muscle.

Muscle spindles – A specialized type of proprioceptor in muscle fibers which aids in managing tension via the detection of tissue length and movement velocity, sending information to the nervous system in response to muscle stretching.

Muscle strains – The stretching or tearing of a muscle or a tendon; the fibrous cord of tissue that connects muscles to bones; occur when muscles are stretched beyond their limits or are forced to contract too strongly.

Muscle tone – Is always present to some degree in skeletal muscle, as motor units are active even when the muscle is not voluntarily contracted; the motor unit activation does not produce enough tension to cause any external movement but provides firmness to the tissue to maintain the integrity of connective structure and force closure in joints.

Muscular endurance – A health-related component of fitness, defined as the measure of muscle force decline over time.

Muscular strength – A health-related component of fitness, defined as the measure of an individual's maximal contractile force production against a resistance.

Myocardial hypertrophy – A disease in which the heart muscle becomes abnormally thick, making it harder for the heart to pump blood. Often goes undiagnosed because many people have few, if any, symptoms.

Myocardial infarction – The medical term for heart attack; it refers to the process by which one or more regions of the heart experience severe or prolonged ischemia due to a blockage of a coronary artery, resulting in the death of the affected cardiac tissue.

Myocardial ischemia – A symptomatic or asymptomatic condition where oxygen supply to the heart muscle does not meet demand; it can occur due to reduced blood flow through the coronary arteries as a result of progressive heart disease and plaque accumulation, and a sudden, severe blockage can lead to a heart attack.

Myocardium – The muscular tissue of the heart that is specialized to allow for continuous contractions; enhanced sarcoplasmic reticulum and calcium delivery systems allow this tissue to manage rapid and non-stop neural impulses: also called cardiac muscle.

Myofibrils – The sectional units found within each muscle fiber which contain bundles of myofilaments.

Myofilaments – The long, cylinder-like protein elements in muscle tissue which operationally set the action of contraction into motion; these are the smallest fiber components in muscle, composed of actin and myosin.

Myoglobin – The oxygen-transporting protein found in muscle that contains heme iron; myoglobin is structurally similar to the hemoglobin found in red blood cells in circulation.

Myosin – The thick myofilament within sarcomeres used to create tension inside muscle cells.

Myostatin – A protein found primarily in skeletal muscle that functions to restrain the growth of muscular tissue; if myostatin were not restrained, muscle growth could theoretically have no limit, creating significant anatomical issues over time.

Needs analysis – The process of identifying an individual's deficiencies, limitations, and aspirations in order to inform decisions for programming.

Nephropathy – A small blood vessel disease of the kidneys which causes damage to the organs, often as a result of diabetes; those with this condition should avoid heavy weightlifting or holding the breath during exercise and should maintain proper hydration.

Neuromuscular junction – This is also known as the motor end plate: a junction where a motor neuron and muscle cells interact via chemo-electrical impulses to facilitate the stimulation of muscle cell contraction.

Neuropathy – A disease that impacts peripheral nerve tissue (often hands or feet) and can result in weakness, numbness, and/or pain; suffers should avoid exercise that causes repetitive impact stress to the hands or feet and should wear proper footwear during exercise.

Neutral spine – A state of proper postural positioning for the spine that includes four major curvatures for shock absorption and efficient movement.

Nitric oxide (NO) – A signaling molecule in the body responsible for vasodilation. Athletes supplement with NO to support the flow of blood and oxygen to skeletal muscle.

Nitrogen balance – A comparison of nitrogen input and nitrogen output; it is widely used to determine recommended dietary intake for protein, as protein is almost the exclusive source of nitrogen to the body.

Nociceptors – Sensory receptors that respond to potentially damaging stimuli and relay a message to higher brain centers, promoting the feeling of pain.

Non-energy-yielding nutrients – Micronutrients (vitamins, minerals) that provide the body with elements necessary for homeostasis.

Non-essential amino acids – Amino acids that are produced by the body.

Non-heme iron – Iron from plant-based foods like beans, fruits, vegetables and nuts. It is absorbed more effectively when eaten with meat, poultry and fish or with food that is high in vitamin C.

Norepinephrine – A catecholamine hormone secreted from the adrenal glands in response to stress by increasing blood pressure and blood glucose levels; it has an affinity to different tissue receptors than epinephrine but facilitates similar responses.

Normal-weight obesity – Classification indicated by normal weight by population norms, but high body fat percentage.

Nucleus-pulposus – A gelatinous, fluid-filled component found in the center of each intervertebral disc.

Nutrient content descriptors – Terms used to describe the relevant aspects of a food source, for example "free," "low," "high," "good source."

Nutritional facts label – A label required on most packaged foods that was updated by the FDA in 2016 to reflect new scientific information, including the link between diet and chronic disease.

Obesity – A complex disease described as an unhealthy quantity of fat mass and quantified by specific physical measurements or stature weight indices.

Octopamine – Biosynthesized sympathomimetic amine used to treat hypotension.

Oligomenorrhea – A condition of infrequent menstruation, with menstrual periods occurring at intervals greater than 35 days.

Open kinetic chain exercise – Exercise in which force is applied to a movable object.

Open skills – Motor skills requiring the participant to react to changes in an unpredictable environment (e.g., playing basketball).

Open-circuit system – This involves the use of two separate (non-connected) loads such as dumbbells when performing an exercise; these systems generally increase peripheral stability requirements and the potential range of motion thereby reducing the potential for loading.

Orthostatic hypotension – A state of low blood pressure commonly caused by rapid changes in position from lying or seated to standing; it can also be caused by other internal factors.

Osteoarthritis – The most common form of arthritis. It involves the degeneration of joint cartilage and the underlying bone, commonly associated with previous injury, but starting during middle age; the condition causes pain and stiffness, especially in the hip, knee, and thumb joints, when bones begin to run directly against each other (a.k.a. degenerative joint disease).

Osteoblasts – A cell responsible for forming new bone.

Osteoclasts – A cell responsible for dissolution and absorption of bone.

Osteopenia – A bone density that is lower than normal peak density but not low enough to be classified as osteoporosis.

Osteophytes – Bony outgrowths, or spurs, associated with the degeneration of cartilage at a joint.

Osteoporosis – A bone disease in which a decrease in mineral density causes skeletal structures to become brittle and fragile, often leading to fractures and disability; this condition is typically caused by negative hormonal changes, sedentary behaviors over the lifespan, and/or a deficiency of energy, calcium and/or Vitamin D.

Overload – A principle of exercise programming, overload is stress applied beyond that which the body is accustomed for the promotion of fitness improvements.

Overreaching (NFO) – A short-term detriment in performance as a result of increased training stress which may take several days or a few weeks to restore.

Overtraining syndrome – A condition caused by an intolerable accumulation of training stress resulting in systemic inflammation, psychologic and neuroendocrinologic symptoms, and performance decrements observed for >2 months.

Oxaloacetate – An intermediate of the Krebs cycle that binds with acetyl-CoA to form citrate; it helps facilitate aerobic energy production.

Oxidative phosphorylation – The formation of ATP energy created by the aerobic breakdown of various substrates, especially the organic compounds involved in the Krebs Cycle.

Oxygen deficit – The difference between total oxygen consumed during the transition to steady state and the actual amount of oxygen required by the working tissues; it must be paid back after work is discontinued, resulting in an elevation in oxygen consumption (e.g., being out of breath after a sprint).

Pancreas – A relatively large gland that secretes digestive enzymes into the small intestines for macronutrient breakdown; it also produces the hormones insulin and glucagon for blood glucose regulation.

Parkinson's disease – A progressive neurodegenerative disease characterized by tremor, muscular rigidity, and slow, imprecise movement capabilities that primarily impacts middle-aged and elderly people; it is associated with degeneration of the basal ganglia of the brain and a deficiency of the neurotransmitter dopamine.

Patellar tendonitis – Commonly referred to as "jumper's knee": an overuse injury to the patellar tendon with the accumulation of microtrauma due to repetitive jumping or rapid changes of direction.

Pelvic floor – The layer of muscles spanning the bottom of the pelvis that support the pelvic organs and stability of the pelvic region.

Perimysium – A layer of tissue below the epimysium that encompasses bundles of fibers.

Periosteum – A dense fibrous membrane covering the surface of bones that serves as an attachment site for tendons to connect muscle to bone.

Peripheral nervous system (PNS) – The portion of the nervous system outside of the brain and spinal cord; the PNS connects the central nervous system to the limbs and organs to regulate sensory and motor control as well as other functions via somatic (voluntary) and autonomic subsystems.

Physical activity – Any purposeful and repeated bodily movement produced by voluntary skeletal muscle actions that increase metabolism.

Phytochemicals – Non-nutritive chemical compounds produced by plants that have various beneficial impacts on health.

Plasma – The clear, liquid portion of blood that contains salts, glucose, amino acids, vitamins, urea, proteins and fats; it is extracted from circulation during dehydration as sweat.

Platelets – Tiny cells responsible for blood coagulation (blood clotting) and the repair of damaged blood vessels.

Plumb line – Linear assessment tool used to evaluate posture and observe variation in anatomical positions.

Plyometrics – A method of training involving repeated rapid lengthening and contracting of muscles for the purpose of increasing power; denotes an amortization phase of <0.03 seconds.

Polypeptide hormones – A chain of amino acids synthesized on the ribosomes of the endoplasmic reticulum of endocrine cells; they attach to membrane receptors in order to activate second messenger systems: examples include insulin and glucagon.

Polysaccharides – Carbohydrate molecules composed of long chains of monosaccharides.

Polyunsaturated fatty acids – "Good" fat: molecules with more than one unsaturated carbon bond in the molecule.

Positive feedback loop – A cyclic process in which the body's response to a stimulus results in a further amplification of the stimulus.

Posterior pelvic tilt – A backward rotational movement of the iliac crests of the pelvis, originating from the lumbosacral joint, which impacts the curvature of the spine.

Post-exercise hypotension (PEH) – A phenomenon of prolonged reduction in resting blood pressure in the minutes and hours following an acute exercise bout.

Postphlebitic syndrome – Also known as post-thrombotic syndrome or venous stress disorder, it involves inflammation within the walls of a vein(s) which manifests as a collection of signs and symptoms: swelling and pain in the legs, skin color changes, and/or sores on the skin; it is caused by damage to venous structures due to a prior blood clot which reduces localized blood flow and can cause discomfort.

Post-traumatic arthritis (PTA) – A type of arthritis where symptoms present acutely in response to a physical injury to a given joint; it can also include the wearing out/overuse of any joint which has had a previous injury, which places it at risk for inflammatory disorder and premature degradation.

Glossary of Terms

Postural syndromes – Static or dynamic malalignment of one or more skeletal segments.

Power – The rate at which work is performed: (force x velocity) = (force * distance/time) = (work/ time).

Pre-eclampsia – The development of elevated blood pressure and protein in the urine after the 20th week of pregnancy.

Premature mortality – A measure of unfilled life expectancy or death before age 75, usually caused by preventable factors.

Prime movers – The muscle required to perform the majority of mechanical work necessary to overcome the load during a given exercise; these may not necessarily contribute more than 50% of the necessary force but will contribute to the greatest extent relative to all tissues involved.

Principles of exercise – Concepts that function to guide exercise programming in order to achieve desired outcomes

Prioritization model – Strategy which dictates that areas/issues of greatest need are addressed as a priority in the training program.

Professional negligence – Failure to take proper care during standard protocol or to use reasonable care, potentially resulting in damage or injury to another person: doing something a reasonable person would not do or the omission of something that a reasonable person would do.

Program matrix – Term used to describe all the necessary components to an exercise prescription which will allow the client to safely and effectively attain their training goals.

Progression – A principle of exercise programming, once the body has adapted to a level of stress, additional or novel stress is needed to promote further adaptations. This principle is normally combined with overload (progressive overload) for ongoing adaptation planning.

Progressive overload – The gradual increase in training stress to elicit a targeted physiological adaptation.

Prohormones – An inactive compound that is converted by enzymes into a biologically active hormone.

Proprioception – The cumulative input to the CNS from receptors that relay body and positional movement: physical awareness of the body's position in space.

Proprioceptive neuromuscular facilitation (PNF) – A group of stretching techniques that utilize autogenic and/or reciprocal inhibition to maximize range of motion.

Proprioceptors – Special sensory receptors found in joints and connective tissues that send signals concerning body position and movement to motor neurons in the spinal cord, thereby effectively managing muscle and tendon tension.

Protein-sparing – The process by which the body derives energy from fat and carbohydrate to avoid converting protein into energy.

Proteolytic enzymes – Function to break down protein compounds and eventually amino acids for energy use or protein recycling.

Pulmonary embolism – A serious, life-threatening type of blood clot that occurs in the pulmonary arteries which oxygenate the lungs themselves; it causes respiratory arrest and sudden death if the clot is big enough, while smaller clots may simply reduce blood flow and damage lung tissue.

Pyruvate – An energy substrate that results as an end-product of sugar metabolism during glycolysis when there is the presence of oxygen.

Range of motion – The full movement potential of a joint measured by linear or angular distance between two limits.

Rate pressure product – An estimate of myocardial oxygen demand and cardiovascular disease risk; it is calculated as systolic blood pressure x heart rate.

Reciprocal inhibition – Describes neuromuscular regulation of agonist-antagonist contraction patterns; reciprocal innervation provides a reduced resistance to opposing muscle contractions.

Recommended dietary allowance (RDA) – The average daily dietary-intake level sufficient to meet the nutrient requirement of nearly all (97-98%) healthy individuals in a particular group.

Recovery period – The period of time in between separate exercise bouts so adaptations may occur.

Red blood cells (RBCs) – The most common type of blood cell and the primary means of delivering oxygen to the tissues: also called erythrocytes.

Renin-angiotensin system – The hormone system which functions to regulate blood pressure and fluid balance throughout the body; improved function of this system can reduce daily workload and stress on the heart.

Re-phosphorylate – The phosphorylation (attachment of a phosphoryl group) of a compound that has been previously dephosphorylated.

Residual adaptations – Physiological training effects that are retained for a period of time after ceasing a particular form of training.

Respiratory exchange ratio (RER) – The ratio of the amount of carbon dioxide (CO_2) produced and oxygen (O_2) consumed, determined by comparing exhaled gasses to that of ambient air; used to estimate the respiratory quotient at sub-maximal intensities.

Respiratory quotient (RQ) – The ratio of carbon dioxide consumed and oxygen produced at the site of the tissue, used to identify the relative oxidation contribution of fat, carbohydrate, and protein.

Rest interval – The period of rest in between sets or structured periods of activity within a single exercise bout; the length of these intervals is dictated by the energy systems involved during the sets of work.

Resting metabolic rate – The energy required to supply bodily functions during resting conditions.

Retinopathy – A small blood vessel disease of the retina in the eye that can result in impairment or loss of vision, often as a result of diabetes; those with this condition should avoid heavy, compressive exercises (e.g., leg press) as well as activities that lower the head below the waist or jar the head.

Return to play – Injury-specific protocols dictate the point in the recovery from an injury when a person is able to return to playing sports or participate in an activity at a pre-injury level

Reversibility principle – Any adaptation that takes place as a result of training will gradually be reversed with the stoppage of training.

Rhabdomyolysis – A potentially life-threatening condition resulting from the destruction of muscle tissue and subsequent release of muscle fiber content into the blood stream which may cause failure of major organs.

Rheumatoid arthritis – A chronic, progressive autoimmune disease that causes notable joint inflammation and results in painful deformities and/or significant immobility over time, especially in the fingers, wrists, feet, and ankles; this condition could be considered the most severe type of arthritis and can create the greatest limits to a client's exercise prescription.

RMR equations – Formulas that incorporate measures of body size and/or body composition used to estimate the caloric expenditure at rest across a 24-hour period.

Rotator cuff – A set of various ligaments and four muscles including the supraspinatus, infraspinatus, teres minor, and subscapularis which function to counteract the relative lack of stability in the shoulder joint and regulate proper movement.

Running economy – Energy demand for a given velocity of submaximal running, represented by the steady-state consumption of oxygen (VO_2) and the respiratory exchange ratio.

Sagittal plane – A plane of movement split by the midline which breaks the body into left and right halves; applicable actions often involve flexion and extension and require a forward-backward movement of the body or joints (e.g., lunge).

Sarcolemma – The external lamina of each single muscle fiber.

Sarcomere – The repeating functional units of a muscle fiber, consisting of contractile myofilaments; sarcomeres are the muscle components which shorten and re-lengthen during contractions.

Sarcopenia – A muscular disease indicated by the loss of total skeletal muscle mass, with particular significance in reductions fast twitch muscle fibers.

Sarcoplasm – The cytoplasm within each single muscle fiber.

Sarcoplasmic reticulum (SR) – The tubular network that surrounds each individual muscle fiber and acts as a storage site for calcium to play its part in facilitating contractions.

Saturated fats – Fats that have no double bonds between carbon molecules because they are saturated with hydrogen molecules.

Sciatica – Refers to pain, numbness, or tingling radiating along the path of the sciatic nerve due to pressure or impingement; a large nerve, it extends from the lower back down to the back of each leg.

Scoliosis – A congenital sideways curvature of the spine that occurs most often around puberty.

Scope of practice – The services that a qualified health care professional is deemed competent to perform and is permitted to undertake in keeping with the terms of his or her professional credential and/or license.

Sedentary – Describes a lifestyle behavioral pattern that includes very little physical activity.

Self-efficacy – A belief in one's ability to be successful in certain situations or accomplish a task.

Serotonin – A hormone-based neurotransmitter which serves various roles, such as regulation of blood pressure, pain perception, the sleep-wake cycle, and even mood; it is released in response to exercise and other stimuli.

Serum lipoproteins – Soluble proteins that combine with and transport fat and other lipids in the blood consisting of four major classes: very-low-density lipoproteins (VLDL), low-density lipoproteins (LDL), high-density lipoproteins (HDL), and chylomicrons.

Shin splints – A common term for medial tibial stress syndrome, a condition characterized by pain along the inner edge of the tibia; caused by an inflammatory response to improper running mechanics or sudden increases in training volume.

Shoulder girdle – A joint complex that includes the articulations between the sternum and clavicle (sternoclavicular joint) and the clavicle and the scapula (acromioclavicular joint).

Simple lipids – Formed primarily from fatty acids: waxes, fats, and oils.

Size principle – The idea that muscle fiber types are recruited sequentially based on their size and force output capacities; recruitment occurs in the following order based on need – type I → type IIa → type IIx.

Skeletal muscle – A type of striated muscle which attaches to the skeleton to facilitate movements by applying force to bones and joints via contractions.

Sleep apnea – A potentially dangerous sleep disorder where the sufferer repeatedly stops breathing for short periods of time during sleep; the airway is intermittently blocked which often results in loud snoring or choking noises – usually waking the person for a quick moment before falling back asleep.

Sliding filament theory – This explains the molecular mechanisms surrounding the multi-step interaction between actin (thin myofilament) and myosin (thick myofilaments) during a muscular contraction.

Smooth muscle – A type of involuntary, non-striated muscle found with the walls of organs and vascular structures.

Sodium-potassium relationship – Electrolytes that control the distribution of fluids throughout the body; a higher potassium intake can cause the excretion of more sodium through urine which can help lower blood pressure.

Soluble fiber – A fiber found in oat bran, barley, nuts, seeds, beans, and some fruits and vegetables; it attracts water and turns to gel during digestion, slowing the digestive process.

Specificity – A principle of exercise programming. A desired adaption must match the specific stresses placed upon the body; controlled stress applied in quantified measures to elicit desirable responses from the body.

Speed – The time to perform a movement in one direction: the rate of positional change.

Spondylitis – Describes several inflammatory conditions affecting the vertebral joints that may, over time, lead to the fusion of vertebrae.

Spondylolithesis – The anterior slipping of one vertebra relative to an adjacent vertebra; seen with bilateral spondylosis in a specific region.

Spondylosis – A stress fracture of a specific portion of the vertebra, the pars interarticularis, usually due to repeated hyperextension of the lumbar spine.

Spotting – This describes various techniques of using verbal/tactile cues and direct manual assistance to help a participant perform a loaded or unloaded movement with proper form; manual assistance should generally function to increase stability rather than to force joint movement.

Stability – The synergistic ability of muscle, nerve, proprioceptors, and connective tissues to maintain firm positioning and offset disruptive forces.

Starch – Chains of sugars that can be digested and metabolized for energy.

Static posture – Biomechanical alignment when standing motionless that is usually assessed via a plumb line; can provide predictions for issues during physical activity and the relative risk of injury or symptomatic conditions due to musculoskeletal malalignment.

Statins – A group of drugs that function to reduce cholesterol and lipid levels in circulation to help lessen the impact and progression of cardiovascular disease, such as atherosclerosis.

Steady state – A condition within the human body which indicates that the current level of oxygen utilization matches demand, signified by a leveling off or steady heart rate; it allows for minimal variance in heart rate (+/- 5 bpm) and other cardiovascular measures if the workload is not changed.

Stenosis – Refers to the abnormal narrowing of a passage in the body, such as a vascular structure.

Steroid hormones – Organic, cholesterol-based hormone compounds that serve various functions related, but not limited to, sexual development, reproduction, tissue synthesis, inflammation regulation, and metabolism: examples include cortisol, aldosterone, estrogen, progesterone, and testosterone.

Sticking point – The specific joint angle where the resistance becomes harder to overcome due to inefficiency in stability during a given lift; usually occurs at a transitional point between working joints.

Stop test indictors – A list of absolute and relative signs that an exercise test should be terminated immediately.

Strength balance – The functional strength ratio of opposing muscle groups across a joint: also referred to as agonist/antagonist muscle ratio or muscle balance ratio.

Stress – A disruptive stimulus eliciting a physiological response.

Stretch reflex – A reflexive contraction of a muscle induced by rapid stretch; triggered by excitation of the muscle spindles and a subsequent feedback loop to the spinal cord resulting in rapid excitation of the stretched muscle and inhibitory signaling of the opposing muscle.

Stroke volume – The volume of blood expelled (to body tissues) per contraction from the left ventricle heartbeat.

Subcutaneous fat – A layer of adipose tissue sitting beneath the skin, comprising the largest compartment of fat storage.

Submaximal tests – A category of assessment methods in which test protocols do not reach the maximal capacities of the systems; maximal measures are predicted by incorporating physiological responses to these submaximal workloads.

Summation – A neuromuscular response that does not allow the muscle to relax between twitches; sequential summation responses lead to complete tetanus.

Supercompensation – The process of adapting to a training stimulus, resulting in an improved performance capacity.

Supplement – Products that are intended to fulfill or complement the diet and may contain one or more ingredients, such as vitamins, herbs, amino acids, or their constituents.

Sympathomimetic – A drug that mimics the effects of sympathetic activation on the heart and circulation, causing vascular smooth-muscle contraction and vasoconstriction.

Synchronicity – The performance of multiple actions in unison, which often results in improved force production.

Synephrine – (Also called bitter orange) A plant in which the peel, flower, fruit and fruit juice are used to create medicinal products for treatment of skin infections, weight loss, chronic fatigue syndrome and many other GI disorders.

Synergistic muscles – Muscles that work together at a given joint or body segment that regulate controlled rotation of the joint and total range of motion so that no compensatory actions occur; these muscles work together to effectively transfer force across the body.

Synovial joint – A type of joint that uses synovial fluid to reduce frictional stresses and allow for considerable movement between the associated articulating bones.

Synovial membrane – A special membrane that lines synovial joints and secretes synovial fluid to lubricate the articulating surfaces.

Systole – The contraction phase of the heart ventricles by which blood is pumped out to the body (systolic phase).

Systolic blood pressure – The pressure within arteries during heart beats via contraction of the left ventricle; it presents as the first value within blood pressure measurements (120/80 mmHg).

Target body weight formula – A computation of healthy or ideal body weight for goal-setting by inputting current weight and desired body fat percentage.

Technology postures – The common positions individuals attain when using technology such as smart phones and computers that contribute to musculoskeletal complications from a forward flexed spinal position.

Telomere – A compound structure at the ends of a chromosome which serves as a protective cap that limits deterioration of DNA in all cells; telomeres have been associated with potential lifespan and longevity.

Tendons – Tough fibrous bands of connective tissue that connect muscles to bones; tendons positively adapt to flexibility and resistance-based exercise.

Test economy – Used to describe the proficiency of the client in performing a given test and their compliance with the testing instructions; can be compromised by choosing an inappropriate test for a given client's fitness level, goal(s), sources of motivation, special needs or limitations.

Test reliability – The ability of a test to allow for consistent reproduction of measures during retesting events; enhanced by duplicating testing conditions every time, using the same protocol every time, ensuring consistency in pretest factors, etc.

Test validity – The ability of a test to accurately measure what it is designed for; enhanced by maintaining proper protocol, tester and testee proficiency, strict scoring discrimination, etc.

Testosterone – An anabolic hormone produced in the gonadal glands of both men and women. Men possess significantly (10x) greater quantities; it stimulates development of male secondary sexual characteristics.

Thermic effect of food (TEF) – The amount of energy expenditure above resting metabolic rate due to the cost of processing food for use as fuel or for storage.

Thermogenesis – The process of heat production; quantified by units of kilocalories in human metabolism.

Thrombosis – The formation of a dangerous blood clot in a major blood vessel, heart, lungs or other body tissue, which can cause various life-threatening issues, such as a stroke or pulmonary embolism.

Thyroid – A gland which serves as the primary regulator for growth and development via the rate of metabolism within the body.

Tibial translation – This describes potentially harmful translational forces created by the tibia that are placed upon the patellar tendon and knee joint due to migration of the knees in front of the toes during lower-body movements, such as stepping and lunging.

Time-under-tension (TUT) – The total amount of time a given muscle experiences tension during structured exercise; maybe calculated in segments (sets) or in totality (bout).

TOFI (Thin-outside-fat-inside) – Term used to describe lean individuals who carry a disproportionate amount of adipose tissue in the abdominal cavity.

Tolerable upper intake level (UL) – The highest average daily-nutrient-intake level that is likely to pose no risk of adverse health effects to almost all individuals in the general population.

Total daily energy expenditure – A measure of the calories expended over a day, often estimated in order to identify daily intake needs.

Total peripheral resistance (TPR) – The resistance to blood flow experienced within peripheral vasculature, which can be modulated by various internal/external factors: systemic vascular resistance (SVR).

Tracking – The act of documenting all applicable testing and program data for a client which allows for an optimized understanding of how they are progression towards their goals; allows the trainer to develop the best exercise prescription possible and make the most appropriate adjustments over time as the client improves, or fails to respond to training.

Training plateau – A decrease in noticeable progress occurring when the body no longer responds to a training stimulus

Training systems – Training methods used to strategically exploit different categories of stress to emphasize specific improvements in strength, power, hypertrophy, or metabolic efficiency.

Training tenure – Genotes the level of training and experience an individual possess related to a stress.

Training volume – A measure of work performed during an exercise bout, taking into consideration the intensity and either the frequency or duration of movement – in resistance training it is calculated by Sets x Reps x Load.

Trans fat – Also known as partially hydrogenated oils, these fats that are created by adding hydrogen molecules to vegetable oils. This process changes the chemical structure of the oil, turning it from liquid to semi-solid. Research has found these fats to significantly increase risk of heart disease.

Transamination – A reversible process involved in both anabolism and catabolism by which excess amino acids are diverted toward energy production, as an amino group is transferred from one molecule to another.

Transverse plane – The plane of movement which breaks the body into top and bottom halves (no dissection line is acknowledged); applicable actions often involve rotational movement of the body or joints (e.g., oblique twists).

Triglycerides – Consist of a glycerol and three fatty acids bound together in a single large molecule; they serve as an important energy source and form much of the body's stored fat.

Troponin-tropomyosin complex – A connection site within separate muscle fibers which allows for the myosin heads to attach to actin and form a cross-bridge for muscular contraction; the attachment site is opened via the unlocking action of calcium ions released from the sarcoplasmic reticulum.

Twitch – A single contraction-relaxation cycle within skeletal muscle fibers

Type 2 diabetes mellitus (T2DM) – A metabolic disorder characterized by high blood sugar, insulin resistance, and relative lack of insulin production; it primarily occurs as a result of obesity and lack of physical activity.

Type I fibers – The slow-twitch oxidative fibers that possess the lowest power output, smallest fiber diameter, and the highest resistance to fatigue; these fibers are well suited for prolonged aerobic work and possess the highest capillary and mitochondrial densities.

Type IIA fibers – The fast-twitch, oxidative-glycolytic fibers that possess intermediate power output capabilities, intermediate fiber diameter, and a moderate resistance to fatigue; these fibers provide support during intense strength/power activities as well as prolonged work, making them the most versatile from a metabolic standpoint.

Type IIX fibers – The fast-twitch glycolytic fibers that possess the highest power output capabilities, largest fiber diameter, and lowest resistance to fatigue; they provide significant support during intense strength and power activities.

Upper cross syndrome – Upper body postural distortion that presents as a forward head, raised, internally-rotated, or rounded shoulders, in addition to an exaggerated thoracic curvature.

Valsalva maneuver – A strain against a closed airway, combined with muscle tightening; it occurs when a person holds his or her breath and tries to move a heavy object; it is contraindicated for those with hypertension, as it creates an immense increase in blood pressure.

Varicose veins – Veins that have become enlarged and twisted; as one ages, vascular structures lose elasticity. Some of the valves may also become weak or dysfunctional, increasing their hyper-dilated appearance.

Vasoconstriction – The constriction or narrowing of a vascular structure due to contraction of the muscular wall, which increases blood pressure and reduces blood flow; it is the opposite of vasodilation.

Vasodilation – The dilation or widening of a vascular structure, which decreases blood pressure and allows for increased blood flow and the potential for improved oxygen and nutrient delivery.

Veins – Any of the blood vessels that are part of the circulatory system and transport deoxygenated blood back to the heart/lungs; they are less muscular than arteries, and are often closer to the skin.

Ventricles – The two lower chambers of the heart. The right ventricle receives blood from the right atrium and pumps it into the lungs via the pulmonary artery, and the left ventricle receives blood from the left atrium and pumps the blood to the rest of the body via the aorta.

Ventricular fibrillation – The most serious form of cardiac rhythm disturbance, where the ventricles essentially quiver or perform erratic mini-contractions; the heart is unable to pump any blood, resulting in cardiac arrest.

Very low-calorie diets – A clinically supervised dietary plan involving intake below 800 kcal per day, usually achieved through liquid meals.

Very-low density lipoproteins (VLDL) – Similar in structure, function, and circulatory impact to low-density lipoproteins, which aid in transporting cholesterol, triglycerides, and other lipids throughout the body; VLDLs were classically considered a component of "bad cholesterol," but contemporary research shows disease risk association is more complicated than originally thought.

Visceral fat – Fat which directly surrounds the internal organs in the abdominal cavity; high quantities are associated with an increased risk for a number of health problems, including type 2 diabetes mellitus and low-grade systemic inflammation.

VO$_2$max – Measure of an individual's cardio-respiratory fitness as indicated by maximal oxygen use – measured by milliliters of oxygen per kilogram of body weight per minute of work.

Volitional failure – Achieved during a set of repetitions when the muscle can no longer perform the action using correct form.

Warmup – A period of preparation for physical activity characterized by gradual increases in heart rate, respiratory rate, metabolism and body temperature

Water-soluble vitamins – Vitamins that travel freely throughout the body, but are not necessarily stored in the body. Excess amounts are excreted by the kidneys and, thus, are not as likely to reach toxic levels as fat-soluble vitamins.

Weight-bearing physical activity – Activities where the skeleton must bear the weight of the body while performing the movement; these activity types are favored for improvements in bone mass, strength, and resilience.

White blood cells (WBC) – A group of immunological cells in the bloodstream which serve various protective functions, such as protection from invasive pathogens.

Winged scapulae – A lifted and outwardly rotated scapula position; the scapula appears to protrude posteriorly away from the ribcage.

Yo-yo dieting – The cyclical loss and gain of weight associated with failing to adhere to strict healthy eating plans.

Index

A

A2-adrenergic receptors 423, 437
Abduction 46-47, 49-50
Acceleration 18-19, 39, 528-530
Acclimation 205-207, 395, 577
Accumulative fatigue................. 630
Acetyl CoA 153-158
    in Krebs Cycle 153-157
Acne vulgaris 419
Acromioclavicular joint 57
Actin 33-36, 143, 592
Action potential 34-35, 39
Active-assisted stretching 604
Activities of daily living (ADLs) 204, 327
Acute angina...................... 206
Acute peripheral fatigue 159-160
Adenosine diphosphate (ADP)....... 143-146
Adenosine monophosphate (AMP) 145
Adenosine triphosphate (ATP)....... 36, 41, 142-155, 166-167, 351, 490, 579
Adequate Intakes (AI)............. 378-379
Adduction 46-47, 49-50
Adductor brevis 62-63
Adductor longus 62-63
Adductor magnus 62-63
Adipocytes 369
Adipokines..................... 244-245
Adipose tissue 153, 244-245, 436
Adrenal cortex 190, 192
Adrenal gland................. 190-191
Adrenal hormones............... 190-191
Adrenal medulla 190-192
Adrenergic 423
Aerobic............................ 41
    effect of hormones 195-196
    fitness...................... 311
    glycolysis 490
    metabolism 151-154
    recommended training intensities .. 562-567
Aerobic system................. 149-150
Aerobic training 557-583
    blood pressure........ 179-180, 241-242
    considerations 576-580, 665, 668
    general guidelines 558-563
    modes 573-575
    types of 565-567
    work to rest ratios................. 497
Afferent stimuli 192
Agility............................ 21
Agonist 37, 119-120, 319
Air displacement plethysmography 272, 443-445

Alanine.................... 373-374, 414
Albumin......................... 153
Aldosterone 190-192
    fluid retention 191
    role of 191-192
Altitude..................... 298, 578
Alveoli.......................... 165
Alzheimer's disease................ 258
Amenorrhea 435
Amino acids.......... 155-156, 372-375
    essential 373-374
    non-essential 373-374
Amortization phase 528
Anabolic hormones........... 183-185, 541
Anaerobic................ 41-42, 142
    training, resistance........ 194, 507-552
    training, work to rest ratio... 497-498, 516, 519, 522, 525, 529
Anaerobic capacity 301
    assessment of.................. 331
    power step test 334-335
Anaerobic metabolism........... 490, 574
Anaerobic glycolysis.......... 146-147, 490
Anaerobic system 150, 154
Anatomical movements............. 48-51
Anatomical positions................. 46
Androgenic hormone 186
Androgenic-anabolic steroids (AAS) 418
    adverse effects of............. 418-419
Android (storage pattern) 436-437
Aneurism....................... 231
Angiogenesis..................... 168
Anorexia nervosa 476-477
Antagonist 37, 119-120, 319
Anterior 45-46
Anterior axillary line 46
Anterior pelvic tilt 55, 130
Anteroposterior axis 46
Antioxidants 380
Aorta...................... 164-165
Apley back scratch test............. 338
Apolipoprotein A-I (ApoA-I).............. 233
Appetite................. 361, 459-460
Appositional growth.................. 28
Aromatization 187
Arrhythmia 206, 235
Arteries 170-173
Arterioles 170-171
Arteriosclerosis................... 174
Articular discs.................... 30
Assessing pulse 173
Asthma 642-645

exercise..................... 642-644
    general recommendations 645
Asymmetrical loading 136
Asynchronous motor unit firing........... 38
Atheroemboli..................... 239
Atherogenic 231
Atherosclerosis 174, 231-234
    exercise 232
Atherothrombotic disease 238
Atria...................... 164-166
Atrioventricular (AV) node 166
Atrium....................... 164
Atrophy....................... 187
Attention-deficit/hyperactivity disorder ... 243
Atwater general factors 349-350
Autogenic inhibition................. 595
Autoimmune disorders................ 230
Autonomic nervous system (ANS) 172
Axial skeleton..................... 27
A-V O_2 difference................... 163

B

β-adrenergic receptors 437
Balance...................... 12, 20
Ballistic stretching 594, 607
Ballistics...................... 528
Baroreceptors 168
Bench press 66, 69, 321
Beta oxidation.................. 153
Beta-blockers 236
Beta-hydroxy beta-methylbutyrate (HMB).. 410
Behavior questionnaire 218-220
Bent-over row 78
Biceps brachii 59
Bicep curls 85
Biceps femoris 63
Bioelectrical impedance analysis (BIA) 449-450
    testing guidelines 450
Bioenergetics 142
Blood lactate 181-182
Blood pooling 172
Blood pressure 168-170, 240-242, 268
    categories of 178-179
    response to exercise 240-242
Blood vessels 163, 171
Blood viscosity 170
Body composition ... 16-17, 270-272, 433-451
    anthropometrics............. 270-271
    assessment 442-450
    continuum 450-451
    girth measurements 272, 441-442
    skinfold 446-448

Body density 443
Body fat 435-437
    distribution 436-437
    role of hormones 437-438
Body mass index (BMI) 439-441
    formulas to calculate 441
    percentage body fat 440
    defining values 440
Bone growth 28-29
Bone mass 28-29, 252-253
Bone mineral density (BMD) 27
Borg scale 534
Brachial artery 171
Brachialis 59
Brachioradialis 59-60
Brain-derived neurotrophic factor (BDNF) . . 258
Branched-chain amino acids (BCAAs) 410
    ergogenic aid 414
Bronchodilator 422
Bulimia nervosa 477
Bundle branches 166
Bursa 30
Bursitis 598

C

Caffeine 421-422
    consumption, effects 422
Calcium 384
    muscle contraction 35-36
Calcium channel blockers 236
Calorie 348-349
Caloric balance 461-462
    negative 462
    positive 462
Caloric restriction 462
Calories-per-kilogram 467
Cancer 254-255
    diet 353, 380
    physical activity 254-255
Capillaries 34, 167, 171
Carbohydrates 351-353, 359-365
    categories of 352
    depletion 362-363
    need 364-365
Carcinogenic, 353
Cardiac arrhythmias 484
Cardiac fibrosis 235
Cardiac muscle 32, 166-167
Cardiac output (CO) 163-164
    peripheral resistance 168
    stroke volume (SV) 163
Cardio-circuit training 575
Cardiomyopathies 419
Cardiorespiratory fitness 14, 557-583
    tests 306-307, 310-318

Cardiovascular disease (CVD) 228
    exercise 649
Carotid pulse 173
Cartilaginous joint 29-30
Casein protein 414
Catabolic 413
    hormones 183
Catecholamines 188, 190-191
Cellular ischemia 489
Cellular permeability 161
Cellulite 449
Center of gravity 289-290
Central fatigue 158, 160
Central nervous system (CNS) 34
Central stability 548
Central-peripheral stability 524
Cerebrovascular disease 248
Chondrocytes 251
Cholesterol 230-232, 269, 369-370
    atherosclerosis 174, 232
    HDL 231
    LDL 231
    lipid screening 269
    VLDL 231
Chondromalacia 581
Chronic dehydration 394
Circuit 487
    kinetic circuits 134-135
Circuit system 536-537
Cardio circuit training 575
Circulation 177-180
Circumduction 47
Circumference measurement . . . 274, 445-446
Closed kinetic chain exercises 134
Closed skills 21
Closed-circuit system 135
Coefficient of digestibility 350
Collagen 26, 593
Common injuries 130, 545, 580
Comorbidities 229, 253, 424, 649, 652
Complete protein 373, 413
Complete tetanus 37-38
Complex carbohydrates 467
Complex system 535
Compliance 173, 174, 182, 235
    exercise 258, 304
    professional 678-679, 682
Composition of bones 26
Compound exercises 51, 631
Compound lipids 365
Compound movements 135, 522
Concentric contraction 39-40
Concurrent training 538
Conducting arteries 170
Conduction 577

Condyloid joint 31
Congestive heart failure (CHF) 239, 241, 654-655
Connective tissue 593
Contractility 158, 162
Contraindications 177, 504, 661
Contralateral 46
Contrast system 535
Convection 577
Cool down 172, 488-489, 608, 625
Coordination 12, 20
Coracobrachialis 57
Core temperature 392
Cori cycle 148
Coronary artery disease (CAD) . 174, 354, 652
Coronary circulation 174, 180
Coronary heart disease (CHD) . . 230, 239, 368
Corrective exercise 132, 134, 136, 138
Cortisol 190-192, 195
Creatine 410-412
Creatine kinase (CK) 144, 552
Creatine phosphate (CP) 144
Creeping obesity 221, 468
Cross bridges 36
Cross-sectional study 257
Cross training 574
Cunningham lean mass equation 467
Cytokines 230, 234, 244
Cytosol 149

D

Daily caloric need 469
Daily fluid intake 389-390
Daily values (DV) 404
Deadlift 91
    modified 92
    Romanian 63, 93
Deaminate 149
Deep vein thrombosis (DVT) 175, 236-237
Dehydration 390, 392-394, 396, 504
Dehydroepiandrosterone (DHEA) 420
Delayed onset muscle soreness (DOMS) . . 162
Deltoids 56-57
Dementia 258
Depression 256-257, 420
    movement 46-47
Derived lipids 366
Detraining 543-544, 580
Diabetes 172
    and exercise 645-649
    and physical activity 245-249
Diaphragm 122
Diastole 165
Diastolic blood pressure 178, 240, 268
Dietary fat and disease 371-372

Dietary reference intakes (DRI) 378
Disaccharides 352, 356
Distal 45-46
Distress 183
Diuretics 236
Dorsal 45-46
Dorsi flexion 46-47, 51, 64, 319
Drop set system 536
Dose response 516
Dual x-ray absorptiometry (DXA) 444
Duty of care 687
Dynamic flexibility 603, 605-606
Dynamic stretching 606-607
Dyslipidemia 219
Dyspnea 292

E

Eating disorders 476-477
Eccentric contraction 39-40
Elasticity 591
Electrolytes 387
Electron transport chain 153
Embolic disease 238
Emergency plan 299, 686-687
Emotion 117, 120
Endocrine system 182-183
Endomysium 33
Endorphins 257
Endothelium 171
Endurance 319
    anaerobic 518-520, 627-629
    assessments 326-330
Energy
    balance 461-462
    expenditure 568
    systems 142-148, 154
    transition 149-151
    value of food 348-350
Energy yielding nutrients 351
Enzymes 143
Ephedra 422, 423
Epidemiological studies 229
Epimysium 33
Epinephrine 190, 192, 195
Epiphyseal plates 28-29
Erector spinae 54
Ergogenic aid 407-408, 410
Essential amino acids 373-374
Essential body fat 435, 450
Estimated average requirement (EAR) . 378-379
Estrogen 187, 192
Ethics 679, 681
Eustress 183
Evaporation 577
Eversion 46-47

Excess post-exercise oxygen consumption
    (EPOC) 150
Excitation-contraction coupling 35
Exercise,
    and asthma 642-644
    and cardiovascular disease 649-657
    and children 662-666
    and diabetes 645-649
    during pregnancy 657-662
    and the elderly 666-670
Exercise-induced asthma (EIA) 643
Exercise considerations 538-544
    age 539-540
    concurrent training 538-539
    detraining 543-544
    gender 540-541
    overtraining 541-542
Exercise order 492-494
Exercise program
    design 482
    components 491
    safety factors 503
Exercise testing 295-297, 306-308
Extension 46-47
Extensor carpi radialis 60
Extensor carpi ulnaris 60
External oblique 54
Exertional-rhabdomyolysis 551
Extensibility 592

F

Fad diets 474
Fartlek training 573, 575
Fascia 33
Fascicle 33
Fat-burning zone 152
Fat-free mass (FFM) 16-17, 451
Fats 366-371
FatMax 152
Fat-soluble vitamins 380
Fatty acids 152, 490
Female athlete triad 385
Fiber 353, 355
Fiber type distribution 43
Fibrinolysis 419
Fibrocartilage 29
Field tests 445
Fight-or-flight response 191
Fitness training 515-516
Fixed compensation 133
Flexibility 588
    assessments 336-345
    benefits 589
    programming 607
    testing 601

    techniques 609-614
    training 602, 609
Flexion 46-47
Flexor carpi radialis 60
Flexor carpi ulnaris 60
Food deserts 457-458
Food labels 403-405
Food recalls 463-464
Force closure 114, 117-119
Force couples 524
Force production 36-39
Form closure 114, 117-119
Free fatty acids 153
Free radicals 248, 380
Frontal plane 44-46
Fructose 355-356
Functional decline 509, 589, 668
Functional range 601
Functional training 485-487
Functional-based activities 124
Functional warm-up 485-487

G

Gait 254
Galactose 352, 355-356
Gastric emptying 395-397
Gastrocnemius 64
Gender 540-541
General peripheral fatigue 157, 160
Genetics 202, 576
Genetic predisposition 202
Geriatric 215
Gestational diabetes mellitus (GDM) .. 646
Girth measurements 445
Global muscle systems 114-115
Glucagon 161, 188
Glucocorticoids 190
Gluconeogenesis 148, 363, 415
Glucose 145-148, 154, 156, 161,
    187-188, 352, 355-357, 360-362
Glutamine 410, 415
Gluteus maximus 61, 116, 123, 129
Gluteus medius 61, 116, 124, 582
Gluteus minimus 61, 124
Glycemic index 355-358
Glycemic load 188, 357, 360
Glycemic response 356-357, 648
Glycogen 145, 148, 157, 160-162, 181,
    245, 352, 359, 362, 364, 406, 490
Glycolysis 145-148, 154, 490
Glycosylated hemoglobin (HbA1c) 647
Goal setting 305
Golgi tendon organs (GTOs) .. 32, 38, 594, 605
Goniometer 336, 601
Gout 270, 600-601

Graded exercise test (GXT) 163, 560
Gross motor activation 484
Growth hormone (GH) 185, 192
Guarana 422
Gynecomastia................... 187, 419
Gynoid (storage pattern) 436, 437

H

Health............................. 5
Health related components of fitness... 12, 13
Heart rate training zone (HRTZ) 560, 563
Health risk appraisal 210, 213
Health screening 208
Health status questionnaire.... 210, 214, 215
Heart attack 180, 236, 652
Heart rate reserve 563-564
Heart rate training zone (HRTZ)..... 560, 563
Heart rate 163, 168, 180, 267, 534, 560-563
Heat stroke....................... 504
Height-weight tables (HWT) 439
Hematocrit 176
Hemoglobin......... 165, 175, 386, 578
Hemorrhagic stroke................. 238
Herniated disc..................... 53
Hexokinase........................ 146
High density lipoprotein (HDL) 230, 231, 233, 269, 369
Hinge joint 31, 59, 62, 64
Hip abductors 124, 130
Hip adductors 116
Hip flexors 127, 130, 137, 138, 319
HMB (Beta-Hydroxy Beta-Methylbutyrate) 410, 417
Homeostasis...................... 27
Homocysteine 380
Horizontal abduction 46, 47, 49, 56
Horizontal adduction 46, 47, 49, 56
Hormones
    adrenal 190
    gonadal...................... 186
    pancreatic...................... 187
    pituitary 185
    thyroid 189
Humidity 504, 577
Hunger.................. 361, 458-460
Hyaline cartilage............... 29, 581
Hydration 389-397
Hydrogenation.................... 369
Hydrostatic weighing............... 444
Hypercapnia 644
Hyperextension 46, 47, 48-50
Hyperglycemia 188, 360
Hyperinsulinemia........... 244, 357, 436
Hyperlipidemia 6, 13, 222, 230, 360
Hypermobility 31, 590
Hyperphagia 459
Hypertension 6, 13, 170, 172, 174, 177, 222, 240-243, 268, 353, 650-651
Hyperthermia 205
Hypertrophy.... 43, 186, 193, 410, 508, 514, 521-523, 526, 533, 630-633
Hypoglycemia 188, 205
Hyponatremia 205
Hypoperfusion 238
Hypothalamus 183, 185, 189-190, 458
Hypothermia 205
Hypothyroidism 189
Hypovolemia 393
Hypoxia................... 238, 577, 578

I

Insulin-dependent diabetes mellitus
    (IDDM)................... 246, 646,
Iliopsoas 129-131, 339, 611
Iliotibial (IT) band syndrome ... 130, 131, 582
Inactivity ... 7, 174, 222, 226, 244, 248, 652
Incomplete protein 374
Incretin 244,
Inflammation 6, 60, 62, 131, 230, 232, 233, 234, 244, 251, 353, 494, 511, 545, 549, 550, 551, 583, 598-601
Informed consent 210-212
Infraspinatus........ 56, 129, 338, 550, 614
Inner unit 118, 122
Insoluble fiber 353
Insulin............ 172, 183-196, 206, 242, 244-249, 356-360, 406, 413, 508, 510-511, 646-652
Insulin-like growth factor 1 (IGF-1) ... 185-186, 194-195, 258, 522
Intensity 482, 496, 497, 498, 500, 565, 566, 618,
Internal oblique 54, 116
Internal rotation 47, 49
Intermittent fasting 462-463
Interstitial spaces 171
Interval training 150, 565, 575, 580, 650, 656
Intervertebral disc..................... 53
Intramuscular fat 436
Inversion.................. 46, 47, 51
Inward rotation 45
Ipsilateral 46, 136, 623
Iron......... 42, 165, 175, 383, 386, 404
Ischemic (ischemia) 147
Ischemic stroke 238
Isocaloric 362, 461, 466

Isokinetic contraction 39, 40
Isometric contraction 39, 40, 115
Isotonic contraction 39

J

Joint capsule 30-32, 250, 593
Joint laxity see "Hypermobility"
Joint.......... 15-16, 20, 32, 46, 114-116, 118-119, 121, 250, 270, 289-291, 319, 336, 338, 486, 524, 551, 581, 588-590, 592-597, 599, 601,
    classifications 29-31

K

Karvonen method see Heart Rate Reserve
Ketosis 249
Kilocalorie........................ 348
Kinetic chain........... 114, 524, 627, 630
Knee extension 51, 319, 343
Knee flexion 51, 319, 342, 546
Krebs cycle 151-154, 155, 157
Kyphosis.......... 53, 126, 128, 138, 289
Kyphotic 52, 128, 129, 131, 138, 252, 290, 549, 623

L

Lactate tolerance 531, 537, 574
Lactate threshold.......... 181, 196, 561, 573, 574, 580
Lactic acid (lactate)..... 147, 148, 158, 162, 178, 415, 490, 537,
Lactose.................. 352, 356, 414
L-arginine 416
Lateral flexion................... 46-48
Latissimus dorsi.......... 56, 57, 67, 123, 338, 345, 623
Leptin........................ 244, 459
Levator scapulae.................. 58, 127
Liability 208, 209, 211, 214, 293, 503, 678, 684, 685, 688
Ligament sprains................... 547
Ligaments 30, 114, 250, 492, 547, 591, 593
Linoleic acids 371, 423
Linolenic acids 371
Lipase...................... 152, 153
Lipids 151-153, 156, 185, 231, 366, 370, 371, 435
    functions....................... 367
    simple, compound, derived.......... 366
Lipogenesis...................... 424
Lipolysis 153, 188, 423
Lipolytic effects 423
Lipoproteins 153, 231, 233, 366, 647
Local muscle systems 114

Long slow distance training 153, 566, 567
Longitudinal axis.................... 45, 46
Longitudinal studies 227
Lordosis 53, 126, 138
Lordotic 52, 55
Low back pain ... 53, 55, 122, 131, 222, 336,
547-548, 581, 582, 590, 602, 666
Low density lipoprotein (LDL) 183,
230-232, 269, 366
Lower cross syndrome 53, 119, 126, 128,
131, 136, 138, 620
Lumbar stenosis 548
Lumen................... 231, 236, 238

M

Maltose 352, 356
Maximal capacity 496
Mean arterial pressure (MAP) 169
Mechanoreceptor 547
Medial........................ 45, 46
Medical clearance 213-215, 292, 293
Medical history questionnaire 210, 214
Metabolic disease................ 244, 425
Metabolic equivalent (MET) 149, 466,
568, 570
Metabolic syndrome............. 188, 219,
292, 353, 511
Metabolism 41, 143, 145, 147, 148,
150, 151, 152, 155, 157, 189, 348,
350, 394, 413, 462, 466-472, 574
Microtrauma...................... 492
Midaxillary line 46, 448
Midline 45, 46
Minerals....... 349-351, 380, 382, 387, 510
Mitochondria 34, 36, 42, 146, 149, 151,
153, 168, 508, 538, 576-578
Mobility, ... 15-16, 31, 132, 136, 336, 344,
484-487, 588-590, 627, 630
Monocytes 232
Monosaccharides 352, 355-357
Monounsaturated fatty acids ... 366-368, 370
Morbidly obese 243, 270, 451
Mortality................ 7, 205, 226-227,
436, 439, 441, 651
Motor learning....................... 120
Motor neuron 35
Motor rehearsal..................... 134
Motor unit 35-42
Movement economy 486
Movement planes................... 44-45
Muscle contraction 34-36, 39-40
Muscle fiber types 41-42
Muscle hypertrophy 412-413, 522
Muscle spindles 37-38, 594
Muscle strains 545-547

Muscle tone...................... 37-38
Muscular endurance 14-15
    tests 326-330
Muscular fitness.............. 14-15, 319
Muscular power 18-19
    tests 332-333
Muscular strength 14-15, 319-320
    tests 321-325
Myocardial hypertrophy 419
Myocardial infarction.................. 180
Myocardial ischemia 235
Myocardium 166
Myofascial release technique....... 594, 603
Myofibrils 34
Myofilaments 34-35
Myoglobin 42
Myosin 34-36
Myostatin 186

N

Needs analysis 133, 222, 292,
303, 491, 619
Negative set system 531, 537
Nephropathy................ 248, 648-649
Nervous system 34-35, 37, 39, 120, 134,
160-161, 193, 387, 500, 525, 595
Neural adaptations 529
Neuromuscular junction............ 35, 160
Neuropathy................ 248, 648-649
Neurotransmitters 188, 257, 460
Neutral spine..................... 53
Neutralizer..................... 64
Nicotinamide adenine dinucleotide (NADH) 152
Nitric oxide (NO) 410, 416
Nitrogen balance........... 191, 374, 377
Nitroglycerin 417
Nociceptors..................... 598
Non-energy-yielding nutrients....... 349, 351
Non-essential amino acids 373-374, 411
Non-heme iron 386,
Non-insulin dependent diabetes mellitus
    (NIDDM) 246
Norepinephrine 188, 190, 192, 257, 423
Normal-weight obesity 17
Nucleus-pulposus.................... 53
Nutrition 6, 202-203, 348, 350,
357, 378, 402-404, 408, 463
Nutrient content descriptors 405
Nutritional facts label 403

O

Obesity......... 17, 219, 221-222, 270-272,
357, 424-425, 434, 451, 468
    physical activity 242-245
    prevalence 3, 243, 439, 456

android 436
    gynoid..................... 436
Octopamine...................... 423
Oligomenorrhea.................... 435
Olympic lifts 18, 145, 529, 635
Omega-3 fatty acids 370-371
Omega-6 fatty acids 368, 371
Open kinetic chain exercise............ 134
Open skills 21
Open-circuit 135-136, 624, 628
Onset of blood lactate accumulation
    (OBLA) 181
Open kinetic chain exercise............ 134
Orlistat 425
Orthostatic hypotension 170, 174
Osmolarity.................. 388, 396
Ossification 28-29
Osteoarthritis ... 250-251, 270, 434, 600-601
Osteoblasts.................. 28, 384
Osteoclasts................... 384
Osteopenia 27-28, 253, 384-385, 510
Osteophytes 250, 600
Osteoporosis 27-28, 207, 252-253,
384-385, 510, 666
    physical activity 207, 252-253
Outer unit...................... 122-124
Outward rotation 45, 128
Overhead press 67, 131, 135
Overload 8-9, 499-502, 637, 639
    principle 8-9, 499-502
Overreaching (NFO) 541-542
Overtraining syndrome 191, 257,
494, 499, 542
Overuse injuries 205, 545, 581-582
Oxaloacetate...................... 157
Oxidative phosphorylation.. 151, 153-154, 157
Oxygen consumption 14, 149-150, 163,
182, 307, 496, 513, 559
Oxygen debt 150, 568
Oxygen deficit................. 149, 150
Oxygen exchange 179
Oxygen uptake 181-182, 307

P

Pancreatic hormones............ 187, 360
Pancreas.......... 183, 187-188, 192,
244-246, 357, 360, 646
Parkinson's disease............. 258, 463
Par-Q 210, 213-214
Participant risk 684
Patellar tendonitis.............. 131, 599
Pectineus 62, 63
Pectoralis major 28, 56-57
Pectoralis minor 58
Pelvic floor 114, 116, 118, 122, 548

Pelvic positioning 55
Performance goals 304, 501
Performance related fitness. 11, 12
Perimysium 33-34
Periodization 482, 501-503, 623, 638
Periosteum 27, 30, 32
Peripheral circulatory system 171
Peripheral fatigue 158-159, 160-161
Peripheral nervous system (PNS). 34, 160
Peripheral neuropathy 649
Peripheral resistance. 168, 169, 179, 241
Peripheral vascular disease 241, 246, 248, 647-648
Peroneus brevis. 64
Peroneus longus 64
Phentermine 425
Phosphagen system . . 144-145, 149, 490, 524
Photosynthesis 149, 348
Physical activity 7
　cancer 10, 254-255
　CVD. 228-229
　diabetes 245, 249
　hypertension. 240
　life quality 204
　mental health. 256-257
　obesity. 242-243, 245
　osteoarthritis 250-251
　osteoporosis. 252-253
　risk for disease. 226-227
　stroke 238-239
Physical fitness 7, 12-13, 21, 202
Phytochemicals. 353, 361
Piriformis 61, 345, 611
Pituitary gland. . . 183, 185-187, 189-190, 195
Pituitary hormones 185
Pivot joint 31, 60
Plantar fasciitis 126, 131, 206, 551, 581-582, 599
Plantar flexion. 51
Plane joint. 31
Planes of movement 609
Plaque 169, 174, 230-232, 234-236, 238, 244, 369, 650, 652
Plasma 153, 170, 176
Plasticity. 543, 591
Platelets. 176, 231, 236, 238
Plumb line 126, 289, 291-292, 621
Plyometrics. 18, 145, 528, 529, 635
Polypeptide hormones 184
Polysaccharides 352
Polyunsaturated fatty acids 367-368, 370
Positive feedback loop. 193, 578, 589
Posterior 45-47
Posterior deltoid 76
Posterior pelvic tilt 55, 100

Post-exercise hypotension (PEH) 651
Postphlebitic syndrome 237
Post-traumatic arthritis (PTA) 251
Postural alignment 126, 289, 291, 588
Postural syndromes. 119
Potassium ions 178
Power. 12, 18-19
　power output. 19, 41, 42, 529
　power training 527-530
Pre-eclampsia 659
Pre-exercise food consumption 407
Pregnancy 246, 377, 384, 386, 391, 596-597, 646, 657-662
Premature mortality 17, 205, 227, 273
PRICE 546-547
Prime movers 40, 43, 52, 127, 533, 622, 628
Principles of exercise 9, 482, 499
　overload 9, 499
　progression 9, 499
　specificity 9, 499
Prioritization model 133, 622
Processed carbohydrates. 17, 359, 465
Professional 676-677
　behavior 677
　ethics 679, 681
　principles 678
Professional negligence. 209, 504, 552
Program matrix 303, 482, 608
Progression. 9
Progressive overload 9, 498, 500-502, 564, 637-639, 666
Prohormones 419-420
Pronation 46-47, 50, 130
Proper breathing technique 654
Proprioception. 20, 486
Proprioceptive neuromuscular facilitation
　(PNF) 603-605
Proprioceptors 15, 20, 31, 37, 594,
Protein 349-351, 358, 362, 367, 372-378, 404, 465, 475
　energy metabolism. 146, 149, 156, 348, 468
　post-exercise recovery 406-407
　supplementation. 408, 412-414, 475
Protein-sparing mechanism 362-363
Proteolytic enzymes 191
Protraction 47
Proximal. 27, 45-46
Psoas major 61-62, 116
Pulmonary disease 6
Pulmonary embolism 175, 230, 236-238
Pulmonary vein 165
Pull-up test 325
Pulse 172-173, 267, 504

Purkinje fibers 166
Push-up. 71, 138, 326, 328
Pyramid training (system) . . 301, 531-532, 536
Pyruvate 147-149, 151, 153, 155-157

Q

Quadratus femoris 61
Quadratus lumborum 54, 116, 124, 129-131, 582
Quadriceps (group) 62, 286, 342

R

Radial deviation 46-47, 50
Radial pulse 173, 267
Radiation 254-255, 577
Range of motion (ROM) 15-16, 31, 289, 336-337, 512, 588-590, 608
　aging 666
　assessing. 336-337
　injury 581
Rate of perceived exertion (RPE) 180, 525, 537, 561, 650
Rate pressure product (RPP) . . . 180, 625, 653
Reaction time 254
Reciprocal inhibition 127, 595, 604
Recommended dietary allowance
　(RDA) 381, 383, 412
Recovery. 145, 159-162, 191, 301, 406-407, 466, 482, 497, 499
Recovery period 145, 159, 194, 301, 482, 499, 522, 656
Rectus abdominis 54, 100-102, 109, 116, 130, 341, 623
Rectus femoris. 62, 63, 131, 339, 342, 611, 621
Red blood cells (RBCs). 27, 42, 165, 176, 363, 381, 577-578
Referral 214-215, 266, 268-270, 292-293, 550, 583, 642
Reinforcement. 639
Reliability 291, 295-298, 320, 336, 446-447, 449, 602
Renin-angiotensin system 235, 242
Repetitions 159, 194-195, 498, 516, 519, 522, 525, 529, 536
Re-phosphorylate 144, 411, 524
Repolarization 166
Residual adaptations. 628, 630
Residual volume 444, 658
Resistance arm 75-76, 100, 105, 624
Resistance training . . 10, 326, 418, 475, 508, 514-515, 541, 625, 654, 670
　benefits. 249, 468, 508-513, 539-540, 597, 647, 669
　blood pressure 169-170, 174, 179

bone density 29, 253, 385, 509-510
    energy pathways 145, 159, 161
    hormones 185, 195, 493
Respiration 181-182, 391,
    561-563, 578, 643-644
Respiratory exchange ratio
    (RER) 512-513, 664
Respiratory quotient (RQ) 513
Respiratory system 444
Rest interval (period) 159, 193, 495,
    497-498, 618
    energy systems 154,
    programming 194, 210, 500, 632
    training guidelines 516, 519,
    522, 525, 529
Resting heart rate 168, 266-267,
    292, 562-564, 620
Resting metabolic rate (RMR) 149, 361,
    462, 466, 513
Retinopathy 241, 248-249, 648-649
Retraction 31, 47, 78-80
Return to play 4, 64, 130, 547
Reversibility principle 544
Rhabdomyolysis 205, 495, 551-552
Rheumatoid arthritis . . 216, 230, 251, 599-601
Rhomboids 58, 78-80, 116, 131,
    345, 549, 621, 623
Ribosomes 184-185
Risk management 293, 683-686, 688
RMR equations 467
Romanian deadlift 63, 91, 93, 517
Rotation 31, 44-50
Rotator cuff . . . 56, 66, 74, 304, 549-550, 559
Running economy 512

S

Sacrum 52, 55, 118, 122, 600
Saddle joint 31
Safety 204, 295, 298, 301, 327,
    497, 503-505, 533-534, 686-688
Sagittal plan 45-46, 51, 60, 67,
    116, 123, 128, 130, 304
Sarcolemma 33, 35, 160
Sarcomere 33-35, 111, 143,
    166, 193, 592, 595-596
Sarcopenia . 19, 385, 509, 511, 539, 596, 667
Sarcoplasm 34-35
Sarcoplasmic reticulum (SR) 35, 41, 166
Sartorius 62-63, 131, 345
Satiety Index 459
Saturated fats 13, 367-369, 374, 475
Scapular protraction 70
Scapular retraction 78-80
Sciatica 548
Scoliosis 548

Scope of practice 2, 4, 68
Screening 249, 292-293, 301, 619,
    645, 648, 680, 684, 687-688
    documents 210-215, 218, 294
    pre-exercise screening . . 208-215, 266, 269,
    risk/injury prevention 205-206
Seated row 57-58, 80, 304, 533, 633
Sedentary 21, 180, 202, 227, 267,
    375, 394, 412, 471, 576
    disease/health risks 125, 214, 226,
    239-240, 245, 249, 257, 646, 666
Self-efficacy . . . 204, 243, 251, 256, 653, 677
Semimembranosus 63, 93, 98, 105
Semitendinosus 63, 93, 98, 105
Serotonin 257
Serum lipoproteins 370
Serratus anterior 58, 129, 131, 345
Shin splints 131, 206, 581, 583
Shoulder abduction 73-76
Shoulder extension 67, 79-80, 109
Shoulder flexion 16, 56, 66, 72, 77,
    85, 104, 109, 549, 668
Shoulder girdle 57-58
Shoulder impingement syndrome 126,
    549, 599
Side raise 57
Signs and symptoms of disease 292
Simple lipids 366
Sinoatrial (SA) node 166
Size principle 42
Skeletal muscle 32
Skill acquisition 299, 492
Skinfold 284-288, 446-448
    guidelines 447
    measurements 443, 446
    sites/locations 448,
    three sites, male/female 286
Sleep apnea 270, 434, 662
Sliding filament theory 34, 36
Slow oxidative fibers 41
Slow-twitch fibers . 37-38, 42-43, 193-194, 566
Smith machine 71, 78, 87, 91, 329
Smooth muscle 32, 170-172
Sodium-potassium relationship 389
Soft tissue 591
Soleus 64, 99, 345
Soluble fiber 353
Somatotropin 185
Spatial terms 44-45
Specificity 9, 499-500
Speed 12, 19-21
Spinal cord 31-32, 34-35
Spine and neck 52
Spondylitis 548

Spondylolisthesis 548
Spondylosis 548
Spot reduction 472
Squat 87-90, 92, 97, 322-323, 344
Stability 15
Stabilizers 116, 122, 533-534
Starch 352-354
Static posture 289, 291
Static stretching 593, 603-604, 668
Statins 232
Steady state . . . 150, 178, 181, 565, 573-575
Step-ups 96
Stenosis 238
Sternoclavicular joint 57
Steroid hormones 184
Sticking point 119
Stop test indicators 308
Strength balance . 20, 289, 304, 519-520, 621
Strength training 524-529, 665, 667
Stress 183, 188, 190-195, 202
Stretching 22, 489, 591-595, 602-604
    active-assisted . 603-604, 609-610, 613-614
    ballistic 594, 607
    dynamic 606-607
    PNF 604-605
    Static 602-603
Stretch reflex 37-38, 603, 607
Stroke 228-230, 238-239
Stroke volume . . 163, 167, 392, 576, 579-580
Subacromial-subdeltoid bursa 599
Subcutaneous fat 436-438, 446-447, 449
Submaximal tests 307, 558-559
Subscapularis 56-57, 338, 550
Sucrose 352, 355-356, 359-360
Sugars 355, 357-359
Summation 37
Supercompensation 502-503
Superficial 46
Superset system 533
Supination 46-47, 50, 65
Supplement
    categories 408, 410, 421
    regulation 408
Supraspinatus 56-57, 550
    tendon 599
Sympathetic nervous system 178-179
Sympathomimetic 422-423
Synchronicity 38-39
Synephrine 423
Synergistic muscles 290
Synovial joint 29-31
Synovial membrane 30, 591
Systole 165
Systolic blood pressure . . . 178, 241, 268, 650